SOUTHMEAD
WITHDRAWN
FROM STOCK
LIBRARY

DIAGNOSTIC PATHOLOGY
HEPATOBILIARY AND PANCREATIC

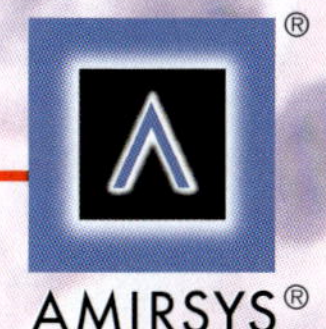

DIAGNOSTIC PATHOLOGY
HEPATOBILIARY AND PANCREATIC

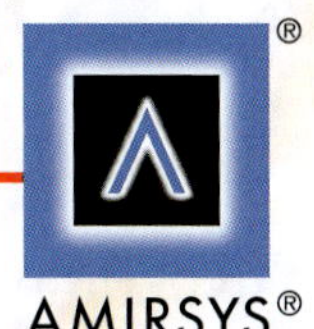

Laura Webb Lamps, MD
Professor and Vice Chair
Director of Diagnostic Laboratories
Department of Pathology
University of Arkansas for Medical Sciences
Little Rock, AR

Joseph Misdraji, MD
Assistant Pathologist
Department of Pathology
Massachusetts General Hospital
Assistant Professor of Pathology
Harvard Medical School
Boston, MA

Lisa Yerian, MD
Director of Hepatopancreaticobiliary Pathology
Director of Surgical Pathology
Assistant Professor of Pathology
Cleveland Clinic Lerner College of Medicine
Cleveland Clinic
Cleveland, OH

Vikram Deshpande, MD
Assistant Pathologist
Department of Pathology
Massachusetts General Hospital
Assistant Professor of Pathology
Harvard Medical School
Boston, MA

Grace E. Kim, MD
Professor of Pathology
Associate Director of Surgical Pathology
Department of Pathology
University of California San Francisco
San Francisco, CA

Mari Mino-Kenudson, MD
Assistant Pathologist
Department of Pathology
Massachusetts General Hospital
Assistant Professor of Pathology
Harvard Medical School
Boston, MA

Sanjay Kakar, MD
Associate Professor and Vice Chair of Anatomic Pathology
University of California San Francisco
Chief of Pathology
San Francisco Veteran Affairs Medical Center
San Francisco, CA

Hanlin L. Wang, MD, PhD
Director of Gastrointestinal Pathology
Department of Pathology and Laboratory Medicine
Cedars-Sinai Medical Center
Los Angeles, CA

Matthew M. Yeh, MD, PhD
Associate Professor of Pathology
University of Washington School of Medicine
Seattle, WA

Kari D. Caradine, MD
Assistant Professor
Department of Pathology
University of Arkansas for Medical Sciences
Little Rock, AR

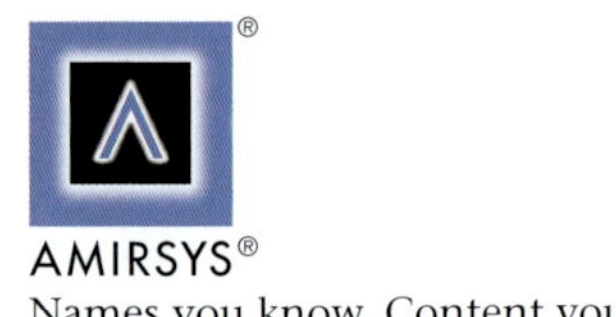

Names you know. Content you trust.®

First Edition

Printed in Canada by Friesens, Altona, Manitoba, Canada

ISBN: 978-1-931884-56-3

Notice and Disclaimer

Library of Congress Cataloging-in-Publication Data

Diagnostic pathology. Hepatobiliary and pancreatic / [edited by] Laura Webb Lamps.
p. ; cm.
Hepatobiliary and pancreatic
Includes index.
ISBN 978-1-931884-56-3
1. Liver--Pathophysiology. 2. Pancreas--Pathophysiology. 3. Bile ducts--Diseases. 4. Liver--Diseases. 5. Pancreas--Diseases. I. Lamps, Laura W. (Laura Webb) II. Title: Hepatobiliary and pancreatic.
[DNLM: 1. Liver--pathology--Atlases. 2. Pancreas--pathology--Atlases. 3. Bile Duct Diseases--diagnosis--Atlases. 4. Biliary Tract--pathology--Atlases. 5. Liver Diseases--diagnosis--Atlases. 6. Pancreatic Diseases--diagnosis--Atlases. WI 17]
RC846.9.D53 2011
616.3'62075--dc22

2010050641

In memory of my mother, Linda Venable Webb, for whom learning was a lifelong joy.

I would also like to thank my coauthors for their wonderful contributions, and Dave Chance, Kellie Heap, Laura Sesto, and Lane Bennion from the Amirsys team for their patience and hard work on behalf of this book.
LWL

To Fiona Graeme-Cook, who began me on this journey, and Greg Lauwers and Robert Young, who guided me along the way.
JM

To my husband, my family, and my colleagues, for all they have taught me.
LY

To my wife, Anita, and my son, Nikhil.
VD

To my loving husband, Jeffrey, and my late grandmother, Hwang, who taught me to persevere.
GEK

To my husband, Cris, and my canine daughters, Chia and Terri, for all their love and support.
MM-K

To my mentors, Larry Bugart and Linda Ferrell, for their inspirational demeanor, for shepherding my way in the world of pathology, and for sharing their penchant for making the correct diagnosis, both in life and in liver biopsies.
SK

To Michelle, Sean, and Jason for their tremendous support and encouragement.
HLW

To my family.
MMY

To Laura Lamps, MD, my mentor and friend.
KDC

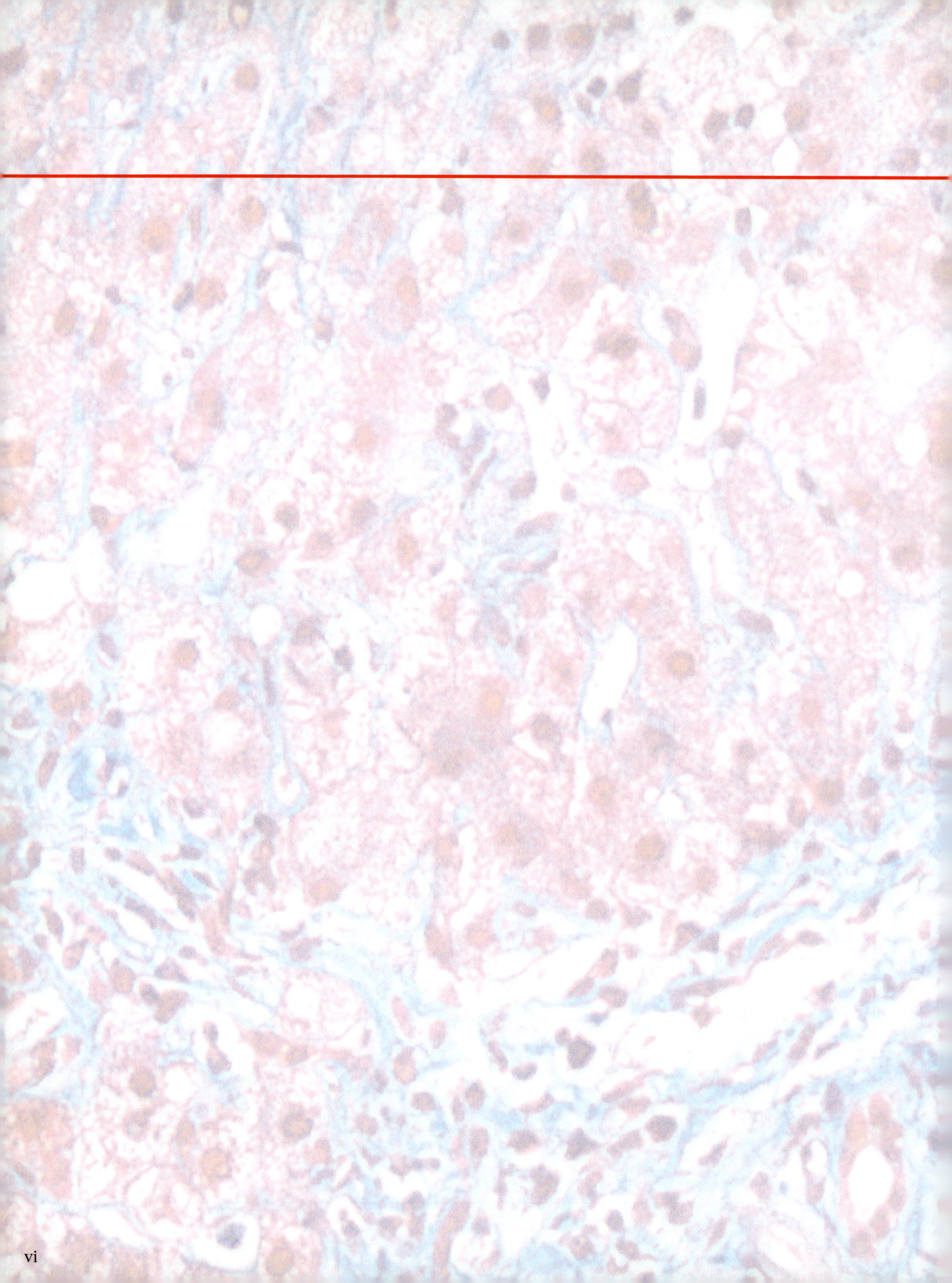

DIAGNOSTIC PATHOLOGY
HEPATOBILIARY AND PANCREATIC

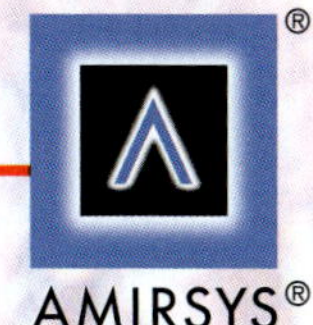

Amirsys, creators of the highly acclaimed radiology series Diagnostic Imaging, proudly introduces its new Diagnostic Pathology series, designed as easy-to-use reference texts for the busy practicing surgical pathologist. Written by world-renowned experts, the series will consist of 15 titles in all the crucial diagnostic areas of surgical pathology.

The newest book in this series, *Diagnostic Pathology: Hepatobiliary and Pancreatic*, contains approximately 500 pages of comprehensive, yet concise, descriptions of more than 120 specific diagnoses. Amirsys's pioneering bulleted format distills pertinent information to the essentials. Each chapter has the same organization providing an easy-to-read reference for making rapid, efficient, and accurate diagnoses in a busy surgical pathology practice. A highlighted Key Facts box provides the essential features of each diagnosis. Detailed sections on Terminology, Etiology/Pathogenesis, Clinical Issues, Macroscopic and Microscopic Findings, and the all important Differential Diagnoses follow so you can find the information you need in the exact same place every time.

Most importantly, every diagnosis features numerous high-quality images, including gross pathology, H&E and immunohistochemical stains, correlative radiographic images, and richly colored graphics, all of which are fully annotated to maximize their illustrative potential.

We believe that this lavishly illustrated series, with its up-to-date information and practical focus, will become the core of your reference collection. Enjoy!

Elizabeth H. Hammond, MD
Executive Editor, Pathology
Amirsys, Inc.

Anne G. Osborn, MD
Chairman and Chief Executive Officer
Amirsys Publishing, Inc.

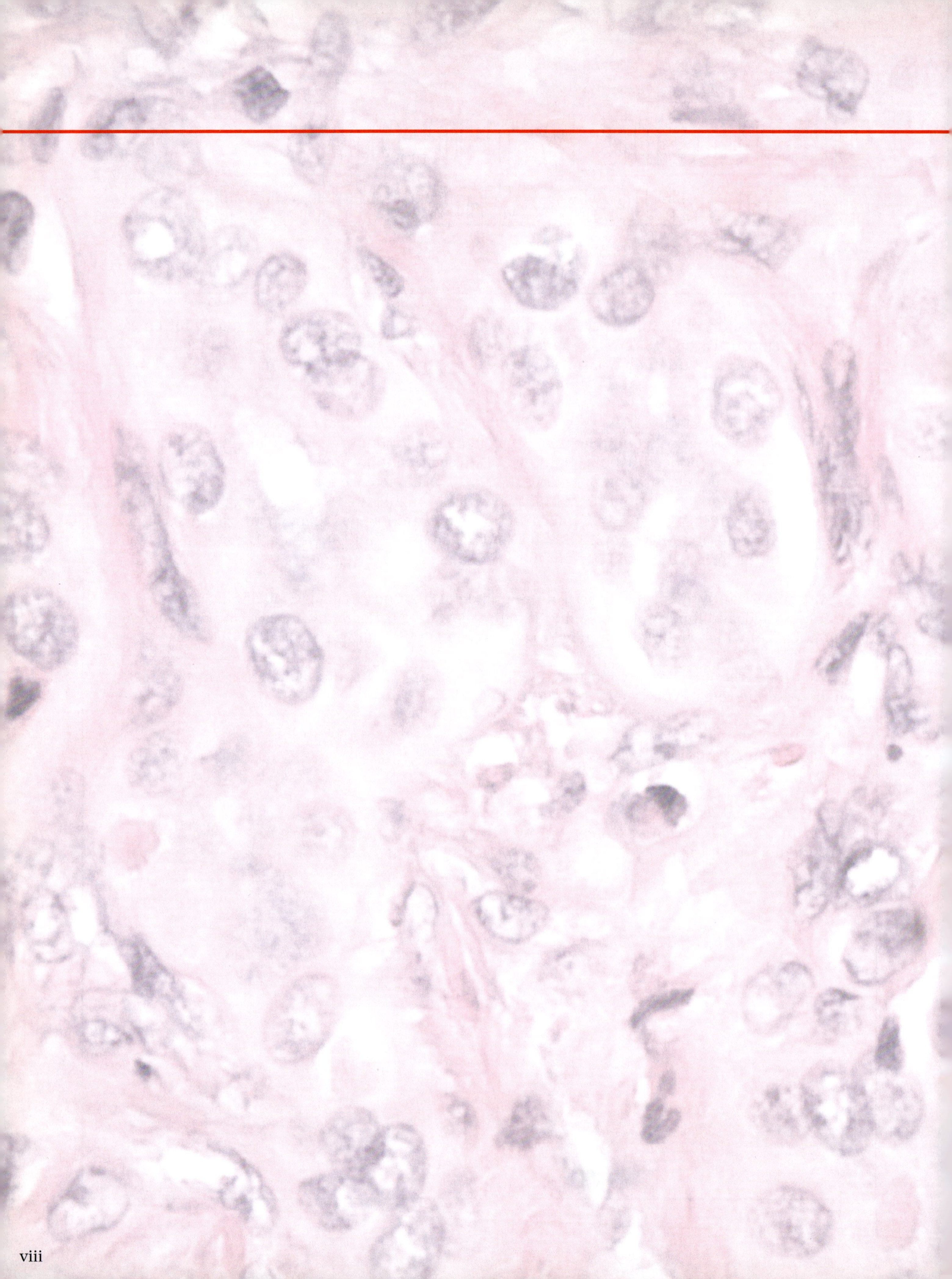

PREFACE

Medical liver disease often poses a challenge for surgical pathologists, for there may be a great deal of overlap among the entities in any given differential diagnosis. Neoplastic lesions of the liver, pancreas, and biliary system may also be difficult to diagnose, especially if infrequently encountered. *Diagnostic Pathology: Hepatobiliary and Pancreatic* is designed to help both practicing pathologists and pathologists in training to address these challenges.

This reference provides clear, concise, up-to-date information on hepatobiliary and pancreatic pathology, along with a wealth of images. (If a picture is worth a thousand words, then there are at least 1,295,000 words' worth of images in this book). The images include photomicrographs, gross photographs, and beautiful medical illustrations, many of which were created especially for this book.

As with all of the books in the Diagnostic Pathology series, the key facts pertaining to each diagnosis are highlighted in a box for ease of use. A list of important entities in the differential diagnosis section is given for each diagnosis. In addition, annotated staging protocols are included for all malignancies, as well as tables of pertinent immunostains and chapters on the gross dissection of specimens.

Given the seemingly exponential speed with which medical knowledge is expanding, any printed book will be fairly rapidly outdated. The Amirsys eBook Advantage™ license included with each printed copy of this book provides fully searchable text and a complete listing of antibodies, which will be regularly updated.

On behalf of all of the authors of this book, we hope that *Diagnostic Pathology: Hepatobiliary and Pancreatic* will prove to be a favorite reference to which pathologists turn again and again in their daily practice.

Laura Webb Lamps, MD
Professor and Vice Chair
Director of Diagnostic Laboratories
Department of Pathology
University of Arkansas for Medical Sciences
Little Rock, AR

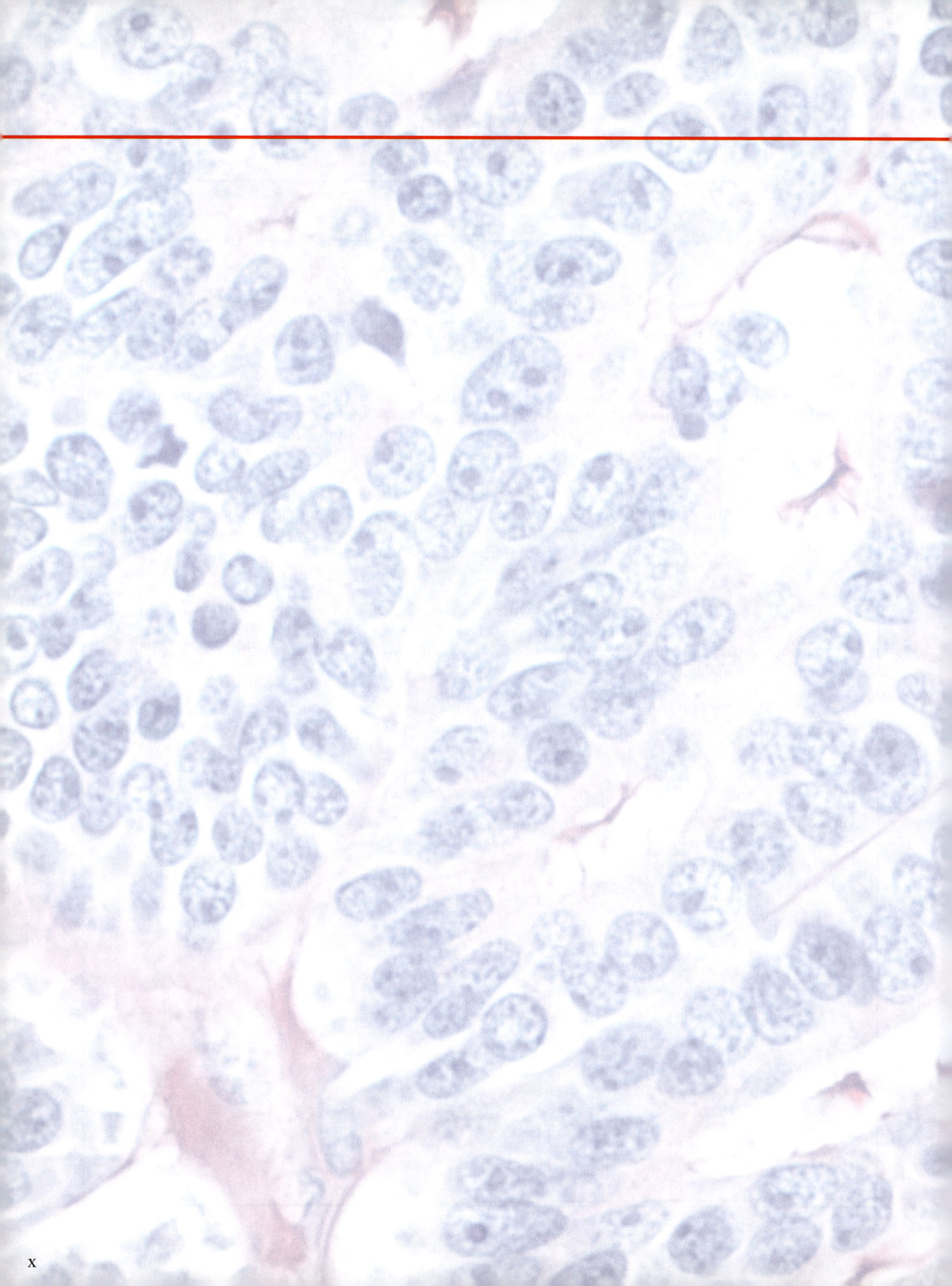

ACKNOWLEDGMENTS

Text Editing

Ashley R. Renlund, MA
Arthur G. Gelsinger, MA
Matthew R. Connelly, MA
Lorna Morring, MS
Alicia M. Moulton

Image Editing

Jeffrey J. Marmorstone
Lisa A. Magar

Medical Text Editing

Shree Gopal Sharma, MD

Illustrations

Lane R. Bennion, MS
Laura C. Sesto, MA
Richard Coombs, MS

Art Direction and Design

Laura C. Sesto, MA

Assistant Editor

Dave L. Chance, MA

Publishing Lead

Kellie J. Heap

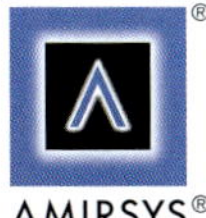

AMIRSYS®

Names you know. Content you trust.®

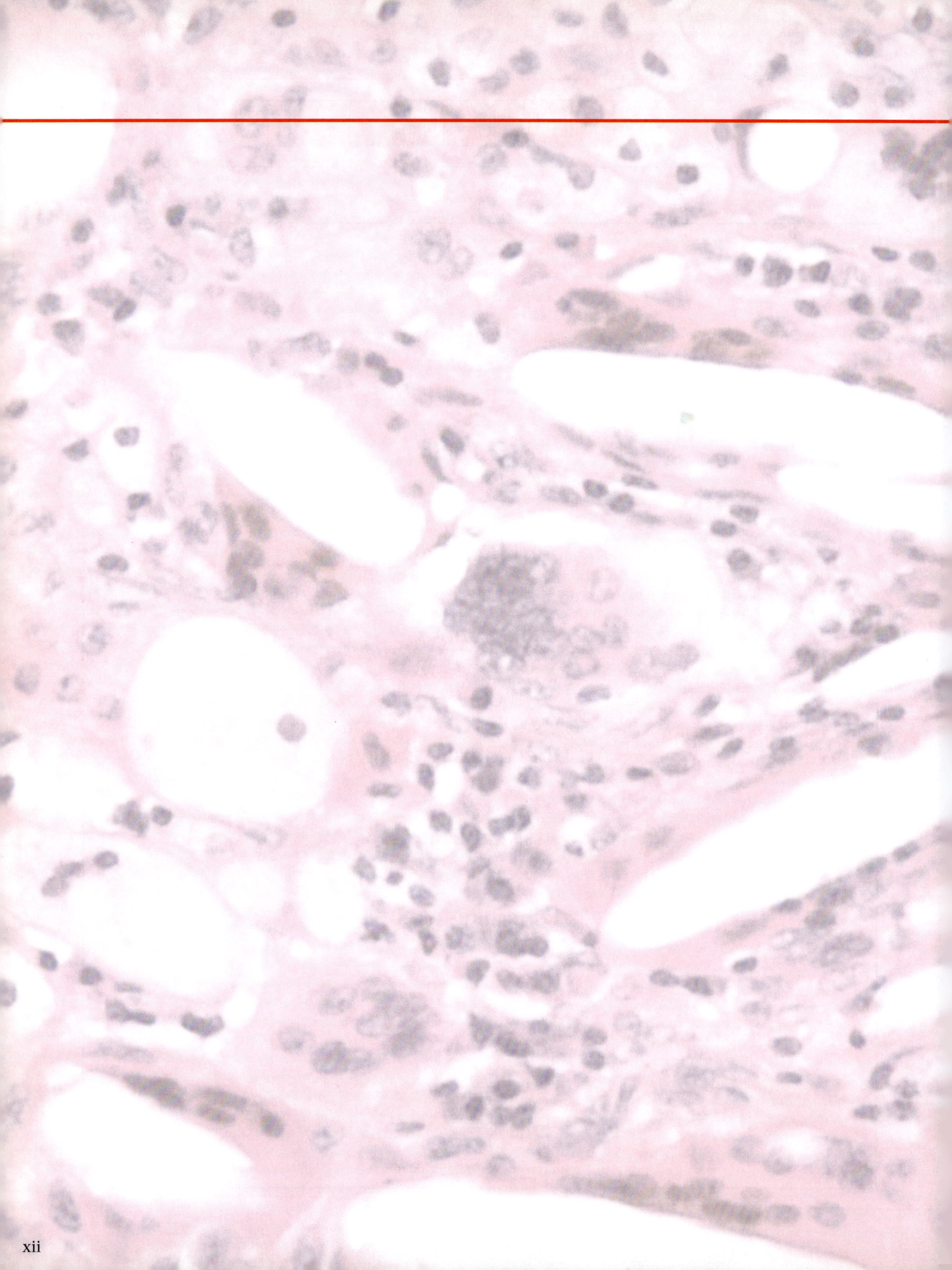

SECTIONS

Liver

Pancreas and Biliary Tract

Reference

TABLE OF CONTENTS

PART I
Liver

SECTION 1
Inherited, Metabolic, and Developmental Disorders

SECTION 2
Infectious Disorders

SECTION 3
Chronic Cholestatic and Autoimmune Disorders

SECTION 4
Pediatric Cholestatic Disorders

SECTION 5
Drug/Toxin-related Hepatitis

SECTION 6
Fatty Liver Diseases

SECTION 7
Vascular Disorders

SECTION 8
Transplantation Pathology

SECTION 9
Tumors of the Liver

SECTION 10
Miscellaneous Hepatic Disorders

PART II
Pancreas and Biliary Tract

SECTION 1
Developmental/Congenital

SECTION 2
Inflammatory Disorders of the Gallbladder and Extrahepatic Biliary Tree

SECTION 3
Nonneoplastic and Inflammatory Disorders of the Pancreas

SECTION 4
Tumors of the Gallbladder and Extrahepatic Biliary Tree

SECTION 5
Tumors of the Pancreas

SECTION 6
Tumors of the Ampulla

SECTION 7
Specimen Handling, Whipple

PART III
Reference

SECTION 1
Antibody Index

DIAGNOSTIC PATHOLOGY
HEPATOBILIARY AND PANCREATIC

AMIRSYS®

Inherited, Metabolic, and Developmental Disorders

GLYCOGEN STORAGE DISEASE

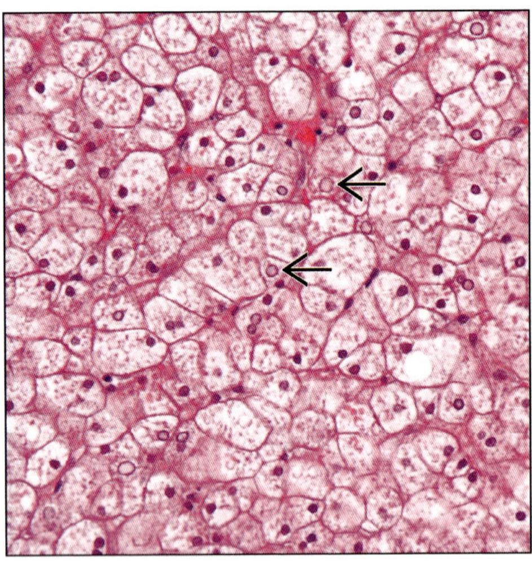

The mosaic pattern results from swollen hepatocytes compressing the sinusoids in this case of GSD Ia. The cell membranes are accentuated, and prominent glycogenated nuclei ➔ are seen.

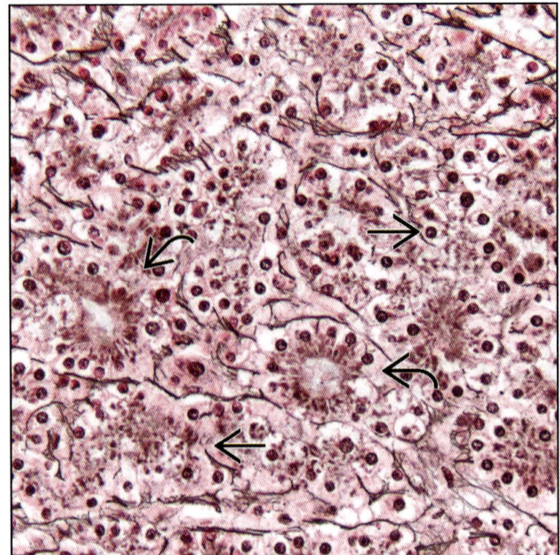

Reticulin stain highlights the abnormal architecture, loss of reticulin fibers ➔, and pseudorosette formation ➚ in this hepatocellular carcinoma arising in a patient with GSD Ia.

TERMINOLOGY

Abbreviations

- Glycogen storage disease (GSD)

Synonyms

- Glycogenoses

ETIOLOGY/PATHOGENESIS

Inborn Error of Carbohydrate Metabolism

- Gene mutation in proteins involved in glycogen synthesis, degradation, or regulation
  - Hepatic enzyme deficiency
    - GSD types 0, I, II, III, IV, VI, and IX
    - 80% of hepatic GSD is types I, III, and IX
  - Abnormal concentration or structure of glycogen
    - GSD 0 results in decreased hepatic glycogen
    - Remaining types of GSD display increased hepatic glycogen
- Inherited as autosomal recessive trait
  - Exception is GSD IX (X-linked disorder)

CLINICAL ISSUES

Presentation

- Hepatomegaly
  - Occurs in GSD I, III, IV, VI, and IX
  - Rarely in GSD II
  - Not in GSD 0
- Hypoglycemia
  - Occurs in GSD 0, I, and III
  - Mild in VI and IX
  - Rarely in GSD IV
  - Not in GSD II

Laboratory Tests

- Confirmation of diagnosis
  - Enzymatic assay on liver
    - GSD 0, I, II, III, VI, and IX
  - DNA mutation analysis

Treatment

- Options, risks, complications
  - Increased incidence of hepatocellular neoplasia
    - Hepatic adenoma is frequent in GSD I and can occur in GSD III
    - Hepatocellular carcinoma occurs in GSD I and is reported in GSD III
  - GSD Ib has been associated with Crohn-like disease
    - Granulomatous colitis
    - Responds to inflammatory bowel disease treatment regimen
  - Dietary intervention
    - Prevent hypoglycemia, particularly for GSD 0 and I, less stringent in GSD III
- Surgical approaches
  - Liver transplantation corrects primary hepatic enzyme defect
    - Has been performed for GSD I, III, and IV
    - Best treatment option for GSD IV

Prognosis

- Variable based on type of GSD
  - GSD II (infantile form) usually results in death in 1st year of life
  - GSD IV (classic hepatic form) has rapid disease progression with liver failure from 3-5 years of age

MICROSCOPIC PATHOLOGY

Histologic Features

- Histologic features are not generally diagnostic of GSD
  - Exception is characteristic cytoplasmic inclusion in GSD IV
    - Weakly basophilic to colorless inclusion, retracts from surrounding cytoplasm
    - PAS positive and partially digested on PAS-D
- Mosaic architecture

GLYCOGEN STORAGE DISEASE

Key Facts

Etiology/Pathogenesis

- Inborn error of carbohydrate metabolism caused by gene mutations in proteins involved in glycogen synthesis, degradation, or regulation
  - Results in different enzymatic defects in liver that are classified as GSD types 0, I, II, III, IV, VI, and IX
  - 80% of hepatic GSD is types I, III, and IX

Clinical Issues

- Most patients present with hepatomegaly and hypoglycemia
- Increased incidence of hepatic adenoma and hepatocellular carcinoma in GSD I and also GSD III
- Liver transplantation corrects primary hepatic enzyme defect and is used primarily for GSD IV

Microscopic Pathology

- Assess liver for mosaic pattern of hepatocytes, glycogenated nuclei, fatty change, and fibrosis
  - GSD 0 has decreased glycogen
  - GSD IV has characteristic cytoplasmic inclusions
- Cirrhosis occurs frequently in GSD IV and can occur in III and IX

Ancillary Tests

- Lysosomal-bound glycogen for GSD II
- Fibrillar glycogen for GSD IV

Top Differential Diagnoses

- Glycogen hepatopathy
- Other entities with ground-glass cytoplasm

  - In GSD I, III, VI, and IX
  - Attributed to enlarged, pale-staining, swollen hepatocytes
  - Compression of sinusoid by expanded hepatocytes
  - Excess glycogen is PAS positive, PAS-D negative
    - Glycogen may wash out with formalin processing
    - Glycogen can be retained with alcohol fixation
- Fibrosis
  - Initially in periportal region
  - GSD III, IV, VI, IX; may occur in GSD I
    - Frequently progresses to cirrhosis in GSD IV
    - Cirrhosis can occur in III and IX
- Features of hepatocytes
  - Glycogenated nuclei
    - In GSD I (prominent) and III (less)
  - Thickened cytoplasmic membrane
    - Resulting from organelles at periphery of cytoplasm
- Cytoplasmic lipid in all GSD
  - More pronounced in GSD I

Ultrastructural Features

- GSD 0
  - Nonspecific with sparse glycogen
- GSD I
  - Cytoplasmic monoparticulate glycogen displaces organelles, large lipid droplets, and prominent intranuclear glycogen
- GSD II
  - Lysosomal monoparticulate glycogen (glycogenosomes)
- GSD III
  - Similar to GSD I, but less lipid and nuclear glycogen
- GSD IV
  - Fibrillar glycogen and glycogen rosettes
- GSD VI
  - Resembles "starry sky" appearance
    - Cytoplasmic monoparticulate glycogen and glycogen rosettes displace organelles
- GSD IX
  - Characteristic "starry sky"
    - Due to dense areas of cytoplasmic glycogen alternating with organelle-free zones
    - Glycogen is mixture of monoparticulated and multiparticulated forms
  - Displacement of organelles to cell margin
- Lipid may be present in all hepatic GSD on ultrastructural studies
- Intracellular collagen has been demonstrated in GSD III and IV

DIFFERENTIAL DIAGNOSIS

Glycogen Hepatopathy

- Histologic overlap with GSD
  - Distinction requires knowledge of clinical history
    - Diabetes mellitus type I
    - Poorly controlled blood sugar
    - Does not usually present in childhood

Treated Urea Cycle Defects

- Can result in hepatocyte glycogen accumulation
  - Nonuniform distribution of glycogen
  - No displacement of organelles by glycogen ultrastructurally
- Glycogen accumulation may be related to therapeutic dietary modification

Lafora Disease

- Lafora bodies are more eosinophilic and stain homogeneously with colloidal iron
- GSD IV can nonspecifically stain with colloidal iron but stains in clumpy granular pattern

Other Entities with Ground-Glass Cytoplasm

- Hepatitis B surface antigen
  - Immunohistochemical stain for HBsAg positive
- Fibrinogen storage disease
  - Eosinophilic spherical and vacuolated inclusions
    - Immunoreactive for fibrinogen
    - Ultrastructurally composed of finger-like pattern inclusion in rough endoplasmic reticulum
- Drug-associated morphologic change

GLYCOGEN STORAGE DISEASE

Enzymatic Defects

Type (Eponym)	Deficient	Chromosome (Gene)
0	Glycogen synthase (hepatic isoform)	12p12.2 (*GYS2*)
Ia (von Gierke)	Glucose-6-phosphate hydrolase	17q21 (*G6PC*)
Ib	Glucose-6-phosphate translocase	11q23 (*G6PT1*)
II (Pompe)	Lysosomal α-1, 4-glucosidase	17q25.2-q25.3 (*GAA*)
III (Cori or Forbes)	Amylo-1, 6 glucosidase (debrancher)	1p21 (*AGL*)
IV (Andersen)	Amylo-1, 4 to 1, 6-transglucosidase (brancher)	3p12 (*GBE1*)
VI (Hers)	Liver phosphorylase	14q21-q22 (*PYGL*)
IXa	Phosphorylase kinase	Xp22.2-p22.1 (*PHKA2*)
IXb	Phosphorylase kinase	16q12-q13 (*PHKB*)
IXc	Phosphorylase kinase	16q12.1-11.2 (*PHKG2*)

Histologic Features

Type	Mosaic Pattern	Glycogenated Nuclei	Fatty Change	Fibrosis
0	No	No	No	No
I	Yes, uniformly	Yes	Yes	Sometimes
II	No	No	No	No
III	Yes, uniformly	Sometimes	Sometimes	Yes
IV	No	No	Sometimes	Yes
VI	Yes, periportal accentuation	Infrequently	Sometimes	Yes
IX	Yes, periportal accentuation	Infrequently	Sometimes	Yes

- Cyanamide-induced injury
  - Large eosinophilic, ground-glass inclusion with artifactual space
  - PAS-D positive
- Other medications
  - Diffuse hypertrophy of smooth endoplasmic reticulum
  - Pseudo-ground-glass cells in immunocompromised or liver transplant patients

DIAGNOSTIC CHECKLIST

Pathologic Interpretation Pearls

- Increased hepatic glycogen in all hepatic GSD except GSD 0
- Diagnostic ultrastructural feature for GSD II
  - Lysosomal-bound glycogen
- Unique cytoplasmic inclusion in GSD IV
  - Pathognomic cytoplasmic inclusions composed of fibrillar glycogen by electron microscopy

SELECTED REFERENCES

1. Heller S et al: Nutritional therapy for glycogen storage diseases. J Pediatr Gastroenterol Nutr. 47 Suppl 1:S15-21, 2008
2. Demo E et al: Glycogen storage disease type III-hepatocellular carcinoma a long-term complication? J Hepatol. 46(3):492-8, 2007
3. Torbenson M et al: Glycogenic hepatopathy: an underrecognized hepatic complication of diabetes mellitus. Am J Surg Pathol. 30(4):508-13, 2006
4. Wisell J et al: Glycogen pseudoground glass change in hepatocytes. Am J Surg Pathol. 30(9):1085-90, 2006
5. Miles L et al: Hepatocyte glycogen accumulation in patients undergoing dietary management of urea cycle defects mimics storage disease. J Pediatr Gastroenterol Nutr. 40(4):471-6, 2005
6. Laberge AM et al: Long-term follow-up of a new case of liver glycogen synthase deficiency. Am J Med Genet A. 120A(1):19-22, 2003
7. Wolfsdorf JI et al: Glycogen storage diseases. Phenotypic, genetic, and biochemical characteristics, and therapy. Endocrinol Metab Clin North Am. 28(4):801-23, 1999
8. Bao Y et al: Hepatic and neuromuscular forms of glycogen storage disease type IV caused by mutations in the same glycogen-branching enzyme gene. J Clin Invest. 97(4):941-8, 1996
9. Jevon GP et al: Reliability of histological criteria in glycogen storage disease of the liver. Pediatr Pathol. 14(4):709-21, 1994
10. Bianchi L: Glycogen storage disease I and hepatocellular tumours. Eur J Pediatr. 152 Suppl 1:S63-70, 1993
11. Phillips MJ et al: The liver. An Atlas and Text of Ultrastructural Pathology. New York: Raven Press, 1987
12. McAdams AJ et al: Glycogen storage disease, types I to X: criteria for morphologic diagnosis. Hum Pathol. 5(4):463-87, 1974

Microscopic Features

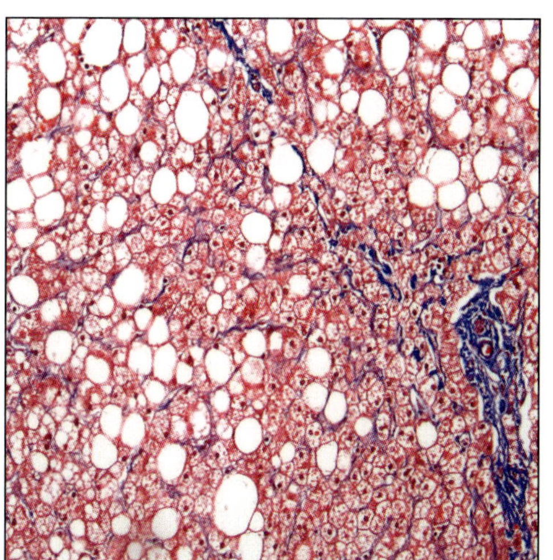

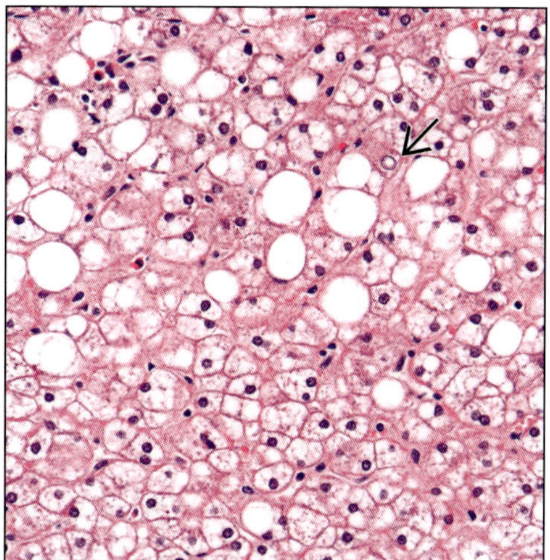

(Left) *Prominent large and small droplet fat as well as periportal fibrosis is depicted in this case of GSD Ia.* ***(Right)*** *The findings in this case of GSD Ib are similar to those observed in GSD Ia. Pale, enlarged hepatocytes with inconspicuous sinusoids contain only a rare glycogenated nucleus ⇒. Fatty change is more apparent in this focus.*

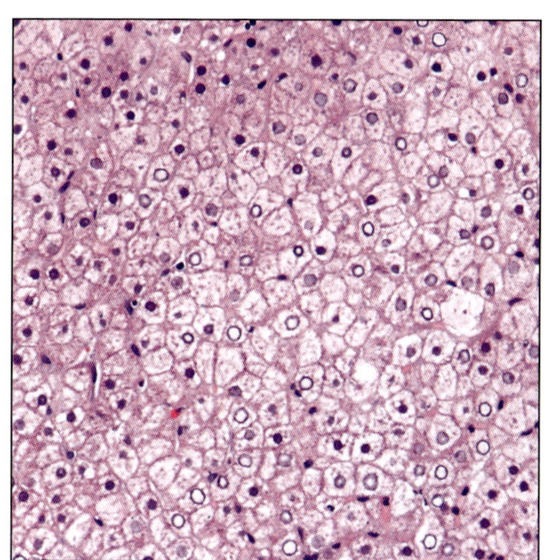

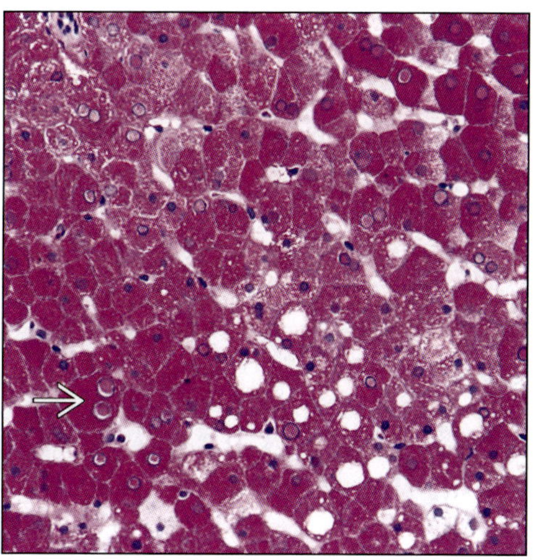

(Left) *In GSD III, the hepatocytes are arranged in a uniform mosaic pattern similar to GSD I but may reveal less fatty change. This focus has many hepatocytes with intranuclear glycogen, a feature that is more frequently observed in GSD I.* ***(Right)*** *This case of GSD III stained with PAS highlights diffuse cytoplasmic glycogen in hepatocytes and occasional intranuclear glycogen ➡. These features can be observed in most hepatic GSD, except in types 0 and IV.*

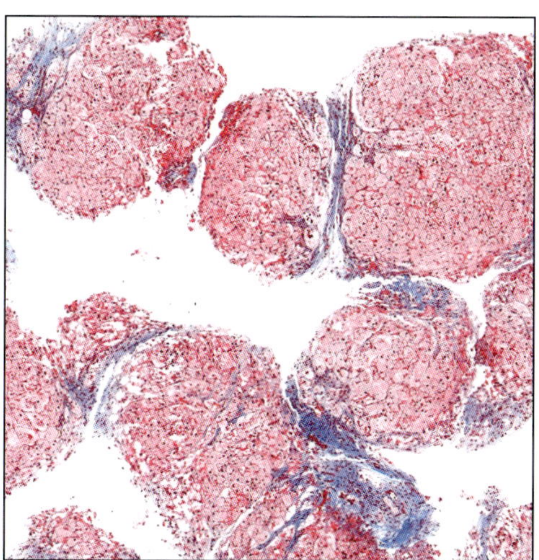

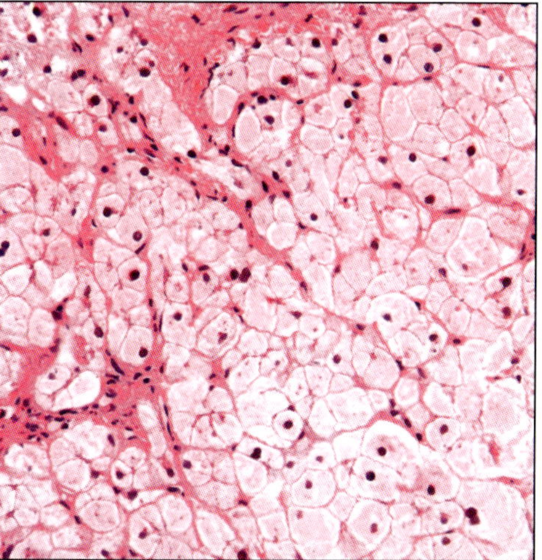

(Left) *This needle core biopsy from a patient with GSD III depicts cirrhosis characterized by nodules of hepatocytes partially surrounded by fibrosis.* ***(Right)*** *The hepatocytes are distended and create a mosaic architecture that is interrupted by fibrosis in this case of GSD III.*

GLYCOGEN STORAGE DISEASE

Microscopic Features

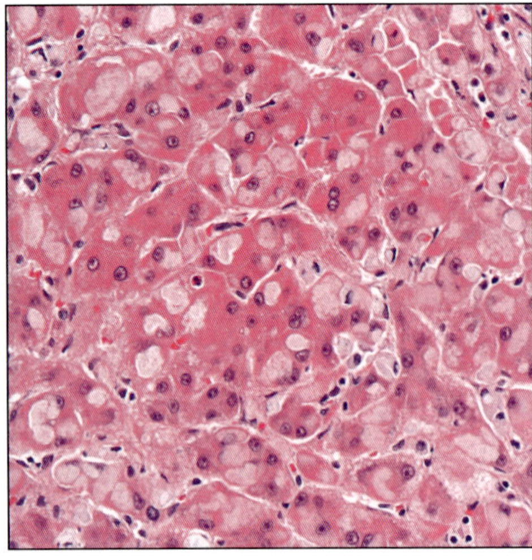

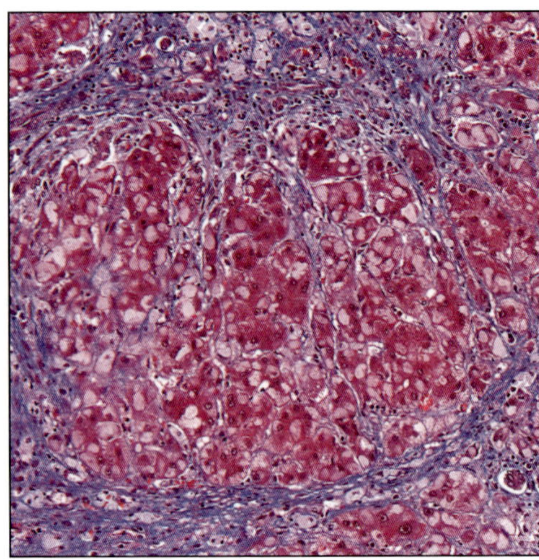

(Left) GSD IV demonstrates characteristic cytoplasmic inclusions within hepatocytes by light microscopy that distinguish it from the other types of GSD. These inclusions are kidney-bean-shaped and lightly basophilic. **(Right)** Trichrome highlights a small cirrhotic nodule completely surrounded by fibrosis in this case of GSD IV that has evolved into cirrhosis.

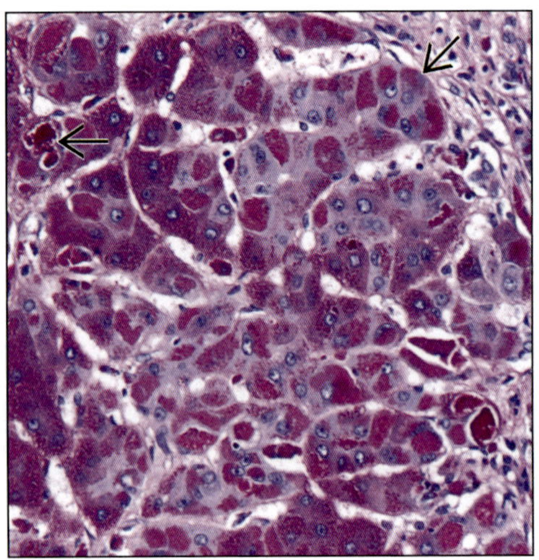

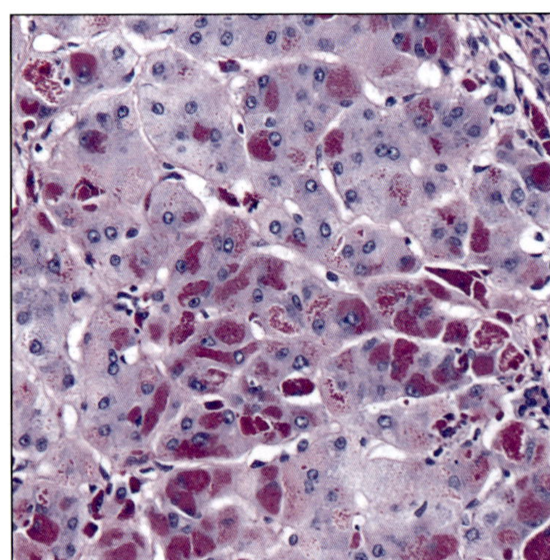

(Left) The characteristic inclusions ⇒ in GSD IV are positive for PAS. These hepatocytes contain both glycogen and amylopectin-like material. **(Right)** The amylopectin-like material that coexists with glycogen in the cytoplasm of hepatocytes results in the inclusions unique to GSD IV. Some positive staining with PAS-D is retained in the amylopectin-like material.

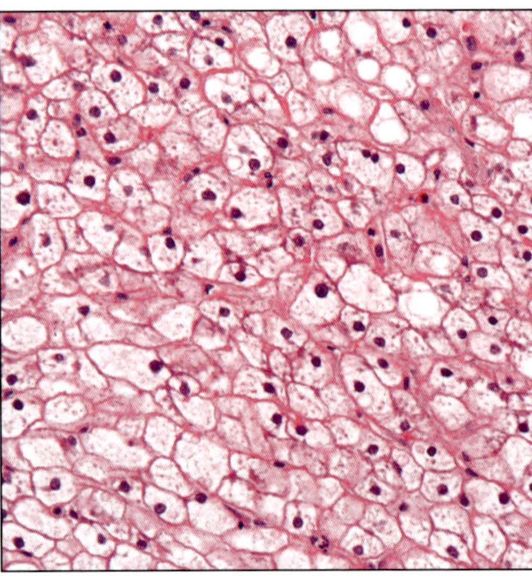

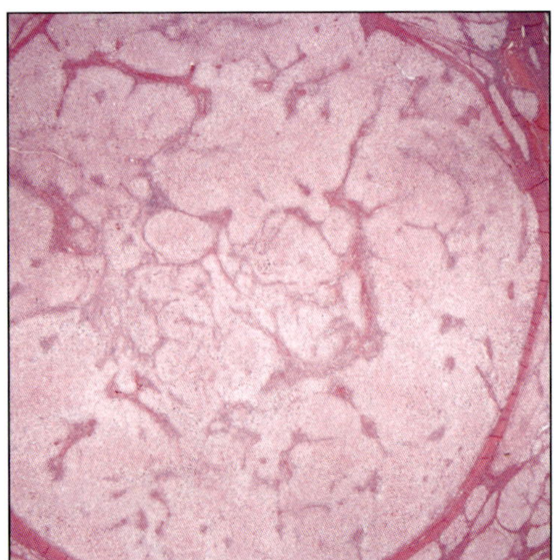

(Left) Unlike the uniform hepatocytes previously noted in GSD I and III, those in GSD IX are irregular in size and only rarely demonstrate nuclear glycogen. **(Right)** A small low-grade dysplastic nodule was incidentally identified in this liver with GSD IX. This well-circumscribed, < 1 cm nodule demonstrated uniform hepatocytes with bland cytologic features.

Ultrastructural Features

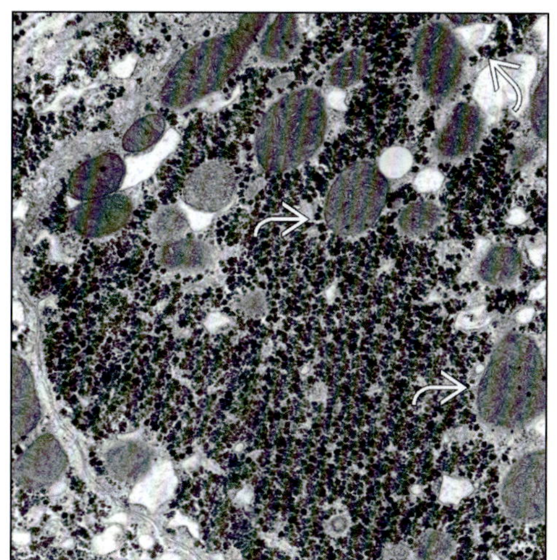

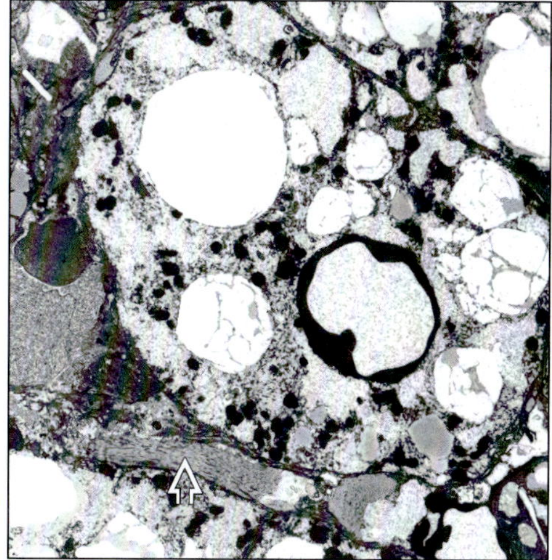

(Left) In GSD I, the increased glycogen occupies most of the cytoplasm and causes mitochondrial disbursement to the cell margin. A lipid vacuole is also present ➡. **(Right)** A hepatocyte from GSD III reveals cytoplasmic and intranuclear glycogen along with cytoplasmic lipid droplets. Fibrosis is characterized by the presence of collagen bundles ➡.

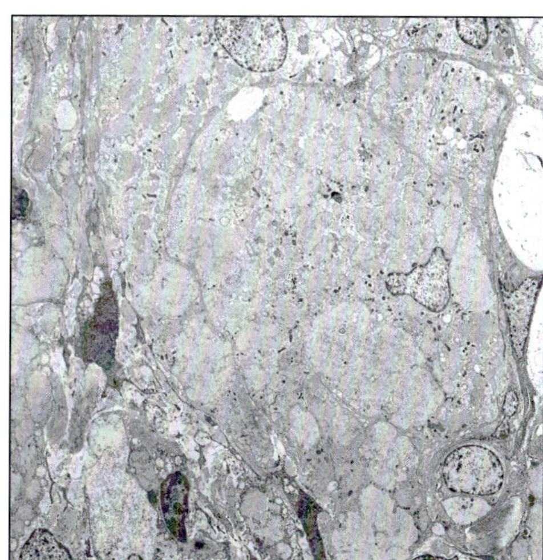

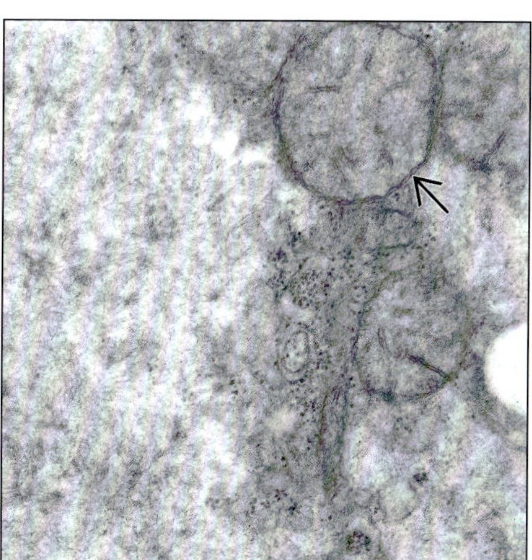

(Left) A hepatocyte in GSD IV with large irregular clusters of pale fibrils of glycogen is shown. (Courtesy J. Hicks, MD.) **(Right)** Higher magnification highlights the fibrillary quality of the glycogen typical of GSD IV and a mitochondria ➡ at the periphery. (Courtesy J. Hicks, MD.)

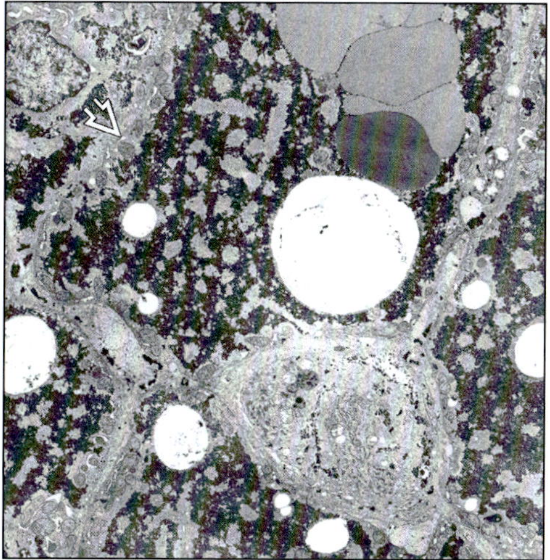

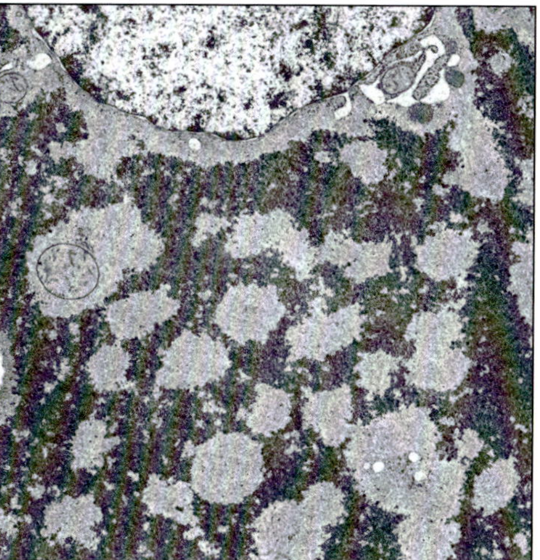

(Left) GSD IX at low magnification depicts displacement of mitochondria ➡ to the periphery of the cytoplasm in these hepatocytes by cytoplasmic glycogen and lipid. **(Right)** GSD IX at higher magnification highlights the "starry sky" appearance. This results from patchy zones of glycogen (dark areas) alternating with organelle-free zones (pale gray areas).

TYROSINEMIA

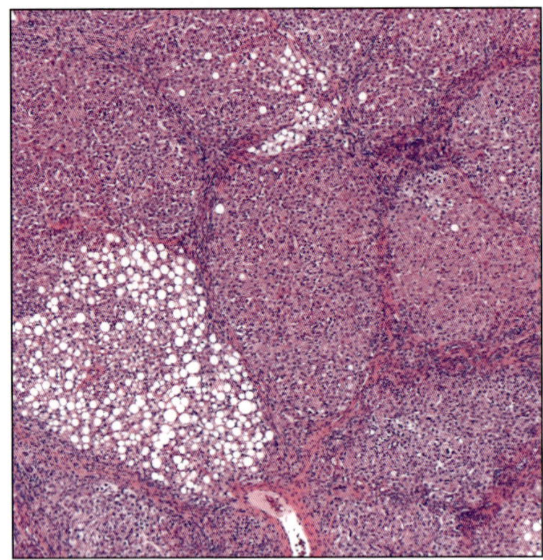

This micronodular cirrhotic liver demonstrates patchy areas of large droplet fatty change in some nodules.

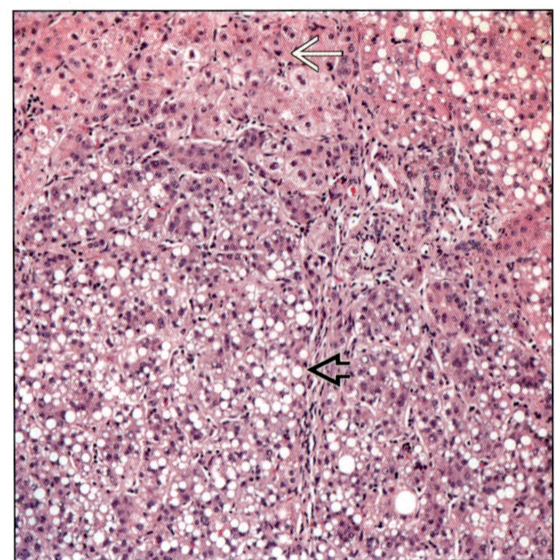

A dysplastic nodule ⮚ displays both small cell change and widened plate architecture. Note the adjacent normal liver ➡. (Courtesy M. J. Finegold, MD.)

TERMINOLOGY

Abbreviations

- Fumarylacetoacetate hydroxylase (FAH) deficiency

Synonyms

- Tyrosinemia, type I
- Hereditary tyrosinemia
- Hepatorenal tyrosinemia

Definitions

- Inborn error of metabolism
  - Autosomal recessive inheritance
  - Tyrosine catabolism pathway
    - Deficiency of fumarylacetoacetate hydroxylase
    - Results in cirrhosis and hepatocellular carcinoma early in life

ETIOLOGY/PATHOGENESIS

Molecular Basis

- Mutations in fumarylacetoacetate hydrolase gene on 15q23-q25
  - Fumarylacetoacetate hydroxylase deficiency
    - Accumulation of toxic and mutagenic metabolites, maleylacetoacetate, and fumarylacetoacetate
    - Excretion of secondary metabolite succinylacetone

CLINICAL ISSUES

Epidemiology

- Incidence
  - 1/100,000 to 1/120,000 worldwide; higher in Scandinavia and Quebec

Presentation

- Highly variable symptoms
  - Acute liver failure with hepatic synthetic dysfunction
  - Renal tubular dysfunction
  - Hypophosphatemic rickets
  - Neurologic crises with episodic paralysis and peripheral neuropathy
  - Positive newborn screening test

Laboratory Tests

- Elevated plasma and urine succinylacetone
- Elevated urinary 5-aminolevulinic acid
- Tyrosinemia and methioninemia on urinary amino acid analysis
- Elevated serum α-fetoprotein
- Decreased fumarylacetoacetate hydrolase enzymatic activity in cultured amniotic cells, fibroblasts, or liver

Natural History

- Prior to early detection, > 90% mortality before 2 years of age
- Progression of fibrosis to cirrhosis
- 15-37% risk of developing hepatocellular carcinoma

Treatment

- Dietary restriction of phenylalanine, tyrosine, and methionine
  - Normalizes plasma amino acids and improves acute symptoms only
- 2-(2-nitro-4-trifluoromethylbenzoyl)-1,3-cyclohexanedione (NTBC) administration
  - Early therapy reduces incidence of hepatocellular carcinoma
- Eventual need for orthotopic liver transplantation

Prognosis

- Good if detected early prior to development of hepatocellular carcinoma and transplanted
- > 90% die before 12 years of age with dietary treatment only

TYROSINEMIA

Key Facts

Terminology
- Synonym: Tyrosinemia, type I

Etiology/Pathogenesis
- Mutations in fumarylacetoacetate hydrolase gene on 15q23-q25
- Fumarylacetoacetate hydroxylase deficiency

Clinical Issues
- Elevated plasma and urine succinylacetone
- Many patients have renal tubular dysfunction
- Liver transplantation is treatment of choice for medical treatment failures
- 15-37% risk of developing hepatocellular carcinoma

Microscopic Pathology
- Variable fatty change and cholestasis
- Pericellular and periportal fibrosis to cirrhosis

MACROSCOPIC FEATURES

General Features
- Macronodular, micronodular, or mixed cirrhosis

MICROSCOPIC PATHOLOGY

Histologic Features
- Cholestasis (variable amounts) and pseudoacinar transformation
- Patchy large or small droplet fatty change
- Hemosiderosis
- Pericellular and periportal fibrosis that may progress to cirrhosis
- Acute form with massive hepatocyte necrosis

Predominant Pattern/Injury Type
- Fibrosis or necrosis

DIFFERENTIAL DIAGNOSIS

Other Metabolic Diseases
- Galactosemia
  - Histologic and ultrastructural findings are similar
    - Requires clinical distinction
- Hereditary fructose intolerance
  - Histologically similar
  - Ultrastructural changes are nearly diagnostic
    - "Fructose holes": Ovoid to irregular lucent, partially membrane-bound areas of cytoplasm up to 2 μm in diameter
    - Distinctive concentric arrays of endoplasmic reticulum with central rarefaction and glycogen particles

Neonatal Hemochromatosis (NH)
- Both can have increased iron stores in liver
- NH characterized by systemic iron deposition

DIAGNOSTIC CHECKLIST

Clinically Relevant Pathologic Features
- High risk of hepatocellular carcinoma

Pathologic Interpretation Pearls
- Fibrosis with variable amounts of steatosis and cholestasis; requires clinical correlation

SELECTED REFERENCES

1. Russo P et al: Visceral pathology of hereditary tyrosinemia type I. Am J Hum Genet. 47(2):317-24, 1990
2. Dehner LP et al: Hereditary tyrosinemia type I (chronic form): pathologic findings in the liver. Hum Pathol. 20(2):149-58, 1989
3. Weinberg AG et al: The occurrence of hepatoma in the chronic form of hereditary tyrosinemia. J Pediatr. 88(3):434-8, 1976

IMAGE GALLERY

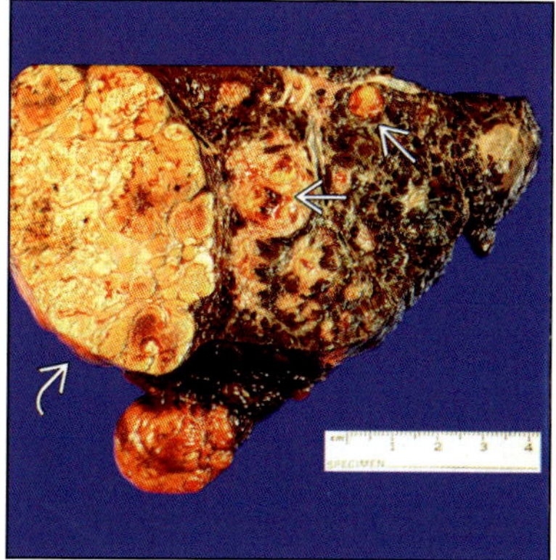
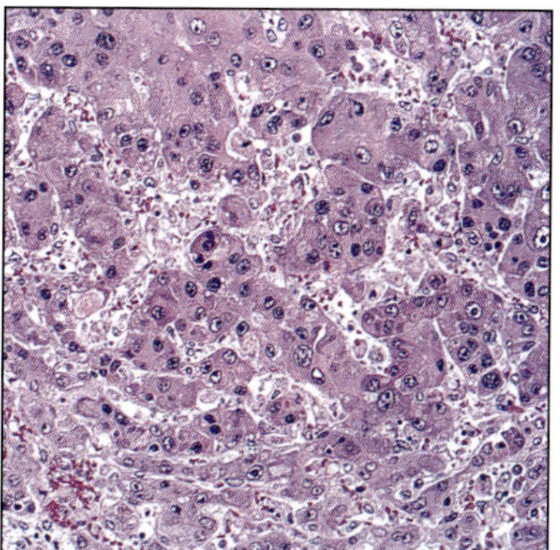
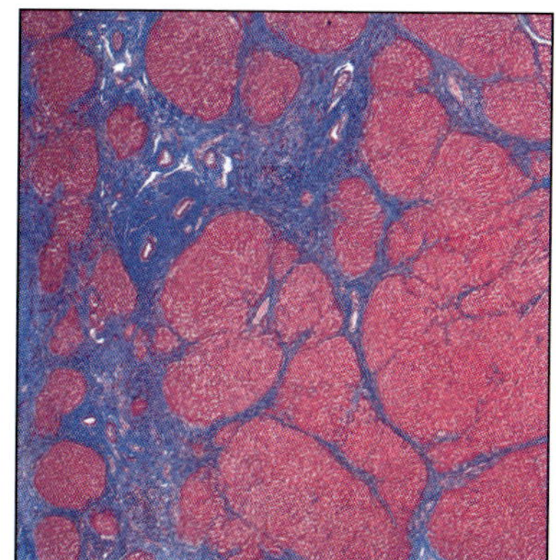

(Left) *Gross photograph of an explanted cirrhotic liver from a 1.5 year old depicts a 7.5 cm multinodular, yellow mass ➡ as well as smaller nodules ➡. (Courtesy M. J. Finegold, MD.)* ***(Center)*** *Histology of a mass from an explanted cirrhotic liver. Note the abnormal plate architecture and enlarged hyperchromatic nuclei typical of hepatocellular carcinoma. (Courtesy M. J. Finegold, MD.)* ***(Right)*** *Trichrome shows wide and narrow bands of fibrosis around variably sized nodules in this cirrhotic liver.*

NIEMANN-PICK DISEASE

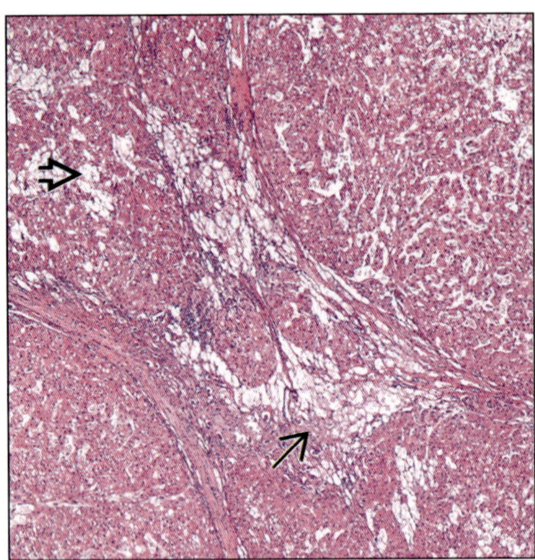

In an explanted liver, the pale-staining Niemann-Pick cells are evident both within cirrhotic nodules ⇨ and in the fibrous septae →.

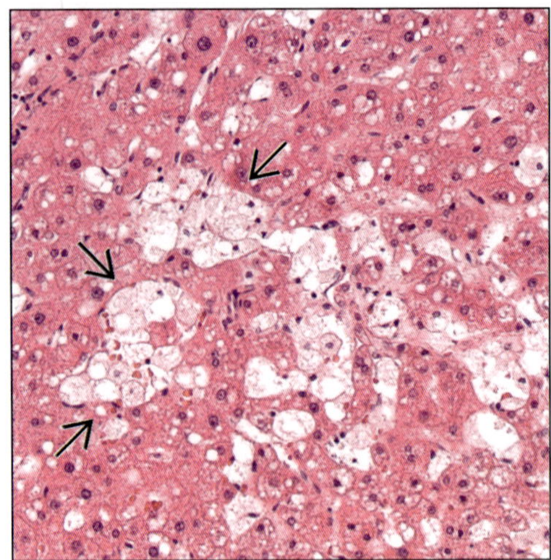

Niemann-Pick cells are pale cells with foamy cytoplasm → that accumulate between hepatocyte cords within the lobular hepatic parenchyma.

TERMINOLOGY

Abbreviations

- Niemann-Pick disease (NPD)

Synonyms

- Sphingomyelin-cholesterol lipidosis

Definitions

- Lysosomal storage disease resulting from defects in lysosomal function
- Disease subtypes
  - Acid sphingomyelinase deficiency
    - Types A and B
  - Cholesterol metabolism defect
    - Types C and D

ETIOLOGY/PATHOGENESIS

Enzyme Deficiency

- Inherited lysosomal hydrolase deficiency leads to accumulation of sphingolipid substrate in lysosomes

Mode of Inheritance

- Autosomal recessive

Disease Subtypes

- Types A and B caused by deficient acid sphingomyelinase activity resulting in sphingomyelin accumulation
  - Acid sphingomyelinase is found in lysosomes and functions in membrane degradation and turnover
  - Sphingomyelin substrate and other lipids accumulate in histiocytes
  - Over 100 mutations described in the *SMPD1* gene encoding acid sphingomyelinase
- Types C and D caused by cholesterol metabolism defect leading to accumulation of cholesterol and sphingomyelin
  - Type D appears to be allelic variant of type C

CLINICAL ISSUES

Epidemiology

- Incidence
  - Estimated 0.5-1 cases in 100,000 newborns
- Ethnicity
  - Types A and B described in Ashkenazi Jews and individuals from North America, Western Europe, North Africa, and Middle East
  - Many patients with NPD type D are Acadians from southwestern Nova Scotia

Presentation

- Hepatosplenomegaly with variable neurodegenerative course
- Type A begins in utero and may present with hydrops fetalis in severe cases
  - Rapidly progressive neurodegeneration
- Type B may present in infancy, childhood, or adulthood
  - Pulmonary compromise occurs due to sphingomyelin deposition in lung parenchyma
  - Little or no neurodegenerative features seen in type B
- Types C and D can present at any age
  - May have infantile cholestasis
  - Slowly progressive but variable neurodegenerative disease

Treatment

- No specific treatment available

Prognosis

- Type A usually fatal by age 3
- Type B leads to progressive liver disease, including cirrhosis, portal hypertension, and ascites
  - Patients with type B frequently survive into adulthood
- Patients with type C or D develop progressive neurological deterioration

NIEMANN-PICK DISEASE

Key Facts

Terminology
- Lysosomal storage disease resulting from defects in lysosomal function

Etiology/Pathogenesis
- Inherited lysosomal hydrolase deficiency leads to accumulation of sphingolipid substrate in lysosomes

Clinical Issues
- Hepatosplenomegaly with variable neurodegenerative course

Microscopic Pathology
- Spotty accumulation of enlarged histiocytes with cytoplasmic inclusions in hepatic lobules and portal tracts

- In severe cases, may lead to death by age 3-5
- Type D follows slower neurodegenerative course than type C

MICROSCOPIC PATHOLOGY

Predominant Pattern/Injury Type
- Storage disease

Predominant Cell/Compartment Type
- Storage cell
- Histiocyte/macrophage

Histologic Features
- Spotty accumulation of enlarged histiocytes in hepatic lobules and portal tracts
  - Histiocyte inclusions rounded and of fairly uniform size, imparting foamy appearance to cytoplasm
  - May lead to hepatic plate atrophy and fibrosis
- Hepatocytes may also accumulate sphingomyelin
- Foamy histiocytes also accumulate in other organs

ANCILLARY TESTS

Electron Microscopy
- Transmission
  - Electron-opaque, concentrically laminated inclusions within histiocyte cytoplasm

DIFFERENTIAL DIAGNOSIS

Gaucher Disease
- Gaucher cells have striated, fibrillary cytoplasmic inclusions within histiocytes

DIAGNOSTIC CHECKLIST

Clinically Relevant Pathologic Features
- Hepatosplenomegaly and variable neurodegenerative disease

Pathologic Interpretation Pearls
- Foamy, vacuolated histiocytes accumulate in liver and other organs

SELECTED REFERENCES

1. Pacheco CD et al: The pathogenesis of Niemann-Pick type C disease: a role for autophagy?. Expert Rev Mol Med. 10:e26, 2008
2. Schuchman EH: The pathogenesis and treatment of acid sphingomyelinase-deficient Niemann-Pick disease. J Inherit Metab Dis. 30(5):654-63, 2007
3. Meikle PJ et al: Prevalence of lysosomal storage disorders. JAMA. 281(3):249-54, 1999
4. Greer WL et al: The Nova Scotia (type D) form of Niemann-Pick disease is caused by a G3097-->T transversion in NPC1. Am J Hum Genet. 63(1):52-4, 1998

IMAGE GALLERY

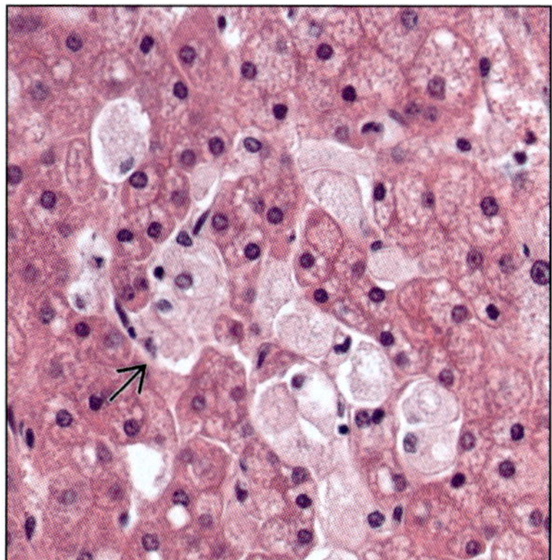

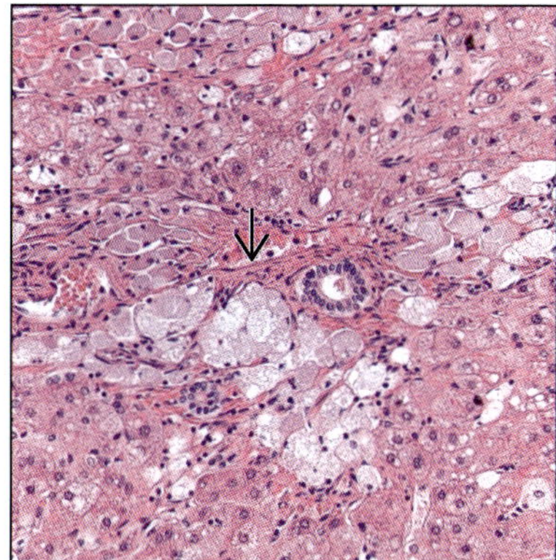

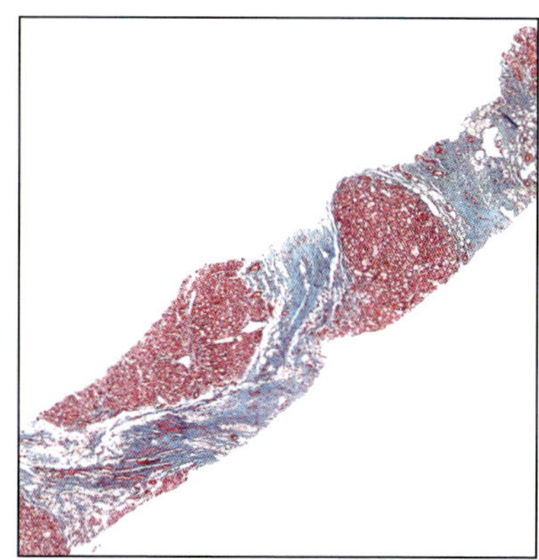

(Left) *Niemann-Pick cells ⇒ are pale-staining, large histocytes with amphophilic, foamy, and vacuolated cytoplasmic inclusions. These cells are distinct from the more deeply eosinophilic hepatocytes.* ***(Center)*** *Large, pale Niemann-Pick cells with vacuolated cytoplasm are easily identified within portal tracts ⇒.* ***(Right)*** *Niemann-Pick disease can cause ongoing liver fibrosis with progression to cirrhosis and complications of end-stage liver disease.*

GAUCHER DISEASE

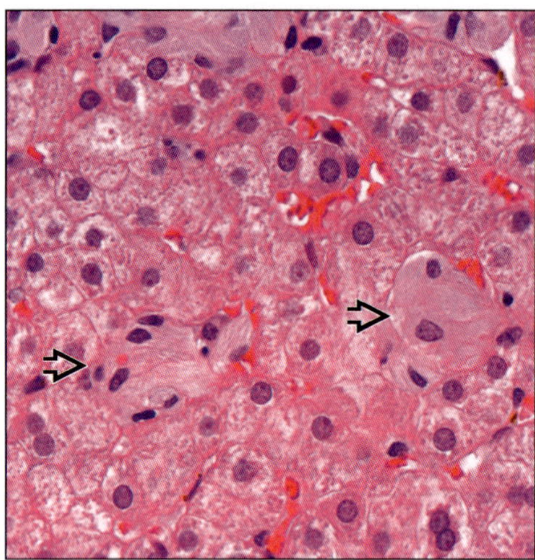

H&E slide shows clusters of enlarged Kupffer cells ➪ with uniquely striated cytoplasm in the lobule.

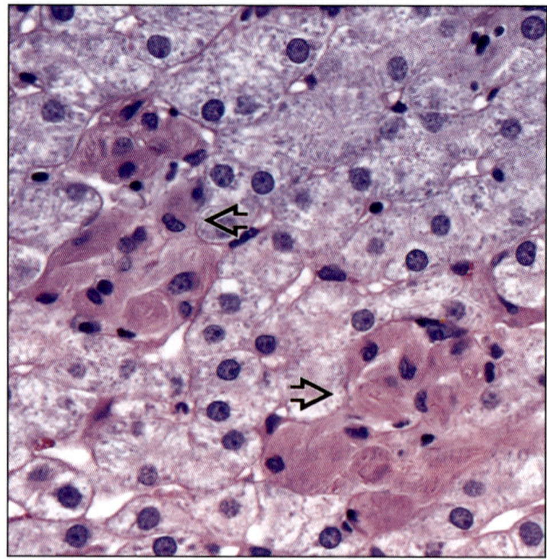

PAS-D positive aggregates of Kupffer cells with striated cytoplasm ➪ fill the sinusoids.

TERMINOLOGY

Synonyms

- Glucocerebrosidase deficiency

Definitions

- Inherited deficiency of lysosomal enzyme glucocerebroside
- 3 clinical forms

ETIOLOGY/PATHOGENESIS

Inborn Error of Metabolism

- Most common lysosomal glycolipid storage disorder
  - Enzyme deficiency
    - Acid β-glucosidase (glucocerebrosidase)
  - Accumulation of glucocerebroside (also called glucosylceramide) in phagocytic cells

Autosomal Recessive Trait

- Mutation in *GBA*, encoding acid β-glucosidase, on 1q21
- Homozygotes are affected

CLINICAL ISSUES

Site

- Visceral organs such as liver, spleen, and lung
- Bone marrow and bone
- With or without central nervous system involvement

Presentation

- Hepatosplenomegaly
- Pancytopenia
  - Anemia
  - Thrombocytopenia
- 3 classic clinical variants
  - Type 1 (nonneuronopathic)
    - Most common form
    - 55-60% diagnosed before 20 years of age
    - 30% diagnosed before 10 years of age
  - Types 2 and 3 (neuronopathic)

Treatment

- Enzyme replacement therapy
- Substrate reduction therapy
- Splenectomy

Prognosis

- Early diagnosis is crucial to improving outcome
- Variable disease progression

MICROSCOPIC PATHOLOGY

Histologic Features

- Accumulation and storage of glucocerebroside
  - In Kupffer cells and macrophages
  - Spares hepatocytes
- Effects secondary to sinusoidal Kupffer cell involvement are rare
  - Atrophic hepatocytes
  - Eventual sinusoidal fibrosis
- Micronodular cirrhosis and hepatocellular carcinoma have been reported

Cytologic Features

- Characteristic linear, tissue paper-like, fibrillary, or corrugated amphophilic cytoplasm
  - Cells are positive for PAS-D

ANCILLARY TESTS

Electron Microscopy

- Enlarged Kupffer cells and portal tract macrophages
    - Cytoplasm expanded by enlarged, irregular, single membrane-bound lysosomes
    - Lysosomes filled with stored glucocerebroside substance

GAUCHER DISEASE

Key Facts

Etiology/Pathogenesis

- Accumulation of glucocerebroside in phagocytic cells
- Autosomal recessive trait with mutation in acid β-glucosidase gene, *GBA*

Clinical Issues

- Primarily involves liver, spleen, bone marrow, and bone
- Results in hepatosplenomegaly, anemia, and thrombocytopenia

Microscopic Pathology

- Accumulation of glucocerebroside in Kupffer cells and portal tract macrophages results in uniquely linear amphophilic cytoplasm
  - Sparing of hepatocytes

Ancillary Tests

- Electron microscopy demonstrates intralysosomal compact long tubular structures

  - Compact long tubular structures or finely reticular to flocculent material

DIFFERENTIAL DIAGNOSIS

Niemann-Pick Disease

- Histological overlap
  - Enlarged Kupffer cells but foamy cytoplasm with small round vacuoles
  - Enlarged pale hepatocytes may be indistinguishable from Kupffer cells
- By electron microscopy
  - Concentric lamellar lipid inclusions in lysosomes of hepatocytes and Kupffer cells in Niemann-Pick disease

Wolman Disease

- Histologically similar to Niemann-Pick disease
  - Frozen section stained slide stained with oil red O reveals abundant lipid, and polarized light highlights needle-shaped cholesterol crystals
- Distinguished by electron microscopy
  - Membrane-bound lipid droplets in hepatocytes and Kupffer cells
  - Cholesterol crystals in hepatocytes and Kupffer cells

Pseudo-Gaucher Cells in Bone Marrow Biopsy

- Resulting from high rate of cell turnover
- Can be found in chronic myelogenous leukemia

DIAGNOSTIC CHECKLIST

Pathologic Interpretation Pearls

- Accumulation of glucocerebroside in Kupffer cells and macrophages but not hepatocytes
- Electron microscopy demonstrates intralysosomal rod-shaped inclusions

SELECTED REFERENCES

1. Chen M et al: Gaucher disease: review of the literature. Arch Pathol Lab Med. 132(5):851-3, 2008
2. Xu R et al: Hepatocellular carcinoma in type 1 Gaucher disease: a case report with review of the literature. Semin Liver Dis. 25(2):226-9, 2005
3. Niederau C et al: Gaucher's disease: a review for the internist and hepatologist. Hepatogastroenterology. 47(34):984-97, 2000
4. Pastores GM: Gaucher's Disease. Pathological features. Baillieres Clin Haematol. 10(4):739-49, 1997
5. Lee RE: The pathology of Gaucher disease. Prog Clin Biol Res. 95:177-217, 1982
6. James SP et al: LIver abnormalities in patients with Gaucher's disease. Gastroenterology. 80(1):126-33, 1981
7. Lee RE et al: Gaucher's disease. I. Modern enzymatic and anatomic methods of diagnosis. Arch Pathol Lab Med. 105(2):102-4, 1981
8. Lee RE et al: Gaucher's disease: clinical, morphologic, and pathogenetic considerations. Pathol Annu. 12 Pt 2:309-39, 1977
9. Hibbs RG et al: A histochemical and electron microscopic study of Gaucher cells. Arch Pathol. 89(2):137-53, 1970

IMAGE GALLERY

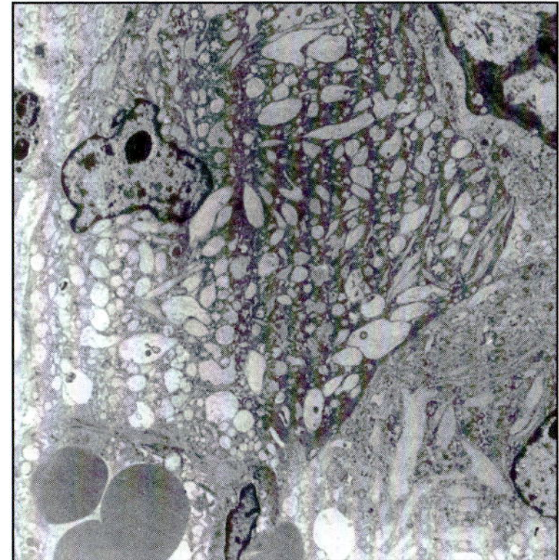

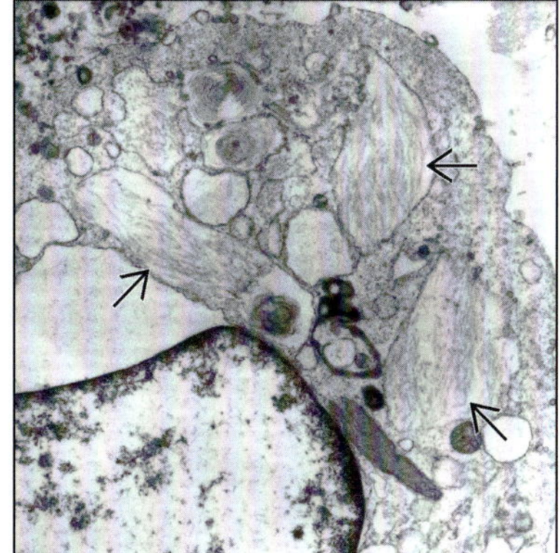

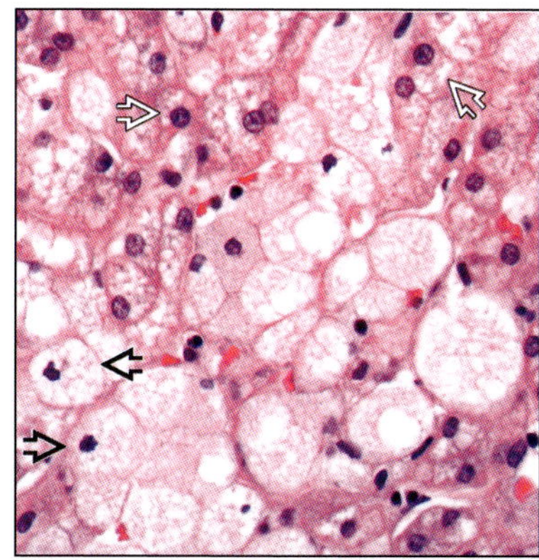

(Left) *An enlarged macrophage with lysosomal inclusions displaces the nucleus. Irregularly shaped single membrane-bound lysosomes are filled with tubular structures. (Courtesy J. Olson, MD.)* ***(Center)*** *Electron microscopy of a Gaucher cell demonstrates lysosomes containing numerous elongated tubular structures ⇒ arranged in compact bundles. (Courtesy Z. Laszik, MD, PhD.)* ***(Right)*** *Clusters of enlarged foamy Kupffer cells ⇨ with microvesicular cytoplasm and eccentric wrinkled nuclei can be difficult to distinguish from hepatocytes ➡.*

NEONATAL HEMOCHROMATOSIS

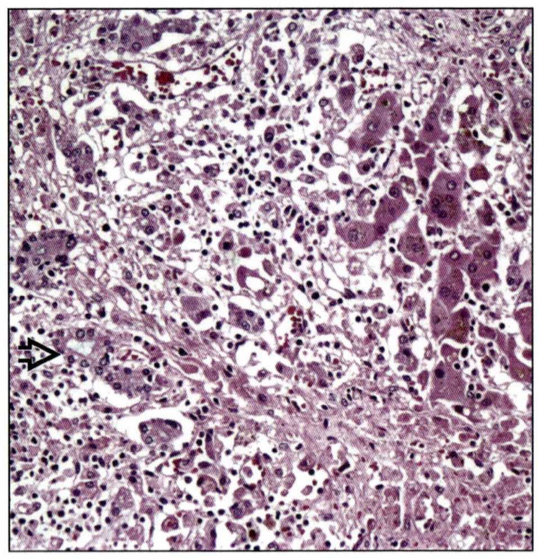

A case of neonatal hemochromatosis shows lobular necrosis and collapse of the hepatocellular cords with residual hepatocytes and bile ductules ⊳.

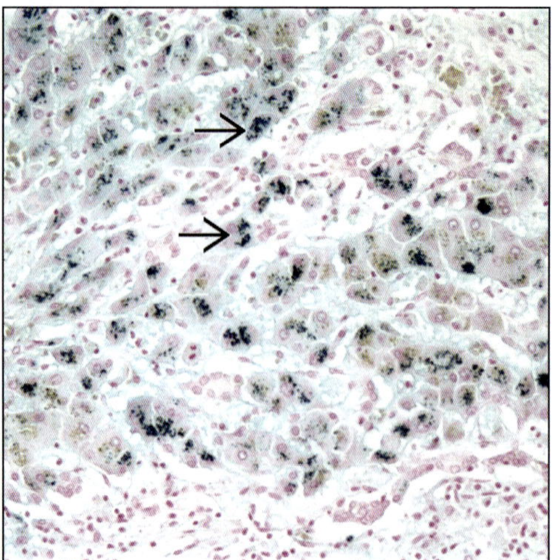

Perl iron stain shows marked iron deposition ⇒ within the hepatocytes.

TERMINOLOGY

Abbreviations

- Neonatal hemochromatosis (NH)

Synonyms

- Congenital hemochromatosis
- Neonatal iron storage disease

Definitions

- Severe liver disease with iron overload in liver and other organs (distribution similar to hereditary hemochromatosis)
  - Fetal or perinatal onset
  - Without hereditary hemochromatosis gene mutation

ETIOLOGY/PATHOGENESIS

Unknown

- Etiology remains unclear though alloimmune liver injury has been suggested

CLINICAL ISSUES

Epidemiology

- Incidence
  - Extremely rare

Site

- Liver
- Pancreas
- Heart
- Thyroid
- Minor salivary glands

Presentation

- Intrauterine growth retardation
- Oligohydramnios
- Stillborn or premature birth
- Severe fetal liver failure
  - Jaundice with elevated bilirubin
  - Coagulopathy
  - Hypoalbuminemia, edema, ascites
  - Very high AFP
    - Disproportionately low aminotransferases
- Multiorgan failure
  - Sepsis
  - Hypoglycemia
  - Oliguria
- Abnormal iron studies
  - Hypotransferrinemia
  - Hyperferritinemia

Laboratory Tests

- Elevated hepatic iron concentration
  - 240 to 38,200 µg/g dry weight (healthy neonate 250 µg/g dry weight)

Treatment

- Drug cocktail containing antioxidants and iron chelator
- Supportive care
- Liver transplantation

Prognosis

- Generally very poor

IMAGE FINDINGS

MR Findings

- Iron deposition may be found on
  - Liver
  - Pancreas
  - Heart

NEONATAL HEMOCHROMATOSIS

Key Facts

Clinical Issues
- Intrauterine growth retardation, oligohydramnios, stillborn or premature birth
- Liver and multiorgan failure
- Abnormal iron studies

Macroscopic Features
- Shrunken liver
- Cirrhosis

Microscopic Pathology
- Marked lobular necrosis with collapse, regenerative nodules
- Giant hepatocytes
- Iron deposition in hepatocytes and ductules as well as in organs outside of liver

Top Differential Diagnoses
- Cytomegalovirus, echovirus, herpes simplex virus infection; neonatal lupus, tyrosinemia

MACROSCOPIC FEATURES

General Features
- Cirrhosis, shrunken liver

MICROSCOPIC PATHOLOGY

Histologic Features
- Marked lobular necrosis
  - Accompanied by parenchymal collapse
- Regenerative nodule formation
- Giant cell transformation of hepatocytes
- Pseudoacinar formation
- Intracanalicular bile plugs
- Iron-laden hepatocytes and ductules
  - Highlighted by iron stain
  - Sparing of reticuloendothelial system
- Also features abnormal iron deposition in other organs

Predominant Pattern/Injury Type
- Abnormal accumulation

Predominant Cell/Compartment Type
- Hepatocytes

DIFFERENTIAL DIAGNOSIS

Viral Infection
- Look for inclusions, evidence of virus on EM

Neonatal Lupus
- Infants have ANA(+), lupoid antibodies on immunofluorescence

Tyrosinemia
- Urinary excretion of toxic metabolites

DIAGNOSTIC CHECKLIST

Clinically Relevant Pathologic Features
- Abnormal hepatic iron accumulation in severely ill neonate

Pathologic Interpretation Pearls
- Abnormal iron accumulation in tissues

SELECTED REFERENCES

1. Whitington PF: Fetal and infantile hemochromatosis. Hepatology. 43(4):654-60, 2006
2. Knisely AS et al: Neonatal hemochromatosis. Gastroenterol Clin North Am. 32(3):877-89, vi-vii, 2003
3. Murray KF et al: Neonatal hemochromatosis. Pediatrics. 108(4):960-4, 2001
4. Kershisnik MM et al: Cytomegalovirus infection, fetal liver disease, and neonatal hemochromatosis. Hum Pathol. 23(9):1075-80, 1992

IMAGE GALLERY

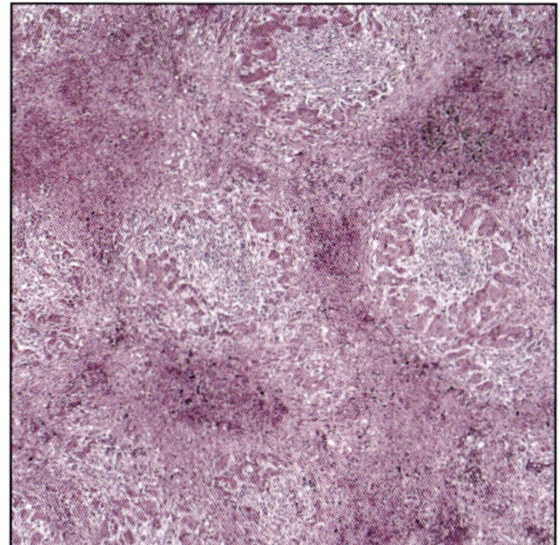

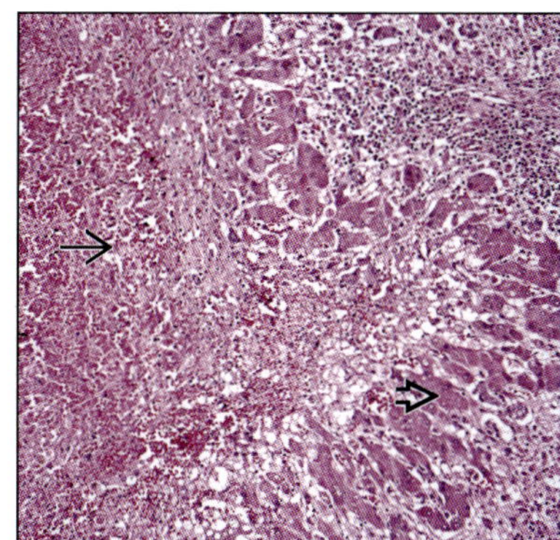

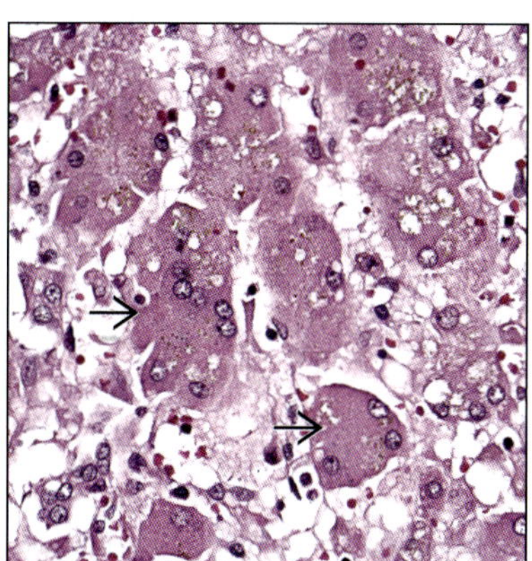

(Left) Low power photomicrograph shows parenchymal collapse and regenerative nodules in a case of neonatal hemochromatosis. ***(Center)*** *Higher power shows submassive hepatocellular necrosis ⇒ with a rim of residual hepatocytes ⇒.* ***(Right)*** *Giant cell transformation of the hepatocytes ⇒ can be seen in neonatal hemochromatosis.*

PORPHYRIN METABOLISM DISORDERS

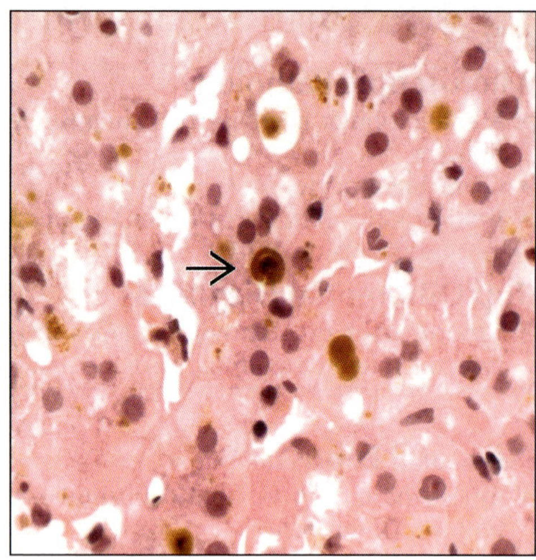

Hematoxylin & eosin section of erythropoietic protoporphyria shows cholestasis and rust-brown deposits ➔ in hepatocytes and canaliculi.

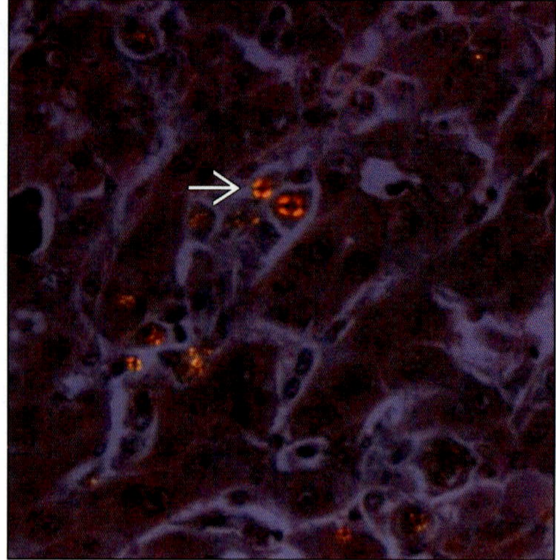

Hematoxylin & eosin section of erythropoietic protoporphyria viewed under polarized light shows birefringent protoporphyrin deposits that are brightly birefringent and have a Maltese cross appearance ➔.

TERMINOLOGY

Abbreviations

- Porphyria cutanea tarda (PCT)
- Erythropoietic protoporphyria (EP)

Synonyms

- EP has also been called erythrohepatic protoporphyria and protoporphyria

Definitions

- Heterogeneous group of inherited and acquired disorders of heme biosynthesis
  - PCT and EP are associated with hepatic pathology
  - "Hepatic" and "erythropoietic" porphyrias are characterized by accumulation of intermediates in liver and erythroid cells, respectively

ETIOLOGY/PATHOGENESIS

Genetic Disorder

- Sporadic PCT is associated with partial deficiency of uroporphyrinogen decarboxylase activity, only in liver
- Familial PCT is due to deficiency of uroporphyrinogen decarboxylase activity in all tissues
- EP is due to partial deficiency of ferrochelatase activity

Sporadic Disease

- Sporadic PCT is primarily an acquired disorder
  - Occurs in patients without genetic defects although partial deficiency of uroporphyrinogen decarboxylase may contribute
  - Associated with genetic conditions that increase iron absorption (e.g., *HFE* mutations)
  - Approximately half of all patients have hepatitis C virus infection (HCV)
  - Other contributory substances or conditions include alcohol, HIV infection, estrogen use, smoking, low vitamin C, and carotenoid status

CLINICAL ISSUES

Epidemiology

- Incidence
  - PCT prevalence: 1 in 25,000 persons in North America and higher in some European countries and among the South African Bantu population
  - EP prevalence: 1 in 75,000-200,000 persons among some Western European populations
- Age
  - Sporadic PCT occurs in patients between 40 and 50 years of age
  - Familial PCT occurs early, sometimes in childhood
  - EP presents with photosensitivity in childhood, but liver disease usually presents after age 30
- Gender
  - Sporadic PCT and EP occur more often in males

Presentation

- PCT: Blistering skin condition on sun-exposed areas and abnormal liver function tests
- EP: Transient cutaneous erythema and swelling immediately after sun exposure
  - Minority of patients develops severe liver disease

Laboratory Tests

- Measuring porphyrins in urine, feces, and, in some cases, erythrocytes

Treatment

- PCT: Phlebotomy, low-dose chloroquine, avoidance of sun exposure, avoidance of alcohol and estrogens
- EP: β-carotene, avoidance of sun exposure, cholestyramine

Prognosis

- PCT: Good prognosis although there is increased risk of cirrhosis and hepatocellular carcinoma (especially with HCV coinfection)

PORPHYRIN METABOLISM DISORDERS

Key Facts

Terminology
- Heterogeneous group of inherited and acquired disorders of heme biosynthesis
  - PCT and EP are associated with hepatic pathology

Etiology/Pathogenesis
- Sporadic PCT is primarily an acquired disorder
  - Precipitating factors include HCV, *HFE* mutations, alcohol, and drugs
- EP due to partial deficiency of ferrochelatase activity

Clinical Issues
- Photosensitivity
- Variable liver disease

Microscopic Pathology
- PCT: Mild to moderate siderosis, steatosis, changes typical of HCV
- EP: Cholestasis; red-brown aggregates of protoporphyrin in canaliculi, hepatocytes, Kupffer cells

Ancillary Tests
- PCT
  - EM
  - Polarization microscopy
  - Ferric ferricyanide stain
  - Laboratory testing for porphyrins
- EP
  - EM
  - Polarization microscopy
  - Laboratory testing for porphyrins

- EP: Prognosis varies according to presence and degree of liver damage
  - Liver transplantation improves survival but is not curative since excess porphyrin is produced in bone marrow and not in liver

MACROSCOPIC FEATURES

General Features
- EP: Black appearance to liver

MICROSCOPIC PATHOLOGY

Histologic Features
- PCT
  - Needle-shaped cytoplasmic inclusions in hepatocytes rarely seen by light microscopy of unstained sections, polarizing light, or ferric ferricyanide stain
  - Steatosis, variable siderosis, and fibrosis
  - Patients with concomitant HCV infection may show chronic hepatitis typical of HCV
- EP
  - Cholestasis and red-brown aggregates of protoporphyrin in canaliculi, hepatocytes, and Kupffer cells
  - Protoporphyrin deposits are birefringent on polarizing microscopy; some show Maltese cross configuration
  - Variable fibrosis or cirrhosis

Predominant Pattern/Injury Type
- Inclusion

Predominant Cell/Compartment Type
- Hepatocyte

ANCILLARY TESTS

Electron Microscopy
- PCT
  - Needle-like structures in hepatocytes
- EP
  - Aggregates of radiating crystals in dilated canaliculi, hepatocyte vacuoles, and Kupffer cells

DIFFERENTIAL DIAGNOSIS

Hepatitis C Infection
- PCT rarely shows needle-like structures in hepatocytes; skin blistering

Hemochromatosis
- PCT associated with skin blistering

Cholestasis
- EP shows more red-brown color of the inspissated material; polarization microscopy shows birefringence and Maltese cross configuration in deposits; cutaneous hypersensitivity

DIAGNOSTIC CHECKLIST

Clinically Relevant Pathologic Features
- Patients have photosensitivity, variable degree of liver disease

Pathologic Interpretation Pearls
- PCT: Nonspecific siderosis, features of HCV; inclusions difficult to identify on H&E
- EP: Look for red-brown inclusions in hepatocytes

SELECTED REFERENCES

1. Gross U et al: Erythropoietic and hepatic porphyrias. J Inherit Metab Dis. 23(7):641-61, 2000
2. Meerman L: Erythropoietic protoporphyria. An overview with emphasis on the liver. Scand J Gastroenterol Suppl. (232):79-85, 2000
3. Pimstone NR: Hematologic and hepatic manifestations of the cutaneous porphyrias. Clin Dermatol. 3(2):83-102, 1985

Gross and Microscopic Features of EP

(Left) Gross specimen of a liver in erythropoietic protoporphyria shows the typical black discoloration. (Right) Trichrome stain shows increased fibrosis with bridging in erythropoietic protoporphyria.

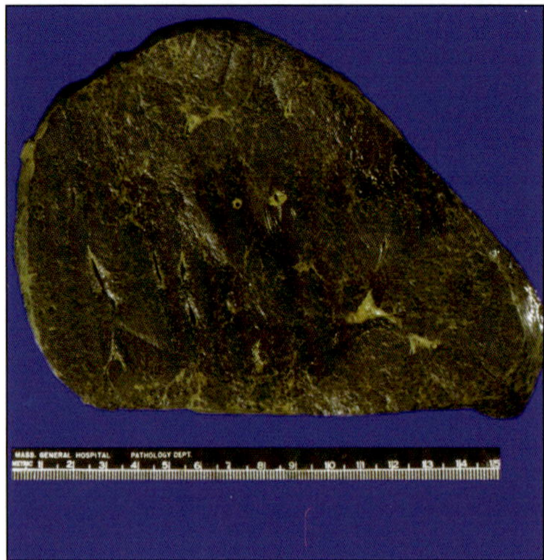

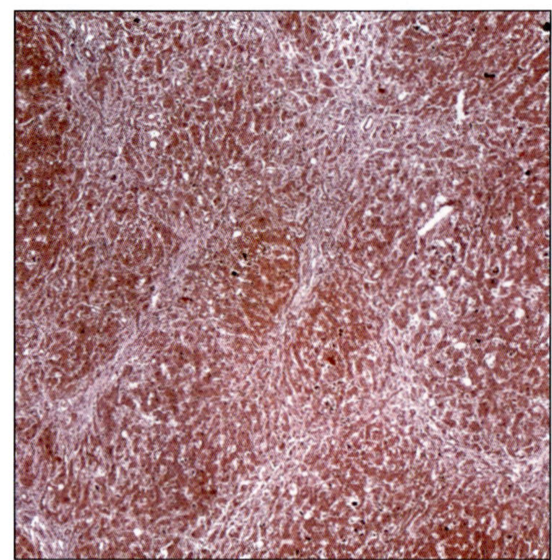

(Left) Hematoxylin & eosin section of erythropoietic protoporphyria shows cholestasis and brown deposits of protoporphyrin in the liver parenchyma with degenerative changes in hepatocytes. (Right) Hematoxylin & eosin section of erythropoietic protoporphyria shows cholestasis and brown protoporphyrin deposits ⇒ in a background of vacuolated and mildly swollen hepatocytes.

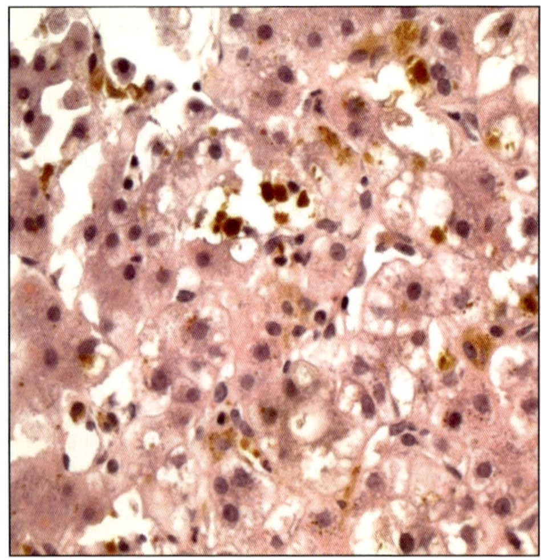

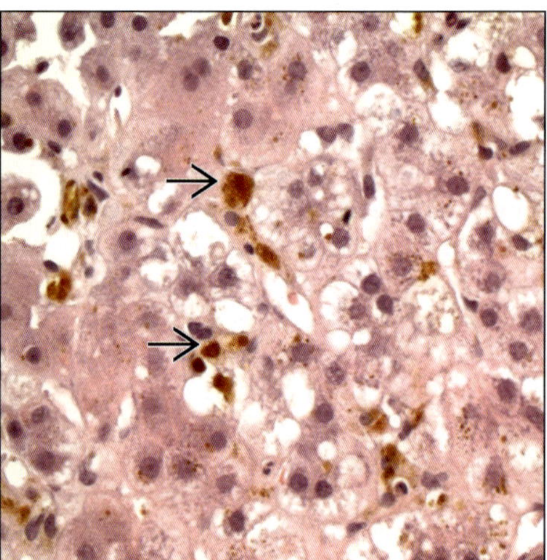

(Left) Hematoxylin & eosin section under polarized light shows a large protoporphyrin deposit with the Maltese cross configuration ➡, whereas other deposits confer a "starry sky" appearance in this case of erythropoietic protoporphyria. (Right) Electron micrograph shows aggregates of crystals of protoporphyrin in a radiating pattern ⇨ in erythropoietic protoporphyria.

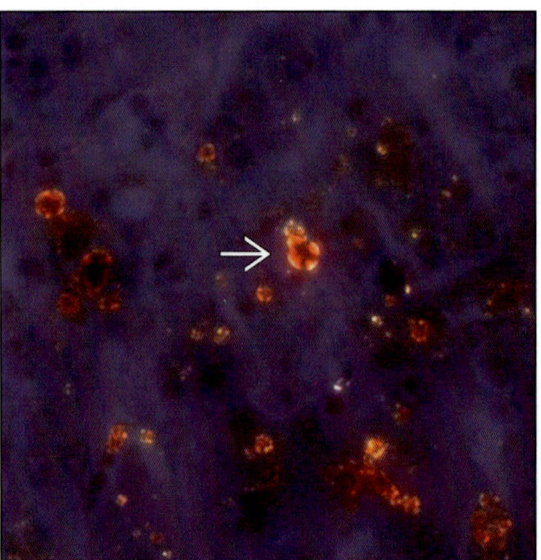

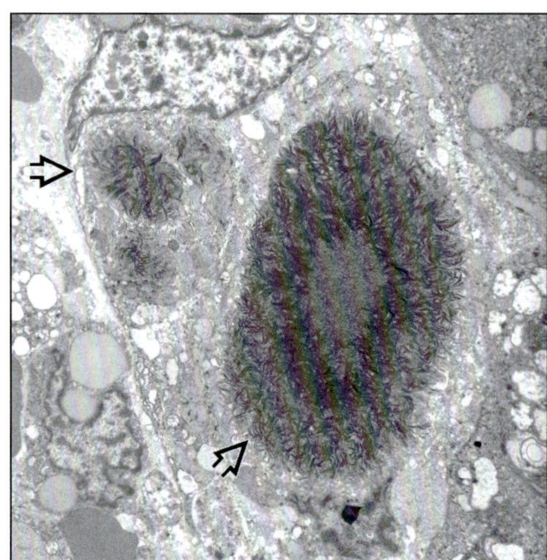

Microscopic and Diagrammatic Features of PCT

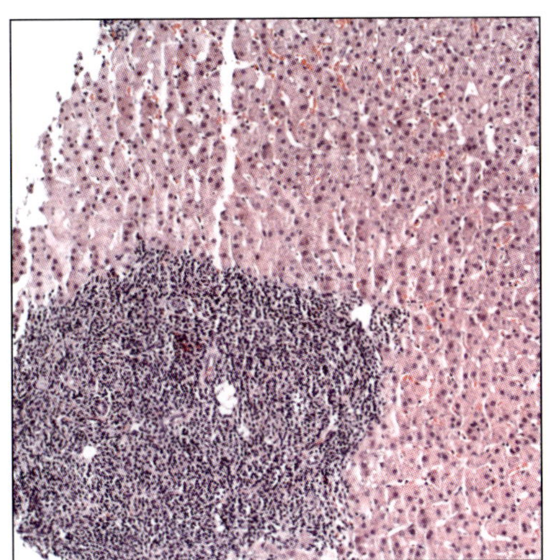

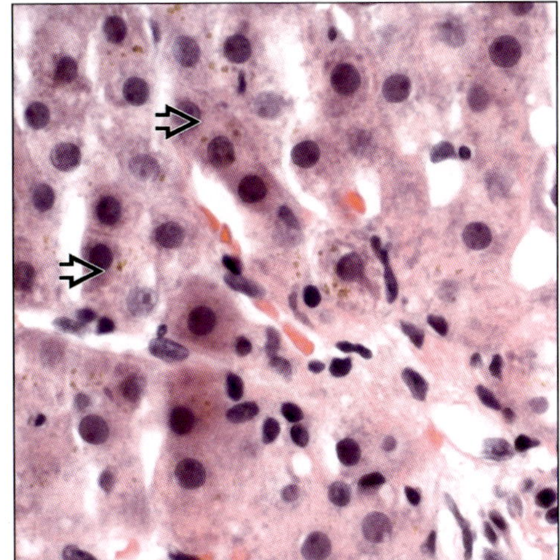

(Left) *Hematoxylin & eosin section shows a dense portal lymphoid aggregate, indicating HCV infection in this patient with porphyria cutanea tarda.* ***(Right)*** *Hematoxylin & eosin section shows subtle pigment granules in periportal hepatocytes ⇨, consistent with hemosiderin in porphyria cutanea tarda.*

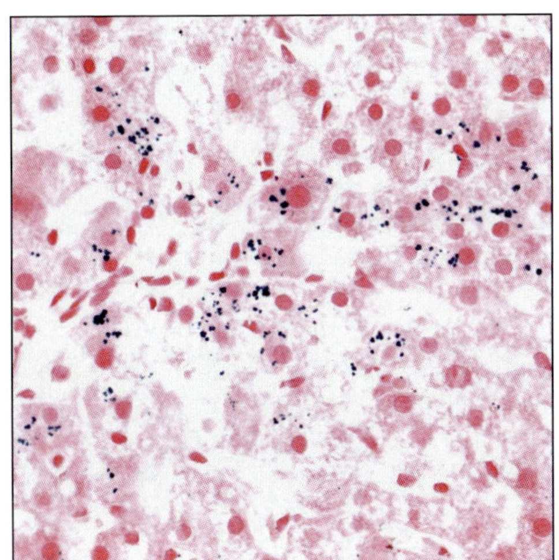

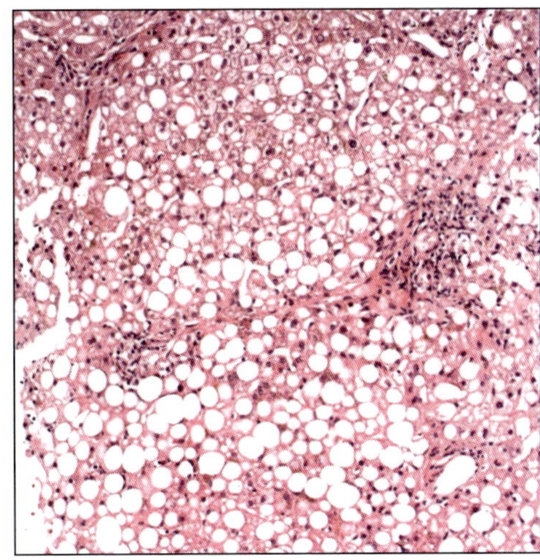

(Left) *Iron stain confirms the presence of coarse hemosiderin deposits in periportal hepatocytes in a patient with porphyria cutanea tarda.* ***(Right)*** *Hematoxylin & eosin stain shows steatosis and mild portal mononuclear infiltrates in porphyria cutanea tarda.*

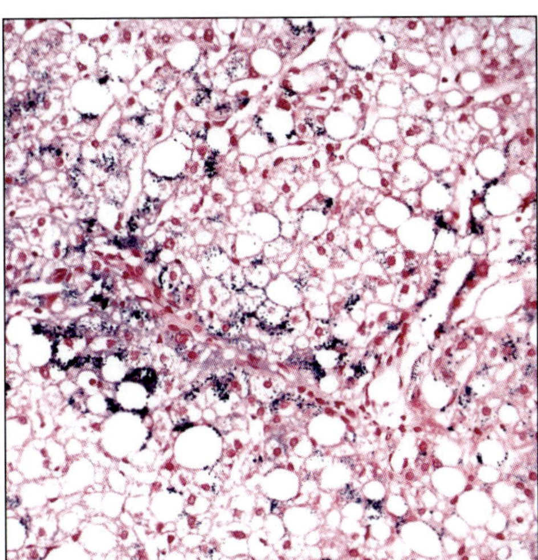

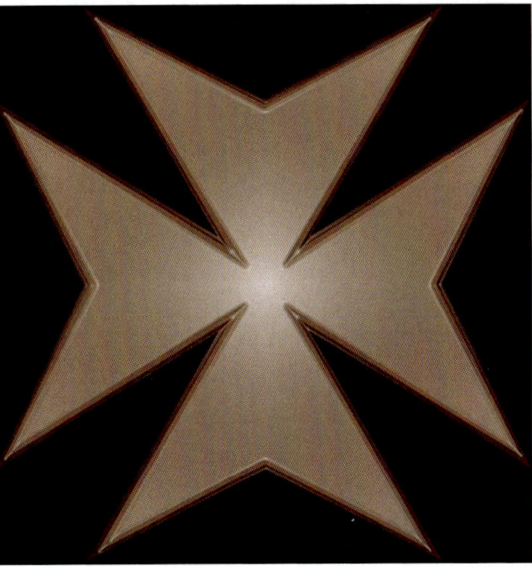

(Left) *Iron stain demonstrates coarse periportal hemosiderin deposition in this patient with porphyria cutanea tarda.* ***(Right)*** *The Maltese cross originated as the symbol of an order of Christian warriors known as the Knights of Malta and became one of the national symbols of Malta.*

DUBIN-JOHNSON SYNDROME

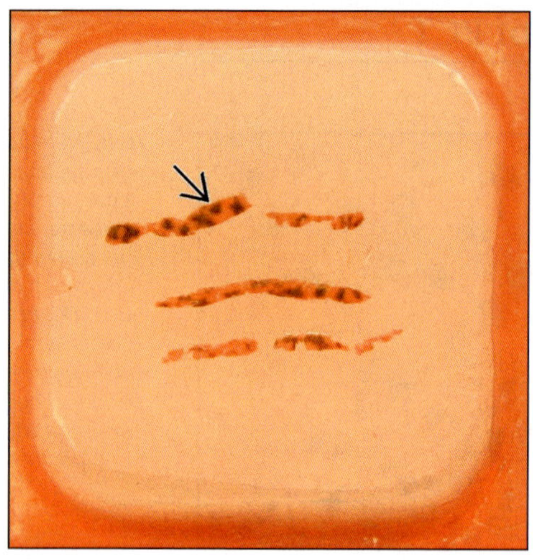

Gross photograph of liver core biopsies embedded in the paraffin block show dark regions ➔ corresponding to the pigment within centrilobular hepatocytes.

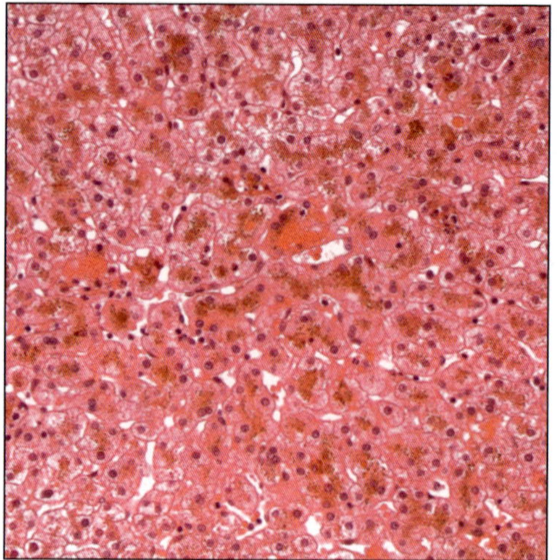

Hematoxylin & eosin section shows coarse granular pigment deposition in centrilobular hepatocytes.

TERMINOLOGY

Definitions

- Defect in hepatocellular secretion of conjugated bilirubin

ETIOLOGY/PATHOGENESIS

Genetic Disorder

- Autosomal recessive
- Mutations in *cMOAT/MRP2/ABCC2* gene, which codes for ATP-dependent organic anion transport localized to canalicular membrane
  - Results in impaired biliary canalicular transport of organic anions including conjugated bilirubin
  - Impaired glutathione excretion reduces bile salt-independent bile flow

CLINICAL ISSUES

Epidemiology

- Incidence
  - Rare
- Age
  - Develop jaundice in teenage years
- Gender
  - Sexes affected equally
- Ethnicity
  - Prevalence highest among Moroccan and Iranian Jews (1:1,300)

Presentation

- Most patients asymptomatic
- Can present as chronic or intermittent jaundice or with mild right upper quadrant abdominal pain
- Serum bile acids are not increased, so pruritus is absent
- Urine may be darker than normal
- Some neonates present with cholestasis
- Jaundice can be precipitated by pregnancy or by drugs that decrease hepatic excretion of organic anions (e.g., oral contraceptives)

Laboratory Tests

- Measurement of urine coproporphyrin isomers shows shift from isomer III to isomer I
- Conjugated hyperbilirubinemia
- Normal alkaline phosphatase and γ-glutamyl transpeptidase

Treatment

- No treatment necessary

Prognosis

- Excellent

MACROSCOPIC FEATURES

General Features

- Grossly, liver is darkly pigmented and can appear green, slate blue, dark gray, or black

MICROSCOPIC PATHOLOGY

Histologic Features

- Coarse granular pigment in centrilobular hepatocytes

Predominant Pattern/Injury Type

- Pigment accumulation

Predominant Cell/Compartment Type

- Centrilobular zone

ANCILLARY TESTS

Histochemistry

- Periodic acid-Schiff with diastase digestion
  - Reactivity: Positive

DUBIN-JOHNSON SYNDROME

Key Facts

Etiology/Pathogenesis
- Mutations in *cMOAT/MRP2* gene causes impaired biliary transport of conjugated bilirubin

Clinical Issues
- Chronic or intermittent jaundice, precipitated by pregnancy or oral contraceptives
- Isolated conjugated hyperbilirubinemia
- Shift in urine coproporphyrin isomers from isomer III to isomer I

Macroscopic Features
- Grossly pigmented liver

Microscopic Pathology
- Coarse granular pigment in centrilobular hepatocytes

Ancillary Tests
- Periodic acid-Schiff with diastase digestion and Fontana-Masson stains highlight pigment

---

  - Staining pattern
    - Cytoplasmic
- Fontana-Masson
  - Reactivity: Positive
  - Staining pattern
    - Cytoplasmic

Immunohistochemistry
- MRP2: Negative staining of canalicular membrane
  - Available through referral centers
  - Helpful in young children whose livers have not accumulated pigment

Electron Microscopy
- Membrane-bound, electron-dense lysosomal granules within cytoplasm of hepatocytes

DIFFERENTIAL DIAGNOSIS

Erythropoietic Protoporphyria
- Can also show grossly pigmented liver but has distinct clinical and histologic features

Gilbert Syndrome
- Pigment in centrilobular hepatocytes is not as coarse
- Unconjugated hyperbilirubinemia

Bilirubinostasis
- Inspissated bile in canaliculi
- Feathery degeneration of hepatocytes in cholestatic area

Hemochromatosis
- Prussian blue positive pigment in periportal hepatocytes

DIAGNOSTIC CHECKLIST

Pathologic Interpretation Pearls
- Coarse pigment in centrilobular hepatocytes in patient with isolated conjugated hyperbilirubinemia
- Pigment may disappear during episode of hepatitis and reaccumulate after recovery

SELECTED REFERENCES

1. Nisa AU et al: Dubin-Johnson syndrome. J Coll Physicians Surg Pak. 18(3):188-9, 2008
2. Jedlitschky G et al: Structure and function of the MRP2 (ABCC2) protein and its role in drug disposition. Expert Opin Drug Metab Toxicol. 2(3):351-66, 2006
3. Lee JH et al: Neonatal Dubin-Johnson syndrome: long-term follow-up and MRP2 mutations study. Pediatr Res. 59(4 Pt 1):584-9, 2006
4. Rastogi A et al: Dubin-Johnson syndrome--a clinicopathologic study of twenty cases. Indian J Pathol Microbiol. 49(4):500-4, 2006
5. Sobaniec-Lotowska ME et al: Ultrastructure of Kupffer cells and hepatocytes in the Dubin-Johnson syndrome: a case report. World J Gastroenterol. 12(6):987-9, 2006

IMAGE GALLERY

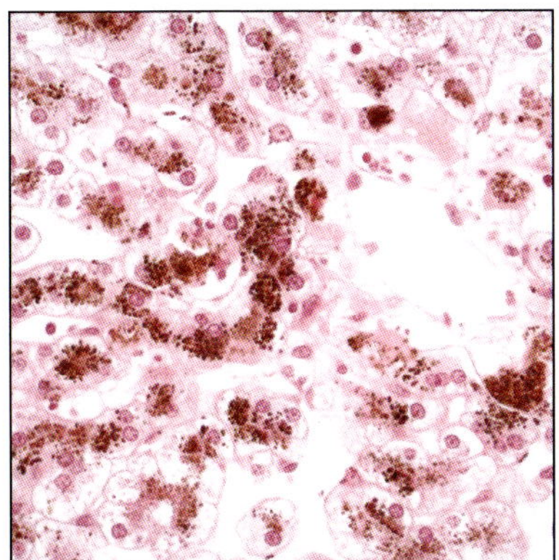

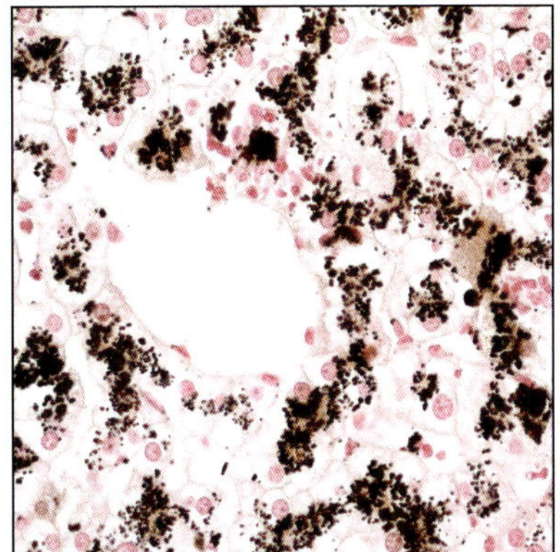

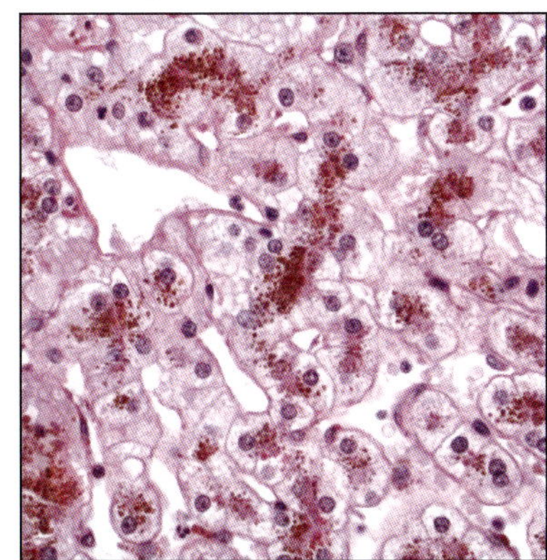

(Left) *Iron stain is negative, confirming that the centrilobular pigment is not hemosiderin.* ***(Center)*** *Fontana-Masson stain highlights the coarse pigment within centrilobular hepatocytes.* ***(Right)*** *Periodic acid-Schiff stain with diastase digestion accentuates the coarse pigment granules within centrilobular hepatocytes.*

GILBERT DISEASE

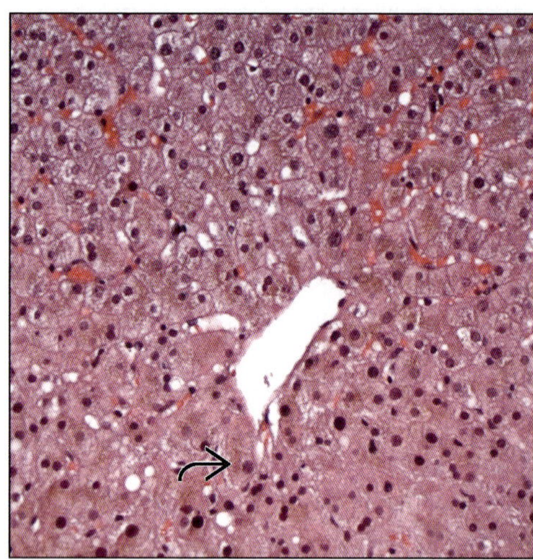

Hematoxylin & eosin shows subtle pigment accumulation in centrilobular hepatocytes ⮫.

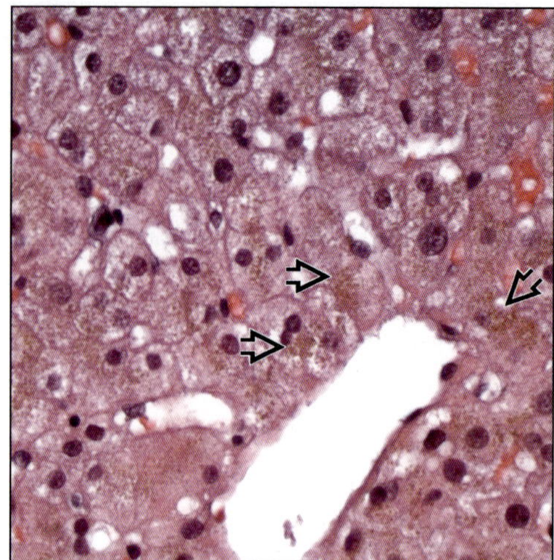

Hematoxylin & eosin at high power confirms the presence of increased lipofuscin pigment ⇨ in centrilobular hepatocytes.

TERMINOLOGY

Definitions

- Inherited unconjugated hyperbilirubinemia due to mutations of bilirubin uridine diphosphate glucuronosyltransferase (*B-UGT* or *UGT1A1)* gene

ETIOLOGY/PATHOGENESIS

Genetic Disorder

- Extra TA in TATAA box of *B-UGT* promoter (this variant is known as *B-UGT*28)*
  - Decreased transcription of gene to 20% of normal
    - Decreased conjugation of bilirubin with glucuronic acid
    - Decreased conjugation of some drugs (irinotecan, atazanavir, TAS-103, indinavir, tolbutamide, rifamycin)
- Affected patients typically have 2nd condition causing increased bilirubin load
  - For example, reduced red blood cell life span or impaired hepatic bilirubin uptake

CLINICAL ISSUES

Epidemiology

- Incidence
  - Among Caucasians, mutation has frequency of 35-40%
    - 11-16% of population homozygous
- Age
  - Often diagnosed at puberty, possibly related to increased hemoglobin turnover and inhibition of bilirubin glucuronidation by endogenous steroid hormones
- Gender
  - Males affected more than females, possible due to higher rate of bilirubin production in males

Presentation

- Mild unconjugated nonhemolytic hyperbilirubinemia, usually fluctuating and less than 3 mg/dL but may increase during illness, stress, or menstrual period
- Otherwise normal liver function
- Jaundice is the only finding on physical examination
- Associated with prolonged neonatal jaundice and development of gallstones in patients with hereditary spherocytosis
- Associated with increased risk of toxicity from drugs metabolized by *B-UGT*
  - Irinotecan has been associated with severe diarrhea and neutropenia
  - Increased risk of hyperbilirubinemia with atazanavir

Laboratory Tests

- Mild unconjugated hyperbilirubinemia with normal alkaline phosphatase, aspartate aminotransferase, alanine aminotransferase, and γ-glutamyl transpeptidase
- Increased proportion of bilirubin glucuronides in bile in Gilbert syndrome is bilirubin monoglucuronide
- Rifampin administration causes disproportionate unconjugated hyperbilirubinemia relative to normal patients
- Caloric restriction causes disproportionate unconjugated hyperbilirubinemia relative to normal patients

Treatment

- No treatment necessary

Prognosis

- Excellent

MACROSCOPIC FEATURES

General Features

- No macroscopic findings

GILBERT DISEASE

Key Facts

Terminology
- Inherited unconjugated hyperbilirubinemia due to mutation of promoter of *B-UGT* gene

Etiology/Pathogenesis
- Decreased transcription of *B-UGT* gene results in decreased conjugation of bilirubin

Clinical Issues
- Up to 16% of population may be homozygous
- No treatment necessary
- Decreased conjugation of some drugs results in increased risk of adverse effect to those drugs

Microscopic Pathology
- Increased lipofuscin in zone 3
- No inflammation, fibrosis, or cirrhosis

MICROSCOPIC PATHOLOGY

Histologic Features
- Increased lipofuscin in zone 3

Predominant Pattern/Injury Type
- Pigment accumulation

Predominant Cell/Compartment Type
- Hepatocyte

DIFFERENTIAL DIAGNOSIS

Lipofuscin Deposition
- Increased lipofuscin can be seen in advancing age, chronic drug ingestion, and as variant of normal

Dubin-Johnson Syndrome
- Pigment is considerably more coarse

Crigler-Najjar, Types 1 and 2
- Severe unconjugated hyperbilirubinemia characterized by total or near total absence of *B-UGT* activity
- Mutations in exons 1-5 of *B-UGT* gene
- Histopathology can show cholestasis or appear normal

DIAGNOSTIC CHECKLIST

Clinically Relevant Pathologic Features
- Does not lead to liver inflammation, fibrosis, cirrhosis, or liver failure
- Testing for *B-UGT*28* often done to identify patients at risk for certain drug toxicities and to tailor dose

Pathologic Interpretation Pearls
- Increased lipofuscin in centrilobular hepatocytes

SELECTED REFERENCES

1. Ehmer U et al: Rapid allelic discrimination by TaqMan PCR for the detection of the Gilbert's syndrome marker UGT1A1*28. J Mol Diagn. 10(6):549-52, 2008
2. Costa E: Hematologically important mutations: bilirubin UDP-glucuronosyltransferase gene mutations in Gilbert and Crigler-Najjar syndromes. Blood Cells Mol Dis. 36(1):77-80, 2006
3. Hallal H et al: A shortened, 2-hour rifampin test: a useful tool in Gilbert's syndrome. Gastroenterol Hepatol. 29(2):63-5, 2006
4. Erdil A et al: Rifampicin test in the diagnosis of Gilbert's syndrome. Int J Clin Pract. 55(2):81-3, 2001
5. Ishihara T et al: Role of UGT1A1 mutation in fasting hyperbilirubinemia. J Gastroenterol Hepatol. 16(6):678-82, 2001
6. Kadakol A et al: Genetic lesions of bilirubin uridine-diphosphoglucuronate glucuronosyltransferase (UGT1A1) causing Crigler-Najjar and Gilbert syndromes: correlation of genotype to phenotype. Hum Mutat. 16(4):297-306, 2000

IMAGE GALLERY

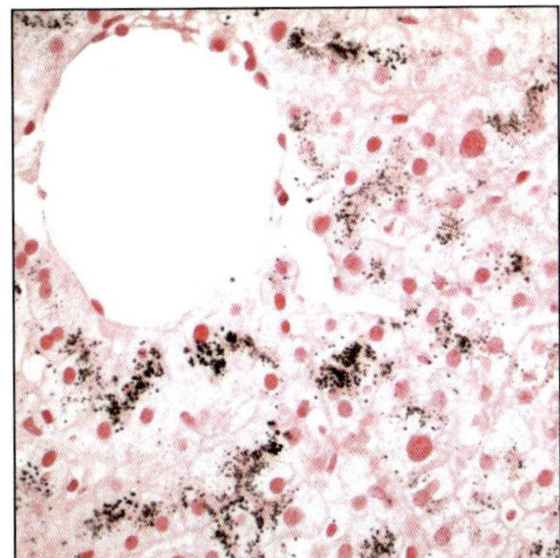

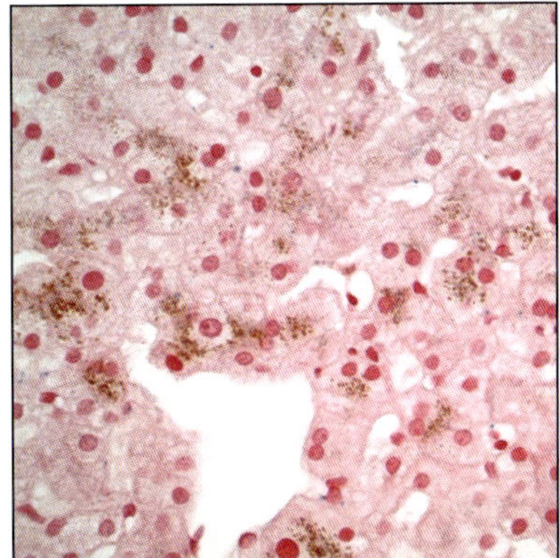

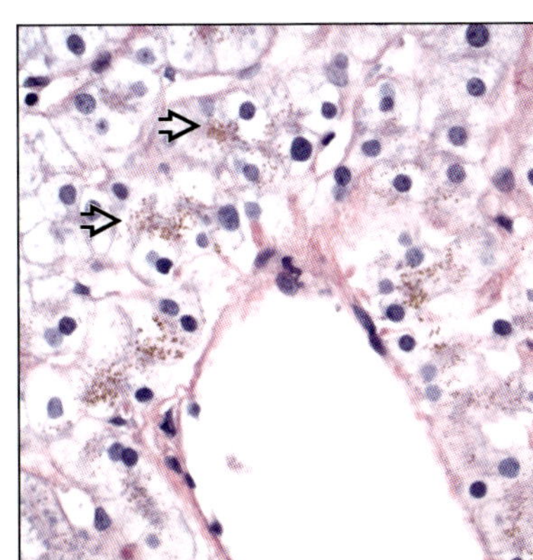

(Left) *Fontana-Masson stain highlights the increased lipofuscin marked by black staining in the centrilobular hepatocytes.* ***(Center)*** *Iron stain is negative, confirming that the pigment is not hemosiderin.* ***(Right)*** *Periodic acid-Schiff with diastase digestion lightly accentuates the granular pigment in centrilobular hepatocytes* ➯.

PROGRESSIVE FAMILIAL INTRAHEPATIC CHOLESTASIS

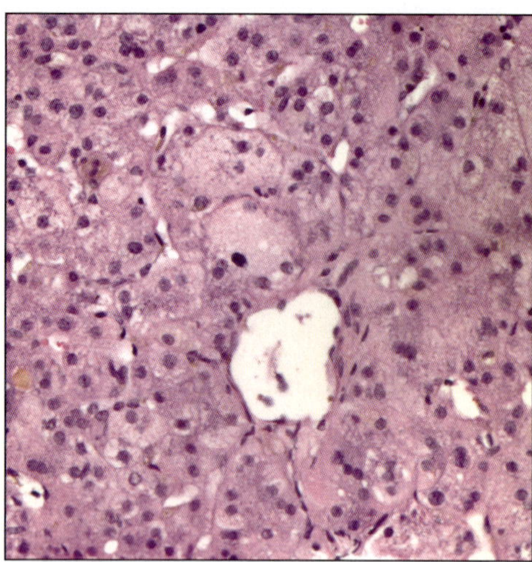

Hematoxylin & eosin stained section of a liver biopsy in a child with PFIC shows giant cell transformation of perivenular hepatocytes, typical of childhood cholestasis syndromes.

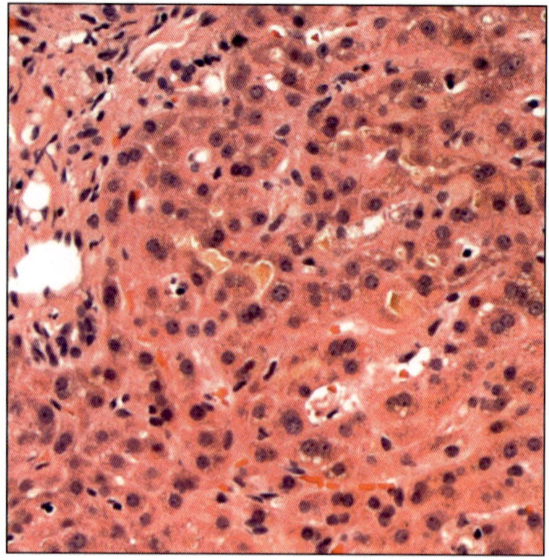

Hematoxylin & eosin stained section of a liver biopsy in an adult patient with BRIC shows bland canalicular cholestasis with mild lobular architectural disarray but minimal inflammation.

TERMINOLOGY

Abbreviations

- Progressive familial intrahepatic cholestasis (PFIC)

Synonyms

- PFIC type 1
  - Familial intrahepatic cholestasis 1 (FIC1) disease
  - Byler disease, Byler syndrome
  - Greenland familial cholestasis (GFC)
- PFIC type 2
  - Bile salt export pump (BSEP) disease
- PFIC type 3
  - Multidrug resistance protein 3 (MDR3) disease

Definitions

- Heterogeneous group of autosomal recessive disorders characterized by chronic cholestasis and progression to cirrhosis and liver failure

ETIOLOGY/PATHOGENESIS

Autosomal Recessive Genetic Disorder

- PFIC1
  - Mutation of *ATP8B1* (*FIC1* gene), located on chromosome 18q21-q22
    - FIC1 is expressed on variety of tissues including liver, intestine, pancreas
    - Functions as aminophospholipid flippase, flipping phosphatidylserine from outer to inner lipid layer of cell membrane
    - Mechanism of cholestasis unclear
- PFIC2
  - Mutations of *ABCB11* gene on chromosome 2q24 that encodes BSEP, an ATP-dependent bile acid transporter on canalicular membrane
- PFIC3
  - Mutation of *ABCB4* gene that encodes MDR3 glycoprotein
    - MDR3 is flippase that flips phosphatidylcholine from inner to outer lipid leaflet of canalicular membrane
    - Phosphatidylcholine in bile reduces its detergent action, and MDR3 deficiency results in bile with more detergent properties
    - Absence of phospholipids destabilizes micelles, promoting lithogenicity of bile with crystallization of cholesterol and leads to small bile duct obstruction

CLINICAL ISSUES

Presentation

- FIC1 deficiency disease
  - Depending on nature of mutation, may present as benign recurrent intrahepatic cholestasis (BRIC1) or progressive and severe form (PFIC1)
  - PFIC1
    - Presents in 1st year of life with intense pruritus and jaundice
    - Systemic disorder with extrahepatic manifestations including pancreatitis, diarrhea, respiratory symptoms, failure to thrive, delayed sexual development, hearing loss
  - BRIC1
    - Recurrent episodes of cholestasis with intense pruritus
    - Episodes resolve spontaneously without histologic progression
- BSEP disease
  - Depending on nature of mutation, may present as BRIC2 or PFIC2
  - PFIC2
    - Presents as severe intrahepatic cholestasis in infancy
  - BRIC2

PROGRESSIVE FAMILIAL INTRAHEPATIC CHOLESTASIS

Key Facts

Etiology/Pathogenesis

- PFIC1 (FIC1 disease) is due to mutations of *ATP8B1* (*FIC1* gene)
- PFIC2 (BSEP disease) is due to mutations of *ABCB11* gene that encodes bile salt export pump
- PFIC3 is due to mutation of *ABCB4* gene that encodes MDR3, a phospholipid flippase

Clinical Issues

- PFIC presents in 1st year of life with intense pruritus and jaundice
- PFIC1 and PFIC2 are characterized by normal serum GGT, whereas PFIC3 is associated with elevated GGT
- Progressive forms lead to liver failure, cirrhosis, and death before adulthood
- Partial external biliary diversion or ileal exclusion may be used with some success, but most patients require liver transplantation

Microscopic Pathology

- PFIC1 is characterized by relatively bland canalicular cholestasis
- PFIC2 is characterized by pattern of neonatal giant cell hepatitis
- PFIC3 is characterized by duct proliferation and bile plugs in ductules

Ancillary Tests

- FIC1 disease reveals coarse, granular bile, referred to as Byler bile
- Immunohistochemistry for canalicular proteins can be used for diagnosis

---

        - Presents as recurrent episodes of pruritus, steatorrhea, nausea, vomiting, anorexia, right upper quadrant abdominal pain, and weight loss
        - Frequently complicated by cholesterol cholelithiasis
- MDR3 disease
    - PFIC3 presents during infancy with pruritus, jaundice, pale stools, hepatomegaly, or complications of portal hypertension, such as splenomegaly or gastrointestinal bleeding
    - MDR3 mutations also seen in patients with intrahepatic lithiasis, cholesterol gallstone disease, intrahepatic cholestasis of pregnancy, transient neonatal cholestasis, cholestatic drug reactions

Laboratory Tests

- GGT
    - Normal in PFIC1 and PFIC2
    - Elevated in PFIC3
- Elevated serum bile acids in all 3 types
- PFIC3 is characterized by low concentrations of phospholipids in bile analysis

Natural History

- Progressive forms can result in worsening hepatic function, liver failure, cirrhosis, and death before adulthood
    - Chronic cholestasis leads to complications of fat malabsorption such as deficiencies of fat-soluble vitamins and weight loss
- BSEP disease is associated with development of hepatocellular carcinoma

Treatment

- Surgical approaches
    - Partial external biliary diversion or cholecystojejunocutaneostomy
        - Short jejunal segment is anastomosed to the dome of gallbladder and terminates as stoma, allowing bile to be discarded
    - Ileal exclusion
        - Approximately 15% of terminal ileum is bypassed, which reduces bile acid reabsorption
    - Liver transplantation
        - May result in intractable diarrhea and steatohepatitis in FIC1 patients
- Drugs
    - Ursodeoxycholic acid (UDCA), rifampin, cholestyramine, and phenobarbital have been used to treat pruritus

MICROSCOPIC PATHOLOGY

Histologic Features

- FIC1 disease
    - BRIC1
        - Bland canalicular cholestasis with variable cholestatic rosettes, compact hepatocytes, hepatocyte multinucleation without prominent giant cell transformation
        - Minimal inflammation
    - PFIC1: Increasing portal fibrosis with eventual cirrhosis
        - Pattern of fibrosis that involves early pericentral sclerosis, central-to-portal fibrosis, and cirrhosis with lacy lobular fibrosis has been described
    - Bile duct injury and paucity may be present as well as bile ductular reaction
- BSEP disease
    - Neonatal hepatitis pattern with giant cell transformation, ballooning, inflammation, and canalicular cholestasis
    - Bile duct injury and paucity may be present as well as bile ductular reaction
    - PFIC2 shows increasing fibrosis and eventual cirrhosis
        - Pattern of fibrosis that involves early pericentral sclerosis, central-to-portal fibrosis, and cirrhosis with lacy lobular fibrosis has been described
- MDR3 disease
    - Expanded portal tracts with ductular proliferation and mixed inflammatory infiltrates
    - Cholestasis and giant cell transformation of hepatocytes may be seen

PROGRESSIVE FAMILIAL INTRAHEPATIC CHOLESTASIS

Comparison of Subtypes of Progressive Familial Intrahepatic Cholestasis

PFIC Subtype	Gene	Extrahepatic Manifestations	GGT	Major Histologic Features	Distinguishing Clinical Features
FIC1 disease	*ATP8B1*	Diarrhea, pancreatitis, cough, wheezing, hearing loss	Normal	Relatively bland cholestasis, coarse granular bile ultrastructurally	Diarrhea worsens after transplant
BSEP disease	*ABCB11*	None	Normal	Inflammatory with pattern of giant cell hepatitis and fibrosis	Higher association with hepatocellular carcinoma
MDR3 disease	*ABCB4*	None	Elevated	Ductular proliferation with bile plugs in small cholangioles, cholesterol clefts in ducts or canaliculi, increasing fibrosis and eventually cirrhosis	More likely to present with complications of portal hypertension

 - Late stages characterized by biliary cirrhosis, bile plugs in ductules, and interlobular bile ducts without periductal fibrosis or epithelial injury
 - May see cholesterol clefts in bile ducts

ANCILLARY TESTS

Immunohistochemistry

- FIC1 disease shows diffuse variable reduction in canalicular expression of CDT3, GGT, and pCEA
- BSEP disease shows absent canalicular staining for BSEP but preserved staining for other canalicular enzymes such as pCEA
- MDR3 disease shows absent canalicular staining for MDR3 but preserved staining for other canalicular proteins such as pCEA and BSEP

Electron Microscopy

- Transmission
  - FIC1 disease reveals coarse, granular bile, referred to as Byler bile
  - MDR3 disease may show cholesterol clefts in bile ducts or canaliculi

DIFFERENTIAL DIAGNOSIS

Bile Acid Synthesis Defect

- Also shows low GGT, but unlike PFIC, serum bile acid concentration is low

Biliary Atresia

- Histology shows obstructive pattern with bile duct proliferation, inspissated bile in ducts
- Hepatobiliary imaging confirms atretic bile duct

Other Childhood Cholestatic Disorders

- Histology of many cholestatic childhood disorders is indistinguishable from PFIC, and their distinction requires wide array of serologic, biochemical, and genetic tests

Primary Sclerosing Cholangitis

- Histology shows periductal fibrosis
- Cholangiogram shows strictures and dilatations

DIAGNOSTIC CHECKLIST

Clinically Relevant Pathologic Features

- BRIC is characterized by cholestasis during attacks but no histologic progression
- PFIC is characterized by increasing fibrosis and may show duct paucity, giant cell hepatitis, or bile ductules with bile plugging, depending on subtype
- Neonatal cholestatic disorder with normal GGT and elevated serum bile acids suggests PFIC1 or PFIC2 whereas elevated GGT suggests possibility of PFIC3

Pathologic Interpretation Pearls

- PFIC1 shows bland cholestasis; PFIC2 shows pattern of giant cell hepatitis; and PFIC3 shows duct proliferation with bile plugs

SELECTED REFERENCES

1. Cai SY et al: ATP8B1 deficiency disrupts the bile canalicular membrane bilayer structure in hepatocytes, but FXR expression and activity are maintained. Gastroenterology. 136(3):1060-9, 2009
2. Alissa FT et al: Update on progressive familial intrahepatic cholestasis. J Pediatr Gastroenterol Nutr. 46(3):241-52, 2008
3. van Mil SW et al: Genetics of familial intrahepatic cholestasis syndromes. J Med Genet. 42(6):449-63, 2005
4. Chen F et al: Progressive familial intrahepatic cholestasis, type 1, is associated with decreased farnesoid X receptor activity. Gastroenterology. 126(3):756-64, 2004
5. Jacquemin E: Role of multidrug resistance 3 deficiency in pediatric and adult liver disease: one gene for three diseases. Semin Liver Dis. 21(4):551-62, 2001
6. Thompson R et al: BSEP: function and role in progressive familial intrahepatic cholestasis. Semin Liver Dis. 21(4):545-50, 2001
7. van Mil SW et al: FIC1 disease: a spectrum of intrahepatic cholestatic disorders. Semin Liver Dis. 21(4):535-44, 2001
8. Alonso EM et al: Histologic pathology of the liver in progressive familial intrahepatic cholestasis. J Pediatr Gastroenterol Nutr. 18(2):128-33, 1994

Microscopic Features of PFIC2 (BSEP Deficiency)

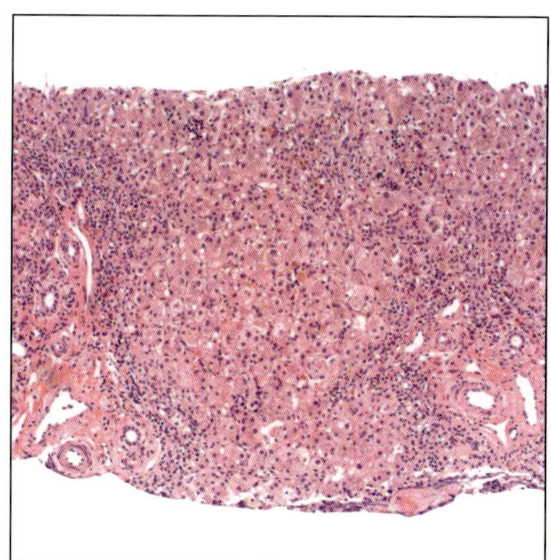

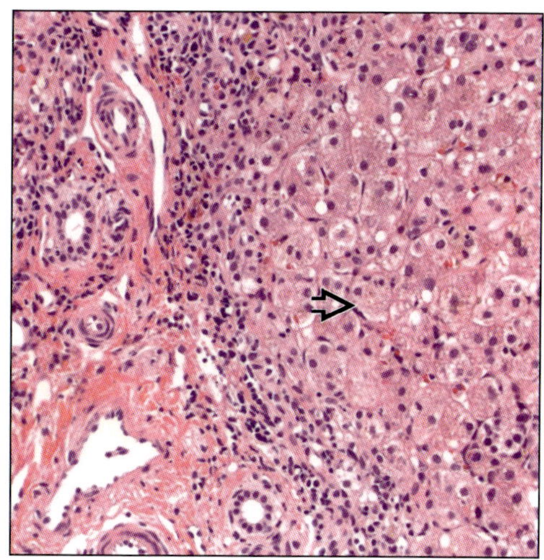

(Left) *Biopsy in an infant with PFIC2 (BSEP deficiency) shows nodule formation and portal inflammation.* ***(Right)*** *Higher magnification of a biopsy in an infant with PFIC2 (BSEP deficiency) shows perinodular inflammation and bile pigment within hepatocytes* ➡.

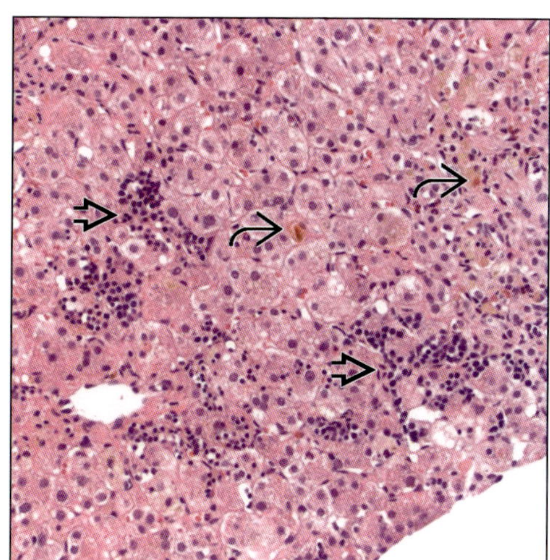

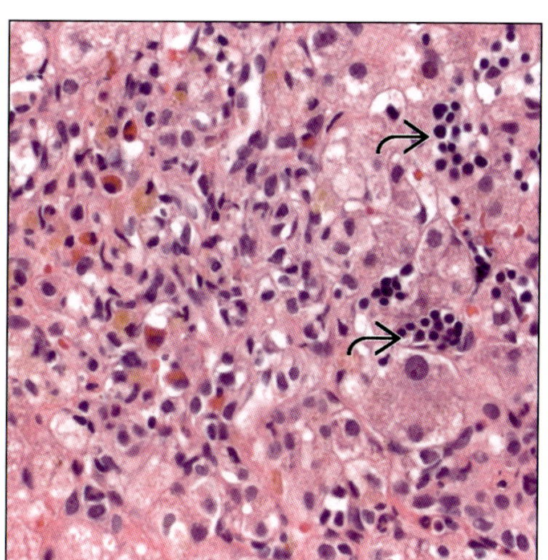

(Left) *Biopsy in an infant with PFIC2 (BSEP deficiency) shows bile plugs within canaliculi* ↪*, inflammation, and extramedullary hematopoiesis* ➡. ***(Right)*** *High magnification of a biopsy in an infant with PFIC2 (BSEP deficiency) shows bile pigment in the liver, mixed inflammatory infiltrates (left), and extramedullary hematopoiesis* ↪.

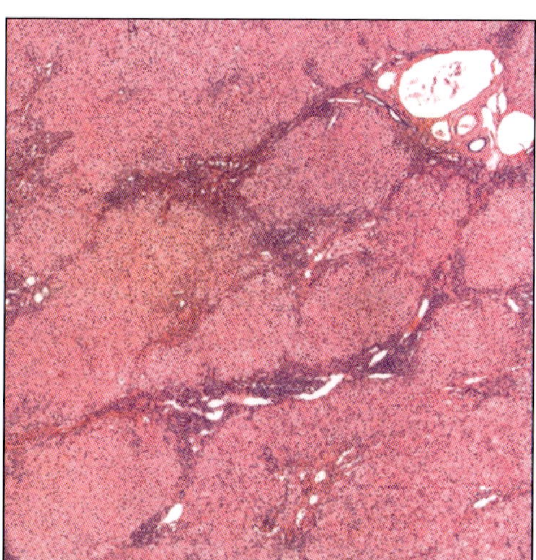

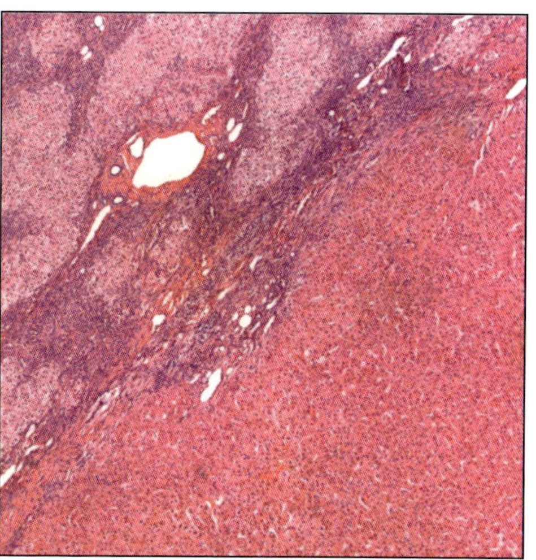

(Left) *Low-power view of an explanted liver in a child with PFIC2 (BSEP deficiency) shows micronodular cirrhosis and septal inflammation.* ***(Right)*** *Hepatocytic neoplasm (lower right) in an explanted liver of a child with PFIC2 (BSEP deficiency) is shown. The tumor is composed of bland hepatocytes. Although PFIC2 is associated with the development of hepatocellular carcinoma, the tumor in this case was interpreted as a hepatic adenoma.*

PROGRESSIVE FAMILIAL INTRAHEPATIC CHOLESTASIS

Microscopic Features of PFIC 2 (BSEP Deficiency)

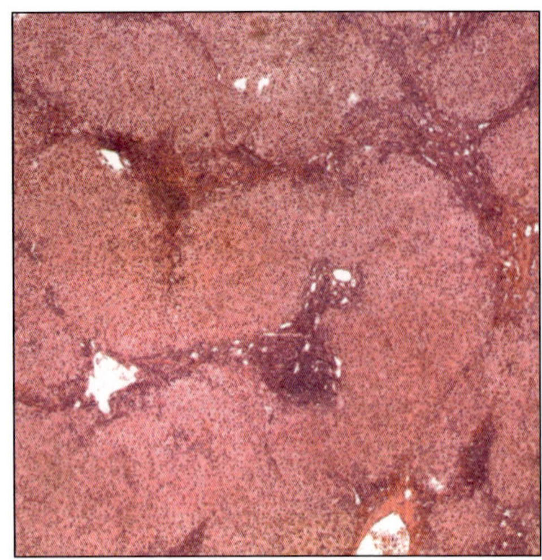

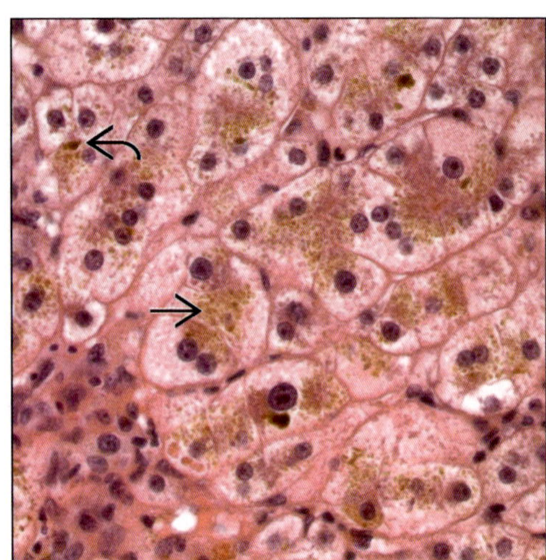

(Left) *Hematoxylin & eosin stained section of liver explant in PFIC2 shows biliary pattern of fibrosis with portal-portal bridging and inflammation in septae.* ***(Right)*** *Hematoxylin & eosin stained section of liver explant in PFIC2 shows pigment in hepatocytes → and canaliculi ↶, consistent with bile. The hepatocytes show rosetting architecture.*

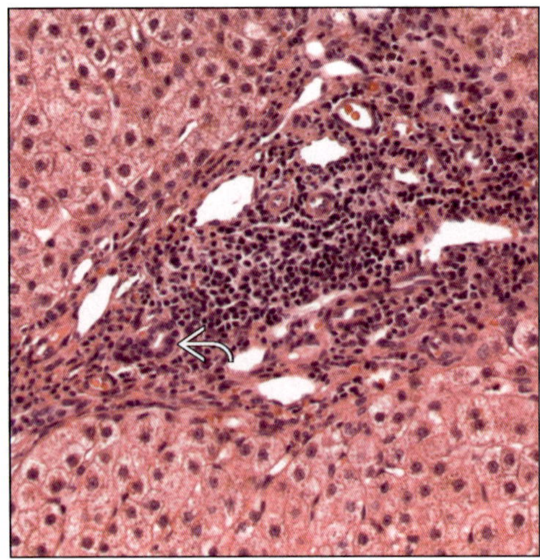

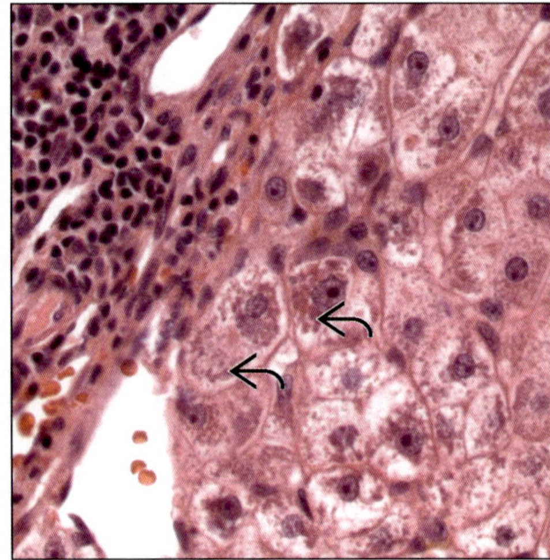

(Left) *Hematoxylin & eosin stained section of a portal tract in PFIC2 shows mononuclear infiltrates. A small duct is visible ↶.* ***(Right)*** *Hematoxylin & eosin stained section of an explant in PFIC2 shows changes of chronic cholestasis with periportal ballooning degeneration and Mallory hyaline ↶.*

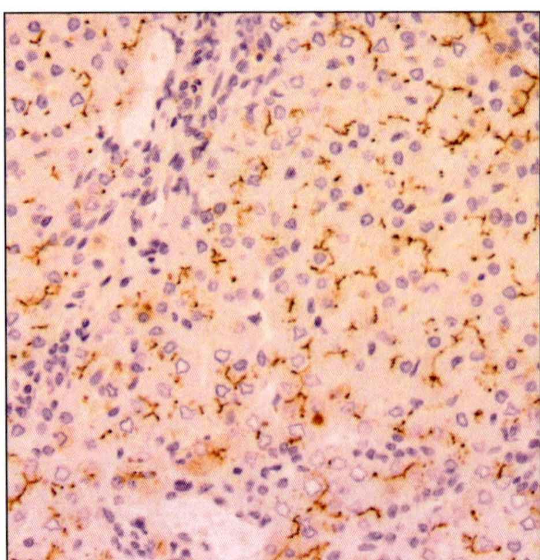

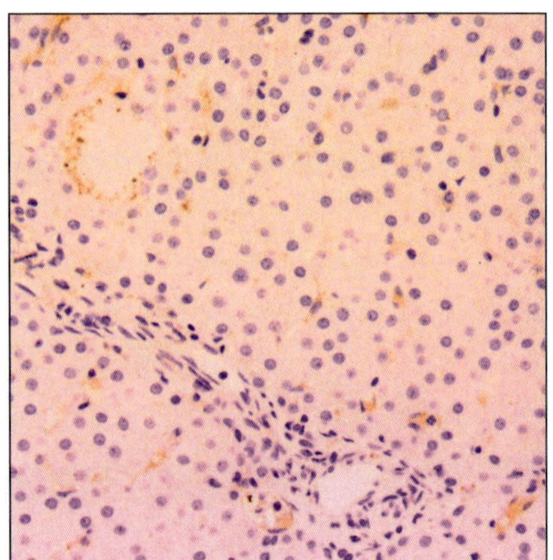

(Left) *Immunohistochemical stain for BSEP in control tissue shows canalicular staining (red-brown).* ***(Right)*** *Immunohistochemical stain for BSEP in a patient explant shows absence of canalicular expression of the bile salt transporter.*

Microscopic Features of PFIC1 and PFIC3

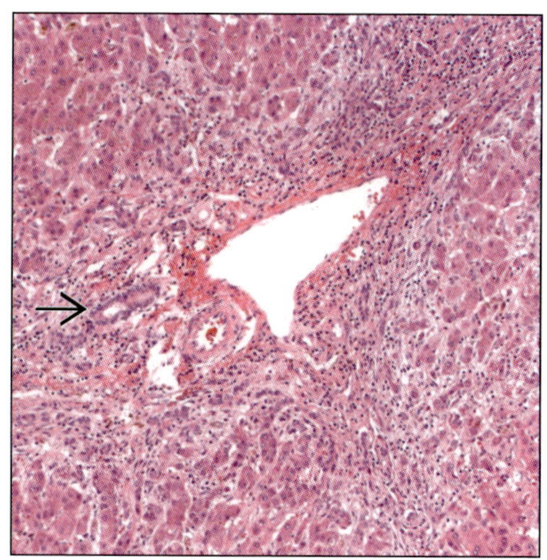

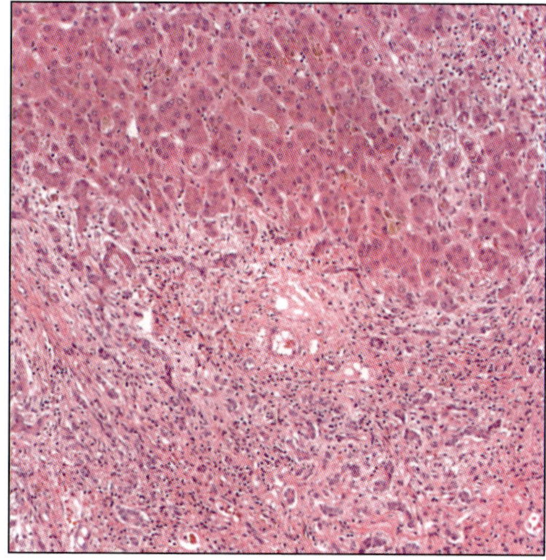

(Left) *Paraffin section of a portal tract in cirrhosis secondary to PFIC1 (FIC1 disease) shows fibrous expansion with bile ductular reaction at the periphery of the septae and pallor at the edge of the nodules, typical of biliary cirrhosis. A native bile duct is present* →. ***(Right)*** *Paraffin section of cirrhosis secondary to PFIC1 (FIC1 disease) shows ductular reaction and inflammation in the septae.*

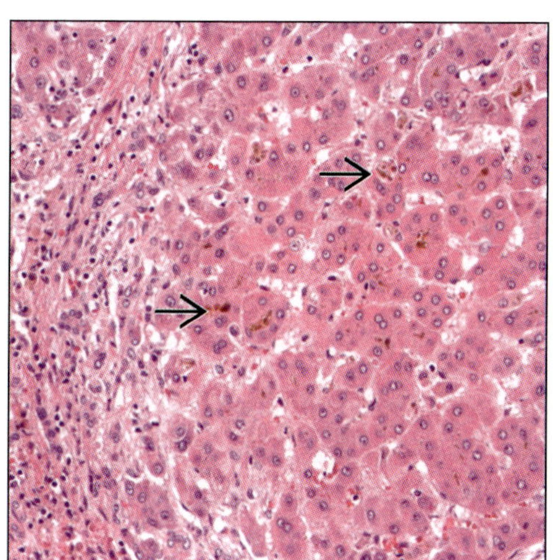

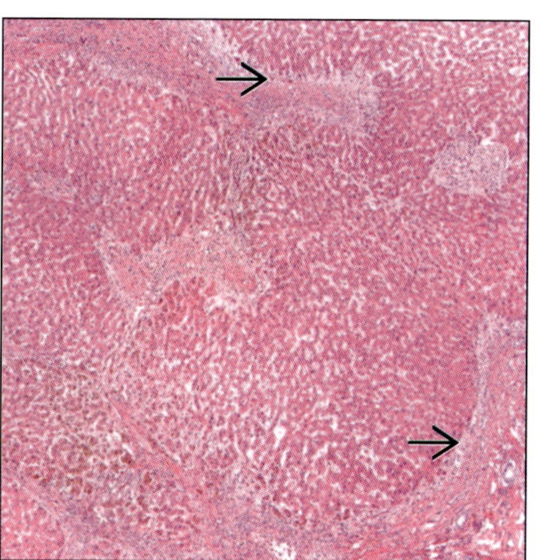

(Left) *Paraffin section of cirrhosis secondary to PFIC1 (FIC1 disease) shows bile stasis in canaliculi* → *and pallor at the edge of the nodule, typical of biliary cirrhosis.* ***(Right)*** *Paraffin section of biliary cirrhosis in PFIC3 (MDR3 deficiency) shows irregular islands of hepatic parenchyma dissected by fibrous bridges. Note the pallor at the edges of the nodule* → *typical of biliary cirrhosis.*

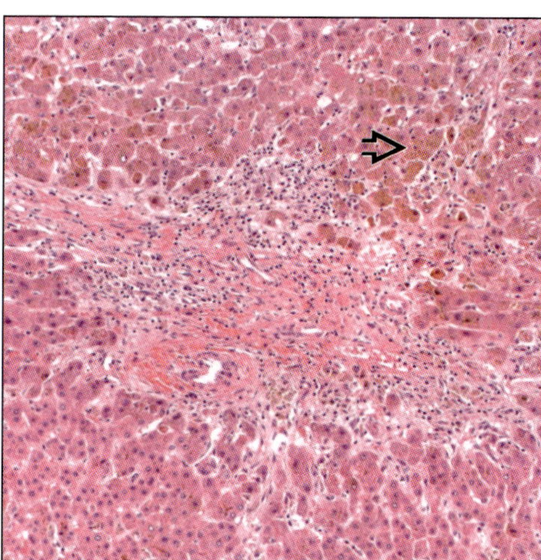

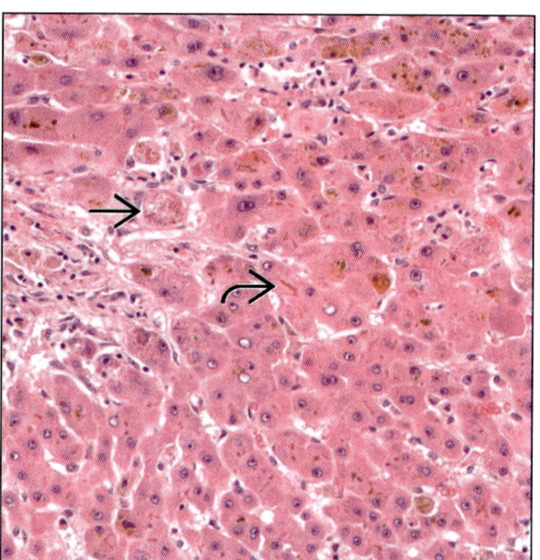

(Left) *Paraffin section of a portal tract in cirrhosis secondary to PFIC3 (MDR3 deficiency) shows bile duct that is absent in this example. There is bile stasis, manifested as pigment in periseptal hepatocytes* ⇨. ***(Right)*** *High-power view of PFIC3 (MDR3 deficiency) shows marked bile stasis within canaliculi* ↗ *as well as Mallory hyaline at the edges of the nodules* →. *Mallory hyaline is a frequent finding in chronic cholestatic disorders.*

CYSTIC FIBROSIS, HEPATIC

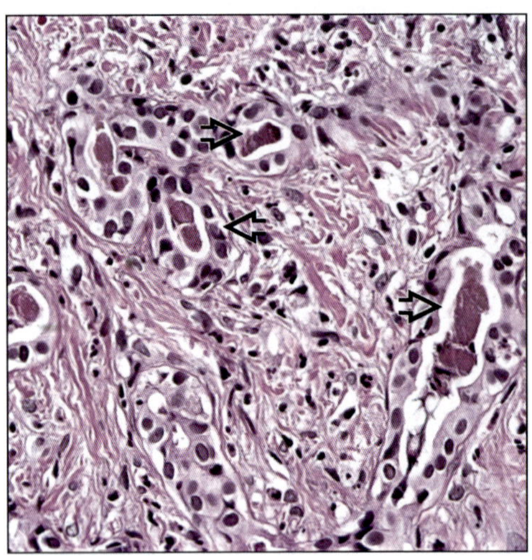

Hematoxylin & eosin shows proliferated bile ductules containing inspissated amorphous, eosinophilic secretions ➪*.*

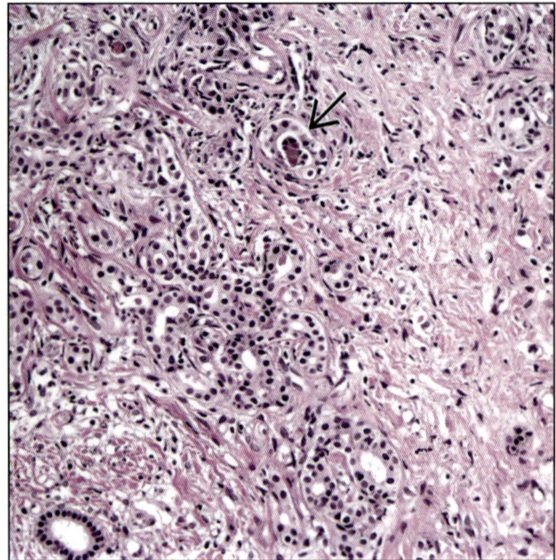

Hematoxylin & eosin section of a liver biopsy in CF shows proliferating bile ductules embedded in an expanded, fibrotic portal tract. Abnormal secretions (concretions) ➔ *can be seen.*

TERMINOLOGY

Abbreviations

- Cystic fibrosis (CF)

Synonyms

- Mucoviscidosis

Definitions

- Generalized inherited disorder of exocrine gland function
  - Impairs clearance of secretions in multiple organs
  - Abnormal chloride transport in apical membrane of epithelial cells
    - Mutation of *CFTR* gene on chromosome 7
  - Up to 40% of affected adolescents have evidence of liver disease
  - As life expectancy increases, hepatobiliary disease in CF more often recognized

CLINICAL ISSUES

Epidemiology

- Incidence
  - Most common autosomal recessive disorder
  - 1 in 2,000-2,500 live births
- Ethnicity
  - Caucasian

Presentation

- Respiratory complaints common
  - Recurrent bronchitis
  - Asthma
  - Recurrent respiratory tract infections
- Infants usually present with steatorrhea, bowel obstruction
- Patients rarely present with liver disease
  - Liver disease appears to peak during late childhood, adolescence

Laboratory Tests

- Intermittent elevation of transaminases, alkaline phosphatase
- Elevated sweat chloride level
- Genetic mutational analysis

Treatment

- No specific therapy for liver disease
  - Cirrhosis accounts for virtually all nonpulmonary deaths in CF
- Ursodeoxycholic acid helps some patients
- Management of portal hypertension, liver transplantation in cirrhotic patients

Prognosis

- Chronic disease, but improved therapy has lengthened survival enormously
- Course of liver disease very variable

MACROSCOPIC FEATURES

General Features

- Depressed white areas of fibrosis in focal biliary fibrosis
- Cirrhosis in patients with end-stage liver disease

MICROSCOPIC PATHOLOGY

Histologic Features

- Focal biliary fibrosis
  - Proliferated, dilated bile ductules
  - Atrophy of biliary epithelium
  - Ductules contain inspissated eosinophilic secretions/concretions
  - Concretions represent abnormal secretions of CF; PAS positive (diastase resistant); mucicarmine and Alcian blue negative
  - Ducts may rupture, producing inflammatory response

CYSTIC FIBROSIS, HEPATIC

Key Facts

Terminology

- Generalized inherited disorder of exocrine gland function
- *CFTR* mutation on chromosome 7
- Most common autosomal recessive inherited disorder

Microscopic Pathology

- Focal biliary fibrosis is characteristic lesion
  - Dilated, proliferated bile ductules
  - Dense secretions/concretions represent abnormal secretions of CF
  - PAS positive (diastase resistant); mucicarmine and Alcian blue negative
- Disease may progress to multilobular biliary cirrhosis
- As life expectancy increases, hepatobiliary disease in CF more often recognized

---

  - Fibrous, expanded portal tracts with variable inflammation
  - Large intrahepatic ducts may contain excessive mucus
  - Steatosis present in up to 1/3 of cases; probably related to malnutrition, fatty acid deficiency
- Focal biliary fibrosis varies in extent, distribution
- With progression, focal lesions become confluent
  - Although not strictly "cirrhosis," the term "multilobular biliary cirrhosis" is used in this context
  - Liver failure, portal hypertension may develop
- Neonatal CF may show features of neonatal (giant cell) hepatitis
- Some patients have extrahepatic biliary strictures, microgallbladder

Predominant Pattern/Injury Type

- Abnormal secretion

Predominant Cell/Compartment Type

- Bile ductule

DIFFERENTIAL DIAGNOSIS

Primary Sclerosing Cholangitis (PSC)

- ERCP findings of CF may mimic PSC
- PSC lacks secretions, other clinical findings of CF

Neonatal Hepatitis of Other Causes

- Rule out infection, neonatal biliary diseases

DIAGNOSTIC CHECKLIST

Clinically Relevant Pathologic Features

- Other clinical features of CF
  - Pulmonary disease
  - Pancreatic insufficiency

Pathologic Interpretation Pearls

- "Focal biliary fibrosis" lesion is virtually pathognomonic
- Eosinophilic secretions/concretions are PAS positive, diastase resistant

SELECTED REFERENCES

1. Lykavieris P et al: Neonatal cholestasis as the presenting feature in cystic fibrosis. Arch Dis Child. 75(1):67-70, 1996
2. Hultcrantz R et al: Morphological findings in the liver of children with cystic fibrosis: a light and electron microscopical study. Hepatology. 6(5):881-9, 1986
3. Oppenheimer EH et al: Pathology of cystic fibrosis review of the literature and comparison with 146 autopsied cases. Perspect Pediatr Pathol. 2:241-78, 1975
4. Craig JM et al: The pathological changes in the liver in cystic fibrosis of the pancreas. AMA J Dis Child. 93(4):357-69, 1957

IMAGE GALLERY

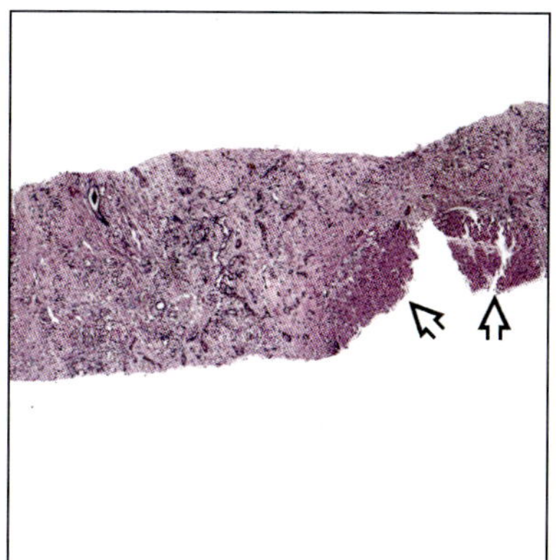

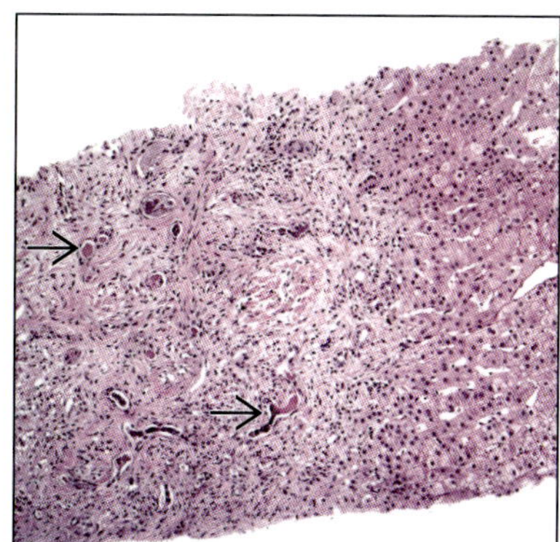

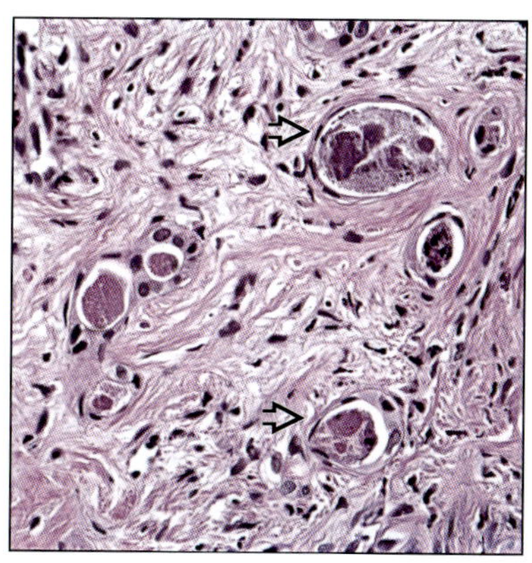

*(**Left**) Hematoxylin & eosin shows irregular, confluent zones of fibrosis with proliferated, dilated bile ductules. A nodule of liver parenchyma ⇨ is seen on the right. This pattern may be referred to as multilobular biliary cirrhosis. (**Center**) Hematoxylin & eosin shows an expanded, irregular portal tract containing proliferating bile ductules. Abnormal secretions within the ductules are visible at low power →. (**Right**) Hematoxylin & eosin shows dilated bile ductules with atrophic epithelium embedded in a fibrous portal tract, containing eosinophilic concretions ⇨.*

HEREDITARY HEMOCHROMATOSIS

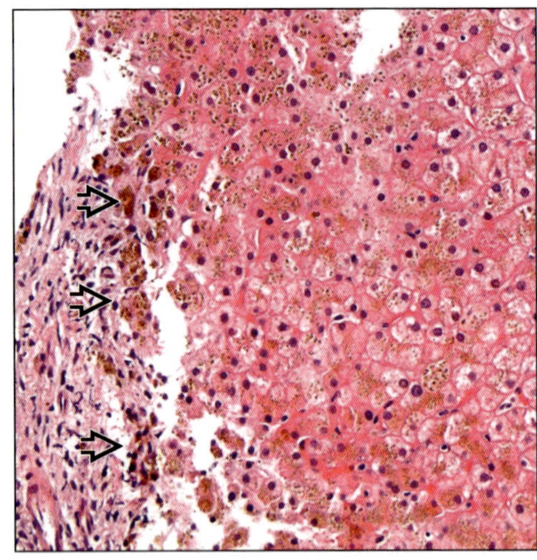

Coarse and refractile iron granules ⇨ are readily discernible within the hepatocytes and bile duct epithelium in a case of hereditary hemochromatosis.

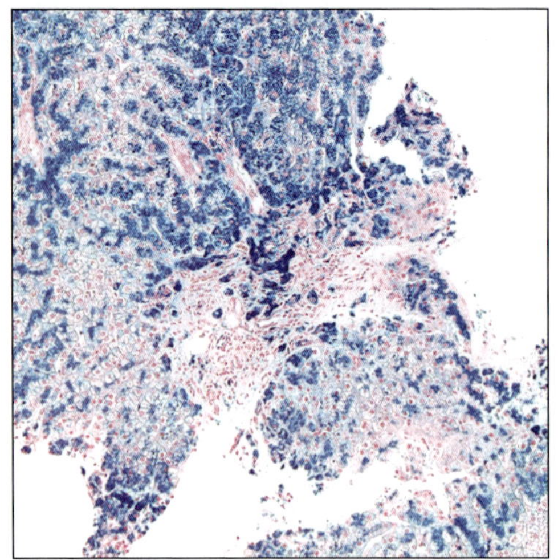

The iron deposition is confirmed by a Perl iron stain.

TERMINOLOGY

Abbreviations

- Hereditary hemochromatosis (HH)

Definitions

- Disorder of iron metabolism inherited as autosomal recessive trait

ETIOLOGY/PATHOGENESIS

Genetic Mutations

- 2 most common mutations are in *HFE* gene
  - C282Y
  - H63D
- Non-*HFE* mutations also occur

CLINICAL ISSUES

Epidemiology

- Incidence
  - C282Y/C282Y genotype
    - 80-85% of phenotypic HH in adults
  - C282Y/H63D genotype
    - 5% of phenotypic HH in adults
  - Mutations in *TfR2* or ferroportin-1 genes
    - 5-10% of phenotypic HH in adults

Presentation

- Classic triad
  - Cirrhosis
  - Diabetes mellitus
  - Increased skin pigmentation
- Arthritis
- Cardiac dysfunction

Treatment

- Phlebotomy
- Chelation therapy
- Liver transplantation

MACROSCOPIC FEATURES

General Features

- Liver has dark, rusty brown discoloration

MICROSCOPIC PATHOLOGY

Histologic Features

- Deposition of iron in periportal hepatocytes in early phases of disease
  - Progressive accumulation in midzonal and centrizonal hepatocytes, biliary epithelium
  - Iron often pericanalicular in distribution
- Deposition of iron in Kupffer cells can be HH or nonhereditary
  - e.g., transfusion
- Portal and lobular chronic inflammation
- Fibrosis is initially portal based
  - Progresses to periportal fibrosis, bridging, and eventually cirrhosis
- Positive iron stain highlights pigment accumulation
- Quantitative iron performed on block can also be useful

Predominant Pattern/Injury Type

- Abnormal accumulation

Predominant Cell/Compartment Type

- Hepatocyte

ANCILLARY TESTS

PCR

- Testing blood for individual mutations

HEREDITARY HEMOCHROMATOSIS

Key Facts

Etiology/Pathogenesis

- Mutation in *HFE* gene (C282Y and H63D) or non-*HFE* gene

Clinical Issues

- Classic triad: Cirrhosis, diabetes, skin pigmentation

Microscopic Pathology

- Deposition of iron in periportal hepatocytes in early phases of disease
- Positive iron stain highlights pigment accumulation
- Fibrosis begins as periportal, may progress to cirrhosis

Top Differential Diagnoses

- Anemia of chronic disease
- Transfusion-related hemosiderosis
- Chronic hemolytic disorders
- Nonspecific iron accumulation in any chronic liver disease

Hereditary Hemochromatosis

Type	Age	Mutated Gene	Genotype	Pattern of Iron Deposition
1	Adult	*HFE*	C282Y/C282Y C282Y/ H63D	Hepatocellular with periportal accentuation
2A	Juvenile	Hemojuvelin		Hepatocellular with periportal accentuation
2B	Juvenile	Hepcidin		Hepatocellular with periportal accentuation
3	Adult	Transferrin receptor-2		Hepatocellular with periportal accentuation
4	Adult	Ferroportin		A. Kupffer cell and hepatocytes B. Predominantly hepatocellular

DIFFERENTIAL DIAGNOSIS

Anemia of Chronic Disease

- Iron deposition in both hepatocytes and Kupffer cells

Transfusion-related Hemosiderosis

- Iron deposition in Kupffer cells in early stages but may accumulate in hepatocytes when excessive

Chronic Hemolytic Disorders

- Iron deposition in both hepatocytes and Kupffer cells

Other Chronic Liver Diseases

- Nonspecific iron accumulation

DIAGNOSTIC CHECKLIST

Clinically Relevant Pathologic Features

- Increased iron in patients with elevated LFTs

Pathologic Interpretation Pearls

- Recommend genetic testing, quantitative iron in patients with histologic iron overload

SELECTED REFERENCES

1. Batts KP: Iron overload syndromes and the liver. Mod Pathol. 20 Suppl 1:S31-9, 2007
2. Brunt EM: Pathology of hepatic iron overload. Semin Liver Dis. 25(4):392-401, 2005

IMAGE GALLERY

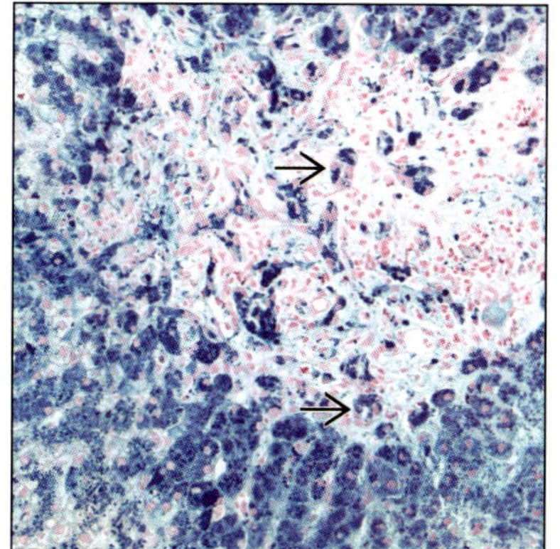

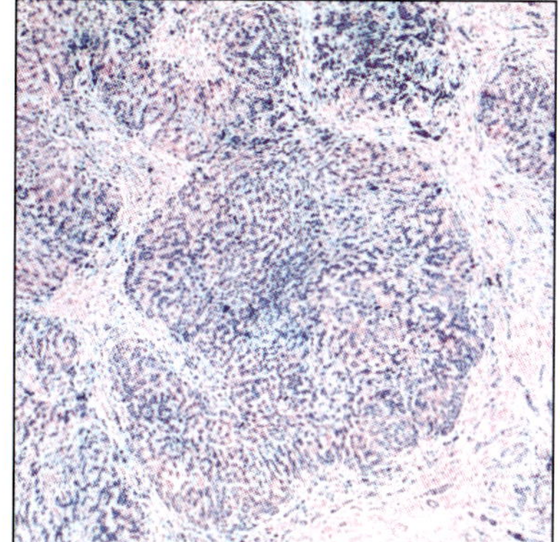

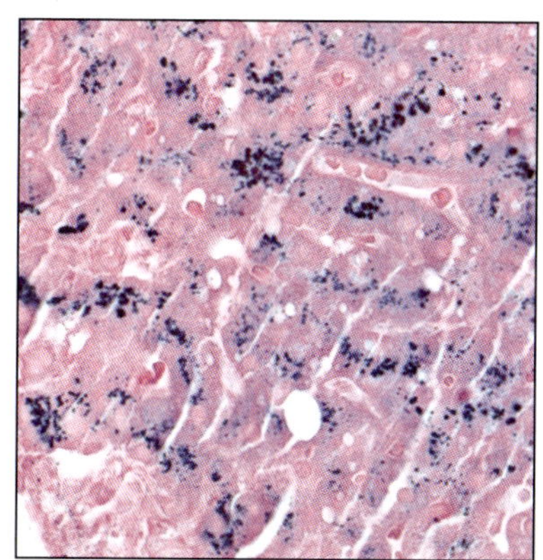

(Left) *Perl iron stain high-power photomicrograph shows the coarse iron granules within the hepatocytes as well as in the bile duct epithelium* ⇒ *and Kupffer cells.* ***(Center)*** *Perl iron stain shows liver cirrhosis due to hereditary hemochromatosis with extensive iron deposition in the hepatocytes of the cirrhotic nodules, as well as in the Kupffer cells, biliary epithelium, and endothelium.* ***(Right)*** *Perl iron stain shows the pericanalicular pattern of iron deposition in the hepatocytes typical of most hereditary hemochromatosis.*

WILSON DISEASE

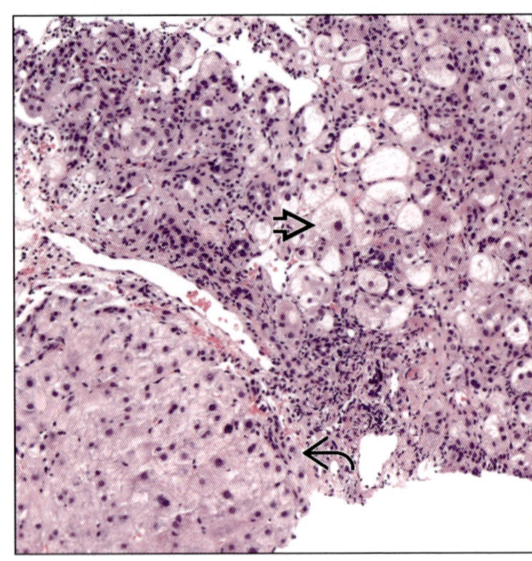

Hematoxylin & eosin stained liver biopsy demonstrates chronic hepatitis with ballooning degeneration of hepatocytes ⇨ and nodule formation ↶.

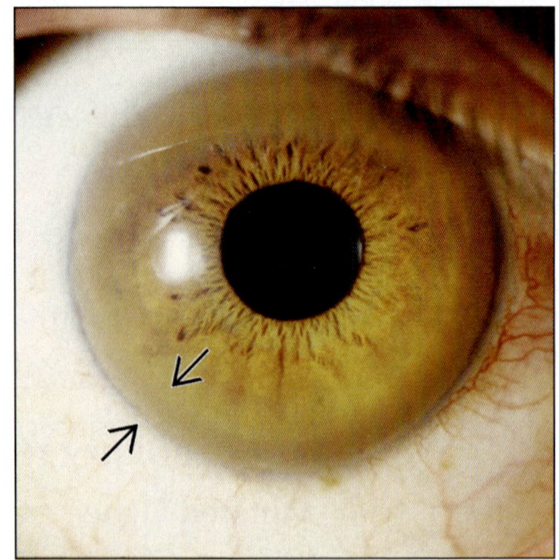

Clinical photograph of Kayser-Fleischer ring shows brown deposits of copper at the periphery of the iris →. (Courtesy S. Uwaydat, MD.)

TERMINOLOGY

Synonyms

- Hepatolenticular degeneration

Definitions

- Autosomal recessive inherited mutation of copper transport protein

ETIOLOGY/PATHOGENESIS

Genetic Defect

- Mutations of *ATP7B* gene, which codes for copper-dependent P-type ATPase, a copper transport protein found on Golgi apparatus and on canalicular membrane
  - Inability to excrete copper in bile leads to its accumulation in liver and various tissues
  - Inability to transport copper into Golgi apparatus makes it unavailable for synthesis of ceruloplasmin, leading to release of apoceruloplasmin into serum and its rapid degradation
    - Ceruloplasmin functions as a plasma ferroxidase, oxidizing ferrous iron for subsequent transfer to plasma apotransferrin, making it available for hemoglobin biosynthesis

CLINICAL ISSUES

Epidemiology

- Incidence
  - 1 in 30,000

Presentation

- Acute liver failure with Coombs negative hemolytic anemia and renal failure
- Chronic liver disease with fibrosis or cirrhosis
- Neurologic/neuropsychiatric signs with Kayser-Fleischer rings

Laboratory Tests

- Low ceruloplasmin is characteristic, but this is neither sensitive nor specific
  - Low ceruloplasmin can also be due to low hepatic synthetic function
  - Normal ceruloplasmin levels can be seen in Wilson diseases since ceruloplasmin is acute phase reactant
- Increased serum-free copper
- Increased urinary copper, typically measured in 24-hour collection specimen
- Increased hepatic copper concentration is most reliable test
  - Best performed on fresh tissue but can be performed on paraffin block
- Genetic testing is difficult due to number of mutations but is definitive
  - Most patients are compound heterozygotes

Treatment

- Drugs
  - Copper chelators
    - Penicillamine binds copper via a free sulfhydryl group, is excreted in urine, and induces metallothionein, leading to sequestration of free intracellular copper
    - Trientine chelates copper by forming stable complexes with 4 constituent nitrogens in planar ring
    - Ammonium tetrathiomolybdate forms complexes with copper and protein in food, inhibiting copper absorption, and with copper and albumin for excretion in bile
- Zinc induces intestinal metallothionein, resulting in binding of copper in enterocytes and its loss when enterocytes are shed, and induces metallothionein in hepatocytes
- Foods high in copper should be avoided, including chocolate, liver, nuts, mushrooms, and shellfish

WILSON DISEASE

Key Facts

Etiology/Pathogenesis
- Mutations of *ATP7B* gene, which codes for copper transport protein found on Golgi apparatus and canalicular membrane
- Inability to excrete copper in bile leads to its accumulation in liver and various tissues

Clinical Issues
- Mainstay of treatment is copper chelators and zinc
- Low serum ceruloplasmin level is characteristic but is neither sensitive nor specific
- Increased serum-free copper and urinary copper are characteristic

Microscopic Pathology
- Early disease is characterized by steatosis, Mallory hyaline, and glycogenated nuclei
- Intermediate stage is characterized by chronic hepatitis with fibrosis or cirrhosis
- Rhodanine or rubeanic acid stains may show copper in periportal hepatocytes but can also be negative
- Orcein or aldehyde fuchsin stains may show granules of copper-associated protein in periportal hepatocytes
- Tissue copper quantification is definitive in most cases

Top Differential Diagnoses
- Nonalcoholic steatohepatitis
- Autoimmune hepatitis

Prognosis
- Without treatment, progresses to cirrhosis and death
- With treatment, can be managed
- Hepatocellular carcinoma is rare complication
- Transplant is option for patients with acute liver failure or chronic disease not responsive to medical therapy

MICROSCOPIC PATHOLOGY

Histologic Features
- Early disease is characterized by steatosis, Mallory hyaline, and glycogenated nuclei, mimicking steatohepatitis
- Intermediate stage is characterized by chronic hepatitis with fibrosis or cirrhosis, mimicking viral or autoimmune hepatitis, but with few plasma cells
- Fulminant cases may have parenchymal necrosis and collapse

Predominant Pattern/Injury Type
- Inflammatory, chronic
- Steatosis

Predominant Cell/Compartment Type
- Portal- and periportal-based inflammation

Histochemical Stains
- Rhodanine or rubeanic acid stains may show varying amounts of copper in periportal hepatocytes but can also be negative
  - Free copper in cytosol is toxic but is washed out in processing and is not detected by histochemical stains
  - Copper bound to metallothionein and sequestered in lysosomes is nontoxic and can be detected by histochemical stains
- Orcein or aldehyde fuchsin stains for copper-associated protein (metallothionein) may show granules in periportal hepatocytes

Ancillary Studies
- Electron microscopy shows mitochondrial abnormalities including widening of intercristal spaces, increased matrix density and granularity, and separation of inner and outer mitochondrial membranes
- Tissue copper quantification of liver is definitive in most cases

DIFFERENTIAL DIAGNOSIS

Nonalcoholic Steatohepatitis
- Clinical features are different
- Tissue copper quantification does not demonstrate elevated copper levels

Autoimmune Hepatitis (AIH)
- Numerous plasma cells in AIH
- Copper stain is negative
- Tissue copper quantification does not demonstrate elevated copper levels

SELECTED REFERENCES

1. Ala A et al: Wilson's disease. Lancet. 369(9559):397-408, 2007
2. Ala A et al: Wilson disease: pathophysiology, diagnosis, treatment, and screening. Clin Liver Dis. 8(4):787-805, viii, 2004
3. Gitlin JD: Wilson disease. Gastroenterology. 125(6):1868-77, 2003
4. Gitlin JD: Aceruloplasminemia. Pediatr Res. 44(3):271-6, 1998
5. Davies SE et al: Hepatic morphology and histochemistry of Wilson's disease presenting as fulminant hepatic failure: a study of 11 cases. Histopathology. 15(4):385-94, 1989
6. Sumithran E et al: Copper-binding protein in liver cells. Hum Pathol. 16(7):677-82, 1985
7. Stromeyer FW et al: Histology of the liver in Wilson's disease: a study of 34 cases. Am J Clin Pathol. 73(1):12-24, 1980

Microscopic Features

(Left) *Hematoxylin & eosin stained liver biopsy demonstrates features of steatohepatitis in Wilson disease, with abundant steatosis and portal expansion.* ***(Right)*** *Hematoxylin & eosin stained liver biopsy in Wilson disease shows mixed large and small droplet steatosis and glycogenated nuclei ⤻.*

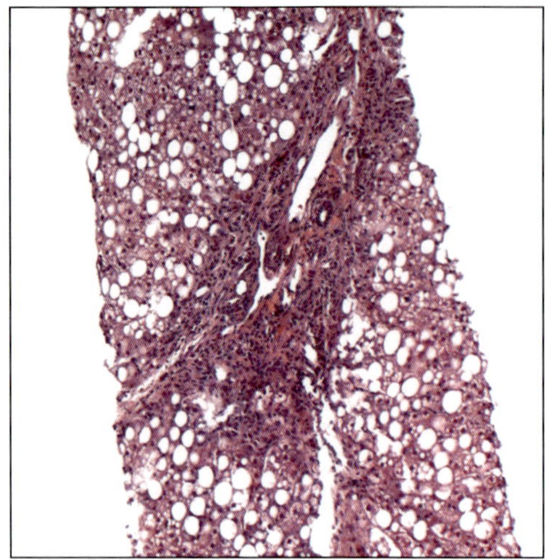

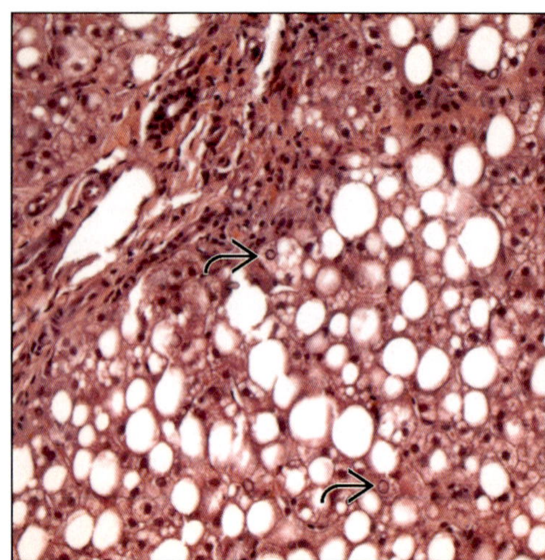

(Left) *Hematoxylin & eosin stained section shows features of steatohepatitis in Wilson disease, with steatosis and glycogenated nuclei ⤻.* ***(Right)*** *Hematoxylin & eosin stained section of liver biopsy in Wilson disease shows portal-based chronic inflammatory infiltrates.*

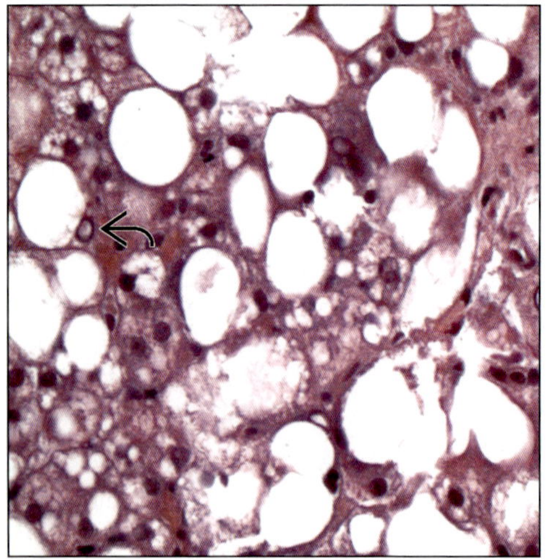

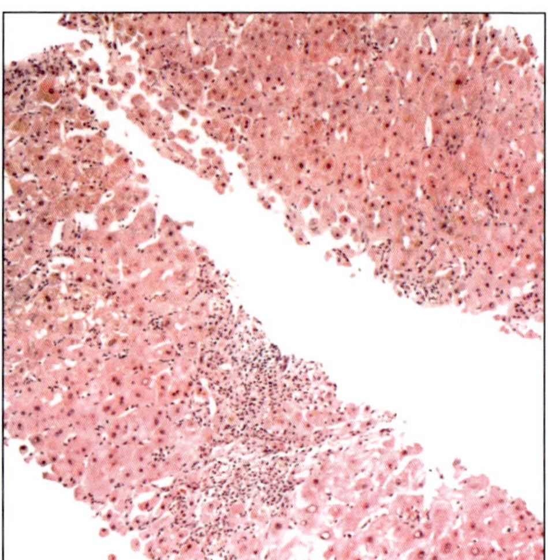

(Left) *Hematoxylin & eosin stained section of liver biopsy in Wilson disease shows portal-based chronic inflammatory cells, necrotic hepatocytes ⤻, and glycogenated nuclei ⇨.* ***(Right)*** *Hematoxylin & eosin stained section of liver biopsy in Wilson disease shows chronic inflammation in periportal parenchyma, increased pigment in hepatocytes, and focal Mallory hyaline →.*

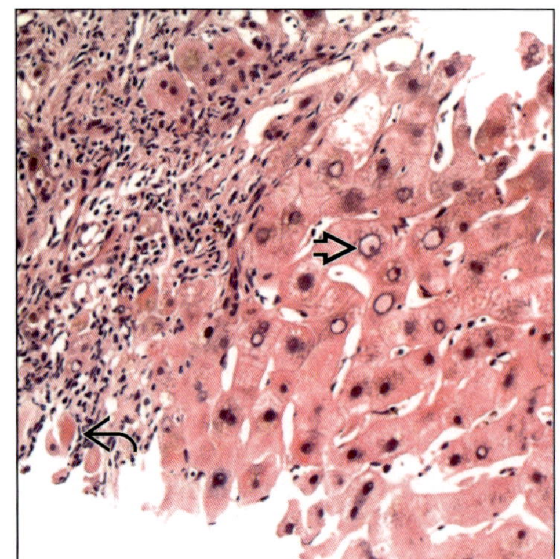

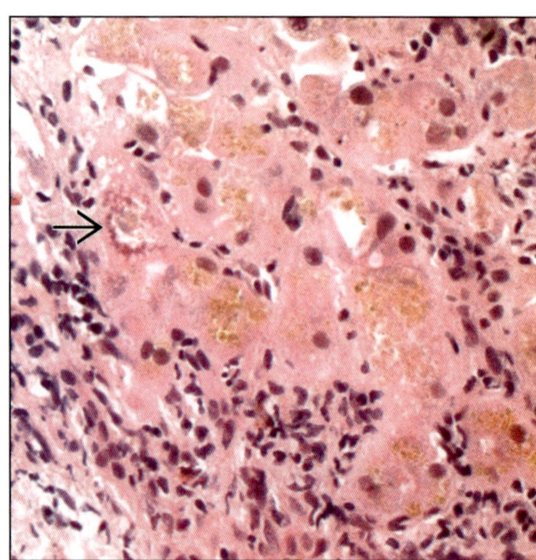

Microscopic Features

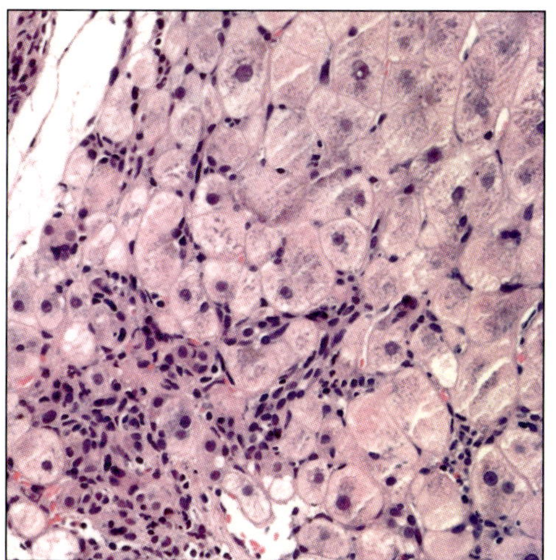

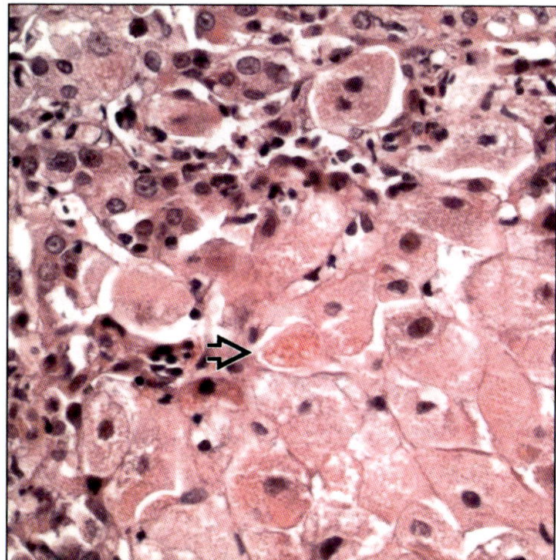

(Left) *Hematoxylin & eosin stained section of liver biopsy in Wilson disease shows chronic inflammatory filtrates, hepatocyte swelling, and oncocytic change of the hepatocytes.* ***(Right)*** *Hematoxylin & eosin stained liver biopsy in Wilson disease shows portal and periportal chronic hepatitis and apoptotic hepatocytes* ⇨.

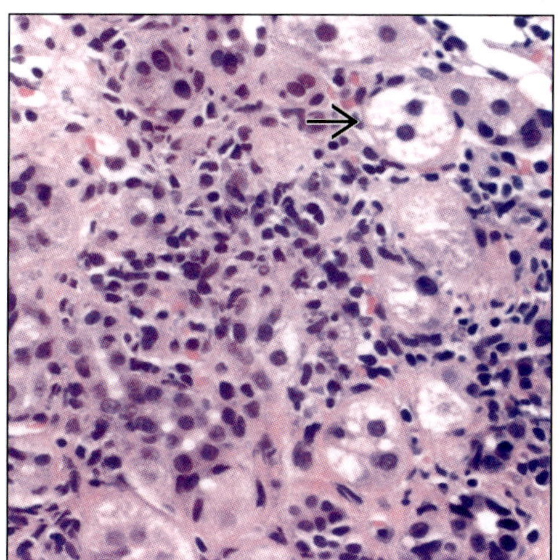

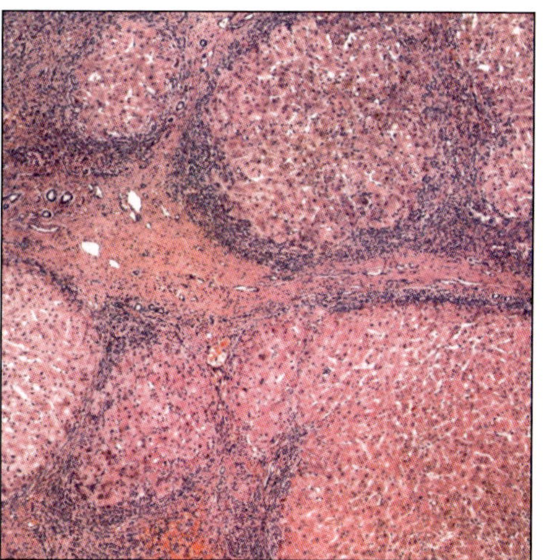

(Left) *Hematoxylin & eosin stained section of liver biopsy in Wilson disease shows severe chronic inflammation and hepatocyte ballooning degeneration* →. ***(Right)*** *Hematoxylin & eosin stained section shows cirrhosis in Wilson disease with chronic inflammatory infiltrates at the edges of the nodules.*

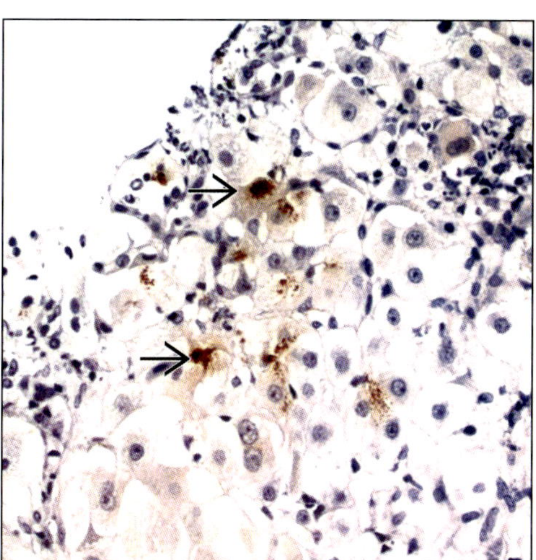

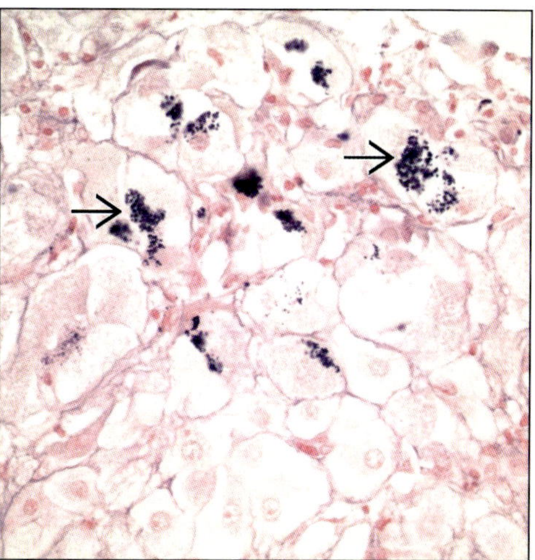

(Left) *Copper stain using the rhodanine method demonstrates granules of copper within periportal hepatocytes* →. ***(Right)*** *Aldehyde fuchsin stain shows darkly staining granules of copper-associated protein (metallothionein) in periportal hepatocytes* →.

ALPHA-1-ANTITRYPSIN DEFICIENCY

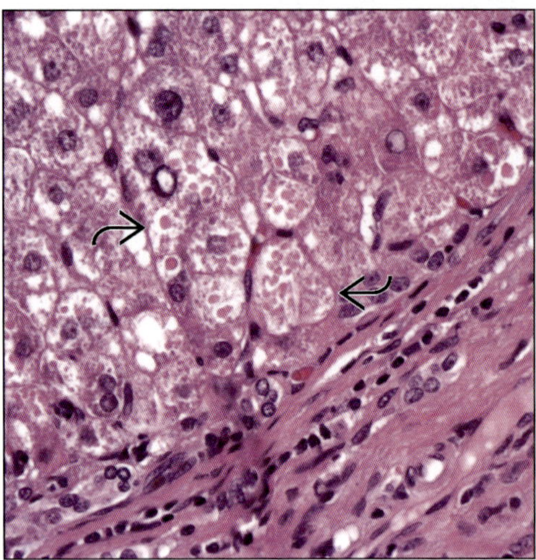

Hematoxylin & eosin section shows numerous eosinophilic globules within the cytoplasm of periportal hepatocytes ⮫.

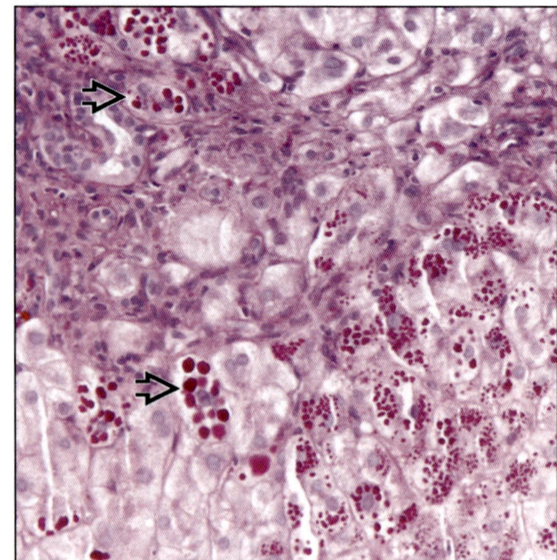

Periodic acid-Schiff with diastase digestion shows numerous periportal PAS positive diastase-resistant globules ⇨.

TERMINOLOGY

Abbreviations

- α-1-antitrypsin disease (A1AT)

Definitions

- Genetic disorder
  - A1AT protein synthesized mainly in liver
    - Protects tissues during acute inflammatory reactions
  - Deficiency is characterized by emphysema and chronic liver disease

ETIOLOGY/PATHOGENESIS

Inherited Metabolic Disorder

- Autosomal recessive
  - Normal gene product is PiM
  - Most common deficiency alleles are PiS and PiZ
  - PiZZ phenotype accounts for most cases of severe A1AT deficiency

Accumulation of Mutant Protein

- Coding sequence defect leads to abnormal polymerization of glycoprotein preventing export from hepatocyte
- Mutant protein accumulates in endoplasmic reticulum of hepatocyte
  - Decrease in serum A1AT
- Direct mechanism of hepatocyte injury is unknown
- Unknown additional genetic factors &/or environmental factors predispose some adults to develop liver disease

CLINICAL ISSUES

Epidemiology

- Incidence
  - Severe A1AT deficiency is found in ~ 1:3,500 live births
- Age
  - Bimodal distribution: Neonatal hepatitis, chronic liver disease in adults
- Gender
  - No predilection until age 50, then male predominance
- Ethnicity
  - Disease most common in Caucasians with northern European ancestry

Presentation

- Pulmonary emphysema, early age, even in nonsmokers
- Liver disease
  - Pediatric population: Neonatal hepatitis and cholestasis (jaundice, hepatomegaly, elevation of liver enzymes)
  - Adults: Variable, from asymptomatic elevation of liver enzymes to advanced cirrhosis

Laboratory Tests

- Serum levels of A1AT < 35% of normal
- Pi phenotyping by polyacrylamide gel isoelectric focusing
- DNA sequencing

Treatment

- No specific therapy
- Liver transplantation has been successful

Prognosis

- Children
  - Majority spontaneously regress by 6 months of age
  - Some have persistent biochemical abnormalities &/or hepatomegaly
  - Minority develop cirrhosis and liver failure
- Adults
  - Poor prognosis after diagnosis of cirrhosis

ALPHA-1-ANTITRYPSIN DEFICIENCY

Key Facts

Terminology
- A1AT protein synthesized mainly in liver
- Protects tissues during acute inflammatory reactions
- Deficiency is characterized by emphysema and chronic liver disease

Etiology/Pathogenesis
- Genetic, autosomal recessive disorder
- PiZZ phenotype accounts for most cases of severe A1AT deficiency
- Accumulation of mutant protein within hepatocyte and decrease in serum A1AT
- Hepatocyte injury is triggered through unknown mechanisms

Clinical Issues
- Bimodal distribution consists of neonatal hepatitis and chronic liver disease in adults (5th decade)
- Disease most common in Caucasians with northern European ancestry
- Characterized by pulmonary emphysema, chronic liver disease, cirrhosis
- No specific therapy

Microscopic Pathology
- Eosinophilic globules within periportal/periseptal hepatocytes
- Globules are strongly PAS positive, diastase-resistant
- Neonatal hepatitis (cholestasis, bile ductular proliferation, paucity of interlobular bile ducts)
- Chronic hepatitis &/or cirrhosis in adults

  - Increased risk of hepatocellular carcinoma ± cirrhosis

MACROSCOPIC FEATURES

General Features
- Hepatomegaly, cirrhosis

MICROSCOPIC PATHOLOGY

Histologic Features
- Eosinophilic round globules within periportal/periseptal hepatocytes
  - Vary in size (1-40 μm in diameter)
  - Strongly PAS positive, diastase resistant
  - Seen in heterozygous (PiMZ, PiSZ) as well as homozygous individuals (PiZZ)
- Neonatal hepatitis
  - Varying degree of hepatocyte injury (ballooning and necrosis), cholestasis, and portal inflammation
  - Paucity of interlobular bile ducts or bile ductular proliferation may be prominent features
  - Globules are difficult to detect in infants < 12 weeks of age
- Adults
  - Variable portal inflammation (with predominance of lymphocytes) and variable fibrosis
  - Cirrhosis (when present), nonspecific mixed micronodular and macronodular pattern
  - Easily identifiable periportal/periseptal A1AT globules

Predominant Pattern/Injury Type
- Cytoplasmic inclusion

Predominant Cell/Compartment Type
- Hepatocyte

Immunohistochemistry
- Stain for A1AT globules

DIFFERENTIAL DIAGNOSIS

Lafora Disease
- Inclusions are pale and round or kidney-shaped; displace nuclei
  - Weakly positive with PAS with diastase; positive with colloidal iron and silver stains

Fibrinogen Storage Disease
- Pale, weakly eosinophilic, PAS negative ground-glass bodies
- Immunohistochemical stain for fibrinogen strongly positive

Congestion-associated Globules
- Centrilobular distribution of PAS positive, diastase-resistant globules
- Associated with sinusoidal congestion and hepatic hypoxia

Extrahepatic Biliary Atresia in Infants
- Abnormal imaging studies and absence of A1AT serum deficiency

DIAGNOSTIC CHECKLIST

Pathologic Interpretation Pearls
- PAS positive, diastase-resistant, eosinophilic globules in periportal/periseptal distribution

SELECTED REFERENCES

1. Fairbanks KD et al: Liver disease in alpha 1-antitrypsin deficiency: a review. Am J Gastroenterol. 103(8):2136-41; quiz 2142, 2008
2. Stoller JK et al: Alpha1-antitrypsin deficiency. Lancet. 365(9478):2225-36, 2005
3. Eriksson S: Alpha 1-antitrypsin deficiency. J Hepatol. 30 Suppl 1:34-9, 1999
4. Birrer P et al: Alpha 1-antitrypsin deficiency and liver disease. J Inherit Metab Dis. 14(4):512-25, 1991

ALPHA-1-ANTITRYPSIN DEFICIENCY

Gross and Microscopic Features

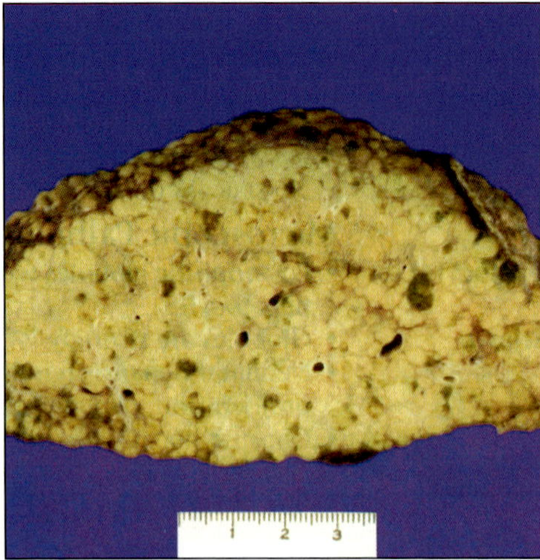

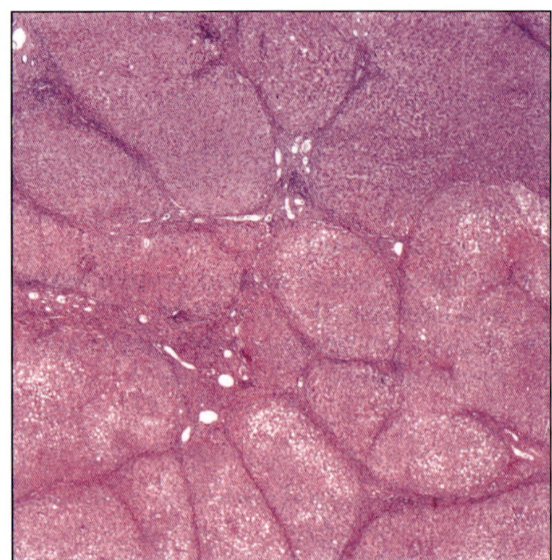

(Left) *Gross photograph of a hepatectomy in an adult with an A1AT deficiency shows nodular capsular and cut surfaces, consistent with cirrhosis. Cirrhosis is frequently established at the time of diagnosis in adults.* ***(Right)*** *Hematoxylin & eosin section shows cirrhosis and mild steatosis. The pattern of cirrhosis in A1AT deficiency is nonspecific and may consist of nodules of varying sizes and shapes.*

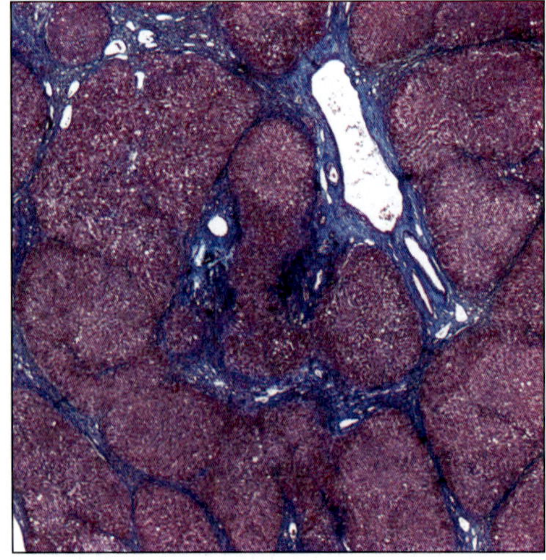

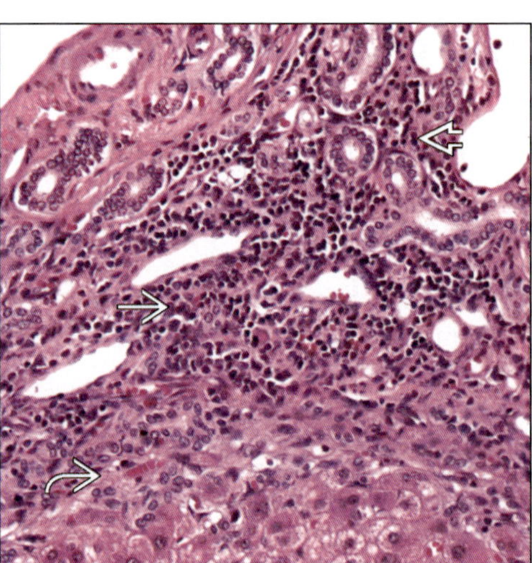

(Left) *Trichrome stain highlights cirrhosis with irregularly shaped nodules (garland- or jigsaw-puzzle-shaped). This biliary pattern of cirrhosis can be seen in patients with A1AT deficiency, especially in pediatric patients and those with homozygous (PiZZ) disease.* ***(Right)*** *Hematoxylin & eosin section shows a portal tract expanded by a predominantly lymphoplasmacytic infiltrate ➔ with proliferation of bile ductules ➪ and mild limiting plate activity ↷.*

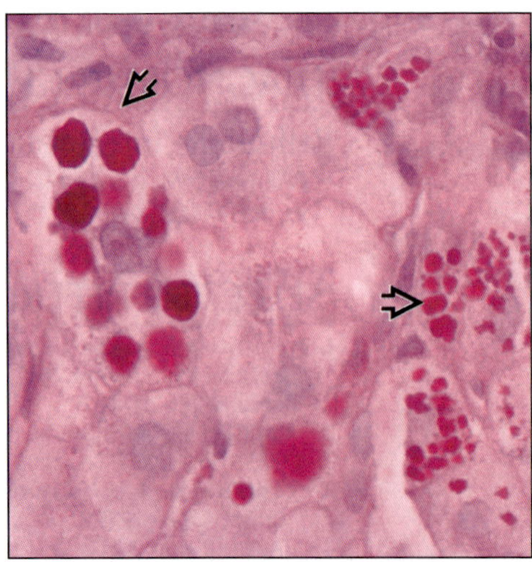

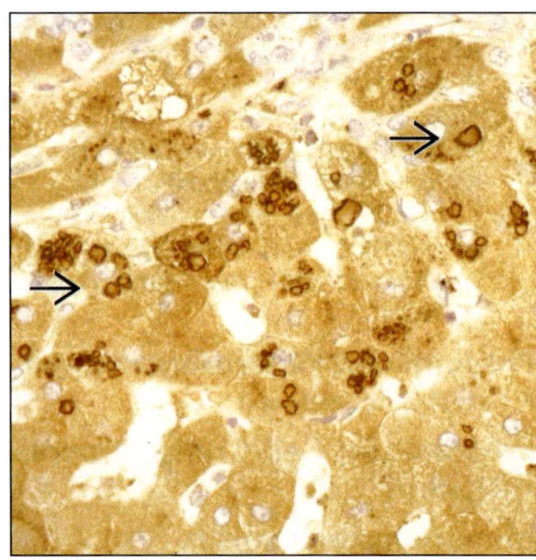

(Left) *Periodic acid-Schiff with diastase digestion shows round, homogeneous, intracytoplasmic inclusions ➪ of varying sizes that are strongly PAS positive and diastase resistant.* ***(Right)*** *α1-antitrypsin immunohistochemical stain confirms the presence of A1AT inclusion bodies within hepatocytes →. The peripheral pattern of staining of each globule is characteristic. In neonates, there is granular cytoplasmic staining since globules are not usually present in this age group.*

Microscopic Features

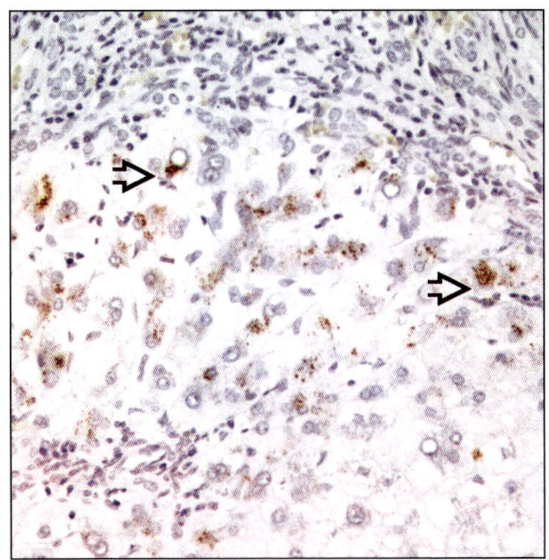

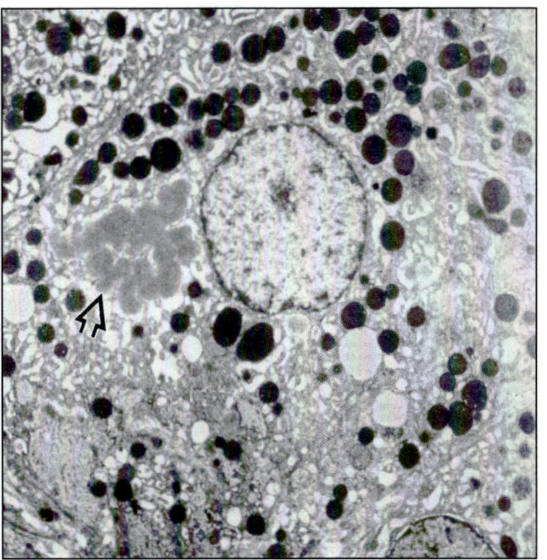

(Left) *Copper stain highlights red-brown granules within periportal hepatocytes ➩, consistent with cholate stasis (chronic cholestasis). This feature is frequently seen in neonates who present with cholestatic hepatitis secondary to A1AT deficiency and in adults with cirrhosis.* ***(Right)*** *Electron micrograph shows round, electron-dense deposits within the endoplasmic reticulum of a hepatocyte ➩.*

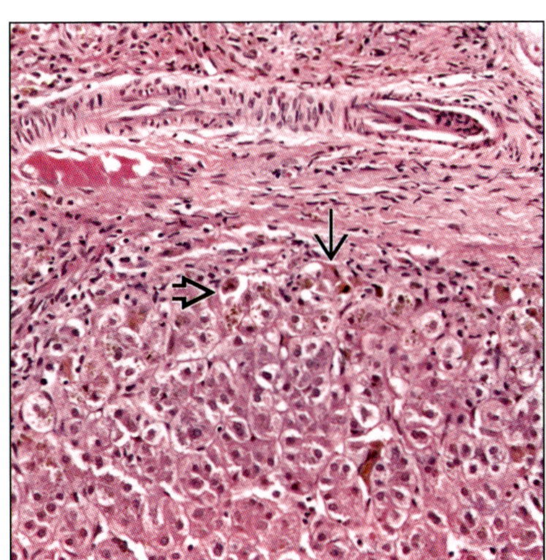

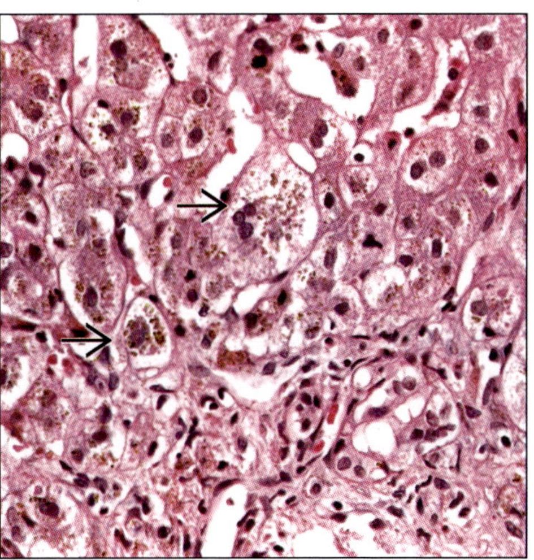

(Left) *Hematoxylin & eosin section of hepatitis in a neonate with an A1AT deficiency shows cholestasis →, predominantly in a periportal distribution, with hepatocyte ballooning and focal hepatocyte necrosis ➩. The amount of portal tract inflammation is variable. In this case, there is minimal portal tract inflammation.* ***(Right)*** *Hematoxylin & eosin section of neonatal hepatitis at higher magnification shows hepatocyte ballooning and cholestasis →.*

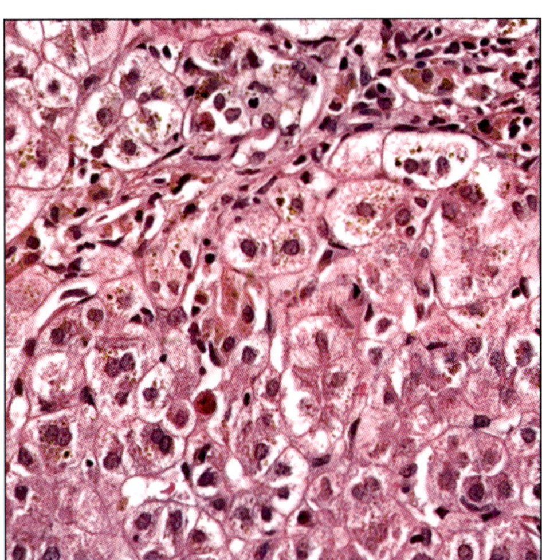

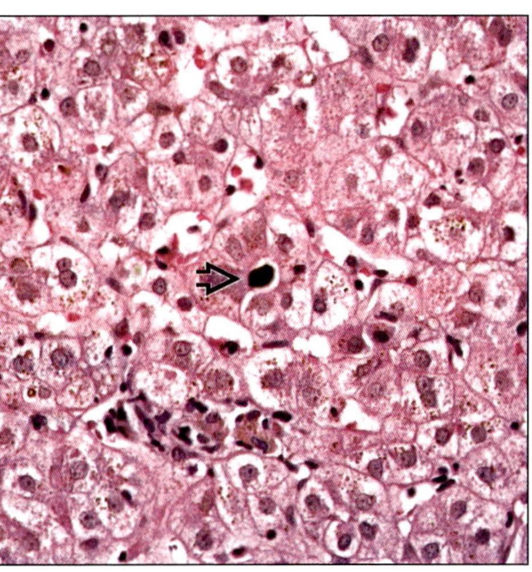

(Left) *Hematoxylin & eosin section of hepatitis in a neonate with A1AT deficiency shows focal hepatocyte necrosis, hepatocellular cholestasis, and canalicular cholestasis. The degree of hepatocyte injury seen secondary to A1AT deficiency is highly variable.* ***(Right)*** *Hematoxylin & eosin section of hepatitis in a neonate with an A1AT deficiency shows a cholestatic rosette containing a bile plug ➩.*

CONGENITAL HEPATIC FIBROSIS

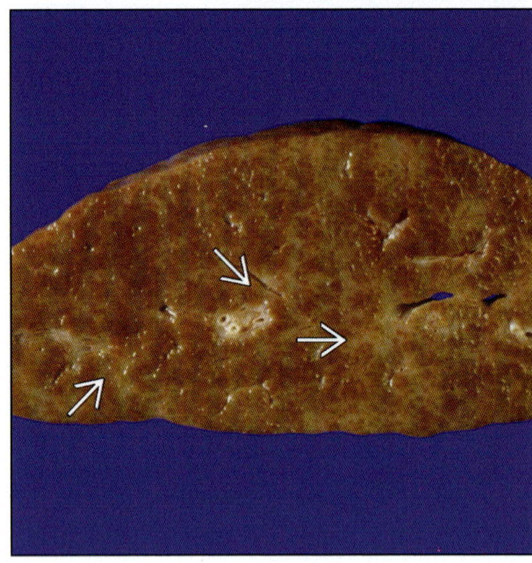

Gross photograph of congenital hepatic fibrosis shows white fibrous bands ➡ that divide the liver parenchyma. There is no definite nodularity as seen in cirrhosis.

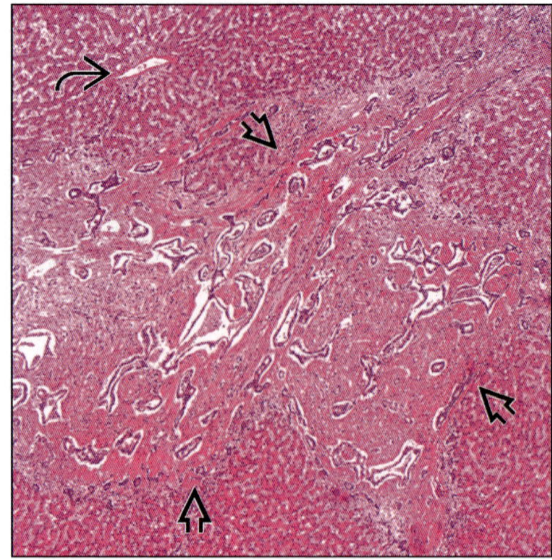

Low-power view shows marked portal expansion and numerous irregularly shaped bile ducts ➢. The lobular architecture in adjacent parenchyma is well maintained with normal central veins ↪.

TERMINOLOGY

Abbreviations

- Congenital hepatic fibrosis (CHF)

Definitions

- Variant of ductal plate malformation
  - Leads to portal and bridging fibrosis, proliferation of aberrant duct profiles, and portal hypertension

ETIOLOGY/PATHOGENESIS

Developmental Anomaly

- Primarily autosomal recessive inheritance
- Rarely autosomal dominant
- Ductal plate malformation at level of small interlobular bile ducts
- Persistence of excess embryonic bile ducts

Disease Associations

- Autosomal recessive polycystic kidney disease
  - Most common coexisting condition
  - Mutations in the *PKHD1* gene encoding fibrocystin
  - Some consider CHF a variant of autosomal recessive polycystic kidney disease
- Caroli syndrome
- Congenital disorder of glycosylation type 1b
- Autosomal dominant polycystic kidney disease
- Meckel-Gruber syndrome
- Joubert syndrome and related disorders, including COACH syndrome
- Bardet-Biedl syndrome
- Jeune syndrome
- Oral-facial-digital syndrome

CLINICAL ISSUES

Epidemiology

- Incidence
  - Rare
    - Exact incidence is unknown
- Age
  - Usually diagnosed during adolescence or young adulthood
    - Range includes early childhood to 6th decade of life
- Gender
  - Equal gender distribution

Presentation

- Portal hypertension and related problems
- Hepatosplenomegaly
- Recurrent cholangitis if it presents as Caroli syndrome
- Rare cases are asymptomatic

Laboratory Tests

- Normal or modestly elevated liver tests

Treatment

- Directed at management of complications of portal hypertension
  - Endoscopic banding or sclerotherapy for varices
  - Transjugular intrahepatic portosystemic shunts
- Antibiotics for cholangitis in Caroli syndrome
- Liver transplantation

Prognosis

- Generally good but can be debilitating
- Occasional evolution into true cirrhosis

IMAGE FINDINGS

General Features

- Hypertrophic left lateral segment and caudate lobe
- Normal or hypertrophic left medial segment
- Atrophic right lobe
- Increased echogenicity with coarse and heterogeneous pattern on ultrasound
- Periportal cuffing, indicative of fibrosis, on CT

CONGENITAL HEPATIC FIBROSIS

Key Facts

Etiology/Pathogenesis
- Primarily autosomal recessive inheritance
- Ductal plate malformation at level of small interlobular bile ducts
- Frequent association with autosomal recessive polycystic kidney disease and Caroli syndrome

Clinical Issues
- Usually diagnosed during adolescence or young adulthood, rarely seen at 5th or 6th decade of life
- Portal hypertension

Microscopic Pathology
- Portal and bridging fibrosis
- Multiple irregularly shaped bile ducts in portal tracts and fibrous septa
- Hypoplastic &/or decreased portal vein branches

Top Differential Diagnoses
- Cirrhosis, idiopathic portal hypertension

- Splenomegaly

MACROSCOPIC FEATURES

General Features
- Enlarged and firm liver
  - Liver may be of normal size
- Entire liver usually involved
  - Irregular white fibrous bands dividing liver parenchyma
  - No definite nodule formation

DIFFERENTIAL DIAGNOSIS

Cirrhosis
- Diffuse nodular regeneration of hepatocytes and remodeling of normal hepatic architecture
- Varying degrees of inflammation
- Compromised liver function

Idiopathic Portal Hypertension
- Lack of bridging fibrosis
- Lack of abnormally proliferative bile ducts
- Characterized by narrowing or obliteration of portal vein branches

von Meyenburg Complexes
- No portal hypertension
- Usually small nodular lesions that are incidental findings
- Also associated with polycystic liver disease

DIAGNOSTIC CHECKLIST

Clinically Relevant Pathologic Features
- Most common associated condition is polycystic kidney disease
- Teenager or young adult with portal hypertension

Pathologic Interpretation Pearls
- Characteristic lesion is combination of portal fibrosis and persistence of excess embryonic bile ducts

SELECTED REFERENCES

1. Shorbagi A et al: Experience of a single center with congenital hepatic fibrosis: a review of the literature. World J Gastroenterol. 16(6):683-90, 2010
2. Gunay-Aygun M: Liver and kidney disease in ciliopathies. Am J Med Genet C Semin Med Genet. 151C(4):296-306, 2009
3. Akhan O et al: Imaging findings in congenital hepatic fibrosis. Eur J Radiol. 61(1):18-24, 2007
4. De Vos M et al: Congenital hepatic fibrosis. J Hepatol. 6(2):222-8, 1988

IMAGE GALLERY

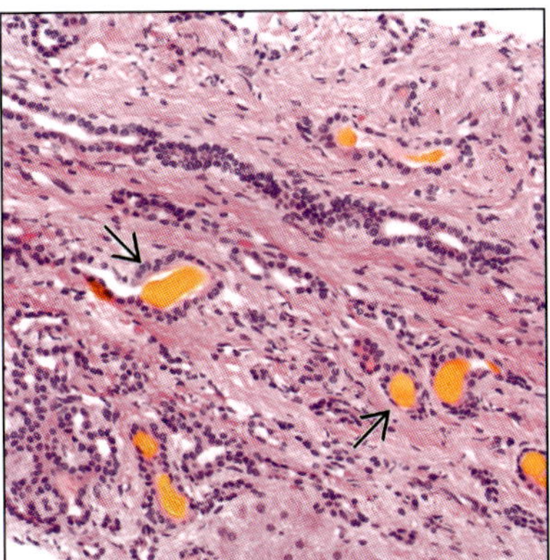

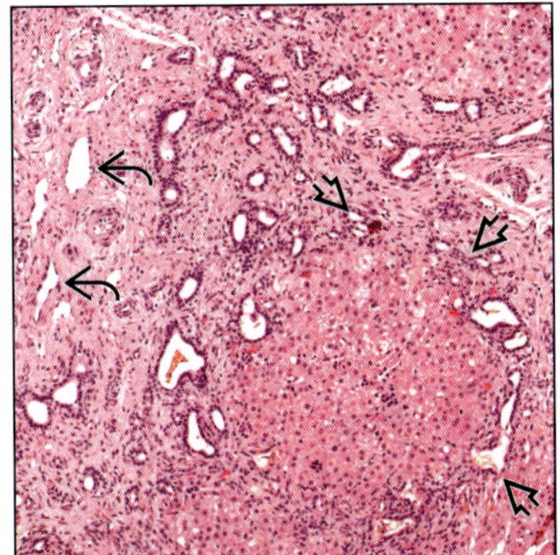

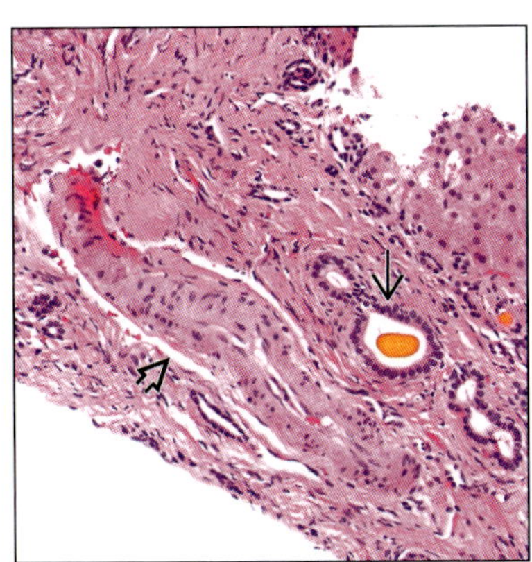

(Left) The aberrantly formed bile ducts are lined by cuboidal or low columnar biliary epithelium, and some contain inspissated bile ➙. (Center) Some of the ducts are characteristically located at the interface with the liver parenchyma ➪. Note the presence of bridging fibrosis. Portal vein branches appear hypoplastic ➚. (Right) A hypertrophic hepatic artery branch ➪ is seen in a case of congenital hepatic fibrosis. Note inspissated bile in a duct ➙.

POLYCYSTIC LIVER DISEASE

Polycystic liver disease features massive involvement by numerous variably sized cysts throughout the liver.

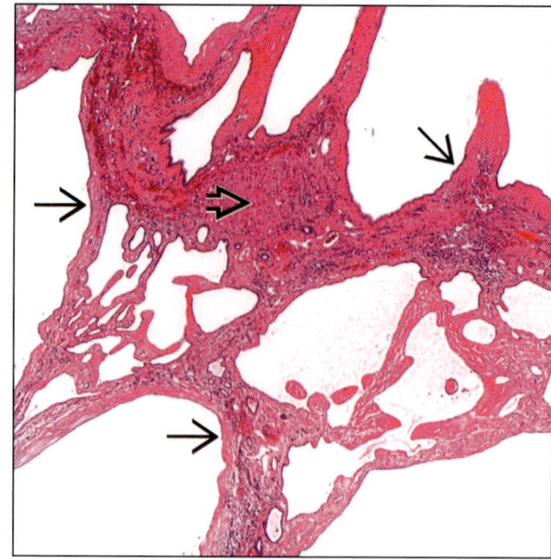

Low-power view shows numerous cystic spaces lined by a single layer of epithelial cells ⇒, supported by variable amounts of connective tissue. Only minimal liver parenchyma remains ➪.

TERMINOLOGY

Abbreviations

- Polycystic liver disease (PLD)
- Autosomal dominant polycystic kidney disease (ADPKD)

Definitions

- Genetic disorder characterized by progressive development of multiple macroscopic liver cysts that lack communication with biliary tree

ETIOLOGY/PATHOGENESIS

Hereditary Anomaly

- Associated with ADPKD
  - Mutations in *PKD1* gene encoding polycystin-1 seen in 80-85% of cases
  - Mutations in *PKD2* gene encoding polycystin-2 seen in 15-20% of cases
- Isolated PLD
  - Mutations in *PRKCSH* gene encoding hepatocystin
  - Mutations in *SEC63* gene encoding Sec63p protein
  - Also autosomal dominant inheritance
- Developing from embryonic ductal plate malformation (von Meyenburg complexes)
- Evolving through overgrowth and dilatation into cysts
- Loss of continuity with biliary tree

CLINICAL ISSUES

Epidemiology

- Incidence
  - ADPKD affecting 1 in 500-1,000 individuals
    - PLD occurring in 30-90% of patients with ADPKD
  - Isolated PLD affecting < 0.01% of population
- Age
  - Age-dependent increase in number and size of cysts in liver in patients with ADPKD
    - 20% in 3rd decade of life
    - 75% by 7th decade
- Gender
  - Higher prevalence of PLD in women with ADPKD
    - 58-75% in women versus 42-62% in men
  - More numerous and larger liver cysts in women, presumably due to stimulatory effects of estrogen
    - After multiple pregnancies
    - Use of oral contraceptives or hormone replacement therapy

Presentation

- Asymptomatic in ~ 80% of patients
- Hepatomegaly with compression of adjacent structures
  - Abdominal pain
  - Early satiety
  - Nausea and vomiting
  - Supine dyspnea
  - Lower body edema and ascites
- Other associated medical conditions
  - Asymptomatic cysts in other organs including pancreas, spleen, ovaries, and lungs
  - Intracranial aneurysm
  - Valvular heart disease

Laboratory Tests

- Usually normal liver tests

Treatment

- Percutaneous aspiration of large dominant cyst
- Sclerosis of cysts
- Cyst fenestration
- Partial hepatectomy
- Liver transplantation

Prognosis

- Rupture of cyst
- Intracystic hemorrhage
- Cyst infection

POLYCYSTIC LIVER DISEASE

Key Facts

Etiology/Pathogenesis
- Frequent association with ADPKD but also occurring in isolated form
- Autosomal dominant inheritance
- Developing from ductal plate malformation

Clinical Issues
- Age-dependent increase in number and size of cysts in liver
- Asymptomatic in ~ 80% of patients
- Symptomatology due to hepatomegaly with compression of adjacent structures
- Treated with fenestration, partial hepatectomy, or liver transplantation

Microscopic Pathology
- Numerous variably sized cysts lined by single layer of cuboidal or flattened biliary epithelium
- Lack of communication with biliary tree
- von Meyenburg complexes commonly present

- Rarely portal hypertension or hepatic failure

IMAGE FINDINGS

CT Findings (3 Types)
- Type 1: Limited number (< 10) of large cysts with large areas of noncystic liver parenchyma
- Type 2: Diffuse involvement by medium-sized cysts with large areas of noncystic liver parenchyma
- Type 3: Massive involvement by small- and medium-sized cysts with only a few areas of noncystic liver parenchyma

MACROSCOPIC FEATURES

General Features
- Hepatomegaly weighing up to 13 kg
- Cysts varying from < 1 mm to > 12 cm in diameter
- Occasionally 1 lobe involved (usually left lobe)
- Clear, colorless, or straw-colored cyst fluid

MICROSCOPIC PATHOLOGY

Histologic Features
- Variably sized cysts lined by single layer of cuboidal or flattened biliary epithelium
- Varying amounts of supporting connective tissue
- von Meyenburg complexes commonly present
- Neutrophil infiltration in infected cysts
- Fibrosis and hyalinization in collapsed cysts
- Dystrophic calcification may be seen in cyst wall

Predominant Pattern/Injury Type
- Cystic

Predominant Cell/Compartment Type
- Ductal plate

DIFFERENTIAL DIAGNOSIS

Multiple Simple Biliary (Unilocular) Cysts
- Fewer in number with abundant liver parenchyma
- Nonhereditary

DIAGNOSTIC CHECKLIST

Clinically Relevant Pathologic Features
- Usually occurring in setting of ADPKD

Pathologic Interpretation Pearls
- Diffuse liver involvement by numerous cysts lined by single layer of biliary epithelium

SELECTED REFERENCES

1. Everson GT et al: Advances in management of polycystic liver disease. Expert Rev Gastroenterol Hepatol. 2(4):563-76, 2008
2. Russell RT et al: Surgical management of polycystic liver disease. World J Gastroenterol. 13(38):5052-9, 2007

IMAGE GALLERY

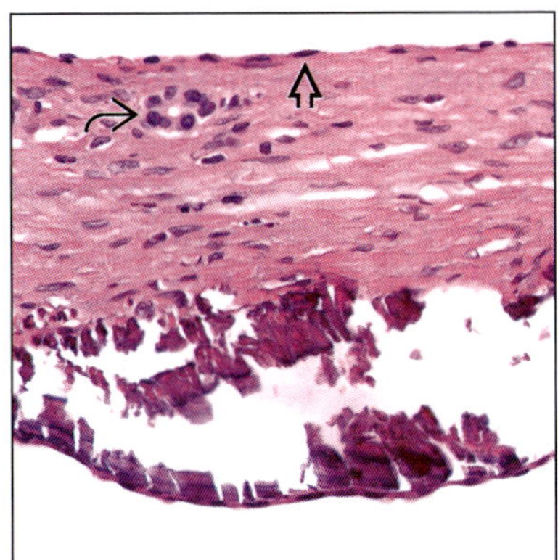
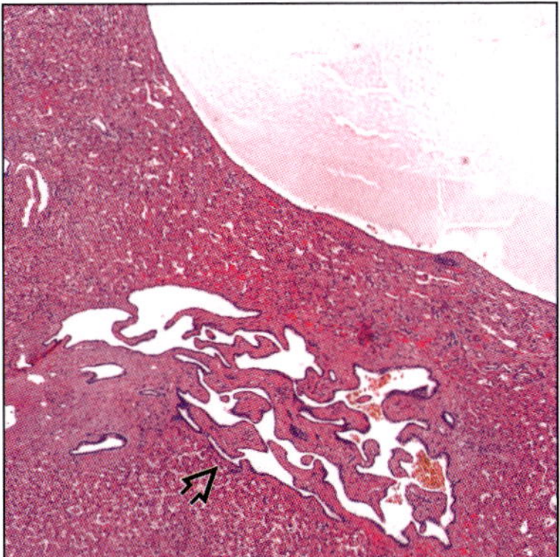
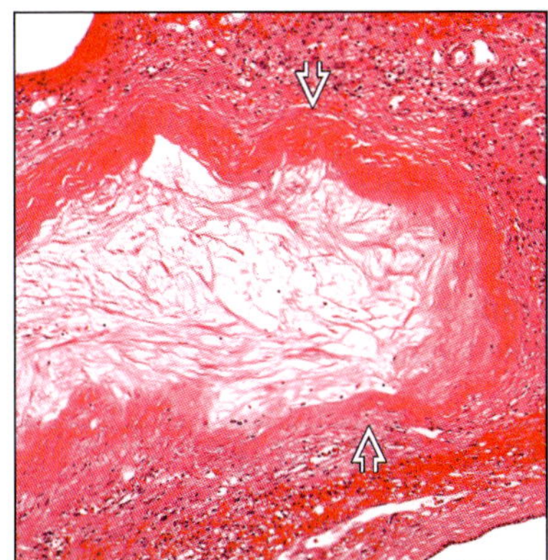

(Left) The biliary epithelium lining the cysts ⇨ is flattened. Note the presence of dystrophic calcification and a residual normal bile duct ↪ in the cyst wall. (Center) A von Meyenburg complex ⇨ is present adjacent to a cyst that contains slightly proteinaceous fluid. (Right) A collapsed cyst consists of a corrugated and hyalinized wall ➡. The lumen is filled with loose connective tissue, resembling a corpus atreticum or fibrosa of the ovary.

CAROLI DISEASE

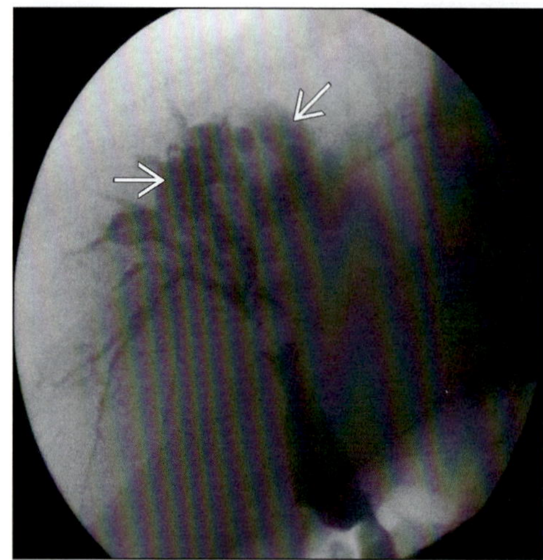

Radiologic image obtained by endoscopic retrograde cholangiopancreatography (ERCP) shows the saccular dilatations of the intrahepatic bile ducts near the hilum ➔.

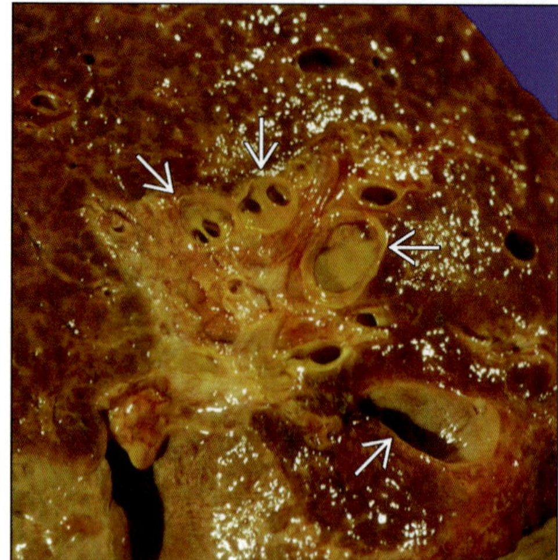

Gross photograph of liver shows clusters of dilated and cystic intrahepatic bile ducts ➔.

TERMINOLOGY

Synonyms

- Congenital cystic dilatation of intrahepatic biliary tree
- Communicating cavernous ectasia

Definitions

- Caroli **disease**: Congenital segmental dilatation of larger intrahepatic bile ducts
- Caroli **syndrome**: Congenital segmental dilatation of larger intrahepatic bile ducts in conjunction with congenital hepatic fibrosis (CHF)

ETIOLOGY/PATHOGENESIS

Developmental Anomaly

- Total or partial arrest of remodeling of ductal plate of larger intrahepatic bile ducts
  - Caroli disease
    - Only larger ducts affected
    - Uncertain; generally considered autosomal recessive although family studies suggest autosomal dominant inheritance pattern
  - Caroli syndrome
    - Defect at level of large and small ducts
    - Autosomal recessive; mutations in *PKHD1* (gene linked to adult recessive polycystic kidney disease) have been identified in some patients

Disease Associations

- Autosomal recessive polycystic kidney disease (ARPKD)
- Autosomal dominant polycystic kidney disease
- Medullary sponge kidney and medullary cystic disease
- Choledochal cyst

CLINICAL ISSUES

Epidemiology

- Incidence
  - Approximately 1:1,000,000 persons; Caroli syndrome is more frequent than pure Caroli disease
- Gender
  - Approximately equal gender distribution

Presentation

- Fever, abdominal pain, jaundice, steatorrhea
- Portal hypertension when associated with CHF

Natural History

- Duct dilatation leads to bile stagnation, hepatolithiasis, repeated episodes of cholangitis, biliary abscess, and death from sepsis
- Cholangiocarcinoma develops in 7-24% of cases
- Amyloidosis is rare complication

Treatment

- Surgical approaches
  - Partial hepatectomy or liver transplant
- Drugs
  - Antibiotics and ursodeoxycholic acid

IMAGE FINDINGS

General Features

- CT and ultrasound can identify intrahepatic saccular or fusiform cysts, but cholangiogram is superior at demonstrating continuity of cysts to biliary tree

CT Findings

- Enhancing fibrovascular bundles in or along margin of dilated ducts results in "central dot" sign

MACROSCOPIC FEATURES

General Features

- Dilated ducts can collapse and be difficult to appreciate unless biliary tree is cannulated and inflated with formalin

CAROLI DISEASE

Key Facts

Terminology

- Congenital segmental dilatation of intrahepatic bile ducts
- Caroli syndrome when associated with congenital hepatic fibrosis

Clinical Issues

- Characterized by cholangitis, hepatolithiasis, abscess, and sepsis
- Associated with ARPKD
- Cholangiocarcinoma develops in 7-24% of cases

Image Findings

- Cholangiogram shows intrahepatic saccular duct dilatation

Microscopic Pathology

- Dilated intrahepatic bile ducts may show periductal fibrosis, inflammation, or frank abscesses
- Background liver can show congenital hepatic fibrosis

- Intrahepatic bile ducts are cystically enlarged and filled with bile, pus, or stones
  - Can affect entire liver or be limited to 1 lobe, more commonly left lobe
- Background liver can show micronodular cirrhosis when associated with congenital hepatic fibrosis

MICROSCOPIC PATHOLOGY

Histologic Features

- Dilated intrahepatic bile ducts may show periductal fibrosis, inflammation, inspissated bile, or frank abscesses
  - Connective tissue containing portal venous and hepatic arterial channels forms polypoid protrusions within lumens of large ducts that may bridge across duct lumen
  - Duct epithelium may show
    - Inflammation
    - Ulceration
    - Dysplasia
- Background liver can show CHF characterized by proliferation of abnormal bile ducts with papillary infolding and inspissated bile embedded in bland fibrous septae

DIFFERENTIAL DIAGNOSIS

Primary Sclerosing Cholangitis (PSC)

- Duct dilatations in PSC are rarely saccular and are more isolated and fusiform
- Associated with inflammatory bowel disease

Recurrent Pyogenic Cholangitis (Oriental Cholangiohepatitis)

- Occurs largely in Far East or among Asian immigrants
- Associated with bile duct parasites in 40% of patients
- Saccular dilatations rare

Polycystic Liver Disease

- Cysts only rarely communicate with bile ducts

SELECTED REFERENCES

1. Yonem O et al: Clinical characteristics of Caroli's disease. World J Gastroenterol. 13(13):1930-3, 2007
2. Yonem O et al: Clinical characteristics of Caroli's syndrome. World J Gastroenterol. 13(13):1934-7, 2007
3. Gupta AK et al: Caroli's disease. Indian J Pediatr. 73(3):233-5, 2006
4. Sgro M et al: Caroli's disease: prenatal diagnosis, postnatal outcome and genetic analysis. Ultrasound Obstet Gynecol. 23(1):73-6, 2004
5. Levy AD et al: Caroli's disease: radiologic spectrum with pathologic correlation. AJR Am J Roentgenol. 179(4):1053-7, 2002

IMAGE GALLERY

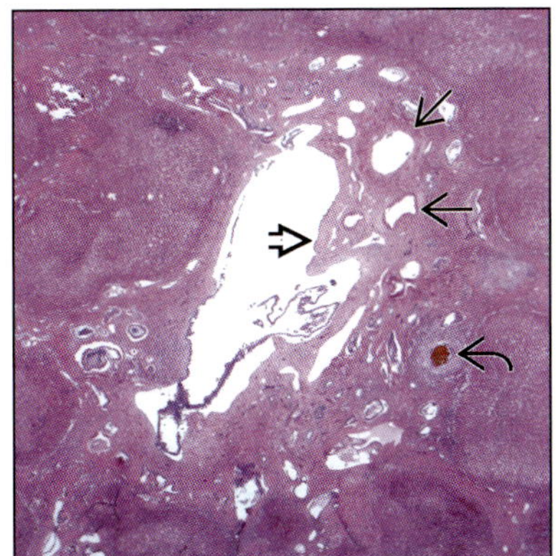

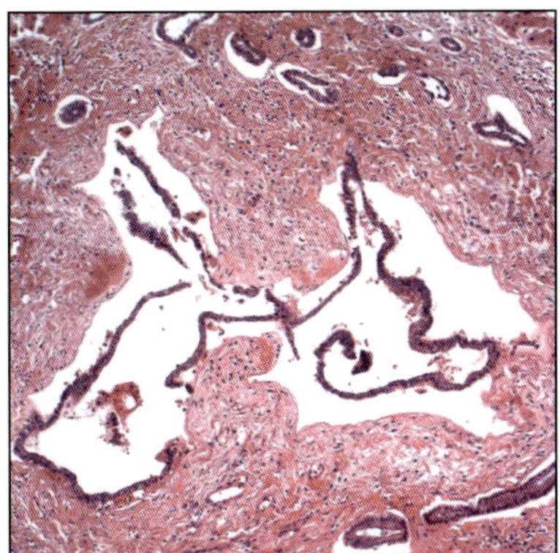

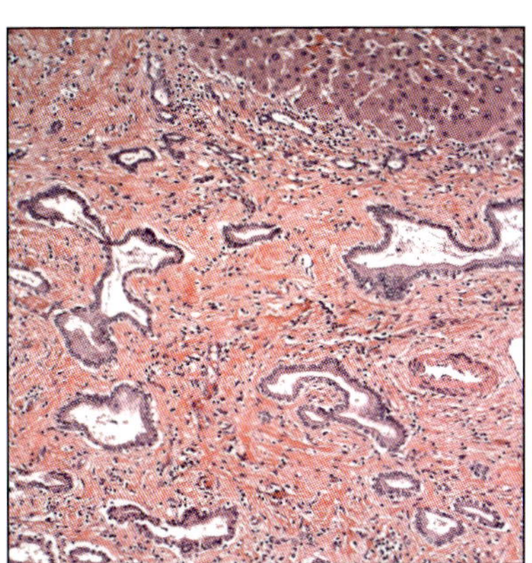

(Left) *H&E shows a very large bile duct out of proportion to its accompanying vessels ⇒. Notice the polypoid protrusion of connective tissue into the duct lumen ⇒. There is a proliferation of small ducts as well, 1 of which is inspissated with bile ⇒.* ***(Center)*** *Polypoid protrusions of connective tissue into the lumen of large ducts is a characteristic feature of Caroli disease.* ***(Right)*** *H&E section of Caroli syndrome shows a background of congenital hepatic fibrosis and a proliferation of abnormal ducts with papillary infolding embedded within collagenous stroma.*

Infectious Disorders

OVERVIEW OF HEPATITIS

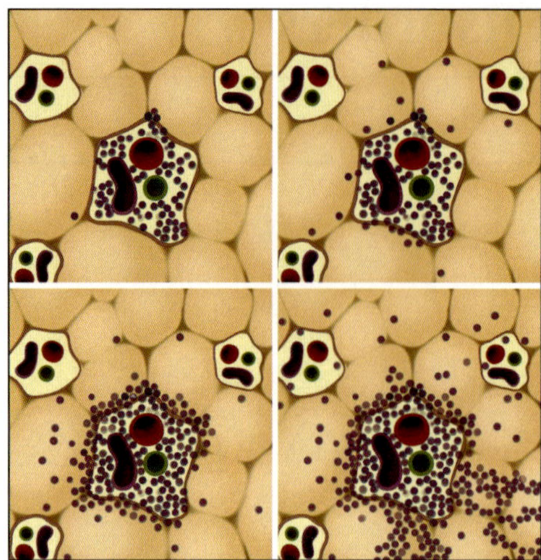

Graphic illustrates grading of chronic hepatitis. Upper left is minimal activity (grade 1), upper right is mild (grade 2), lower left is moderate (grade 3), and lower right is severe (grade 4).

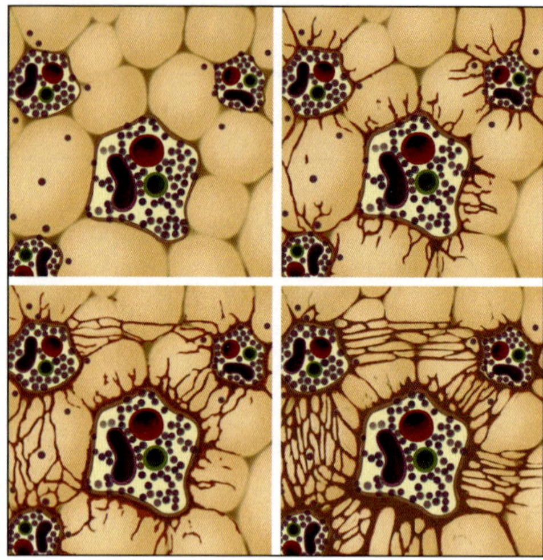

Graphic illustrates staging of fibrosis. Upper left is portal fibrosis (stage 1), upper right is periportal (stage 2), lower left is bridging (stage 3), and lower right is cirrhosis (grade 4).

TERMINOLOGY

Definitions

- General classification
  - Chronic hepatitis: Persistent, often progressive inflammatory process characterized by lymphocytic inflammation of portal tracts with varying degrees of parenchymal inflammation, hepatocellular injury, and fibrosis
    - Chronicity judged in several ways: Clinical, laboratory, morphologic
    - May be difficult to determine chronicity
    - Practically defined as 6 months or more of elevated transaminases
  - Acute hepatitis: Active hepatocellular damage and necrosis, usually of short &/or self-limited duration
    - Usually due to viral infection or adverse drug reaction
    - Rarely biopsied because diagnosis usually made by clinical or laboratory data

ETIOLOGY/PATHOGENESIS

Viral Hepatitis

- Hepatotropic viruses (A, B, C, E)
- Other viruses such as EBV, CMV

Autoimmune Hepatitis

- Type 1: ANA/SMA(+), hypergammaglobulinemia, concurrent autoimmune diseases
- Type 2: Anti-LKM antibodies, more likely to develop cirrhosis
- Type 3: Less well characterized; anti-SLA/LP antibodies; may have positive AMA

Drug-associated Hepatitis

- Necroinflammatory
  - Acetaminophen, phenytoin, macrodantin, sulphonamides
- Cholestatic
  - Many antibiotics, steroids
- Granulomatous
  - Allopurinol, many antibiotics, phenytoin

Other

- Wilson disease
- α-1-antitrypsin deficiency
- Nonspecific reactive hepatitis
  - Reaction to extrahepatic infection or neoplasm or to adjacent mass lesion in liver

CLINICAL IMPLICATIONS

Clinical Presentation

- Fatigue
- Malaise
- Jaundice
- Anorexia
- Fever
- Nausea
- Abdominal pain
- Signs and symptoms of liver failure
- Many patients asymptomatic

Laboratory Findings

- Elevated transaminases
- Alkaline phosphatase may be mildly elevated
- Viral serologies positive in viral hepatitis
- Autoimmune serologies usually positive in autoimmune hepatitis

MICROSCOPIC FINDINGS

General Features

- Broad range of histologic appearances with some features in common
  - Portal inflammation

        - Infiltrate consists primarily of lymphocytes, may have admixed plasma cells, histiocytes, and granulocytes
        - Lymphoid follicles common in hepatitis C
        - Nonspecific cholangiolar proliferation may be present at periphery of portal tract
    - Lobular inflammation/necrosis
        - Necrosis may be mild and spotty or confluent and bridging
        - May be accompanied by ballooning degeneration, reactive hepatocellular changes
    - Piecemeal necrosis (interface activity)
        - Defined as extension of inflammation into adjacent parenchyma with destruction of individual hepatocytes at interface
        - Results in ragged interface between portal tract and hepatic parenchyma
    - Fibrosis
- Predominant pattern of inflammation in a given case may be portal, periportal, lobular, or a combination
    - Acute hepatitis usually diffusely involves lobule and is not confined to portal area
- Lesions may be sporadically distributed within liver, resulting in sampling bias

Grading

- Grade 1 (minimal activity): Mild portal inflammation with scant piecemeal necrosis and no lobular necrosis
- Grade 2 (mild activity): Mild portal inflammation with piecemeal necrosis but scant lobular spotty necrosis
- Grade 3 (moderate activity): Moderate portal inflammation, piecemeal necrosis, spotty lobular necrosis
- Grade 4 (severe activity): Marked portal inflammation, brisk piecemeal necrosis, significant spotty lobular necrosis, areas of confluent necrosis resulting in bridging necrosis

Staging

- Stage 1 (portal fibrosis): Mild fibrous expansion of portal tracts
- Stage 2 (periportal fibrosis): Fine periportal strands of connective tissue with only rare portal-portal septa
- Stage 3 (septal or bridging fibrosis): Connective tissue bridges that link portal tracts to other portal tracts and to central veins
- Stage 4 (cirrhosis): Established bridging fibrosis with regenerative nodules

Histologic Patterns and Clinical Associations

- Predominantly portal-based hepatitis
    - Autoimmune hepatitis
    - Chronic hepatitis C
    - Nonspecific reactive hepatitis
- Predominantly periportal hepatitis
    - Autoimmune hepatitis
    - Chronic viral hepatitis
    - Drug-associated hepatitis
    - α-1-antitrypsin deficiency
    - Wilson disease
    - Nonspecific reactive hepatitis
- Predominantly lobular hepatitis
    - Acute viral hepatitis
    - Chronic or unresolved viral hepatitis
    - Autoimmune hepatitis
    - Drug-associated hepatitis
    - Nonspecific reactive hepatitis
- Some etiologies may occasionally have prominent cholestatic features
    - Acute or unresolved viral hepatitis
    - Autoimmune hepatitis
    - Drug-associated hepatitis

Differential Diagnoses

- Chronic biliary disease
    - Copper deposition
    - Bile duct damage or loss
    - Elevation of alkaline phosphatase out of proportion to transaminases
    - Appropriate serologic studies &/or imaging studies may be helpful
- Large bile duct obstruction
    - Elevated alkaline phosphatase, GGT, and bilirubin
    - Usually lacks increased fibrosis
    - Imaging studies helpful
- Lymphoma
    - Infiltrates composed of atypical lymphocytes
    - Immunohistochemistry, gene rearrangement studies may be required

Reporting

- Chronic hepatitis must be graded and staged in pathology report
    - "Chronic persistent" and "chronic active" hepatitis should no longer be used
- Comments regarding etiology, if possible

SELECTED REFERENCES

1. Lefkowitch JH: Liver biopsy assessment in chronic hepatitis. Arch Med Res. 38(6):634-43, 2007
2. Theise ND: Liver biopsy assessment in chronic viral hepatitis: a personal, practical approach. Mod Pathol. 20 Suppl 1:S3-14, 2007
3. Scheuer PJ: Liver biopsy size matters in chronic hepatitis: bigger is better. Hepatology. 38(6):1356-8, 2003
4. Batts KP et al: Chronic hepatitis. An update on terminology and reporting. Am J Surg Pathol. 19(12):1409-17, 1995
5. Burgart LJ et al: Recent-onset autoimmune hepatitis. Biopsy findings and clinical correlations. Am J Surg Pathol. 19(6):699-708, 1995
6. Desmet VJ et al: Classification of chronic hepatitis: diagnosis, grading and staging. Hepatology. 19(6):1513-20, 1994
7. Lefkowitch JH et al: Pathological diagnosis of chronic hepatitis C: a multicenter comparative study with chronic hepatitis B. The Hepatitis Interventional Therapy Group. Gastroenterology. 104(2):595-603, 1993
8. Scheuer PJ et al: The pathology of hepatitis C. Hepatology. 15(4):567-71, 1992
9. Schlichting P et al: Liver biopsy in chronic aggressive hepatitis. Diagnostic reproducibility in relation to size of specimen. Scand J Gastroenterol. 18(1):27-32, 1983
10. Peters RL: Viral hepatitis: a pathologic spectrum. Am J Med Sci. 270(1):17-31, 1975
11. Popper H et al: The vocabulary of chronic hepatitis. N Engl J Med. 284(20):1154-6, 1971

OVERVIEW OF HEPATITIS

Examples of Grading and Staging

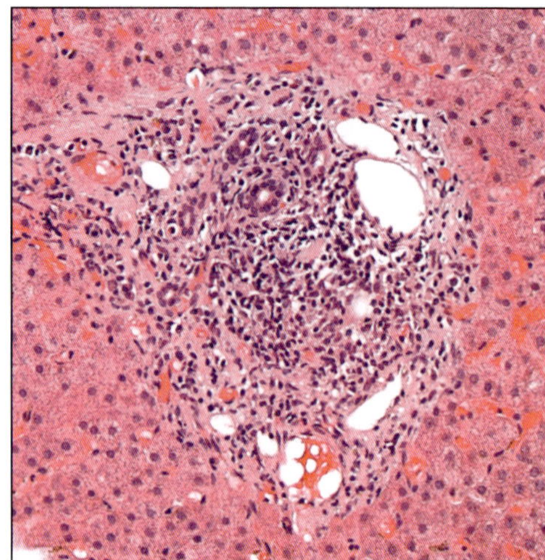

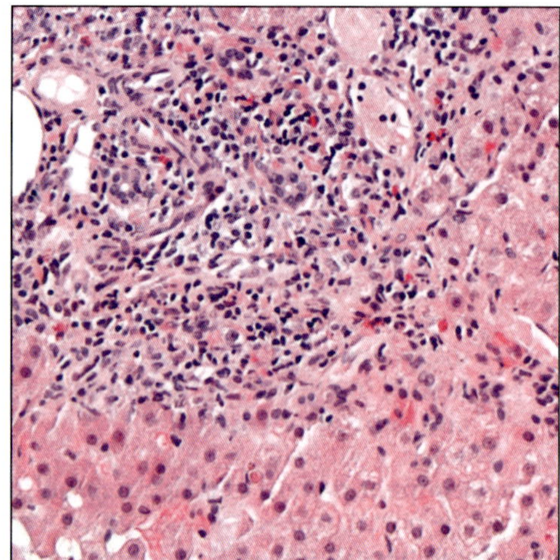

(Left) *This case of hepatitis C shows minimal (grade 1) portal inflammation without piecemeal necrosis or significant lobular activity.* ***(Right)*** *This case of hepatitis C shows moderate portal inflammation and piecemeal necrosis. Spotty lobular necrosis was also seen in the biopsy, making this a grade 3 lesion.*

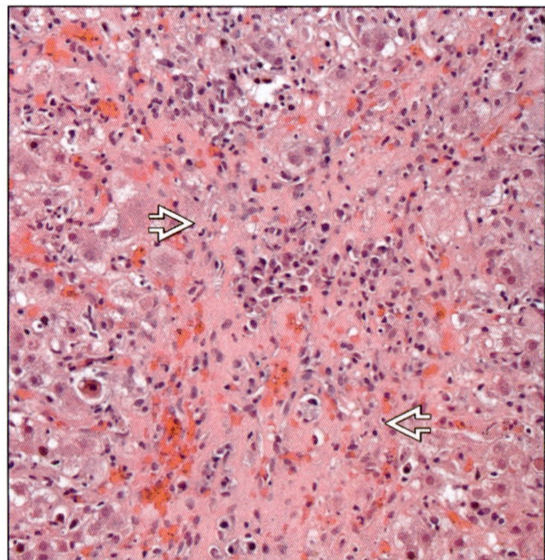

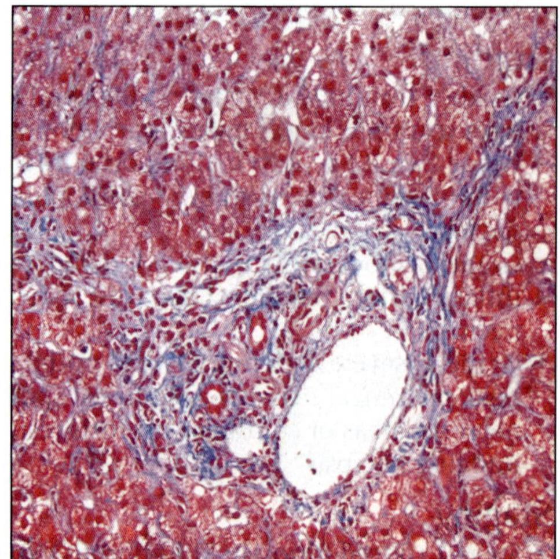

(Left) *This case of autoimmune hepatitis shows bridging necrosis ➡, a hallmark of severe (grade 4) activity.* ***(Right)*** *Stage 2 (periportal) fibrosis shows fine strands of periportal connective tissue. Rare portal-portal septa may be present.*

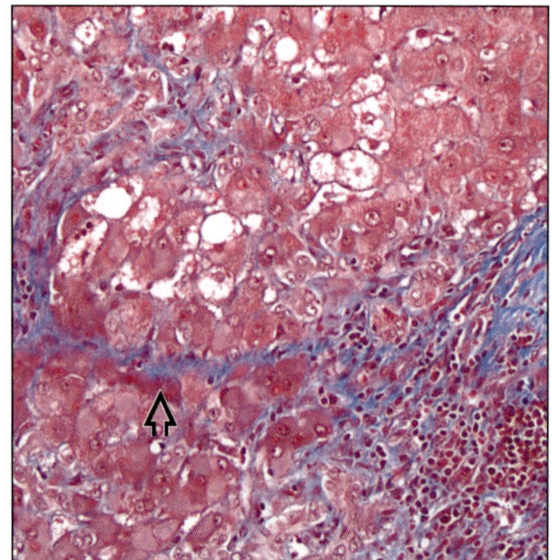

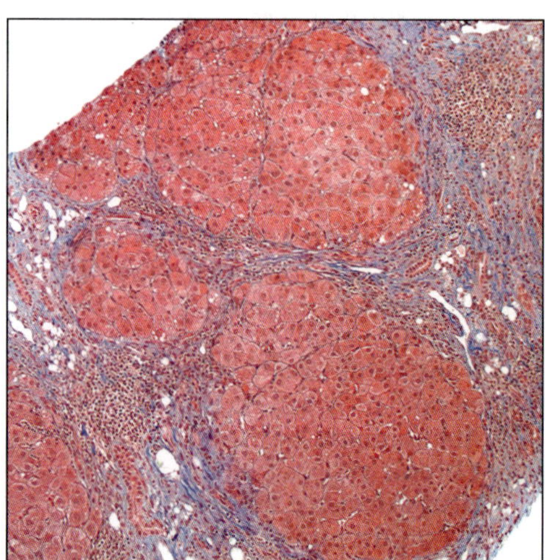

(Left) *Bridging or septal fibrosis (stage 3) consists of connective tissue bridges ➡ that link portal tracts to each other or to central veins. Architecture may be mildly distorted, but there are no regenerative nodules.* ***(Right)*** *Cirrhosis (stage 4 fibrosis) consists of established bridging fibrosis and regenerative nodules.*

Microscopic Features

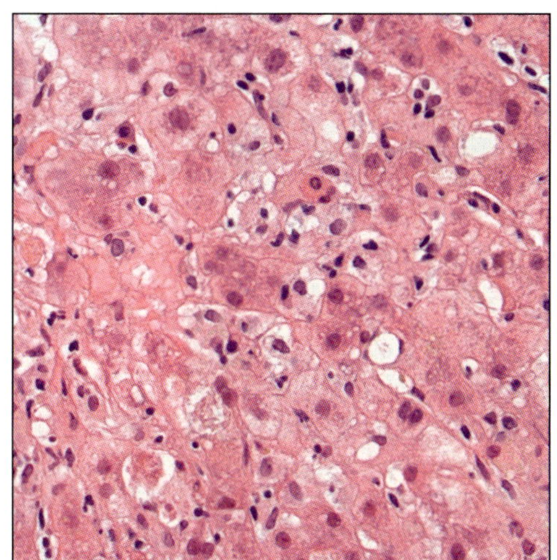

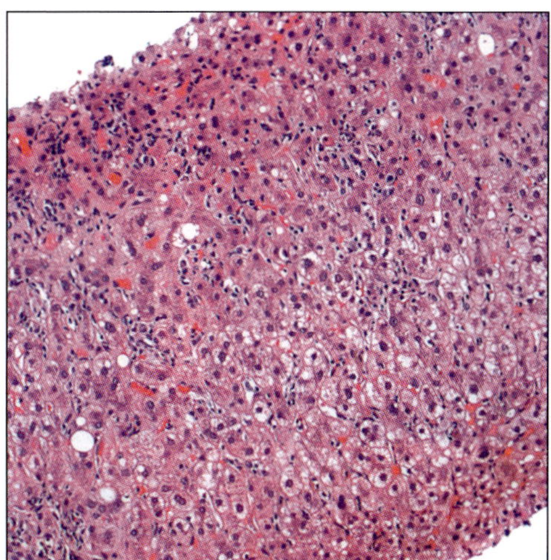

(Left) *This case of acute viral hepatitis shows a mild lobular lymphocytic infiltrate along with increased Kupffer cells and reactive hepatocellular changes.* ***(Right)*** *A more severe lobular hepatitis is seen in this case of autoimmune hepatitis, featuring a marked lymphocytic infiltrate with hepatocyte necrosis and lobular disarray.*

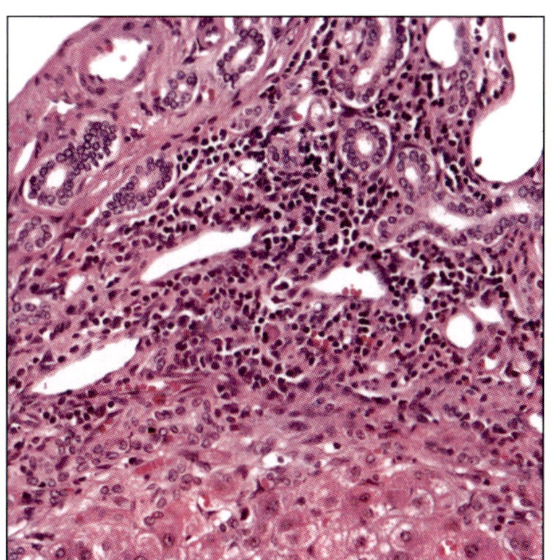

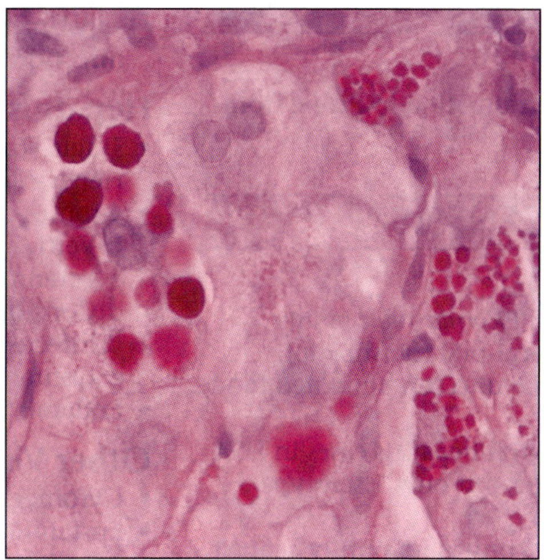

(Left) *This case of α-1-antitrypsin deficiency shows a chronic hepatitis-like pattern featuring a portal/periportal lymphocytic infiltrate with cholangiolar proliferation.* ***(Right)*** *This PAS with diastase demonstrated PAS positive, diastase-resistant globules in the periportal region in α-1-antitrypsin deficiency.*

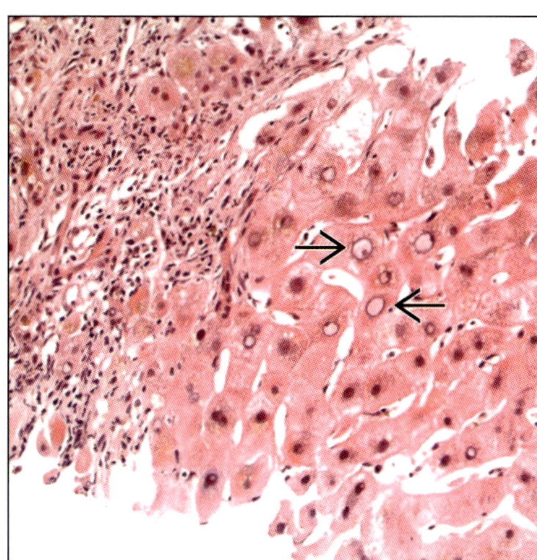

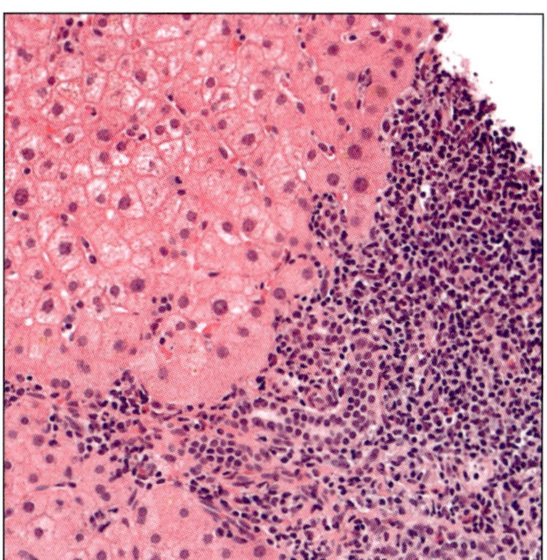

(Left) *This case of Wilson disease shows a portal and periportal lymphocytic infiltrate. Note the prominent glycogenated nuclei* ⇒*.* ***(Right)*** *This case of primary biliary cirrhosis shows portal-based inflammation without florid duct lesions, mimicking chronic hepatitis of other causes.*

ACUTE VIRAL HEPATITIS

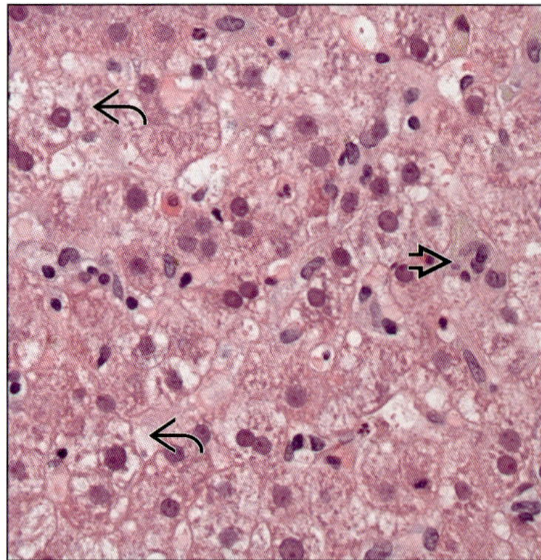

Hematoxylin & eosin demonstrates lobular disarray characterized by hepatocyte swelling ⇗, Kupffer cell hyperplasia ⇨, and lobular inflammation in a case of acute viral hepatitis.

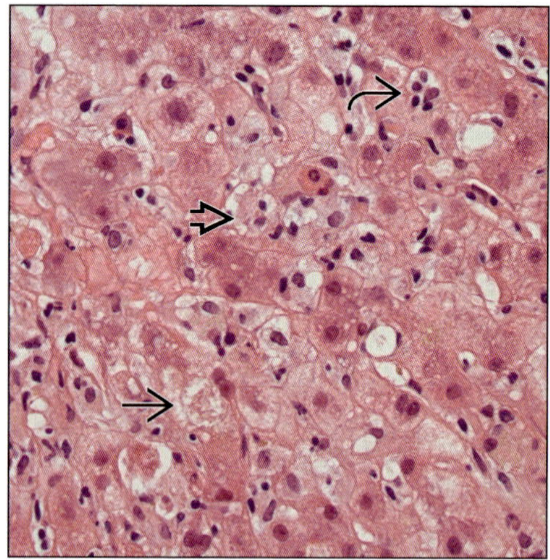

Hematoxylin & eosin demonstrates mild hepatocyte swelling ⇨, Kupffer cell hyperplasia ⇨, and lobular inflammation ⇗ in a case of acute viral hepatitis.

TERMINOLOGY

Definitions

- Hepatocyte necrosis and inflammation resulting from acute viral infection

ETIOLOGY/PATHOGENESIS

Hepatitis A Virus

- Single-stranded RNA virus in *Picornaviridae* family
- Usually spreads via oral or fecal-oral transmission
  - Community outbreaks related to contaminated food or water
- Accounts for ~ 1/2 of acute viral hepatitis cases in USA
- At least 4 genotypes described, but only 1 serotype exists
  - Infection with 1 genotype confers immunity against all genotypes
- Never results in chronic infection

Hepatitis B Virus

- Partially double-stranded DNA virus in *Hepadnaviridae* family
- Parenteral, perinatal, and sexual transmission
- Up to 40% of acute hepatitis cases in USA attributable to hepatitis B
- ~ 10% of infected patients develop chronic infection

Hepatitis C Virus

- RNA virus of the Flaviviridae family
- Parenteral, perinatal, and sexual transmission
- Accounts for ~ 20% of cases of acute hepatitis
- Only 10-15% of infected individuals develop symptomatic acute hepatitis
- ~ 85% of infected patients develop chronic infection

Hepatitis D Virus (Delta Agent)

- Defective RNA virus
- Parenteral transmission
- Requires coinfection with hepatitis B virus or superinfection in patient with chronic hepatitis B virus infection

Hepatitis E Virus

- Single-stranded, nonenveloped RNA virus in Hepeviridae family
- 4 routes of infection
  - Vertical transmission
  - Parenteral transmission
  - Consumption of raw or undercooked meat of infected animals
  - Contaminated water supply
- Endemic in parts of Asia, Africa, and India

Other Viruses

- Cytomegalovirus
- Epstein-Barr virus

CLINICAL ISSUES

Presentation

- Malaise
- Fatigue
- Vomiting
- Nausea
- Anorexia
- Right upper quadrant pain
- Hepatomegaly
- Jaundice
- Low-grade fever
- Rarely, fulminant hepatic failure

Laboratory Tests

- Elevated transaminases at 5-10x normal values
- Hepatitis A virus
  - Detection of anti-hepatitis A virus IgM (anti-HAV) in patient with hepatitis or elevated serum aminotransferases is diagnostic of acute hepatitis A virus infection

ACUTE VIRAL HEPATITIS

Key Facts

Etiology/Pathogenesis

- Hepatitis A virus infection accounts for ~ 1/2 of acute viral hepatitis cases in USA

Clinical Issues

- Generally mild or asymptomatic
- Elevated transaminases at 5-10x normal values
- Supportive care is mainstay of treatment for patients with acute hepatitis A or acute hepatitis E
- Hospitalization recommended for severe or persistent nausea and for patients with signs of developing liver failure
- No specific drug therapy available for acute hepatitis A virus infection
- Liver transplantation considered for patients with acute liver failure
- Most patients with acute hepatitis A virus infection fully recover within 2 months of disease onset

Microscopic Pathology

- Lobular disarray characterized by diffuse lobular inflammation and hepatocyte swelling, necrosis, and regeneration
- May see mild portal and periportal inflammation, particularly in acute hepatitis A virus infection

Diagnostic Checklist

- Lobular inflammation and injury exceed portal inflammation
- Usually recognized clinically, so liver biopsy seldom performed

- Hepatitis B virus
  - Hepatitis B surface antigen (HBsAg) positivity
  - Markers of virus replication (HBeAg and hepatitis B virus DNA)
  - Anti-hepatitis B core antigen IgM (anti-HBcAg) detectable at symptom onset
- Hepatitis C virus
  - Hepatitis C RNA detectable in serum within 2 weeks after exposure
- Hepatitis D virus
  - Detection of anti-hepatitis D virus IgM (anti-HDV)
- Hepatitis E virus
  - Usually diagnosis of exclusion
  - Detection of anti-hepatitis E virus IgM (anti-HEV) available in some settings

Treatment

- Drugs
  - No specific drug therapy available for acute hepatitis A virus infection or acute hepatitis E virus infection
  - Antiviral therapy (lamivudine) or immune modulators (interferon) may be beneficial to select patients with acute hepatitis B
  - Pegylated interferon is beneficial and cost effective for acute hepatitis C
- Supportive care is mainstay of treatment for patients with acute hepatitis A or acute hepatitis E
- Hospitalization recommended for severe or persistent nausea and for patients with signs of developing liver failure
- Liver transplantation considered for patients with acute liver failure

Prognosis

- Most patients with acute hepatitis A virus infection fully recover within 2 months of disease onset
  - 85% of patients with acute hepatitis A virus infection improve with supportive care
    - Patients with chronic liver disease at increased risk of complications and death
  - Fulminant hepatic failure with coagulopathy and encephalopathy is rare
  - Disease severity related to patient age
    - Increased mortality in patients > 40 years of age
  - Atypical variants are well recognized
    - Relapsing variant in 3-20% of patients in whom recovery is followed by relapse at 4-15 weeks after initial episode
    - ~ 10% develop prolonged cholestasis lasting > 2 weeks
    - Possible extrahepatic manifestations include leukocytoclastic vasculitis, arthritis, and glomerulonephritis
  - Infection confers lifelong immunity
- ~ 90% of patients with acute hepatitis B virus infection recover fully
  - 1% of acutely infected patients develop fulminant hepatic failure
- Acute hepatitis C may last 2-12 weeks
  - Almost never fulminant
  - Disease is self-limiting in 15% of patients infected with hepatitis C
- Acute hepatitis E follows 2-10-week incubation period
  - Illness usually lasts 1-4 weeks
  - Pregnant women and infants at increased risk of mortality

MACROSCOPIC FEATURES

General Features

- In severe cases with massive necrosis, liver is shrunken, and capsule is flaccid
- Islands of regenerating hepatocytes may form grossly visible nodules that cause concern for malignancy

MICROSCOPIC PATHOLOGY

Histologic Features

- Lobular disarray
  - Diffuse, mixed lobular inflammatory cell infiltrates
    - Predominantly mononuclear inflammatory cell infiltrates
  - Hepatocyte necrosis

    - Foci of parenchymal collapse evident on trichrome or reticulin stains
  - Hepatocyte swelling
  - Hepatocyte regeneration
  - Kupffer cell hyperplasia
- May see mild portal and periportal inflammation, particularly in acute hepatitis A virus infection
  - Portal inflammation usually less prominent than lobular inflammation and injury
- Pigment-laden macrophages may be seen on periodic acid-Schiff stain
- Areas of confluent hepatocyte necrosis in severe cases
- Canalicular cholestasis present in some cases

Cytologic Features

- Hepatocyte swelling

Predominant Pattern/Injury Type

- Inflammatory

Predominant Cell/Compartment Type

- Hepatic lobules

DIFFERENTIAL DIAGNOSIS

Autoimmune Hepatitis

- Although priori chronic disease, initial clinical presentation may reflect acute or fulminant hepatitis
- Characterized clinically by positive autoimmune serologies
  - Anti-nuclear antibodies
  - Anti-smooth muscle antibodies
  - Anti-liver-kidney-microsomal antibodies
- Polyclonal hypergammaglobulinemia often seen
- Portal and periportal hepatitis often present in addition to lobular hepatitis
- Plasma cell infiltrates may be prominent
- Fibrosis often present at presentation
- Most cases highly responsive to immunosuppressive therapy

Drug- or Toxin-induced Hepatitis

- Usually cannot be reliably distinguished from acute viral hepatitis based on histology
- Eosinophils may be prominent but are not sensitive or specific feature
- Generally self-limited and resolves after withdrawal of drug
- Requires clinical history of exposure for diagnosis

Wilson Disease

- Can present clinically as fulminant hepatitis
- Usually presents chronic hepatitis with fibrosis
- Quantitative copper testing shows elevated liver copper level
  - Most helpful diagnostic test
- Rarely presents as massive liver necrosis

Ischemia

- Characterized clinically by sharp rise in serum aminotransferases
  - Aminotransferases also decline quickly with recovery
- Focal or diffuse centrilobular hepatocyte necrosis
- Lobular inflammation and hepatocyte swelling are not major features
- Often associated with vascular injury or hypercoagulable state

Idiopathic Hepatitis or Hepatic Failure

- Subset of cases in which etiology cannot be determined

DIAGNOSTIC CHECKLIST

Clinically Relevant Pathologic Features

- Positive viral hepatitis serologies in many cases
  - Antibodies unreliable in diagnosis of acute hepatitis C virus infection
    - Antibody production may be delayed
  - Hepatitis E virus diagnosed by ELISA or RNA detection by real-time PCR

Pathologic Interpretation Pearls

- Lobular hepatitis with hepatocyte swelling and necrosis
- Lobular inflammation and injury exceed portal inflammation
- Usually recognized clinically, so liver biopsy seldom performed

SELECTED REFERENCES

1. Liang TJ: Hepatitis B: the virus and disease. Hepatology. 49(5 Suppl):S13-21, 2009
2. Fabris P et al: Acute hepatitis C: clinical aspects, diagnosis, and outcome of acute HCV infection. Curr Pharm Des. 14(17):1661-5, 2008
3. Ichai P et al: Etiology and prognosis of fulminant hepatitis in adults. Liver Transpl. 14 Suppl 2:S67-79, 2008
4. Kamal SM: Acute hepatitis C: a systematic review. Am J Gastroenterol. 103(5):1283-97; quiz 1298, 2008
5. Turner J et al: Hepatitis e: a UK perspective. Br J Hosp Med (Lond). 69(9):517-9, 2008
6. Cuthbert JA: Hepatitis A: old and new. Clin Microbiol Rev. 14(1):38-58, 2001
7. Krawczynski K et al: Hepatitis E: an overview. Minerva Gastroenterol Dietol. 45(2):119-30; discussion 130-5, 1999
8. Kobayashi K et al: Liver biopsy features of acute hepatitis C compared with hepatitis A, B, and non-A, non-B, non-C. Liver. 13(2):69-72, 1993
9. Sciot R et al: Cholestatic features in hepatitis A. J Hepatol. 3(2):172-81, 1986

Microscopic Features

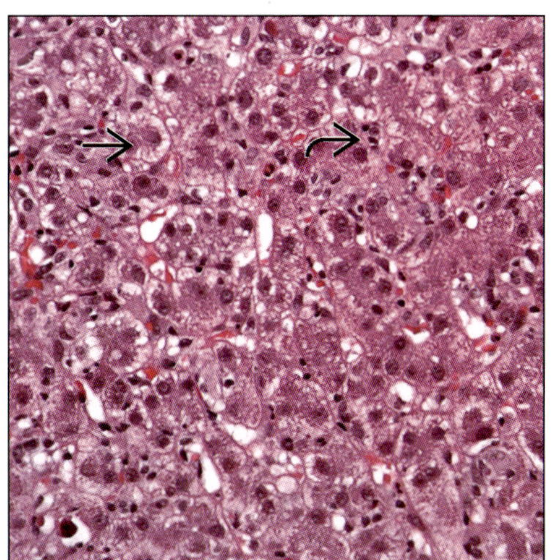

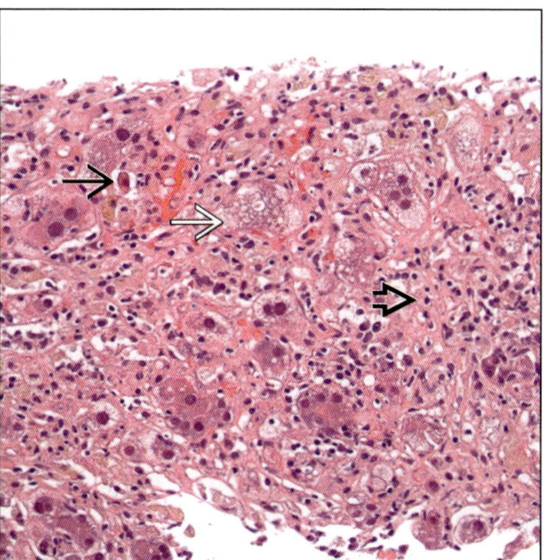

(Left) *Hematoxylin & eosin shows diffuse hepatocyte swelling ➔ and scattered inflammatory cells ➔ in acute hepatitis.* ***(Right)*** *Hematoxylin & eosin shows diffuse lobular disarray characterized by hepatocyte swelling ➔, single-cell necrosis ➔, and areas of hepatocyte dropout ➔ in a background of lobular inflammation.*

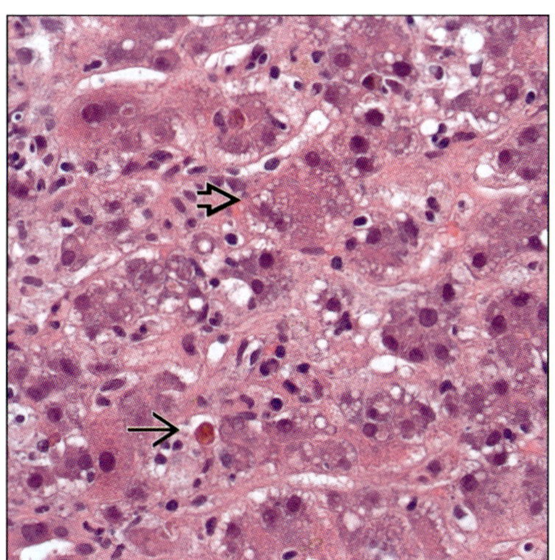

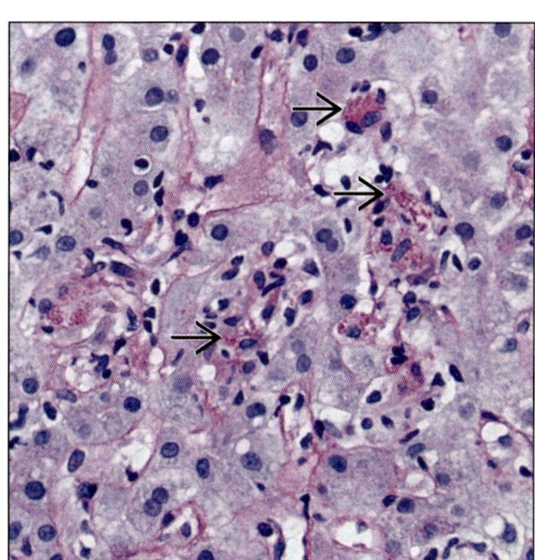

(Left) *Hematoxylin & eosin shows hepatocyte swelling ➔ and necrosis ➔ associated with mild lobular inflammation.* ***(Right)*** *Periodic acid-Schiff with diastase digestion highlights Kupffer cell hyperplasia with granular staining ➔ in pigment-laden Kupffer cells.*

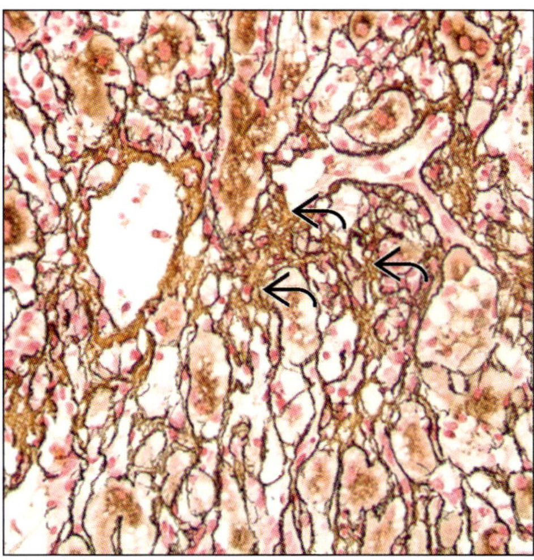

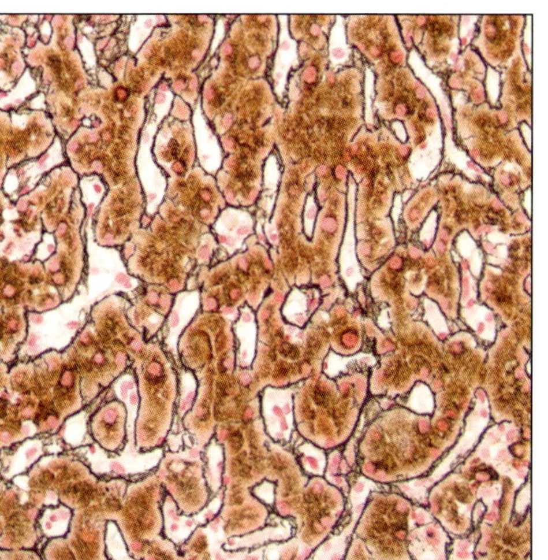

(Left) *Reticulin stain highlights areas of collapse ➔ of the reticulin framework secondary to hepatocyte necrosis.* ***(Right)*** *This normal liver demonstrates an intact reticulin framework. This stain highlights in black the normal reticulin fibers surrounding the hepatocyte trabeculae.*

HEPATITIS B

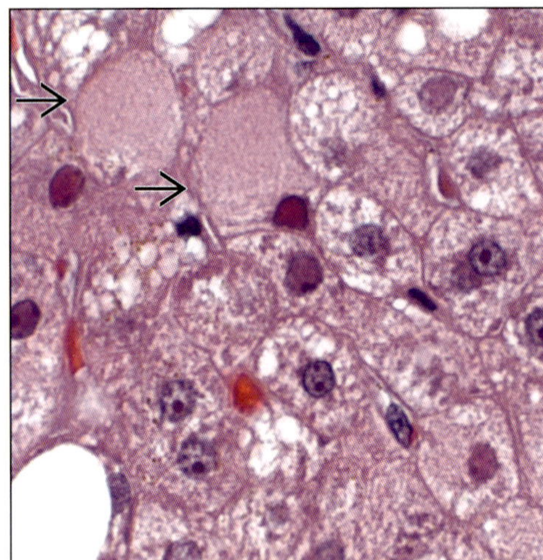

Ground-glass hepatocytes ⇒ have glassy eosinophilic cytoplasm representing proliferation of smooth ER in response to HBsAg.

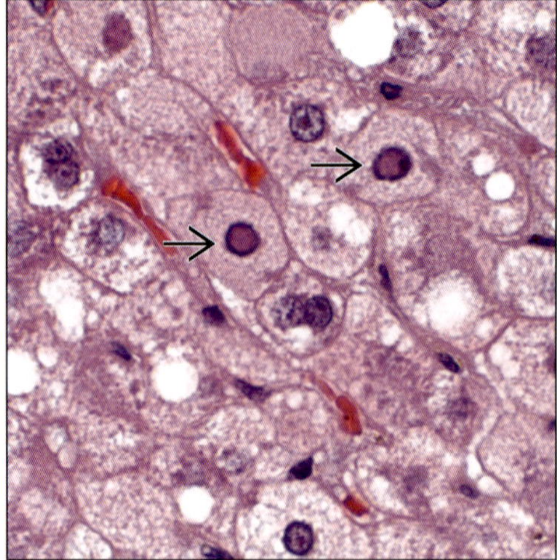

Hepatitis B-infected hepatocytes have pale pink, finely granular intranuclear inclusions (sanded nuclei ⇒) representing nuclear accumulation of HBcAg.

TERMINOLOGY

Abbreviations

- Hepatitis B virus (HBV)

Synonyms

- Australia antigen: Hepatitis B surface antigen (HBsAg)

Definitions

- Infection by hepatitis B virus
  - Member of Hepadnaviridae family
  - Genome comprises a partially double-stranded DNA virus

ETIOLOGY/PATHOGENESIS

Infectious Agents

- Transmitted parenterally
  - Vertical transmission: Mothers to newborn infants
  - Horizontal transmission: Between young children
  - Sexual contact
- Liver injury appears to be immune mediated
  - HBV-specific T cells play key role in pathogenesis and viral clearance

CLINICAL ISSUES

Epidemiology

- Incidence
  - 400 million people worldwide are chronically infected with HBV

Presentation

- Acute hepatitis B
  - More than 50% are asymptomatic
  - Symptoms include mild flu-like syndrome, nausea, vomiting, jaundice
  - Less than 1% develop fulminant liver failure leading to death or liver transplantation
  - Serum HBsAg and anti-HBc virus IgM Ab positive
- Chronic hepatitis B
  - Serum HBsAg positive and anti-HBc virus IgM Ab negative

Laboratory Tests

- Serology for HBV viral antigens: HBsAg, HBcAg, HBeAg
- Serology for anti-HBV antibodies: Anti-HBs, anti-HBc, anti-HBe
- Serum HBV DNA and viral load
- Liver function tests

Natural History

- 10% of infected individuals become chronically infected
- Life-long risk of developing cirrhosis &/or HCC in chronic hepatitis B
  - Cirrhosis is not prerequisite for developing HCC
    - HBV viral genome can act as oncoprotein and intergrade into host genome
- Coinfection with HIV, HCV, and HDV is common, as they share common transmission route

Treatment

- Drugs
  - Nucleoside analogue therapy: Lamivudine, adefovir, entecavir
  - Interferon

MACROSCOPIC FEATURES

Cirrhosis

- Nodularity (macronodular or mixed macro- and micronodular) and scarring

MICROSCOPIC PATHOLOGY

Histologic Features

- Acute hepatitis B

HEPATITIS B

Key Facts

Etiology/Pathogenesis

- Partially double-stranded DNA virus
- Vertical transmission
- Horizontal transmission
- Sexual contact

Clinical Issues

- 10% become chronically infected
- Risk of cirrhosis &/or HCC
- Cirrhosis is not prerequisite for developing HCC

Microscopic Pathology

- Acute hepatitis B
  - Hepatocytic swelling, mononuclear cell infiltrates, spotty necrosis, apoptotic bodies, confluent and bridging necrosis, collapse of hepatocytic cords, hepatocytic regeneration
- Chronic hepatitis B
  - Portal inflammation, interface hepatitis, lobular hepatitis, fibrosis
- Ground-glass hepatocytes
- Sanded nuclei of hepatocytes
- Grading denotes inflammatory activity while staging indicates degree of fibrosis
- Fibrosing cholestatic hepatitis B
  - Unique histology and more progressive course following orthotopic liver transplantation and in other immunosuppression status

Top Differential Diagnoses

- Hepatitis A, autoimmune hepatitis, chronic hepatitis C, drug hepatitis, other viral infections (CMV, EBV, HSV, yellow fever virus), PBC
  - Correlation with history and serology is crucial

  - Hepatocytic swelling
  - Inflammatory cell infiltrates
    - Mainly mononuclear, including lymphocytes, plasma cells, and Kupffer cells
  - Spotty necrosis
  - Many apoptotic bodies
  - Confluent necrosis
  - Bridging necrosis
  - Collapse of hepatocytic cords
    - Best demonstrated by reticulin stain
  - Hepatocytic regeneration
- Chronic hepatitis B
  - Portal inflammation
    - Mononuclear inflammatory cells infiltrates, composed predominantly of lymphocytes admixed with Kupffer cells and plasma cells
    - May expand portal tracts
  - Interface hepatitis
    - Mononuclear inflammatory cells and apoptotic hepatocytes beyond limiting plate
    - Previously termed piecemeal necrosis
  - Lobular hepatitis
    - Aggregates of mononuclear inflammatory cells, apoptotic hepatocytes, hepatocytic debris, &/or confluent necrosis
  - Fibrosis
    - Begins in portal regions, extends beyond limiting plate, and then forms bridging septa between portal-portal and portal-central regions
    - Cirrhosis is final stage
    - Stage of fibrosis indicates disease progression and is important therapeutic and prognostic indicator
  - Ground-glass hepatocytes
    - Finely granular cytoplasmic inclusion
    - Pushes cellular contents and nucleus to side due to proliferation of smooth ER in response to abundant HBsAg
    - Can be highlighted by Shikata Orcein stain, Victoria Blue stain, and anti-HBs immunohistochemical stain
    - Indicate chronic hepatitis B infection
    - Not specific for hepatitis B
  - Sanded nuclei of hepatocytes
    - Pale pink granular inclusions in hepatocytic nuclei containing HBcAg
    - Can be highlighted by anti-HBc immunohistochemical stain
    - Extensive nuclear staining for anti-HBc indicates active HBV viral replication and may suggest immunosuppression status
- Fibrosing cholestatic hepatitis B
  - Variant of viral hepatitis B that often has more progressive course and worse outcome
  - Pathogenesis is thought to be due to viral cytopathic effect
  - Occurs following orthotopic liver transplantation
  - Also occurs in other immunosuppression status, such as chemotherapy
  - Occurrence is less common nowadays due to better prevention and antiviral regimens
  - Unique histopathology
    - Hepatocytic swelling due to cholestasis
    - Canalicular and bile ductal cholestasis
    - Marked bile ductular reaction
    - Extensive fibrosis beginning from portal tracts, surrounding hepatocytes within sinusoidal spaces, with "serpiginous pattern"

Semiquantitative Grading and Staging

- Grading denotes inflammatory activity while staging indicates degree of fibrosis
  - Ishak score
    - Modified from Knodell (histologic activity index) scoring system
    - Composite score of portal inflammation, interface hepatitis, parenchymal injury, and confluent necrosis appropriate for evaluation of large cohorts of patients
    - Fibrosis score from 1-6
  - Batts and Ludwig system
    - Simple scoring system appropriate for management of individual patients
    - Grading activity from 1-4 based on overall portal and lobular inflammatory activity combined

HEPATITIS B

- Staging fibrosis from 1-4

DIFFERENTIAL DIAGNOSIS

Hepatitis A

- Positive hepatitis A serology (anti-HAV IgM)
- Negative HBV serology
- Often positive travel or food poisoning history

Autoimmune Hepatitis

- Positive autoimmune serology (ANA, anti-SMA, LKM, SLA)
- Negative HBV serology (HBsAg, anti-core IgM, anti-core IgG)
- More prominent plasma cells
- Responds to steroids

Chronic Hepatitis C

- Positive anti-HCV antibody and HCV RNA in serum
- Negative HBV serology
- Portal lymphoid aggregates, Poulsen (bile duct) lesion, and steatosis more common in hepatitis C

Drug-associated Hepatitis

- Medication history that corresponds to onset of liver disease
  - Symptoms ideally resolve after drug withdrawal
- Negative HBV serologies
- Eosinophils may be prominent

Hepatitis E

- Positive travel history and anti-HEV serology

Other Viral Hepatitides

- CMV hepatitis
  - Neutrophilic microabscesses typical
  - Characteristic viral inclusions
- EBV hepatitis
  - Atypical lymphocytes in lobules, especially those lining sinusoidal space in bead-like appearance
- Herpes simplex virus hepatitis
  - Confluent necrosis mimicking ischemia
  - Typical syncytial cell virus inclusion
- Yellow fever
  - Positive travel history and virologic studies
- Dengue fever
  - Positive travel history and virologic studies
- Syphilitic hepatitis
  - Positive serology
  - Warthin-Starry stain or immunostain for *Treponema pallidum*

Primary Biliary Cirrhosis

- Elevated antimitochondrial antibody
- Elevated alkaline phosphatase and GGT
- Predominantly affecting middle-aged women
- Bile ductular reaction and cholestatic picture with pseudoxanthomatous change in periportal region
- Florid duct lesion (granuloma) destroying interlobular bile duct is diagnostic

Other Causes of Ground-Glass Cells

- Lafora disease
- Cyanamide toxicity
- Fibrinogen storage disease
- Glycogen pseudo-ground-glass cell change
  - Commonly seen in immunosuppressed individuals and post liver transplant

DIAGNOSTIC CHECKLIST

Pathologic Interpretation Pearls

- Purpose of liver biopsy is to grade and stage HBV-induced liver disease and exclude concomitant liver diseases
- HBV coinfection with other viruses, such as HCV, HDV, and HIV, is common
  - Correlation with clinical history and serology is important
- Unlike hepatitis C, recurrent hepatitis B after liver transplantation is rare due to advent of antiviral prophylaxis
  - Be cautious not to overcall recurrent hepatitis B in post-transplant biopsy

SELECTED REFERENCES

1. Liang TJ: Hepatitis B: the virus and disease. Hepatology. 49(5 Suppl):S13-21, 2009
2. Mani H et al: Liver biopsy findings in chronic hepatitis B. Hepatology. 49(5 Suppl):S61-71, 2009
3. McMahon BJ: The natural history of chronic hepatitis B virus infection. Hepatology. 49(5 Suppl):S45-55, 2009
4. Goodman ZD: Grading and staging systems for inflammation and fibrosis in chronic liver diseases. J Hepatol. 47(4):598-607, 2007
5. Harrison TJ: Hepatitis B virus: molecular virology and common mutants. Semin Liver Dis. 2006 May;26(2):87-96. Review. Erratum in: Semin Liver Dis. 26(3):304-5, 2006
6. Wisell J et al: Glycogen pseudoground glass change in hepatocytes. Am J Surg Pathol. 30(9):1085-90, 2006
7. Brunt EM: Grading and staging the histopathological lesions of chronic hepatitis: the Knodell histology activity index and beyond. Hepatology. 31(1):241-6, 2000
8. Batts KP et al: Chronic hepatitis. An update on terminology and reporting. Am J Surg Pathol. 19(12):1409-17, 1995
9. Ishak K et al: Histological grading and staging of chronic hepatitis. J Hepatol. 22(6):696-9, 1995
10. Harrison RF et al: Recurrent hepatitis B in liver allografts: a distinctive form of rapidly developing cirrhosis. Histopathology. 23(1):21-8, 1993
11. Ishak KG: Light microscopic morphology of viral hepatitis. Am J Clin Pathol. 65(5 Suppl):787-827, 1976

Microscopic Features

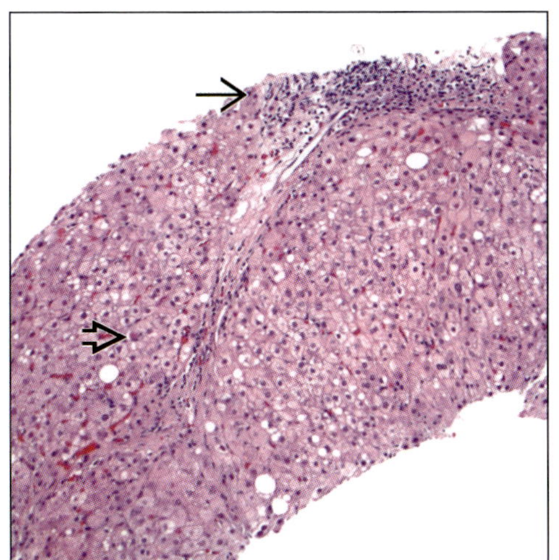

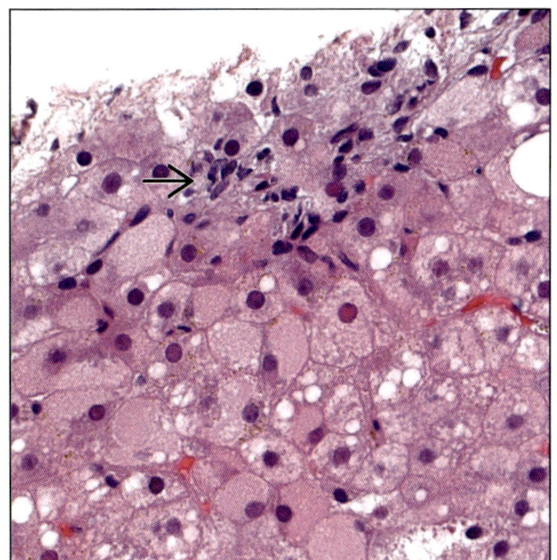

(Left) *Hematoxylin & eosin section illustrates chronic hepatitis B with portal inflammatory infiltrates* ⇒ *and apoptotic bodies* ⇨ *in the lobule.* ***(Right)*** *Hematoxylin & eosin section demonstrates a focus of lobular inflammation composed of lymphocytes and Kupffer cells* ⇒.

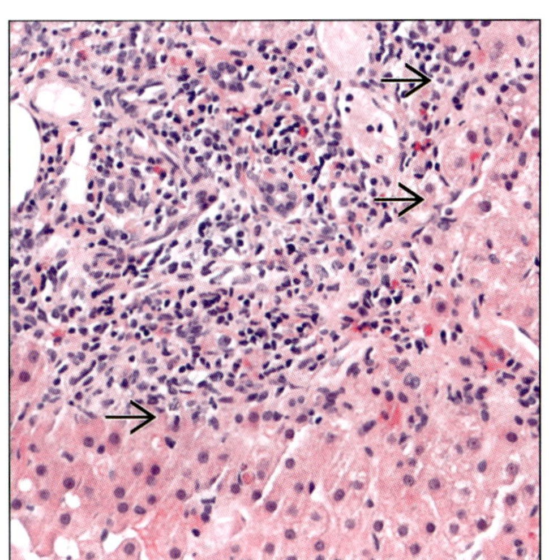

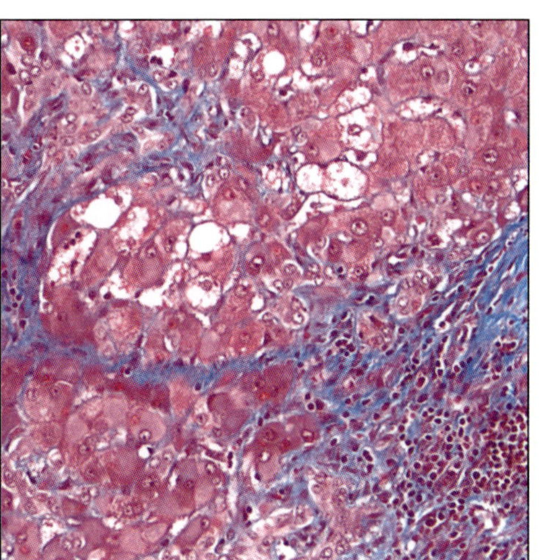

(Left) *Hematoxylin & eosin section shows interface hepatitis in chronic hepatitis B consisting of chronic inflammatory cells that extend beyond the limiting plate* ⇒ *and replace dead hepatocytes.* ***(Right)*** *Masson trichrome stain shows collagen strands that extend beyond portal tracts to reach the central region and form bridging septa in chronic hepatitis B.*

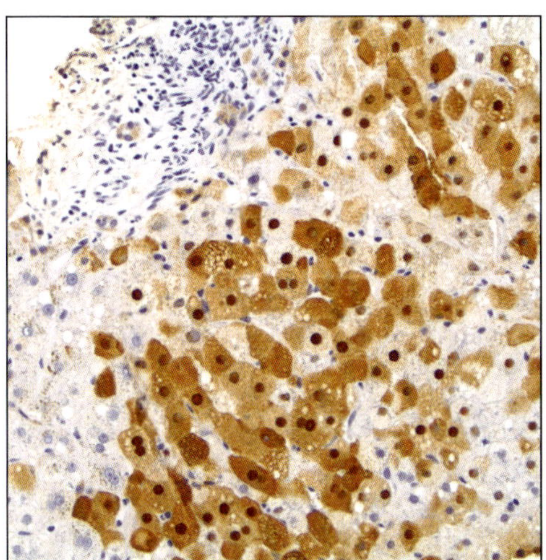

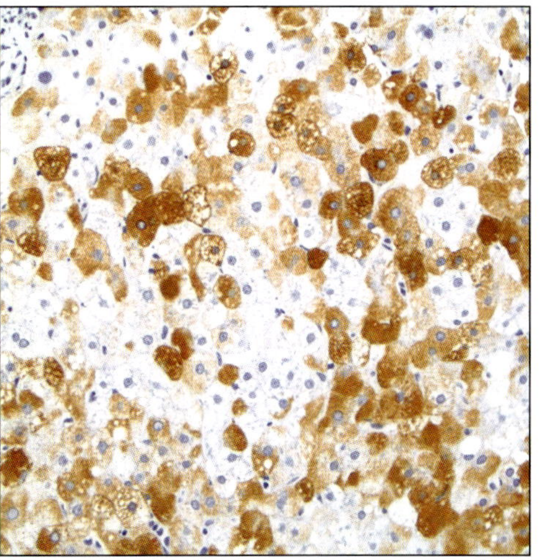

(Left) *Immunohistochemical stain for anti-HBc (core antigen) shows both cytoplasmic and nuclear staining.* ***(Right)*** *Immunohistochemical stain for anti-HBs (surface antigen) shows cytoplasmic staining.*

HEPATITIS C

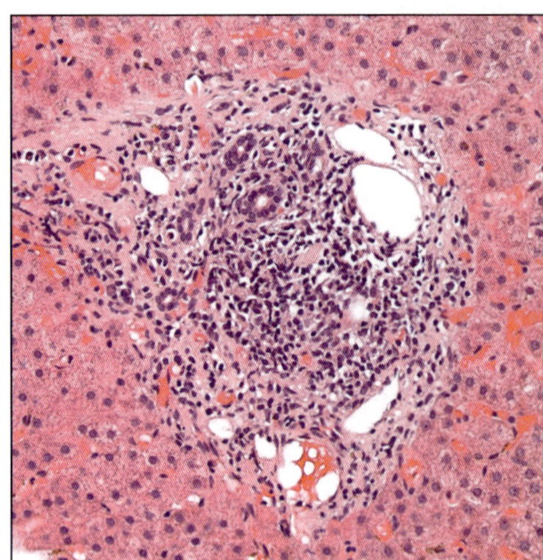

Hematoxylin & eosin stain shows dense portal inflammation composed primarily of lymphocytes.

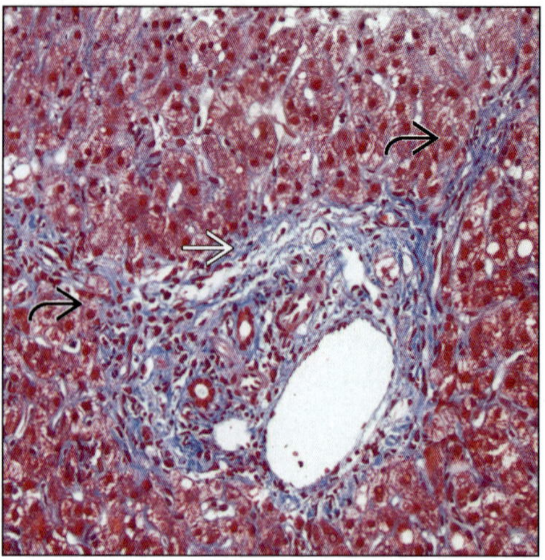

Trichrome stain demonstrates portal fibrous expansion ➡ and periportal fibrous extension ↪.

TERMINOLOGY

Abbreviations

- Hepatitis C virus infection (HCV)

Definitions

- Hepatitis, usually chronic, secondary to hepatitis C virus infection

ETIOLOGY/PATHOGENESIS

Infectious Agents

- Enveloped, single-stranded RNA virus of Flaviviridae family
  - Positive-sense RNA encodes a single polypeptide
  - Polypeptide post-translationally cleaved to form structural, nonstructural, and envelope proteins
- Inherent high mutation rate generates viral heterogeneity
  - 6 viral genotypes and over 50 subtypes
    - Vary in geography, mode of transmission, and response to treatment

Modes of Transmission

- Blood transfusion
- Needlestick inoculation
- Perinatal exposure probably occurs with low efficiency
- Efficiency of sexual transmission is controversial but probably low

Pathogenesis

- Virus is directly cytopathic and induces immune-mediated cellular injury

CLINICAL ISSUES

Epidemiology

- Incidence
  - Worldwide seroprevalence of HCV antibodies (anti-HCV) estimated at 3%
  - Estimated 3-4 million persons infected in United States

Presentation

- Fatigue
- Nausea and anorexia
- Depression and difficulty concentrating
- May be asymptomatic

Laboratory Tests

- Antibodies (anti-HCV) indicate exposure
- Detection of HCV RNA indicates virus persistence
- Liver biopsy performed to grade and stage disease and exclude other liver diseases

Natural History

- Acute infection is often subclinical
- Fulminant hepatitis is rare
- Produces persistent (chronic) infection in 85% of infected persons
  - Defined as failure to clear virus in 6 months
  - Remaining 15% have self-limited infection

Treatment

- Drugs
  - Standard therapy is pegylated interferon-α in combination with ribavirin

Prognosis

- Chronic HCV is progressive disease
  - Progression usually slow (over decades) and clinically silent
  - Disease progression leads to cirrhosis and liver failure
- Risk of hepatocellular carcinoma, usually developing after progression to cirrhosis

HEPATITIS C

Key Facts

Terminology
- Hepatitis, usually chronic, secondary to hepatitis C virus infection

Clinical Issues
- Liver biopsy is performed to grade and stage disease and exclude other liver diseases
  - Grade indicates degree of necroinflammatory activity
  - Stage indicates extent of fibrosis
- Standard therapy is pegylated interferon-α in combination with ribavirin
- Chronic HCV is slowly progressive disease, ultimately leading to cirrhosis, liver failure, and risk of hepatocellular carcinoma

Microscopic Pathology
- Variably dense portal inflammatory cell infiltrates composed mostly of lymphocytes
  - Periportal interface activity usually present but tends to be relatively mild
- Scattered lobular collections of inflammatory cells with or without acidophil bodies
- Progressive fibrosis begins in portal areas and extends outward in stellate fashion

Top Differential Diagnoses
- HCV enters differential diagnosis for many forms of portal hepatitis
  - Can be confirmed or excluded by laboratory testing for hepatitis C antibodies (anti-HCV) or viral RNA

MICROSCOPIC PATHOLOGY

Histologic Features
- Variably dense portal inflammatory cell infiltrates
  - Portal inflammation includes predominantly lymphocytes
  - Periportal interface activity
    - Lymphocytes disrupt limiting plate and surround nearby hepatocytes, causing hepatocyte injury and necrosis
- Scattered lobular collections of inflammatory cells with or without acidophil bodies
- Cholestatic hepatitis in some cases
- Mild duct injury dubbed "Paulsen lesions"
- Mild, patchy steatosis may be seen, particularly in genotype 3b
- Progressive fibrosis begins in portal areas and extends outward in stellate fashion
- Histologic features are scored
  - Grade: Extent and severity of interface activity and lobular inflammation and injury
  - Stage: Extent of fibrosis
  - Several grading and staging systems available
- Acute infection rarely recognized clinically and rarely biopsied
  - Usually relatively mild lobular hepatitis

DIFFERENTIAL DIAGNOSIS

Hepatitis B Virus Infection
- Ground-glass hepatocytes are seen in hepatitis B but are not present in all cases
- Distinguished by serologic testing

Autoimmune Hepatitis
- Usually more severe hepatitis with more extensive interface activity and hepatocyte injury
- May exhibit more plasma cells
- Distinguished by serologic testing for autoantibodies
  - False-positive anti-HCV can occur in autoimmune hepatitis, and autoantibodies may be expressed in HCV

Wilson Disease
- Elevated liver copper levels

Drug-induced Hepatitis
- Exclusion of HCV and identification of causative agent

Biliary Diseases
- More prominent bile duct injury or duct loss and less hepatocellular injury
- Portal edema and bile infarcts favor biliary obstruction

α-1-Antitrypsin Deficiency
- PAS-positive, diastase-resistant inclusions in periportal hepatocytes

Other Portal-based Hepatitides
- Exclude with laboratory testing for anti-HCV and HCV RNA

DIAGNOSTIC CHECKLIST

Pathologic Interpretation Pearls
- Usually relatively mild chronic hepatitis
- Predominantly portal-based inflammation and fibrosis

SELECTED REFERENCES

1. Bedossa P: Assessment of hepatitis C: non-invasive fibrosis markers and/or liver biopsy. Liver Int. 29 Suppl 1:19-22, 2009
2. Burra P: Hepatitis C. Semin Liver Dis. 29(1):53-65, 2009
3. Diepolder HM: New insights into the immunopathogenesis of chronic hepatitis C. Antiviral Res. 82(3):103-9, 2009
4. Lavanchy D: The global burden of hepatitis C. Liver Int. 29 Suppl 1:74-81, 2009
5. Nash KL et al: Managing hepatitis C virus infection. BMJ. 338:b2366, 2009

HEPATITIS C

Microscopic Features

*(**Left**) Hematoxylin & eosin demonstrates the portal tract inflammatory cell infiltrate to be composed of lymphocytes with occasional histiocytes and plasma cells. A few eosinophils and neutrophils may be seen but are generally not prominent. (**Right**) Hematoxylin & eosin shows a portal tract with focal disruption of the limiting plate ➔ by inflammatory cells, or "interface activity." The lymphocytes surround hepatocytes, inciting hepatocyte injury and death.*

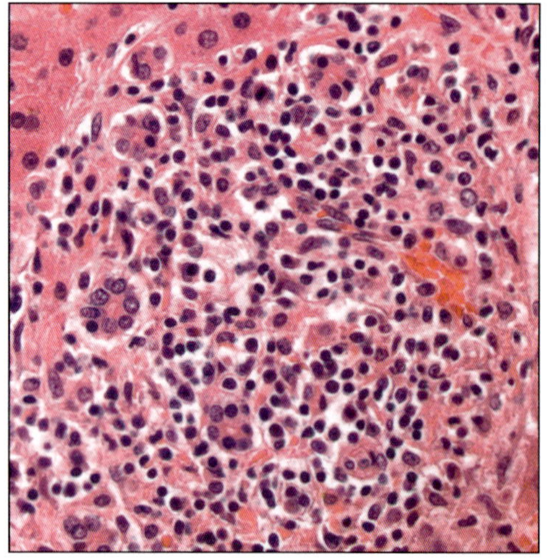

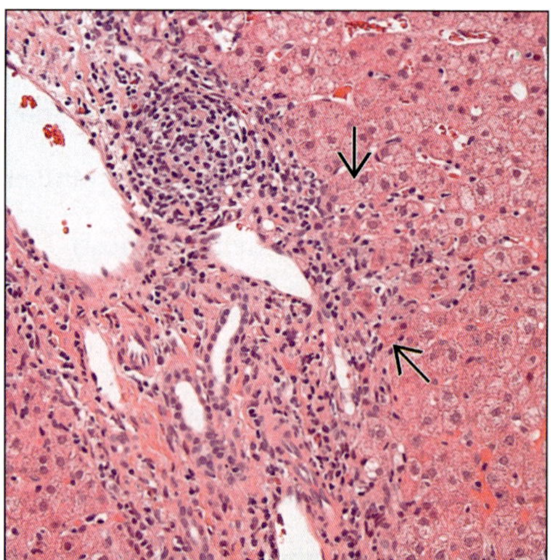

*(**Left**) Hematoxylin & eosin shows an inflamed portal tract with focal disruption of the limiting plate by interface activity ➔. Also present is a lymphoid aggregate ➲. (**Right**) At higher power, this hematoxylin & eosin stained slide demonstrates lymphocytes passing beyond the limiting plate and surrounding hepatocytes. Mild hepatocyte swelling, eosinophilia, and necrosis are often evident, reflecting the resultant hepatocyte injury.*

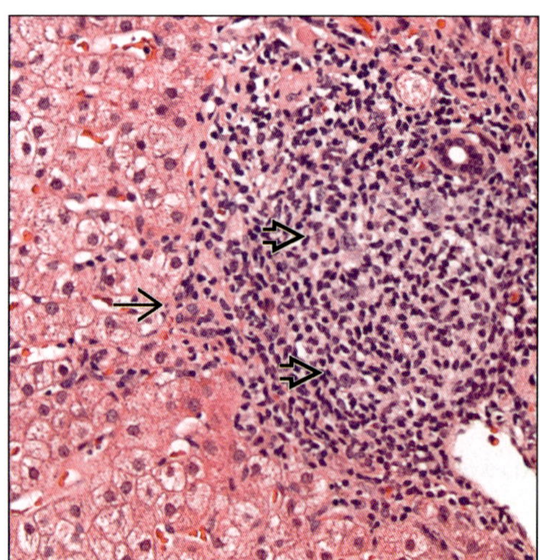

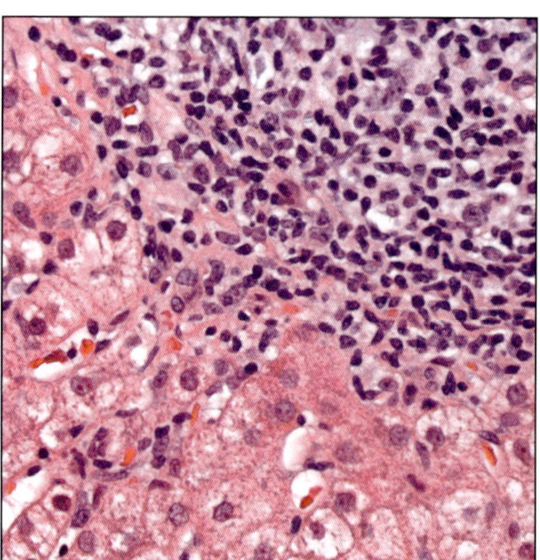

*(**Left**) Hematoxylin & eosin stain demonstrates a lobular collection of inflammatory cells ➲ in a case of chronic hepatitis C virus infection. (**Right**) Hematoxylin & eosin stain demonstrates a focus of necroinflammatory activity in chronic hepatitis C. There is a collection of inflammatory cells ➲ and a single acidophil body ➔, a.k.a. a Councilman body or necrotic hepatocyte.*

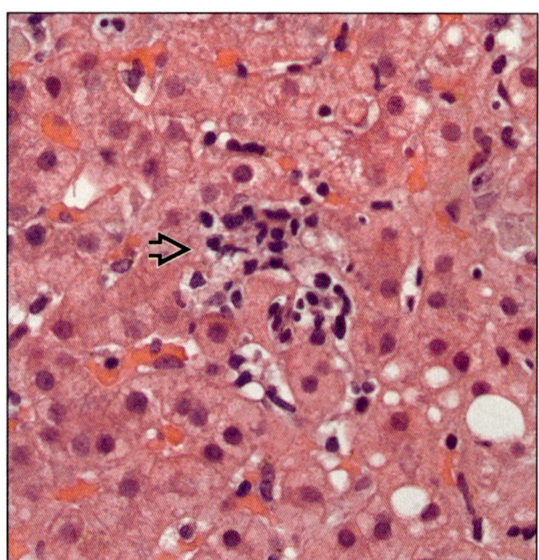

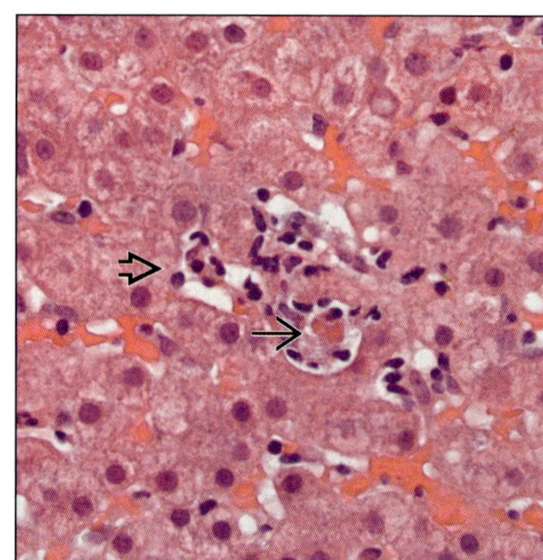

Microscopic Features

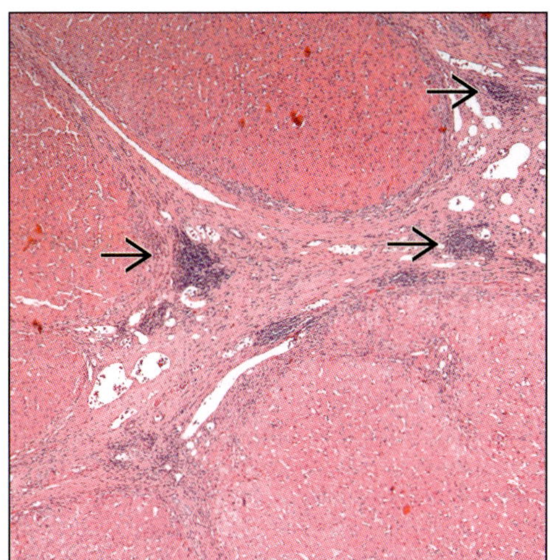

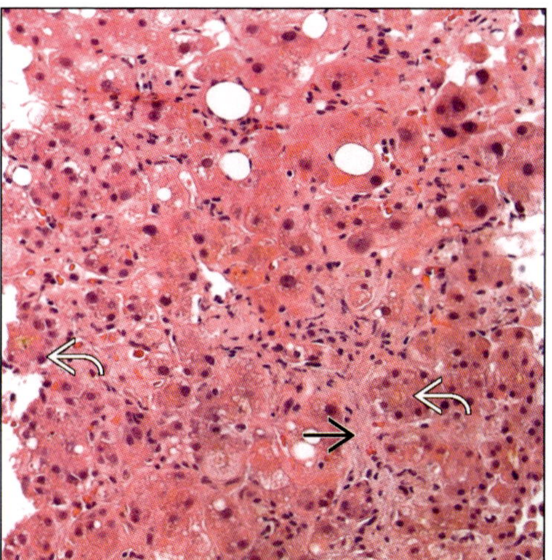

(Left) *Hematoxylin & eosin shows scattered lymphoid aggregates ⇒ in portal areas and fibrous bands in this case of burned-out hepatitis C cirrhosis. These lymphoid aggregates should not be considered in determination of the grade.* ***(Right)*** *Hematoxylin & eosin stain shows cholestasis ⇒, inflammation, and fibrosis ⇒ in a severe, cholestatic form of recurrent hepatitis C in a liver transplant recipient.*

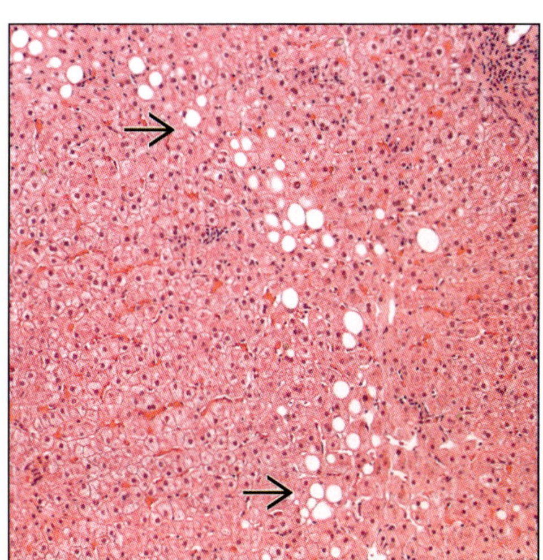

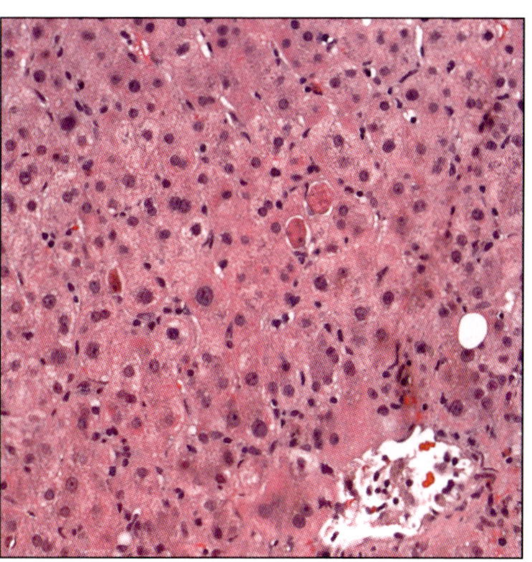

(Left) *Hematoxylin & eosin stain shows mild, patchy steatosis ⇒ in a patient with chronic hepatitis C virus infection. The steatosis lacks a zonal distribution.* ***(Right)*** *Hematoxylin & eosin shows numerous acidophil bodies in a case of early recurrent hepatitis C after liver transplantation. Acute hepatitis C infection is rarely biopsied in native livers, but an early or acute phase is often recognized with hepatitis C recurrence after liver transplantation.*

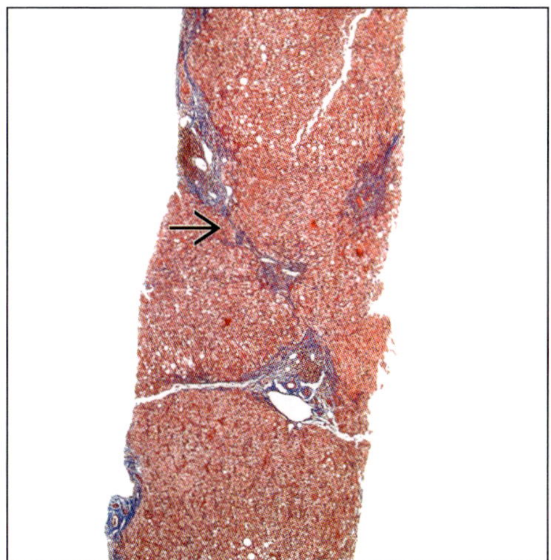

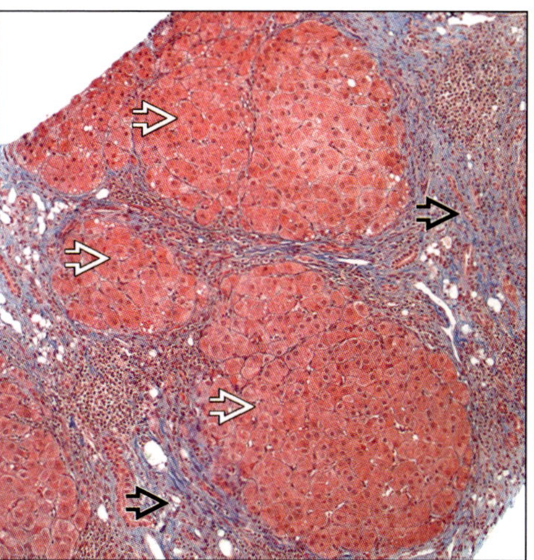

(Left) *Trichrome stain highlights the portal-based fibrosis that extends outward from the portal tracts and, with progression, forms bridging fibrous septa ⇒ between portal tracts.* ***(Right)*** *Trichrome stain demonstrates rounded cirrhotic nodules ⇒ in a background of fibrous stroma ⇒. Cirrhosis represents the final stage of chronic hepatitis C virus progression.*

EPSTEIN-BARR VIRUS

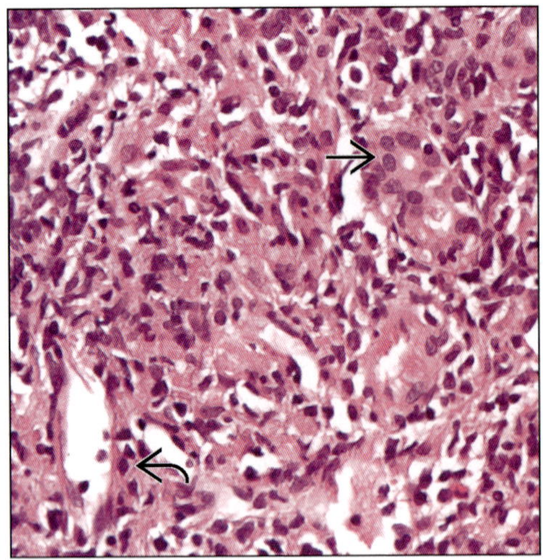

EBV hepatitis causes predominantly lymphocytic infiltrates in the portal tracts. Note the presence of mild endophlebitis ⮫ and mild bile duct damage ⮕.

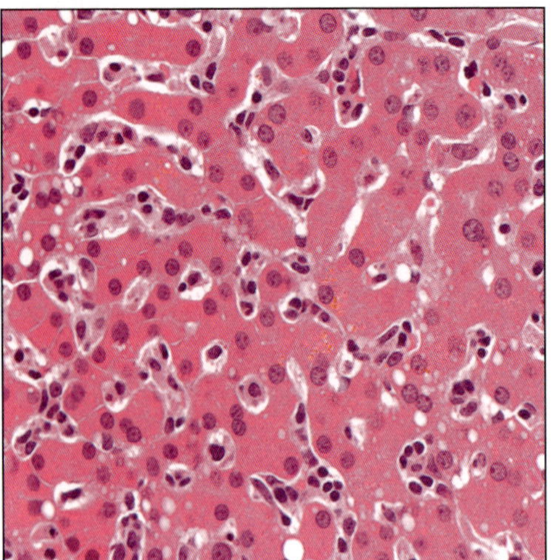

EBV hepatitis is characterized by sinusoidal lymphocytic infiltrates with an "Indian file" or "string of beads" pattern.

TERMINOLOGY

Abbreviations

- Epstein-Barr virus (EBV)
- Post-transplant lymphoproliferative disorder (PTLD)

Synonyms

- Human herpesvirus-4

Definitions

- Hepatitis and lymphoproliferative disorders caused by EBV infection

ETIOLOGY/PATHOGENESIS

Infectious Agents

- Member of herpesvirus family
- Transmission via intimate contact with saliva of infected person
- Asymptomatic lifelong infection in > 90% of world adult population
- Dormant in memory B lymphocytes in healthy individuals at concentration of ~ 1 in 1 x 10^5 to 1 x 10^6 cells

CLINICAL ISSUES

Presentation

- Infectious mononucleosis
  - New infection typically occurs during adolescence or young adulthood
  - Occasionally seen in middle-aged and elderly persons
  - Incubation time of 4-6 weeks
  - Fever, fatigue, malaise, sore throat, arthralgia, jaundice, lymphadenopathy, splenomegaly, and hepatomegaly
  - Usually resolves in 1-2 months
- EBV hepatitis
  - Usually represents liver involvement by infectious mononucleosis
  - Primary infection or reactivation of latent infection
  - Seen in immunocompetent and immunocompromised individuals
  - Hepatomegaly seen in 10-15% of patients
  - Jaundice seen in ~ 5% of patients
  - Elevated serum transaminase, alkaline phosphatase, and bilirubin levels
- EBV-associated lymphoproliferative disorders
  - In immunocompromised individuals due to uncontrolled EBV replication
    - PTLD in solid organ transplant recipients
    - Occurs in 1-2.8% of liver transplants
    - Accounts for > 50% of all tumors in children and ~ 15% of all tumors in adults following liver transplantation
    - Approximately 80% of cases occur in the first 2 years after transplantation
    - Host origin in majority of cases, rarely donor origin
    - Heavy immunosuppression for treatment of rejection is major risk factor

Laboratory Tests

- Peripheral lymphocytosis with > 10% atypical lymphocytes
- Serologic studies
  - Positive monospot test for heterophile antibody
  - Primary infection
    - Elevated IgM titer to viral capsid antigen (VCA)
    - Rising IgG titer to VCA
    - Absent antibody to nuclear antigen (EBNA)
    - Positive antibody to early antigen (EBEA)
  - Reactivation of latent infection
    - Elevated antibody titer to EBEA in presence of antibody to EBNA
  - Past infection
    - Presence of antibodies to both VCA and EBNA
- Molecular tests

EPSTEIN-BARR VIRUS

Key Facts

Clinical Issues

- Fever, fatigue, malaise, sore throat, arthralgia, jaundice, lymphadenopathy, splenomegaly, and hepatomegaly
- Elevated serum transaminase, alkaline phosphatase, and bilirubin levels
- Self limited in majority of cases
- Lymphoproliferative disorders in immunocompromised individuals due to uncontrolled EBV replication
- Associated with a number of human malignancies

Microscopic Pathology

- EBV hepatitis
  - Diffuse sinusoidal lymphocytic infiltration in "Indian file" or "string of beads" pattern
  - Mixed inflammatory cell infiltrates in portal tracts, consisting predominantly of lymphocytes
  - Scattered large and irregular (atypical) lymphocytes in sinusoids and portal tracts
- Hepatic PTLD
  - Early lesions, polymorphic PTLD, and monomorphic PTLD (lymphomas)

Ancillary Tests

- Detection of EBV early RNA (EBER) on tissue sections by in situ hybridization

Top Differential Diagnoses

- Hepatic involvement by leukemia
- Acute cellular rejection of allograft
- Recurrent hepatitis C viral infection in allograft
- Drug-induced mononucleosis-like hepatitis

  - Detection of viral DNA in peripheral blood by polymerase chain reaction
  - Detection of EBV early RNA (EBER) on tissue sections by in situ hybridization
  - Gene arrangement for immunoglobulins and T-cell receptors for cases suspicious for PTLD
- Immunohistochemistry
  - Detection of EBV latent membrane proteins (LMP) on tissue sections
  - Immunohistochemical stains for B- and T-cell markers as well as κ and λ light chains in cases suspicious for PTLD

Treatment

- EBV hepatitis
  - Symptomatic &/or supportive treatment
  - Use of corticosteroids and antiviral agents remains controversial
- PTLD lacks general treatment paradigm due to disease heterogeneity
  - Restoration of cellular immunity
    - Reduction of immunosuppression
    - Interferon-α
  - Antitumor therapies
    - Surgical resection for localized disease
    - Radiation therapy for localized disease
    - Chemotherapy
    - Rituximab for CD20(+) disease
    - Anti-IL-6 antibody
  - Antiviral agents

Prognosis

- Self-limited in majority of EBV hepatitis cases
  - Does not progress to chronic hepatitis or cirrhosis
- Serious complications of EBV hepatitis occur in < 5% of cases
  - Fulminant hepatic failure
  - Splenic rupture
  - Hemolytic anemia
  - Hemophagocytic syndrome
  - Guillain-Barré syndrome
  - Malignancies
- PTLD
  - Varies from benign lymphoproliferation to aggressive lymphoma

MACROSCOPIC FEATURES

General Features

- Hepatomegaly
- Liver mass in patients with PTLD

MICROSCOPIC PATHOLOGY

Histologic Features

- EBV hepatitis
  - Diffuse sinusoidal lymphocytic infiltration in "Indian file" or "string of beads" pattern
  - Moderate to marked mixed inflammatory cell infiltrates in portal tracts, consisting predominantly of lymphocytes
    - Scattered large and irregular (atypical) lymphocytes in sinusoids and portal tracts
    - Scattered foci of interface activity
  - Focal lobular disarray with focal hepatocyte ballooning and scattered acidophil bodies
  - Small noncaseating epithelioid granulomas (microgranulomas) or fibrin-ring granulomas in lobules
  - Varying degree of steatosis with no particular zonal distribution
  - Cholestasis not prominent
  - Mild bile duct damage
    - No significant ductular reaction
  - Focal endophlebitis
  - No fibrosis
- Hepatic PTLD
  - 3 major disease categories
  - Early lesions characterized by reactive plasmacytic hyperplasia or infectious mononucleosis-like lesions
    - Mixed mononuclear cell infiltrates in portal tracts, including small- and medium-sized lymphocytes,

atypical lymphocytes, immunoblasts, and plasma cells
- Sinusoidal lymphocytic infiltration similar to that seen in EBV hepatitis
- Infiltrative lymphocytes are predominantly B cells, in contrast to predominantly T cells in EBV hepatitis

- Polymorphic PTLD characterized by mixed lymphoplasmacytic proliferation
  - More frequent atypical lymphoid cells (blast forms)
  - Either polyclonal or monoclonal
- Monomorphic PTLD is same as lymphoma seen in immunocompetent hosts
  - Classified according to standard lymphoma classification
  - > 80% derive from B-cell proliferation; most common subtype is diffuse large B-cell lymphoma
  - Rare subtypes include Burkitt or Burkitt-like lymphoma, plasma cell myeloma, peripheral T-cell lymphoma, γ/δ T-cell lymphoma, T/NK-cell lymphoma, Hodgkin lymphoma, and Hodgkin lymphoma-like PTLD
  - Proliferation of neoplastic lymphoid cells form solitary mass or multiple masses
  - Diffuse infiltration of portal tracts &/or sinusoids by neoplastic lymphoid cells less common
  - Destruction of normal hepatic architecture

DIFFERENTIAL DIAGNOSIS

Hepatic Involvement by Leukemia

- Sinusoidal and portal infiltration by monotonous lymphoid or myeloid cells
- Flow cytometry and immunohistochemical stains are helpful

Hepatosplenic T-cell Lymphoma

- Sinusoidal infiltration by monotonous, medium-sized cytotoxic T-cells expressing γ/δ receptor
- Characteristic CD3(+), CD4(-), and CD8(-) immunophenotype
- Clonal γ/δ T-cell receptor rearrangement
- Clonal α/β T-cell receptor rearrangement seen in occasional cases
- Presence of isochromosome 7q

Acute Cellular Rejection

- More pronounced bile duct damage &/or endophlebitis
- Less prominent sinusoidal lymphocytic infiltrates
- Negative EBER by in situ hybridization

Recurrent Hepatitis C Post-transplant

- Less prominent sinusoidal lymphocytic infiltrates
- Portal lymphoid aggregates
- Portal and periportal fibrosis
- Negative EBER by in situ hybridization

CMV Hepatitis

- Occasionally produces mononucleosis-like picture
- Intranuclear and intracytoplasmic viral inclusions with or without microabscesses
- Immunohistochemical stains and in situ hybridization are helpful

Drug-induced Lobular Hepatitis

- May produce mononucleosis-like picture
- History of drug use (phenytoin, sulfonamides, dapsone, minocycline, etc.)
- May show confluent lobular necrosis occasionally
- Portal eosinophils may be more prominent
- Cholestasis may be more pronounced
- Negative EBER by in situ hybridization

DIAGNOSTIC CHECKLIST

Clinically Relevant Pathologic Features

- Elevated liver function tests in patients with symptoms and signs of infectious mononucleosis
- Development of PTLD in organ transplant recipients

Pathologic Interpretation Pearls

- Characteristic diffuse and beaded sinusoidal lymphocytic infiltrates
- Predominantly lymphocytic infiltrates in portal tracts
- Presence of atypical lymphocytes
- Positive EBER by in situ hybridization

SELECTED REFERENCES

1. Shah KM et al: Epstein-Barr virus and carcinogenesis: beyond Burkitt's lymphoma. Clin Microbiol Infect. 15(11):982-8, 2009
2. Frey NV et al: The management of posttransplant lymphoproliferative disorder. Med Oncol. 24(2):125-36, 2007
3. Suh N et al: Epstein-Barr virus hepatitis: diagnostic value of in situ hybridization, polymerase chain reaction, and immunohistochemistry on liver biopsy from immunocompetent patients. Am J Surg Pathol. 31(9):1403-9, 2007
4. Kremers WK et al: Post-transplant lymphoproliferative disorders following liver transplantation: incidence, risk factors and survival. Am J Transplant. 6(5 Pt 1):1017-24, 2006
5. LaCasce AS: Post-transplant lymphoproliferative disorders. Oncologist. 11(6):674-80, 2006
6. Gershburg E et al: Epstein-Barr virus infections: prospects for treatment. J Antimicrob Chemother. 56(2):277-81, 2005
7. Taylor AL et al: Post-transplant lymphoproliferative disorders (PTLD) after solid organ transplantation. Crit Rev Oncol Hematol. 56(1):155-67, 2005
8. Young LS et al: Epstein-Barr virus: 40 years on. Nat Rev Cancer. 4(10):757-68, 2004
9. Goodman ZD: Drug hepatotoxicity. Clin Liver Dis. 6(2):381-97, 2002
10. Macon WR et al: Hepatosplenic alphabeta T-cell lymphomas: a report of 14 cases and comparison with hepatosplenic gammadelta T-cell lymphomas. Am J Surg Pathol. 25(3):285-96, 2001

Microscopic Features and Differential Diagnosis

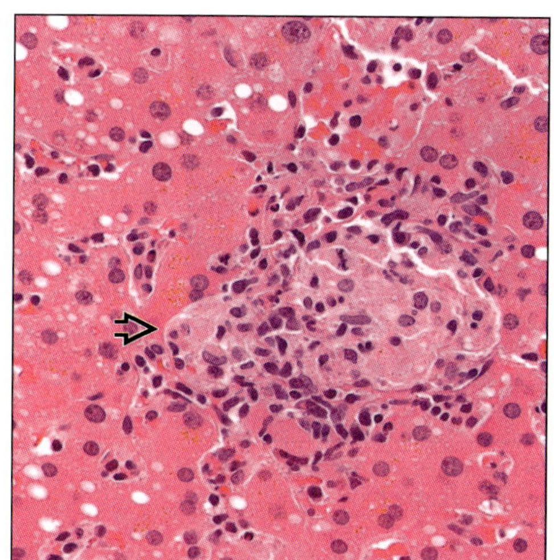

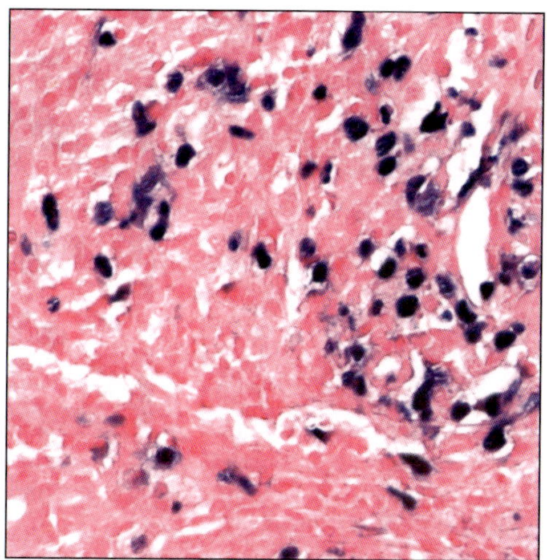

(Left) *EBV hepatitis can produce granulomas. This photomicrograph shows a microgranuloma ⇨ in the lobule. Note the presence of small droplet steatosis in hepatocytes.* ***(Right)*** *EBER in situ hybridization shows that infiltrative lymphocytes in the portal tracts and sinusoids are positive for EBV early RNA (EBER) in EBV hepatitis.*

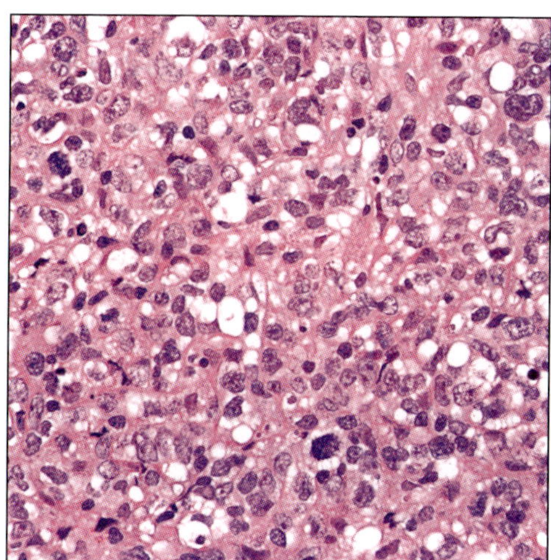

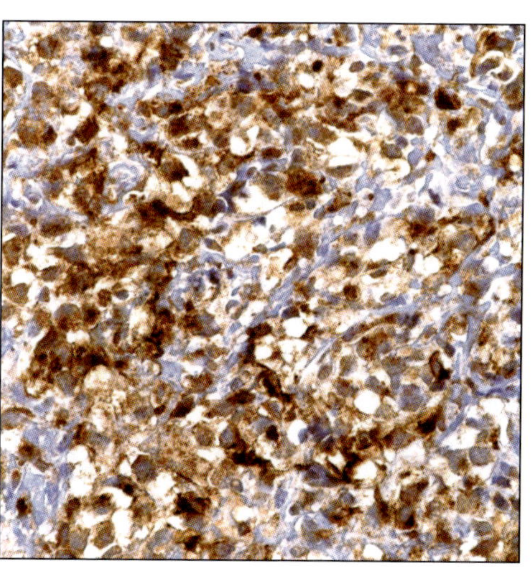

(Left) *This photomicrograph shows a case of EBV-associated diffuse large B-cell lymphoma in a liver allograft (monomorphic post-transplant lymphoproliferative disorder).* ***(Right)*** *This immunohistochemical stain for EBV-LMP shows positive cytoplasmic staining in neoplastic cells in a case of hepatic monomorphic post-transplant lymphoproliferative disorder (diffuse large B-cell lymphoma).*

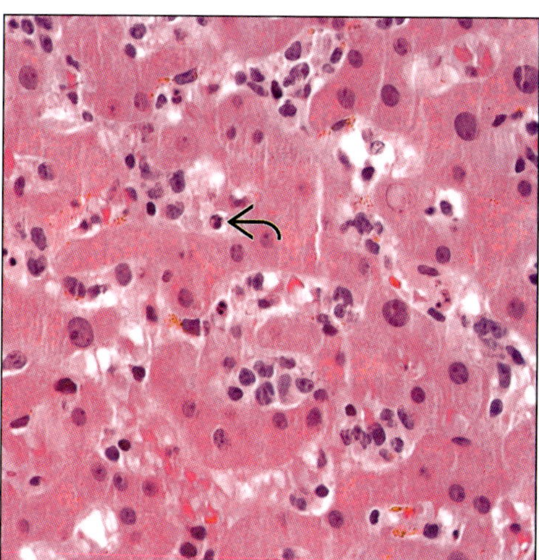

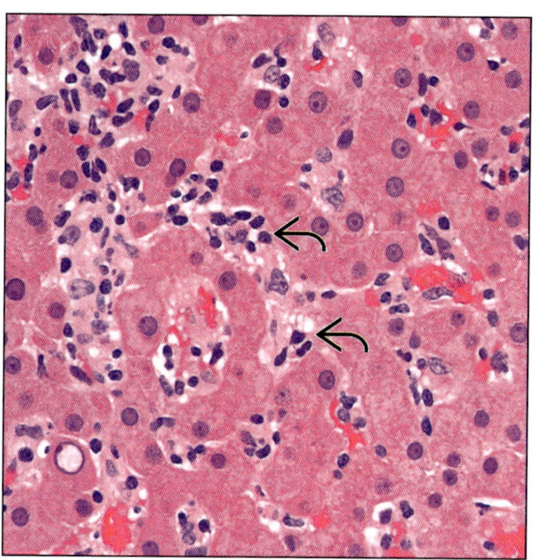

(Left) *This case of hepatosplenic T-cell lymphoma also shows monotonous, medium-sized lymphoid cells infiltrating the sinusoids and mimicking mononucleosis-like hepatitis. However, note the presence of frequent mitotic figures in the tumor cells ↩.* ***(Right)*** *This case of phenytoin-induced, mononucleosis-like hepatitis also shows diffuse sinusoidal infiltration by lymphocytes ↩, thus mimicking EBV hepatitis.*

CYTOMEGALOVIRUS

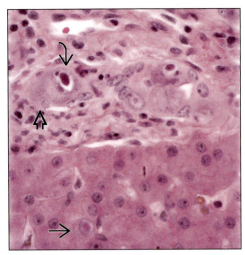

Hematoxylin & eosin shows characteristic cytomegaly with intranuclear ⇨ and intracytoplasmic ⇨ CMV inclusions within biliary epithelial cells and hepatocytes →.

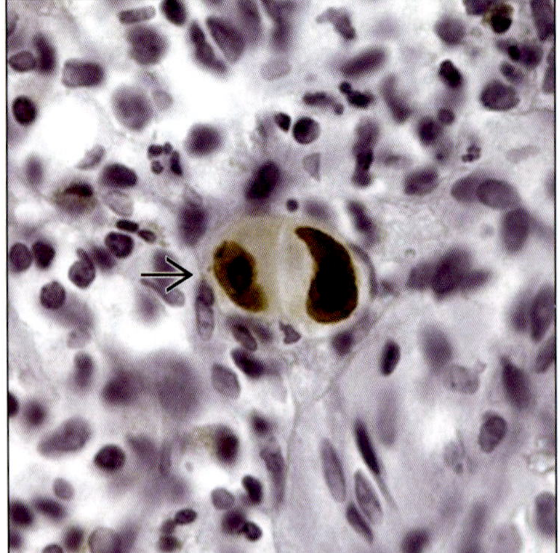

CMV immunohistochemical stain highlights 2 viral inclusions within endothelial cells →.

TERMINOLOGY

Abbreviations

- Cytomegalovirus (CMV)

Definitions

- CMV is a member of the family Herpesviridae
- At least 50% of adults in USA have serologic evidence of past infection
- Most clinically significant infections are seen in setting of immunosuppression
  - Organ transplantation, acquired immunodeficiency syndrome (AIDS), congenital infection

ETIOLOGY/PATHOGENESIS

Infectious Agent: CMV

- CMV has been identified in numerous body fluids
- Infection can be acquired before birth, at time of birth, or later in life
- After active infection, latent infection may persist for years
  - Reactivation may occur, usually when normal immunity is lost or impaired
- Pathogenesis of CMV hepatitis is unclear
  - Direct viral damage &/or host inflammatory response may play roles in producing functional liver abnormalities

CLINICAL ISSUES

Presentation

- Most infections are clinically silent
- Intact immune function: Mononucleosis-like illness (similar to Epstein-Barr virus)
  - Malaise, fever, atypical lymphocytosis
- Immunocompromised patients: Highly variable
  - Fever, malaise, myalgias, arthralgias, nausea, abdominal pain
  - Allograft recipients' symptoms usually develop from 2 weeks to 4 months after transplantation
- Congenital infection: Asymptomatic to severe infection with jaundice, hepatosplenomegaly, encephalitis, chorioretinitis

Treatment

- Antiviral therapy with ganciclovir &/or reduce immunosuppression

Prognosis

- Mononucleosis-like pattern: Usually resolves within several weeks without chronic liver disease
- Only congenital infection leads to development of chronic liver disease (rare)

MICROSCOPIC PATHOLOGY

Histologic Features

- Characteristic cytopathic effects of CMV
  - Cytoplasmic and nuclear enlargement (2-4x normal)
  - Intranuclear inclusions: Large glassy round to oval masses within nucleus separated by clear halo from thickened nuclear membrane
  - Intracytoplasmic inclusions: Basophilic or amphophilic granules that stain positive with PAS and GMS stains
  - Changes can be seen in hepatocytes, biliary epithelium, endothelial cells, and Kupffer cells
  - Positive immunohistochemical stain for CMV inclusions
- Mononucleosis-like pattern
  - Prominent mononuclear infiltrate within portal tracts and sinusoids ("string of beads" arrangement)
  - Possible granulomas
  - Absence of viral inclusions; immunohistochemistry may not be helpful
- Immunosuppressed patients

CYTOMEGALOVIRUS

Key Facts

Terminology

- At least 50% of adults in USA have serologic evidence of past infection

Clinical Issues

- Expected clinical and histological presentation of CMV hepatitis depends on age and immune status of patient

Microscopic Pathology

- Characteristic cytoplasmic and nuclear enlargement with intranuclear and intracytoplasmic inclusions
- Immunocompetent patients: Mononucleosis-like pattern with sinusoidal lymphocytic infiltrate and absence of viral inclusions
- Immunocompromised and neonatal patients: Variable portal and lobular inflammation and characteristic viral inclusions

  - Presence of typical CMV cytopathic effects (enlargement, inclusions)
  - Other nonspecific alterations: Mild lobular hepatitis, hepatocellular necrosis, patchy portal inflammation by mononuclear cells
  - Viral inclusions may be accompanied by neutrophilic microabscesses or inflammation may be absent
- Congenital infections
  - Resemble those of immunosuppressed patients (including presence of viral cytopathic effects)
  - Some have neonatal hepatitis-like pattern (cholestasis, hepatocyte necrosis) or features that simulate biliary atresia (bile ductular proliferation and portal fibrosis)
  - Extramedullary hematopoiesis is common finding

Predominant Pattern/Injury Type

- Viral inclusion

Predominant Cell/Compartment Type

- Hepatocyte

DIFFERENTIAL DIAGNOSIS

Epstein-Barr-associated Lobular Hepatitis

- Positive heterophil antibodies with EBV infection

Other Viral Infections

- i.e., herpes simplex and Varicella-Zoster
- Immunohistochemical stains for HSV1/2 and CMV &/ or serological assays are helpful

Graft Rejection in Liver Transplant Patients

- Absence of characteristic viral inclusions; immunohistochemical stain for CMV is negative

DIAGNOSTIC CHECKLIST

Clinically Relevant Pathologic Features

- CMV infection may be systemic and affect multiple organ systems, especially in immunocompromised patients
  - i.e., pneumonitis, retinitis, or gastrointestinal ulceration

Pathologic Interpretation Pearls

- Cytomegaly with characteristic intranuclear and intracytoplasmic viral inclusion bodies

SELECTED REFERENCES

1. Varani S et al: Cytomegalovirus as a hepatotropic virus. Clin Lab. 48(1-2):39-44, 2002
2. Jeffries DJ: The spectrum of cytomegalovirus infection and its management. J Antimicrob Chemother. 23 Suppl E:1-10, 1989
3. Griffiths PD: Cytomegalovirus and the liver. Semin Liver Dis. 4(4):307-13, 1984

IMAGE GALLERY

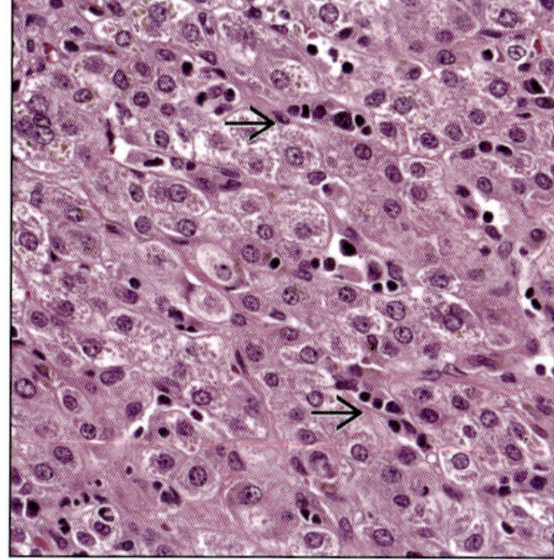

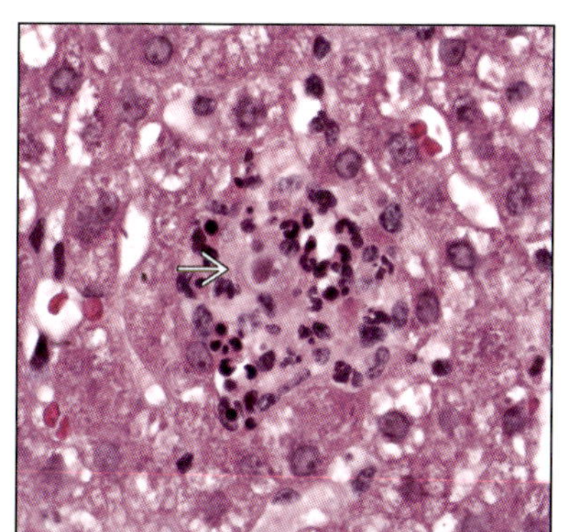

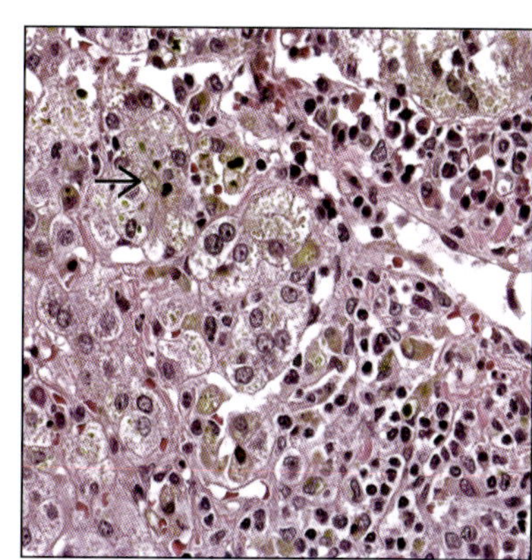

(Left) *H&E stain demonstrates the mononucleosis-like pattern of CMV infection with a mononuclear lymphocytic infiltrate within the hepatic sinusoids in a "string of beads" configuration ⇒.* ***(Center)*** *H&E stain shows a hepatocyte containing intranuclear and intracytoplasmic viral inclusions surrounded by a neutrophilic microabscess ➡.* ***(Right)*** *Hematoxylin & eosin stain shows liver parenchyma with cholestasis ⇒ and a mononuclear infiltrate. Congenital CMV infections can show a neonatal hepatitis-like pattern with cholestasis.*

HERPES SIMPLEX VIRUS

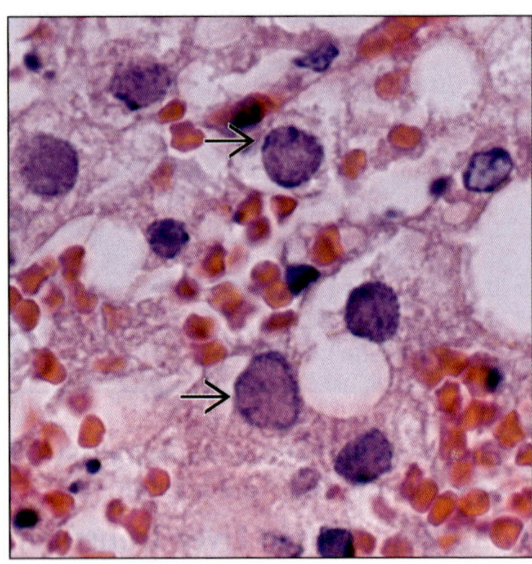

Hematoxylin & eosin shows viral inclusions ➔ with smudged hepatocyte nuclei and margination of nuclear chromatin. The inclusions are typically located at the edge of necrotic zones.

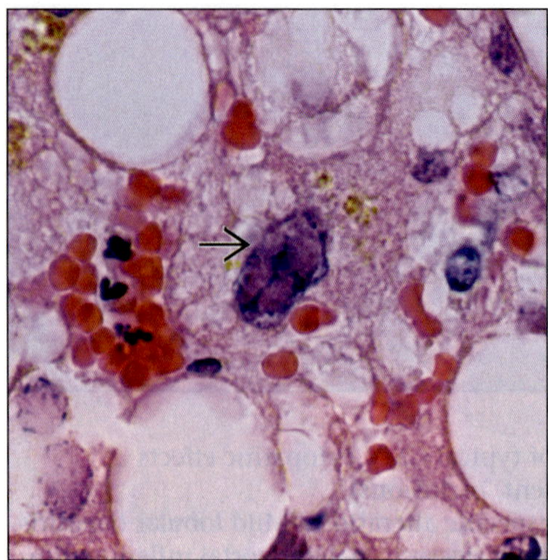

Hematoxylin & eosin shows a multinucleated cell ➔ with nuclear molding. These cells are commonly observed in herpetic mucosal lesions but are uncommon in HSV hepatitis.

TERMINOLOGY

Abbreviations

- Herpes simplex virus (HSV) hepatitis

ETIOLOGY/PATHOGENESIS

Infectious Agents

- Hepatitis is result of disseminated infection and can occur with both HSV1 and HSV2
- Dissemination may occur due to immunosuppression, large initial inoculum, enhanced virulence at reactivation, or hepatovirulence of certain strains

CLINICAL ISSUES

Epidemiology

- Incidence
  - Risk factors
    - Immunosuppression
    - Neonates
    - 3rd trimester of pregnancy
  - Fulminant infections rare in immunocompetent individuals

Presentation

- Nonspecific flu-like symptoms
  - Fever
  - Headache
  - Abdominal/muscle pain
- Oropharyngeal or genital manifestations in 30-50% of cases
- Acute decompensation occurs 3-21 days after nonspecific symptoms
  - Anicteric
  - No hepatomegaly
  - Marked elevation of transaminases (AST > ALT)
  - Leukopenia, thrombocytopenia
  - Encephalitis, renal failure, and disseminated intravascular coagulation can occur
- Neonatal HSV typically presents at 5-7 days after birth with symptoms that mimic bacterial sepsis (poor feeding, lethargy, fever)

Laboratory Tests

- Viral culture from mucocutaneous lesions, urine, stool, or blood
- Polymerase chain reaction for viral DNA using plasma, body fluids, tissue

Treatment

- Antiviral drugs: Acyclovir and adenine arabinoside
- Early treatment is crucial as disease can follow rapidly progressive course

Prognosis

- High mortality (80-90%) in untreated cases
- Survival is better in pregnant patients compared with other groups

MICROSCOPIC PATHOLOGY

Histologic Features

- Extensive nonzonal coagulative hemorrhagic necrosis
- Inflammatory response is inconspicuous
- Viral inclusions in hepatocyte nuclei at interface of necrotic and viable areas
  - Inclusions characterized by ground-glass or smudged nuclei with margination of chromatin
  - Eosinophilic intranuclear inclusions surrounded by halo (Cowdry type A) can be present
  - Multinucleated cells with nuclear molding are less common compared with mucocutaneous HSV infections
- Immunohistochemistry with antibodies directed against both HSV1 and HSV2 should be obtained to confirm diagnosis

HERPES SIMPLEX VIRUS

Key Facts

Clinical Issues
- Anicteric hepatitis with marked elevation of transaminases
- Mucocutaneous or genital manifestations in 30-50% of cases
- Early treatment is crucial as disease can follow rapidly progressive course
- Antiviral therapy with acyclovir

Microscopic Pathology
- Extensive nonzonal coagulative necrosis with negligible inflammation
- Viral inclusions in hepatocyte nuclei at interface of necrotic and viable areas
  - Characterized by ground-glass or smudged nuclei with margination of chromatin

Predominant Pattern/Injury Type
- Necrosis

Predominant Cell/Compartment Type
- Hepatocyte

DIFFERENTIAL DIAGNOSIS

Acetaminophen Toxicity
- Necrosis, often perivenular, without significant inflammation
- History of drug intake, elevated blood levels of drug, and absence of viral inclusions

Toxin-induced Liver Injury
- Mushroom poisoning, cocaine, herbal medications, carbon tetrachloride
- Necrosis without significant inflammation
- History of exposure and absence of viral inclusions

Adenovirus Hepatitis
- Usually affects immunosuppressed patients
- Immunohistochemistry necessary to distinguish from HSV; inclusions very similar

Wilson Disease
- Rarely presents as fulminant hepatitis with necrosis and no significant inflammation
- Elevated hepatic copper, urinary copper, low ceruloplasmin
- No viral inclusions

Acute Vascular Injury
- Acute ischemia (circulatory shock) or venous outflow obstruction (Budd-Chiari syndrome)
- Hemorrhagic necrosis around central vein
- Sinusoidal dilatation in venous outflow obstruction
- No viral inclusions

DIAGNOSTIC CHECKLIST

Pathologic Interpretation Pearls
- Look for inclusions at interface between necrotic zones and viable parenchyma

SELECTED REFERENCES

1. Czartoski T et al: Fulminant, acyclovir-resistant, herpes simplex virus type 2 hepatitis in an immunocompetent woman. J Clin Microbiol. 44(4):1584-6, 2006
2. Verma A et al: Neonatal herpes simplex virus infection presenting as acute liver failure: prevalent role of herpes simplex virus type I. J Pediatr Gastroenterol Nutr. 42(3):282-6, 2006
3. Sharma S et al: Herpes simplex hepatitis in adults: a search for muco-cutaneous clues. J Clin Gastroenterol. 38(8):697-704, 2004
4. Peters DJ et al: Herpes simplex-induced fulminant hepatitis in adults: a call for empiric therapy. Dig Dis Sci. 45(12):2399-404, 2000

IMAGE GALLERY

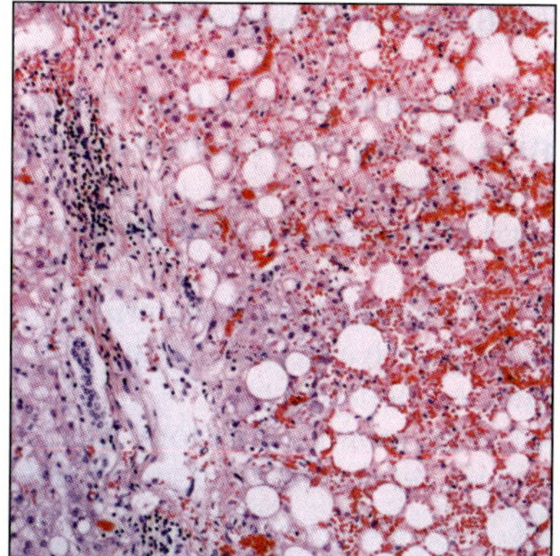

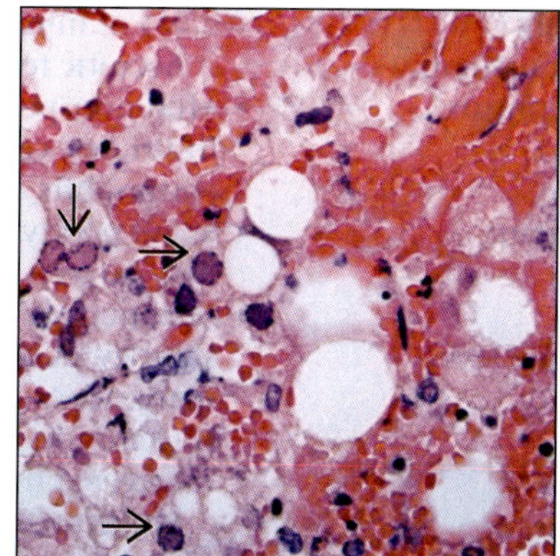

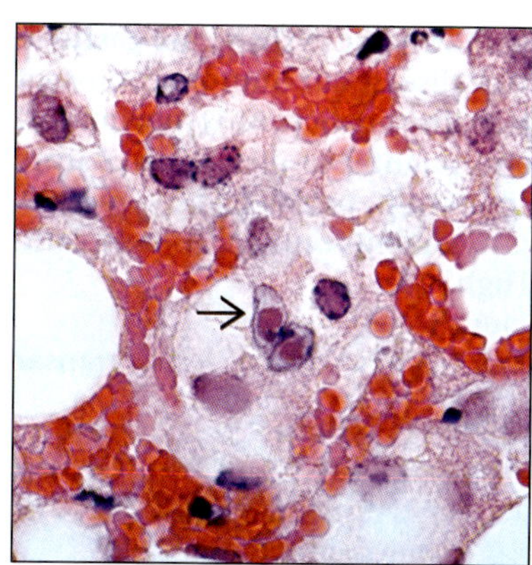

(Left) *Hematoxylin & eosin shows extensive hemorrhagic necrosis with negligible inflammation.* ***(Center)*** *Hematoxylin & eosin shows HSV inclusions at the interface of necrotic and viable areas. In most cells, the inclusions appear as eosinophilic ground-glass areas in the nucleus with margination of nuclear chromatin ⇒.* ***(Right)*** *Hematoxylin & eosin shows typical Cowdry type A (or type 1) viral inclusions ⇒ in some hepatocytes. These are characterized by a prominent eosinophilic inclusion surrounded by a clear halo.*

ADENOVIRUS

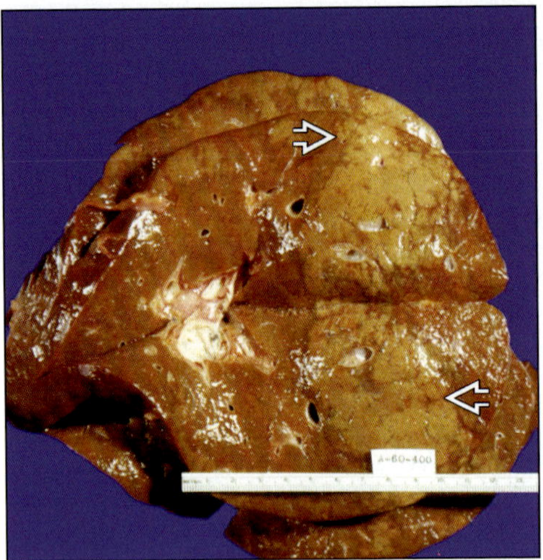

Gross photograph shows variably sized yellow-tan foci of necrosis ➪.

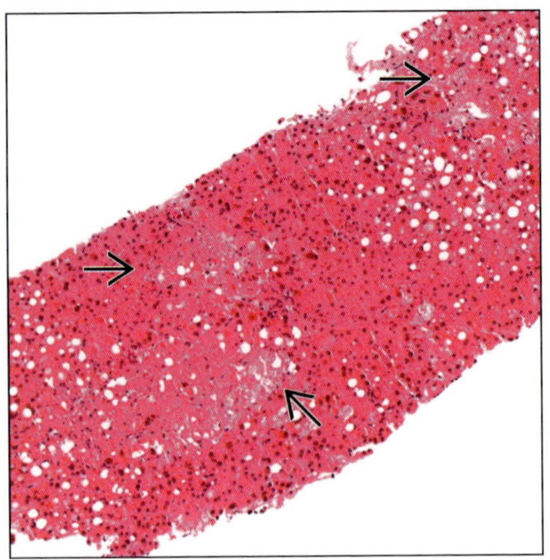

Hematoxylin & eosin stain shows foci of coagulative necrosis →. Mild steatosis is also noted, which may or may not be related to adenovirus infection.

TERMINOLOGY

Definitions

- Hepatitis caused by adenoviruses

ETIOLOGY/PATHOGENESIS

Infectious Agents

- Nonenveloped double-stranded DNA viruses that include 53 serotypes known to infect humans
- Serotypes 1, 2, and 5 are most common hepatic isolates
- Primary infection or reactivation of latent infection
- Spread by aerosolized droplets, water, fomites, and donor organs as well as fecal-oral, ocular, and nosocomial routes
- Incubation time of 2-14 days for new infection

CLINICAL ISSUES

Presentation

- Mild self-limited illnesses in immunocompetent individuals
  - Respiratory infection, keratoconjunctivitis, hemorrhagic cystitis, and gastroenteritis
- Severe diseases in immunocompromised patients
  - Hepatitis, pancreatitis, pneumonia, nephritis, encephalitis, or disseminated disease
- Fulminant hepatitis typically occurs in immunocompromised or transplant patients
  - High fever
  - Jaundice
  - Marked elevation of serum transaminase levels

Laboratory Tests

- Detection of viral DNA by polymerase chain reaction
- Direct viral antigen detection
- Viral isolation by culture
- Serology

Treatment

- No virus-specific therapy
  - Successful treatment with cidofovir, ribavirin, or serum immunoglobulin containing high titers of neutralizing antibody to adenovirus has been reported
- Symptomatic treatment
- Reduction of immunosuppression

Prognosis

- Fulminant hepatitis is usually fatal with > 50% mortality rate

MACROSCOPIC FEATURES

General Features

- Hepatomegaly with mottled foci of necrosis

MICROSCOPIC PATHOLOGY

Histologic Features

- Random small or large foci of coagulative necrosis of hepatocytes
  - No or minimal inflammatory response around necrotic foci
- Mild nonspecific lobular and portal inflammatory cell infiltrates, consisting of lymphocytes, neutrophils, and eosinophils, may be present
- Small poorly formed granulomas and microabscesses may be seen
- Intranuclear viral inclusions with characteristic smudgy nuclear appearance and chromatin margination in infected hepatocytes
  - Commonly seen at periphery of necrotic foci
  - Infected hepatocytes do not exhibit cytomegaly or multinucleation

ADENOVIRUS

Key Facts

Clinical Issues

- Fulminant hepatitis occurring in setting of severe immunosuppression

Microscopic Pathology

- Random small or large foci of coagulative necrosis of hepatocytes
- No or minimal inflammatory response around necrotic foci
- Intranuclear viral inclusions with characteristic smudgy nuclear appearance and chromatin margination in infected hepatocytes commonly seen at periphery of necrotic foci

Ancillary Tests

- Immunohistochemistry

Top Differential Diagnoses

- Herpes simplex virus hepatitis

- Rarely infect biliary tree with viral inclusions noted in biliary epithelium, causing necrotizing cholangitis and bile duct loss

Predominant Pattern/Injury Type

- Coagulative necrosis

Predominant Cell/Compartment Type

- Hepatocytes

DIFFERENTIAL DIAGNOSIS

Herpes Simplex Virus Hepatitis

- Infected hepatocytes may be slightly enlarged and multinucleated
- May show hemorrhagic appearance in areas of necrosis
- Immunohistochemical stain is helpful

Varicella-Zoster Virus Hepatitis

- Histologically indistinguishable from herpes simplex virus hepatitis
- Presence of typical skin lesions
- Immunohistochemical stain and polymerase chain reaction are helpful

Cytomegalovirus Hepatitis

- Large eosinophilic nuclear viral inclusions typically surrounded by clear halo
- Presence of cytoplasmic viral inclusions
- Typically lack large foci of coagulative necrosis
- Immunohistochemical stain is helpful

Drug-induced Hepatitis

- May show more pronounced cholestasis &/or steatosis
- Lack of characteristic viral inclusions

DIAGNOSTIC CHECKLIST

Clinically Relevant Pathologic Features

- Jaundice and hepatic failure in setting of severe immunosuppression

Pathologic Interpretation Pearls

- Foci of coagulative necrosis with no particular zonal distribution
- Characteristic nuclear viral inclusions

SELECTED REFERENCES

1. Engelmann G et al: Adenovirus infection and treatment with cidofovir in children after liver transplantation. Pediatr Transplant. 13(4):421-8, 2009
2. Echavarría M: Adenoviruses in immunocompromised hosts. Clin Microbiol Rev. 21(4):704-15, 2008
3. Hough R et al: Fatal adenovirus hepatitis during standard chemotherapy for childhood acute lymphoblastic leukemia. J Pediatr Hematol Oncol. 27(2):67-72, 2005
4. Wang WH et al: Fulminant adenovirus hepatitis following bone marrow transplantation. A case report and brief review of the literature. Arch Pathol Lab Med. 127(5):e246-8, 2003

IMAGE GALLERY

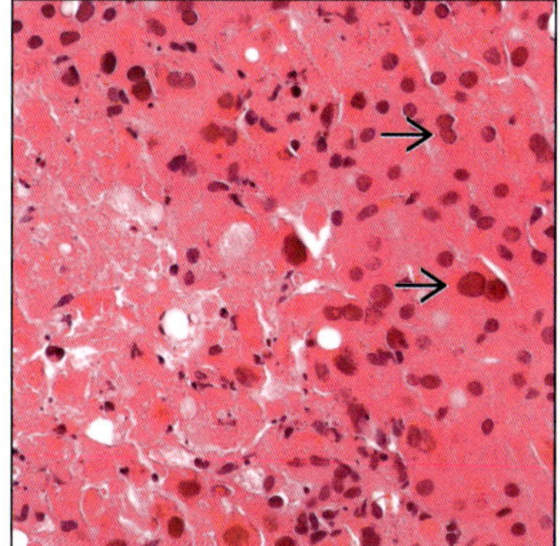

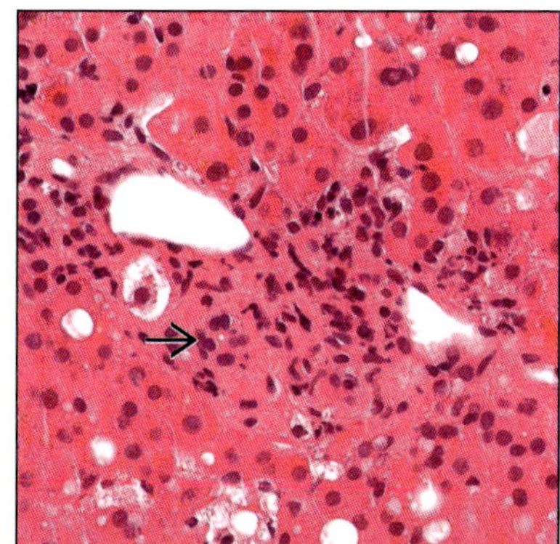

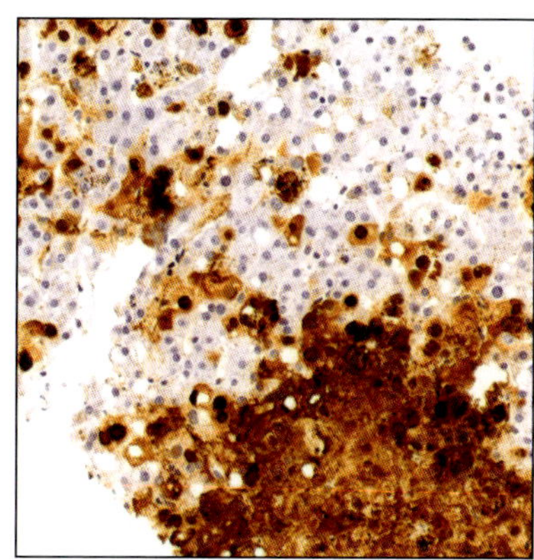

(Left) *Hematoxylin & eosin stain shows coagulative necrosis (left lower corner) with no significant inflammatory response. The infected hepatocytes exhibit smudgy nuclei and chromatin margination ⇒.* ***(Center)*** *Hematoxylin & eosin stain shows mild inflammatory cell infiltrates in the portal tract. The bile duct ⇒ is not damaged.* ***(Right)*** *Immunohistochemical stain for adenovirus highlights infected hepatocytes with nuclear, and some cytoplasmic, reactivity.*

PYOGENIC ABSCESS

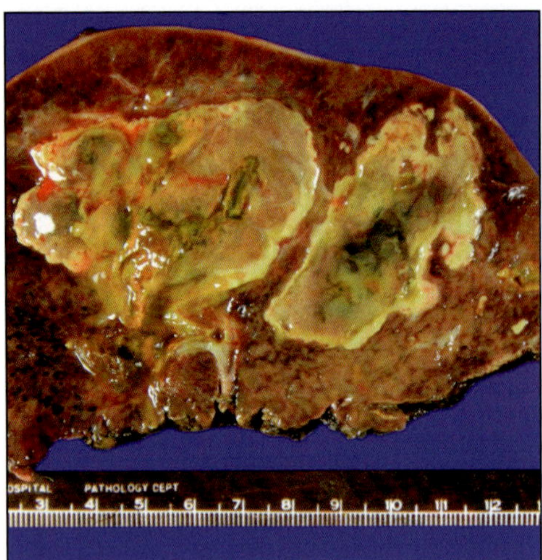

Gross photograph of a hepatectomy specimen shows large, irregular, yellow-tan soft abscesses with central green bile-stained necrosis.

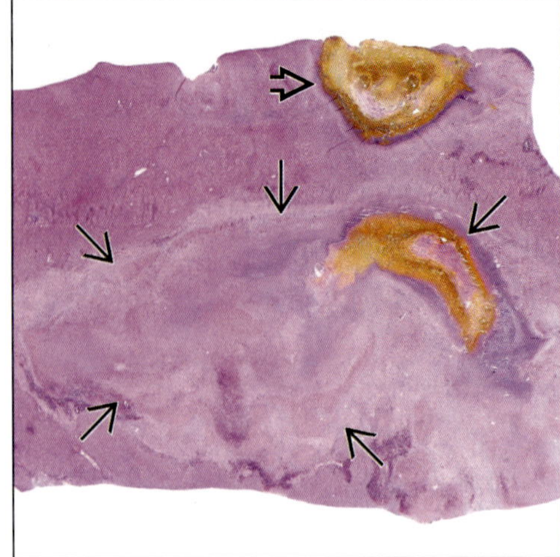

Whole mount of a paraffin section of liver abscesses shows irregular necrotic lesions ➔ with bile and inflammation. Another abscess is present at the top of the section ➩.

TERMINOLOGY

Definitions

- Localized accumulation of pus in liver with surrounding inflammation

ETIOLOGY/PATHOGENESIS

Infectious Agents

- Most commonly isolated organisms: *Escherichia coli*, *Klebsiella pneumonia*, *Enterococcus* spp., *Streptococcus* spp., and *Pseudomonas* spp.
  - Organisms that produce formic hydrogenylase (*Klebsiella* spp. and *E. coli*) can convert acids in abscess into carbon dioxide and hydrogen gas
    - Gas-forming pyogenic abscess carries higher risk of septic shock, bacteremia, and death
- Anaerobes are isolated in up to 25% of cases
  - Most commonly microaerophilic *Streptococci*, *Bacteroides fragilis*, *Fusobacterium necrophorum*, and *Clostridia* spp.
  - *Actinomyces* spp. can be associated with formation of sinus tracts
- Rare isolates include *Francisella tularensis*, *Burkholderia pseudomallei* (cause of melioidosis), *Brucella* spp. (particularly *B. suis*), and *Listeria monocytogenes*
- Fungi, such as *Candida* and *Aspergillus*, are found in 15% of cases
- At least 1/3 of cases are polymicrobial

Predisposing Conditions

- Historically associated with acute appendicitis or intraabdominal infection, particularly in children
- Biliary disease has emerged as most common etiology

CLINICAL ISSUES

Epidemiology

- Age
  - 55-60 years old
- Gender
  - Males affected more often than females

Site

- Most abscesses occur in right lobe (70%); left lobe or bilateral disease is less common

Presentation

- Symptoms include fever, chills, right upper quadrant pain, and elevated alkaline phosphatase

Laboratory Tests

- Culture of aspirated purulent material
- Culture of peripheral blood; may not correlate with pus culture results

Natural History

- Complications include metastatic infections such as endophthalmitis, meningitis, osteomyelitis, pyelonephritis, and pneumonia
  - Main risk factors for metastatic infection are diabetes and infection with *K. pneumonia*

Treatment

- Surgical approaches
  - Percutaneous drainage
  - Resection
- Drugs
  - Antibiotics

Prognosis

- Mortality from 5-31%

Associated Conditions

- Diabetes mellitus is major risk factor

PYOGENIC ABSCESS

Key Facts

Etiology/Pathogenesis

- Most commonly isolated organisms are *Escherichia coli, Klebsiella pneumonia, Enterococcus* spp., *Streptococcus* spp., and *Pseudomonas* spp.
- Anaerobes are isolated in up to 25% of cases
- Fungi, such as *Candida* and *Aspergillus*, are found in 15% of cases
- At least 1/3 of cases are polymicrobial

Clinical Issues

- Major causes include biliary disease and intraabdominal infection
- Risk factors: Diabetes mellitus, malignancy, alcohol abuse, cirrhosis, hypertension, recent surgery, and immunosuppression
- Percutaneous drainage and antibiotics are mainstay of therapy
- Main risk factors for metastatic infection are diabetes mellitus and infection with *K. pneumonia*
- Mortality ranges from 5-31%

Macroscopic Features

- Most abscesses are solitary; multiple abscesses occur in 25-45% of cases
- Right lobe most frequent site

Microscopic Pathology

- Abundant neutrophils, fibrin, and bile
- Aerobic and anaerobic culture of abscess contents and histochemical stains for organisms are required to determine cause

- Also associated with malignancy, alcohol abuse, cirrhosis, hypertension, recent surgery, and immunosuppression
- Abscesses secondary to *Yersinia enterocolitica* or *Y. pseudotuberculosis* are often associated with hemochromatosis
- Significant number are cryptogenic

MACROSCOPIC FEATURES

General Features

- Most are solitary; multiple abscesses occur in 25-45% of cases
- Appear as irregular area of softening with central liquefactive necrosis and green discoloration with variable surrounding fibrosis

MICROSCOPIC PATHOLOGY

Histologic Features

- Collection of neutrophils with fibrin, bile, or necrotic debris
- Surrounding fibrosis variable
- Additional findings may be seen depending on causative organism, such as sulfur granules in *Actinomyces* infection
- Cholangitis may be seen

Ancillary Studies

- Histochemical stains for organisms
  - Tissue Gram stain, fungal silver stain, acid-fast stain, PAS stain, and Steiner stain
- Aerobic and anaerobic culture of abscess contents

DIFFERENTIAL DIAGNOSIS

Tuberculous Abscess

- Immunocompromised patient
- Numerous acid-fast bacilli on acid-fast stain

Recurrent Pyogenic Cholangitis

- Patients from the Far East or Asian immigrants
- Recurrent attacks of suppurative cholangitis with hepatic stones
- Associated with biliary parasites, usually *Clonorchis sinensis* or *Ascaris lumbricoides*

Ascariasis

- Patient from endemic area with biliary abnormalities or prior sphincterotomy
- Dead or dying worms, or ova, can be found in abscess along with bile and bacteria

Amebiasis

- Amoebic trophozoites imbedded in necrotic rim of abscess; positive serology

DIAGNOSTIC CHECKLIST

Pathologic Interpretation Pearls

- Steiner is good screening stain as it stains dead or degenerated organisms

SELECTED REFERENCES

1. Fang CT et al: Klebsiella pneumoniae genotype K1: an emerging pathogen that causes septic ocular or central nervous system complications from pyogenic liver abscess. Clin Infect Dis. 45(3):284-93, 2007
2. Ruiz-Hernández JJ et al: Pyogenic liver abscesses: mortality-related factors. Eur J Gastroenterol Hepatol. 19(10):853-8, 2007
3. Thomsen RW et al: Diabetes mellitus and pyogenic liver abscess: risk and prognosis. Clin Infect Dis. 44(9):1194-201, 2007
4. Rahimian J et al: Pyogenic liver abscess: recent trends in etiology and mortality. Clin Infect Dis. 39(11):1654-9, 2004
5. Bergmann TK et al: Multiple hepatic abscesses due to Yersinia enterocolitica infection secondary to primary haemochromatosis. Scand J Gastroenterol. 36(8):891-5, 2001
6. Zibari GB et al: Pyogenic liver abscess. Surg Infect (Larchmt). 1(1):15-21, 2000

PYOGENIC ABSCESS

Microscopic Features

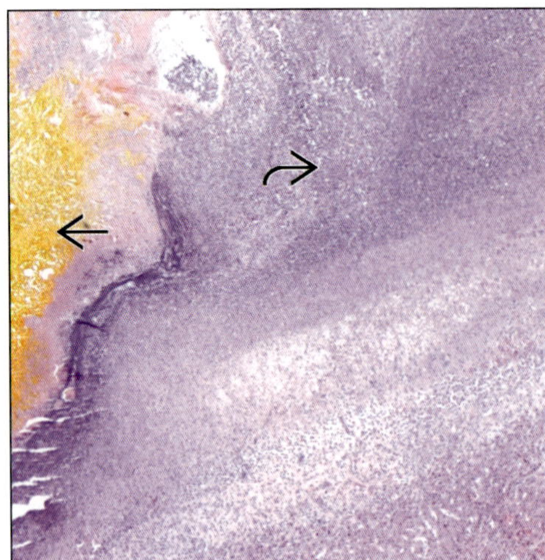

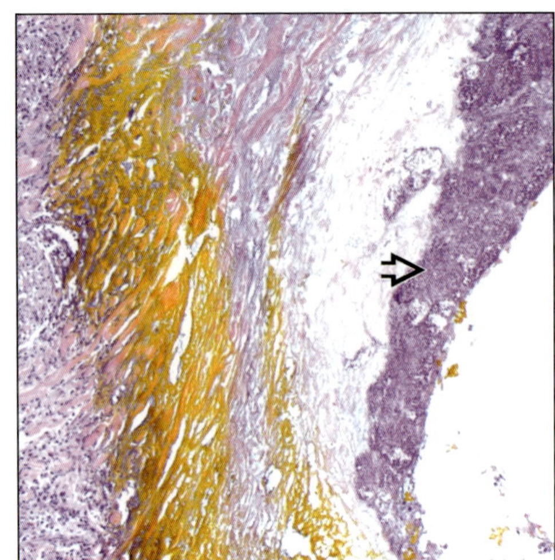

(Left) Paraffin section of a large liver abscess shows a large amount of pus ⮫, fibrin, and bile →. Uninvolved liver parenchyma is seen in lower right corner. **(Right)** Higher magnification of a liver abscess shows bile, fibrin, and bacteria ⇨ within the abscess.

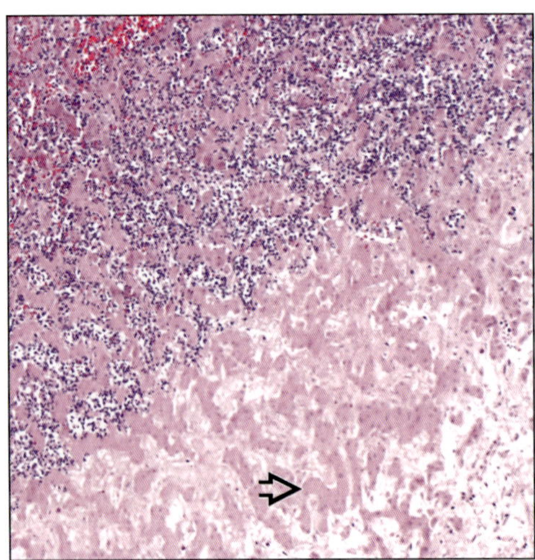

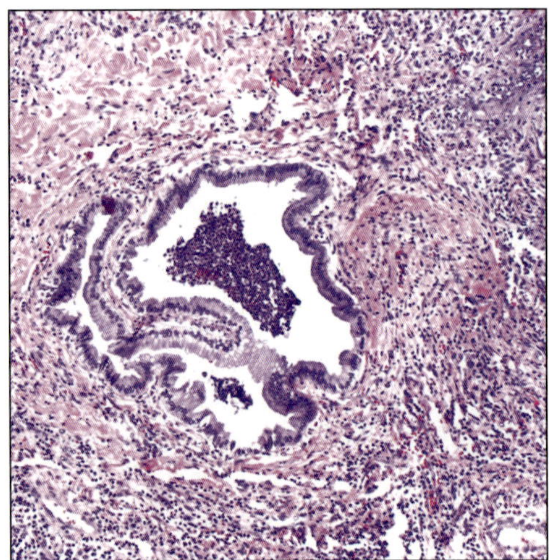

(Left) In this region of the abscess, necrotic liver parenchyma is identifiable by the hepatic plate architecture ⇨. The necrotic parenchyma is infiltrated with neutrophils (upper left). **(Right)** Paraffin section adjacent to a large liver abscess shows areas of suppurative cholangitis with accumulation of neutrophils and fibrin within a duct. Cholangitis may occur secondary to the inflammation in the liver, but many abscesses result from suppurative cholangitis.

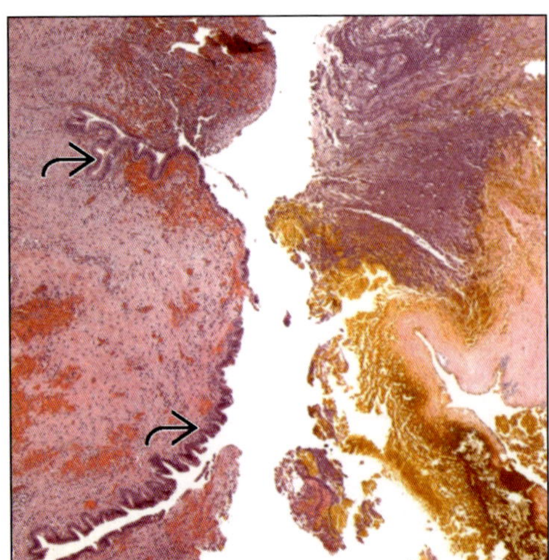

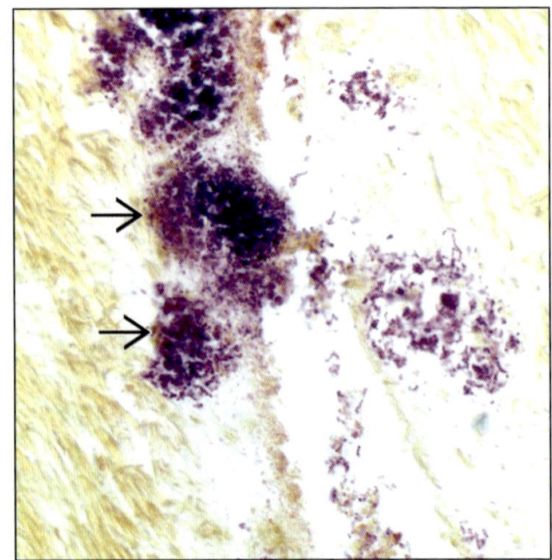

(Left) Paraffin section of a large liver abscess with bile, fibrin, and neutrophils (right) shows residual duct lining focally ⮫, suggesting origin from suppurative cholangitis. **(Right)** Tissue Gram stain shows clusters of gram-positive cocci → in this liver abscess that proved to be Enterococcus on microbiologic culture of purulent material.

Microscopic Features

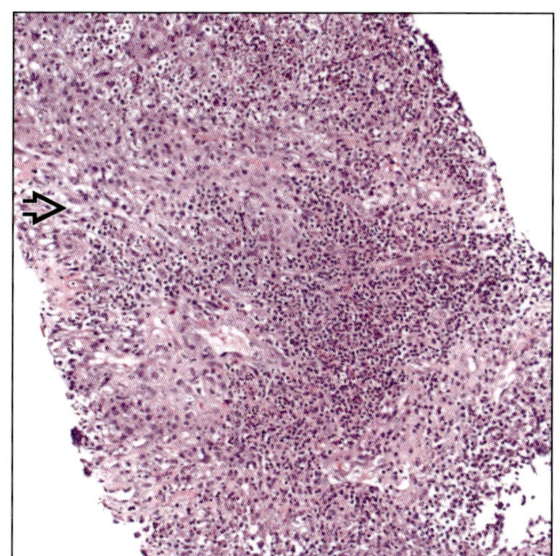

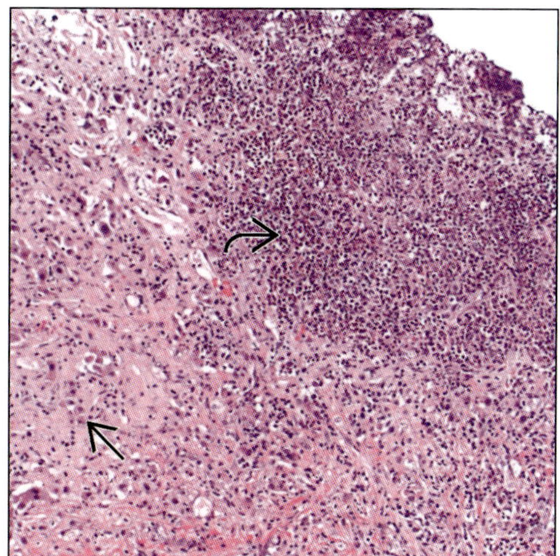

(Left) *Biopsy of a liver with pyogenic abscess shows dense neutrophilic infiltration and entrapped hepatocytes ⇨.* ***(Right)*** *Medium-power view of a liver biopsy with pyogenic abscess shows a dense neutrophil accumulation ↷ surrounded by inflammatory cells, edema, and entrapped hepatocytes →.*

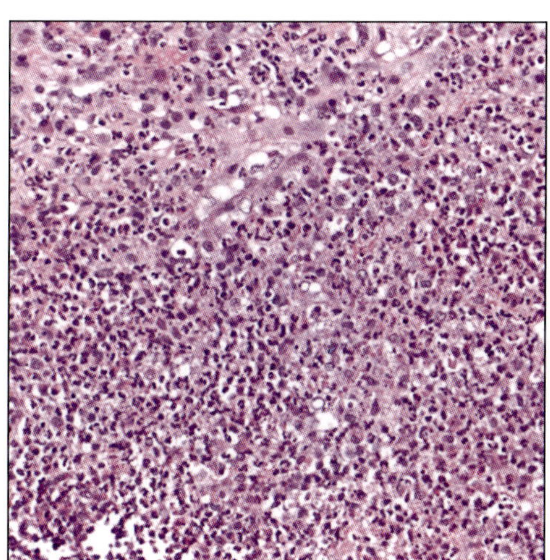

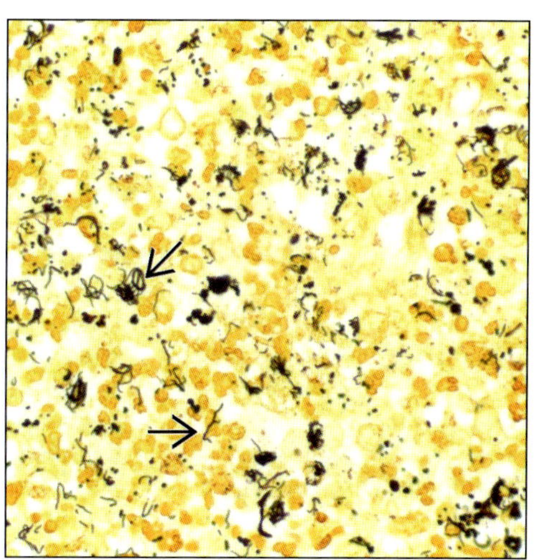

(Left) *Dense neutrophilic inflammation characterizes pyogenic liver abscess.* ***(Right)*** *Steiner stain shows a mixture of bacteria, including long slender rod-shaped bacteria → consistent with polymicrobial abscess; culture showed mixed anaerobes.*

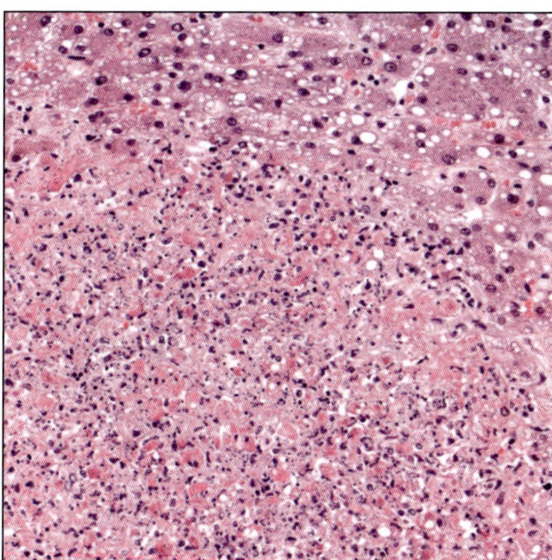

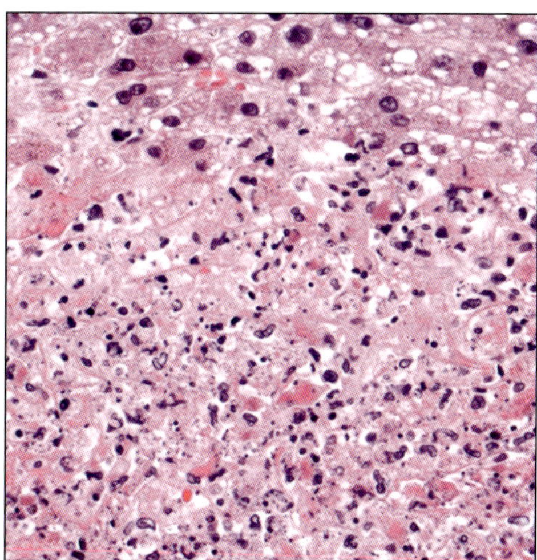

(Left) *Necrotic abscess in the lower 1/2 of the field is adjacent to hepatocytes with steatosis in pyogenic abscess secondary to listeria.* ***(Right)*** *High-power view of hepatic abscess in listeriosis shows abundant necrosis admixed with histiocytes and debris (lower 1/2 of field). The viable hepatocytes in this case show steatosis (upper 1/2).*

SEPSIS IN THE LIVER

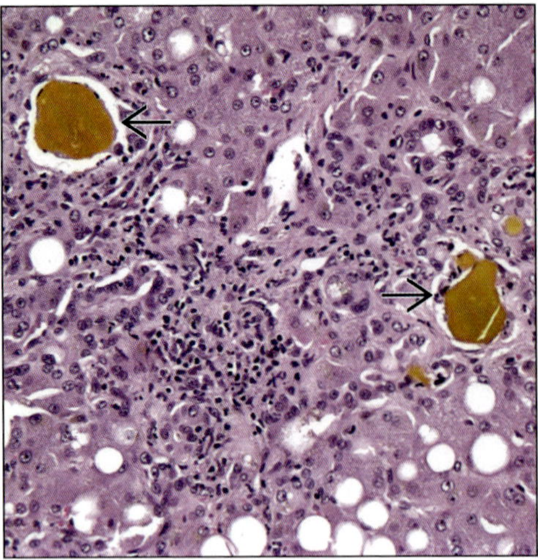

Hematoxylin & eosin shows proliferated bile ductules at the periphery of the portal tract that contain dense, inspissated bile ⇒ (ductular cholestasis).

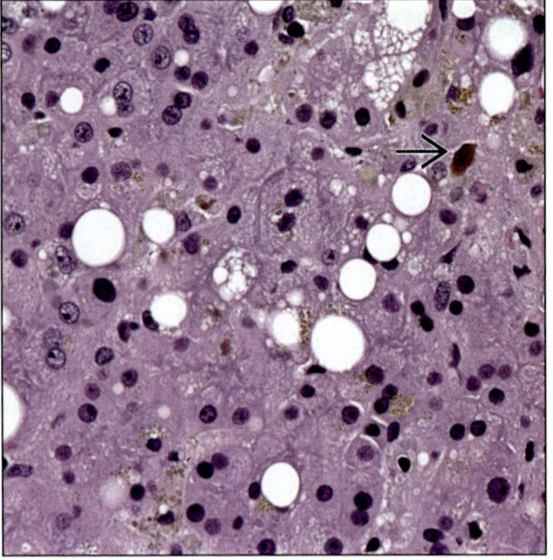

Hematoxylin & eosin shows canalicular cholestasis ⇒ without significant accompanying inflammation. "Pure" cholestasis is common in infants and children.

TERMINOLOGY

Definitions

- Spectrum of hepatic injury in patients with sepsis or bacteremia

ETIOLOGY/PATHOGENESIS

Infectious Agents

- Systemic infection, usually bacterial
  - Most common underlying infectious processes
    - Bacterial pneumonia
    - Intraabdominal suppurative infection
- Mechanism uncertain
  - Presumably, bacterial endotoxins interfere with normal ductular secretory activity and resorption

CLINICAL ISSUES

Presentation

- Patients are systemically ill from sepsis/bacteremia
  - May be in shock
- Jaundice is common

Laboratory Tests

- Enzyme elevations
  - Hepatitis pattern
  - Cholestatic pattern
  - Mixed hepatitic and cholestatic enzyme elevations
- Blood cultures may reveal infectious organism

Treatment

- Treat underlying infection

Prognosis

- Depends on severity of underlying infection
- Patients are often severely ill with poor prognosis

MACROSCOPIC FEATURES

General Features

- Variably present hepatomegaly

MICROSCOPIC PATHOLOGY

Histologic Features

- Neutrophilic inflammation
  - May be portal &/or lobular
  - Variably present microabscesses
  - Clusters of bacteria occasionally seen within microabscesses
- Cholestatic pattern
  - Centrilobular canalicular cholestasis
  - Proliferated bile ductules at perimeter of portal tracts with inspissated bile ("ductular cholestasis")
  - Periductular neutrophilic infiltrate
  - Ductules may be dilated, with atrophic and flattened epithelium
  - "Pure" cholestasis with no significant inflammation is fairly common in sepsis, especially in infants and children
- Additional findings
  - Focal hepatocyte necrosis
  - Centrilobular &/or midzonal fatty change, usually microvesicular
  - Kupffer cell hyperplasia
- Many cases have mixed features of several of above patterns
- Patients in septic shock may have ischemic necrosis, particularly in perivenular distribution

Predominant Pattern/Injury Type

- Inflammatory, acute
- Cholestasis

Predominant Cell/Compartment Type

- Hepatocyte

SEPSIS IN THE LIVER

Key Facts

Terminology
- Spectrum of hepatic injury in patients with sepsis or bacteremia

Etiology/Pathogenesis
- Usually caused by sepsis from underlying bacterial pneumonia or intraabdominal infection

Clinical Issues
- Patients are systemically ill from sepsis/bacteremia
- Jaundice is common
- Enzyme elevations may be hepatitic, cholestatic, or mixed

Microscopic Pathology
- Ductular cholestasis pattern strongly associated with sepsis
  - Proliferated bile ductules at perimeter of portal tracts with inspissated bile
- Neutrophilic inflammation also common

- Bile ductule

DIFFERENTIAL DIAGNOSIS

Large Bile Duct Obstruction
- Histologic features may be very similar
- Obstruction generally shows ductal rather than ductular cholestasis
- May need clinical history to differentiate

Adverse Drug Reaction
- May show ductular cholestasis or "pure" cholestasis, both of which can mimic sepsis

Total Parenteral Nutrition
- May also show ductular cholestasis

Other Infectious Processes
- Viral, fungal, or bacterial infections of liver

Biliary Atresia in Newborns
- May also show ductular cholestasis

DIAGNOSTIC CHECKLIST

Clinically Relevant Pathologic Features
- Elevated liver enzymes in patients who are septic/ bacteremic

Pathologic Interpretation Pearls
- Sepsis produces many different histologic patterns in liver
- Cholestatic pattern may mimic large bile duct obstruction
- Ductular cholestasis pattern is strongly associated with sepsis
- Caveat
  - Many entities in differential diagnosis above can coexist along with sepsis
  - May confound histologic picture

SELECTED REFERENCES

1. Hawker F: Liver dysfunction in critical illness. Anaesth Intensive Care. 19(2):165-81, 1991
2. Cone LA et al: Clinical and bacteriologic observations of a toxic shock-like syndrome due to Streptococcus pyogenes. N Engl J Med. 317(3):146-9, 1987
3. Banks JG et al: Liver function in septic shock. J Clin Pathol. 35(11):1249-52, 1982
4. Caruana JA Jr et al: Functional and histopathologic changes in the liver during sepsis. Surg Gynecol Obstet. 154(5):653-6, 1982
5. Lefkowitch JH: Bile ductular cholestasis: an ominous histopathologic sign related to sepsis and "cholangitis lenta". Hum Pathol. 13(1):19-24, 1982
6. Jaundice due to bacterial infection. Gastroenterology. 77(2):362-74, 1979

IMAGE GALLERY

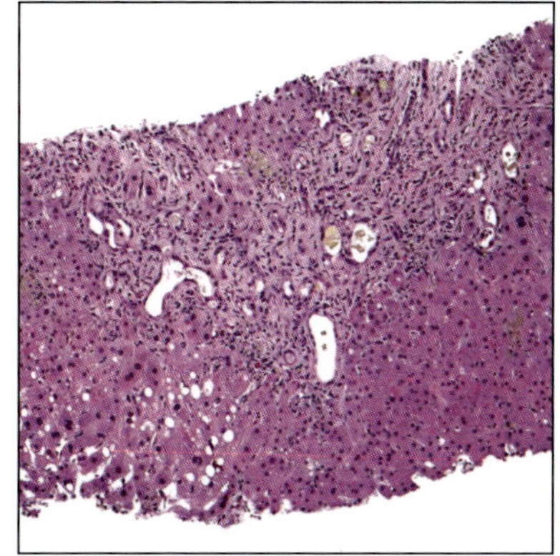

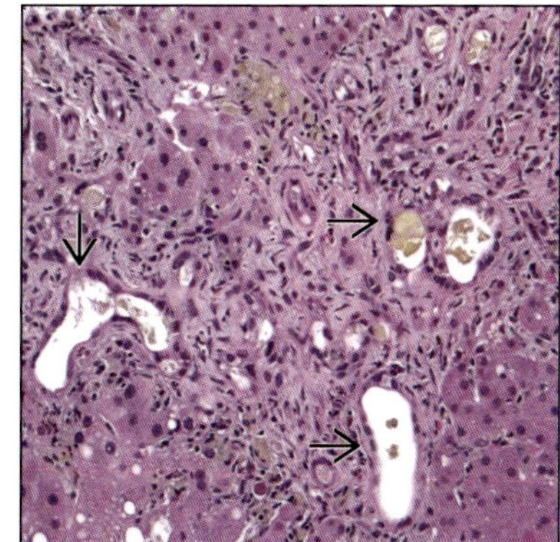

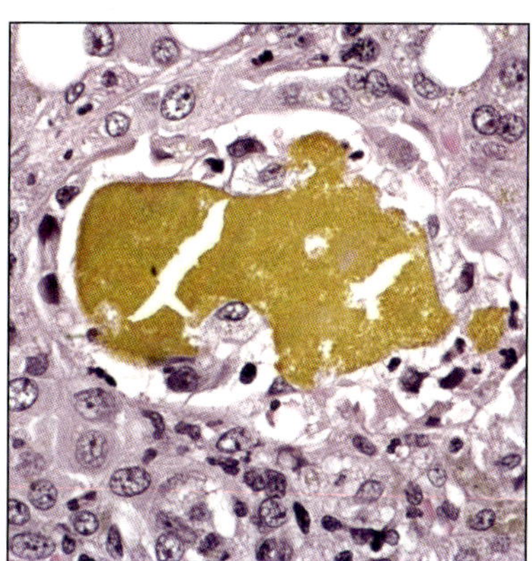

(Left) A low-power photograph of a liver biopsy specimen in a septic patient shows expanded portal tracts with proliferated bile ductules, which contain inspissated bile, at the edges. (Center) Hematoxylin & eosin shows a portal tract containing mixed inflammation with numerous eosinophils. Proliferated bile ductules are present at the edge of the portal tract, containing inspissated bile ⇒. (Right) Hematoxylin & eosin shows a high-power view of a bile ductule with flattened, atrophic epithelium. The ductule contains dense, inspissated bile.

MYCOBACTERIUM TUBERCULOSIS

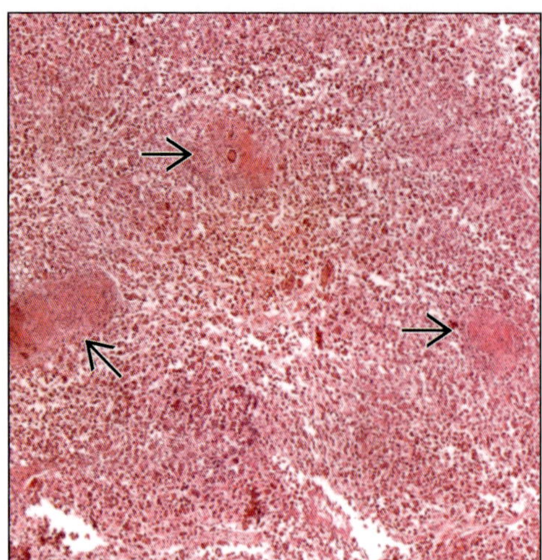

Paraffin section of the liver from an autopsy of a patient who died of miliary TB shows multiple necrotizing granulomas ⇒.

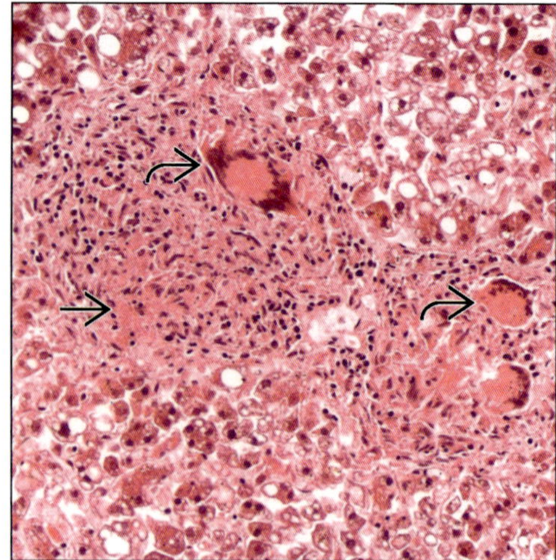

High-power view of hepatic miliary tuberculosis shows a granuloma with focal eosinophilic granular necrotic material ⇒ and several multinucleated giant cells ↪.

TERMINOLOGY

Abbreviations

- *Mycobacterium tuberculosis* (MTB)
- Tuberculosis (TB)

Definitions

- Infection by *M. tuberculosis*

ETIOLOGY/PATHOGENESIS

Infectious Agents

- *Mycobacterium tuberculosis*
  - Cell wall rich in mycolic acid makes organism impervious to Gram staining
  - Acid-fast staining demonstrates bacterium

CLINICAL ISSUES

Epidemiology

- Incidence
  - Hepatic TB accounts for 1% of TB infections

Presentation

- In primary TB, liver is usually involved as part of disseminated TB
  - Elevated alkaline phosphatase and hyponatremia are common
- In reactivation TB, liver can be involved as part of multiorgan involvement (typically lungs) or alone
- Tuberculoma can occur from coalescence of granulomas
  - Mimics neoplasm
  - Can cause obstructive jaundice from compression of bile ducts
  - Can cause portal hypertension from compression of portal vein
- In immunocompromised patients, TB can present as generalized wasting syndrome
  - Can develop tuberculous abscesses
- Tuberculous cholangitis (infection of biliary tree) is rare
  - Presents with biliary strictures and obstructive jaundice

Natural History

- Respiratory symptoms or chest radiographs suggestive of pulmonary TB seen in 65-78% of patients

Treatment

- Drugs
  - Antituberculous regimens similar to those used to treat TB infecting other sites

Prognosis

- Mortality ranges from 10-40%

IMAGE FINDINGS

CT Findings

- Hepatic calcifications in 1/2 of cases

MACROSCOPIC FEATURES

General Features

- In most cases, hepatic TB is not grossly visible
- Tuberculomas appear as cheesy or chalky white, irregular nodules

MICROSCOPIC PATHOLOGY

Histologic Features

- Primary TB is characterized by numerous granulomas with central amorphous granular necrotic debris (caseating necrosis)
- Reactivation TB that involves liver is characterized by numerous granulomas, more often without central necrosis

MYCOBACTERIUM TUBERCULOSIS

Key Facts

Clinical Issues
- In primary TB, liver is usually involved as part of disseminated TB
- Reactivation TB can involve liver along with lungs or liver alone
- Evidence of pulmonary TB in 65-78% of patients

Microscopic Pathology
- Numerous granulomas with or without central necrosis
  - Coalescence of granulomas can produce tuberculoma
- Immunocompromised patients have poorly developed granulomas or abscesses

Ancillary Tests
- Acid-fast stains positive in 60% of cases
- Culture is more likely to be positive in cases with caseating necrosis
- PCR has 53-88% sensitivity and 96-100% specificity

- Tuberculomas are composed of confluent granulomas and contain few organisms
- TB in immunocompromised patients shows poorly formed granulomas or collections of foamy histiocytes with innumerable organisms
  - Tuberculous abscesses are centrally suppurative and contain numerous organisms

Ancillary Techniques
- Acid-fast stains positive in up to 60% of cases
- Culture is more likely to be positive in cases with caseating necrosis
- PCR has sensitivity of 53-88% and specificity of 96-100%

DIFFERENTIAL DIAGNOSIS

Sarcoidosis
- Numerous granulomas that may be aggregated in fibrotic mass
- Typically nonnecrotizing

Drug-induced Liver Injury
- Nonnecrotizing granulomas, often associated with cholestatic hepatitis and duct injury

Fungal Infection
- Requires methenamine silver stain for diagnosis
- Fungal culture

Bacterial Infection
- Depending on organism, can be associated with necrotizing granulomas
- Requires culture, histochemical stain, &/or PCR for diagnosis depending on organism

Mycobacterial Infection
- Other mycobacterial species (e.g., leprosy, atypical mycobacteria) can look similar
- Clinical features, mycobacterial culture, or PCR

DIAGNOSTIC CHECKLIST

Pathologic Interpretation Pearls
- Mycobacterial infection must always be considered in cases of granulomatous hepatitis, particularly when granulomas show central necrosis

SELECTED REFERENCES

1. Chong VH: Hepatobiliary tuberculosis: a review of presentations and outcomes. South Med J. 101(4):356-61, 2008
2. Wang JY et al: Disseminated tuberculosis: a 10-year experience in a medical center. Medicine (Baltimore). 86(1):39-46, 2007
3. Maharaj B et al: A prospective study of hepatic tuberculosis in 41 black patients. Q J Med. 63(242):517-22, 1987
4. Essop AR et al: Tuberculosis hepatitis: a clinical review of 96 cases. Q J Med. 53(212):465-77, 1984

IMAGE GALLERY

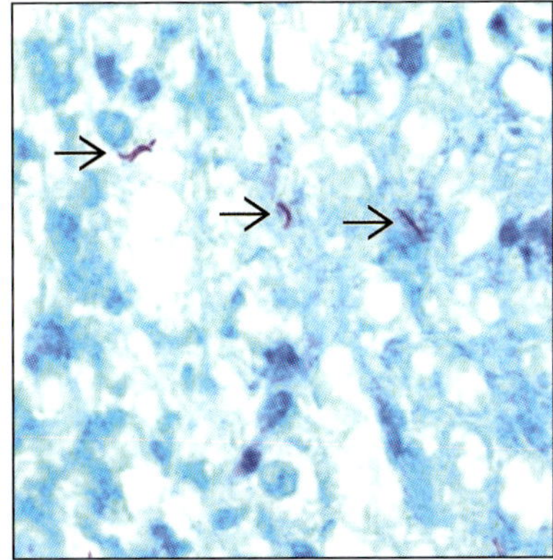

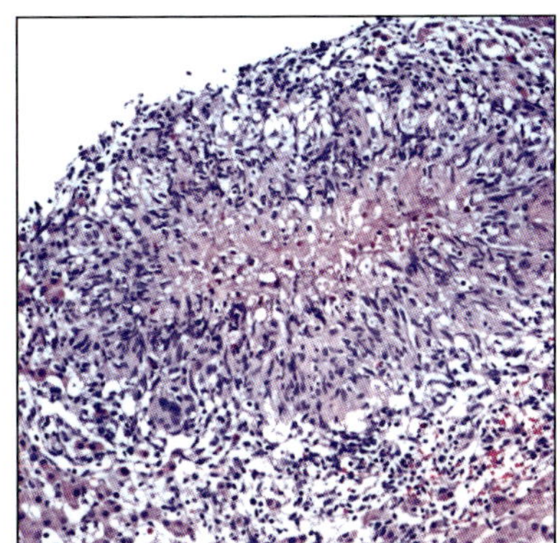

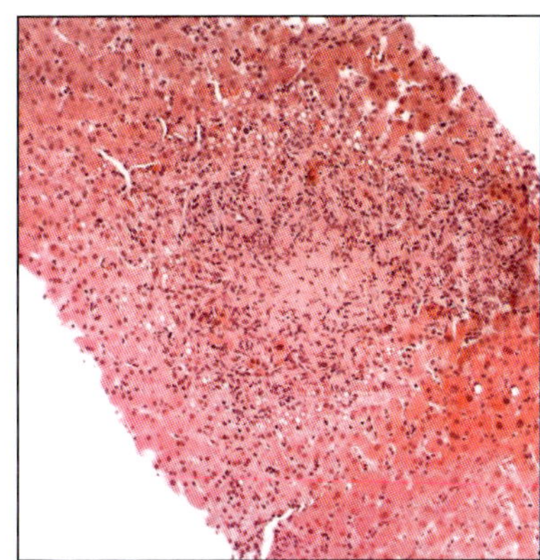

*(**Left**) Acid-fast stain shows a few acid-fast bacteria ⇒ with a slender, beaded appearance, consistent with M. tuberculosis. (**Center**) A necrotizing granuloma features central necrosis surrounded by a rim of palisading histiocytes and lymphocytes. (**Right**) Liver biopsy in hepatic TB shows an expansile granuloma with central amorphous granular material, typical of caseating necrosis.*

ATYPICAL MYCOBACTERIA

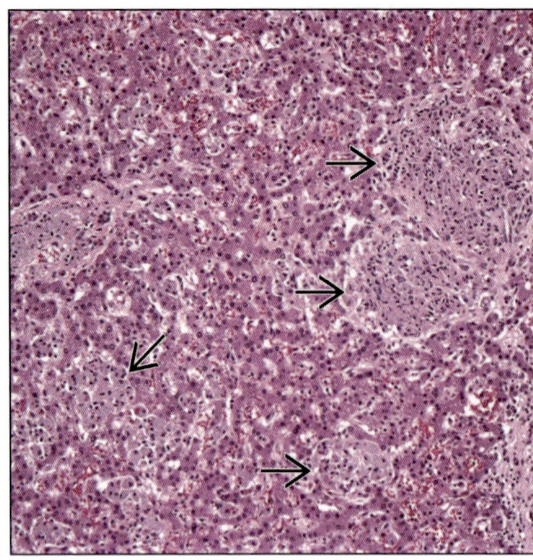

Paraffin section of liver in MAC infection shows several loose aggregates of histiocytes and poorly formed granulomas ➔.

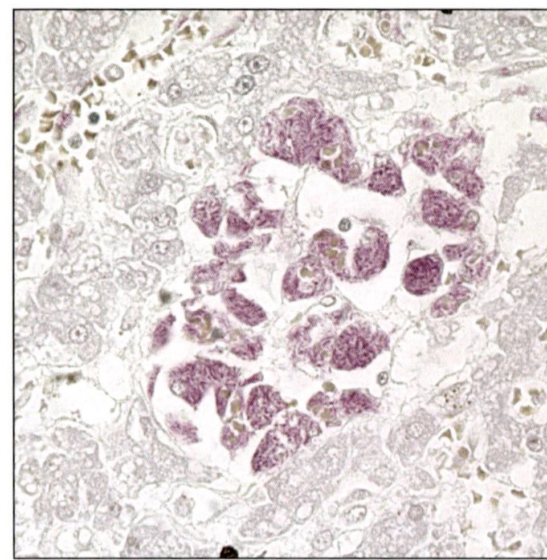

Acid-fast stain shows innumerable acid-fast bacteria within clustered histiocytes in a patient with MAC infection.

TERMINOLOGY

Abbreviations

- *Mycobacterium avium-intracellulare* complex (MAC)

Definitions

- Infection by any one of many species of mycobacteria that does not cause tuberculosis or leprosy

ETIOLOGY/PATHOGENESIS

Infectious Agents

- Atypical mycobacteria are potentially pathogenic environmental mycobacteria (a.k.a. mycobacteria other than tuberculosis)
  - Includes *M. avium, M. intracellulare, M. kansasii, M. marinum, M. gordonae, M. chelonae, M. scrofulaceum, M. szulgai, M. malmoense, M. xenopi, M. abscessus,* and *M. fortuitum*
  - Classified according to growth rate, presence or absence, and type of pigment
  - *M. avium* and *M. intracellulare*, known together as *M. avium-intracellulare* complex (MAC), are nonchromogens and the most common of atypical mycobacteria to cause hepatic disease
  - Next to MAC, *M. kansasii* is most common cause of nontuberculous mycobacterial infection in HIV patients

CLINICAL ISSUES

Epidemiology

- Incidence
  - Up to 35% of all AIDS patients develop disseminated MAC eventually
    - 1-year incidence is 3% among patients with CD4 counts between 100 and 199 cells/μL and 39% for patients with CD4 counts less than 10 cells/μL
    - Frequency is decreasing with widespread use of highly active antiretroviral therapy (HAART)
  - Worldwide distribution
- Gender
  - More common in males, mirroring HIV prevalence

Site

- Most commonly causes pulmonary disease, lymphadenitis, skin and soft tissue infection

Presentation

- Fever
- Hepatomegaly
- Elevated alkaline phosphatase
- Patients treated with HAART may develop clinical manifestations of disseminated MAC due to immune reconstitution inflammatory syndrome (IRIS)

Laboratory Tests

- Mycobacterial blood culture establishes diagnosis in 86-98% of patients with MAC confirmed at autopsy

Treatment

- Drugs
  - 2 or more antibiotics with activity against atypical mycobacteria

Prognosis

- Median survival is 6 months, with only 24% of patients surviving for 1 year
  - Poor survival is often function of advanced AIDS rather than disseminated MAC infection

Risk Factors

- AIDS, malignancy, chronic renal disease, chronic pulmonary disease, cystic fibrosis, and alcoholism
  - In AIDS, most patients have CD4 counts less than 50 cells/μL

ATYPICAL MYCOBACTERIA

Key Facts

Terminology
- Infection by mycobacteria other than tuberculosis or leprosy

Etiology/Pathogenesis
- Exposure is almost inevitable due to ubiquitous presence of atypical mycobacteria as environmental saprophytes
- *M. avium* and *M. intracellulare*, known together as *M. avium-intracellulare* complex (MAC), are most common atypical mycobacteria to cause hepatic disease

Clinical Issues
- Common opportunistic infection in AIDS patients, particularly those that have CD4 counts less than 50 cells/µL
- Presents with fever, hepatomegaly, and elevated alkaline phosphatase
- Median survival is 6 months

Microscopic Pathology
- Poorly formed granulomas, loose aggregates of histiocytes or of foamy histiocytes with numerous acid-fast organisms on acid-fast bacterial stain
- Areas of necrosis with nuclear debris surrounded by loose collections of histiocytes and liver abscesses
- Fibrin ring granulomas are rare

Ancillary Tests
- Histochemical stain for acid-fast bacteria
- PCR can be performed on paraffin-embedded tissue
- Blood mycobacterial culture

IMAGE FINDINGS

CT Findings
- Hepatomegaly, uniform attenuation of lymph nodes, and clustered pattern of lymph nodes

MICROSCOPIC PATHOLOGY

Histologic Features
- Poorly formed granulomas, aggregates of histiocytes or foamy histiocytes
  - Numerous acid-fast organisms on acid-fast bacterial stain in histiocytes and nearby Kupffer cells
- Necrotic areas filled with inflammatory cells and nuclear debris or liver abscess
- In patients with preserved T-cell function, granulomas can be well formed and nonnecrotizing with few organisms on acid-fast bacterial stain, similar to tuberculosis
- Fibrin ring granulomas have been described

ANCILLARY TESTS

Histochemistry
- Acid-fast bacterial stain
  - Reactivity: Positive

PCR
- Can be performed on paraffin-embedded tissue
- Can distinguish atypical mycobacteria from tuberculosis

DIFFERENTIAL DIAGNOSIS

Tuberculosis
- Granulomas more apt to be well formed with caseating necrosis and fewer organisms
- Clinical setting, culture, or PCR specific for atypical mycobacteria may be necessary

Histoplasmosis
- Can also cause aggregates of foamy histiocytes in immunocompromised patients
- Methenamine silver stain demonstrates yeast in histiocytes
  - Caveat: GMS stain will also stain rapidly dividing atypical mycobacteria
- Fungal culture yields *H. capsulatum*

Q Fever
- Prototypical disease associated with fibrin ring granulomas
- Rickettsial disease that usually manifests as pneumonitis or endocarditis
- Complement-fixing antibodies to *C. burnetii* antigen in serum

Leprosy
- Lepromatous leprosy shows aggregates of foamy histiocytes
- Clinical setting, culture, PCR

DIAGNOSTIC CHECKLIST

Pathologic Interpretation Pearls
- Aggregates of foamy histiocytes in liver biopsy from patient with AIDS warrants stains for acid-fast organisms

SELECTED REFERENCES

1. Flegg PJ et al: Disseminated disease due to Mycobacterium avium complex in AIDS. QJM. 88(9):617-26, 1995
2. Chin DP: Mycobacterium avium complex and other nontuberculous mycobacterial infections in patients with HIV. Semin Respir Infect. 8(2):124-38, 1993
3. Inderlied CB et al: The Mycobacterium avium complex. Clin Microbiol Rev. 6(3):266-310, 1993
4. Farhi DC et al: Pathologic findings in disseminated Mycobacterium avium-intracellulare infection. A report of 11 cases. Am J Clin Pathol. 85(1):67-72, 1986

ATYPICAL MYCOBACTERIA

Microscopic Features

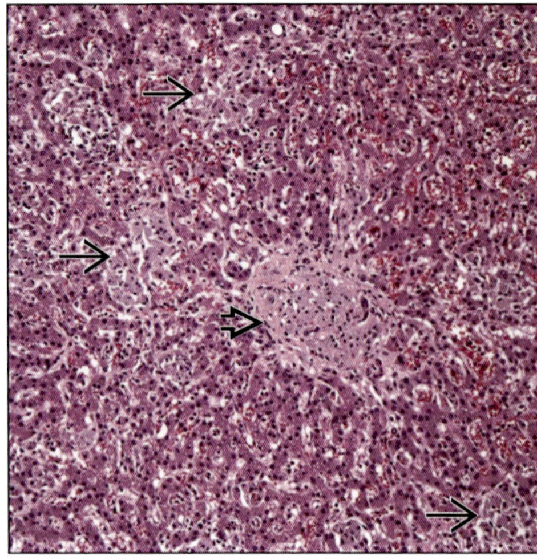

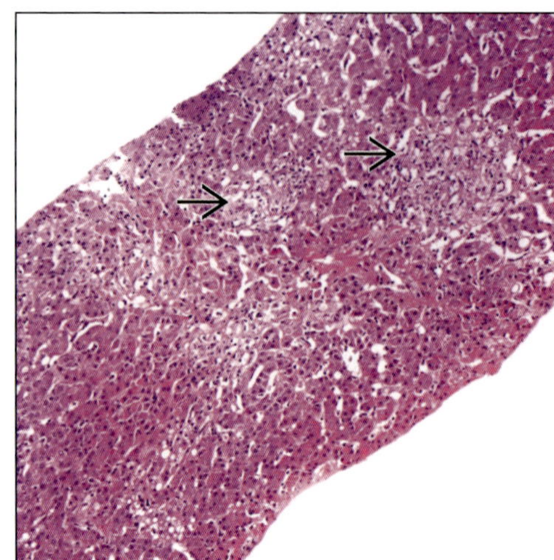

(Left) *Paraffin section of liver with MAC infection shows a large aggregate of histiocytes forming a loose granuloma ⇨ as well as several clusters of histiocytes that are not forming granulomas at all →.* ***(Right)*** *Paraffin section of a liver biopsy in a patient with MAC infection shows poorly formed granulomas →.*

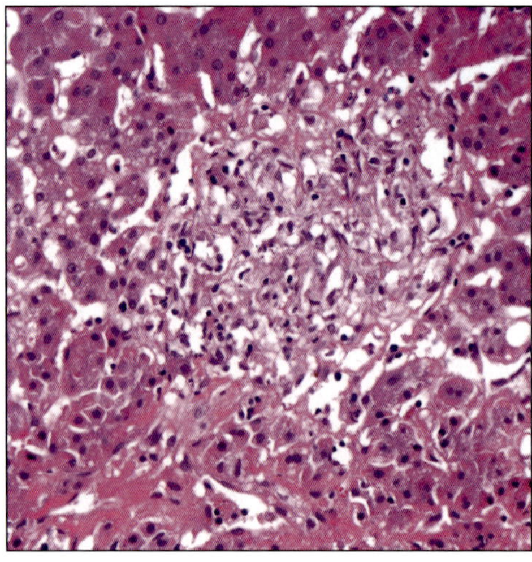

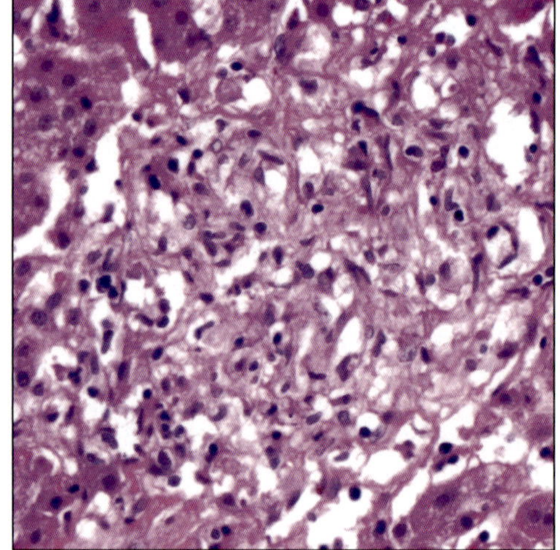

(Left) *High magnification of a poorly formed granuloma in MAC infection shows a rounded, loose collection of histiocytes.* ***(Right)*** *A poorly formed granuloma in MAC infection appears as a rounded cellular aggregate of histiocytes with ill-defined borders.*

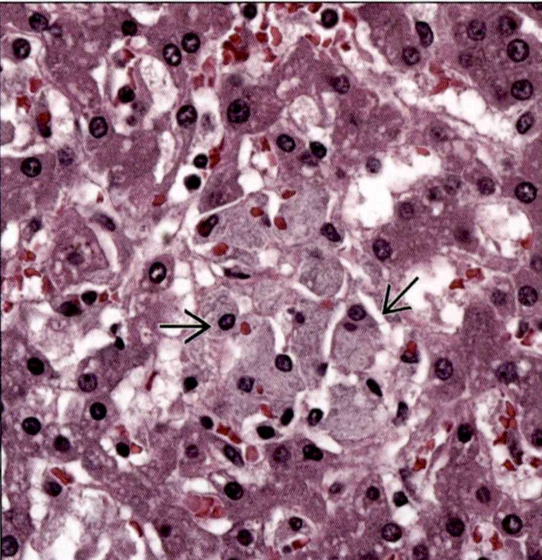

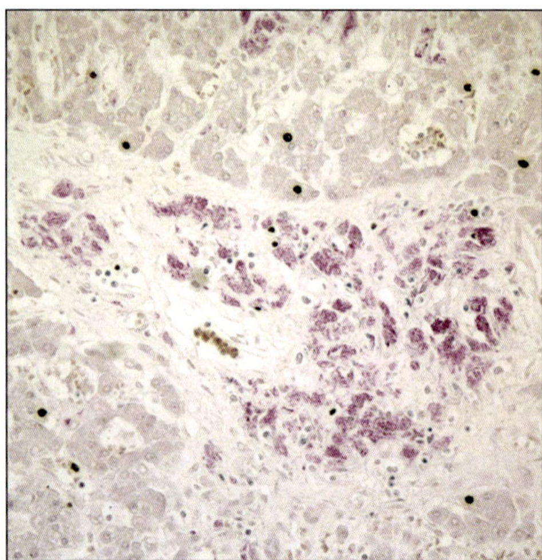

(Left) *An aggregate of foamy histiocytes → is shown in the hepatic lobule in a patient with MAC infection.* ***(Right)*** *Acid-fast stain shows numerous acid-fast bacilli in portal macrophages in an immunocompromised patient with MAC infection.*

ATYPICAL MYCOBACTERIA

Microscopic Features

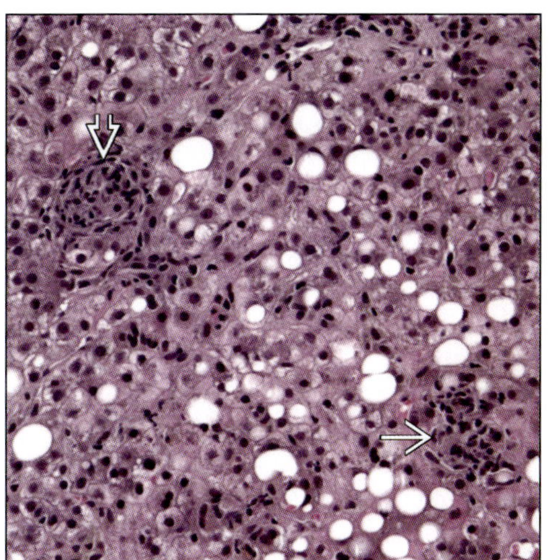
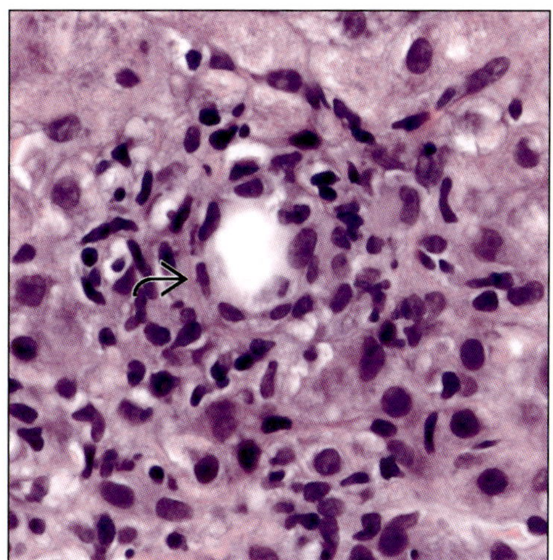

(Left) *In this case of MAC infection, there are several clusters of histiocytes ➡ and loose granulomas ⇨ in a steatotic background.* ***(Right)*** *A fibrin ring granuloma is present in a patient with MAC infection. Note the central lipid vacuole surrounded by a layer of histiocytes, a ring of fibrin ↷, and more peripheral histiocytes.*

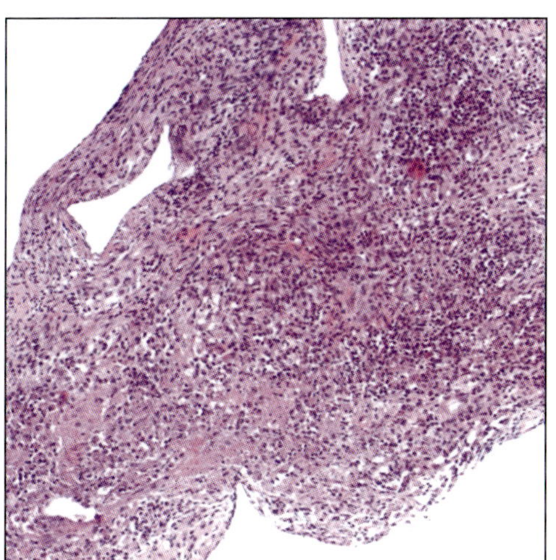
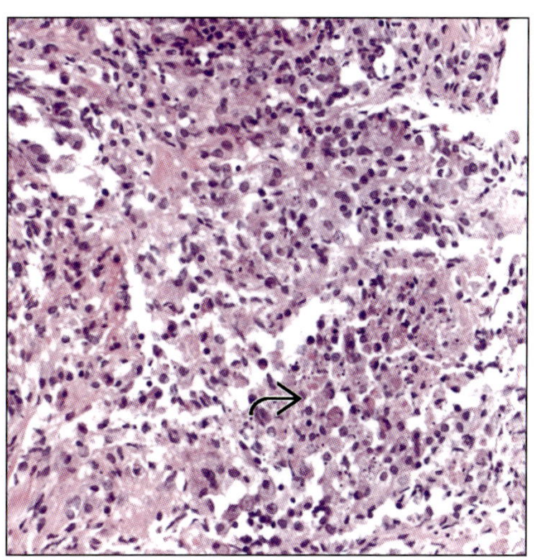

(Left) *Liver biopsy in a patient with M. kansasii infection shows a mixture of necrosis, histiocytes, and acute inflammation without well-formed granulomas.* ***(Right)*** *Higher magnification of liver biopsy in M. kansasii infection shows areas of necrosis and nuclear debris ↷ surrounded by loose sheets of histiocytes without well-formed granulomas.*

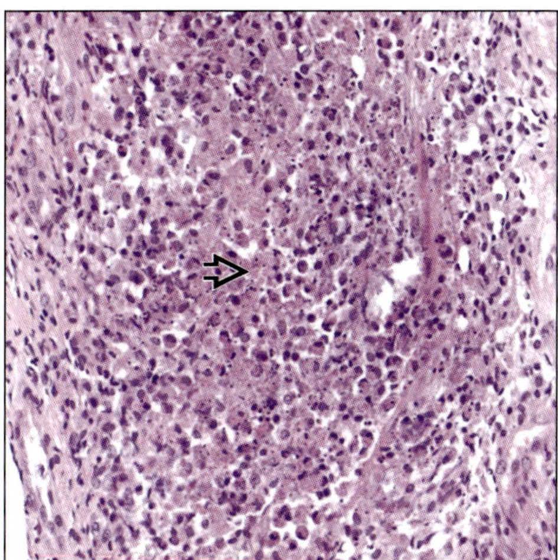
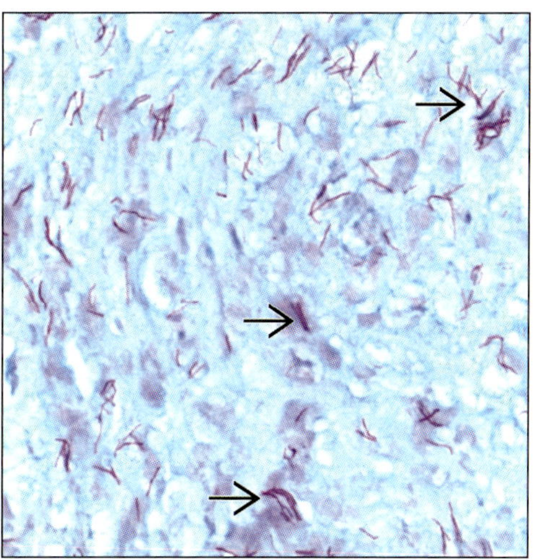

(Left) *Another area from the biopsy in M. kansasii infection shows a collection of necrotic debris ⇨ surrounded by histiocytes without well-formed granulomas.* ***(Right)*** *Acid-fast stain in liver biopsy from a patient with M. kansasii infection shows a large number of acid-fast bacilli → that are long, slender, and beaded.*

CAT SCRATCH DISEASE

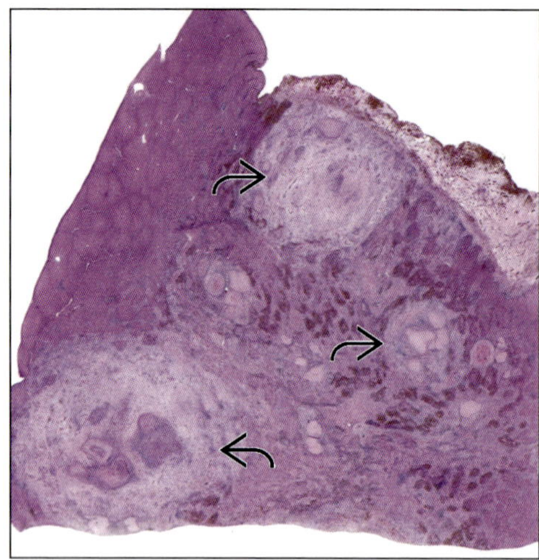

Hematoxylin & eosin stained section of a liver wedge excision shows several nodules of granulomatous inflammation ➔ with stellate abscesses and fibrosis.

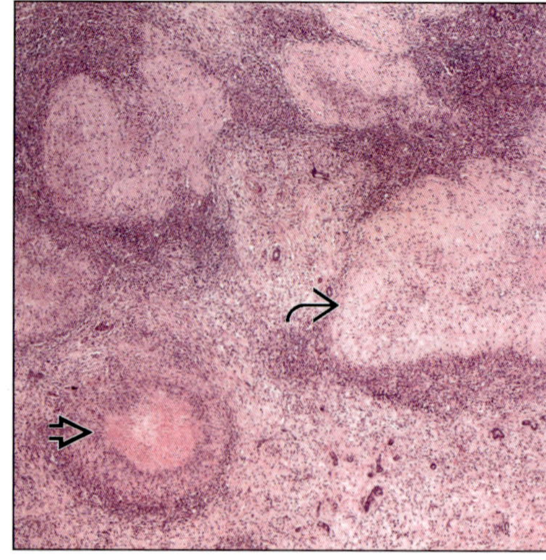

Hematoxylin & eosin stained section shows stellate microabscesses at various stages of evolution, including young lesions with central necrosis ➔ and older, more fibrotic lesions ➔.

TERMINOLOGY

Abbreviations

- Cat scratch disease (CSD)

Synonyms

- Bartonellosis

Definitions

- Self-limited infection by *Bartonella* species after inoculation by cat
  - Usually presents as local skin reaction and lymphadenopathy
  - Visceral involvement is rare

ETIOLOGY/PATHOGENESIS

Infectious Agents

- Most cases are attributed to *B. henselae* but *B. quintana* has been implicated in some

CLINICAL ISSUES

Epidemiology

- Age
  - Most cases are children 5-10 years of age

Presentation

- Approximately 1-2% of patients with CSD develop severe systemic disease with involvement of liver, spleen, bone, central nervous system, or lung
- Nonspecific symptoms, including fever, abdominal pain, chills, headache, malaise, and weight loss
- About 25% of patients with hepatic CSD have lymphadenopathy, but often, classical skin papule of CSD is absent in visceral disease
- Presence of hepatic nodules, with splenic nodules and lymphadenopathy in some cases, raises concern for neoplasia

Laboratory Tests

- Serology, PCR, skin testing confirm diagnosis

Treatment

- Drugs
  - Rifampin, erythromycin, or doxycycline

Prognosis

- Self-limited without long-term hepatic dysfunction

MACROSCOPIC FEATURES

General Features

- Liver may be studded with hard nodules of varying sizes

MICROSCOPIC PATHOLOGY

Histologic Features

- Irregular, stellate microabscesses
  - Surrounded by layers of palisading histiocytes, lymphocytes, and outer rim of fibrous tissue
- Temporal heterogeneity
  - Younger lesions may show more necrosis with less organization of inflammatory granulomatous response
  - Older lesions may show confluent granulomas with scarring and scant residual necrosis
- Occasional small rounded granulomas with giant cells and small foci of central necrosis, similar to caseating granulomas in mycobacterial or fungal infections

Predominant Pattern/Injury Type

- Inflammatory, granulomatous

ANCILLARY TESTS

Histochemistry

- Warthin-Starry stain

CAT SCRATCH DISEASE

Key Facts

Terminology

- Self-limited infection by *Bartonella* species after inoculation by cat

Clinical Issues

- Most cases are children 5-10 years of age
- 25% of patients with hepatic CSD have lymphadenopathy, but often classical skin papule is absent
- Presence of hepatic nodules, with splenic nodules and lymphadenopathy in some cases, raises concern for neoplasia

Microscopic Pathology

- Irregular, stellate microabscesses surrounded by layer of palisading histiocytes, lymphocytes, and rim of fibrous tissue

- Reactivity: Positive in some cases
- Staining pattern
  - Organism often clusters around vessels and between collagen

Immunohistochemistry

- Recently developed IHC antibody

PCR

- PCR or Southern blot for *Bartonella* DNA on tissue can confirm diagnosis

DIFFERENTIAL DIAGNOSIS

Granulomatous Infections of Liver

- *Yersinia enterocolitica, Francisella tularensis*, lymphogranuloma venereum, mycobacterial species, candidiasis, and actinomyces infection may look similar
  - Culture and identification of organism in tissue using histochemical stains or molecular studies is necessary to distinguish these infections

Sarcoidosis

- Necrotizing inflammation, young patient age, exposure to cat favor cat scratch disease

DIAGNOSTIC CHECKLIST

Clinically Relevant Pathologic Features

- Stellate microabscesses in liver of child being investigated for hepatic neoplasia

SELECTED REFERENCES

1. Laham FR et al: Hepatosplenic cat-scratch fever. Lancet Infect Dis. 8(2):140, 2008
2. Scolfaro C et al: Prolonged follow up of seven patients affected by hepatosplenic granulomata due to cat-scratch disease. Eur J Pediatr. 167(4):471-3, 2008
3. Ventura A et al: Systemic *Bartonella henselae* infection with hepatosplenic involvement. J Pediatr Gastroenterol Nutr. 29(1):52-6, 1999
4. Lamps LW et al: The histologic spectrum of hepatic cat scratch disease. A series of six cases with confirmed Bartonella henselae infection. Am J Surg Pathol. 20(10):1253-9, 1996
5. Liston TE et al: Granulomatous hepatitis and necrotizing splenitis due to Bartonella henselae in a patient with cancer: case report and review of hepatosplenic manifestations of bartonella infection. Clin Infect Dis. 22(6):951-7, 1996
6. Malatack JJ et al: Cat-scratch disease without adenopathy. J Pediatr. 114(1):101-4, 1989
7. Lenoir AA et al: Granulomatous hepatitis associated with cat scratch disease. Lancet. 1(8595):1132-6, 1988

IMAGE GALLERY

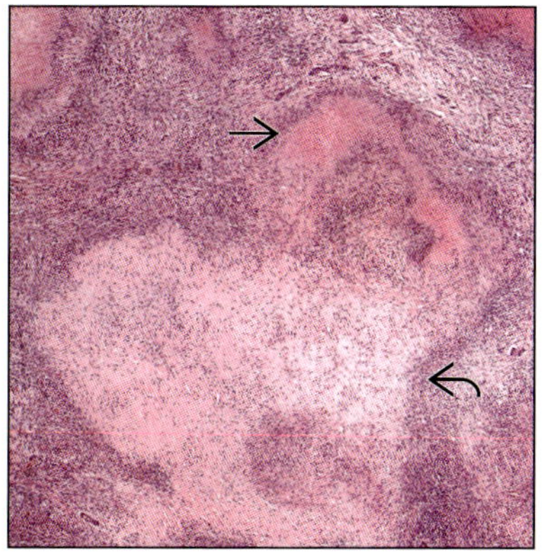

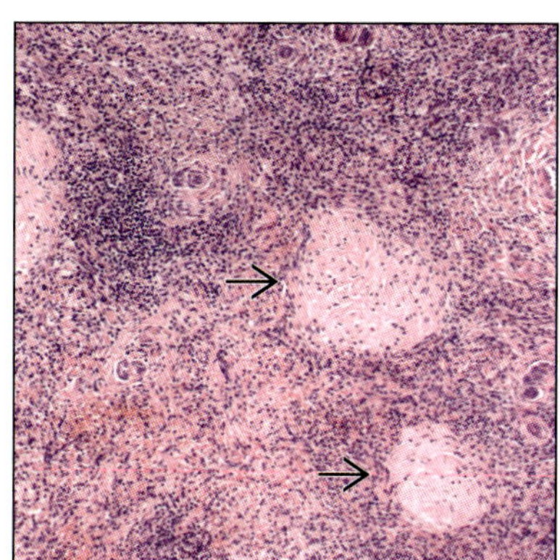

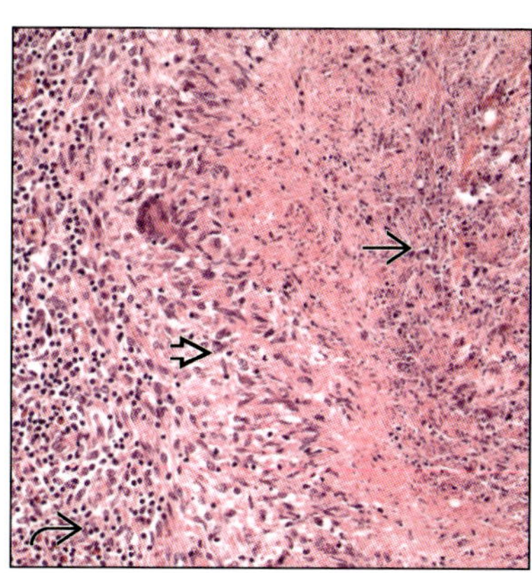

(Left) *Hematoxylin & eosin stained section shows stellate abscess with central necrosis lined by palisading histiocytes and lymphocytes ➔ in continuity with fibrotic areas ➔.* ***(Center)*** *Hematoxylin & eosin stained section shows fibrotic nodules consistent with organization and healing of granulomatous lesions ➔.* ***(Right)*** *Hematoxylin & eosin stained section at high magnification shows a stellate microabscess with central necrotic region ➔ surrounded by a rim of palisaded histiocytes ➔ and lymphocytes ➔.*

CANDIDIASIS

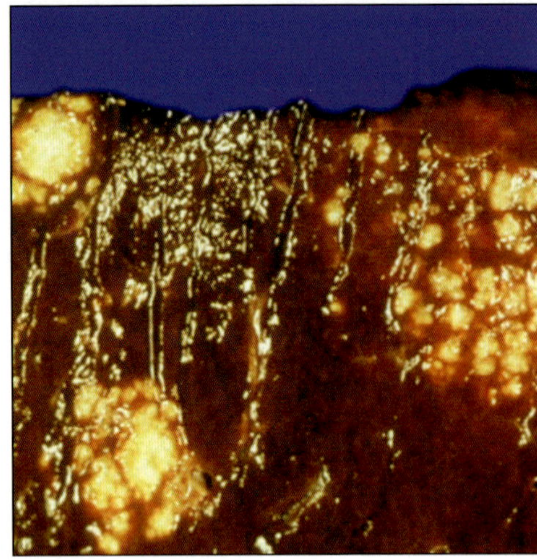

Gross photograph of a liver from an autopsy showing multiple yellow-white Candida lesions.

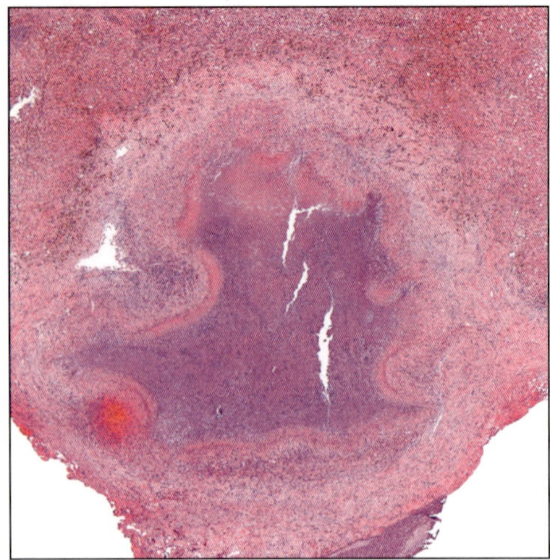

Hematoxylin & eosin sections shows a stellate Candida abscess with central necrosis and peripheral fibrosis in a liver wedge biopsy.

TERMINOLOGY

Definitions

- Infection of liver by *Candida* fungus
  - Candidiasis is most common disseminated fungal infection in immunocompromised hosts
  - Liver involvement is common in disseminated infection

ETIOLOGY/PATHOGENESIS

Infectious Agents

- *Candida* species
  - *Candida albicans* most common
    - Endogenous commensal that is part of normal flora of GI tract, mouth, respiratory tract, vagina
  - Other pathogenic *Candida* include *C. tropicalis, C. parapsilosis, C. krusei*
    - Saprophytic yeasts present in both humans and environment
  - *Candida (Torulopsis) glabrata*
    - Normal flora of skin, GI tract, GU tract, respiratory tract
- Patients with hepatic infection almost always immunocompromised
  - Rarely described in immunocompetent persons
- Liver transplant patients
  - Associated with ischemic/necrotic bile ducts, hepatic artery thrombosis

Risk Factors

- Disruption of mucosal or cutaneous barriers
- Broad-spectrum antibiotics
- Metabolic abnormalities
- Indwelling catheters/vascular devices
- Neutropenia, immunosuppression
- Steroids
- Neonates

CLINICAL ISSUES

Presentation

- Hepatomegaly
- Abdominal pain
- Systemic febrile illness

Laboratory Tests

- Elevated transaminases
- Elevated bilirubin

Treatment

- Drugs
  - Antifungal therapy

Prognosis

- Depends on underlying immune status of patient
  - Difficult to eliminate fungus
  - Persistent lesions may produce scarring

MACROSCOPIC FEATURES

General Features

- Yellow-white nodules
- Usually multiple
- 1-2 cm in size

MICROSCOPIC PATHOLOGY

Histologic Features

- Typical inflammatory reaction is granulomatous
  - Giant cells may be present
  - Palisading histiocytes and peripheral scarring may be seen
- Usually suppurative center
  - Variable necrosis
- Nonspecific reactive findings, usually near fungal lesion
  - Cholestasis

CANDIDIASIS

Key Facts

Terminology

- Candidiasis is most common disseminated fungal infection in immunocompromised hosts
  - Rarely seen in immunocompetent patients

Macroscopic Features

- Yellow-white nodules
  - Usually multiple

Microscopic Pathology

- Typical inflammatory reaction is granulomatous
  - Frequently with suppurative/necrotic center
- Mixture of budding yeast, hyphae, and pseudohyphae
- All are GMS, PAS positive

Diagnostic Checklist

- Fungi can sometimes be speciated by morphology, but culture is gold standard

---

  - Portal inflammation
  - Ductular proliferation
  - Sinusoidal dilatation
- Morphologic features of fungus
  - Mixture of budding yeast, hyphae, and pseudohyphae
    - *Candida albicans*
    - *Candida tropicalis*
  - Budding yeast only
    - *Candida (Torulopsis) glabrata*
  - All are GMS, PAS positive

DIFFERENTIAL DIAGNOSIS

Cat Scratch Disease

- Similar palisading histiocytes and central stellate suppuration
- GMS stain, culture negative for fungi
- PCR, silver impregnation stains to confirm *Bartonella*

Other Fungi

- *Aspergillus*
  - True hyphae that branch at acute angles
  - Usually vasocentric
- Zygomycetes
  - Broad, pauciceptate, ribbon-like hyphae
  - Usually vasocentric
- Histoplasmosis
  - More uniform than *C. (Torulopsis) glabrata*
  - "Halo" effect around organism in tissue

Necrotic Tumor

- GMS stain negative in malignancy

Bacterial Abscess

- No fungi seen on GMS
- Usually lacks granulomatous features

DIAGNOSTIC CHECKLIST

Pathologic Interpretation Pearls

- Consider in any immunocompromised patient with multiple liver lesions
- Fungi can sometimes be speciated by morphology, but culture is gold standard

SELECTED REFERENCES

1. Fung JJ: Fungal infection in liver transplantation. Transpl Infect Dis. 4 Suppl 3:18-23, 2002
2. Johnson TL et al: Candida hepatitis. Histopathologic diagnosis. Am J Surg Pathol. 12(9):716-20, 1988
3. Thaler M et al: Hepatic candidiasis in cancer patients: the evolving picture of the syndrome. Ann Intern Med. 108(1):88-100, 1988
4. Maksymiuk AW et al: Systemic candidiasis in cancer patients. Am J Med. 77(4D):20-7, 1984
5. Hughes WT: Systemic candidiasis: a study of 109 fatal cases. Pediatr Infect Dis. 1(1):11-8, 1982

IMAGE GALLERY

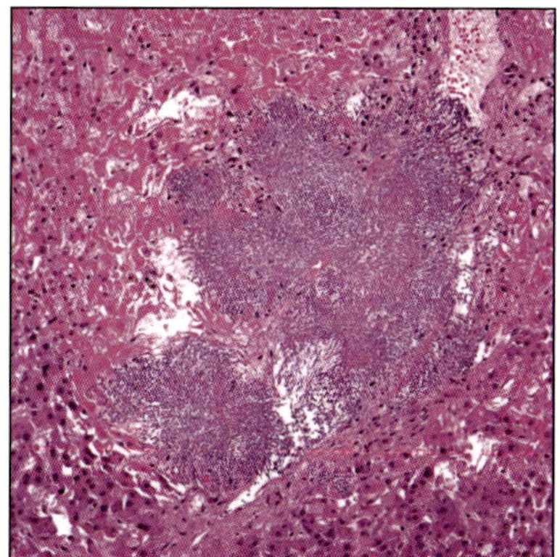

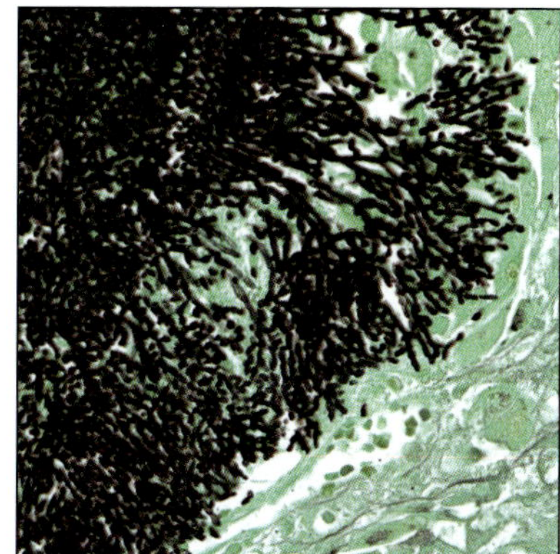

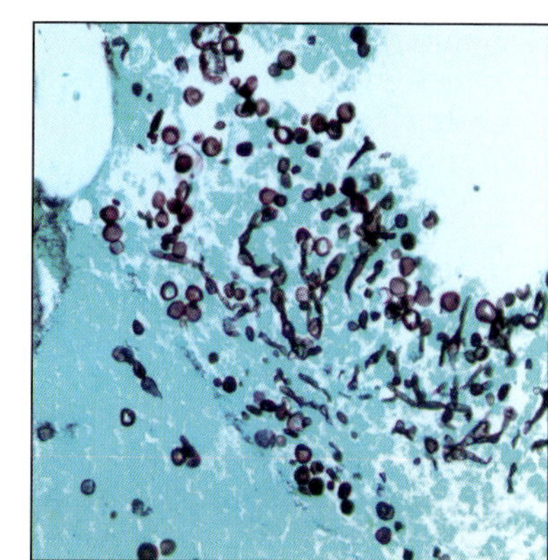

(Left) *Hematoxylin & eosin section shows a Candida abscess with associated necrosis but minimal inflammation in a severely immunocompromised patient. (Courtesy D. Milner, MD.)* ***(Center)*** *GMS (Gomori methenamine silver) stain highlights the Candida within the hepatic abscess. (Courtesy D. Milner, MD.)* ***(Right)*** *GMS (Gomori methenamine silver) stain shows budding yeast and pseudohyphae in a Candida liver abscess.*

HISTOPLASMOSIS

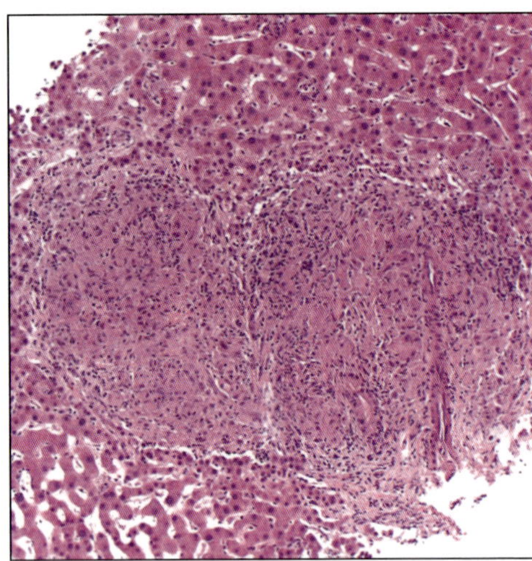

Liver biopsy in a patient with disseminated histoplasmosis shows large, coalescent, loosely formed granulomas.

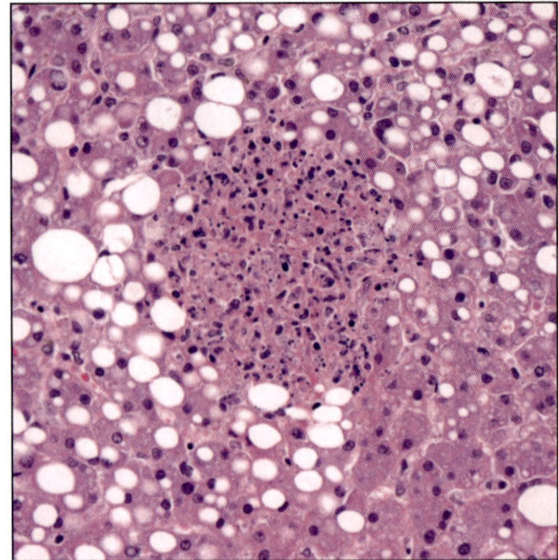

The liver in an immunocompromised patient who died of disseminated histoplasmosis shows foci of necrotic debris, lymphocytes, and histiocytes; the surrounding liver shows steatosis.

TERMINOLOGY

Definitions

- Infection by fungus *Histoplasma capsulatum*

ETIOLOGY/PATHOGENESIS

Infectious Agents

- *H. capsulatum:* Dimorphic fungus that exists as mycelial form at room temperature and as yeast form at body temperature
  - Found in soil, particularly when contaminated with bird or bat droppings

CLINICAL ISSUES

Epidemiology

- Incidence
  - Endemic in Ohio, Missouri, and Mississippi River valleys, Central and South America, and parts of eastern United States, southern Europe, Africa, and southeastern Asia
  - Outbreaks associated with demolition of buildings, moving soil, and spelunking
  - Disseminated histoplasmosis occurs in approximately 55% of infected immunocompromised patients and 4% of infected immunocompetent patients

Site

- Liver is involved in up to 90% of cases of disseminated histoplasmosis

Presentation

- Symptomatic acute disseminated infection
  - Occurs in immunosuppressed patients
  - Common symptoms include chills, fever, anorexia, weight loss, mucous membrane ulcers, and skin lesions
  - Hepatosplenomegaly and elevated liver enzymes, especially alkaline phosphatase
- Chronic progressive disseminated histoplasmosis
  - Occurs in older patients without immunosuppression who are unable to control organism
  - Fever, night sweats, weight loss, fatigues, and oral ulcers are common
  - Adrenal insufficiency with destruction of adrenal glands
- Can present as reactivation years after initial exposure and outside endemic area if cell-mediated immunity is compromised

Laboratory Tests

- Fungal culture of tissue or blood
- Antibody assays include complement fixation (CF) and immunodiffusion (ID) assays
  - Not useful in patients with acute disseminated infection who might not have developed antibody
- Antigen detection assays include enzyme immunoassay (EIA) in urine, serum, or other body fluids
  - High sensitivity (80-90%)

Natural History

- Aerosolized microconidia are inhaled and survive within macrophages as yeast form
- Organism disseminates throughout reticuloendothelial cell system
- Sensitized T cells activate macrophages, which then are able to kill organism

Treatment

- Drugs
  - Antifungal agents: Itraconazole, amphotericin B

Prognosis

- With treatment, death rate is < 10%
- Immunocompromised patients have worse prognosis than immunocompetent

HISTOPLASMOSIS

Key Facts

Etiology/Pathogenesis

- *H. capsulatum:* Dimorphic fungus found in soil contaminated with bird or bat droppings

Clinical Issues

- Endemic in Ohio and Mississippi River valleys
- Disseminated infection is more likely in infants, AIDS patients with CD4 count below 150 cells per μL, patients on steroids or immunosuppressive drugs, or with TNF antagonists
  - Adrenal insufficiency is more common in disseminated histoplasmosis than with other fungal infections
- Fungal culture of tissue or blood
- Antibody assays include complement fixation and immunodiffusion assays
- Antigen detection assays include enzyme immunoassay in urine, serum, or other body fluids

Microscopic Pathology

- Portal and lobular lymphohistiocytic inflammation
- Discrete granulomas in portal and lobular regions
- Large numbers of yeast organisms in macrophages
- Might have limited or no inflammatory response
- Yeast are 2-4 μm, oval, with narrow-based budding

Ancillary Tests

- GMS and PAS-diastase positive

Top Differential Diagnoses

- Sarcoidosis: Similar epithelioid discrete granulomas
- Leishmaniasis: Kinetoplast and GMS negative
- Candidiasis: Larger yeast, more budding

Risk Factors for Disseminated Disease

- Exposure in infancy before cell-mediated immunity is well developed
- AIDS with CD4 cell count less than 150 cells per μL
- Use of corticosteroids or other immunosuppressive drugs
- Hematologic malignancies
- Solid organ transplantation
- Use of tumor necrosis factor (TNF) antagonists: Etanercept, infliximab, and adalimumab

MACROSCOPIC FEATURES

General Features

- Enlarged liver appears congested or mottled
- Can demonstrate nodules up to 1 cm in diameter

MICROSCOPIC PATHOLOGY

Histologic Features

- Portal and lobular lymphohistiocytic inflammation and Kupffer cell hyperplasia
- Discrete granulomas in portal and lobular regions may be seen regardless of immune status
- Large numbers of fungal organisms in portal and sinusoidal macrophages
  - Yeast are uniformly small (2-4 μm) and oval with narrow-based budding
- Might have limited or no inflammatory response
- Nodules may contain caseous necrotic material with histocytic or fibroblastic rim

ANCILLARY TESTS

Histochemistry

- GMS (Gomori methenamine silver)
  - Reactivity: Positive
- PAS-diastase
  - Reactivity: Positive

DIFFERENTIAL DIAGNOSIS

Pneumocystosis

- Lack of budding, extracellular location, characteristic internal structure

Candidiasis

- Slightly larger yeast than *H. capsulatum*, more frequent budding, extracellular location, different clinical features

Cryptococcosis

- Mucicarmine-positive capsule

Leishmaniasis

- Presence of kinetoplast, GMS negative

Penicilliosis

- Endemic in southeast Asia, yeast forms accompanied by elongated and septal fungal forms

Sarcoidosis

- Histoplasmosis may cause discrete epithelioid granulomas, indistinguishable from sarcoidosis by morphology alone

DIAGNOSTIC CHECKLIST

Clinically Relevant Pathologic Features

- Liver biopsies from patients known to be immunosuppressed should be screened with PAS-diastase or GMS for histoplasmosis

SELECTED REFERENCES

1. Kauffman CA: Histoplasmosis. Clin Chest Med. 30(2):217-25, v, 2009
2. Lamps LW et al: The pathologic spectrum of gastrointestinal and hepatic histoplasmosis. Am J Clin Pathol. 113(1):64-72, 2000

HISTOPLASMOSIS

Microscopic Features

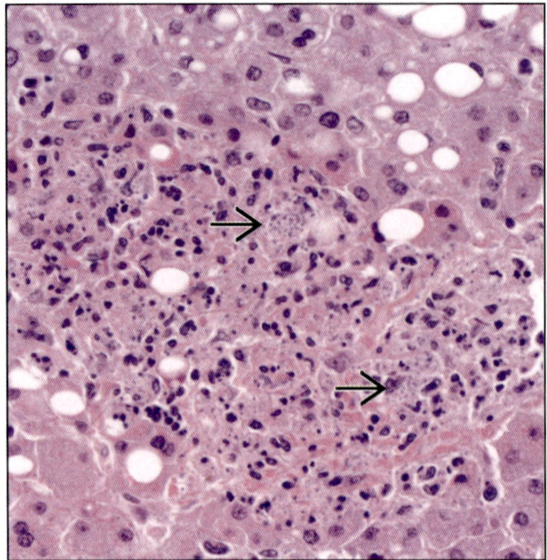

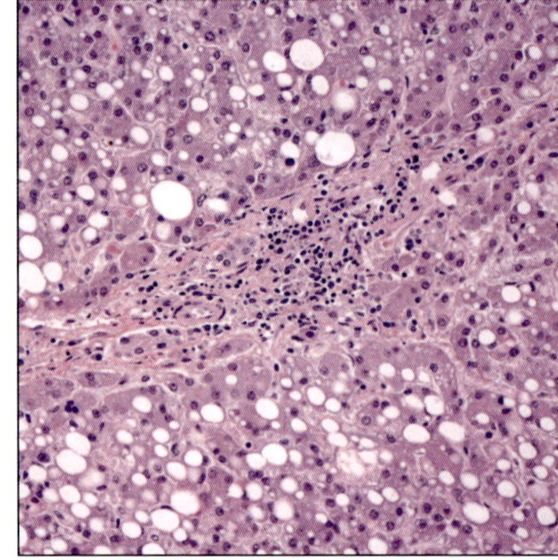

(Left) *Necrotic lesion in an immunocompromised woman with disseminated histoplasmosis shows lymphocytes and histiocytes that are filled with organisms →.* ***(Right)*** *The portal tract in this case shows a sparse lymphohistiocytic infiltrate without granuloma formation, which might not compel the pathologist to examine a fungal stain.*

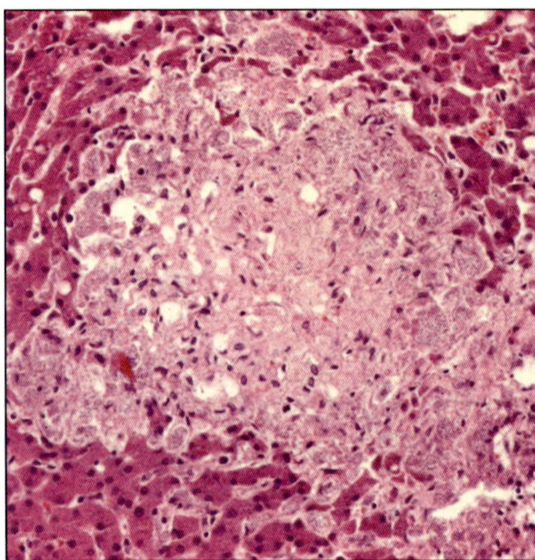

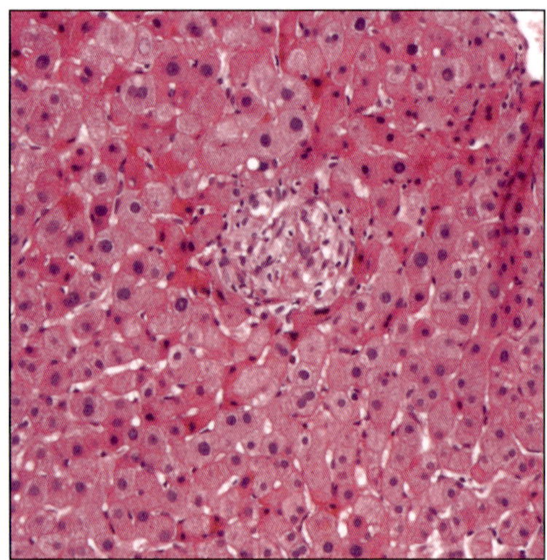

(Left) *In this example of disseminated histoplasmosis, clusters of histiocytes are present in the lobule.* ***(Right)*** *An isolated, well-formed granuloma in the liver of a patient with hepatosplenic histoplasmosis is shown. The differential diagnosis for this case includes many granulomatous processes, including noninfectious causes.*

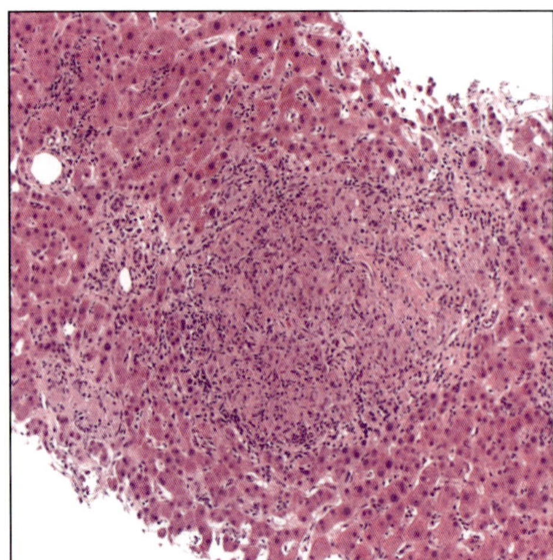

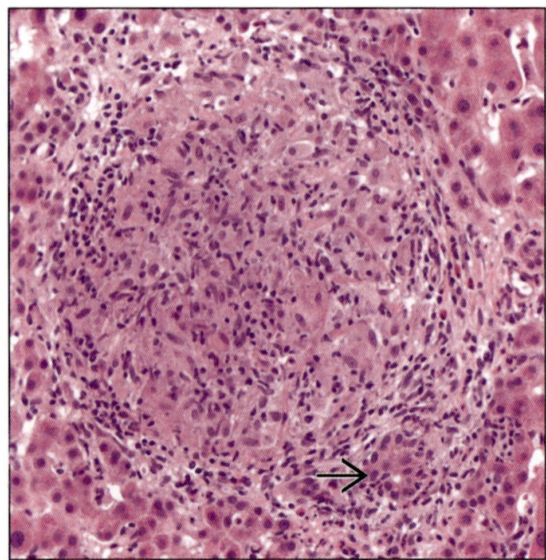

(Left) *Liver biopsy in an older man with adrenal histoplasmosis shows an expansile large granuloma with surrounding lymphocytic inflammation and sinusoidal mononuclear cells.* ***(Right)*** *Higher magnification of the biopsy in a patient with adrenal histoplasmosis shows a portal-based large epithelioid granuloma with admixed lymphocytes. A bile duct is at lower right →.*

Microscopic Features

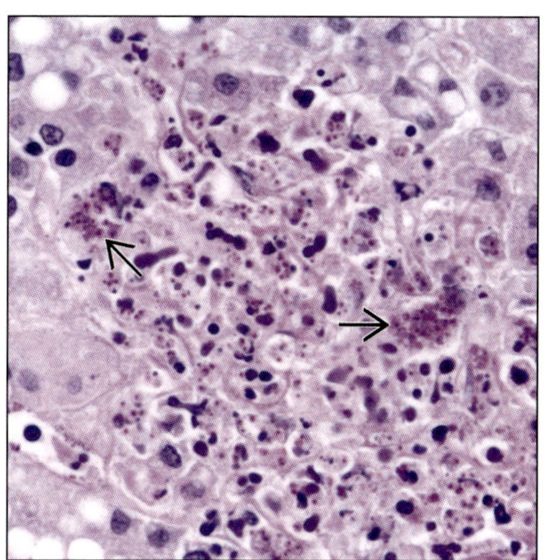

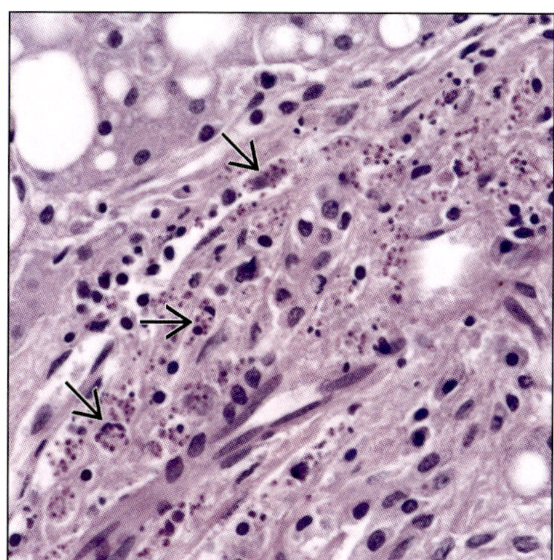

(Left) *PAS-diastase stain of the liver biopsy shows macrophages filled with yeast* ➔ *in the necrotic foci.* ***(Right)*** *PAS-diastase stain shows yeast within macrophages in portal areas* ➔ *despite the minimal inflammation and absence of granulomas.*

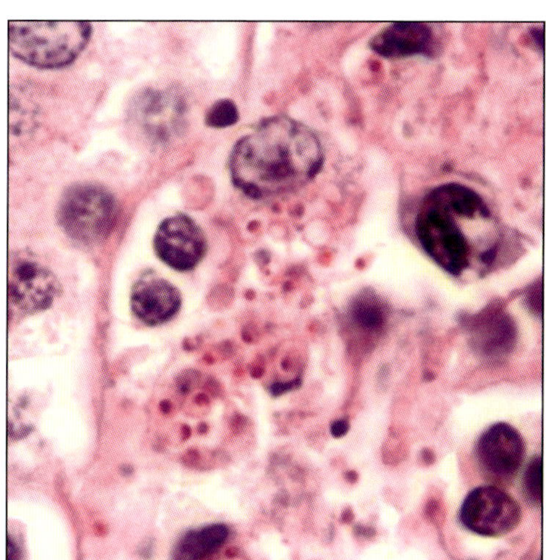

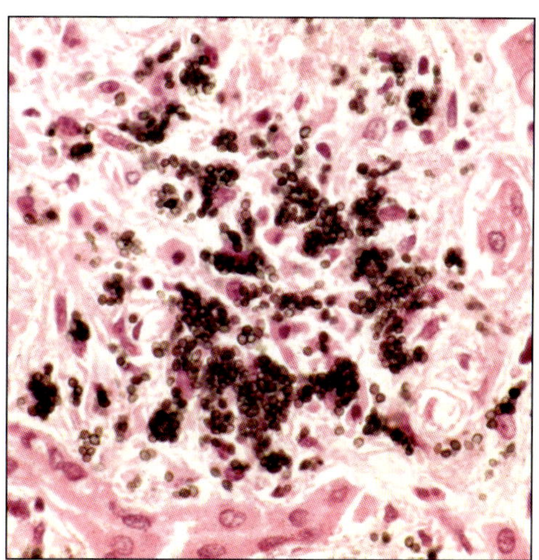

(Left) *PAS-diastase stain at very high magnification shows macrophages with numerous intracellular yeast that appear as small oval organisms with a distinctive "halo" effect that is typical of histoplasmosis.* ***(Right)*** *Methenamine silver with hematoxylin and eosin counterstain nicely demonstrates the yeast within a collection of portal macrophages in the liver.*

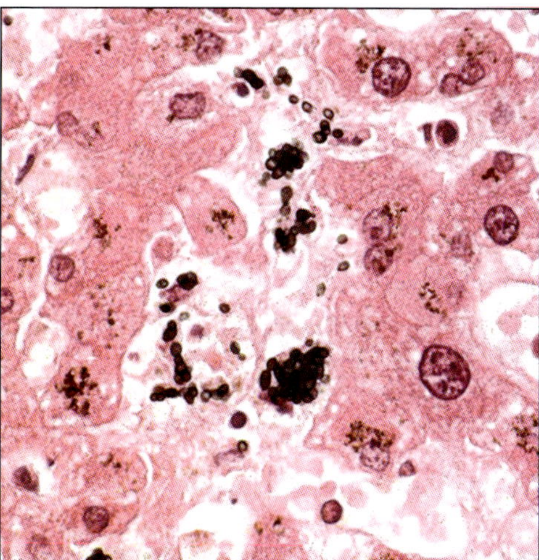

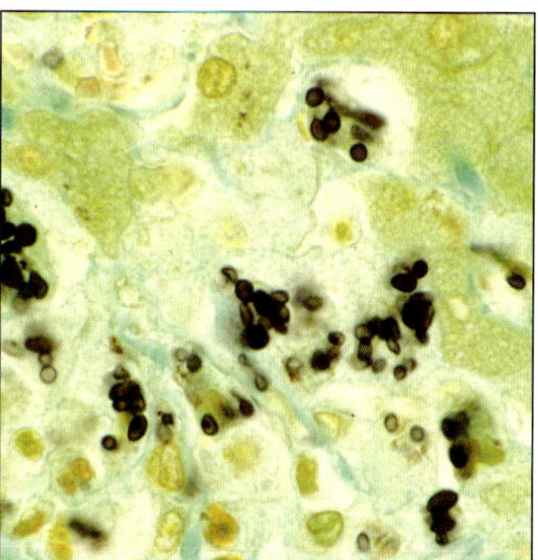

(Left) *High-power view of a GMS with H&E counterstain shows small budding yeast within macrophages in the sinusoids.* ***(Right)*** *Histoplasma are uniformly small with narrow-based buds at the more pointed end of the organism.*

CRYPTOCOCCOSIS

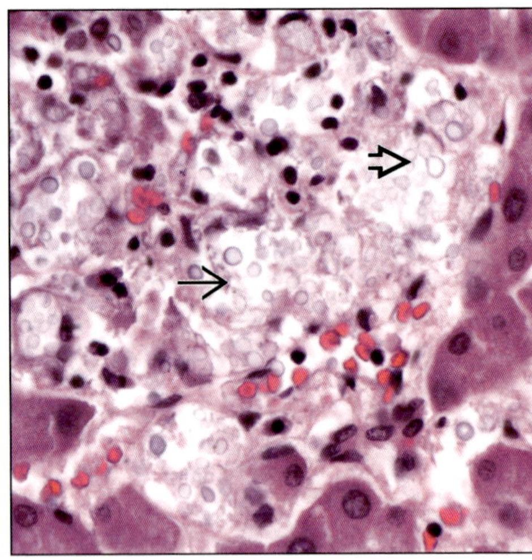

Hematoxylin & eosin stain shows numerous Cryptococci expanding the hepatic sinusoids. Note narrow-based bud ⇨ and variation in size →.

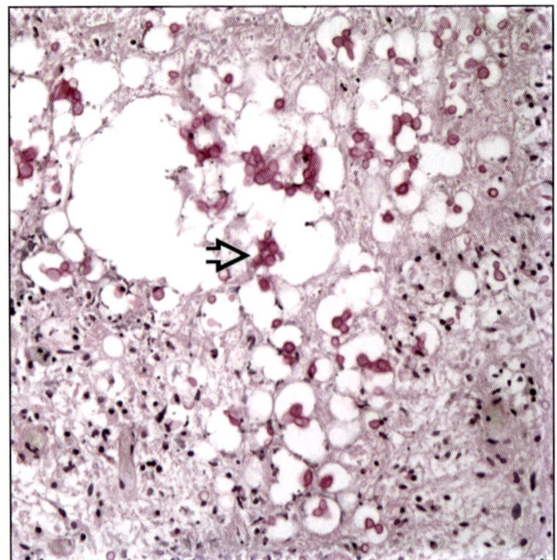

Mucicarmine stain highlights the mucopolysaccharide capsule characteristic of Cryptococcus ⇨. (Courtesy B. Smoller, MD.)

TERMINOLOGY

Synonyms

- Cryptococcosis, torulosis, European blastomycosis, Busse-Buschke disease

Definitions

- Infection by fungus *Cryptococcus neoformans*
- Most common cause of systemic mycosis in patients with AIDS
- Usually hematogenously disseminated disease with multiorgan system involvement

ETIOLOGY/PATHOGENESIS

Environmental Exposure

- Widespread in nature
  - Ubiquitous saprophyte of soil; acquired by inhalation
  - Most abundant in avian habitats, especially those with pigeon excreta
- Worldwide distribution

CLINICAL ISSUES

Site

- Most common sites of involvement are lungs and cerebral meninges with hematogenous or lymphatic dissemination to other sites

Presentation

- Most often encountered as opportunistic infection in immunosuppressed patients (AIDS, malignancies, corticosteroid therapy, etc.)

Laboratory Tests

- Definite speciation requires culture

Treatment

- Drugs
  - Antifungal medication (intravenous amphotericin B and oral 5-fluorocytosine)

Prognosis

- Duration of disease from days to years
- Untreated disease is almost always fatal

MACROSCOPIC FEATURES

General Features

- Usually unremarkable
  - Rarely there are multiple foci of necrosis
- Extrahepatic biliary tree may be involved, mimicking sclerosing cholangitis

MICROSCOPIC PATHOLOGY

Histologic Features

- Fungal morphology
  - Round to oval yeast
  - Narrow-based buds
  - Considerable variation in size from 2-20 μm in diameter
  - Halo around organisms representing mucopolysaccharide capsule
    - "Soap bubble" appearance at low magnification
    - Capsule may have a diameter up to 5x that of fungal cells they surround
    - Some cryptococci may be capsule deficient and mucicarmine negative, making diagnosis more difficult
  - Occasionally may produce hyphae and pseudohyphae
- Inflammatory response
  - Kupffer cells or portal macrophages contain engulfed yeast

CRYPTOCOCCOSIS

Key Facts

Terminology
- Infection by fungus *Cryptococcus neoformans*
- Usually hematogenously disseminated disease with multiorgan system involvement

Etiology/Pathogenesis
- Found in soil, most abundant in avian habitats, especially those with pigeon excreta

Microscopic Pathology
- Round to oval yeast with narrow-based budding
- Considerable variation in size from 2-20 μm in diameter
- Halo around organisms representing mucopolysaccharide capsule

Top Differential Diagnoses
- *Blastomyces dermatitidis*
- *Histoplasma capsulatum*

  - Usually minimal accompanying inflammation, especially in immunocompromised patients
  - Occasionally epithelioid granulomas develop, and large multinucleated giant cells containing yeast are present
- Histochemical stains
  - GMS positive
  - Capsule will stain with Alcian blue, mucicarmine, colloidal iron, and Fontana-Masson

DIFFERENTIAL DIAGNOSIS

Other Fungal Infections
- *Blastomyces dermatitidis*
  - Larger in size than *Cryptococcus*
  - More uniform in size
  - Broad-based buds
  - Occasionally mucicarmine positive
- *Histoplasma capsulatum*
  - Smaller than *Cryptococcus*
  - More uniform in size
  - Mucicarmine negative

Other Suppurative and Granulomatous Processes
- Bacterial and mycobacterial infections
- Noninfectious causes of hepatic granulomas

DIAGNOSTIC CHECKLIST

Clinically Relevant Pathologic Features
- Often represents part of a disseminated infection
- Lungs and meninges are most common sites of involvement
- Patients are usually immunocompromised

Pathologic Interpretation Pearls
- Mucin-positive capsule is highly suggestive of *Cryptococcus* species
- Capsule-deficient *Cryptococcus* usually has at least some weakly positive cells when mucin stains are examined carefully

SELECTED REFERENCES

1. Patel NC et al: Disseminated Cryptococcus neoformans: case report and review of the literature. Cutis. 84(2):93-6, 2009
2. Lazcano O et al: Combined histochemical stains in the differential diagnosis of Cryptococcus neoformans. Mod Pathol. 6(1):80-4, 1993
3. Bonacini M et al: Gastrointestinal, hepatic, and pancreatic involvement with Cryptococcus neoformans in AIDS. J Clin Gastroenterol. 12(3):295-7, 1990
4. Kovacs JA et al: Cryptococcosis in the acquired immunodeficiency syndrome. Ann Intern Med. 103(4):533-8, 1985
5. Sabesin SM et al: Hepatic failure as a manifestation of cryptococcosis. Arch Intern Med. 111:661-9, 1963

IMAGE GALLERY

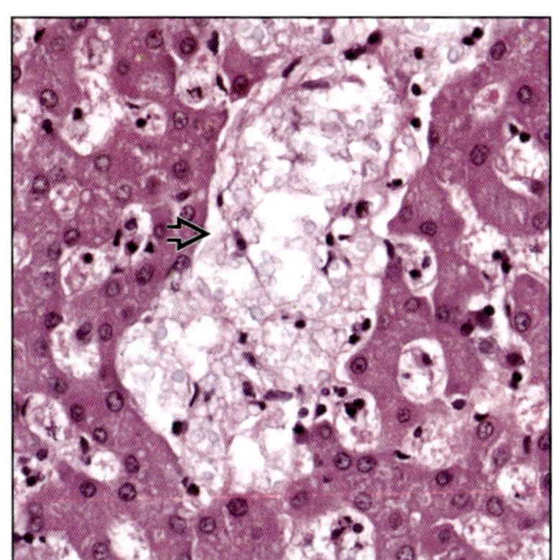
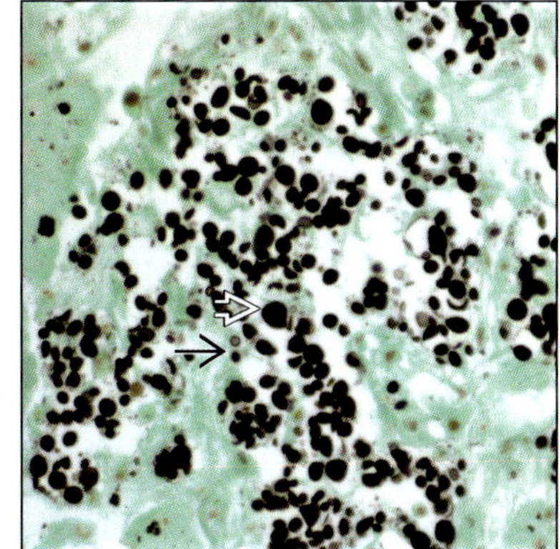
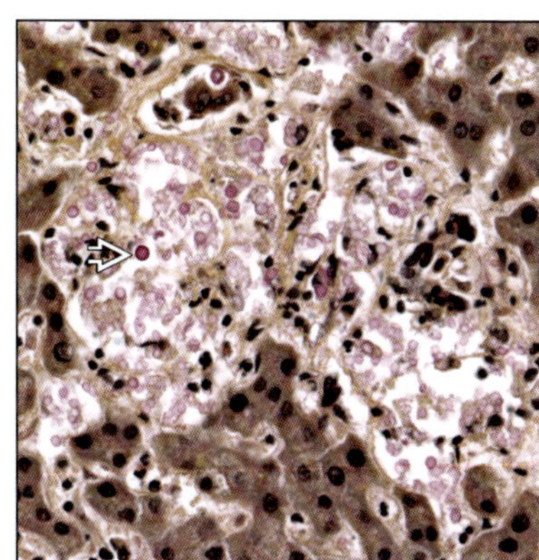

(Left) *Hematoxylin & eosin stain shows the low-power "soap bubble" appearance of Cryptococcus* ⇨*.* ***(Center)*** *GMS (Gomori methenamine silver) stain highlights the pleomorphic nature of Cryptococcus. Note the presence of both small* → *and large* ➡ *fungi.* ***(Right)*** *Mucicarmine stain of capsule-deficient Cryptococcus shows rare mucicarmine-positive organisms* ➡*.*

AMEBIASIS

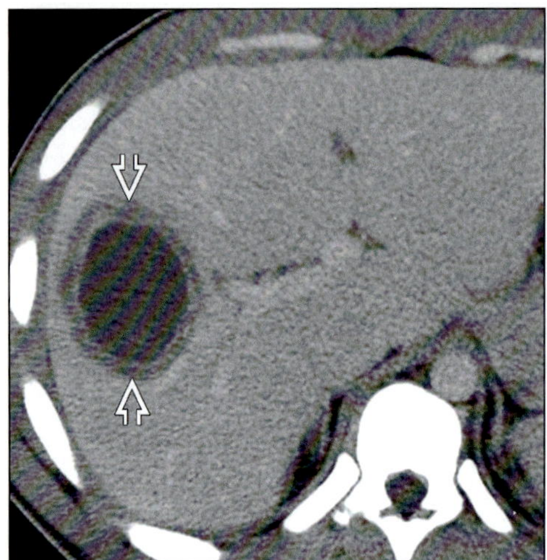

Contrast enhanced CT of the liver shows an amebic abscess with a surrounding rim ➡. This cavity was filled with thick, tenacious necrotic debris ("anchovy paste").

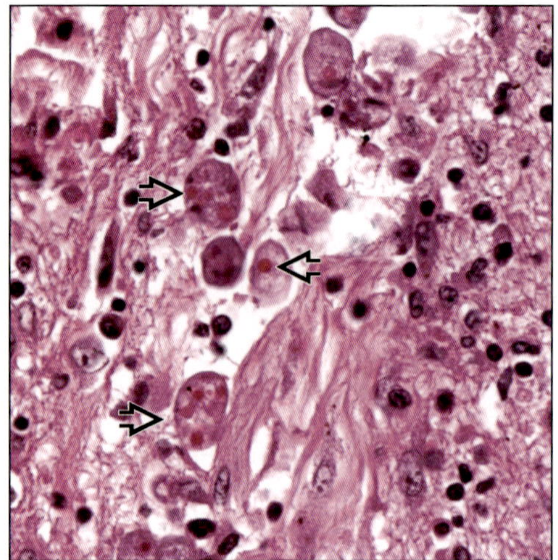

Ingested red blood cells are virtually pathognomonic of E. histolytica ➡.

TERMINOLOGY

Synonyms

- *Entamoeba histolytica*

Definitions

- Infection of liver by protozoa *E. histolytica*

ETIOLOGY/PATHOGENESIS

Environmental Exposure

- Most common in poor communities with inadequate sanitation
- Human carriers are main reservoir

Infectious Agents

- Liver abscess is most frequent complication of invasive amebiasis
- Portal vein is major route by which ameba get from intestine to liver

CLINICAL ISSUES

Presentation

- Fever
  - Profuse afternoon and night sweats
- Right upper quadrant pain
  - Radiates to scapular region/shoulder
  - Worse with coughing, deep inspiration, exertion
- Abdominal tenderness
- Hepatomegaly
- Weight loss
- Malaise
- Jaundice (rare)
- Complications
  - Rupture of abscess into peritoneum
  - Fistulize with other organs or skin
- Most patients with amebic liver abscess do not have gastrointestinal symptoms

Laboratory Tests

- Elevated alkaline phosphatase in over 50%
- Elevated transaminases (rare)
- Leukocytosis in > 90%
- Serologic assays available as well

Treatment

- Drugs
  - Amebicides
    - Especially metronidazole
- Guided percutaneous drainage when
  - Rupture is concern
  - Response to drugs is slow/inadequate
  - Bacterial superinfection

Prognosis

- Excellent with modern amebicidal therapy

MACROSCOPIC FEATURES

General Features

- Solitary or multiple lesions
- Usually right lobe
- Wide range of size
  - Barely visible to > 20 cm
- Often irregularly shaped
- May have prominent fibrous capsule
- Frequently contain necrotic debris
  - Necrotic contents often compared to "anchovy paste"

MICROSCOPIC PATHOLOGY

Histologic Features

- Early lesion
  - Trophozoites within sinusoids
  - Focal necrosis
  - Neutrophilic infiltrate with edema
- Later lesion

AMEBIASIS

Key Facts

Etiology/Pathogenesis
- Liver abscess is most frequent complication of invasive amebiasis

Clinical Issues
- Elevated alkaline phosphatase, leukocytosis common
- Fever and RUQ pain

Macroscopic Features
- Irregular solitary or multiple lesions
- Often contain necrosis resembling "anchovy paste"

Microscopic Pathology
- Abundant nuclear debris but few intact inflammatory cells
- Organisms have foamy cytoplasm; round, eccentric nuclei
  - Ingested red blood cells essentially pathognomonic of *E. histolytica*
- Trophozoites may mimic macrophages

  - Necrotic material
    - Abundant nuclear debris but few intact inflammatory cells
  - Organisms most often at advancing edge; may be hard to find
  - Mononuclear cells at advancing edge, along with edema
  - Eventually develop fibrosis and granulation tissue
- Morphologic features of organism
  - Foamy cytoplasm
  - Distinct cell membrane
  - Nuclear features
    - Eccentric
    - Round
    - Peripheral margination of chromatin
    - Central karyosome
  - Ingested red blood cells essentially pathognomonic of *E. histolytica*
  - Trophozoites are PAS, trichrome positive

DIFFERENTIAL DIAGNOSIS

Neoplasms
- May mimic amebic abscess radiographically

Pyogenic Liver Abscess
- Pyogenic abscess usually has more neutrophils
- Aspiration with culture invaluable in resolving this differential

Macrophages
- Macrophages are CD68 positive
- Amebic nuclei rounder, more open chromatin pattern than macrophages

Entamoeba dispar
- Morphologically identical but noninvasive

Balantidium coli
- Large ciliate with kidney-bean-shaped nucleus

DIAGNOSTIC CHECKLIST

Pathologic Interpretation Pearls
- Look for protozoa in amorphous necrotic material with few intact inflammatory cells
- Ameba may closely resemble macrophages

SELECTED REFERENCES

1. Sharma MP et al: Amoebic liver abscess. Trop Gastroenterol. 14(1):3-9, 1993
2. Maltz G et al: Amebic liver abscess: a 15-year experience. Am J Gastroenterol. 86(6):704-10, 1991
3. Greenstein AJ et al: Pyogenic and amebic abscesses of the liver. Semin Liver Dis. 8(3):210-7, 1988
4. Brandt H et al: Pathology of human amebiasis. Hum Pathol. 1(3):351-85, 1970

IMAGE GALLERY

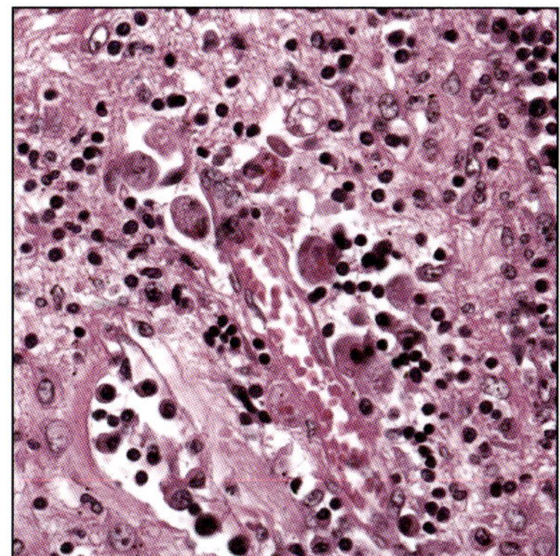

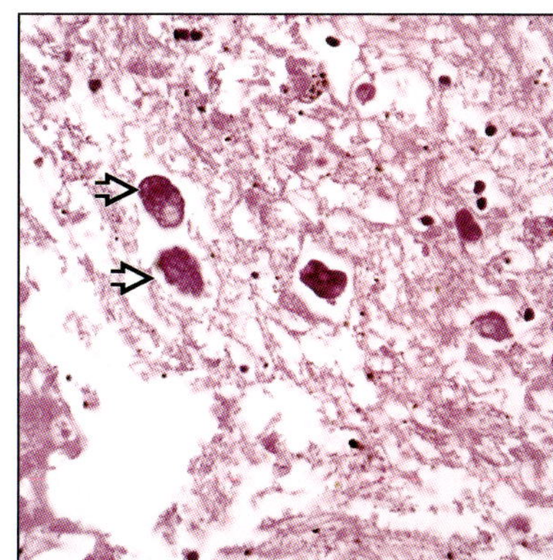

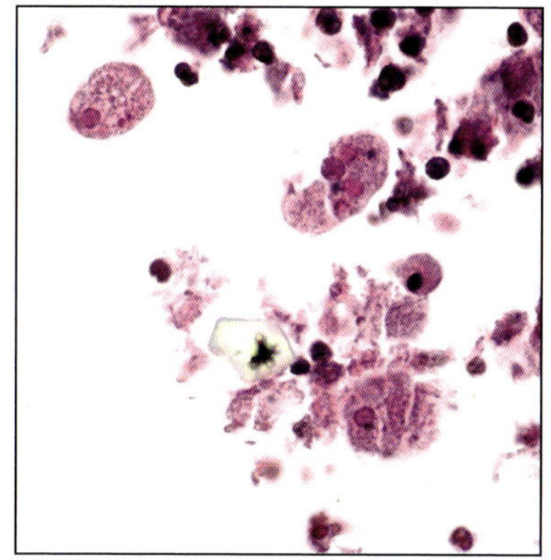

(Left) *Hematoxylin & eosin section shows amebae with admixed mononuclear cells and necrotic debris.* ***(Center)*** *Periodic acid-Schiff stain highlights amebae ⇨ within amorphous necrotic debris. Note that there is nuclear debris present but no intact neutrophils.* ***(Right)*** *High-power view of amebic trophozoites shows distinct cell membrane, foamy cytoplasm, and round, eccentric nucleus with open chromatin pattern.*

SCHISTOSOMIASIS

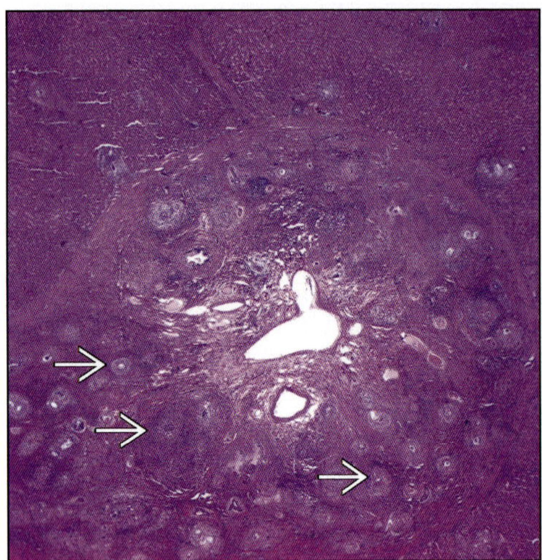

Paraffin section of liver with schistosomiasis shows a markedly enlarged portal tract without septae formation. The numerous rounded nodules ➔ are ova with granulomatous reaction.

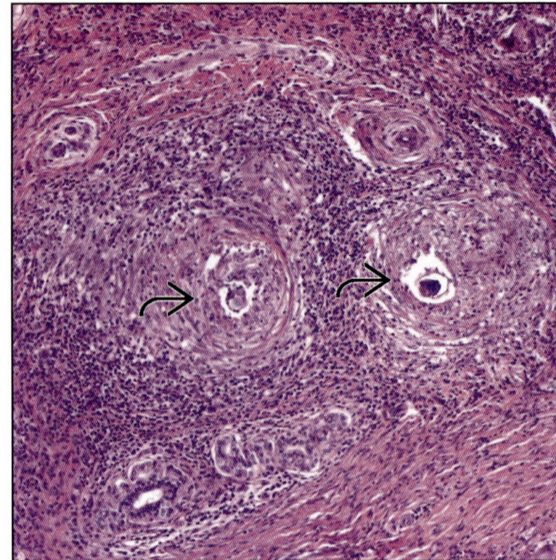

An expanded portal tract shows chronic inflammation and several granulomas containing degenerate ova ➔.

TERMINOLOGY

Synonyms

- Bilharzia, bilharziosis, or snail fever
- Katayama fever (acute schistosomiasis)

Definitions

- Parasitic infection caused by flukes of genus *Schistosoma*

ETIOLOGY/PATHOGENESIS

Infectious Agents

- Of schistosomes, *Schistosoma japonicum* and, to lesser degree, *Schistosoma mansoni* are most commonly associated with hepatic pathology
  - Morbidity is related to inflammatory response to ova trapped in host tissue

CLINICAL ISSUES

Epidemiology

- Age
  - In endemic areas, children are infected as soon as they begin to have contact with freshwater, and prevalence peaks in older school-age children
- Ethnicity
  - Tropical countries in Africa, Caribbean, eastern South America, southeast Asia, and Middle East
    - Intermediate host is population of snails that are not found in North America or Europe

Presentation

- Acute presentation (Katayama fever)
  - Abdominal pain, cough, diarrhea, eosinophilia, fever, hepatosplenomegaly, and rash of feet
- Chronic presentation
  - Portal hypertension with esophageal varices, splenomegaly, and thrombocytopenia
  - Colonic polyposis with bloody diarrhea
  - Cystitis and hematuria
  - Pulmonary hypertension

Laboratory Tests

- Stool or urine examination for ova
- Serology to detect antischistosomal antibodies

Natural History

- Infection occurs when cercariae exit snail and penetrate skin of vertebrate host
- Cercaria transforms into migrating schistosomulum and migrates to lungs, where they mature
- After maturing, they reach left side of heart and are carried to mesenteric venous plexus where male occupies gynecophoric canal of female
- Adult flukes live 3-5 years on average, during which they feed on host blood and release eggs into mesenteric venous plexus
- Eggs released into environment through intestine hatch into miracidium, which infect freshwater snails
- Some eggs migrate into liver where they lodge in small portal vein tributaries
  - Inflammation induced by eggs leads to pyelophlebitis, periportal fibrosis, and portal hypertension

Treatment

- Drugs
  - Praziquantel

Prognosis

- 10% of patients progress to severe hepatic fibrosis

MICROSCOPIC PATHOLOGY

Histologic Features

- Portal fibrosis with partial or complete destruction of main branches of portal vein and sparing of arteries and ducts

SCHISTOSOMIASIS

Key Facts

Terminology

- Hepatosplenic schistosomiasis is caused primarily by *S. japonicum* and *S. mansoni*

Clinical Issues

- Cercariae exit snail, penetrate skin of vertebrate host, mature in lungs, and travel via blood to mesenteric veins
- Adult flukes release ova into mesenteric venous plexus, some of which migrate into liver
- Inflammation induced by ova leads to pyelophlebitis, periportal fibrosis, and noncirrhotic portal hypertension

Microscopic Pathology

- Portal fibrosis with partial or complete destruction of main branches of portal vein and sparing of arteries and ducts
- Ova with refractile shell and lateral spine

- Symmers pipe stem fibrosis characterized by marked portal fibrosis but preserved lobular architecture
- Ova with refractile shell and lateral spine
  - May be associated with granuloma formation, foreign body giant cell reaction, eosinophilia
  - Degenerate eggs may be calcified
- Pigment in sinusoids and portal tracts caused by adult worms metabolizing hemoglobin and regurgitating hematin pigment

DIFFERENTIAL DIAGNOSIS

Sarcoidosis

- Numerous granulomas without ova; eosinophils not a feature

Primary Biliary Cirrhosis

- Duct centric granulomas (florid duct lesions); lymphoplasmacytic infiltrate; lymphocytes in duct epithelium

Drug-induced Granulomatous Hepatitis

- May show cholestatic hepatitis; timing of hepatitis with ingestion of offending drug

DIAGNOSTIC CHECKLIST

Clinically Relevant Pathologic Features

- Granulomatous hepatitis in patient from endemic area warrants search for ova
- Important cause of presinusoidal portal hypertension in patients from endemic areas
  - Liver function is maintained, so patients lack stigmata of liver insufficiency

Pathologic Interpretation Pearls

- Granulomas in portal tracts, ± eosinophils, reacting to oval refractile bodies that represent ova

SELECTED REFERENCES

1. Gryseels B et al: Human schistosomiasis. Lancet. 368(9541):1106-18, 2006
2. Kibiki GS et al: Hepatosplenic schistosomiasis: a review. East Afr Med J. 81(9):480-5, 2004
3. Vennervald BJ et al: Morbidity in schistosomiasis: an update. Curr Opin Infect Dis. 17(5):439-47, 2004
4. Bica I et al: Hepatic schistosomiasis. Infect Dis Clin North Am. 14(3):583-604, viii, 2000
5. Elliott DE: Schistosomiasis. Pathophysiology, diagnosis, and treatment. Gastroenterol Clin North Am. 25(3):599-625, 1996
6. Da Silva LC et al: Hepatosplenic schistosomiasis. Pathophysiology and treatment. Gastroenterol Clin North Am. 21(1):163-77, 1992

IMAGE GALLERY

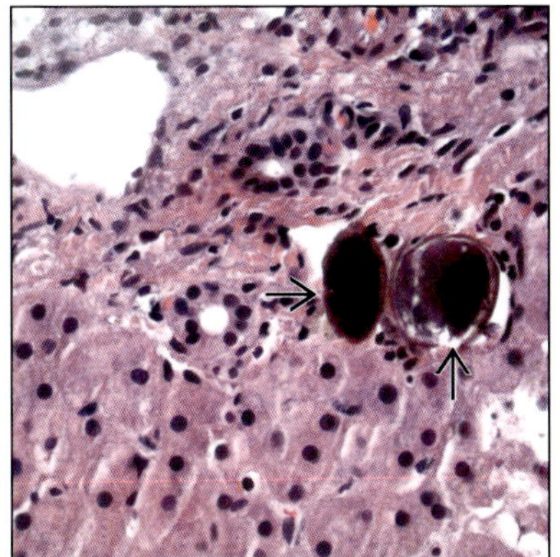

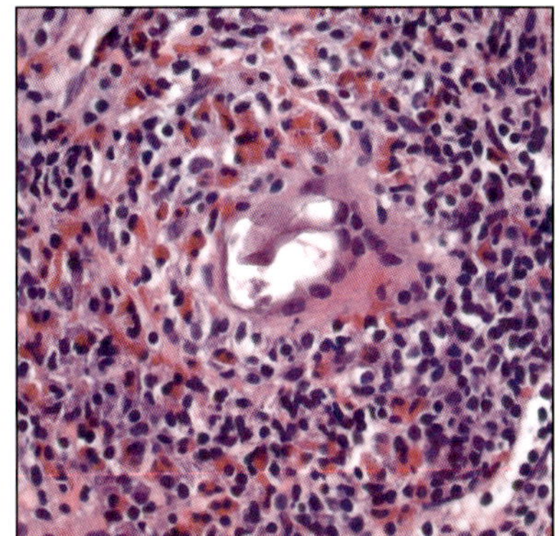

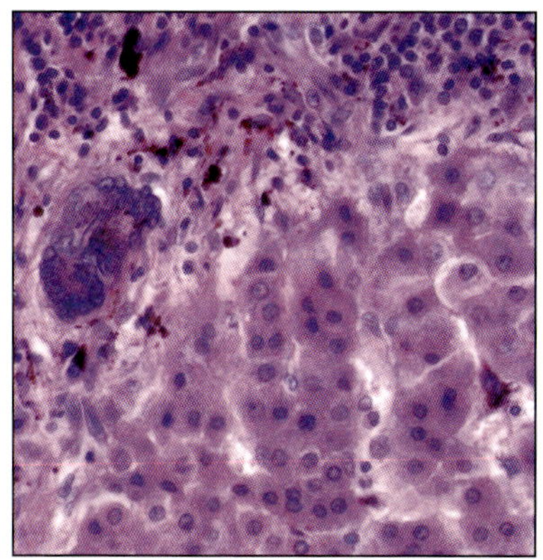

(Left) *Two ova are present in a portal tract ⇒, possibly in a small venule; the spines are not visible. In this case, a granulomatous reaction is not present.* ***(Center)*** *A giant cell engulfing degenerate egg fragments is surrounded by numerous eosinophils and mononuclear cells.* ***(Right)*** *Macrophages within the portal tract and lobule are laden with dark brown pigment, consistent with hematin, which is regurgitated by the flukes after metabolizing hemoglobin.*

ECHINOCOCCOSIS

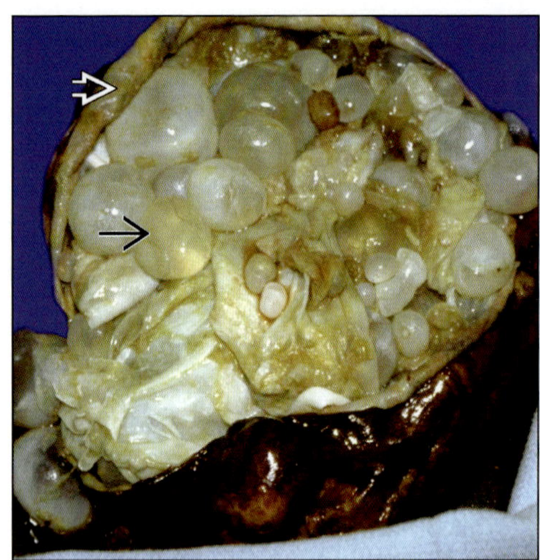

Gross photograph of liver shows a hydatid cyst containing multiple daughter cysts ➔. The fibrous rim can be seen surrounding the cyst ➔.

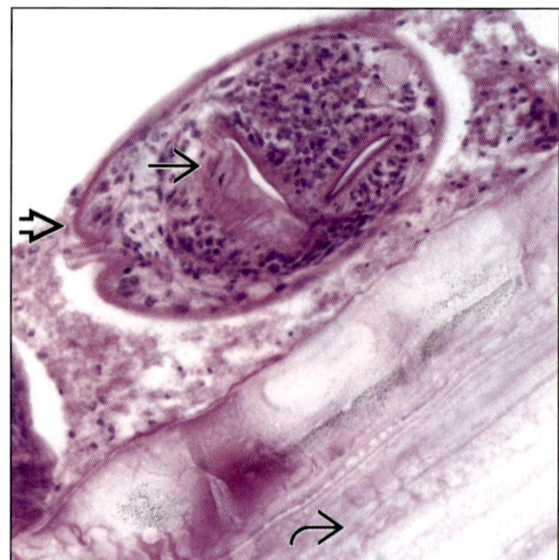

The inner lining of the echinococcal cyst gives rise to the brood capsule ➔ containing the developing scolices ➔. The next layer is composed of acellular, hyalinized material ➔.

TERMINOLOGY

Synonyms

- Hydatidosis, hydatid disease

Definitions

- Zoonosis caused by larval stages of cestodes of genus *Echinococcus*
- *E. granulosus* and *E. multilocularis* are the 2 most common species that infect humans

ETIOLOGY/PATHOGENESIS

Infectious Agents

- Echinococcosis is widely distributed worldwide
  - Tapeworm attaches to small intestinal mucosa in definitive hosts, usually dogs
  - Humans infected accidentally by exposure to contaminated feces
  - After ingestion, eggs hatch, and larval oncospheres pass to liver by portal vein
  - Oncosphere then develops into a metacestode
  - Cyst grows slowly, about 1 mm in diameter per month in liver

CLINICAL ISSUES

Site

- Right lobe of liver is most common site
- May also involve lung, kidneys, spleen, brain, and musculoskeletal system

Presentation

- Often asymptomatic
- Symptoms usually due to space-occupying repression or displacement of vital host tissue
  - Bile duct compression, bacterial infection, rupture with cholangitis, rupture into peritoneal or pleural cavities
  - Rarely can compress portal vein and cause portal hypertension
- Cyst fluid is highly antigenic, and leakage can result in urticaria or anaphylaxis

Laboratory Tests

- Serologic techniques are more specific but less sensitive than most imaging modalities
- Most commonly used serologic methods are indirect hemagglutination and ELISA

Treatment

- Primarily surgical with complete cystectomy is procedure of choice
- Liver transplantation attempted in recent cases
- Chemotherapy with long-term albendazole, although this is not definitive
- Puncture, aspiration, injection, reaspiration (PAIR)
  - Puncture with radiologic guidance, aspiration, infusion of protoscolicidal agent, reaspiration

IMAGE FINDINGS

General Features

- Ultrasound or CT scan shows internal septations and calcifications

MACROSCOPIC FEATURES

General Features

- *E. granulosus* cysts
  - Usually single, unilocular, spherical
  - Diameters ranging up to 35 cm
  - Fibrous rim present
- *E. multilocularis* liver lesions are multilocular, necrotic, fibrous rim absent

ECHINOCOCCOSIS

Key Facts

Terminology
- Zoonosis caused by larval stages of cestodes of genus *Echinococcus*

Etiology/Pathogenesis
- Humans infected accidentally by exposure to contaminated feces

Clinical Issues
- Right lobe of liver is most common site

Microscopic Pathology
- Viable cysts of *E. granulosus* are composed of 3 layers
  - Innermost layer is delicate germinal membrane with protoscolices
  - Middle layer is hyalinized, laminated, acellular material secreted by parasite
  - Outer peripheral layer is granulation tissue and fibrosis

MICROSCOPIC PATHOLOGY

Histologic Features
- Viable cysts of *E. granulosus* are composed of 3 layers
  - Innermost layer is delicate germinal membrane
    - Thin lining of nucleated cells from which brood capsules and their enclosed protoscolices develop
    - Protoscolices represent incipient heads of adult tapeworms, are ovoid, contain 2 circles of hooklets and a sucker
  - Middle layer is hyalinized, white membrane of laminated, acellular material secreted by parasite
  - Outer peripheral layer is granulation tissue and fibrosis
- Larger lesions may have daughter cysts
  - Daughter cysts are structurally identical to primary cyst
  - May be produced by protoscolices released from germinal membrane or ruptured brood capsules
- Cysts may degenerate and contain only shed hooklets and calcifications
- Eosinophils are not conspicuous, but if cyst has died or ruptured, they may be more evident, along with giant cell granulomas
- *E. multilocularis*
  - Multilocular cysts with fragmented laminated membranes but no nucleated germinal membrane or protoscolices
  - Invades necrotic liver tissue much like a malignant tumor

Cytologic Features
- Fine needle aspiration fluid can be spun down and searched for protoscolices or hooklets

Histological Stains
- Hooklets are partially acid-fast on Ziehl-Neelsen stain, stain with GMS, and are birefringent

DIFFERENTIAL DIAGNOSIS

Other Cystic Lesions
- Amebic abscess, pyogenic abscess, noninfectious processes such as fibropolycystic liver disease
- Presence of protoscolices distinguishes *Echinococcus*

SELECTED REFERENCES

1. Chrieki M: Echinococcosis--an emerging parasite in the immigrant population. Am Fam Physician. 66(5):817-20, 2002
2. Gottstein B: Molecular and immunological diagnosis of echinococcosis. Clin Microbiol Rev. 5(3):248-61, 1992
3. Maltz G et al: Amebic liver abscess: a 15-year experience. Am J Gastroenterol. 86(6):704-10, 1991

IMAGE GALLERY

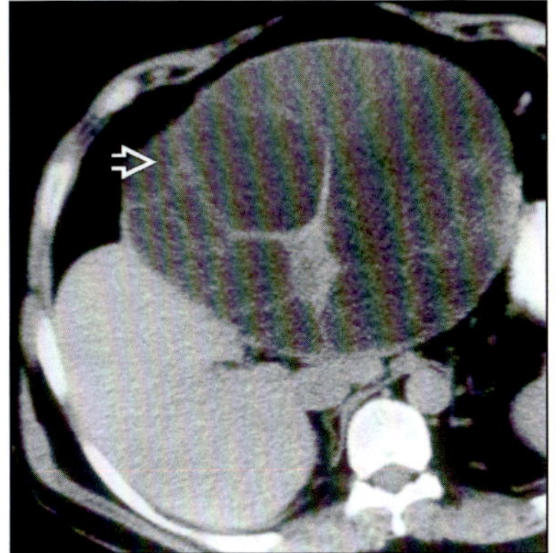

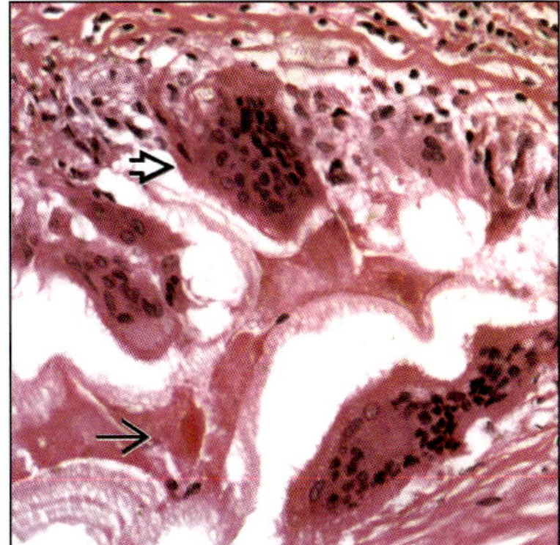

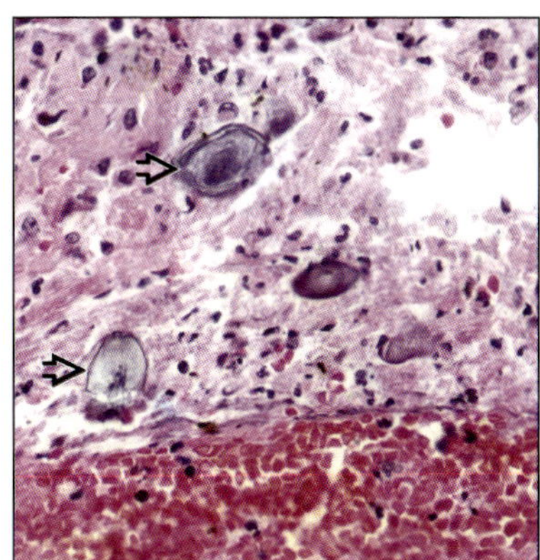

(Left) *A radiograph shows a large hydatid cyst within the liver with internal septations ⇨.* ***(Center)*** *Occasionally a cyst may die or rupture → and incite a host response consisting of inflammation and a granulomatous reaction with giant cells ⇨.* ***(Right)*** *Many echinococcal cysts are partially or completely degenerated and may only show debris with fragments of degenerated protoscolices ⇨.*

Chronic Cholestatic and Autoimmune Disorders

AUTOIMMUNE HEPATITIS

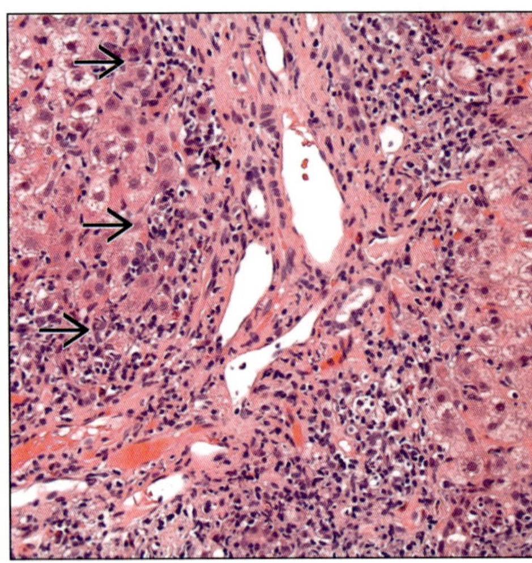

Hematoxylin and eosin stain shows typical portal inflammatory cell infiltrate containing large numbers of plasma cells with periportal interface activity ⇒, or "piecemeal necrosis."

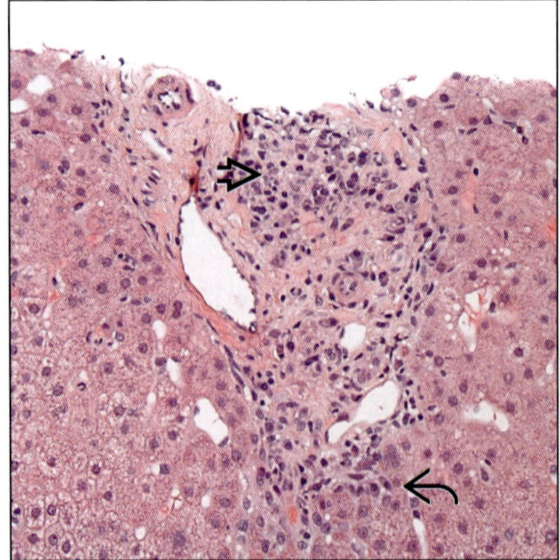

Hematoxylin and eosin stain shows mild portal inflammation including lymphocytes and numerous plasma cells ⇒ in a patient with autoimmune hepatitis. There is also interface activity ⇒.

TERMINOLOGY

Abbreviations

- Autoimmune hepatitis (AIH)

Synonyms

- Lupus hepatitis
- Autoimmune chronic active hepatitis
- Plasma cell hepatitis
- Active juvenile cirrhosis

Definitions

- Ongoing hepatitis presumed autoimmune in etiology
- 3 types described based on identification of serum autoantibodies
  - Type 1
    - Most common form
    - Antinuclear antibodies (ANA) &/or antismooth muscle antibodies (SMA)
    - Bimodal age distribution with peaks from 10-20 and 45-70 years of age
  - Type 2
    - Anti-liver/anti-kidney microsomal antibodies (anti-LKM-1)
    - Most commonly affects children (ages 2-14) but also affects adults
    - More severe disease with greater frequency of relapse
  - Type 3
    - Soluble liver antigen (anti-SLA) or liver pancreas antigen (LP) antibodies
    - Usually affects adults, ages 30-50
  - Subtyping of AIH is of descriptive value only and has no bearing on disease management

ETIOLOGY/PATHOGENESIS

Inciting Event Unknown

- May include infectious agents, drugs, or toxins
- Ongoing immune-mediated liver cell destruction

CLINICAL ISSUES

Epidemiology

- Incidence
  - 0.1 to 1 per 100,000 per year in North American and European populations
- Age
  - Affects patients of all ages
- Gender
  - Predominantly affects females
    - M:F = 1:4
- Ethnicity
  - All ethnicities affected

Presentation

- Defined as priori chronic disease
  - But may present clinically as acute onset or fulminant hepatitis
    - Patients with acute onset of symptoms often found to have clinical, laboratory, &/or histologic signs of chronic liver disease
    - Acute presentation may represent flare of previously subclinical disease
    - Some patients have no evidence of chronic liver disease, appear clinically similar to acute viral or drug-related hepatitis
- Common signs and symptoms
  - Fatigue and lethargy
  - Upper abdominal discomfort
  - Hepatomegaly
  - Jaundice
- Many patients have concurrent autoimmune diseases affecting other organs

Laboratory Tests

- Elevated transaminases
- Hyperbilirubinemia may be seen but is usually mild
- Serum autoantibodies

AUTOIMMUNE HEPATITIS

Key Facts

Clinical Issues

- Affects patients of all ages, predominantly women
- First-line therapy is immunosuppression with corticosteroids in combination with azathioprine
  - Most patients improve dramatically with treatment
  - Reduces disease activity and improves survival
- Elevated transaminases
- Serum autoantibodies
  - ANA, SMA, LKM-1
  - Perinuclear antineutrophil cytoplasm (p-ANCA) in type 1 AIH only
- Polyclonal hypergammaglobulinemia

Microscopic Pathology

- Untreated AIH usually presents chronic hepatitis with marked interface activity and lobular injury
- Plasma cells may be prominent but are not constant feature of AIH
- Treated disease may present with normal biopsy or mild chronic hepatitis without specific histologic features
- Severe AIH may mimic acute viral hepatitis
- Extent of inflammation and injury ("grade") and scarring ("stage") may be scored

Diagnostic Checklist

- Look for serum autoantibodies, hypergammaglobulinemia, history of other autoimmune diseases, and prior treatment to help establish diagnosis

  - ANA
  - SMA
  - LKM-1
  - Perinuclear antineutrophil cytoplasm (p-ANCA) in type 1 AIH only
- Polyclonal hypergammaglobulinemia

Natural History

- Progressive disease
  - Characterized by ongoing hepatic injury and scarring with development of cirrhosis and end-stage liver disease

Treatment

- Surgical approaches
  - Liver transplantation indicated for patients with fulminant hepatitis or end-stage disease with decompensation
    - Recurrent AIH occurs in 20-30% of patients
- Drugs
  - First-line therapy is corticosteroids in combination with azathioprine
  - Treatment reduces disease activity and improves survival
    - 65% of patients achieve clinical, biochemical, and histologic remission within 3 years
  - Over time, treatment regimen managed to minimize disease activity and mitigate medication side effects

Prognosis

- Prognosis mainly relates to severity of hepatitis at initial presentation
- 90% of patients improve dramatically with immunosuppressive therapy
  - Failure to respond is associated with early age at onset, acute or fulminant presentation, and hyperbilirubinemia
- Decompensated liver disease, ascites, or hepatic encephalopathy predicts poor prognosis
- Progressive disease associated with increasing fibrosis, ultimately leading to cirrhosis and liver failure

MICROSCOPIC PATHOLOGY

Histologic Features

- Dense portal inflammatory cell infiltrates
  - Mostly comprised of lymphocytes and plasma cells
  - Plasma cells may be prominent, present in large sheets or clusters
    - Plasma cells are typical but are not constant feature of AIH
- Interface activity
  - Also termed "piecemeal necrosis" because hepatocytes undergo necrosis in piecemeal fashion
  - Defined as inflammation extending beyond portal tract, crossing limiting plate, and inciting hepatocyte injury and necrosis
  - Often prominent feature in untreated AIH but usually improves with immunosuppressive therapy
- Lobular inflammation and hepatocyte necrosis
  - May be severe, particularly in untreated patients
    - May see single-cell apoptosis ("acidophil bodies") or confluent necrosis
    - Areas of confluent hepatocyte necrosis may extend between adjacent lobules as "bridging necrosis"
  - Plasma cells may be prominent component of lobular inflammatory cell infiltrates
    - Not invariable feature
- Fibrosis
  - Portal-based fibrosis similar to that in other forms of chronic hepatitis
  - Fibrosis progresses in stellate or periportal fashion
  - Progressive fibrosis results in bridging fibrous septa between lobules, and ultimately, cirrhosis
  - In cases with extensive necrosis, collapse of reticulin framework should not be misinterpreted as fibrosis
    - Type 3 collagen of reticulin fibers stains pale gray-blue with trichrome
    - Type 1 collagen in fibrosis stains intense blue with trichrome

- Residual areas of viable or regenerating hepatocytes should not be misinterpreted as cirrhotic nodules
- Perivenular parenchymal necrosis
  - Foci of inflammation and hepatocyte necrosis around central veins very characteristic of AIH
  - Termed "centrilobular piecemeal necrosis"
- Cholestasis
  - AIH may present as cholestatic hepatitis
    - Particularly in patients who present with acute onset of symptoms
  - Bile duct damage or ductopenia are not features of AIH
- Giant cell transformation of hepatocytes
  - Numerous large multinucleated hepatocytes seen in selected cases
  - a.k.a. postinfantile giant cell hepatitis
  - Not specific to any etiology
    - Probably reflection of extensive hepatocyte injury and regeneration
- Severity of inflammation and injury and degree of scarring may be scored
  - Multiple scoring systems available for describing grade and stage
  - Grade: Severity and extent of necroinflammatory activity, defined as periportal interface activity and lobular inflammation and injury
  - Stage: Extent of fibrosis, as assessed with Masson trichrome stain

DIFFERENTIAL DIAGNOSIS

Chronic Viral Hepatitis

- Distinguished by laboratory testing for viral vs. autoimmune markers
- Typically exhibits less severe interface activity and hepatocyte necrosis than untreated AIH

Primary Biliary Cirrhosis

- Antimitochondrial antibody positive in over 90% of cases of primary biliary cirrhosis
- Bile duct injury, often with granulomas and ductopenia
- Absence of hepatocyte injury or necrosis
- Important to distinguish from AIH because therapies differ

Drug-induced Hepatitis

- Clinically distinguished based on autoimmune markers and presence of offending agent
- Medications may incite AIH, which may or may not abate after removal of drug

Overlap Syndromes

- Diagnosis requires clinical and histologic evidence of both diseases, either simultaneously or in succession
- Minimal diagnostic criteria not well defined
- Primary biliary cirrhosis: Autoimmune hepatitis overlap syndrome
  - Histologic evidence of bile duct damage in addition to hepatocyte injury and necrosis
  - Clinical evidence of both diseases may include transaminase elevation, alkaline phosphatase elevation, and serologic markers of both diseases
- Autoimmune hepatitis: Primary sclerosing cholangitis overlap syndrome
  - More common in pediatric patients

DIAGNOSTIC CHECKLIST

Clinically Relevant Pathologic Features

- International Autoimmune Hepatitis Group proposed scoring system that reflects certainty of diagnosis
  - Weighted scoring system based on combination of histologic, clinical, and laboratory findings that either provide evidence in support of or against diagnosis of AIH
  - Largely used for research purposes
  - Rarely required for diagnosis in clinical practice

Pathologic Interpretation Pearls

- Untreated AIH usually presents chronic hepatitis with marked interface activity and lobular injury
  - Plasma cells may be prominent
- Severe AIH may exhibit more prominent lobular inflammation and injury, mimicking acute viral hepatitis
- Treated disease may present with normal biopsy or mild chronic hepatitis without specific histologic features

SELECTED REFERENCES

1. Czaja AJ et al: Non-classical phenotypes of autoimmune hepatitis and advances in diagnosis and treatment. World J Gastroenterol. 15(19):2314-28, 2009
2. Czaja AJ: Features and consequences of untreated type 1 autoimmune hepatitis. Liver Int. 29(6):816-23, 2009
3. Mehendiratta V et al: Serologic markers do not predict histologic severity or response to treatment in patients with autoimmune hepatitis. Clin Gastroenterol Hepatol. 7(1):98-103, 2009
4. Ramakrishna J et al: Long-term minocycline use for acne in healthy adolescents can cause severe autoimmune hepatitis. J Clin Gastroenterol. 43(8):787-90, 2009
5. Verma S et al: Liver failure as initial presentation of autoimmune hepatitis: clinical characteristics, predictors of response to steroid therapy, and outcomes. Hepatology. 49(4):1396-7, 2009
6. Hennes EM et al: Simplified criteria for the diagnosis of autoimmune hepatitis. Hepatology. 48(1):169-76, 2008
7. Washington MK: Autoimmune liver disease: overlap and outliers. Mod Pathol. 20 Suppl 1:S15-30, 2007

Microscopic Features

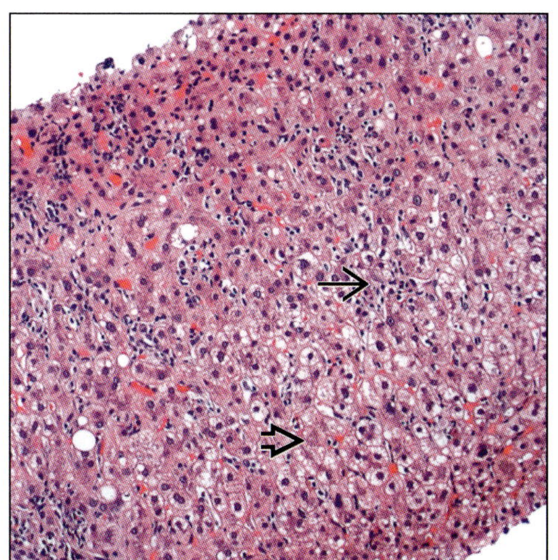

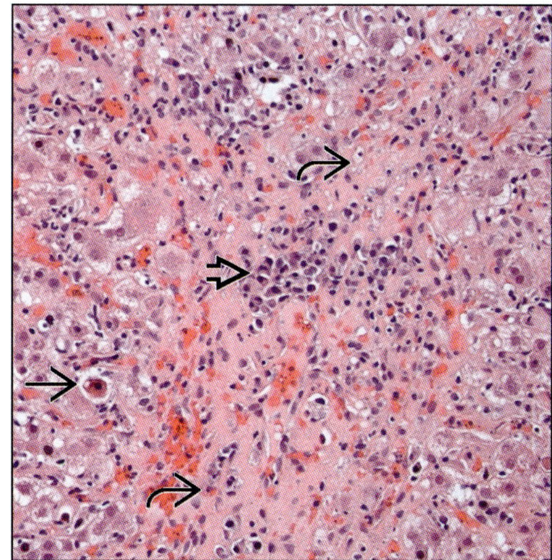

(Left) *Hematoxylin and eosin stain demonstrates diffuse lobular injury with inflammation ➙, hepatocyte swelling ➙, and necrosis in a patient presenting with severe autoimmune hepatitis.* ***(Right)*** *Hematoxylin and eosin stain demonstrates both single-cell necrosis ➙ and areas of confluent necrosis ➙. Plasma cells ➙ are prominent.*

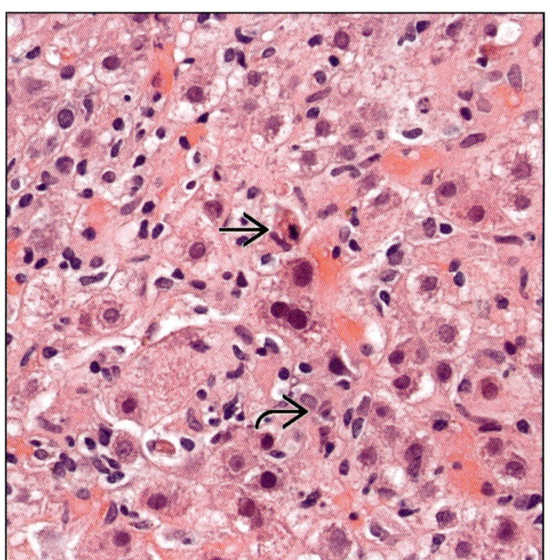

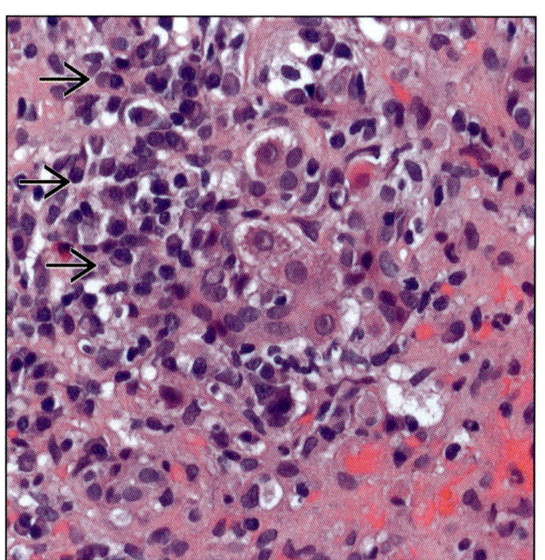

(Left) *Hematoxylin and eosin stain demonstrates spotty lobular inflammation ➙ and necrosis ➙, a common finding in autoimmune hepatitis.* ***(Right)*** *Hematoxylin and eosin stain shows prominent lobular inflammatory cell infiltrates with large numbers of plasma cells ➙ in a case of autoimmune hepatitis.*

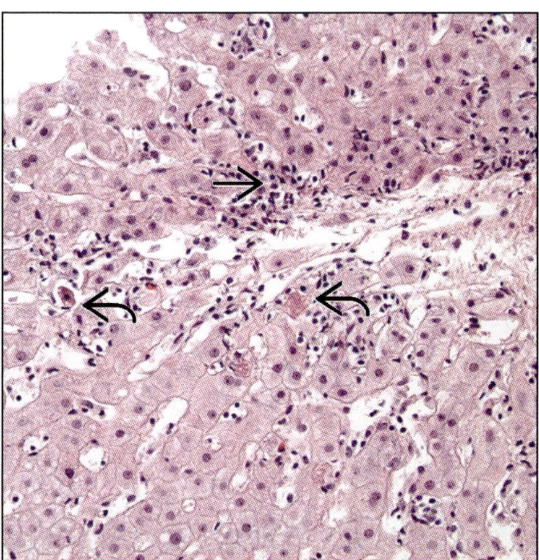

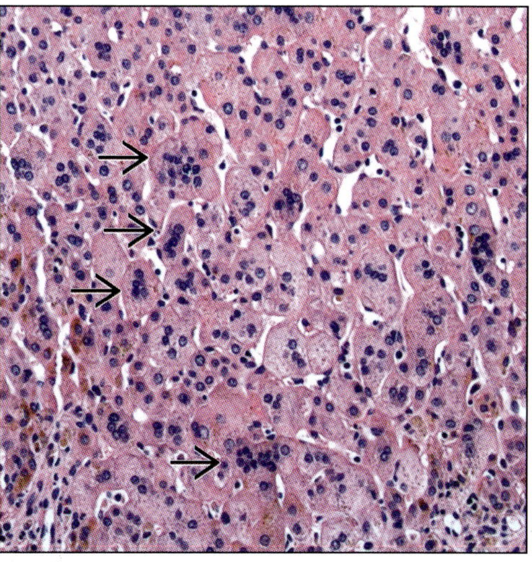

(Left) *Hematoxylin and eosin stain shows inflammation ➙ and necrosis ➙ clustered around the central vein, often referred to as "centrilobular piecemeal necrosis." This finding is characteristic of autoimmune hepatitis.* ***(Right)*** *Hematoxylin and eosin stain demonstrates numerous multinucleated hepatocytes ➙ in a case of autoimmune hepatitis. Also termed "postinfantile giant cell hepatitis," this probably represents a nonspecific response to extensive injury.*

PRIMARY BILIARY CIRRHOSIS

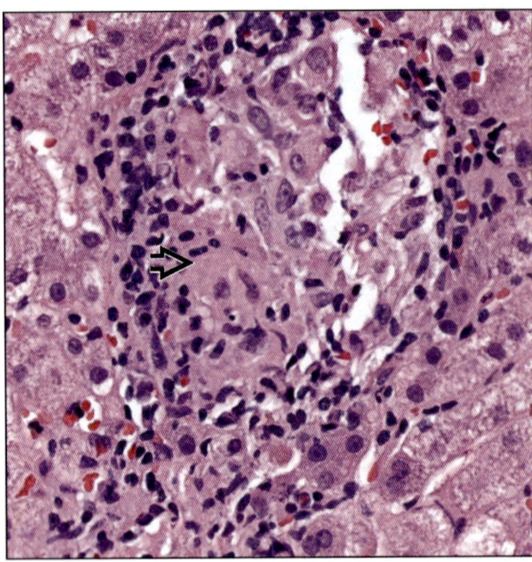

The florid duct lesion with nonnecrotizing granulomas ➪ is typical of primary biliary cirrhosis.

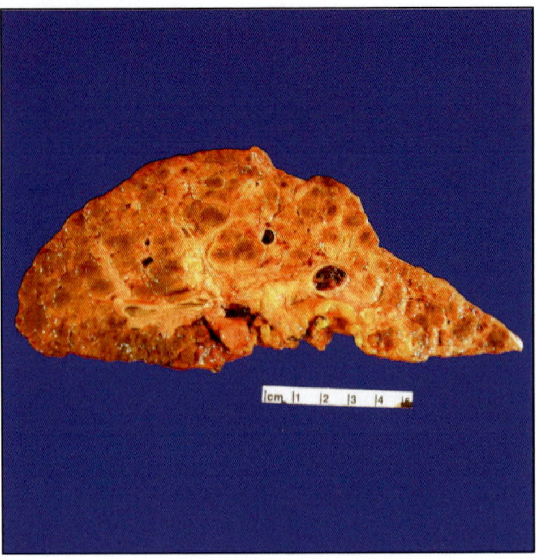

Primary biliary cirrhosis may require liver transplantation. This cholestatic explanted liver is from a patient with primary biliary cirrhosis.

TERMINOLOGY

Abbreviations

- Primary biliary cirrhosis (PBC)

Definitions

- Chronic cholestatic autoimmune disease in which intrahepatic bile ducts are progressively destroyed by nonsuppurative inflammation

ETIOLOGY/PATHOGENESIS

Unknown

- Most likely multifactorial

CLINICAL ISSUES

Epidemiology

- Incidence
  - Up to 30/100,000 in Scandinavia and parts of North America
    - Much more prevalent among individuals of North European descent
  - Distinctly rare in Asians
- Age
  - Middle-aged to elderly (40-60 years old)
- Gender
  - Predominantly women (F:M = 9:1)

Presentation

- Insidious onset with pruritus (most common), fatigue, jaundice, associated autoimmune disorders

Laboratory Tests

- Positive antimitochondrial antibodies (AMA)
- Elevation of GGT &/or alkaline phosphatase
- Elevated bilirubin
- Elevated IgM
- Mildly elevated transaminases

Treatment

- Surgical approaches
  - Liver transplantation
- Drugs
  - Ursodeoxycholic acid (UDCA)

Prognosis

- Chronic, progressive disease

MICROSCOPIC PATHOLOGY

Histologic Features

- Florid duct lesion
  - Inflammatory infiltrates
    - Lymphocytes, eosinophils, macrophages, plasma cells
    - Interface hepatitis may be present and may spill over into lobules (hepatitic phase), resembling chronic hepatitis
  - Bile duct injury
    - Irregularly sized and pseudostratified nuclei
    - Vacuolated, swollen cytoplasm
    - Lymphocytic infiltrate of bile ductal epithelium
    - Disrupted basement membrane
    - Eventually there is loss of interlobular bile ducts
  - Variably present nonnecrotizing granulomas
- Bile ductular reaction
- Portal-based fibrosis
  - Extends beyond portal tracts and eventually forms portal-portal bridging
  - Eventually develop biliary-type (so-called "jigsaw puzzle" pattern) cirrhosis
- Chronic cholestasis
  - Swollen and rarefied hepatocytes adjacent to portal tracts (cholate stasis)
    - Copper stain highlights accumulated copper in hepatocytes (copper is normally excreted in bile)
- Histologic staging
  - Scheuer staging system

PRIMARY BILIARY CIRRHOSIS

Key Facts

Terminology

- Idiopathic chronic cholestatic autoimmune liver disease in which intrahepatic bile ducts are progressively destroyed by nonsuppurative inflammation

Clinical Issues

- Middle-aged to elderly women
- Insidious onset with pruritus
- Fatigue, jaundice, associated autoimmune disorders
- Positive antimitochondrial antibodies (AMA)
  - Minority of cases are AMA(-)
- Elevation of GGT, alkaline phosphatase, bilirubin
- Ursodeoxycholic acid (UDCA) is treatment of choice

Microscopic Pathology

- Florid duct lesion
- Bile duct injury
- Bile ductular reaction
- Chronic cholestasis
- Portal-based fibrosis
- Copper stain highlights accumulated copper in hepatocytes (copper is normally excreted in bile)

Top Differential Diagnoses

- Primary sclerosing cholangitis (PSC)
- Secondary biliary obstruction
- Drug-induced chronic cholestasis
- Sarcoidosis
- Autoimmune hepatitis
  - Some patients have autoimmune hepatitis-PBC overlap syndrome with features of both

    - Stage 1: Florid duct lesion
    - Stage 2: Ductular proliferation (reaction)
    - Stage 3: Bridging fibrosis; loss of ducts
    - Stage 4: Cirrhosis
  - Ludwig system
    - Stage 1: Portal hepatitis
    - Stage 2: Periportal hepatitis
    - Stage 3: Bridging fibrous septa
    - Stage 4: Cirrhosis

DIFFERENTIAL DIAGNOSIS

Primary Sclerosing Cholangitis (PSC)

- Predominantly men
- Commonly associated with inflammatory bowel disease, especially ulcerative colitis
- Negative AMA
- Typical endoscopic retrograde cholangiopancreatography (ERCP) or magnetic resonance retrograde cholangiopancreatography (MRCP) findings
  - Beading, strictures at branch points, peripheral pruning

Secondary Biliary Obstruction

- AMA negative, lack of florid duct lesion

Drug-induced Chronic Cholestasis

- Positive medication history

Infection

- Special stains (AFB and fungal stains) necessary to exclude infection when granulomas are present

Sarcoidosis

- Has systemic involvement

Chronic Viral Hepatitis

- Bile duct damage/lymphocytic cholangitis is common
  - So-called Poulsen lesion, especially in chronic hepatitis C, may mimic PBC
- AMA negative
- Cholestasis is not known feature
- Positive viral serology or molecular test

Autoimmune Hepatitis

- Lack of florid duct lesion; bile duct damage/ lymphocytic cholangitis not a common feature

Autoimmune Hepatitis-PBC Overlap Syndrome

- < 10% of PBC patients
- Both laboratory and histologic features of autoimmune hepatitis and PBC
- Combination therapy with UDCA and immunosuppression may be indicated

Autoimmune Cholangitis/AMA-Negative PBC

- Negative AMA, otherwise histology resembles PBC

DIAGNOSTIC CHECKLIST

Pathologic Interpretation Pearls

- Florid duct lesion
- Loss of interlobular bile ducts

SELECTED REFERENCES

1. Washington MK: Autoimmune liver disease: overlap and outliers. Mod Pathol. 20 Suppl 1:S15-30, 2007
2. Kaplan MM et al: Primary biliary cirrhosis. N Engl J Med. 2005 Sep 22;353(12):1261-73. Review. Erratum in: N Engl J Med. 354(3):313, 2006
3. Chazouillères O et al: Primary biliary cirrhosis-autoimmune hepatitis overlap syndrome: clinical features and response to therapy. Hepatology. 28(2):296-301, 1998
4. Taylor SL et al: Primary autoimmune cholangitis. An alternative to antimitochondrial antibody-negative primary biliary cirrhosis. Am J Surg Pathol. 18(1):91-9, 1994

PRIMARY BILIARY CIRRHOSIS

Microscopic Features

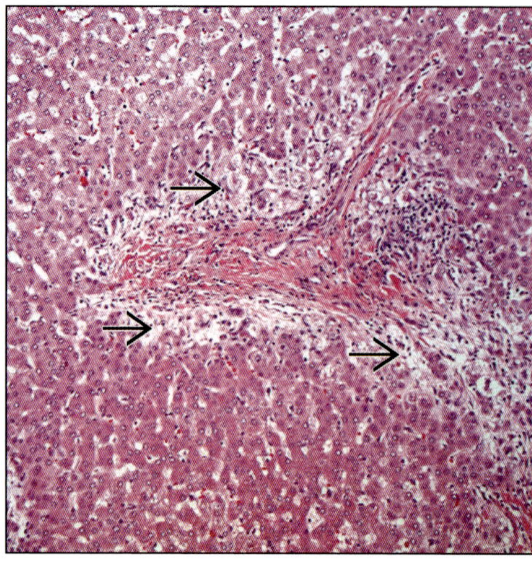
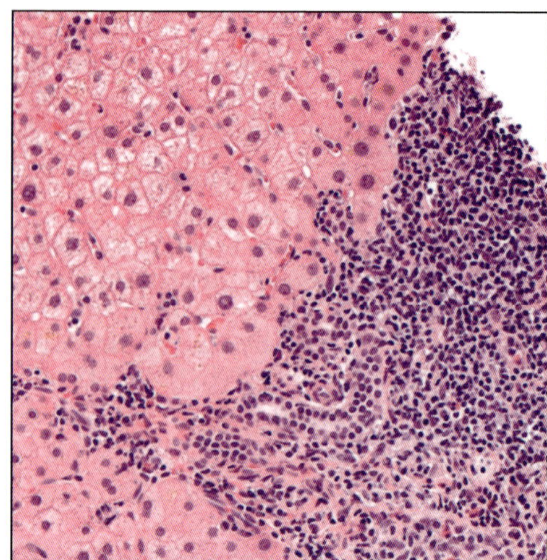

(Left) *Cholate stasis in primary biliary cirrhosis is characterized by rarefied and swollen hepatocytes* ⇨ *adjacent to the portal tracts.* ***(Right)*** *Both primary biliary cirrhosis and autoimmune cholangitis (AMA-negative primary biliary cirrhosis) may have florid duct lesions, bile duct injury, and ductular reaction.*

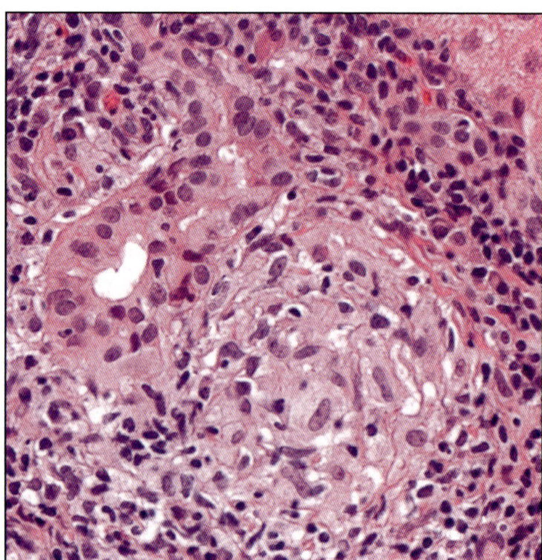
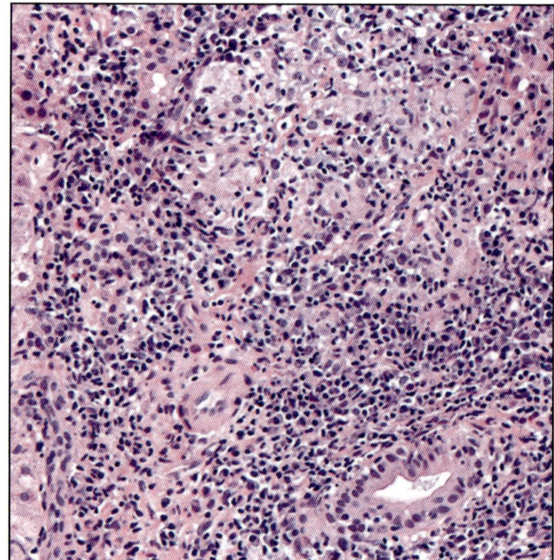

(Left) *Hematoxylin & eosin illustrates a typical florid duct lesion with granulomatous inflammation.* ***(Right)*** *Hematoxylin & eosin of autoimmune cholangitis (AMA-negative primary biliary cirrhosis) illustrates a florid duct lesion with inflammatory cell infiltrate and abundant plasma cells.*

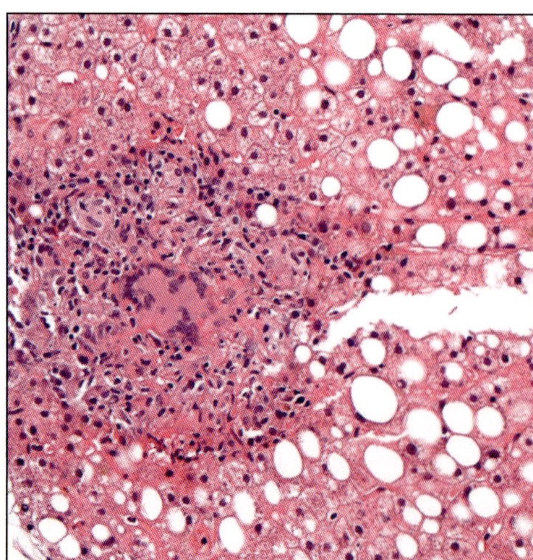
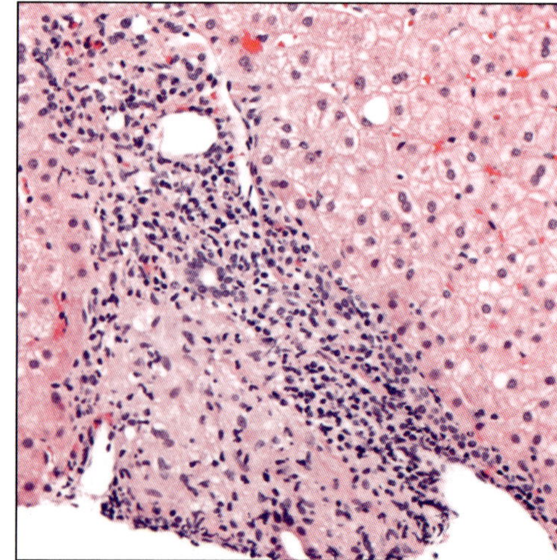

(Left) *Changes of PBC in the portal tract include a granuloma centered on a bile duct with associated portal inflammation and ductular reaction. There is a background of fatty liver.* ***(Right)*** *Stage 1 primary biliary cirrhosis is characterized by florid duct lesions and portal hepatitis.*

Microscopic Features

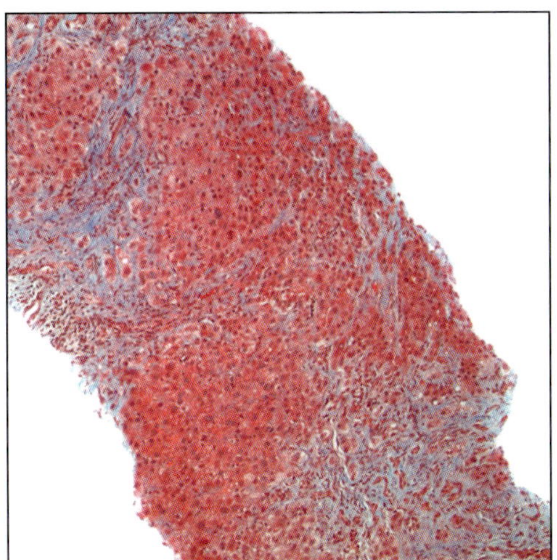

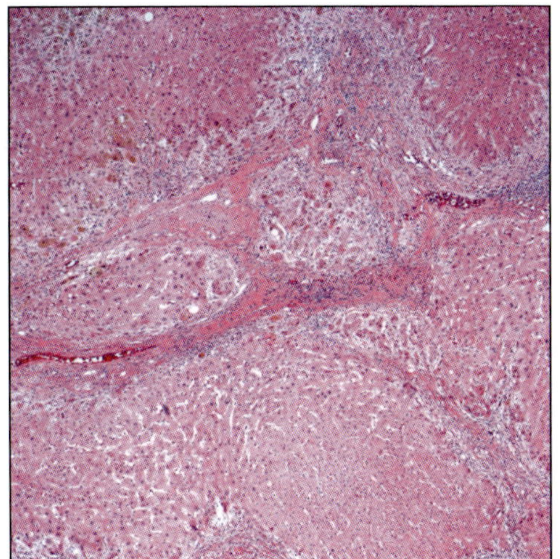

*(**Left**) Stage 3 primary biliary cirrhosis is characterized by bridging fibrosis (Masson trichrome stain). (**Right**) Biliary-type cirrhosis (stage 4) secondary to primary biliary cirrhosis shows the typical "jigsaw puzzle" pattern fibrosis.*

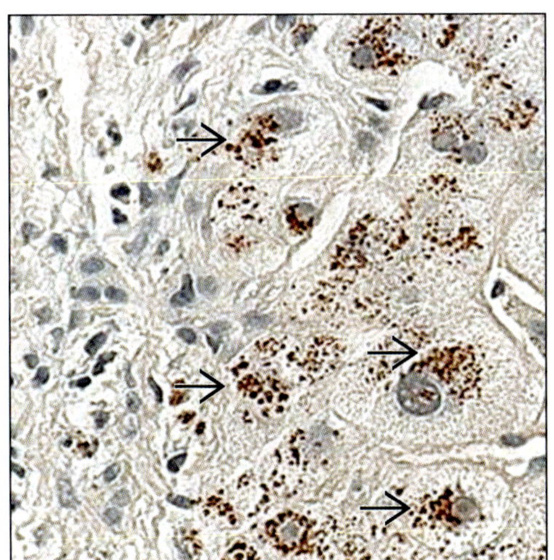

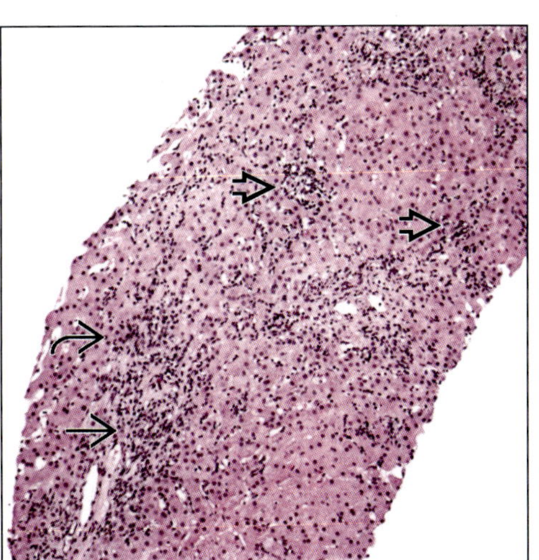

*(**Left**) Copper stain shows cholestasis with positive periportal orange-red granules ➔ in the hepatocytes in primary biliary cirrhosis. (**Right**) Florid duct lesions ➔, interface hepatitis ➔, and marked lobular hepatitis ➔ are seen in this biopsy of PBC-autoimmune hepatitis overlap syndrome.*

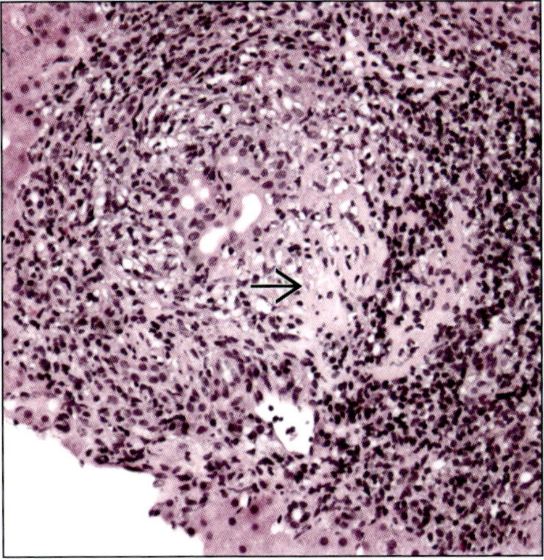

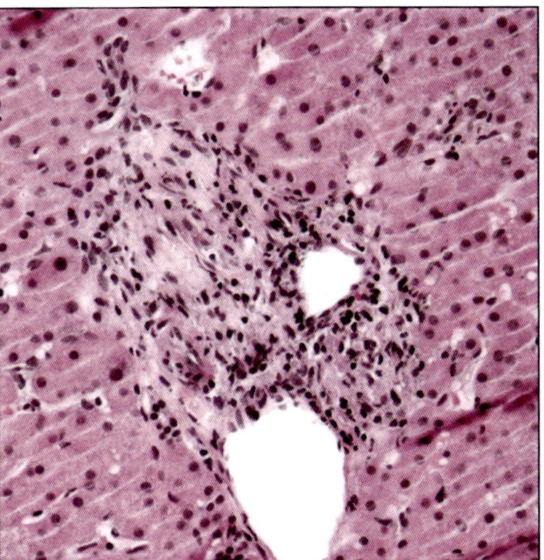

*(**Left**) A high-power view of PBC-autoimmune hepatitis overlap syndrome features a florid duct lesion with granulomatous inflammation ➔ and marked interface hepatitis. (**Right**) This case of PBC-autoimmune hepatitis overlap syndrome shows loss of the interlobular bile duct in the portal tract with mild inflammation.*

PRIMARY SCLEROSING CHOLANGITIS

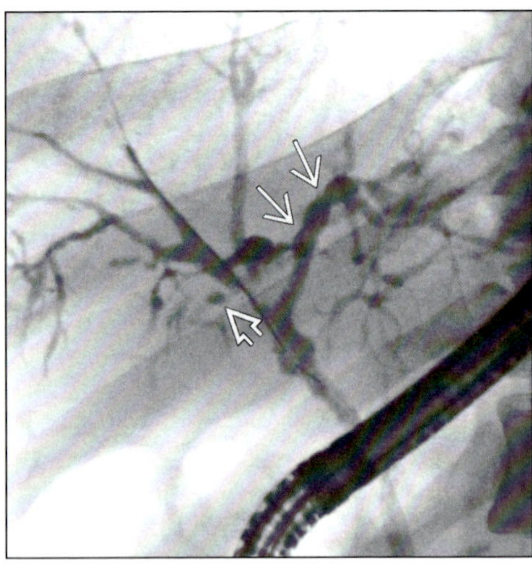

A classic ERCP image of PSC shows multiple segmental strictures of the biliary tree, resulting in a "beaded" appearance ➡. There are also diverticular outpouchings of dilated bile ducts ➡.

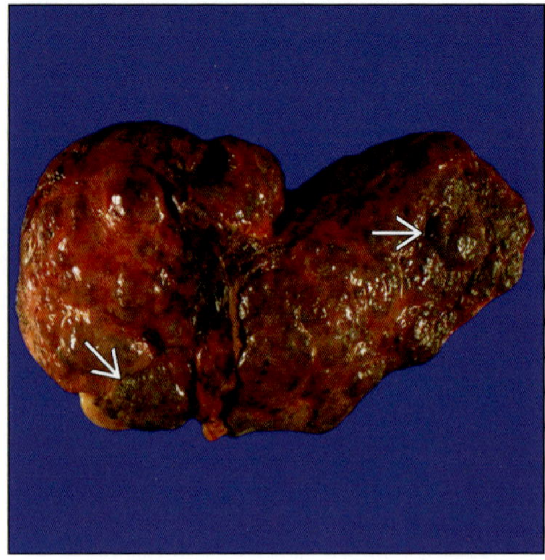

An explanted liver from a patient with PSC shows biliary cirrhosis. The liver contour is irregular, shrunken, and firm and shows diffuse, variably sized green nodules ➡.

TERMINOLOGY

Abbreviations

- Primary sclerosing cholangitis (PSC)

Definitions

- Fibroinflammatory disorder that affects intrahepatic and extrahepatic biliary tree leading to biliary strictures and cirrhosis

ETIOLOGY/PATHOGENESIS

Unknown

- Autoimmune versus nonimmune
  - No specifically associated autoantibodies
- Genetic predisposition
  - Frequent association with HLA B8 and DR3

Disease Associations

- Inflammatory bowel disease, mainly ulcerative colitis
  - ~ 70% of patients with PSC have ulcerative colitis
  - 2-7.5% of patients with ulcerative colitis have PSC

CLINICAL ISSUES

Epidemiology

- Incidence
  - 0.9-13.6 in 100,000 people
- Age
  - Any age, common from 20-50 years
- Gender
  - Male predominance (M:F = 2:1)

Presentation

- Fatigue, vague upper abdominal pain, pruritus, jaundice
  - May be asymptomatic

Laboratory Tests

- Elevated serum alkaline phosphatase activity

Natural History

- Protracted indolent but progressive course

Treatment

- Ursodeoxycholic acid (UDCA)
- Endoscopic balloon dilation or stenting
- Liver transplantation for end-stage liver disease

Prognosis

- Progresses to biliary cirrhosis
- Cholangiocarcinoma in 3.3-36.4% of patients

IMAGE FINDINGS

Cholangiography (ERCP or MRCP)

- Characteristic "beaded" appearance of intrahepatic and extrahepatic biliary tree, attributed to segmental strictures and saccular dilations of affected bile ducts
- Virtually diagnostic except for small duct variant

MACROSCOPIC FEATURES

General Features

- Irregularly nodular and green at cirrhotic stage
- Annular scars and saccular dilation of large ducts, with or without ulceration, abscesses, bile sludge, or stones

MICROSCOPIC PATHOLOGY

Histologic Features

- Fibrosing cholangitis
  - Concentric fibrosis around affected bile ducts with "onion skin" appearance
  - Degeneration and atrophy of duct epithelium
  - Lymphocytic infiltration of bile ducts
  - Mild ductular reaction

PRIMARY SCLEROSING CHOLANGITIS

Key Facts

Etiology/Pathogenesis

- Idiopathic fibroinflammatory disorder that affects intrahepatic & extrahepatic biliary tree, leading to biliary strictures & cirrhosis
- Frequent association with inflammatory bowel disease, particularly ulcerative colitis
- Lack of specific autoimmune antibodies

Clinical Issues

- Predilection for young and middle-aged men
- Increased risk for cholangiocarcinoma

Image Findings

- Characteristic "beaded" appearance of biliary tree

Microscopic Pathology

- Concentric fibrosis around affected bile ducts with "onion skin" appearance
- Degeneration and atrophy of duct epithelium
- Replacement of bile ducts by fibro-obliterative scar
- Biliary cirrhosis with "jigsaw puzzle" nodular pattern and ductopenia
- Overlapping with autoimmune hepatitis in small fraction of PSC cases
- Recurring in ~ 10% of PSC patients after liver transplantation

Top Differential Diagnoses

- Secondary sclerosing cholangitis
  - Chronic biliary obstruction
  - Ischemia
  - Immunodeficiency and infections
- IgG4-associated cholangitis
  - Association with autoimmune pancreatitis
  - Good response to steroid therapy

  - Mild portal lymphocytic infiltrates with occasional small lymphoid aggregates
  - Occasional portal eosinophils and plasma cells
  - Progressive portal, periportal, and bridging fibrosis
  - Narrowing and eventual obliteration of duct lumen with complete loss of duct epithelium, leaving a round fibro-obliterative scar
- Biliary cirrhosis
  - Highly irregular, "geographic" or "jigsaw puzzle" nodular pattern
  - Ductopenia with or without round fibrous scar
  - Ductular reaction may become more prominent
  - Cholate stasis characterized by periseptal hepatocyte swelling, Mallory hyaline, and copper deposition
- Histologic staging
  - Stage 1: Portal inflammation and cholangitis
  - Stage 2: Periportal fibrosis
  - Stage 3: Bridging fibrosis, ductopenia
  - Stage 4: Biliary cirrhosis
- Variants
  - Small duct PSC
    - Pure form seen in ~ 5% of PSC patients
    - Lacks characteristic cholangiographic findings
    - More frequently associated with Crohn disease
    - Diagnosis based on histologic findings
    - More favorable clinical course and outcome
  - Overlap syndrome
    - Overlap with autoimmune hepatitis in 1.4-8% of patients with PSC
    - More common in pediatric patients (up to 49%)
    - Has additional clinical, laboratory, and histologic features of autoimmune hepatitis
    - Immunosuppressive therapy is beneficial
  - Recurrent PSC after liver transplant
    - Recurring in ~ 10% of transplant recipients
    - Usually occurs after 1 year post transplantation, incidence increases with time thereafter

DIFFERENTIAL DIAGNOSIS

Secondary Sclerosing Cholangitis

- Chronic mechanical obstruction
  - Cholelithiasis, tumors of pancreatic head or ampulla, prior biliary surgery
- Ischemic cholangiopathy
  - History of impaired blood supply to biliary system, such as hepatic artery thrombosis
- Immunodeficiency and infections
  - Congenital or acquired immunodeficiency, such as HIV cholangiopathy
  - CMV infection &/or cryptosporidiosis
  - Recurrent pyogenic cholangitis

IgG4-associated Cholangitis

- Associated with other IgG4-related fibrosclerosing diseases including autoimmune pancreatitis
- No association with inflammatory bowel disease
- Primarily involves extrahepatic bile ducts
- Large number of IgG4(+) cells
- Good response to steroids

DIAGNOSTIC CHECKLIST

Pathologic Interpretation Pearls

- Diagnostic features may not be evident in needle biopsy due to patchy nature of disease

SELECTED REFERENCES

1. Karlsen TH et al: Update on primary sclerosing cholangitis. Dig Liver Dis. 42(6):390-400, 2010
2. Alderlieste YA et al: Immunoglobulin G4-associated cholangitis: one variant of immunoglobulin G4-related systemic disease. Digestion. 79(4):220-8, 2009
3. Silveira MG et al: Primary sclerosing cholangitis. Can J Gastroenterol. 22(8):689-98, 2008
4. Weismüller TJ et al: The challenges in primary sclerosing cholangitis--aetiopathogenesis, autoimmunity, management and malignancy. J Hepatol. 48 Suppl 1:S38-57, 2008

PRIMARY SCLEROSING CHOLANGITIS

Gross and Microscopic Features

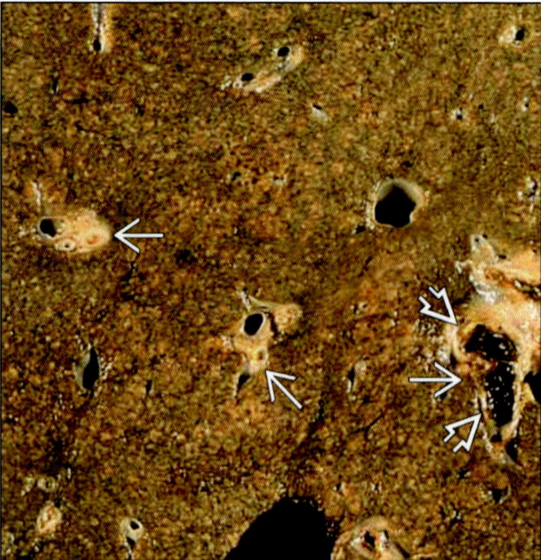

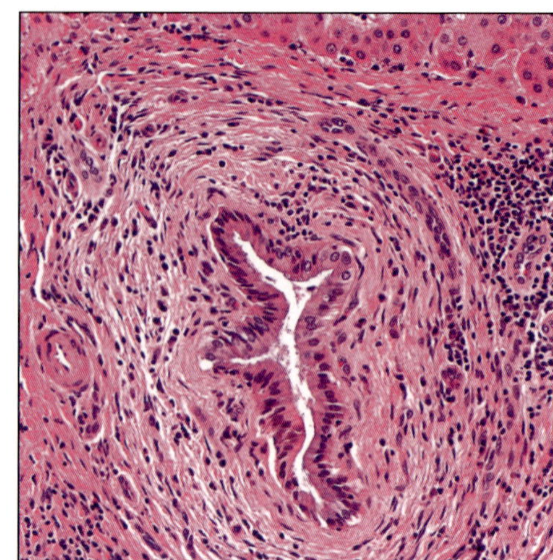

(Left) Cut surface of an explanted liver shows biliary cirrhosis with diffuse nodularity. There is thickening of the walls of the large- and medium-sized bile ducts ➔ attributed to concentric periductal fibrosis. Inspissated bile sludge is present in dilated ducts ➔. **(Right)** Concentric fibrosis around a bile duct produces an "onion skin" appearance. There is mild lymphocytic infiltration of the portal tract and the duct epithelium.

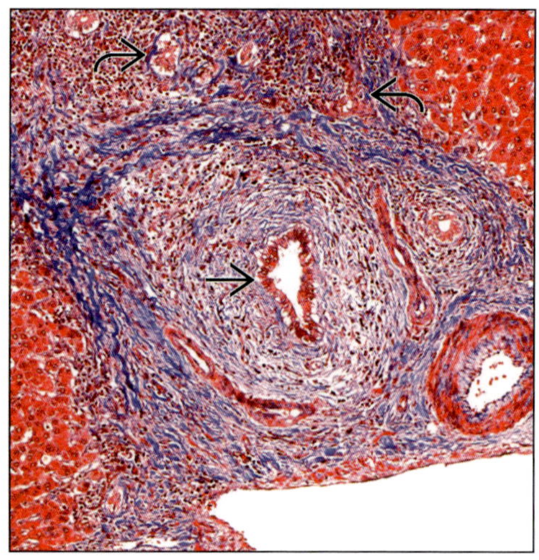

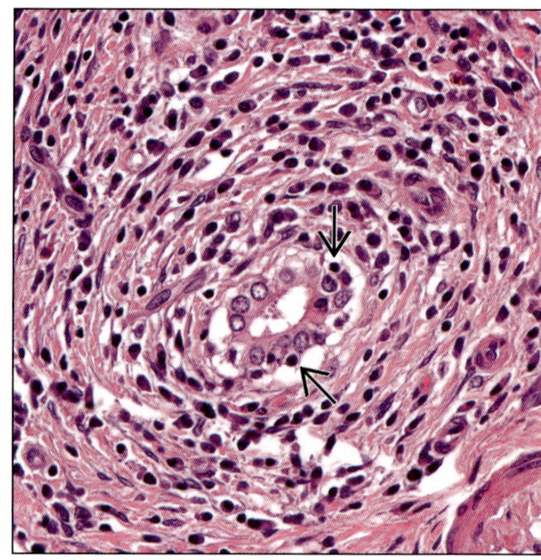

(Left) Trichrome stain highlights "onion skin"-type periductal fibrosis, characteristic of PSC. The duct epithelium is atrophic ➔. There are mild inflammatory cell infiltrates and mild ductular reaction ➔ in the portal tracts. **(Right)** Degenerative changes of the duct epithelium are seen, including cytoplasmic vacuolation and intraepithelial lymphocytes ➔. Portal lymphoplasmacytic infiltrates and periductal laminar collagen deposition are evident.

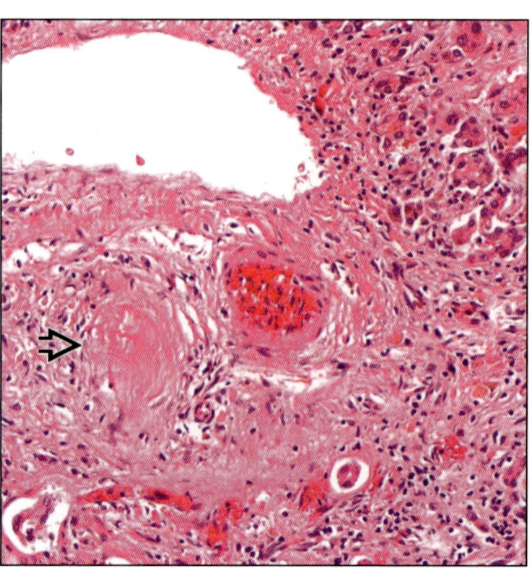

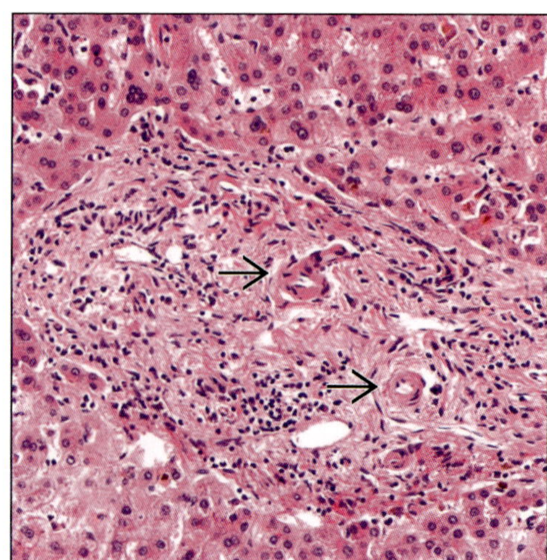

(Left) The bile duct has been entirely replaced by a round fibro-obliterative scar ➔. The hepatic artery and portal vein branches are unremarkable. Mild ductular reaction and mononuclear inflammatory cell infiltrates are noted. **(Right)** The bile duct is absent in this portal tract, but a distinct round fibro-obliterative scar is not seen. Note the presence of unremarkable hepatic artery branches ➔ and mild inflammatory cell infiltrates. Ductular reaction is not prominent.

Microscopic Features and Differential Diagnosis

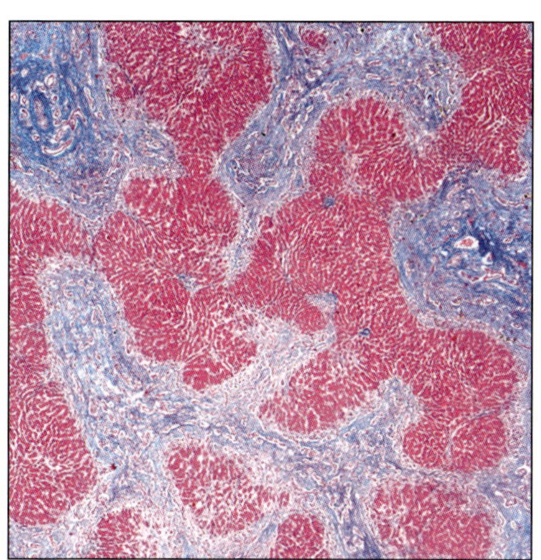

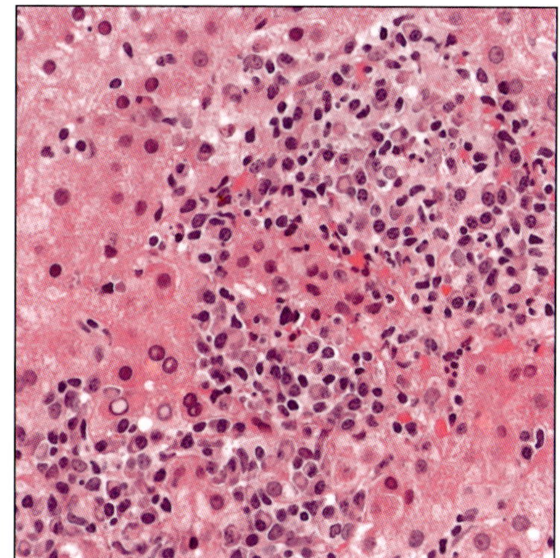

(Left) *End-stage PSC shows characteristic biliary cirrhosis with a "geographic" nodular pattern. The irregular fibrous septa are highlighted by trichrome stain.* ***(Right)*** *A case of clinically confirmed autoimmune hepatitis-PSC overlap syndrome shows more pronounced interface and lobular activity than that seen in regular PSC. Note the presence of abundant plasma cells. Characteristic "onion skin" fibrosis is present in the same case (not shown in this field).*

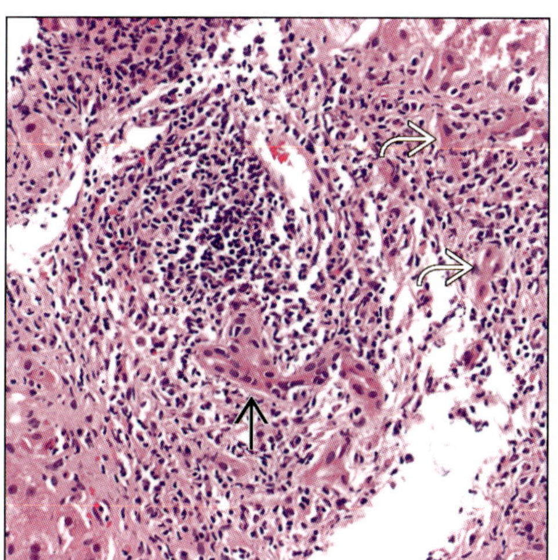

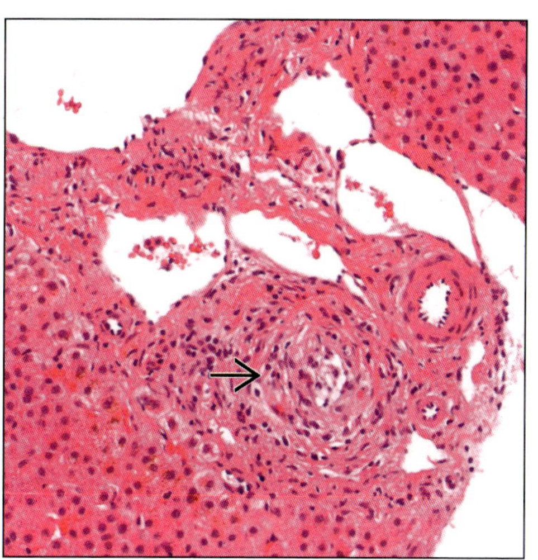

(Left) *A case of recurrent PSC (3 years post liver transplantation) shows bile duct degeneration with lymphocytic infiltration ➔ and portal inflammatory cell infiltrates. The presence of ductular reaction ➔ and the lack of definite endotheliitis help differentiate PSC from acute cellular rejection.* ***(Right)*** *A case of HIV cholangiopathy shows ductopenia with mild laminar fibrosis ➔. No infectious agents are demonstrated in this biopsy. Only rare inflammatory cells are present.*

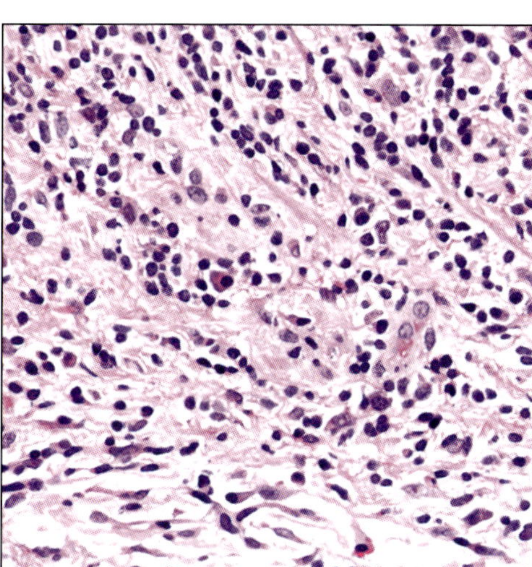

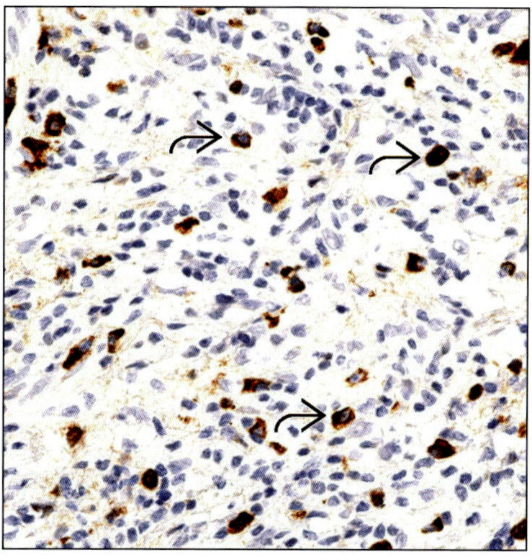

(Left) *A biopsy of a strictured extrahepatic bile duct shows dense lymphoplasmacytic infiltrates, typical histologic findings of IgG4-associated cholangitis. A pancreatic mass was also detected in this case, and the biliary stricture was thought to be malignant endoscopically.* ***(Right)*** *Numerous IgG4(+) plasma cells ➔ are demonstrated by immunohistochemical stain performed on a bile duct biopsy, confirming the diagnosis of IgG4-associated cholangitis.*

ISCHEMIC CHOLANGITIS

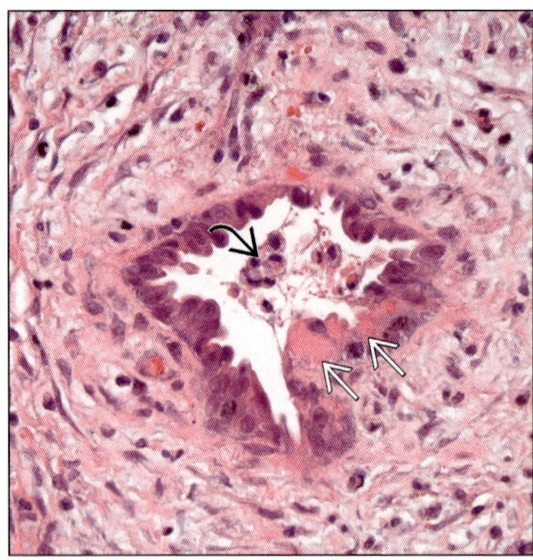

Hematoxylin and eosin section demonstrates bile duct epithelial cell necrosis ➔ and sloughing into the bile duct lumen ➔ to form biliary casts in acute ischemic cholangitis.

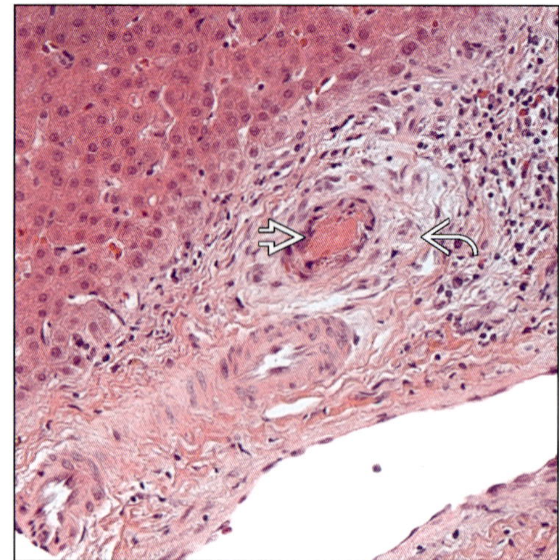

Hematoxylin & eosin section demonstrates an injured bile duct with an eosinophilic biliary cast ➔ in acute ischemic cholangitis. There is also mild portal inflammation and periductal edema ➔.

TERMINOLOGY

Synonyms

- Ischemic cholangiopathy

Definitions

- Bile duct injury due to impaired blood supply

ETIOLOGY/PATHOGENESIS

Ischemic Bile Duct Injury

- Unlike hepatocytes, biliary system is entirely dependent on arterial blood supply
- Impairment of hepatic artery or peribiliary vascular plexus blood flow results in ischemic bile duct injury
- Risk factors: Hepatic artery thrombosis, liver transplantation, previous biliary surgery

CLINICAL ISSUES

Presentation

- Abdominal pain
- Fever
- Jaundice, cholestasis
- Biliary sepsis

Natural History

- Progressive bile duct obliteration leading to biliary cirrhosis, liver failure, and cholangiocarcinoma

Treatment

- Surgical approaches
  - Revision of hepatic artery anastomosis to improve perfusion
  - Biliary drainage or reconstruction
  - Liver transplantation
- Thrombolysis
- Often not treatable

Prognosis

- Varies depending on rapidity and extent of ischemic insult
  - In severe cases, may lead to acute hepatic failure
- Consequences lessened by presence or development of collateral circulation

IMAGE FINDINGS

Radiographic Findings

- Acute ischemic injury results in dilated bile ducts with filling defects due to biliary casts
- Intrahepatic bilomas may be seen
- In chronic setting, diffuse stricturing and segmental dilatation of biliary tree seen by CT, MR, MRCP, or ERCP

MICROSCOPIC PATHOLOGY

Histologic Features

- Vary with location, timing, and extent of injury
- Acute
  - Bile duct epithelial cell necrosis and desquamation with formation of biliary casts
  - Bile duct contents spill over into portal tract or parenchyma, causing necrosis and biloma formation
- Chronic
  - Atrophy and erosion of large duct epithelium
  - Periductal fibrosis with progressive bile duct loss
  - Biliary strictures and cholangiectases
  - Secondary features of biliary obstruction, including cholestasis, portal edema, and bile infarcts
  - Portal inflammation usually mild
  - Development of biliary fibrosis or cirrhosis

ISCHEMIC CHOLANGITIS

Key Facts

Etiology/Pathogenesis

- Impairment of hepatic artery or peribiliary vascular plexus blood flow results in ischemic bile duct injury

Clinical Issues

- Prognosis varies depending on rapidity and extent of ischemic insult
  - Severe acute injury may lead to hepatic failure
  - Chronic ischemia leads to progressive obliteration of bile ducts, biliary cirrhosis, liver failure

Microscopic Pathology

- Acute ischemia causes bile duct epithelial cell necrosis and desquamation with formation of biliary casts
- Chronic ischemic injury results in periductal fibrosis with progressive bile duct loss, stricturing, and fibrosis

Top Differential Diagnoses

- Primary sclerosing cholangitis
- Other forms of cholangitis

Causes of Ischemic Cholangiopathy

Iatrogenic	Systemic Diseases
Obliterative arteriopathy of ductopenic allograft rejection after liver transplantation	Many forms of vasculitis, including polyarteritis nodosa, Kawasaki disease
Arterial stenosis or occlusion secondary to abdominal surgery or trauma	AIDS-related cholangiopathy
Chemotherapy infusion into hepatic artery	Hereditary hemorrhagic telangiectasia
	Septic shock

DIFFERENTIAL DIAGNOSIS

Primary Sclerosing Cholangitis

- Primary sclerosing cholangitis associated with ulcerative colitis and absence of risk factors for ischemia or other etiology of bile duct injury

Cholangiocarcinoma

- Usually produces more focal bile duct narrowing than ischemic cholangitis

Other Forms of Secondary Sclerosing Cholangitis

- Choledocholithiasis
- Recurrent pyogenic cholangitis
- Congenital disorders (choledochal cyst, Caroli disease)
- Fungal infection with invasion or colonization of biliary tree
- Biliary parasites

SELECTED REFERENCES

1. Ruemmele P et al: Secondary sclerosing cholangitis. Nat Rev Gastroenterol Hepatol. 6(5):287-95, 2009
2. Deltenre P et al: Ischemic cholangiopathy. Semin Liver Dis. 28(3):235-46, 2008
3. Zilkens C et al: Hepatic failure after injury - a common pathogenesis with sclerosing cholangitis? Eur J Med Res. 13(7):309-13, 2008
4. Kaczmarek B et al: Ischemic cholangiopathy after liver transplantation from controlled non-heart-beating donors-a single-center experience. Transplant Proc. 39(9):2793-5, 2007
5. Lee HW et al: Classification and prognosis of intrahepatic biliary stricture after liver transplantation. Liver Transpl. 13(12):1736-42, 2007

IMAGE GALLERY

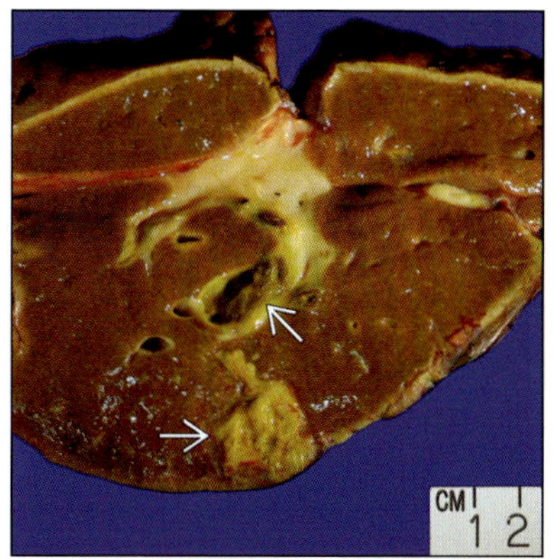

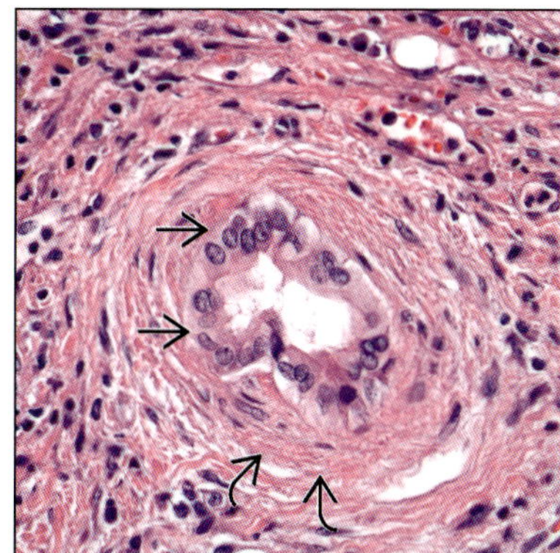

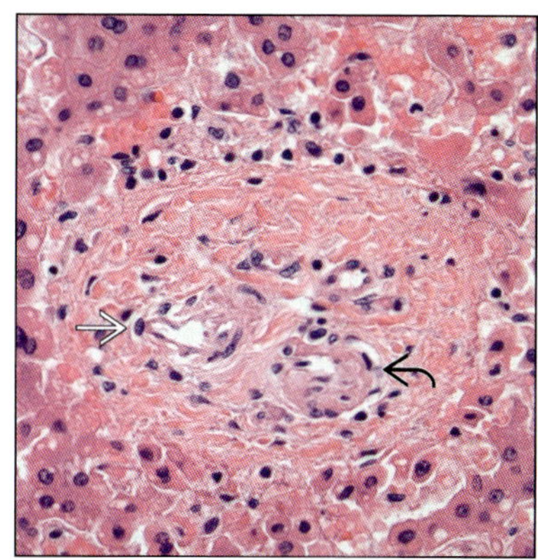

(Left) *Acute ischemic bile duct injury-induced necrosis ➡ is shown in this liver.* ***(Center)*** *Hematoxylin and eosin section demonstrates bile duct injury ⇨ (uneven nuclear spacing and loss of polarity) and periductal fibrosis ⬀ in chronic ischemic cholangitis.* ***(Right)*** *Hematoxylin and eosin section demonstrates bile duct loss in chronic ischemic cholangitis. This portal tract contains hepatic artery ⬀ and portal vein ➡ branches but lacks an identifiable bile duct profile.*

LARGE BILE DUCT OBSTRUCTION

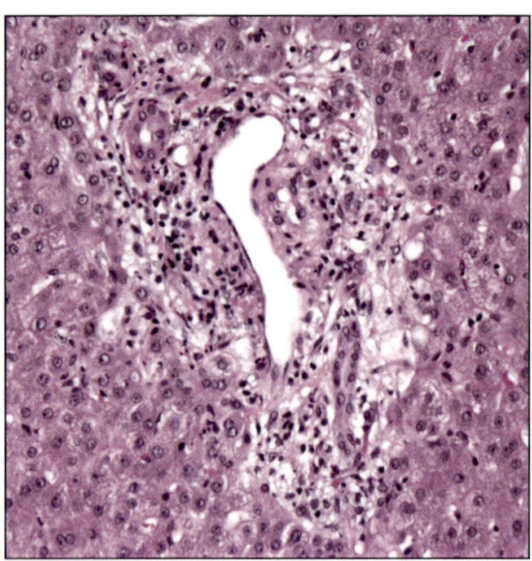

This portal tract in a case of large bile duct obstruction shows edema, proliferating cholangioles, and a mixed inflammatory infiltrate.

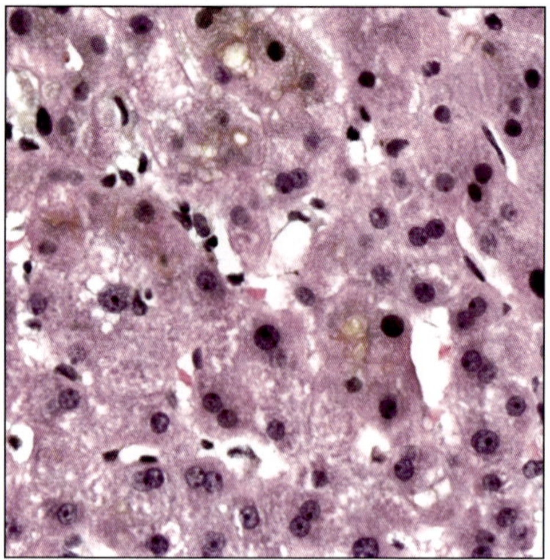

Cholestasis is often the earliest feature of large bile duct obstruction.

TERMINOLOGY

Abbreviations

- Large bile duct obstruction (LDO)

Definitions

- Mechanical blockage of extrahepatic or large intrahepatic bile ducts
  - Changes on liver biopsy are secondary to process occurring in bile ducts

ETIOLOGY/PATHOGENESIS

Multifactorial

- Gallstones
- Neoplasms/masses
- Strictures
- Sclerosing cholangitis, primary or secondary
- Biliary atresia
- Bile duct anomalies
- Parasitic infection

CLINICAL ISSUES

Presentation

- Abdominal pain
- Jaundice
  - May be absent in partial or low-grade obstruction
- Pruritis
- Steatorrhea
- Complications
  - Bacterial cholangitis/sepsis
  - Cirrhosis
  - Fat-soluble vitamin deficiencies

Laboratory Tests

- Elevated bilirubin and alkaline phosphatase

Treatment

- Diagnose and treat cause of obstruction

Prognosis

- Depends on underlying cause of LDO

IMAGE FINDINGS

General Features

- Ultrasound and CT can noninvasively confirm dilated bile ducts
  - May be absent in early or intermittent obstruction, or if ducts are fibrotic
- Cholangiography is invasive but allows direct visualization of duct lumen, defines site, and often reveals cause of obstruction

MICROSCOPIC PATHOLOGY

Histologic Features

- Histologic findings nonspecific and affected by duration, severity, and cause of LDO
- Portal tract alterations
  - Edema
  - Mixed portal inflammation with prominent neutrophils and variably present eosinophils
  - Bile ductular proliferation at edges of portal tracts
    - Neutrophils often admixed with proliferating cholangioles
    - Nonspecific but frequent finding in LDO
  - Reactive changes in interlobular bile ducts
    - Neutrophils may infiltrate ductal epithelium; does not necessarily imply biliary tree infection
- Cholestasis
  - Canalicular cholestasis typically earliest change
    - Often accompanied by inflammation, hepatocellular injury
    - May be absent if blockage is partial or intermittent

LARGE BILE DUCT OBSTRUCTION

Key Facts

Clinical Issues

- Elevated bilirubin and alkaline phosphatase very common
- Jaundice variably present depending on severity of obstruction

Microscopic Pathology

- Histologic findings nonspecific, affected by duration, severity, and cause of LDO
  - Portal edema, mixed inflammation, ductular proliferation
  - Reactive epithelial changes in interlobular bile ducts ± neutrophils
  - Canalicular cholestasis typically earliest change
  - Copper deposition, fibrosis can develop if process is chronic

- ○ Ductal cholestasis rarely seen
- ○ Bile lakes may form from leakage of bile from ducts/ductules
- ○ Large &/or periportal bile infarcts imply high-grade obstruction
- ○ Features of chronic cholestasis
  - ▪ Periportal cholate stasis (swollen, vacuolated hepatocytes) ± Mallory bodies
  - ▪ Copper staining
  - ▪ Expansion of portal areas by fibrosis, inflammation, ductular proliferation
- ○ Fibrosis
  - ▪ Irregular expansion of portal tract yields portal/portal septa in chronic LDO
  - ▪ Eventually progresses to biliary cirrhosis if untreated

DIFFERENTIAL DIAGNOSIS

Sepsis

- Look for ductular reaction with presence of inspissated ductular bile ("ductular cholestasis")
- Other clinical features of infection

Drug-induced Cholestasis

- History of offending drug
- Absence of ductular reaction

Total Parenteral Nutrition (TPN)

- History of TPN use
- Presence of steatosis

Acute Viral Hepatitis

- May have severe cholestatic features and ductular reaction
- Look for parenchymal changes of viral hepatitis
- Transaminases elevated in addition to bilirubin, alkaline phosphatase
- Viral serologic studies helpful

Chronic Hepatitis

- Can mimic chronic biliary obstruction
- Chronic BO favored by copper staining, obstructive enzymes, radiographic findings

DIAGNOSTIC CHECKLIST

Clinically Relevant Pathologic Features

- Usually clinical and radiographic diagnosis
  - Liver biopsy often unnecessary unless clinical findings/radiographic studies equivocal or misleading

SELECTED REFERENCES

1. Lefkowitch JH: Histological assessment of cholestasis. Clin Liver Dis. 8(1):27-40, v, 2004
2. Morris JS et al: Percutaneous liver biopsy in patients with large bile duct obstruction. Gastroenterology. 68(4 Pt 1):750-4, 1975
3. Christoffersen P et al: Histological changes in human liver biopsies following extrahepatic biliary obstruction. Acta Pathol Microbiol Scand Suppl. 212:Suppl 212:150+, 1970

IMAGE GALLERY

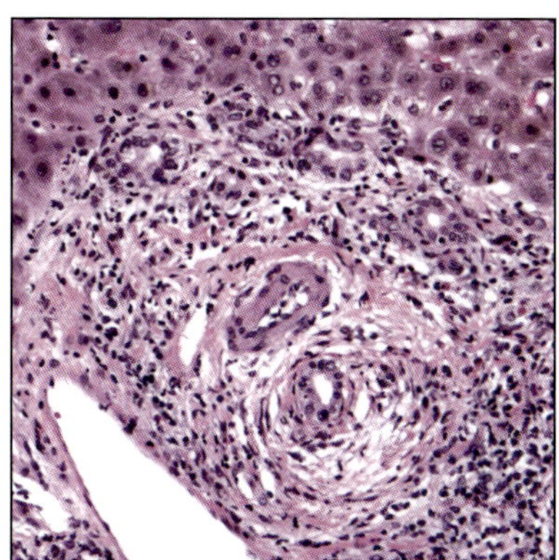

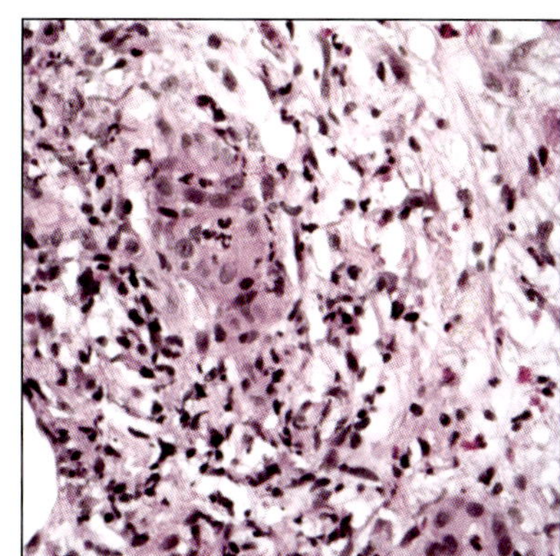

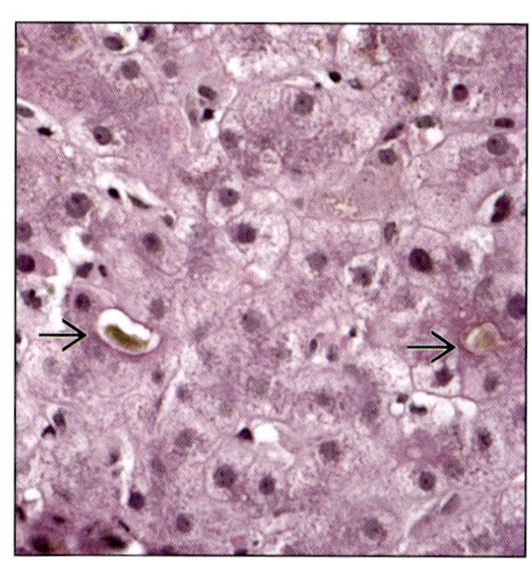

(Left) *This case of large bile duct obstruction shows marked periductal edema, proliferating cholangioles, and a mixed portal inflammatory infiltrate.* ***(Center)*** *High-power view of a portal tract in large bile duct obstruction shows neutrophilic cholangitis and marked portal edema. Numerous neutrophils and eosinophils are seen within the inflammatory infiltrate.* ***(Right)*** *Prominent canalicular bile plugs may be seen in large bile duct obstruction* ⇒.

IDIOPATHIC ADULTHOOD DUCTOPENIA

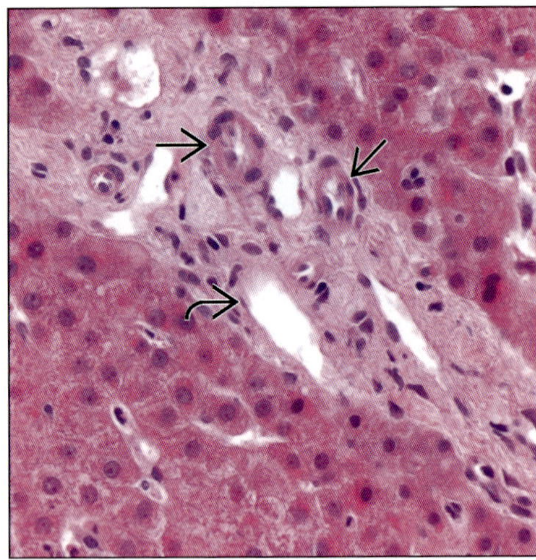

Portal tract in a young woman with idiopathic adulthood ductopenia shows arterioles ⇒ and portal veins ⇒ but no bile duct. The patient presented with persistent alkaline phosphatase elevation.

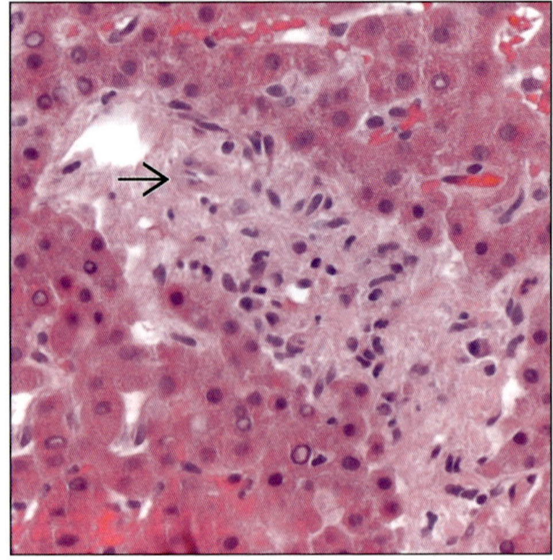

A portal tract of a young woman with idiopathic adulthood ductopenia shows an arteriole ⇒ unaccompanied by a bile duct.

TERMINOLOGY

Abbreviations

- Idiopathic adulthood ductopenia (IAD)

Definitions

- Ductopenia in adult without known cause or clinicopathologic features of specific etiology

ETIOLOGY/PATHOGENESIS

Developmental Anomaly

- Some cases may represent late onset of nonsyndromic paucity of intrahepatic bile ducts
- Familial cases may be related to mutation of canalicular transporter bile salt export protein (BSEP) or multidrug resistance protein (MDR3)

Infectious Agents

- Some cases may represent sequelae of destructive viral cholangitis

Autoimmune Condition

- Some cases may represent small duct primary sclerosing cholangitis (PSC) in patients without inflammatory bowel disease
- Autoimmune cholangitis in patients without autoantibodies might be diagnosed as IAD

CLINICAL ISSUES

Epidemiology

- Age
  - Young or middle-aged adults
- Gender
  - Male predominance

Presentation

- Episodic jaundice and pruritus
- Can be asymptomatic with biochemical evidence of cholestasis

Laboratory Tests

- Elevated alkaline phosphatase, γ-glutamyltransferase (GGT), and bilirubin

Treatment

- Surgical approaches
  - Liver transplant for patients who progress to liver failure
- Drugs
  - Ursodeoxycholic acid

Prognosis

- Ranges from nonprogressive to liver failure

IMAGE FINDINGS

Cholangiogram

- Normal extrahepatic bile ducts

MICROSCOPIC PATHOLOGY

Histologic Features

- Loss of interlobular or septal bile ducts
  - Bile ducts, which travel with hepatic artery, must be distinguished from bile ductules, which proliferate at edge of portal tract near limiting plate
  - Ductopenia is defined as absence of bile ducts in 50% of portal tracts since up to 25% of normal portal tracts may lack a duct
    - Requires at least 10 portal tracts, and preferably 20, to diagnose ductopenia, although diagnosis can be suggested on fewer portal tracts
  - Patients with loss of bile ducts in < 50% of portal tracts have been described

IDIOPATHIC ADULTHOOD DUCTOPENIA

Key Facts

Terminology
- Ductopenia in adult without known cause or clinicopathologic features of specific etiology

Clinical Issues
- Presents with episodic jaundice and pruritus
- Can be asymptomatic with elevated alkaline phosphatase, γ-glutamyltransferase (GGT), and bilirubin
- Prognosis varies from nonprogressive to liver failure

Microscopic Pathology
- Loss of interlobular or septal bile ducts
- Ductopenia is defined as absence of bile ducts in 50% of portal tracts although some patients have milder forms
- Remaining ducts may show mononuclear or mixed inflammation
- Other features include biliary fibrosis, cholate stasis, ductular reaction, and copper in periportal hepatocytes

Top Differential Diagnoses
- PBC, PSC, sarcoidosis, cystic fibrosis, drug-induced vanishing bile duct syndrome, Hodgkin lymphoma, ischemia

Diagnostic Checklist
- Liver biopsy evaluation in patient with persistent alkaline phosphatase elevation should include careful assessment of portal tracts for absence of bile ducts

- Remaining ducts may show mononuclear or mixed inflammation, but granulomatous cholangitis excludes IAD
- Consequences of ductopenia may be seen including biliary fibrosis, cholate stasis, ductular reaction, and copper in periportal hepatocytes

ANCILLARY TESTS

Histochemistry
- Copper
  - Reactivity: Positive in periportal hepatocytes

Immunohistochemistry
- Cytokeratin 7 or cytokeratin 19 can be performed to highlight ducts

DIFFERENTIAL DIAGNOSIS

Primary Biliary Cirrhosis (PBC)
- Female preponderance, antimitochondrial or antinuclear antibodies, florid duct lesions

Primary Sclerosing Cholangitis (PSC)
- Abnormal cholangiogram, inflammatory bowel disease, "onion skin" periductal fibrosis

Sarcoidosis
- Epithelioid granulomas, extrahepatic sarcoidosis, elevated angiotensin converting enzyme

Cystic Fibrosis
- Bile duct proliferation with PAS(+) inspissated secretion, sweat test, pancreatic insufficiency

Cholestatic Drug Reaction
- Exposure to drug known to cause vanishing bile duct syndrome (e.g., ibuprofen, carbamazepine, chlorpromazine, several antibiotics such as amoxicillin-clavulanate)

Hodgkin Lymphoma
- Granulomas, cholestasis, &/or ductopenia can occur whether or not liver is involved by lymphoma

Ischemia
- Hepatic artery injury, hepatic artery infusion chemotherapy, or vasculitis can cause bile duct loss

Graft-vs.-Host Disease
- Bone marrow transplant patients, mild lymphocyte infiltration of portal tracts and bile duct epithelium, vacuolization of bile duct epithelium

Chronic Allograft Rejection
- Liver transplant recipient, foam cell arteriopathy, bile duct epithelial degeneration

DIAGNOSTIC CHECKLIST

Pathologic Interpretation Pearls
- Liver biopsy evaluation in patient with persistent alkaline phosphatase elevation should include careful assessment of portal tracts for absence of bile ducts

SELECTED REFERENCES

1. Burak KW et al: Familial idiopathic adulthood ductopenia: a report of five cases in three generations. J Hepatol. 32(1):159-63, 2000
2. Ludwig J: Idiopathic adulthood ductopenia: an update. Mayo Clin Proc. 73(3):285-91, 1998
3. Moreno A et al: Idiopathic biliary ductopenia in adults without symptoms of liver disease. N Engl J Med. 336(12):835-8, 1997
4. Bruguera M et al: Nonsyndromic paucity of intrahepatic bile ducts in infancy and idiopathic ductopenia in adulthood: the same syndrome? Hepatology. 15(5):830-4, 1992
5. Ludwig J et al: Idiopathic adulthood ductopenia. A cause of chronic cholestatic liver disease and biliary cirrhosis. J Hepatol. 7(2):193-9, 1988

IDIOPATHIC ADULTHOOD DUCTOPENIA

Differential Diagnosis

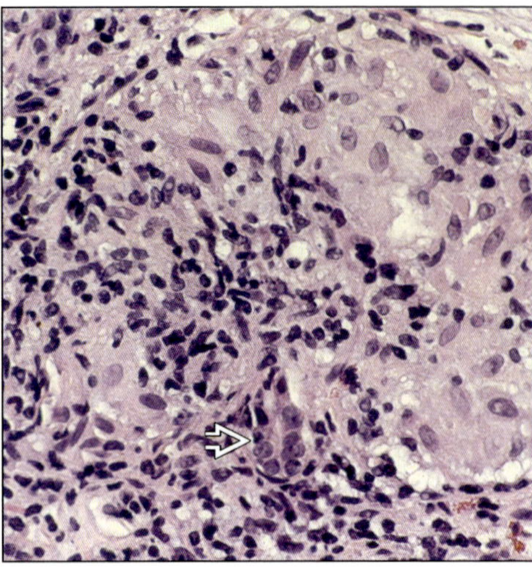

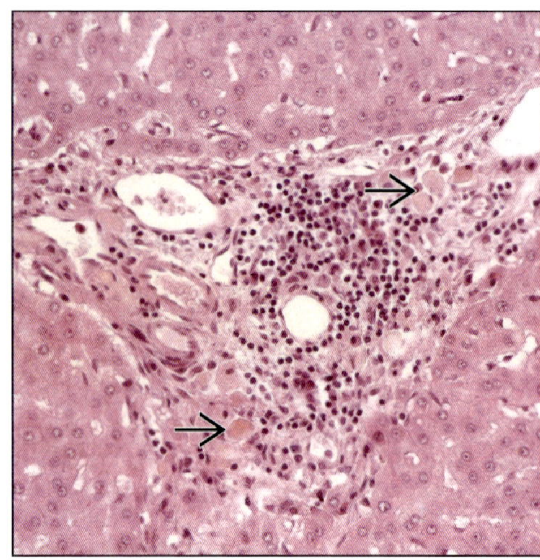

(Left) *Primary biliary cirrhosis typically shows florid duct lesions characterized by granulomatous cholangitis. Note the injured bile duct ➡ surrounded by the granulomatous reaction.* ***(Right)*** *This case of ductopenia in primary biliary cirrhosis shows a portal tract with a collection of lymphocytes marking the site previously occupied by the bile duct. Note the pigmented macrophages ➔ denoting injury.*

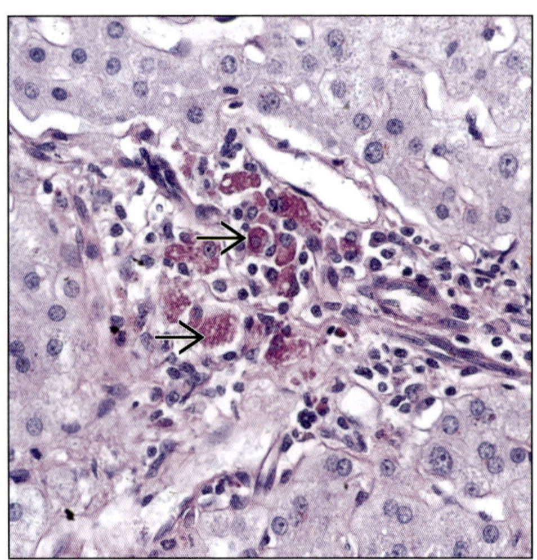

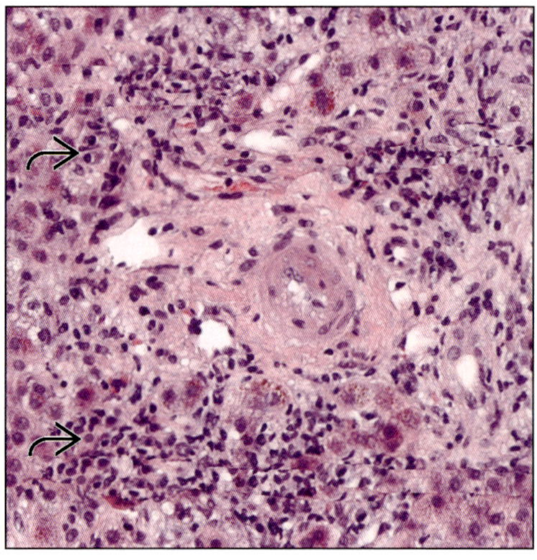

(Left) *PAS-diastase stain in primary biliary cirrhosis highlights ceroid laden macrophages ➔ in this portal tract that lacks a bile duct.* ***(Right)*** *An arteriole is not accompanied by a bile duct, and there is extensive periportal infiltration with plasma cells ➚ in this case of ductopenia in overlap syndrome (primary biliary cirrhosis and autoimmune hepatitis).*

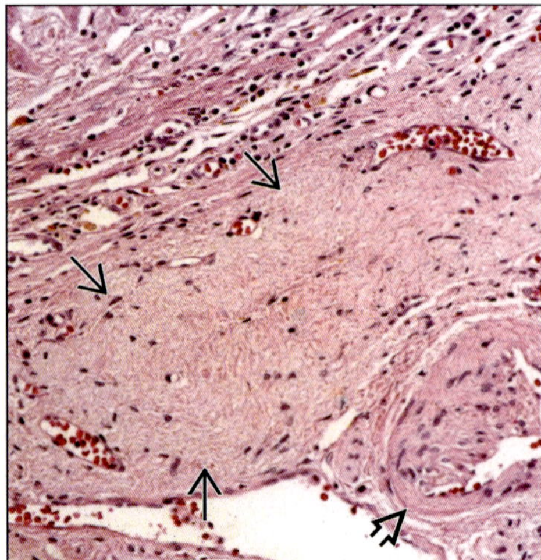

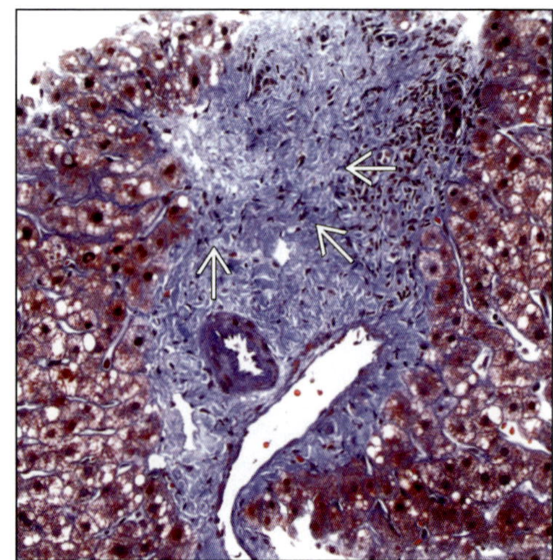

(Left) *Primary sclerosing cholangitis with fibrous obliteration of a septal bile duct features a rounded scar ➔ that marks the site once occupied by the duct traveling with the adjacent artery ➡.* ***(Right)*** *Trichrome stain in primary sclerosing cholangitis highlights a portal scar ➡ where the bile duct resided.*

Differential Diagnosis

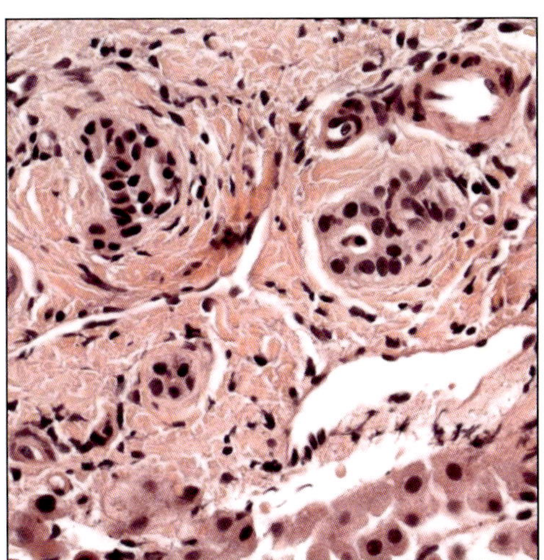

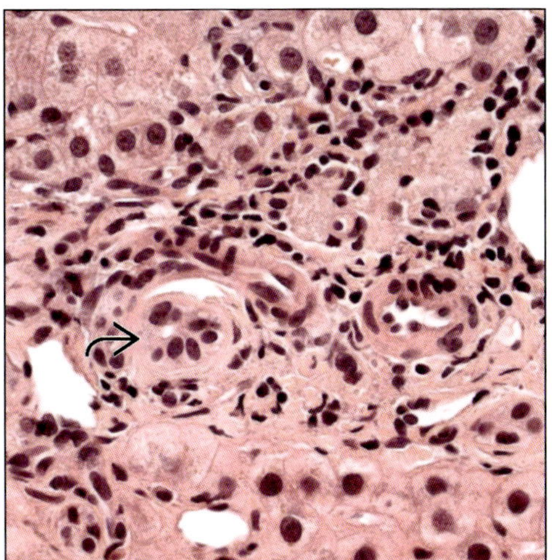

(Left) *This case of small duct primary sclerosing cholangitis in a patient with inflammatory bowel disease shows several ducts with nuclear hyperchromasia, nuclear jumbling, periductal fibrosis, and mild portal mononuclear infiltrate.* ***(Right)*** *A portal tract from a patient with small duct primary sclerosing cholangitis shows mononuclear infiltrates and a small bile duct with jumbled nuclei and nuclear dropout* ⮫.

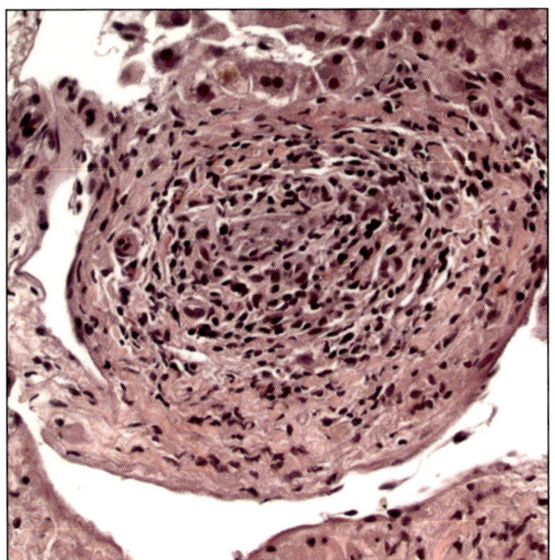

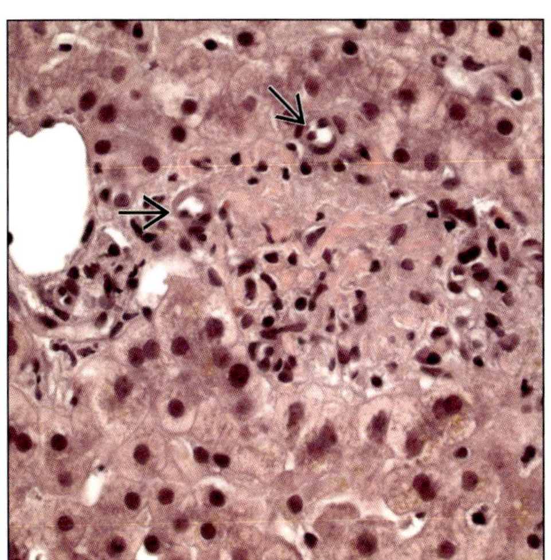

(Left) *Liver biopsy in a patient who developed cholestatic hepatitis secondary to amoxicillin-clavulanate shows destructive cholangitis with intense periductal mononuclear inflammation.* ***(Right)*** *Another portal tract in amoxicillin-clavulanate-induced vanishing bile duct syndrome shows small arterioles* → *but no bile duct.*

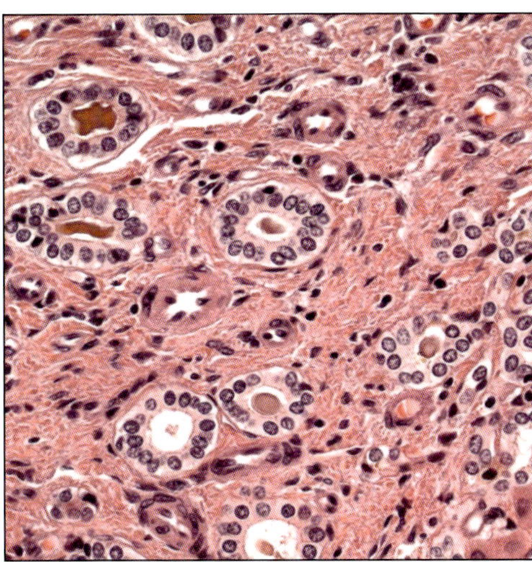

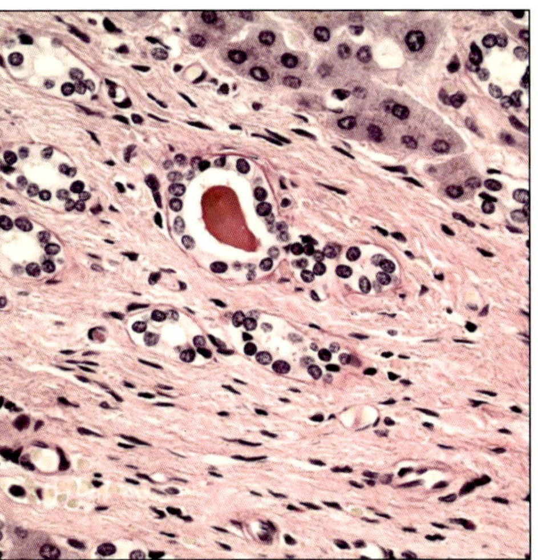

(Left) *Cystic fibrosis classically shows bile duct proliferation with inspissated secretions.* ***(Right)*** *PAS-diastase stain in cystic fibrosis highlights the inspissated mucoid material within proliferated bile ducts.*

Differential Diagnosis

(Left) In this fibrous septum, a medium-sized artery is present ➪, but the accompanying bile duct is absent in a case of sarcoidosis with duct loss. **(Right)** Elsewhere in that same biopsy of sarcoidosis with duct loss, the portal tract is expanded with marked bile ductular reaction.

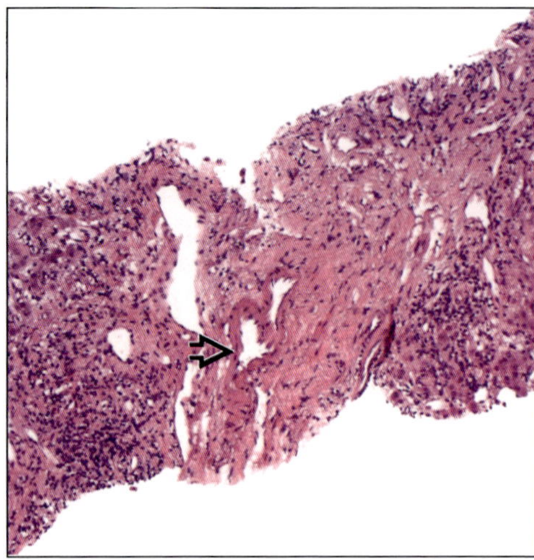

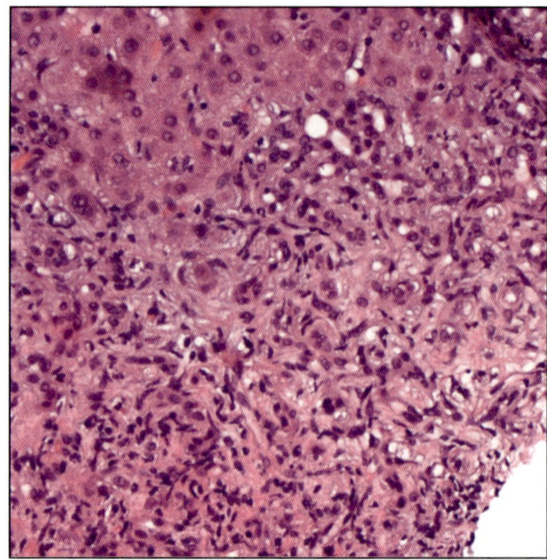

(Left) A large epithelioid granuloma is seen in a liver biopsy from a case of sarcoidosis with ductopenia. **(Right)** Cholestatic reaction in Hodgkin lymphoma features parenchymal cholestasis ➦, mild lobular inflammation, and degenerative changes to the hepatocytes.

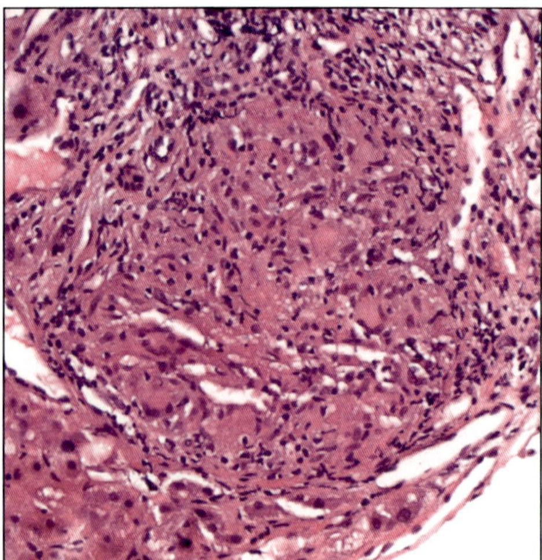

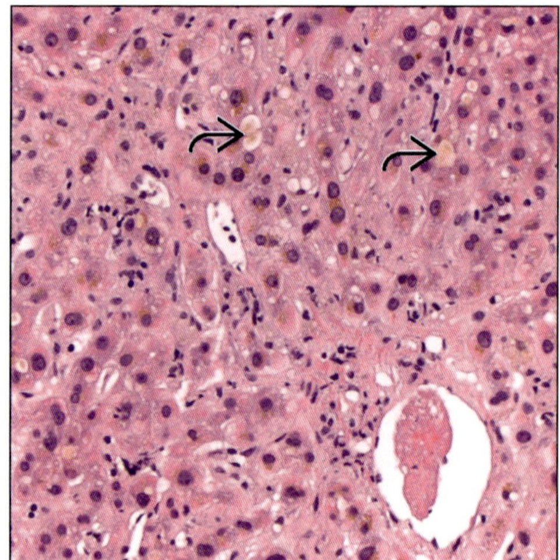

(Left) High-power view of the lobule in Hodgkin lymphoma shows obvious cholestasis ➔ with mild lobular inflammation, and reactive hepatocyte changes, including nuclear anisonucleosis. **(Right)** A portal tract in a patient with Hodgkin lymphoma shows the absence of a bile duct.

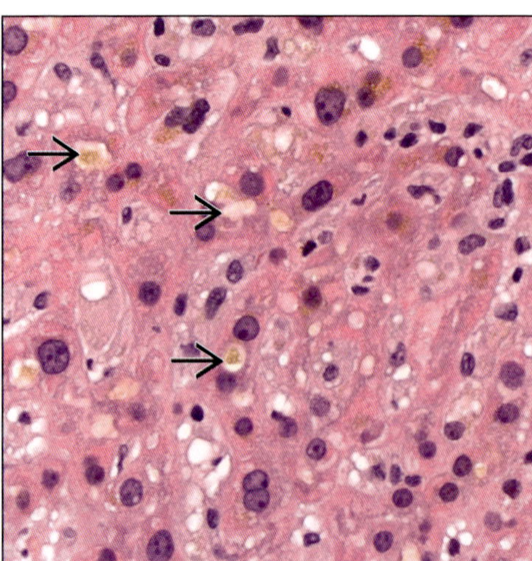

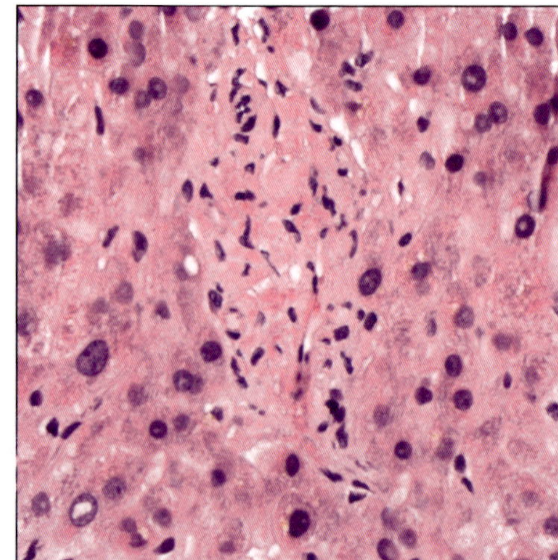

Differential Diagnosis

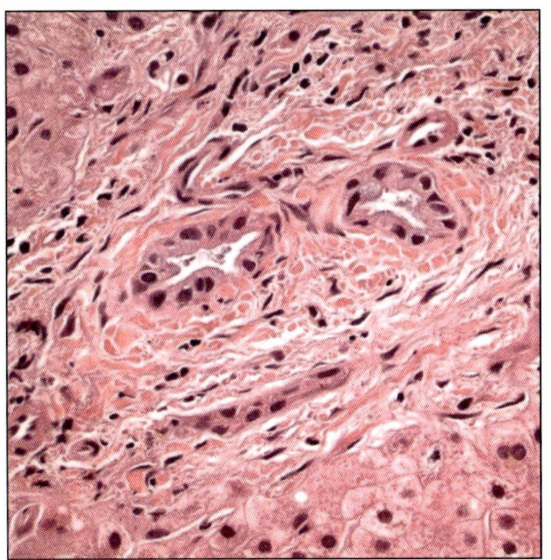

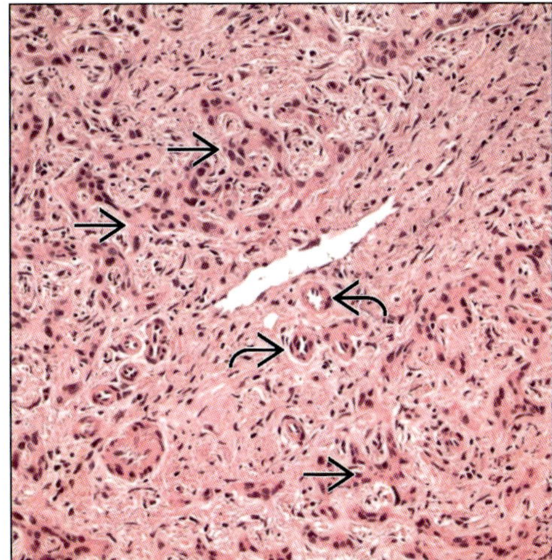

(Left) *Hepatic artery chemotherapy infusion with bile duct injury is characterized by nuclear smudginess and hyperchromasia.* ***(Right)*** *An area of a biopsy in a patient status post hepatic artery chemotherapy infusion shows arteries ↪ unaccompanied by a bile duct. Note the marked ductular reaction →.*

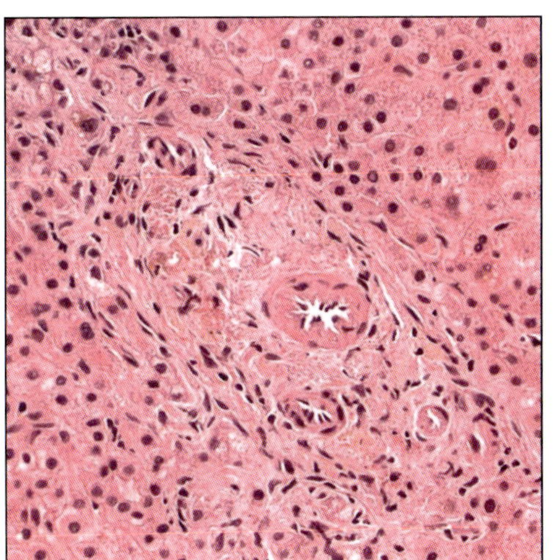

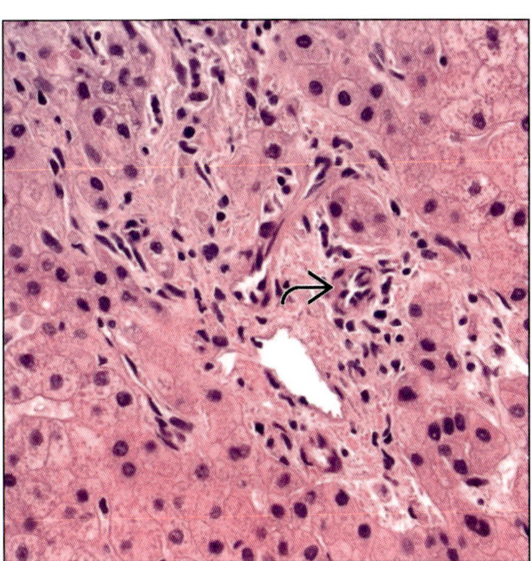

(Left) *Another portal tract in hepatic artery chemotherapy infusion shows arteries but no bile duct.* ***(Right)*** *Again, this portal tract in hepatic artery chemotherapy infusion shows small arterioles ↪ but no bile duct.*

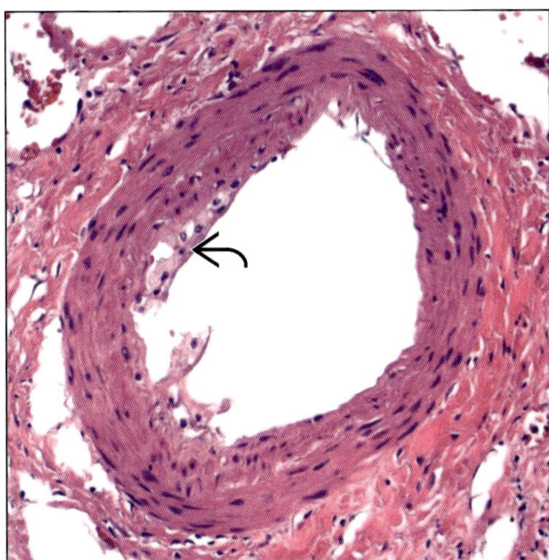

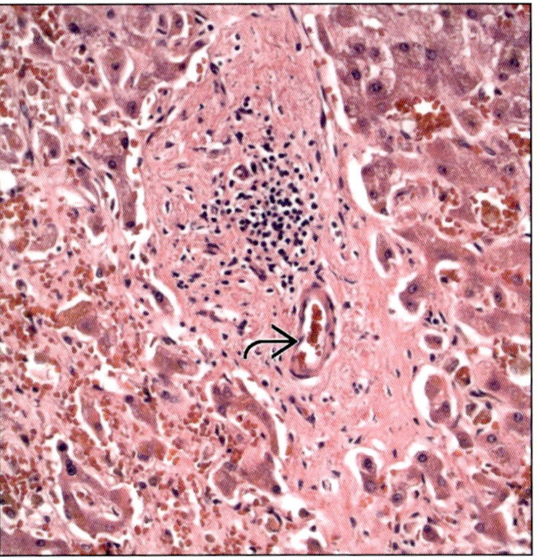

(Left) *Chronic rejection, a well-known cause of ductopenia, shows foam cell arteriopathy characterized by intimal collections of foamy macrophages ↪ within a large muscular artery.* ***(Right)*** *This portal tract in chronic rejection shows a sparse mononuclear infiltrate and an artery ↪ but no bile duct.*

Pediatric Cholestatic Disorders

BILIARY ATRESIA

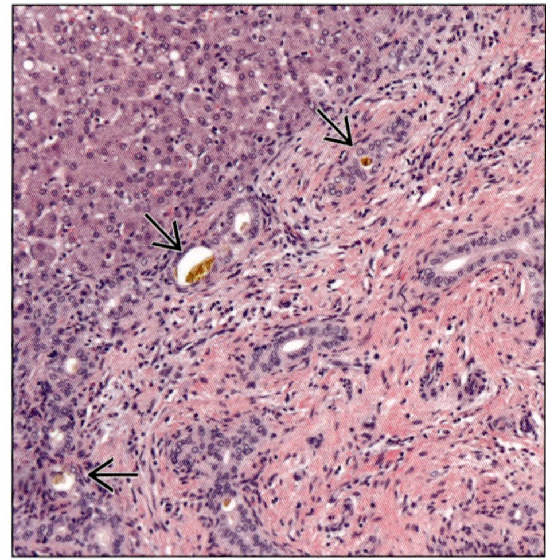

This wedge liver biopsy specimen from an 8-week-old infant shows an expanded portal tract with ductular reaction. The ductules along the periphery contain bile plugs ➙.

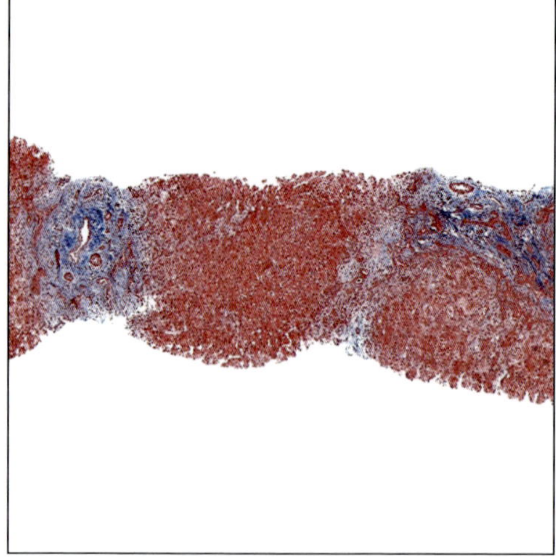

Trichrome stain highlights the expanded portal tracts with associated ductular reaction in a liver biopsy specimen from a 7-week-old infant.

TERMINOLOGY

Abbreviations

- Biliary atresia (BA)

Synonyms

- Extrahepatic biliary atresia
  - Involves both extrahepatic and intrahepatic biliary tree
    - Thus, best classified simply as "biliary atresia"

Definitions

- Idiopathic necroinflammatory fibrosing process of bile ducts
  - May culminate in ductopenia and biliary cirrhosis

ETIOLOGY/PATHOGENESIS

Unknown

- Probable multiple disease mechanisms
  - Possible roles for viral infection, genetic factors, congenital malformations
  - Genetic/chromosomal conditions associated with biliary atresia
    - Trisomy 18 and 21
    - Cateye and Kabuki syndromes

CLINICAL ISSUES

Epidemiology

- Incidence
  - 1:5,000 to 1:19,000 newborns
  - Most common in East Asian countries

Presentation

- Most common cause of pathologic infant jaundice
- Clinical triad
  - Persistent neonatal jaundice, beyond 2 weeks of life
  - Dark urine and acholic pale stools
  - Hepatomegaly
- Associated extrahepatic congenital anomalies
  - Present in up to 20% of BA cases
  - Most common is biliary atresia splenic malformation syndrome
- 2 general clinical patterns
  - Prenatal, embryonal/fetal, congenital, or early form
    - Accounts for 15-35% of all BA cases
    - Infants have low birth weight and jaundice at birth
  - Perinatal, postnatal, infantile, acquired, or late form
    - Accounts for 65-85% of all BA cases
    - Healthy anicteric, average weight neonates
    - Jaundice usually becomes apparent after 2 weeks of age

Laboratory Tests

- Similar to other forms of neonatal cholestasis
  - Conjugated hyperbilirubinemia
  - Variably elevated alkaline phosphatase
  - Variably elevated transaminases
  - γ-glutamyl transpeptidase typically > 200 U/L

Treatment

- Most frequent surgical cause of neonatal cholestatic jaundice that requires surgery
  - Hepatoportoenterostomy (Kasai procedure)
    - Palliative procedure to reestablish some bile flow
    - Best if performed before 45-60 days of age
  - Liver transplantation
    - Biliary atresia most frequent indication for pediatric liver transplantation
    - For infants without bile drainage procedure, transplant within 6 months to 2 years of age

Prognosis

- Fatal by age 2 if untreated
  - Prenatal form has worse outcome than postnatal form
- 25-35% of patients with Kasai survive > 10 years without liver transplantation

BILIARY ATRESIA

Key Facts

Terminology
- Idiopathic necroinflammatory fibrosing process of both extrahepatic and intrahepatic bile ducts

Clinical Issues
- Conjugated hyperbilirubinemia
- Surgical intervention required
  - Kasai procedure to reestablish bile flow has best outcome if performed before 45-60 days of age
  - Biliary atresia most frequent indication for pediatric liver transplantation

Macroscopic Features
- Level of extrahepatic duct obliteration is most common within portal hepatis
- Associated with hypoplastic or atretic gallbladder

Microscopic Pathology
- Best indicator of obstructive features
  - Ductular reaction, duct/ductular bile plugs, and portal and periportal fibrosis
  - Associated with lobular cholestasis, focal giant cell transformation, and extramedullary hematopoiesis
- Must be clinically correlated to exclude differential diagnosis

Top Differential Diagnoses
- Idiopathic neonatal hepatitis
- α-1-antitrypsin deficiency
- Total parenteral nutrition-associated cholestasis
- Cytomegalovirus infection
- Choledochal cyst

- 1/3 of patients develop complications of cirrhosis and require transplantation before age 10
- Native cirrhotic liver at risk for malignancy
  - Hepatocellular carcinoma, hepatoblastoma, and cholangiocarcinomas have all been described

IMAGE FINDINGS

Radiographic Findings
- Ultrasound
  - Absent or abnormal gallbladder
  - Evaluate for cystic biliary atresia and other congenital anatomic abnormalities of prenatal biliary atresia
  - Exclude other causes, such as choledochal cyst
- Hepatobiliary scan demonstrates failure of excretion of radiotracer into duodenum
  - Nonspecific; other etiologic causes result in false-positive scans
  - Excretion excludes diagnosis of biliary atresia
    - High sensitivity (~ 100%) but specificity of 87%
- Cholangiography to assess morphology and patency of biliary tree
  - Endoscopic retrograde cholangiopancreatography
    - Invasive procedure, requires general anesthesia and is technically difficult
  - Intraoperative cholangiogram

MACROSCOPIC FEATURES

Surgical Classification
- Based on level of extrahepatic duct obliteration
  - Type I (5-10%)
    - Within common bile duct
  - Type II (3-5%)
    - Within common hepatic duct
  - Type III (> 85-90%)
    - Within portal hepatis

MICROSCOPIC PATHOLOGY

Histologic Features
- Obstructive-type pattern of injury
  - Nonspecific
  - Clinical correlation required to exclude other entities in differential diagnosis
- Should have at least 5-7 evaluable portal tracts
  - Portal edema and inflammation
  - Expanded portal tracts with ductular reaction
  - Bile plugs within ducts/ductules
  - Periportal and bridging fibrosis with eventual biliary cirrhosis
  - Bile duct loss and ductopenia can develop
- Lobular features
  - Canalicular cholestasis with variable pseudoacinar transformation
  - Focal giant cell transformation
  - Scattered foci of extramedullary hematopoiesis
  - No significant necrosis
- Biliary atresia is dynamic process that evolves over time
  - Histologic timing of various stages is an approximation at best
- Stages of biliary atresia in patients who have not undergone surgery; timing of stages is only an approximation
  - Early stage: 1-4 weeks
    - Nonspecific, features are not diagnostic
    - Cholestasis with minimal inflammation
    - Few lobular multinucleated hepatocytes (giant cell transformation)
  - 2nd stage: 4-7 weeks
    - Characteristic obstructive features
    - Ductular reaction, best developed at or after 6 weeks, is most reliable criterion
    - Portal tract edema and variable inflammation
    - Interlobular duct epithelial damage
    - Cholestasis with bile plugs
  - 3rd stage: 7-8 weeks
    - Portal and periportal fibrosis

- 4th stage: 10 weeks
  - Portal to bridging fibrosis
  - Inflammation decreases
  - Variable periductal fibrosis
- Last stage: > 12 weeks
  - Biliary cirrhosis
  - Ductular reaction may not be prominent
  - Variable paucity of interlobular bile ducts
- Histologic features of biliary remnant
  - Variable histology
  - Single-duct or multiple-duct/ductule profiles that may have narrowed lumen
    - Dense fibrosis, granulation-like tissue, or active fibroplasia ± inflammation
    - Squamous metaplasia of ductal epithelium has been described
    - Cartilage rarely seen
  - No ductal lumen, just fibrous cord

DIFFERENTIAL DIAGNOSIS

Idiopathic Neonatal Hepatitis

- Primarily lobular process
  - Hepatocyte disarray with giant cell transformation predominates
  - Absent to minimal ductular reaction

Choledochal Cyst or Cholelithiasis

- Radiographic imaging studies needed

Total Parenteral Nutrition-associated Cholestasis

- History of total parenteral nutrition (TPN)

α-1-Antitrypsin Deficiency

- Decreased levels of serum α-1-antitrypsin
  - Confirmation by protease inhibitor typing
- Typical periportal PAS-D(+) cytoplasmic globules may not be evident before 12 weeks of age
- Electron microscopy shows stored protein in dilated endoplasmic reticulum

Cytomegalovirus Infection

- Cytomegalovirus in endothelial cells, hepatocytes, or bile duct epithelium
  - Important to examine every section and use immunohistochemistry because inclusions often focal

Alagille Syndrome

- Can mimic BA histologically and radiographically
  - Ductular reaction without decreased ducts can occur and will resemble BA
  - Common bile duct hypoplasia without visualization of intrahepatic biliary tree on cholangiogram further mimics BA
- Absence of decreased interlobular ducts, especially < 6 months of age, does not exclude diagnosis of Alagille
  - Immunohistochemical stain for CK7 is useful in assessing ducts/ductules
- Kasai procedure is unnecessary in these patients
- Clinical manifestation can be useful in arriving at diagnosis early in disease
  - Congenital heart disease, usually peripheral pulmonary stenosis
  - Butterfly-shaped vertebral arch defects
  - Typical facies (may not be evident in early neonatal period)
  - Posterior embryotoxon

Cholestasis-associated Sepsis

- Sepsis may cause dilated ductules with bile plugs
- Interlobular bile ducts usually intact and free of injury
- Need history of sepsis

Progressive Familial Intrahepatic Cholestasis Type 3

- Mutation of MDR3, multidrug resistance protein 3, coded by *ABCB4* gene
- Early in course has expanded portal tracts with ductular reaction
- Elevated γ-glutamyl transpeptidase
- 1/3 to 1/2 of patients present during infancy

Cystic Fibrosis

- Dilated ductules with luminal amorphous pink secretion
- Mutation in *CFTR*

Langerhans Cell Histiocytosis

- CD1a(+) Langerhans cells, may be focal

DIAGNOSTIC CHECKLIST

Pathologic Interpretation Pearls

- 1st distinguish neonatal hepatitis-like pattern of injury from obstructive-type pattern of injury
  - If obstructive-type pattern of injury is favored, in addition to biliary atresia, consider other etiologies that can cause this pattern
    - Variable amount of ductular reaction can be seen in many conditions

SELECTED REFERENCES

1. Hartley JL et al: Biliary atresia. Lancet. 374(9702):1704-13, 2009
2. Sokol RJ et al: Screening and outcomes in biliary atresia: summary of a National Institutes of Health workshop. Hepatology. 46(2):566-81, 2007
3. Kahn E: Biliary atresia revisited. Pediatr Dev Pathol. 7(2):109-24, 2004
4. Azar G et al: Atypical morphologic presentation of biliary atresia and value of serial liver biopsies. J Pediatr Gastroenterol Nutr. 34(2):212-5, 2002
5. Lefkowitch JH: Biliary atresia. Mayo Clin Proc. 73(1):90-5, 1998
6. Nietgen GW et al: Intrahepatic bile duct loss in biliary atresia despite portoenterostomy: a consequence of ongoing obstruction? Gastroenterology. 102(6):2126-33, 1992
7. Raweily EA et al: Abnormalities of intrahepatic bile ducts in extrahepatic biliary atresia. Histopathology. 17(6):521-7, 1990

Microscopic Features

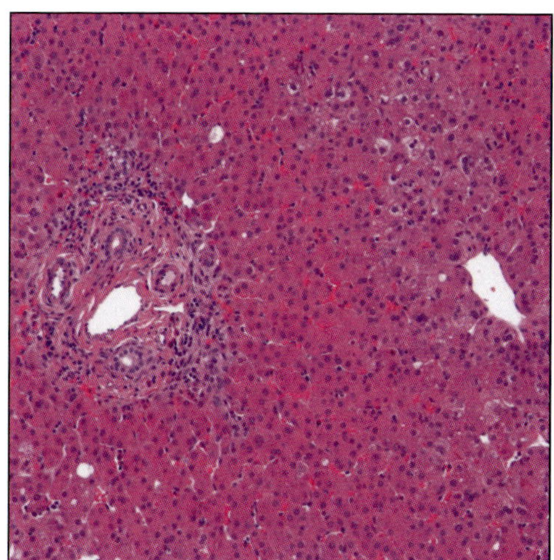

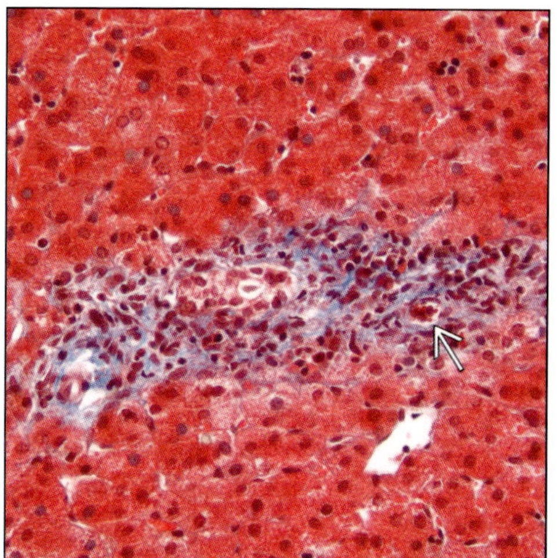

(Left) *This infant's biopsy at 4 weeks was not diagnostic of BA. Only minimal ductular reaction is seen in this portal tract, along with lobular cholestasis and a few centrizonal multinucleated giant cells.* ***(Right)*** *Most of the portal tracts in this liver biopsy were unremarkable except for this single focus with a bile plug ➔ on the trichrome stain. In the appropriate clinical context, as in this liver biopsy from a 4 week old, this finding suggests an obstructive pattern of injury.*

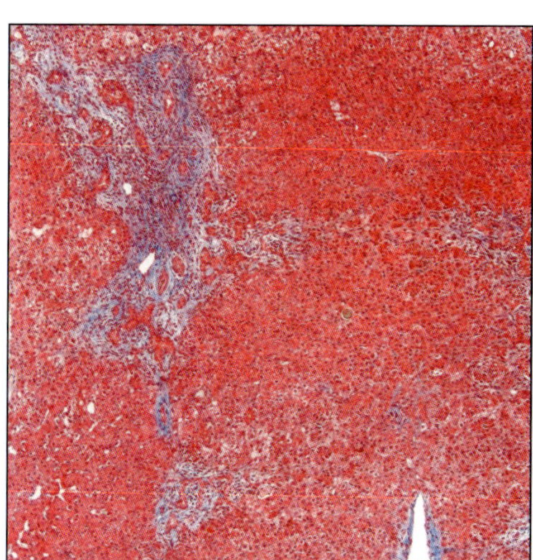

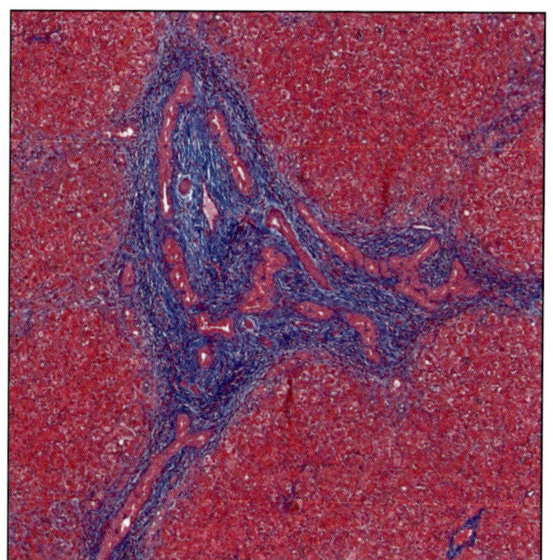

(Left) *This portal tract in a 5-week-old infant already shows marked expansion by fibrosis and early septal formation as well as ductular reaction supportive of an obstructive pattern of injury.* ***(Right)*** *This discontinuous, semicircumferential configuration of bile ducts with a central fibrovascular core, reminiscent of ductal plate malformation, can be found in BA. Its presence does not distinguish between the 2 clinical forms (prenatal vs. postnatal) of BA.*

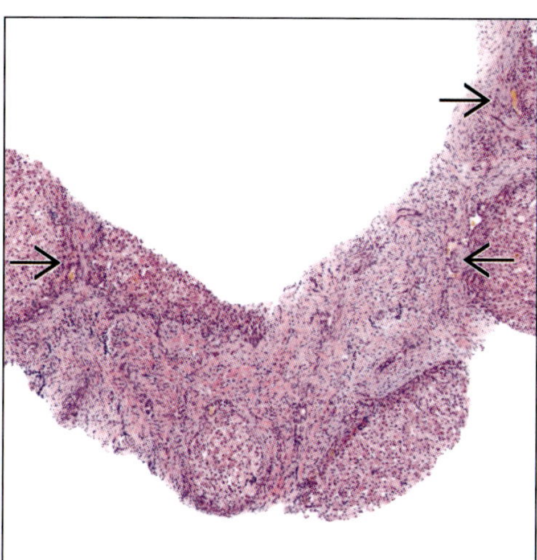

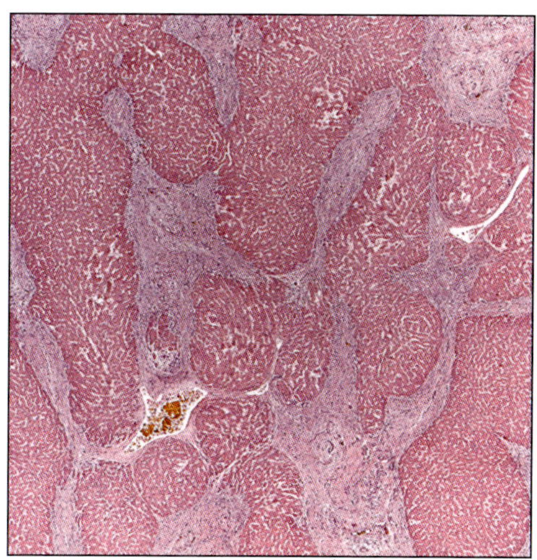

(Left) *This liver biopsy from a 9-week-old infant is cirrhotic with wide bands of fibrosis between the nodules of remaining hepatocytes. Note the bile plugs in the ductules ➔. This infant was clinically diagnosed as BA.* ***(Right)*** *Liver explanted from a 7 month old with BA shows irregular nodules of parenchyma separated by portal-to-portal bridging fibrosis, resulting in the architectural distortion typical of biliary cirrhosis.*

BILIARY ATRESIA

Microscopic and Gross Features

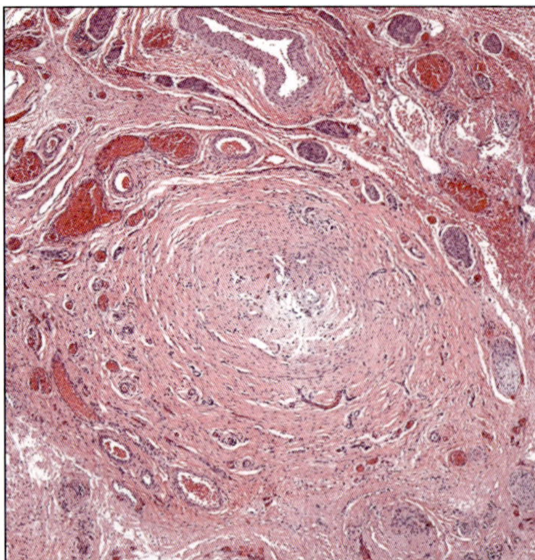

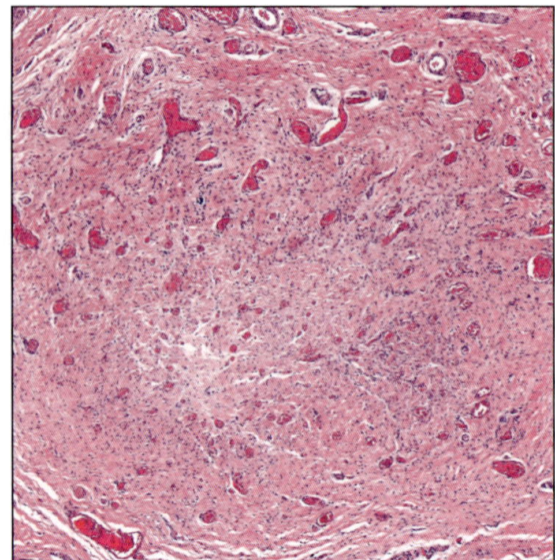

***(Left)** A section of biliary remnant removed during Kasai procedure demonstrates a markedly narrowed bile duct-like structure with a nearly absent lumen surrounded by fibrosis. Distal to this section, a patent bile duct lumen was identified. **(Right)** A biliary remnant from a 9 week old shows no bile duct lumen but rather fibrovascular tissue cuffed by a vascular plexus. This section was taken near the hilum of the liver. Distal to this section, a single patent bile duct lumen was found.*

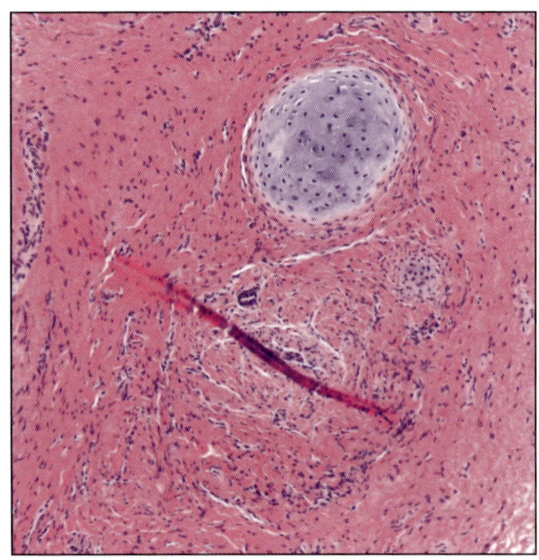

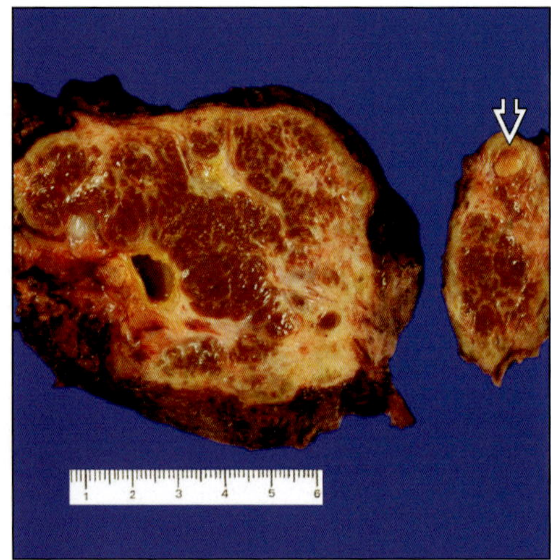

***(Left)** This section from portal hepatis shows focal hyaline cartilage, an unusual finding in biliary atresia. **(Right)** This explanted liver from a 12 year old with BA is cirrhotic. In the left lobe of the liver, a 0.9 cm yellow nodule ➔ was discovered. Histologically, this was a well-differentiated hepatocellular carcinoma.*

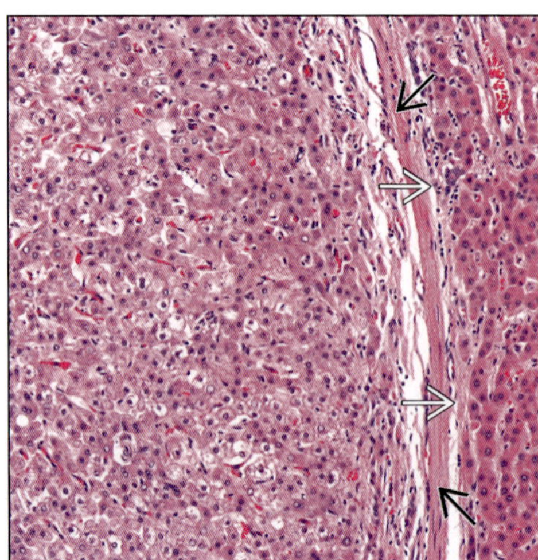

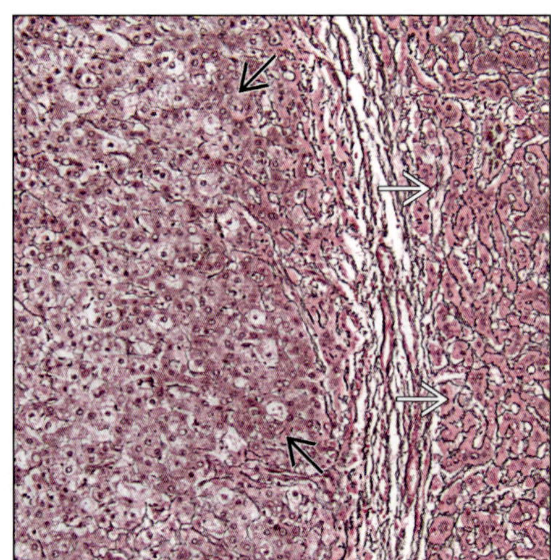

***(Left)** This incidentally identified 0.9 cm well-differentiated hepatocellular carcinoma ⇨ in an explanted liver from a 12 year old is partially encapsulated. The adjacent cirrhotic hepatic parenchyma is on the right side ➔ for comparison. **(Right)** Reticulin stain reveals a loss of reticulin fibers ⇨ in this well-differentiated hepatocellular carcinoma, in contrast to the intact reticulin framework ➔ in the adjacent hepatic parenchyma on the right side for comparison.*

Differential Diagnosis

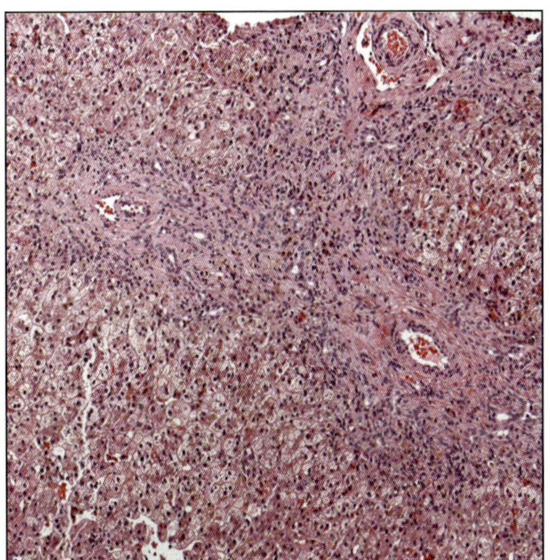

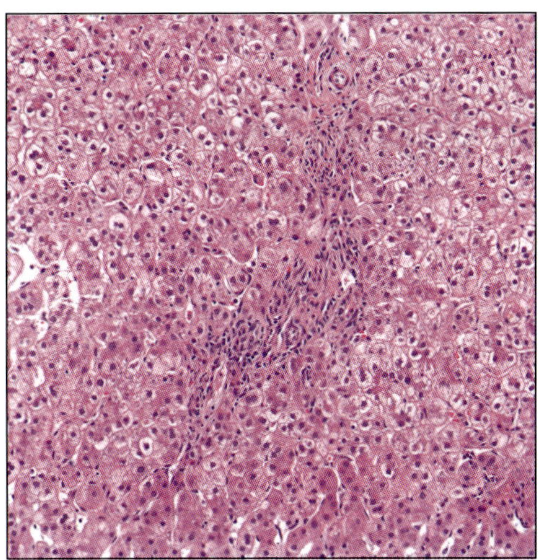

(Left) *In a 9-week-old infant who had been on total parenteral nutrition (TPN) since birth, the liver displays portal tract expansion with extensive ductular reaction. The differential diagnosis includes BA, TPN hepatopathy, and α-1-antitrypsin deficiency.* ***(Right)*** *Only focal and minimal ductular reaction is seen in this portal tract from liver biopsy from an 8 week old who was on total parenteral nutrition since birth. A diagnosis of BA is unlikely with this morphology.*

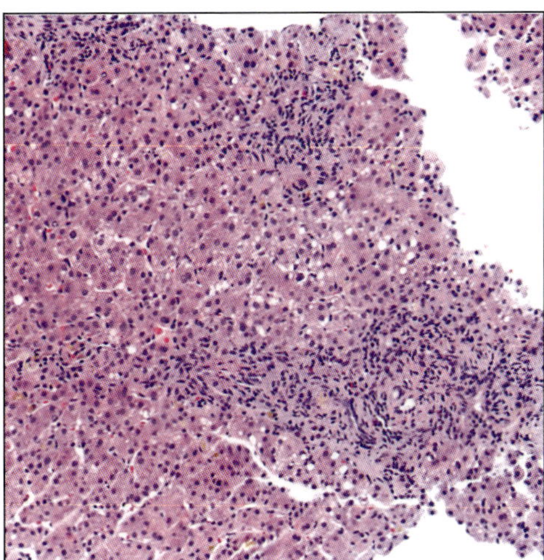

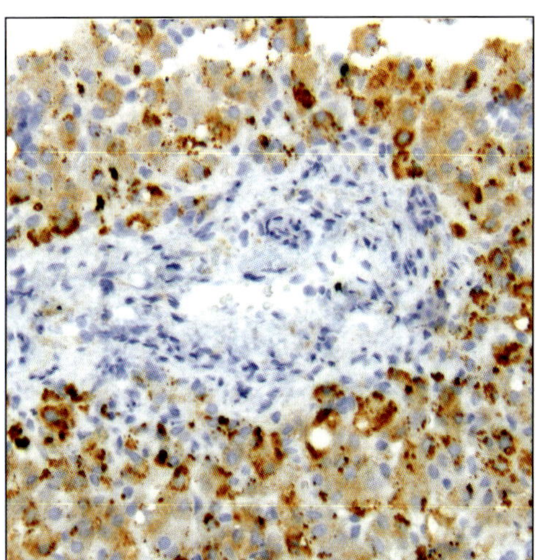

(Left) *The liver biopsy specimen from a 7-week-old infant with α-1-antitrypsin deficiency has cholestasis and mildly expanded portal tracts with ductular reaction. These changes in the liver can be indistinguishable from BA patients.* ***(Right)*** *α-1-antitrypsin staining is seen in periportal hepatocytes in this biopsy specimen from a 7 week old with α-1-antitrypsin deficiency. Cytoplasmic globules were not apparent on H&E stain and are not typically visible until >12 weeks of age.*

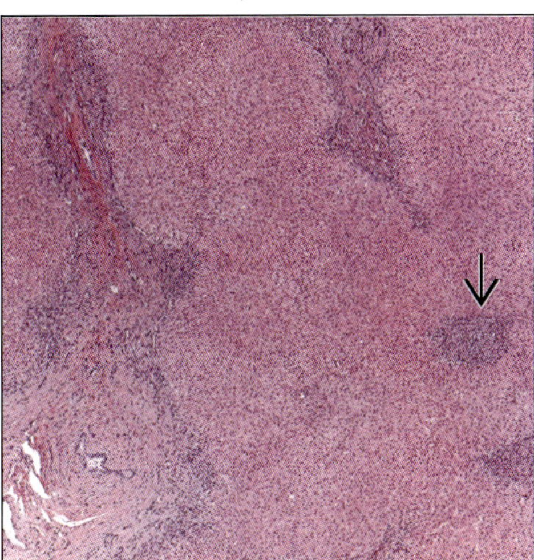

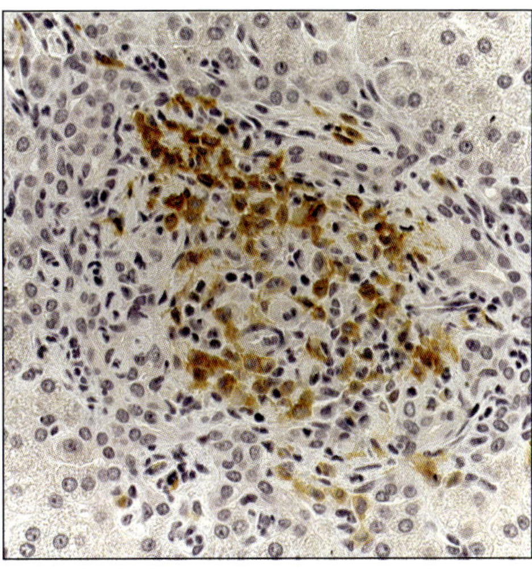

(Left) *Langerhans cell histiocytosis at low power features expanded portal tracts with significant ductular reaction, mimicking the obstructive pattern of injury seen in BA. However, in a focal small portal tract ➙, a mononuclear infiltrate is also present.* ***(Right)*** *Positive CD1a staining in a small portal tract with a mononuclear infiltrate provides support for the diagnosis of Langerhans cell histiocytosis. The infiltrate was very focal, however.*

IDIOPATHIC NEONATAL HEPATITIS

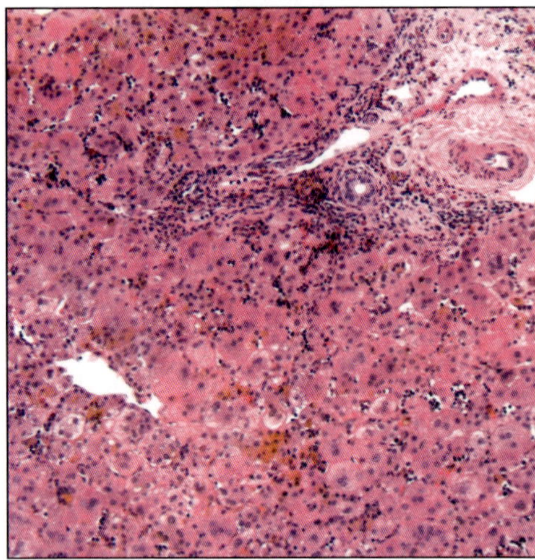

The characteristic features of INH include lobular giant cell transformation and extramedullary hematopoiesis. Ductular reaction is absent, and hepatocyte necrosis may not be apparent.

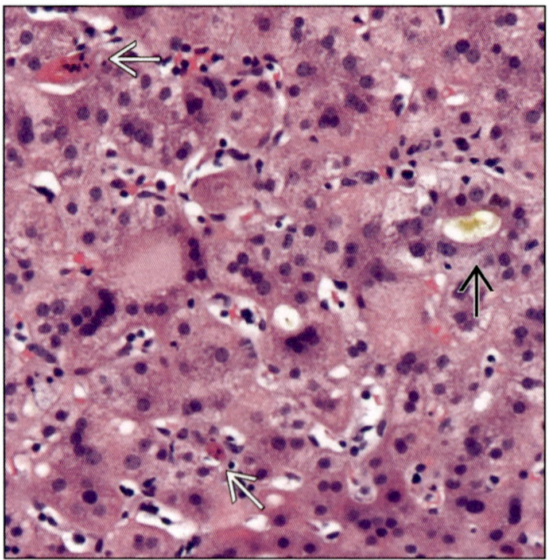

INH is primarily a lobular process with hepatocytes showing giant cell change and necrosis ➡ along with cholestasis ➡.

TERMINOLOGY

Abbreviations

- Idiopathic neonatal hepatitis (INH)

Definitions

- General term for clinical condition manifested by prolonged jaundice in neonates with variable but definable histologic picture
  - Clinicopathologic picture is termed "neonatal hepatitis syndrome"
  - Uniform clinical presentation but broad spectrum of causative disease processes
  - INH is diagnosis of exclusion

ETIOLOGY/PATHOGENESIS

Unknown

- Many different insults linked to this pattern of injury; if known etiologies are excluded, then idiopathic

CLINICAL ISSUES

Epidemiology

- Incidence
  - In early 1970s, 65% of neonatal cholestasis cases were attributed to INH
  - By mid-2000s, INH comprised only 15-30% of neonatal cholestasis due to
    - Increased knowledge of hepatobiliary physiology, specifically in hepatic metabolic and excretory function
    - Advances in molecular genetics techniques

Presentation

- Jaundice, cholestatic
- Hepatomegaly ± splenomegaly

Laboratory Tests

- Elevated serum total and conjugated bilirubin
- Elevated or near normal alanine transaminase

Treatment

- Supportive

MICROSCOPIC PATHOLOGY

Histologic Features

- Predominately lobular histological changes with syncytial giant cell hepatocytes
- Minimal alterations in portal tracts
  - Mild to absent portal inflammation
  - May have portal extramedullary hematopoiesis
  - Bile ducts not absent or decreased in number
- Diffuse lobular changes
  - Lobular disarray with giant cell transformation
  - Canalicular cholestasis ± pseudorosettes
  - Prominent extramedullary hematopoiesis, both myelopoiesis and erythropoiesis
  - Mild to absent lobular inflammation
  - Scattered to absent necrotic hepatocytes
- Not specific for etiology

DIFFERENTIAL DIAGNOSIS

Biliary Atresia

- Early in disease course, obstructive-type pattern of injury with ductular reaction may not be evident
- Less predominant or focal giant cell transformation
- Lacks patency of extrahepatic bile duct on imaging studies
- Very important to exclude because it requires early surgical intervention

Hypopituitarism

- Histologically indistinguishable from INH but may have small hypoplastic bile ducts

IDIOPATHIC NEONATAL HEPATITIS

Key Facts

Terminology
- Convenient term for clinical condition manifested by prolonged jaundice in neonates with variable but definable histologic picture

Microscopic Pathology
- Predominately lobular histological changes
  - Syncytial giant cell hepatocytes with extramedullary hematopoiesis
  - Canalicular cholestasis and scattered to absent necrotic hepatocytes

Top Differential Diagnoses
- Exclude biliary atresia right away because it requires early surgical intervention
- If neonatal hepatitis-like pattern of injury present, use clinical information and molecular tests to exclude known disorders
  - INH is diagnosis of exclusion

- Clinical features
  - Dysmorphic features including frontal bossing and hypertelorism
  - Nystagmus may suggest optic nerve hypoplasia
  - Micropenis in males
  - Hypotonia
  - Hypoglycemia
- Septo-optic dysplasia: Patients can have hypopituitarism and neonatal hepatitis

Paucity of Intrahepatic Bile Ducts
- Reduction of bile duct numbers

α-1-Antitrypsin Deficiency
- Low serum α-1-antitrypsin level
- Abnormal protease inhibitor (PiZZ or PiSZ) phenotype
- Cytoplasmic globules not apparent on H&E at < 12 weeks of age

Infections
- "TORCH" infections (evaluate with serologic tests or culture)
  - Carefully examine liver biopsy for viral inclusion indicative of cytomegalovirus or herpes simplex

Bile Acid Synthetic Defects
- Giant cell hepatitis is pattern of injury that may be seen
- Normal levels of serum γ-glutamyl transpeptidase
- Low or normal levels of serum bile acids
- Identification of specific metabolic defect by analysis of urine by fast atom bombardment-mass spectrometry & gas chromatography-mass spectrometry

BSEP Deficiency (Progressive Familial Intrahepatic Cholestasis Type 2)
- Lobular fibrosis along with giant hepatocytes
- Mutations in *ABCB11* gene encoding bile salt export protein (BSEP)
  - Negative BSEP canalicular staining
- Normal levels of serum γ-glutamyl transpeptidase

DIAGNOSTIC CHECKLIST

Pathologic Interpretation Pearls
- When neonatal liver biopsy demonstrates neonatal hepatitis-like pattern of injury
  - INH syndrome has uniform clinical presentation but broad spectrum of causative disease processes
  - Histologic features alone cannot reliably determine etiology
    - INH is diagnosis of exclusion
  - Use clinical manifestations and molecular genetic techniques to exclude recognizable disorders

SELECTED REFERENCES

1. Balistreri WF et al: Whatever happened to "neonatal hepatitis"? Clin Liver Dis. 10(1):27-53, v, 2006
2. Roberts EA: Neonatal hepatitis syndrome. Semin Neonatol. 8(5):357-74, 2003

IMAGE GALLERY

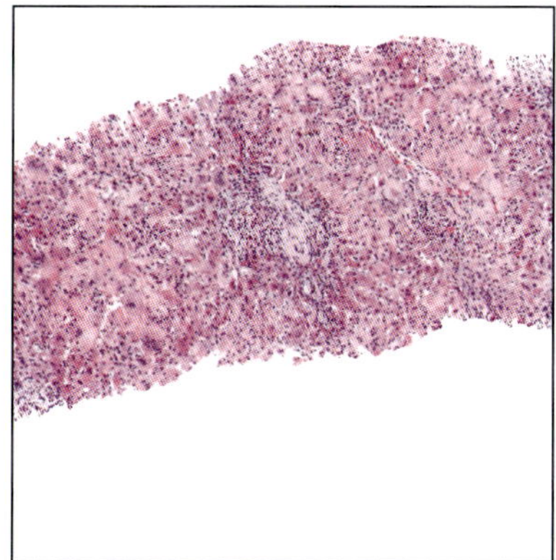

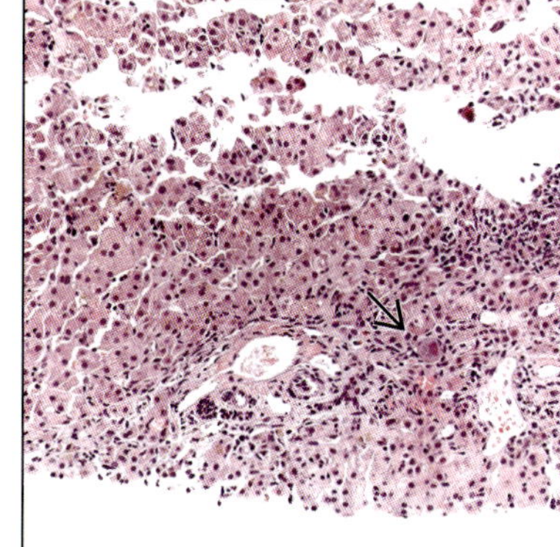

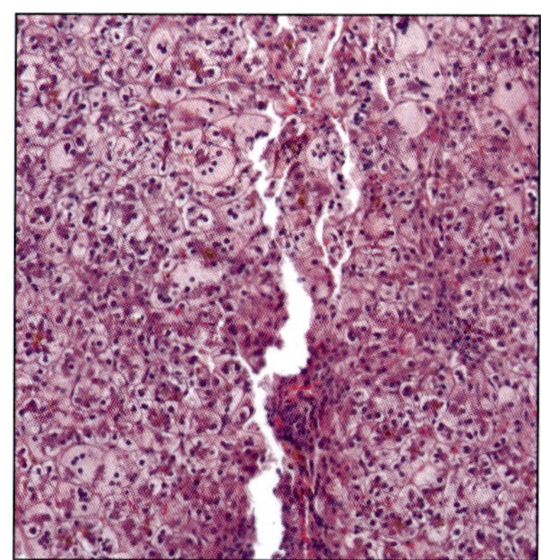

(Left) *This biopsy from a 9 week old with biliary atresia has features similar to INH but also contains expanded portal tracts with ductular reaction.* ***(Center)*** *This case of neonatal hepatitis due to CMV shows a few giant cell hepatocytes along with extramedullary hematopoiesis. A single CMV inclusion ➔ was identified.* ***(Right)*** *This case of neonatal hepatitis with syncytial giant cells, lobular cholestasis, and no necrosis is shown in an infant with septo-optic dysplasia.*

PAUCITY OF INTRAHEPATIC BILE DUCTS (SYNDROMIC)

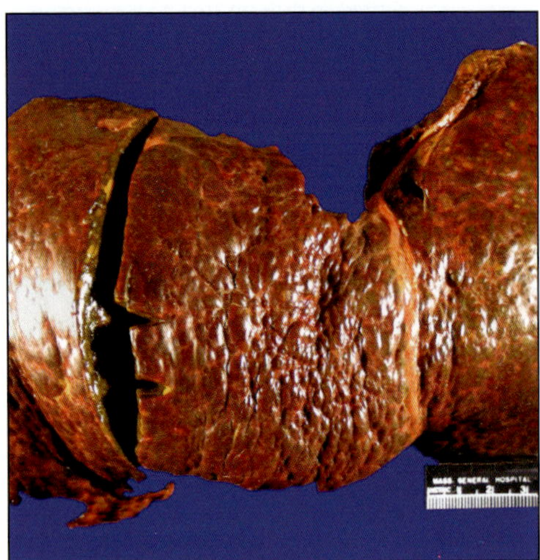

Explanted cirrhotic liver from an adult with Alagille syndrome shows a nodular distorted surface.

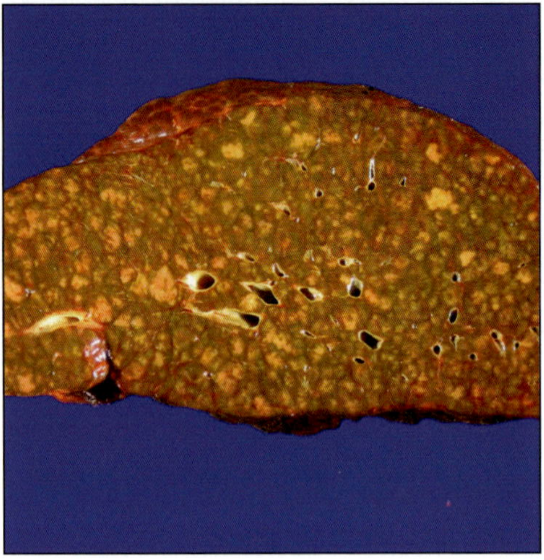

Cut surface of cirrhotic liver from an adult with Alagille syndrome shows micronodular cirrhosis, extensive fibrosis, and green discoloration.

TERMINOLOGY

Synonyms

- Alagille syndrome
- Arteriohepatic dysplasia

Definitions

- Syndrome characterized by intrahepatic bile duct hypoplasia and loss, along with at least 3 of the following major clinical features or 2 features in patients with family history
  - Chronic cholestasis
  - Cardiac abnormalities: Peripheral pulmonary stenosis, pulmonary valve stenosis, tetralogy of Fallot, aortic stenosis, ventricular septal defects
  - Skeletal abnormalities: Butterfly vertebrae, curved phalanges, short ulna
  - Ocular abnormalities: Posterior embryotoxon, optic nerve drusen
  - Characteristic facies: Broad forehead, deep set eyes, straight nose, pointed chin

ETIOLOGY/PATHOGENESIS

Genetic Disorder

- Mutations in *Jagged1* gene that encodes ligand for Notch receptor are seen in 70% of patients
  - Interaction between *Jagged1* and *Notch2* may be important in bile duct formation and maturation to more differentiated state
    - Mutations lead to impaired ductal plate remodeling and subsequent impaired postnatal intrahepatic bile duct development
  - Alternatively, interaction between *Jagged1* and *Notch4* may be involved in vascular remodeling, and abnormal portal blood vessel remodeling could lead to ductopenia
  - Autosomal dominant inheritance with variable expressivity
- Patients without *Jagged1* mutations may have mutations of *Notch2* gene

CLINICAL ISSUES

Epidemiology

- Incidence
  - 1 in 100,000
- Age
  - Typically presents in childhood
- Gender
  - Affects sexes equally
- Ethnicity
  - Found in all ethnic groups

Presentation

- Jaundice before age of 6 months
  - Consequences of cholestasis, including xanthomas, fat-soluble vitamin deficiency, pruritus
- Hepatomegaly
- Splenomegaly in 50% of cases
- Symptoms related to cardiac defects

Laboratory Tests

- Conjugated hyperbilirubinemia
- Increased GGT, alkaline phosphatase, and serum bile acids
- Increased cholesterol

Natural History

- Progresses to cirrhosis in approximately 20% of patients
- Associated with risk of hepatocellular carcinoma

Treatment

- Surgical approaches
  - Partial external biliary diversion
  - Liver transplantation
- Drugs

PAUCITY OF INTRAHEPATIC BILE DUCTS (SYNDROMIC)

Key Facts

Terminology

- Alagille syndrome: Intrahepatic bile duct hypoplasia progressing to ductopenia that results in chronic cholestasis, associated with other congenital abnormalities
  - Cardiac abnormalities, particularly pulmonary stenosis
  - Skeletal abnormalities, particularly butterfly vertebrae
  - Ocular abnormalities, particularly posterior embryotoxon
  - Characteristic facies

Etiology/Pathogenesis

- Mutations in *Jagged1* gene, which encodes ligand for *Notch* receptor
- Interaction between *Jagged1* and *Notch2* may be necessary for bile duct maturation

Clinical Issues

- Presents as jaundice before age of 6 months

Microscopic Pathology

- Early in life, bile duct destruction, bile ductular proliferation, and inspissated bile in ductules can be confused with biliary atresia
- As patient ages, liver shows evolving ductopenia

Top Differential Diagnoses

- Extrahepatic biliary atresia
- Paucity of intrahepatic bile ducts (nonsyndromic)

  - Ursodeoxycholic acid, rifampin, phenobarbitone, cholestyramine to manage cholestasis and pruritus

Prognosis

- In era before liver transplantation, survival to age 20 was 75%
- About 25% of all patients require liver transplantation
- Presentation with neonatal cholestasis carries worse prognosis, with 50% requiring liver transplantation before age of 10 years
- Patients who do not present with neonatal cholestasis may develop liver-related complications later in life
- Presence of cardiac disease predicts increased mortality

Additional Manifestations

- Vascular anomalies
  - Intracranial bleeds account for 25% of deaths
- Renal abnormalities

IMAGE FINDINGS

Hepatobiliary Scan

- Excretion of technetium labeled iminodiacetic dye is typically absent, mimicking extrahepatic biliary atresia

Cholangiography

- May show bile duct hypoplasia

MICROSCOPIC PATHOLOGY

Histologic Features

- Early in life (< 3 months), bile duct destruction may be associated with bile ductular proliferation, causing confusion with biliary atresia
- As patient ages, liver shows evolving ductopenia, which may be patchy
- Later in life, fibrosis and biliary cirrhosis may develop

DIFFERENTIAL DIAGNOSIS

Extrahepatic Biliary Atresia

- Similar presentation to Alagille with conjugated hyperbilirubinemia, small gallbladder, and hypoplasia of common bile duct
- Bile duct proliferation with bile plugs and portal fibrosis on liver biopsy
- Careful examination of hepatobiliary scan and laparotomy may be necessary to distinguish the 2 conditions
- Stigmata of syndromic disorder favors Alagille

Paucity of Intrahepatic Bile Ducts (Nonsyndromic)

- Liver biopsy does not distinguish between syndromic and nonsyndromic paucity of intrahepatic bile ducts
- Stigmata of syndromic disorder favors Alagille

DIAGNOSTIC CHECKLIST

Clinically Relevant Pathologic Features

- Bile duct paucity in infant is indication for slit lamp examination and dorsal spine radiograph examination

Pathologic Interpretation Pearls

- Liver biopsies in infants with neonatal cholestasis due to Alagille syndrome may be indistinguishable from biliary atresia

SELECTED REFERENCES

1. Kodama Y et al: The role of notch signaling in the development of intrahepatic bile ducts. Gastroenterology. 127(6):1775-86, 2004
2. Kamath BM et al: Heritable disorders of the bile ducts. Gastroenterol Clin North Am. 32(3):857-75, vi, 2003
3. Crosnier C et al: Alagille syndrome. The widening spectrum of arteriohepatic dysplasia. Clin Liver Dis. 4(4):765-78, 2000

PAUCITY OF INTRAHEPATIC BILE DUCTS (SYNDROMIC)

Pediatric Microscopic Features

*(Left) Trichrome stain of a liver explant from a 5-year-old boy with Alagille syndrome shows micronodular cirrhosis with small regenerative nodules separated by bands of fibrous tissue. **(Right)** Portal tract in Alagille syndrome in a child shows an arteriole ➔ unaccompanied by a bile duct, consistent with bile duct paucity, and bile ductule proliferation with inspissated bile at the portal edge ➚.*

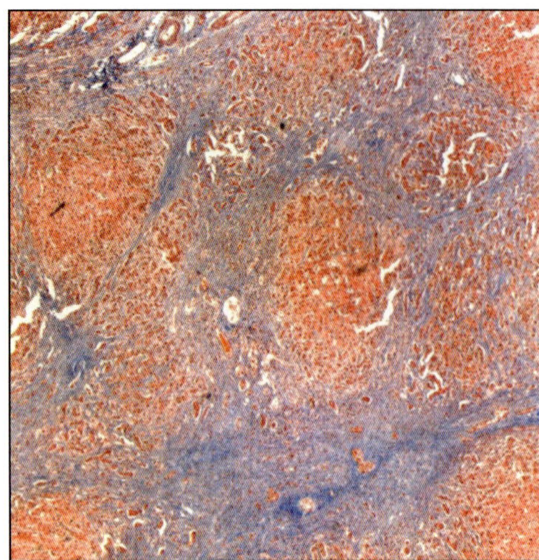

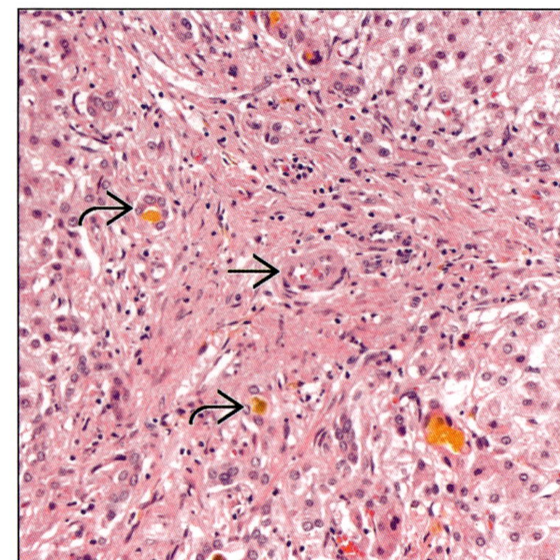

*(Left) The edge of a large portal area shows vascular structures (top) but no bile duct. Notice the ductular reaction at the edge of the portal area ➢. **(Right)** High magnification of the portal area in Alagille syndrome shows proliferation of bile ductular structures.*

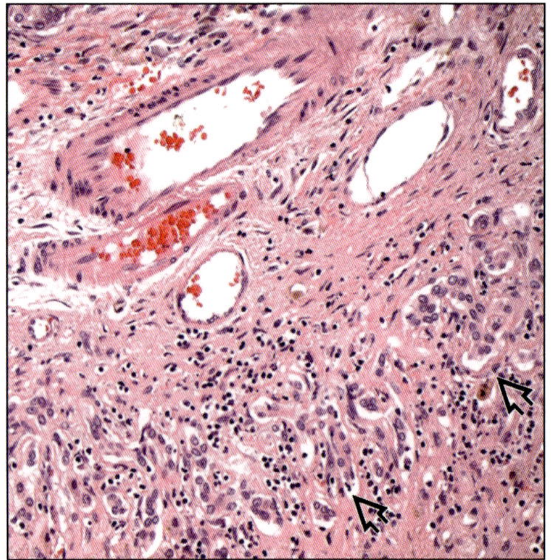

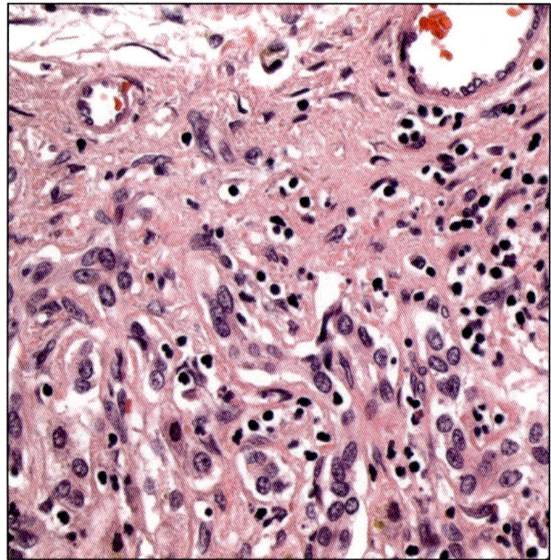

*(Left) The edge of a fibrous septum in cirrhotic liver in Alagille syndrome shows bile ductular proliferation with inspissated bile in bile ductules ➔ that can lead to a misdiagnosis of extrahepatic biliary atresia. **(Right)** Bile ductular proliferation in Alagille syndrome with bile inspissated in ductules ➚ can cause confusion with biliary atresia.*

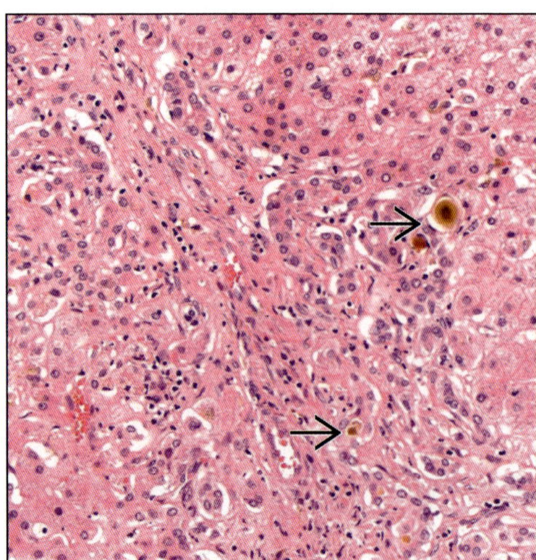

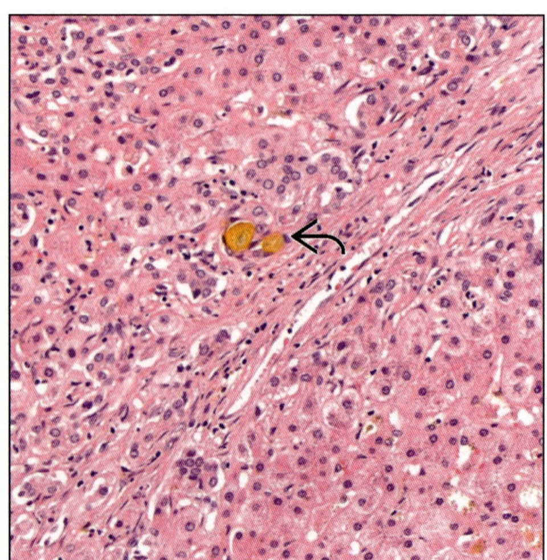

Adult Microscopic Features

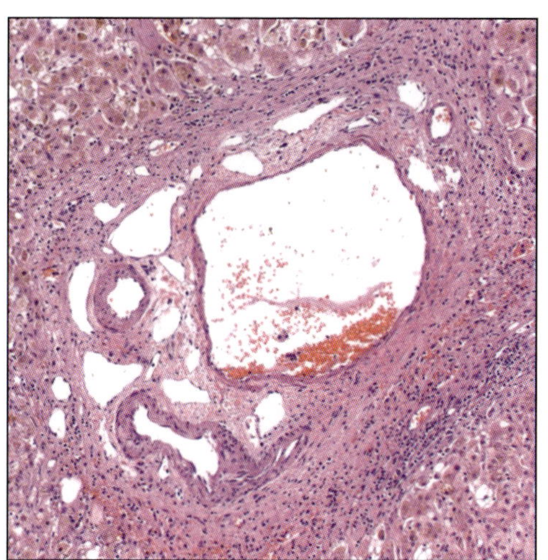

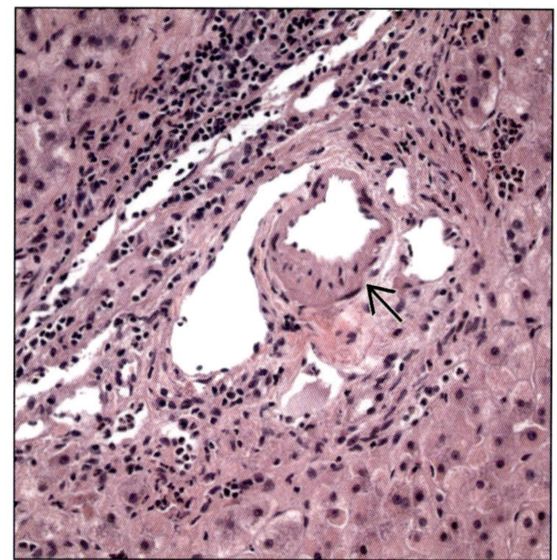

*(**Left**) A large portal region in an explant from an adult patient with Alagille syndrome shows large vascular structures without bile ducts. (**Right**) A smaller portal tract in an adult patient with Alagille syndrome shows a small artery ➙ and vein but no bile duct. Note the absence of bile ductular reaction.*

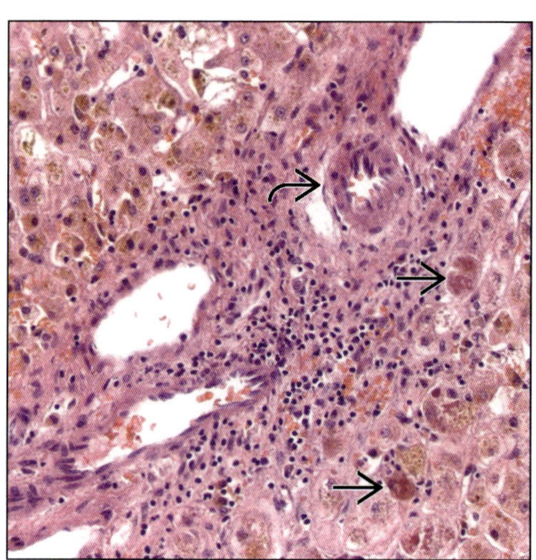

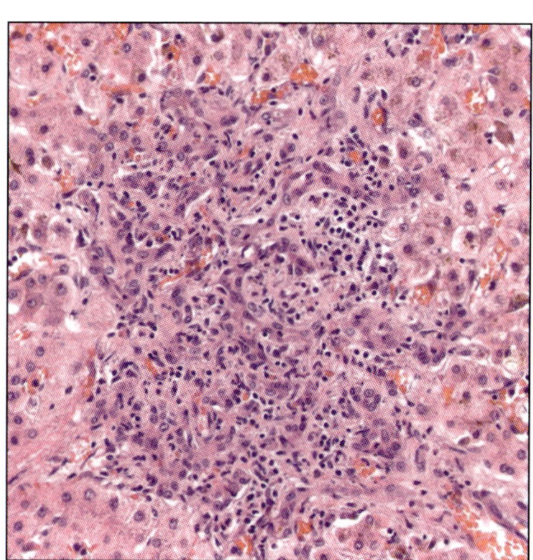

*(**Left**) A portal area in Alagille syndrome is shown. The surrounding liver is cholestatic with Mallory-Denk bodies ➙. The portal tract contains a small artery ➚ but no duct. (**Right**) Explanted liver in an adult patient with Alagille syndrome shows ductular proliferation in a portal tract.*

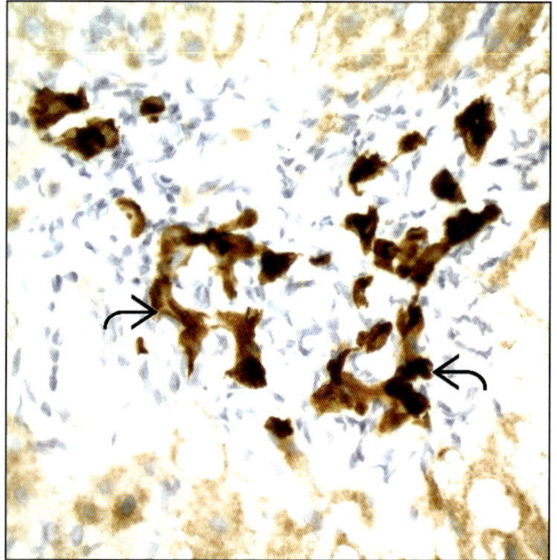

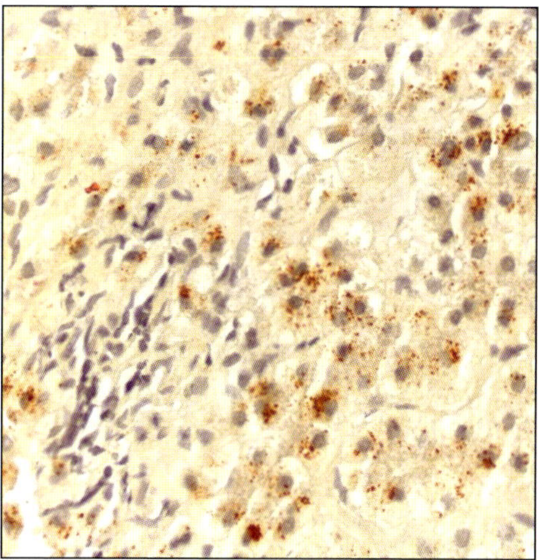

*(**Left**) CK19 immunohistochemical stain in a liver biopsy from an adult patient with Alagille syndrome shows ductular proliferation ➚ in a portal tract without a native duct. (**Right**) Copper stain in a liver biopsy from an adult patient with Alagille syndrome shows copper deposition in periportal hepatocytes (red-brown granules), consistent with chronic cholestasis.*

PAUCITY OF INTRAHEPATIC BILE DUCTS (NONSYNDROMIC)

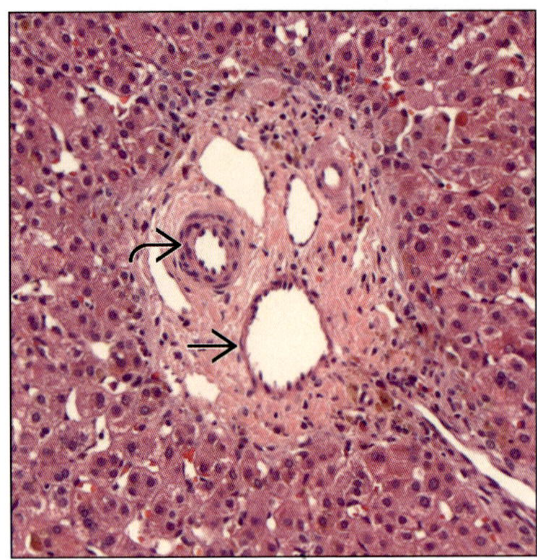

A portal tract in an infant with nonsyndromic paucity of intrahepatic bile ducts shows arteries ⇗ and veins ⇒ but no bile ducts. The hepatocytes are compact and clustered.

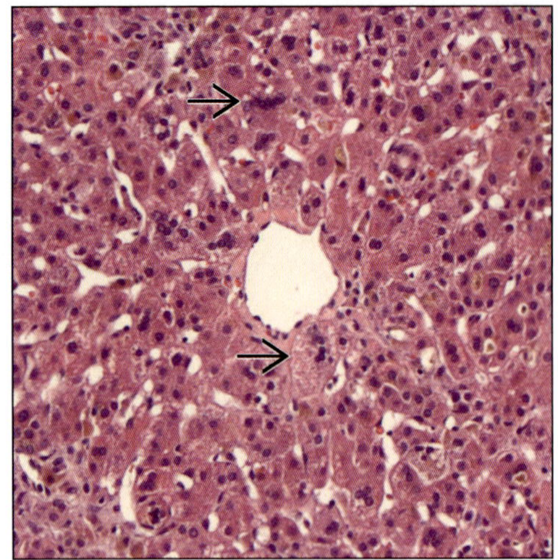

The centrilobular region in nonsyndromic bile duct paucity shows cholestasis and giant cell transformation of hepatocytes ⇒, nonspecific features of many neonatal cholestatic disorders.

TERMINOLOGY

Synonyms

- Hypoplasia of intrahepatic bile ducts
- Intrahepatic biliary atresia

Definitions

- Heterogeneous group of disorders that causes bile duct paucity or ductopenia in patients without congenital abnormalities indicative of Alagille syndrome
  - Ductopenia is defined as significant decrease in number of interlobular bile ducts
    - Ratio of number of interlobular bile ducts to number of portal tracts is < 0.4, with normal between 0.9 and 1.8
    - Alternatively, ductopenia is diagnosed when > 50% of portal tracts lack bile ducts; normally, 80-100% of portal tracts contain ducts

ETIOLOGY/PATHOGENESIS

Developmental Anomaly

- Congenital disorders: Extrahepatic biliary atresia
- Metabolic disorders: α-1-antitrypsin deficiency, cystic fibrosis, progressive familial intrahepatic cholestasis (PFIC), peroxisomal disorders, disorders of bile acid synthesis, Niemann-Pick type C, arthrogryposis-renal dysfunction-cholestasis syndrome (ARC)
- Chromosomal abnormalities: Turner syndrome, monosomy X, trisomies

Infectious Agents

- Intrauterine infections: Cytomegalovirus (CMV), rubella, syphilis

Idiopathic

- Accounts for variable percentage of total cases, depending on population studied
- Idiopathic group has been diminishing as metabolic and genetic mechanisms of ductopenia are elucidated
- Diagnosis of exclusion

CLINICAL ISSUES

Epidemiology

- Incidence
  - Varies according to population evaluated but increased in regions of world where consanguineous marriage is common
- Age
  - Generally considered disease of childhood since adults with ductopenia are classified in different disease categories
  - Some patients with idiopathic adulthood ductopenia may represent late presentation of disorder that began in childhood

Presentation

- Jaundice and acholic stools
- Pruritus
- Hepatomegaly

Laboratory Tests

- Increased alkaline phosphatase, γ-glutamyl transpeptidase, and serum bilirubin
- Increased serum cholesterol may be seen

Natural History

- Complications of fat malabsorption and deficiency of fat-soluble vitamins: Prolonged prothrombin time, rickets, vitamin E-responsive hemolytic anemia, corneal ulcers

Treatment

- Surgical approaches
  - Liver transplantation may be necessary for patients who progress to cirrhosis and liver failure
- Drugs
  - Ursodeoxycholic acid, cholestyramine, phenobarbital

PAUCITY OF INTRAHEPATIC BILE DUCTS (NONSYNDROMIC)

Key Facts

Terminology
- Heterogeneous group of disorders that causes bile duct paucity in patients without congenital abnormalities indicative of Alagille syndrome
- Ductopenia is diagnosed when > 50% of portal tracts lack bile ducts

Etiology/Pathogenesis
- Congenital disorders: Extrahepatic biliary atresia
- Metabolic disorders: α-1-antitrypsin deficiency, cystic fibrosis, PFIC, peroxisomal disorders, disorders of bile acid synthesis, Niemann-Pick type C, ARC
- Chromosomal abnormalities: Turner syndrome, monosomy X, trisomies
- Intrauterine infections: CMV, rubella, syphilis
- Idiopathic: Diagnosis of exclusion

Clinical Issues
- Prognosis varies depending on underlying cause and ranges from liver failure to complete resolution
- Treated with ursodeoxycholic acid and drugs to combat pruritus
- About 45% progress to cirrhosis, requiring liver transplantation

Microscopic Pathology
- Native bile ducts absent in > 1/2 of portal tracts
- Intracellular cholestasis and giant cell transformation of hepatocytes
- Fibrosis ranging from portal fibrosis to cirrhosis

Prognosis
- Ranges from liver failure requiring transplant to complete resolution, depending on underlying cause
  - Progression to cirrhosis is seen in approximately 45% of patients
- Prognosis is worse than for patients with syndromic paucity of intrahepatic bile ducts
- Many patients die of progressive liver failure without transplantation

MICROSCOPIC PATHOLOGY

Histologic Features
- Native bile ducts are absent in > 1/2 of portal tracts
  - Ductular proliferation may be present and may hinder evaluation of duct loss
  - To reliably determine ductopenia, at least 10 portal tracts must be evaluated
- Intracellular cholestasis and giant cell transformation of hepatocytes may be present
- Fibrosis is variable, ranging from mild portal fibrosis to cirrhosis

DIFFERENTIAL DIAGNOSIS

Paucity of Intrahepatic Bile Ducts (Syndromic)
- Presence of congenital abnormalities indicative of Alagille syndrome, including skeletal, ocular, and cardiac abnormalities, and characteristic facies
- *JAG1* mutations

Extrahepatic Biliary Atresia
- Hepatobiliary scanning shows absent common bile duct
- Ultrasound shows absent or small gallbladder
- Liver biopsy shows ductular proliferation with bile plugs in cholangioles

α-1-Antitrypsin Deficiency
- PAS-diastase globules in hepatocytes often present although may be absent in early life
- Proteinase inhibitor phenotyping, measurement of serum α-1-antitrypsin

Cystic Fibrosis
- Bile duct proliferation with PAS(+) inspissated secretion in the duct lumen

Progressive Familial Intrahepatic Cholestasis
- Identification of genetic mutation, immunohistochemistry for deficiency of responsible canalicular protein

Adulthood Idiopathic Ductopenia
- Ductopenia in adult without specific disease that results in ductopenia
- May be same disorder as childhood nonsyndromic paucity of intrahepatic bile ducts

DIAGNOSTIC CHECKLIST

Clinically Relevant Pathologic Features
- As peripheral bile ducts are last to undergo remodeling, biopsies from premature infants or even superficial biopsies from near-term infants can give false impression of paucity

SELECTED REFERENCES

1. Yehezkely-Schildkraut V et al: Nonsyndromic paucity of interlobular bile ducts: report of 10 patients. J Pediatr Gastroenterol Nutr. 37(5):546-9, 2003
2. Koçak N et al: Nonsyndromic paucity of interlobular bile ducts: clinical and laboratory findings of 10 cases. J Pediatr Gastroenterol Nutr. 24(1):44-8, 1997
3. Hadchouel M: Paucity of interlobular bile ducts. Semin Diagn Pathol. 9(1):24-30, 1992

PAUCITY OF INTRAHEPATIC BILE DUCTS (NONSYNDROMIC)

Differential Diagnosis

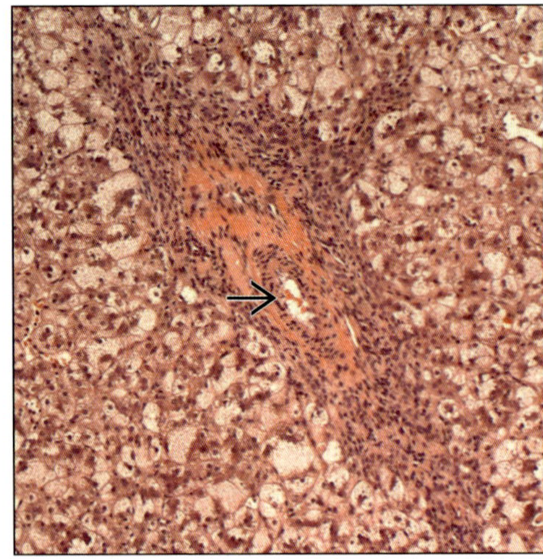

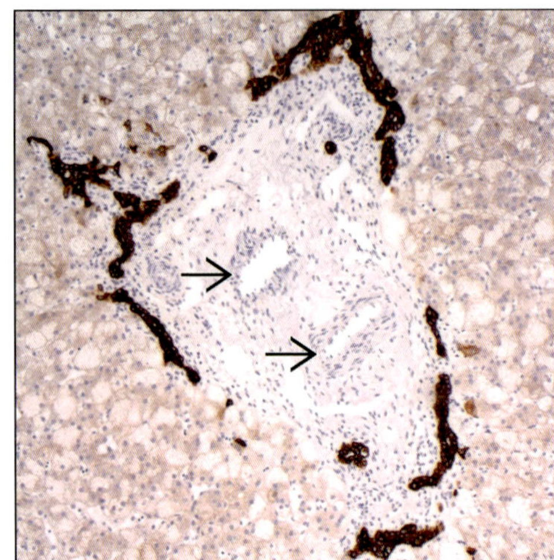

(Left) *A portal tract in an infant with ductopenia shows a muscular artery ➔ without an accompanying bile duct. Ductular reaction is evident at the portal edge. The hepatocytes show giant cell transformation.* ***(Right)*** *Cytokeratin 19 immunohistochemical stain shows peripheral ductules surrounding this portal tract, reminiscent here of ductal plate malformation, but the muscular arteries in the center of the portal tract ➔ lack a similarly sized accompanying bile duct.*

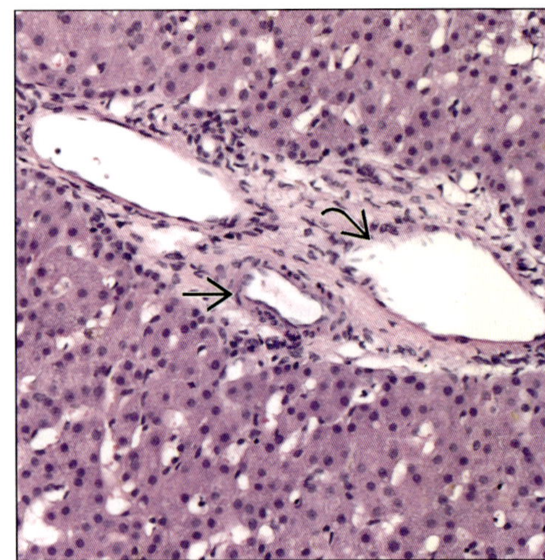

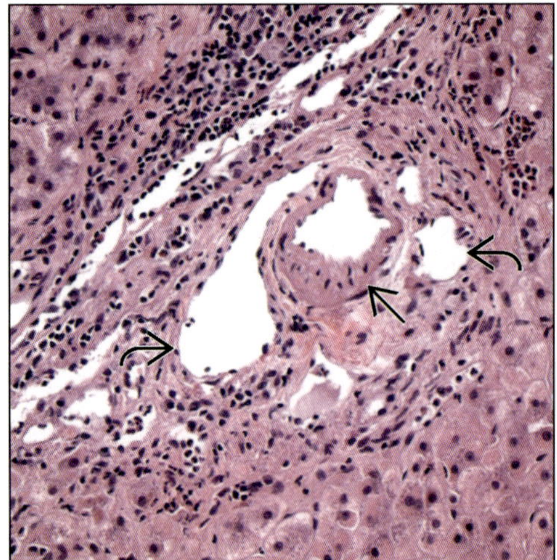

(Left) *A portal tract in an infant carrying a diagnosis of progressive familial intrahepatic cholestasis shows arteries ➔ and veins ↷ but no bile duct.* ***(Right)*** *A portal tract in an infant with syndromic bile duct paucity (Alagille syndrome) shows an artery ➔ and veins ↷ but no bile duct. There is also a mild portal lymphocytic infiltrate.*

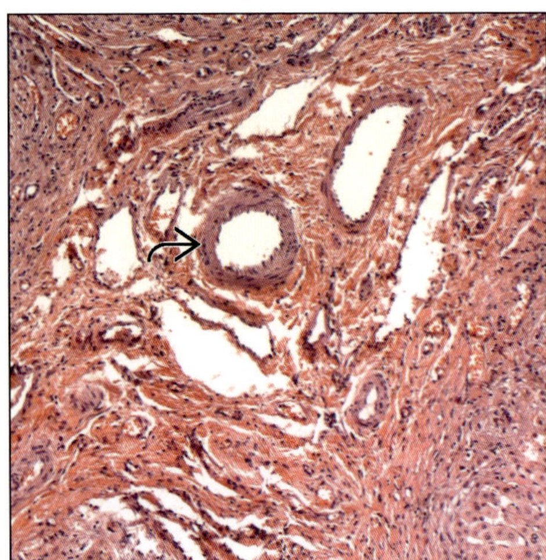

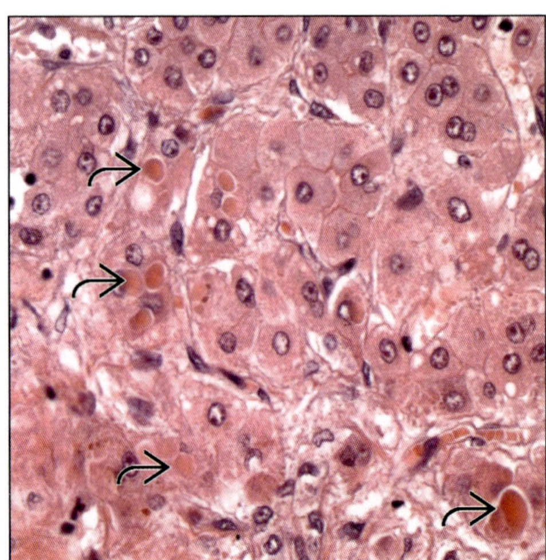

(Left) *A large portal area in an explant from a child with α-1-antitrypsin deficiency shows several vascular structures including a medium-sized muscular artery ↷, but no bile duct.* ***(Right)*** *High-power examination of the liver in a child with α-1-antitrypsin deficiency shows eosinophilic globules in periseptal hepatocytes ↷ consistent with abnormal accumulation of α-1-antitrypsin.*

Differential Diagnosis

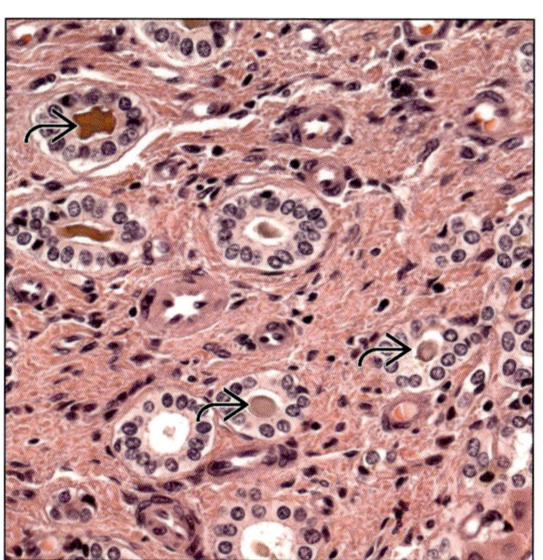

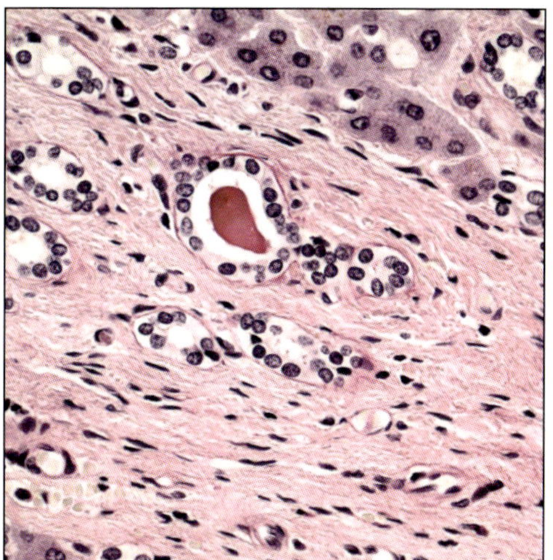

(Left) *Cystic fibrosis can lead to ductopenia secondary to chronic ductal obstruction due to inspissated intraductal secretions, which appear here as yellow-pink dense material* ⮫ *within proliferated bile duct.* ***(Right)*** *The inspissated secretion in cystic fibrosis is highlighted on PAS-diastase stain.*

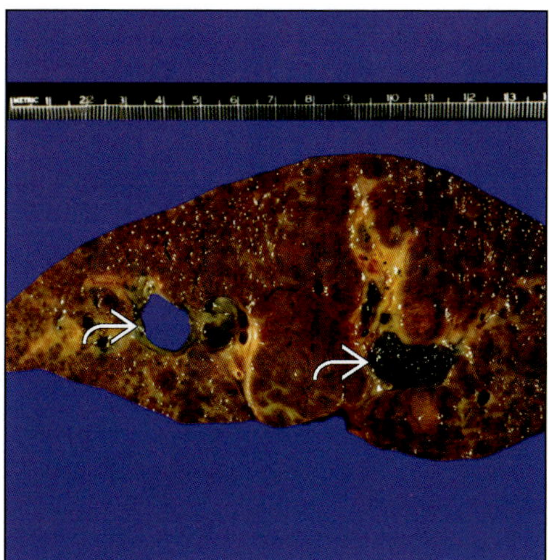

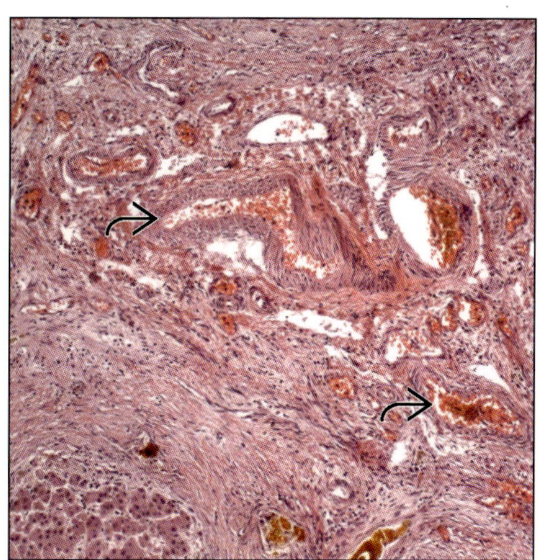

(Left) *An explanted liver from a child with extrahepatic biliary atresia shows large cystic ducts filled with inspissated bile* ⮫*, which can mimic Caroli disease.* ***(Right)*** *A large portal area in an explant from a child with extrahepatic biliary atresia shows large muscular arteries* ⮫ *and veins but no similarly sized bile ducts. At the bottom of the field are bile duct structures with inspissated bile.*

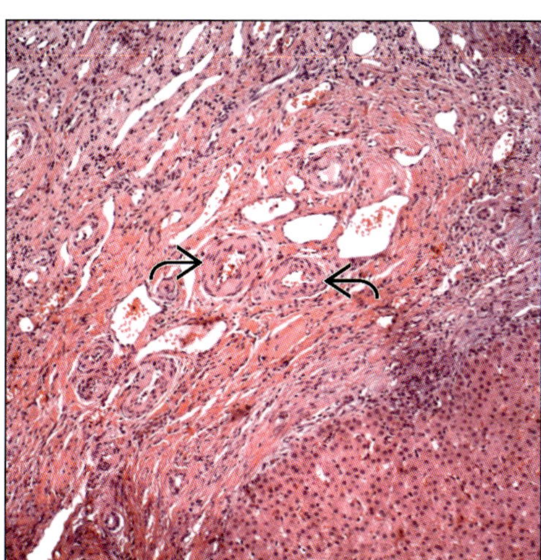

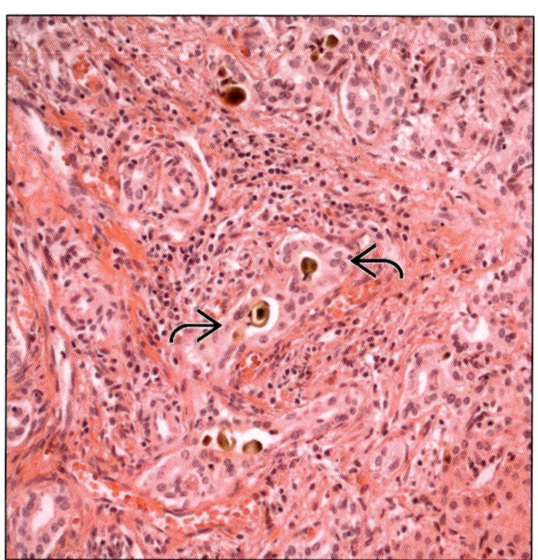

(Left) *Another portal area from the same liver shows smaller arteries* ⮫ *and veins yet no accompanying bile ducts.* ***(Right)*** *The classic picture of extrahepatic biliary atresia features bile duct proliferation with inspissated bile within the proliferated ducts* ⮫*.*

Drug/Toxin-related Hepatitis

DRUG-RELATED ACUTE HEPATITIS

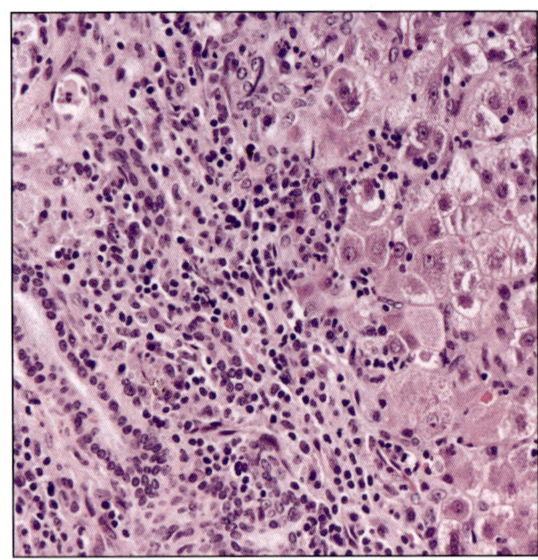

The inflammation-predominant pattern of drug-related acute hepatitis features dense lymphoplasmacytic infiltrate and interface hepatocellular injury.

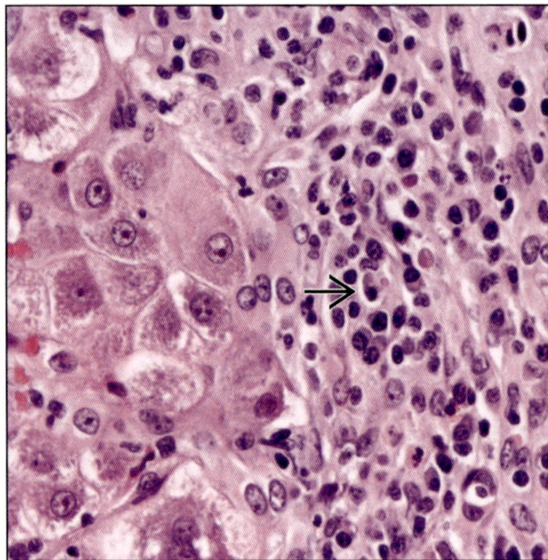

Numerous plasma cells ➔ can be seen in DILI and do not necessarily indicate autoimmune hepatitis.

TERMINOLOGY

Abbreviations

- Drug-induced liver injury (DILI)

ETIOLOGY/PATHOGENESIS

Two Chief Mechanisms

- Intrinsic hepatotoxicity
  - Predictable, dose-dependent hepatocellular damage by drug or its metabolite
    - Industrial, household, or environmental toxins
  - Typical histological feature is necrosis with negligible inflammation
- Idiosyncratic hepatotoxicity
  - Majority of adverse drug reactions fall in this category
  - Further classified into metabolic and immunological categories
    - Metabolic: Drug is metabolized into toxic metabolite in predisposed individuals
    - Immunological: "Drug allergy" or hypersensitivity following sensitization to drug
  - Typical histological feature is inflammation-predominant liver injury

Herbals/Botanicals

- Important but often overlooked cause of hepatotoxicity
- Not regulated by Food and Drug Administration and hence not subject to rigorous testing
- Nearly 20% of American adults have used herbal remedies, and more than 5 billion dollars are spent on these annually
- Contaminants in herbal supplements, including heavy metals such as arsenic, cadmium, lead, or mercury, can also lead to liver toxicity

CLINICAL ISSUES

Presentation

- Clinical patterns of injury classified based on pattern of liver enzyme abnormalities
  - Hepatitic
    - Acute hepatitis with autoimmune markers may mimic autoimmune hepatitis (AIH)
    - May have features of hypersensitivity like rash, arthralgia, and peripheral eosinophilia
    - Progression to chronic hepatitis with fibrosis and even cirrhosis can occur
  - Cholestatic
  - Mixed
- Classified into acute or chronic based on duration of injury
- Establishing drug as causative agent is key
  - Temporal profile of onset of liver dysfunction is crucial
  - Liver toxicity may manifest weeks or months after drug ingestion and even after drug has been stopped
  - Systematic literature search for each drug that patient has been taking is necessary
  - If observed and reported patterns of clinical and histological injury are similar, case for DILI is strengthened
  - Rechallenge can help confirm drug etiology but is rarely done

Laboratory Tests

- Measurement of serum levels of drug or its metabolite can be helpful in diagnosis (e.g., acetaminophen toxicity)
- Antinuclear &/or antismooth muscle antibodies may be present
- Transaminase elevations may be marked

Treatment

- Drug withdrawal
- Steroids may be necessary

DRUG-RELATED ACUTE HEPATITIS

Key Facts

Etiology/Pathogenesis

- 2 chief mechanisms: Intrinsic and idiosyncratic
- Herbal and botanical drugs are important but often overlooked cause of hepatotoxicity

Clinical Issues

- Classified into hepatitic, cholestatic, or mixed based pattern of enzyme elevation
- DILI with autoimmune markers can be indistinguishable from de novo AIH
- Symptomatic and biochemical improvement in most cases on withdrawal of drug
  - Minority of cases progress to chronic hepatitis and rarely cirrhosis
  - Jaundice, high AST levels, and preexisting chronic liver disease are adverse prognostic factors

Microscopic Pathology

- Most medications produce inflammation-predominant pattern
- Most toxins & a few medications like acetaminophen produce necrosis-predominant pattern
- Concomitant bile duct injury, eosinophils, granulomas, perivenular necrosis, and cholestasis out of proportion to hepatocellular injury suggest DILI, but none of these are specific

Top Differential Diagnoses

- Inflammation-predominant pattern: Acute viral hepatitis, autoimmune hepatitis, Wilson disease
- Necrosis-predominant pattern: Herpes/adenoviral hepatitis, ischemic necrosis, acute venous outflow obstruction

Prognosis

- Symptomatic and biochemical improvement in most cases on withdrawal of drug
- Liver enzymes can remain elevated for up to several months after discontinuation of drug
- Minority of cases progress to chronic hepatitis, and rarely, cirrhosis (despite drug withdrawal)
- Jaundice, high AST levels, and preexisting chronic liver disease are adverse prognostic factors

MICROSCOPIC PATHOLOGY

Histologic Features

- Acute hepatitis: Inflammation-predominant pattern
  - Portal and parenchymal inflammation with hepatocellular injury
  - Necrosis can affect single hepatocyte (spotty necrosis) or groups of hepatocytes (confluent necrosis)
  - By definition, fibrosis is absent
  - Regenerative features like binucleate hepatocytes and thick cell plates
  - Prominent Kupffer cells often are present in sinusoids
- Acute hepatitis: Necrosis-predominant pattern
  - Necrosis with minimal inflammation
  - Periportal (zone 1): Cocaine, ferrous sulphate
  - Midzonal (zone 2): Beryllium
  - Centrizonal (zone 3): Acetaminophen, halothane, carbon tetrachloride
  - When extensive, confluent necrosis can lead to acute hepatic failure
- Resolving hepatitis pattern
  - Minimal-mild hepatocellular injury & inflammation
  - Numerous macrophages in sinusoids highlighted by PAS-D stain
- Syncytial giant cell hepatitis pattern
  - Uncommon pattern of hepatic DILI
  - Severity can range from mild to fulminant

Predominant Pattern/Injury Type

- Inflammatory

Predominant Cell/Compartment Type

- Hepatocyte

DIFFERENTIAL DIAGNOSIS

Acute Hepatitis: Inflammation-Predominant Pattern

- Acute viral hepatitis, autoimmune hepatitis, Wilson disease
- Clinical and serological information necessary for final diagnosis
- Concomitant bile duct injury, eosinophils, granulomas, perivenular necrosis, and cholestasis out of proportion to hepatocellular injury suggest DILI, but none of these are specific
- Autoantibodies, elevated IgG levels, and prominent plasma cells favor autoimmune hepatitis

Acute Hepatitis: Necrosis-Predominant Pattern

- Herpes and adenoviral hepatitis, ischemic necrosis, acute venous outflow obstruction
- Viral inclusions at periphery of necrotic zones in herpes and adenoviral hepatitis
- Clinical information necessary to distinguish DILI from necrosis due to vascular etiologies

Resolving Hepatitis Pattern

- Nonspecific reactive hepatitis in systemic diseases
- Viral hepatitis

Syncytial Hepatitis Pattern

- Autoimmune hepatitis, paramyxovirus, hepatitis C, human immunodeficiency virus hepatitis
- Distinction based on clinical and serological features

DRUG-RELATED ACUTE HEPATITIS

CIOMS Consensus Criteria for Terminology in Drug-induced Liver Injury

Terminology	Criteria
Hepatocellular injury	Isolated increase in ALT > 2x normal, or ALT/ALP ratio > 5
Cholestatic injury	Isolated increase in ALP > 2x normal, or ALT/ALP ratio < 2
Mixed injury	Both ALT and ALP are increased; ALT/ALP ratio between 2 and 5
Acute injury	Above changes present for < 3 months
Chronic injury	Above changes present for > 3 months
Chronic liver disease	This term is used only after histologic confirmation

Drugs Associated with Acute Hepatitis Pattern of Injury

Class of Drugs	Individual Drugs
Inflammation-Predominant Pattern	
Nonsteroidal anti-inflammatory drugs	Indomethacin, tolmetin, sulindac, ibuprofen, ketoprofen, mefenamic acid, celecoxib
Anticonvulsants	Phenytoin, valproic acid
Antibacterial agents	Ampicillin, amoxicillin-clavulanic acid, oxacillin, cephalosporins, tetracycline, sulfonamides, erythromycin, trimethoprim-sulfamethoxazole
Antifungal	Griseofulvin, fluconazole, ketoconazole
Antiparasitic	Albendazole, thiabendazole, Fansidar
Anti-tuberculous	Isoniazid, rifampin
Antiviral	Zidovudine, ribavirin
Antitumor	6-mercaptopurine, azathioprine, L-asparaginase, mithramycin, vincristine, cyclophosphamide, carmustine
Antihypertensive	Methyldopa, hydralazine, lisinopril, labetalol
Antiarrhythmic	Quinidine, procainamide
Hypolipidemics	Statins, clofibrate, nicotinic acid
Hypoglycemics	Rosiglitazone, troglitazone
Others	Sulfonylureas, troglitazone, dantrolene, chlorzoxazone, dextropropoxyphene, allopurinol, gold
Herbal agents	Chapparal leaf, mistletoe, germander, kava, lycopodium
Necrosis-Predominant Pattern	
Drugs and toxins	Drugs: Acetaminophen, halothane; toxins: Aflatoxin, death cap mushroom (*Amanita phalloides*), carbon tetrachloride, ethylene dichloride, allyl compounds, ferrous sulfate phosphorus, MDMA (ecstasy)
Herbal agents	Pennyroyal, glue thistle, germander
Autoimmune markers positive	
AIH type 1-like disease	Minocycline, nitrofurantoin, alpha-methyl dopa
AIH type 2-like disease	Hydralazine
Syncytial giant cell hepatitis	
Drugs	Methotrexate, p-aminosalycilic acid, 6-mercaptopurine, clomethacin, ticlopidine
Herbal agents	Isabgol

DIAGNOSTIC CHECKLIST

Clinically Relevant Pathologic Features

- Elevated liver enzymes in variety of patterns temporally associated with drug

Pathologic Interpretation Pearls

- Multiple patterns of enzyme elevation and liver injury
- Careful review of medication history, including herbal/botanical drugs, is critical

SELECTED REFERENCES

1. Andrade RJ et al: Outcome of acute idiosyncratic drug-induced liver injury: Long-term follow-up in a hepatotoxicity registry. Hepatology. 44(6):1581-8, 2006
2. Watkins PB et al: Drug-induced liver injury: summary of a single topic clinical research conference. Hepatology. 43(3):618-31, 2006
3. Andrade RJ et al: Drug-induced liver injury: an analysis of 461 incidences submitted to the Spanish registry over a 10-year period. Gastroenterology. 2005 Aug;129(2):512-21. Erratum in: Gastroenterology. 129(5):1808, 2005

Microscopic Features

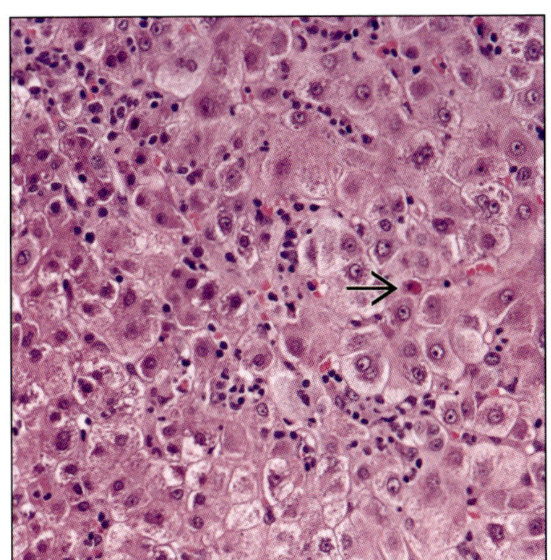

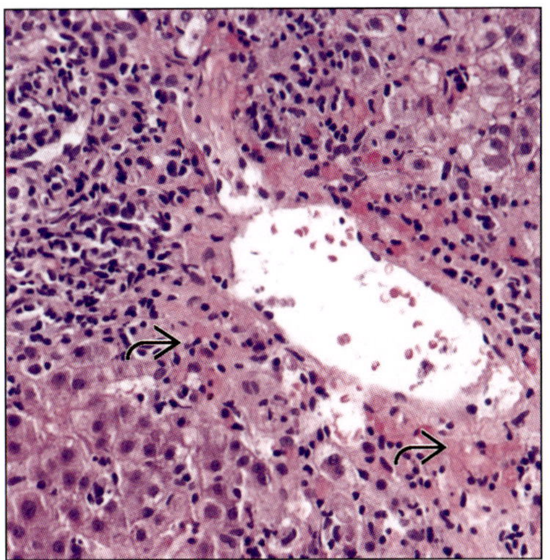

(Left) *Lobular hepatitis in a case of drug-induced hepatitis features mild inflammation, swollen hepatocytes, and occasional hepatocyte dropout ➡. The features are indistinguishable from other etiologies of acute hepatitis.* ***(Right)*** *Centrizonal necrosis ↪ with lymphoplasmacytic inflammation is not a specific finding but is highly suggestive of drug-induced liver injury.*

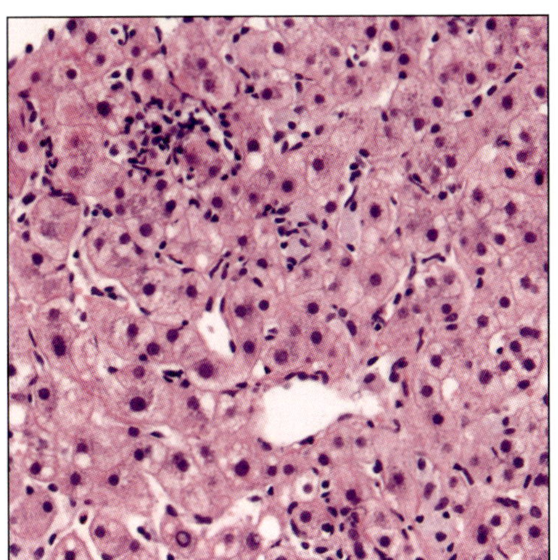

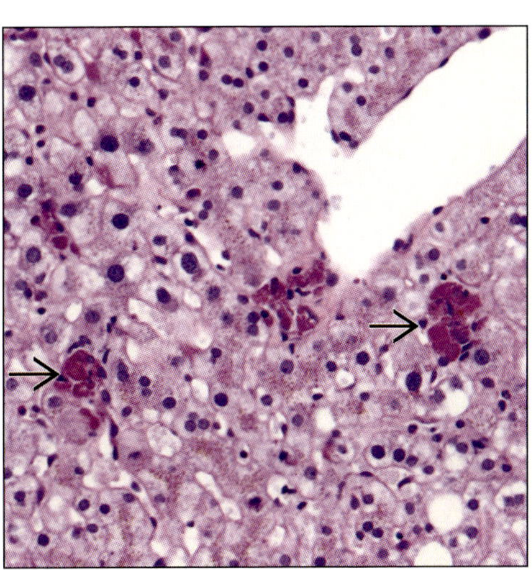

(Left) *Resolving drug-induced hepatitis shows mild lobular inflammation, minimal hepatocellular injury, and scattered macrophages along the sinusoids.* ***(Right)*** *Macrophages in the sinusoids ➡ in resolving drug-induced hepatitis are highlighted by PAS-D stain.*

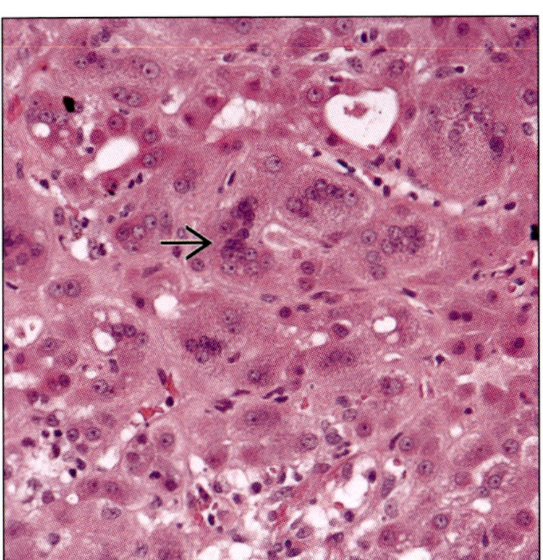

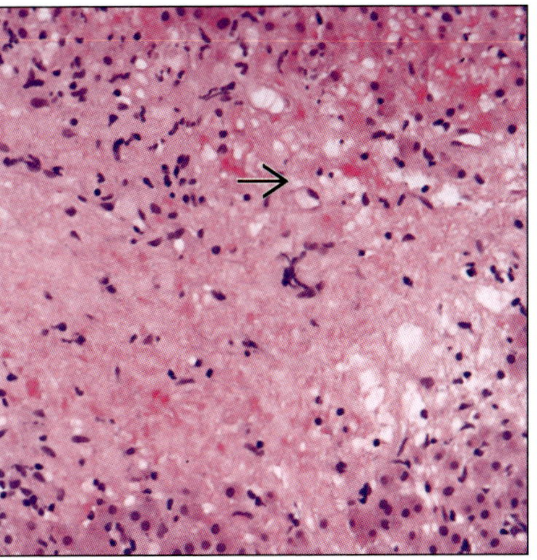

(Left) *Syncytial giant cell hepatitis, characterized by numerous multinucleated hepatocytes ➡, is a rare pattern of acute drug-induced liver injury.* ***(Right)*** *Necrosis-predominant drug-induced liver injury ➡ with minimal inflammation is difficult to histologically distinguish from ischemic injury.*

DRUG-INDUCED ACUTE HEPATIC FAILURE

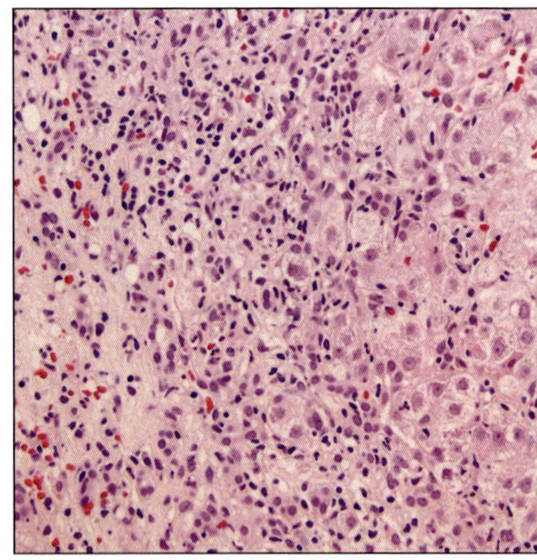

H&E of acute liver failure shows confluent necrosis with lymphoplasmacytic inflammation (left). Swelling and inflammation are seen in the remaining parenchyma (right).

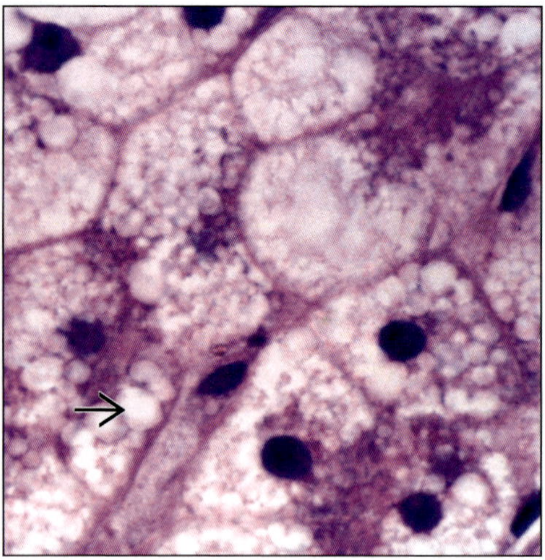

Diffuse microvesicular steatosis is characterized by multiple small fat droplets filling the cytoplasm ⇒. There is no necrosis or inflammation.

TERMINOLOGY

Abbreviations

- Acute liver failure (ALF)

Definitions

- Hepatic encephalopathy and reduced synthetic function evidenced by INR > 1.5
- Duration of disease less than 26 weeks
- Absence of chronic liver disease
  - Corresponding pathologic term is massive/submassive necrosis or fulminant hepatitis

ETIOLOGY/PATHOGENESIS

Mechanisms of Injury

- Massive/submassive necrosis due to intrinsic hepatotoxins
  - Most toxins fall in this category
    - Carbon tetrachloride, mushroom poisoning, recreational drugs like cocaine and MDMA (ecstasy)
  - Very few drugs cause this pattern of injury
    - Acetaminophen, halothane
    - Herbal medications: Pennyroyal, glue thistle, germander
- Massive/submassive necrosis due to idiosyncratic injury
  - Most drugs fall in this category
    - Drugs used for treatment of tuberculosis such as isoniazid are one of leading culprits of ALF in developing world
    - Other implicated drugs: Monoamine oxidase inhibitors, anticonvulsants (valproate, phenytoin), antimicrobial agents (sulfonamides, co-trimoxazole, ketoconazole)
- Diffuse microvesicular steatosis due to acute mitochondrial injury
  - Presents as ALF without histological necrosis
  - Commonly implicated drugs: Tetracycline, zidovudine, valproic acid, amineptine

CLINICAL ISSUES

Presentation

- Depends on specific drug or toxin
- Acetaminophen is most common cause of ALF in USA accounting for 40-50% of cases
  - Dose-dependent toxicity occurs with accidental (1/3 of cases) or suicidal (2/3 of cases) overdose
  - Minimum toxic dose in adults is 7.5-10 g, but severe liver damage occurs with ingestion of 15-25 g
  - Chronic alcohol consumption, obesity, and drugs that induce P-450 cytochrome system can lower toxic threshold of acetaminophen
  - Gastrointestinal symptoms for first 12-24 hours and latent phase of 24-48 hours is followed by ALF 72-96 hours after drug ingestion

Treatment

- Drug withdrawal, supportive care, and liver resuscitation (hypothermia, albumin dialysis, artificial liver support)
- Liver transplantation is often necessary
- Acetaminophen hepatotoxicity can be prevented with acetyl-cysteine therapy within 12 hours of drug ingestion

Prognosis

- Severe encephalopathy and older age are adverse prognostic factors for spontaneous recovery
- For acetaminophen toxicity, blood levels 4-16 hours after ingestion are best predictor of outcome; highest mortality is encountered in late presenters

DRUG-INDUCED ACUTE HEPATIC FAILURE

Key Facts

Terminology

- Onset of hepatic encephalopathy within 8 weeks of onset of symptoms
  - INR is > 1.5, and there is no evidence of chronic liver disease
- Corresponding pathologic terms: Massive/submassive necrosis, fulminant hepatitis

Clinical Issues

- Acetaminophen is most common cause of ALF in USA, accounting for 40-50% of cases

Microscopic Pathology

- Massive/submassive necrosis with little or no inflammation: Acetaminophen, most toxins
- Massive/submassive necrosis with prominent inflammation: Most idiosyncratic drug reactions
- Microvesicular steatosis: Tetracycline, zidovudine
- Regenerative nodules can be seen later in course of disease and can be mistaken for cirrhosis
- Unlike fibrous septa of cirrhosis, necrotic areas show pale staining with trichrome stain and lack elastic fibers on elastic stain

Top Differential Diagnoses

- Necrosis with inflammation: Acute viral hepatitis A and B, autoimmune hepatitis, Wilson disease
- Necrosis with minimal inflammation: Herpes simplex and adenoviral hepatitis, acute ischemia, acute Budd-Chiari syndrome
- Microvesicular steatosis: Alcoholic foamy degeneration, acute fatty liver of pregnancy, Reye syndrome, Jamaican vomiting sickness, rare metabolic disorders like carnitine deficiency

MICROSCOPIC PATHOLOGY

Histologic Features

- Based on pattern of injury, drug-induced ALF can be divided into 4 categories
- Massive/submassive necrosis with little or no inflammation
  - Extensive confluent hepatocellular necrosis
  - Necrosis may be nonzonal, centrizonal (acetaminophen, halothane, carbon tetrachloride), midzonal (beryllium), or periportal (cocaine, ferrous sulphate)
  - Concomitant steatosis, often microvesicular, can be present (carbon tetrachoride poisoning, cocaine)
  - Mild or absent inflammation
- Massive/submassive necrosis with prominent inflammation
  - Portal and often panacinar inflammation, predominantly lymphocytic, with variable number of eosinophils and plasma cells
  - Confluent necrosis common
- Extensive microvesicular steatosis
  - Diffuse accumulation of small fat droplets in hepatocyte cytoplasm
  - Inconspicuous inflammation and necrosis
- Massive/submassive necrosis with regenerative nodules
  - Regenerative nodules can be seen later in course of disease and mistaken for cirrhosis
  - Area between nodules is not fibrous septa of cirrhosis but bridging necrosis with collapse of liver parenchyma
  - Necrotic areas show pale staining with trichrome stain in contrast to coarse, densely staining collagen in fibrous septa of cirrhosis
  - Elastic stain demonstrates lack of elastic fibers in necrotic areas; fibrous septa of cirrhosis are typically richly endowed with elastic fibers
    - Trichrome stain is more reliable than elastic stain to distinguish necrosis and fibrosis

DIFFERENTIAL DIAGNOSIS

Acute Viral Hepatitis

- Hepatotropic viruses
  - In USA and Europe, only accounts for 10-15% of cases (5-10% each by hepatitis A and B)
  - Hepatitis C has been reported to cause ALF in Asia but rarely in western world
  - Coinfection or superinfection with hepatitis D can lead to ALF
  - Hepatitis E has been associated with ALF in Indian subcontinent, especially in pregnant women
- Nonhepatotropic viruses
  - Herpes simplex and adenovirus infection can lead to ALF with necrosis-predominant pattern of injury
  - Less common infections: Cytomegalovirus, Epstein-Barr virus, yellow fever, dengue fever, Ebola fever
  - Parvovirus B19 can cause fulminant hepatitis in children

Autoimmune Hepatitis

- Rapid deterioration of liver function can lead to ALF
- Extensive necroinflammatory activity with plasma cell-rich infiltrate
- Histologically indistinguishable from idiosyncratic drug reaction
- Autoantibodies, elevated serum IgG, and presence of fibrosis on biopsy favor autoimmune hepatitis

Ischemic Liver Injury

- Causes
  - Cardiogenic or septic shock
  - Variceal hemorrhage
- Inflammation is typically mild or absent, mimicking toxic pattern of drug-induced injury
- Histologic features favoring ischemia
  - Centrizonal or panacinar necrosis with congestion and pooling of blood in zone 3 sinusoids
  - Periportal cholangiolar bile plugs in cholangioles (cholangitis lenta) in absence of demonstrable biliary obstruction

DRUG-INDUCED ACUTE HEPATIC FAILURE

Histological Patterns of Injury in Acute Liver Failure

Histological Pattern	Drugs Implicated	Differential Diagnosis
Massive/submassive necrosis with minimal inflammation	Acetaminophen, cocaine, MDMA (ecstasy), carbon tetrachloride	Herpes simplex or adenoviral hepatitis, acute ischemic injury, acute Budd-Chiari syndrome, Wilson disease
Massive/submassive necrosis with prominent inflammation	Isoniazid, monoamine oxidase inhibitors, anticonvulsants (phenytoin, valproate), antimicrobials (sulfonamides, co-trimoxazole, ketoconazole)	Autoimmune hepatitis, viral hepatitis, Wilson disease
Microvesicular steatosis	Tetracycline (antibiotic), zidovudine (nucleoside analogue), valproic acid (anticonvulsant), amineptine (antidepressant)	Acute alcohol intoxication, Reye syndrome, acute fatty liver of pregnancy

Acute Budd-Chiari Syndrome

- Acute presentation is rare, can mimic ischemia or toxic pattern of drug injury
- Centrizonal or panacinar necrosis with hemorrhage, congestion, and sinusoidal dilatation

Wilson Disease

- Rare but important cause of ALF in young patients (presentation after 50 years is rare)
  - Recovery of hepatic function is rare in fulminant Wilson disease, and transplantation is only viable option
- Can mimic toxic as well as idiosyncratic drug reaction
  - Hemolytic anemia, if present, favors Wilson disease
  - AST:ALT > 2.2, high bilirubin (> 20 mg/dL), and low alkaline phosphatase has high specificity for Wilson disease
  - Serum ceruloplasmin, urinary copper, or quantitative determination of hepatic copper from paraffin block helps in establishing diagnosis

Malignant Neoplasms

- Infiltration of liver by malignant neoplasms rarely leads to ALF
  - Implicated tumors include leukemia/lymphoma, metastatic carcinoma, and melanoma
- Identification of tumor as underlying etiology is important to avoid transplantation as prognosis is poor

Pregnancy-related ALF

- HELLP syndrome
  - Hemolysis (H), elevated liver (EL) enzymes, and low platelets (LP)
  - Serious complication of preeclampsia, occurs in 3rd trimester
  - ALF is rare complication
  - Histologically shows focal necrosis, periportal hemorrhage, and fibrin deposits
- Acute fatty liver of pregnancy
  - Occurs in 3rd trimester, often associated with preeclampsia
  - Hyperbilirubinemia and elevations of ALT and AST are modest compared to other causes of ALF
  - Increase in blood pressure, hyperuricemia, and intense thirst favor this diagnosis
  - Liver biopsy is often not done due to risk of bleeding
  - Histologically shows microvesicular steatosis, hepatocellular swelling, inconspicuous necrosis

DIAGNOSTIC CHECKLIST

Clinically Relevant Pathologic Features

- Acute liver failure in patient who has been exposed to drug or toxin

Pathologic Interpretation Pearls

- Necrosis that may be significantly out of proportion to inflammation

SELECTED REFERENCES

1. Lee NM et al: Liver disease in pregnancy. World J Gastroenterol. 15(8):897-906, 2009
2. Korman JD et al: Screening for Wilson disease in acute liver failure: a comparison of currently available diagnostic tests. Hepatology. 48(4):1167-74, 2008
3. Polson J et al: False positive acetaminophen concentrations in patients with liver injury. Clin Chim Acta. 391(1-2):24-30, 2008
4. Larson AM et al: Acetaminophen-induced acute liver failure: results of a United States multicenter, prospective study. Hepatology. 42(6):1364-72, 2005
5. Schiødt FV et al: Viral hepatitis-related acute liver failure. Am J Gastroenterol. 98(2):448-53, 2003
6. Ostapowicz G et al: S. Acute Liver Failure Study Group. Results of a prospective study of acute liver failure at 17 tertiary care centers in the United States. Ann Intern Med. 137(12):947-54, 2002
7. Rowbotham D et al: Acute liver failure secondary to hepatic infiltration: a single centre experience of 18 cases. Gut. 42(4):576-80, 1998
8. Bhaduri BR et al: Fulminant hepatic failure: pediatric aspects. Semin Liver Dis. 16(4):349-55, 1996
9. Williams R: Classification, etiology, and considerations of outcome in acute liver failure. Semin Liver Dis. 16(4):343-8, 1996
10. Powell-Jackson PR et al: Budd-Chiari syndrome presenting as fulminant hepatic failure. Gut. 27(9):1101-5, 1986

Microscopic Features

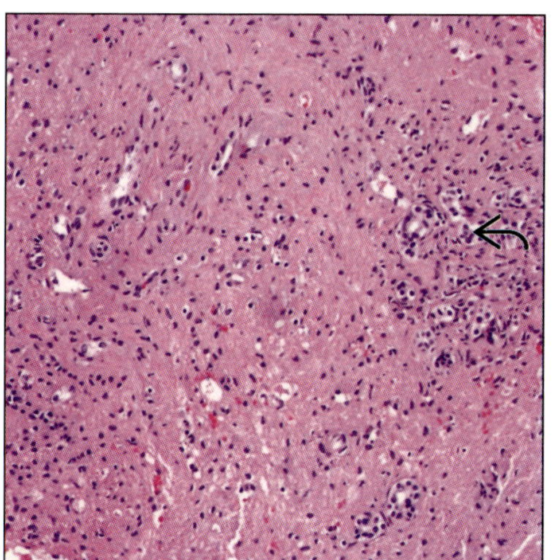

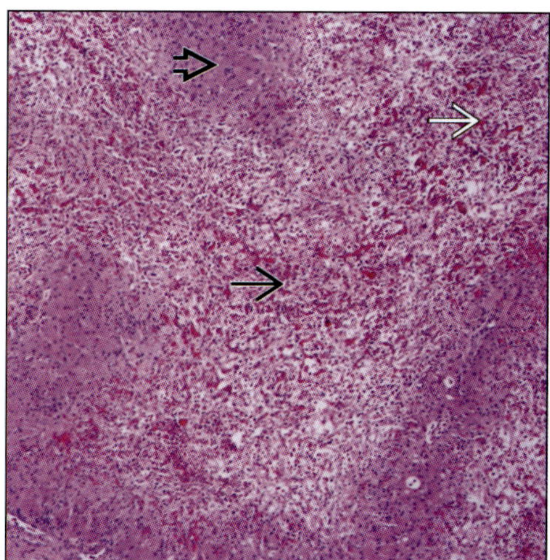

(Left) *Extensive panacinar necrosis with negligible inflammation is seen in the parenchyma. Note a residual portal tract ➔. These findings are typical of the "toxic pattern" of drug injury.* ***(Right)*** *Multiacinar hemorrhagic necrosis ➔, congestion ➔, and lack of inflammation with sparing of periportal hepatocytes ➔ are typical of acetaminophen toxicity but can also be seen in acute ischemia and acute Budd-Chiari syndrome.*

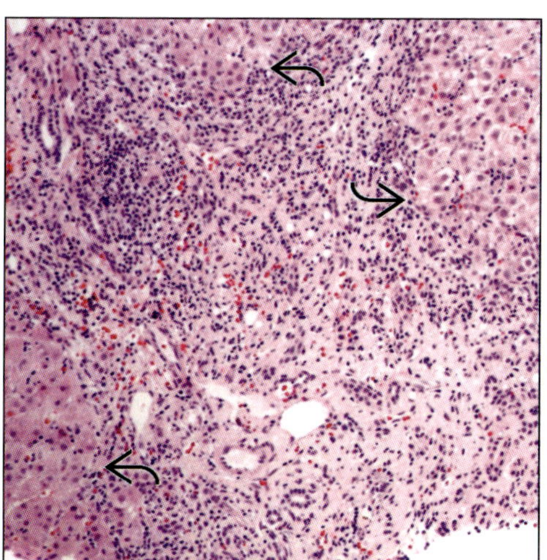

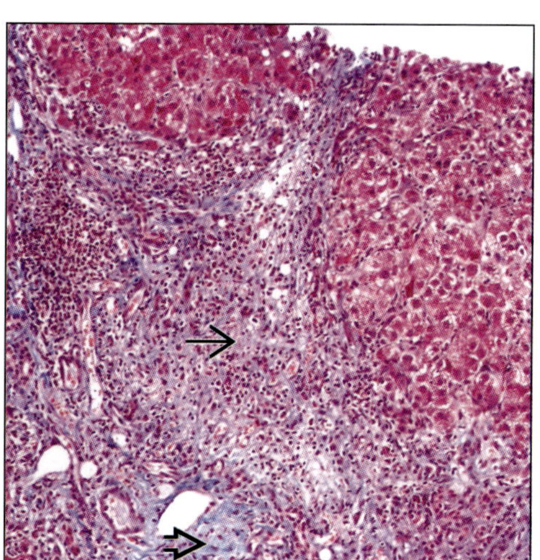

(Left) *Regenerative nodules of liver parenchyma ➔ are separated by areas of bridging necrosis, mimicking cirrhosis.* ***(Right)*** *Trichrome stain shows pale staining in the areas of bridging necrosis ➔ in contrast to the darkly stained collagen in the portal tract ➔. Fibrous septa in cirrhosis also show coarse, darkly stained collagen similar to portal tracts.*

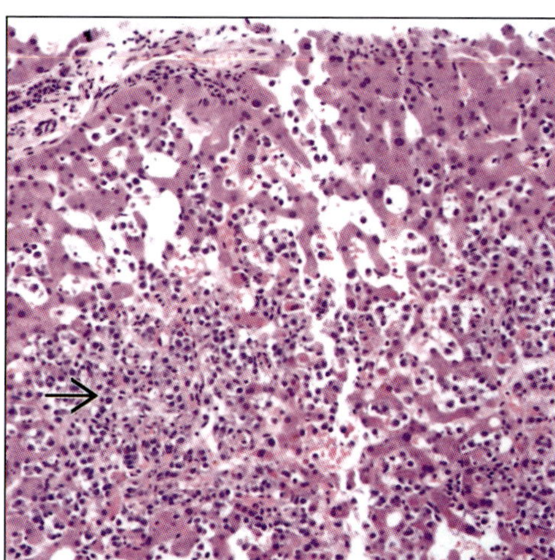

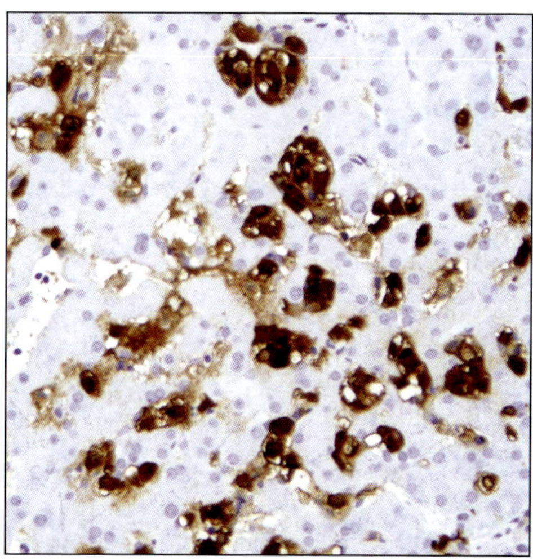

(Left) *The hepatic sinusoids in this biopsy are extensively infiltrated by tumor cells ➔, leading to acute liver failure. Inflammation and necrosis are minimal or absent.* ***(Right)*** *Immunohistochemistry for S100 highlights the infiltrating tumor cells in the sinusoids. HMB-45 and melan-A were also positive. Malignant melanoma with liver involvement is a rare cause of ALF.*

DRUG-INDUCED CHOLESTATIC LIVER INJURY

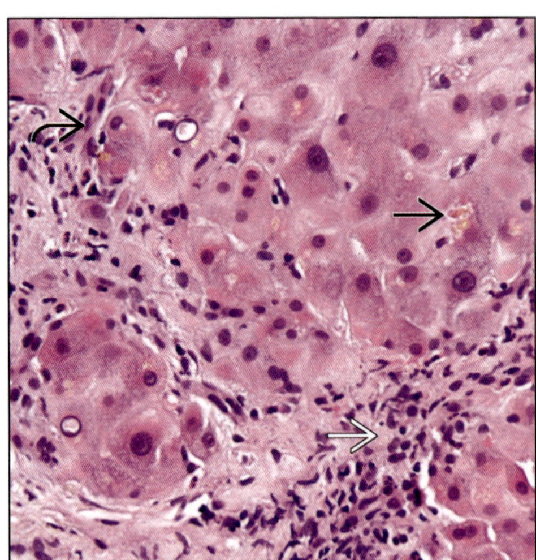

Cholestatic hepatitis is characterized by cholestasis ➙, mild lymphocytic inflammation ➡, and focal hepatocellular damage ⇨.

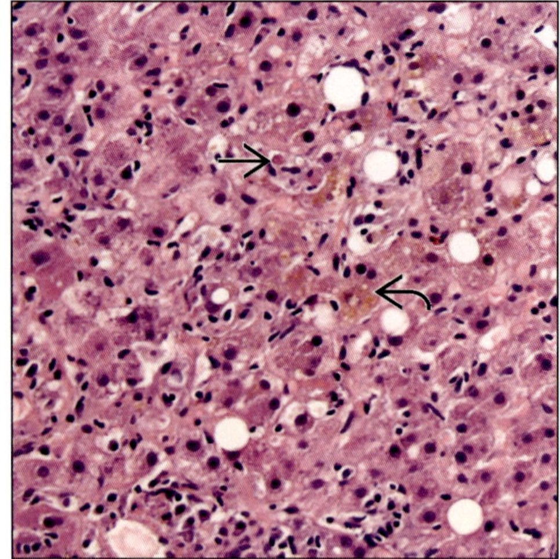

Cholestatic hepatitis is characterized by lobular inflammation, hepatocyte dropout ➙, and cholestasis ↪. This is the most common histologic pattern observed in drug-induced liver injury.

TERMINOLOGY

Abbreviations

- Cholestatic drug-induced liver injury (DILI)

ETIOLOGY/PATHOGENESIS

Four General Categories

- Based on symptom duration and histologic pattern of injury

Pure Cholestasis

- Cholestasis with minimal hepatocellular injury
- Commonly implicated drugs: Anabolic steroids, oral contraceptives, prochlorperazine, thiabendazole, warfarin

Cholestatic Hepatitis

- Most common pattern of DILI
- Cholestasis with hepatocellular injury
- Macrolide antibiotics (erythromycin), antipsychotics (chlorpromazine), numerous other drugs

Prolonged Cholestasis and Ductopenia

- Antibiotics, antifungals, anticonvulsants, antipsychotics, NSAIDs; rarely oral contraceptives, amiodarone

Sclerosing Bile Duct Injury

- 5-fluorodeoxyuridine (intraarterial infusion for metastatic colorectal carcinoma), formaldehyde, and sodium chloride (injected into hydatid cysts)

CLINICAL ISSUES

Presentation

- Jaundice, pruritus, dark urine, pale stools

Laboratory Tests

- Elevated alkaline phosphatase and GGT
- Transaminases minimally elevated in pure cholestasis; modest to marked elevation in cholestatic hepatitis

Prognosis

- Most cases resolve with cessation of offending drug
- Prolonged cholestasis (> 3 months) and ductopenia occurs in rare instances

MICROSCOPIC PATHOLOGY

Histologic Features

- Pure (bland) cholestasis
  - Bile plugs in hepatocytes &/or canaliculi
    - Most prominent in centrizonal region
  - Portal/lobular inflammation, bile ductular reaction, and hepatocellular injury are minimal or absent
  - No bile duct damage
- Cholestatic hepatitis (cholangiolitic or hypersensitivity cholestasis)
  - Bile plugs in hepatocytes &/or canaliculi
  - Portal &/or lobular inflammation, predominantly lymphocytic, with variable plasma cells and eosinophils
  - Bile ductular reaction with associated neutrophilic infiltrate may be present
  - Bile duct epithelial injury and lymphocytic cholangitis may be present
    - No ductopenia
  - Variable degree of hepatocellular injury ranging from isolated hepatocellular dropout to confluent necrosis
- Prolonged cholestasis (> 3 months) and ductopenia
  - Variable inflammation, bile duct injury, ductular reaction, and hepatocellular damage
  - Some cases progress to loss of bile ducts and overt ductopenia (vanishing bile duct syndrome)
  - Rare cases progress to cirrhosis
- Sclerosing bile duct injury

DRUG-INDUCED CHOLESTATIC LIVER INJURY

Key Facts

Etiology/Pathogenesis

- Most common histologic pattern of DILI

Microscopic Pathology

- Pure cholestasis: Cholestasis with minimal inflammation or hepatocellular damage
- Cholestatic hepatitis: Cholestasis with inflammation and hepatocellular damage
- Prolonged cholestasis/ductopenia: Cholestasis > 3 months, bile duct loss
- Sclerosing duct injury: Fibrosis affecting large bile ducts similar to PSC

Top Differential Diagnoses

- Pure cholestasis: Sepsis, shock, BRIC
- Cholestatic hepatitis: Other causes of hepatitis, large duct obstruction
- Obstructive biliary disease
- Prolonged cholestasis/ductopenia: PBC and PSC

  - Fibrosis and strictures affecting extrahepatic and intrahepatic bile ducts similar to primary sclerosing cholangitis

DIFFERENTIAL DIAGNOSIS

Pure Cholestasis

- Systemic disorders (sepsis, cardiac failure, shock)
- Postoperative cholestasis, intrahepatic cholestasis of pregnancy, benign recurrent intrahepatic cholestasis (BRIC)
- Clinical information is necessary to exclude these etiologies
- Early obstructive biliary disease can lack portal edema, ductular reaction, and inflammation, mimicking pure cholestasis

Cholestatic Hepatitis

- Autoimmune hepatitis, acute viral hepatitis, Wilson disease
  - Serological tests for hepatitis viruses, autoantibodies, and work-up for Wilson disease
- Obstructive biliary disease
  - Ductular reaction, bile duct injury, and cholestasis similar to cholestatic DILI
  - Imaging necessary to evaluate bile ducts
- Primary biliary cirrhosis (PBC) and primary sclerosing cholangitis (PSC)
  - Hepatocellular injury minimal or absent, transaminases modestly elevated (typically less than 300 U/L)
  - Histological cholestasis in early disease (without fibrosis) does not occur in PBC and PSC
  - Antimitochondrial antibodies (AMA) in PBC
  - Characteristic abnormalities in large ducts on cholangiography in PSC

Prolonged Cholestasis and Vanishing Bile Duct Syndrome

- PBC and PSC: AMA and cholangiography essential to exclude these possibilities
- Rare causes of ductopenia: Ischemic bile duct injury, chronic hepatitis C

Sclerosing Bile Duct Injury

- Indistinguishable from primary or secondary sclerosing cholangitis
- Cholangiographic findings, history of ischemic injury, drug history necessary to establish etiology

SELECTED REFERENCES

1. Ramachandran R et al: Histological patterns in drug-induced liver disease. J Clin Pathol. 62(6):481-92, 2009
2. Levy C et al: Drug-induced cholestasis. Clin Liver Dis. 7(2):311-30, 2003

IMAGE GALLERY

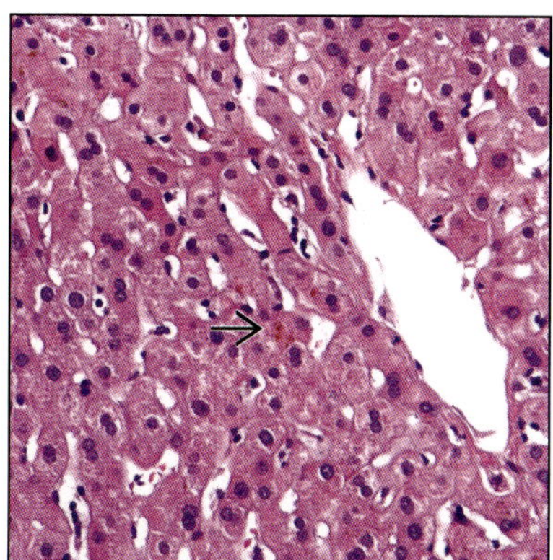

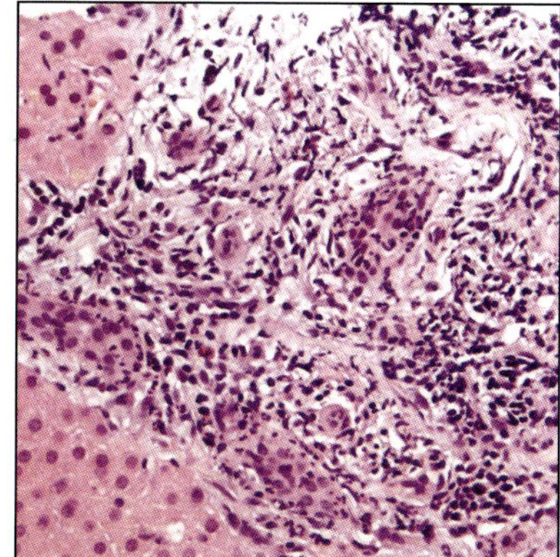

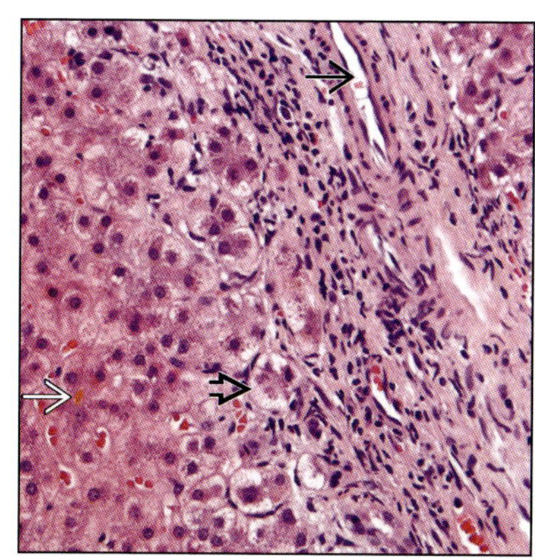

(Left) *Pure cholestasis is characterized by bile in hepatocytes and canaliculi ⇒ with no hepatocellular injury or inflammation. Portal tracts and bile ducts are also normal in this pattern of injury.* ***(Center)*** *Portal edema, inflammation, and bile ductular reaction in DILI may be indistinguishable from obstructive biliary disease on histologic grounds.* ***(Right)*** *Prolonged cholestasis with ductopenia features mild portal inflammation, loss of bile ducts (note arteriole ⇒ unaccompanied by interlobular bile duct), focal cholestasis ➡, and cholate stasis ⇒.*

DRUG-RELATED GRANULOMATOUS HEPATITIS

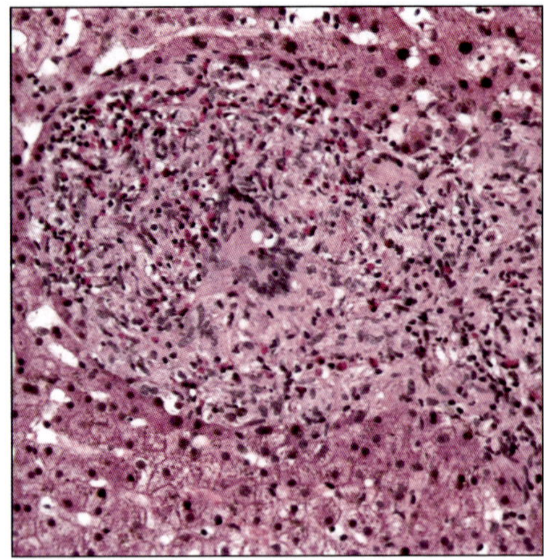

This portal tract contains an epithelioid granuloma with numerous associated eosinophils as well as a central giant cell in a patient with granulomatous hepatitis associated with echinacea tea.

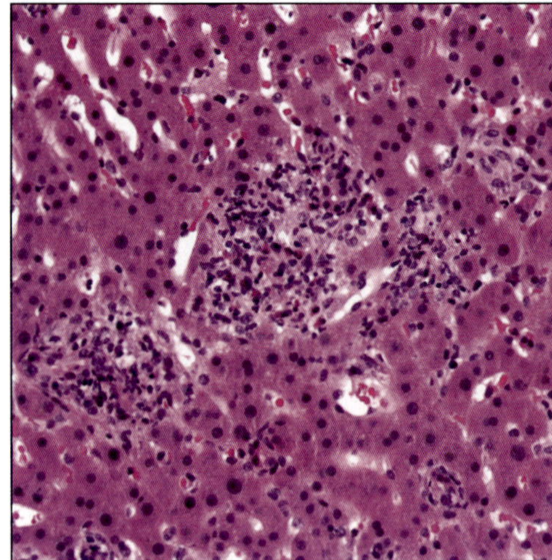

Microgranulomas, shown here with admixed lymphocytes and eosinophils, are often seen in drug reactions. This patient had a reaction to propylthiouracil.

TERMINOLOGY

Definitions

- Granulomatous inflammation caused by drug or toxin
  - Important mechanism of drug-related hepatotoxicity
  - Drugs reportedly responsible for up to 30% of hepatic granulomas
  - Many implicated drugs, including over-the-counter and herbal preparations

ETIOLOGY/PATHOGENESIS

Probable Hypersensitivity Reaction

- Common offenders
  - Antimicrobials
    - Penicillins
    - Sulfa drugs
    - Cephalexin
    - Sulfadoxine (antimalarial)
    - Dapsone (antibacterial)
  - Anticonvulsants
    - Carbamazepine
    - Phenytoin (anticonvulsant)
  - Cardiac drugs
    - Diltiazem (calcium channel blocker)
    - Procainamide (antiarrhythmic)
    - Trichlormethiazide (diuretic)
  - Other
    - Allopurinol (antihyperuricemic)
    - Diazepam (benzodiazepine)
    - Glyburide (hypoglycemic)
    - Gold (antiarthritic)
    - Interferon
    - Procarbazine (antineoplastic)
    - Propylthiouracil (antithyroidal)

CLINICAL ISSUES

Presentation

- Vary with offending drug
  - Fever
  - Hepatomegaly
  - Clinical signs of hypersensitivity
    - Rash
    - Lymphadenopathy
- Drug-induced hepatic injury can mimic any other form of liver disease
- Some patients are asymptomatic

Laboratory Tests

- Elevated transaminases, sometimes markedly so
- Elevated alkaline phosphatase
- Variably elevated bilirubin
- May have peripheral eosinophilia
- May have hypergammaglobulinemia
- Variably present autoantibodies

Treatment

- Remove offending drug
- Steroids may be necessary

Prognosis

- Histology usually improves with cessation of offending drug
  - Usually does not result in progressive liver disease or fibrosis if drug is stopped

MICROSCOPIC PATHOLOGY

Histologic Features

- Vary with implicated drug
  - Noncaseating granulomas
    - Vary in number and size
    - May be compact or loose
    - Both portal and lobular

Key Facts

Clinical Issues
- Drug-induced hepatic injury can mimic any other form of liver disease

Microscopic Pathology
- Noncaseating granulomas
  - Presence of granulomas, ± eosinophils, does not prove drug-related etiology
- Combination of microgranulomas and hepatocyte injury is very suggestive of granulomatous drug reaction

Diagnostic Checklist
- Drugs responsible for up to 30% of hepatic granulomas
- Careful drug history and temporal correlation between drug administration and liver disease are useful

---

    - Granulomas infiltrated by lymphocytes, plasma cells, and most notably eosinophils
    - Multinucleate giant cells often present
  - Fibrin ring granulomas may be seen with allopurinol
- Unless eosinophils are present, very difficult to distinguish drug-induced granulomas from granulomas of other causes
  - However, presence of granulomas, with or without eosinophils, does not prove drug-related etiology
- Granulomas may be sole alteration or accompanied by
  - Hepatocyte reactive changes
  - Apoptotic hepatocytes
  - Steatosis
  - Cholestasis
  - Cytoplasmic ballooning
  - Cholangitis (usually associated with portal granulomas)
  - Vasculitis

DIFFERENTIAL DIAGNOSIS

Sarcoidosis
- Abnormal chest x-ray, elevated serum angiotensin converting enzyme (ACE) favor sarcoidosis

Infection
- Special stains, immunohistochemistry, microbiological cultures useful to exclude infection

DIAGNOSTIC CHECKLIST

Clinically Relevant Pathologic Features
- Diagnosis requires high level of suspicion
- Need careful drug history and temporal correlation between drug administration and liver disease

Pathologic Interpretation Pearls
- Combination of microgranulomas and hepatocyte injury is very suggestive of granulomatous drug reaction

SELECTED REFERENCES

1. Wainwright H: Hepatic granulomas. Eur J Gastroenterol Hepatol. 19(2):93-5, 2007
2. Kleiner DE: Granulomas in the liver. Semin Diagn Pathol. 23(3-4):161-9, 2006
3. Anderson CS et al: Hepatic granulomas: a 15-year experience in the Royal Adelaide Hospital. Med J Aust. 148(2):71-4, 1988
4. Al-Kawas FH et al: Allopurinol hepatotoxicity. Report of two cases and review of the literature. Ann Intern Med. 95(5):588-90, 1981
5. Irani SK et al: Hepatic granulomas: review of 73 patients from one hospital and survey of the literature. J Clin Gastroenterol. 1(2):131-43, 1979

IMAGE GALLERY

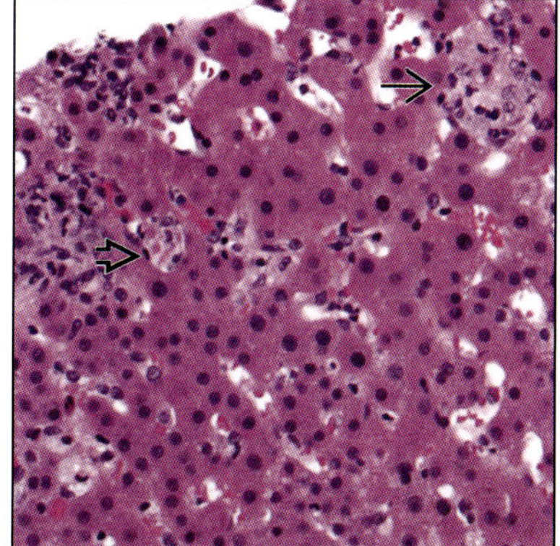

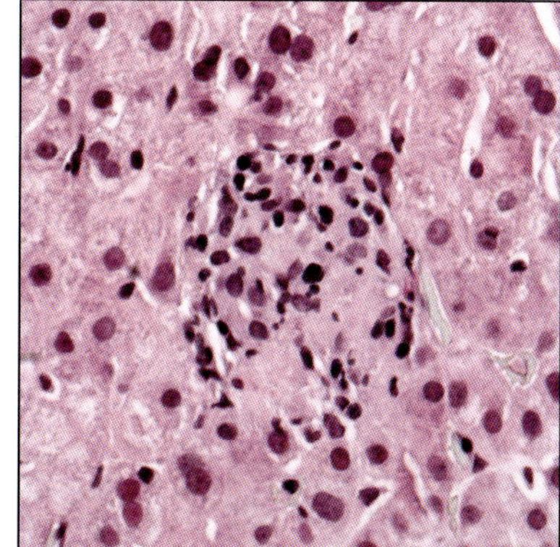

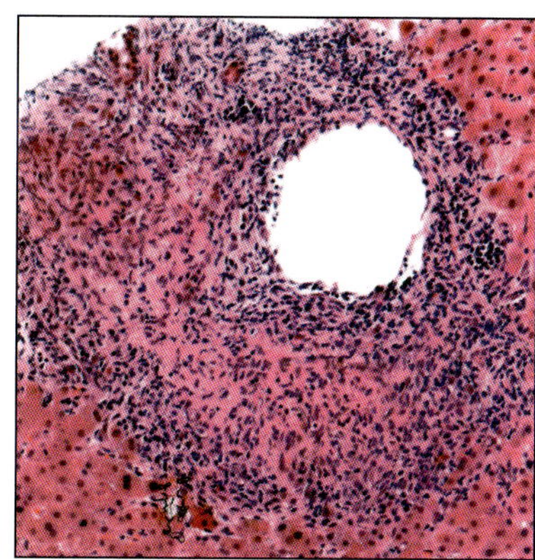

(Left) *A microgranuloma ➔ with associated apoptotic hepatocytes ⇨ and lobular inflammation is seen in a case of granulomatous drug reaction secondary to propylthiouracil.* ***(Center)*** *A small portal epithelioid granuloma with associated lymphocytes is seen in this case of Tegretol-related granulomatous hepatitis.* ***(Right)*** *Fibrin ring granulomas with a central lipid vacuole are associated with Allopurinol.*

DRUG-RELATED STEATOHEPATITIS/PHOSPHOLIPIDOSIS

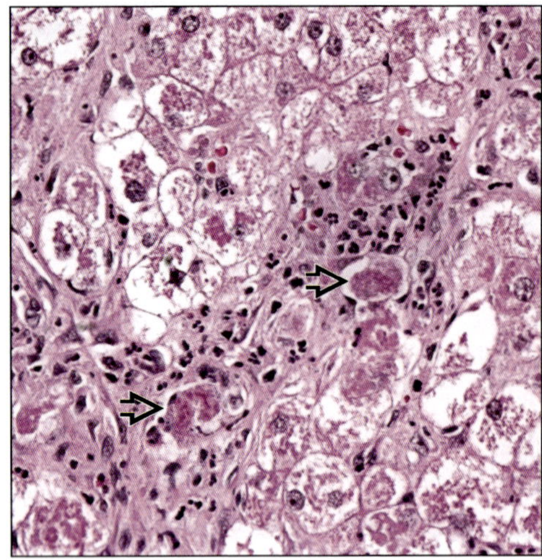

Features of amiodarone hepatotoxicity include foamy, ballooned hepatocytes and abundant Mallory hyaline ➔ with surrounding neutrophils.

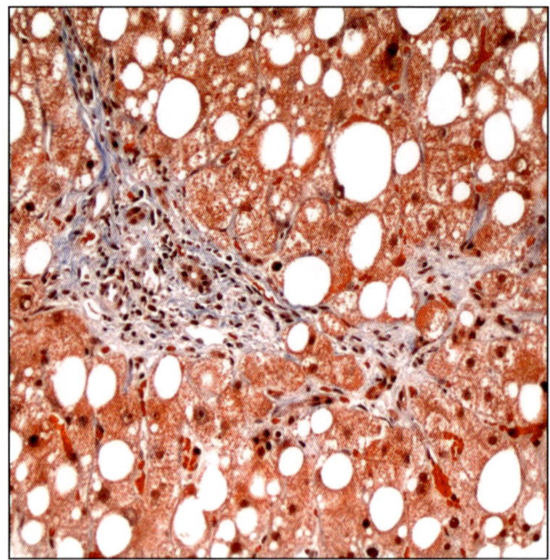

Trichrome stain shows delicate spurs of periportal fibrosis, as well as steatosis, in methotrexate toxicity.

TERMINOLOGY

Definitions

- Steatohepatitis as consequence of drug exposure
  - Some seem to produce their effect by exacerbating underlying nonalcoholic steatohepatitis

ETIOLOGY/PATHOGENESIS

Commonly Implicated Drugs

- Amiodarone (antiarrhythmic)
  - Strongly tissue-bound, becomes concentrated in liver
- Nifedipine (calcium channel blocker)
- Perhexiline maleate (calcium channel blocker)
- Methotrexate (immunosuppressant/antineoplastic)
  - Hepatic injury usually occurs after long-term use
- Tamoxifen (estrogen antagonist)
- Steroids
- Naproxen (NSAID)
- Trimethoprim-Sulfa (antibiotic)
- Total parenteral nutrition
  - Steatosis particularly seen in adults
- Anti-HIV drugs
  - Induce syndrome of dyslipidemia, fat maldistribution, insulin resistance
    - Known as HIV-associated lipodystrophy syndrome or HIV-associated metabolic and morphological abnormality syndrome (HAMMAS)

CLINICAL ISSUES

Presentation

- Variably present constitutional complaints, hepatomegaly, jaundice
  - May be asymptomatic (especially methotrexate injury)
- Symptoms may present after months to years of therapy

Laboratory Tests

- Elevated transaminases
  - May be normal despite hepatic injury, especially in patients on methotrexate

Prognosis

- Amiodarone
  - Cessation of therapy should lead to regression of injury
  - Due to long half-life of drug, may take months to see improvement
  - If drug is not withdrawn, process can progress to cirrhosis, hepatic failure
- Methotrexate
  - Risk of liver damage depends on duration of therapy and dose
  - Exacerbated by concomitant obesity, alcohol use
  - May progress to fibrosis or cirrhosis
  - Periodic liver biopsy recommended for surveillance

MICROSCOPIC PATHOLOGY

Histologic Features

- Amiodarone and other drugs causing phospholipidosis
  - Phospholipidosis: Granular, foamy appearance of hepatocytes corresponding to lamellar lysosomal inclusions by EM
    - Corresponds to entrapment of amiodarone in lysosomes, with subsequent binding of phospholipids
  - Hepatocyte swelling
  - Abundant Mallory hyaline
    - Often with associated neutrophils known as satellitosis
    - Occasionally, abundant Mallory hyaline but fatty changes absent
  - Steatosis

DRUG-RELATED STEATOHEPATITIS/PHOSPHOLIPIDOSIS

Key Facts

Terminology

- Definition: Steatohepatitis as consequence of drug exposure

Etiology/Pathogenesis

- Commonly implicated drugs
  - Amiodarone
  - Methotrexate
  - Antiretroviral drugs
  - Nifedipine

Clinical Issues

- Symptoms may present after months to years of therapy
- May be asymptomatic despite liver injury
  - Especially methotrexate injury
- Due to long half-life of amiodarone, may take months to see improvement
- Risk of liver damage with methotrexate use depends on duration of therapy and dose
  - Exacerbated by concomitant obesity, alcohol use

Microscopic Pathology

- Amiodarone
  - Steatosis
  - Phospholipidosis
  - Mallory hyaline, often with associated neutrophils (satellitosis)
- Methotrexate
  - Steatosis
  - Reactive changes
  - Fibrosis

  - Fibrosis/cirrhosis with progressive disease
- Methotrexate
  - Steatosis
    - Usually macrovesicular
    - Occasionally microvesicular
    - Variably present hypertrophic Ito cells
  - Nonspecific reactive changes
    - Hyperchromasia and anisocytosis of hepatocyte nuclei
    - Spotty hepatocyte necrosis with associated Kupffer cells
  - Portal inflammation
  - Fibrosis
    - Begins as irregular periportal spurs
    - Progresses to portal/portal and portal/central bridging
    - Pericellular fibrosis may also be present
  - Grading scheme exists for purposes of clinical decision making
    - Grade I: Normal or only mild fatty or reactive changes
    - Grade II: Moderate to severe fatty or reactive changes
    - Grade III: Mild periportal fibrosis (IIIA) or moderate to marked fibrosis (IIIB)
    - Grade IV: Cirrhosis
  - Methotrexate should be stopped in IIIB or IV cases; cautiously continued with rebiopsy in 6 months in IIIA biopsies

DIFFERENTIAL DIAGNOSIS

Alcoholic Hepatitis

- Need history of alcohol use to distinguish from drug-related steatohepatitis

Nonalcoholic Steatohepatitis (NASH)

- NASH may lack abundant Mallory bodies
- May need history of obesity, diabetes, hyperlipidemia, and lack of exposure to offending drugs to distinguish from drug-related steatohepatitis

Niemann-Pick Disease

- Hereditary disorder of lipid metabolism
- Diminished sphingomyelinase activity
- May mimic amiodarone-induced phospholipidosis

Preexisting Hepatitis Treated with Steroids

- Most commonly seen in treated autoimmune hepatitis
  - Autoimmune serologies, medication history help to distinguish from drug-related steatohepatitis

Wilson Disease

- Ceruloplasmin, urinary copper, medication history may be needed to resolve differential diagnosis

Malabsorption/Malnutrition

- Clinical history and medication history necessary to resolve differential diagnosis
- May lack abundant Mallory hyaline

DIAGNOSTIC CHECKLIST

Pathologic Interpretation Pearls

- Appropriate history of exposure to offending drug is necessary for diagnosis

SELECTED REFERENCES

1. Loulergue P et al: Hepatic steatosis as an emerging cause of cirrhosis in HIV-infected patients. J Acquir Immune Defic Syndr. 45(3):365, 2007
2. Lewis JH et al: Histopathologic analysis of suspected amiodarone hepatotoxicity. Hum Pathol. 21(1):59-67, 1990
3. Kremer JM et al: Liver histology in rheumatoid arthritis patients receiving long-term methotrexate therapy. A prospective study with baseline and sequential biopsy samples. Arthritis Rheum. 32(2):121-7, 1989
4. Lewis JH et al: Amiodarone hepatotoxicity: prevalence and clinicopathologic correlations among 104 patients. Hepatology. 9(5):679-85, 1989
5. Roenigk HH Jr et al: Methotrexate in psoriasis: revised guidelines. J Am Acad Dermatol. 19(1 Pt 1):145-56, 1988
6. Nyfors A et al: Morphogenesis of fibrosis and cirrhosis in methotrexate-treated patients with psoriasis. Am J Surg Pathol. 1(3):235-43, 1977

Microscopic Features

*(**Left**) Low-power photomicrograph of amiodarone toxicity shows lobular disarray with foamy, ballooned hepatocytes containing Mallory hyaline and a neutrophilic infiltrate. (**Right**) Ballooned hepatocytes containing abundant Mallory hyaline are surrounded by neutrophils, known as satellitosis ➩. This is a frequent feature of amiodarone toxicity. Steatosis may or may not be present.*

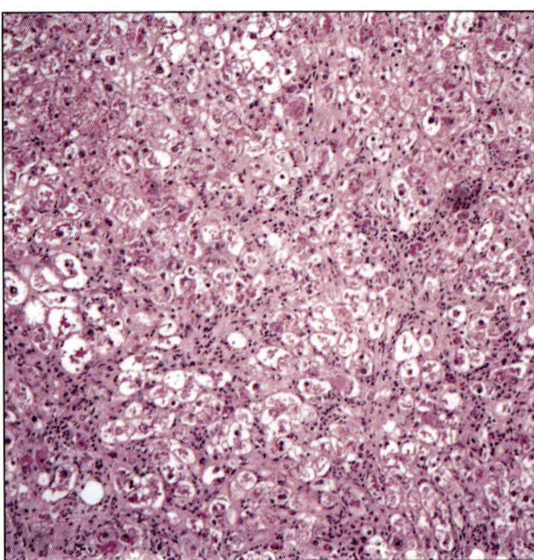

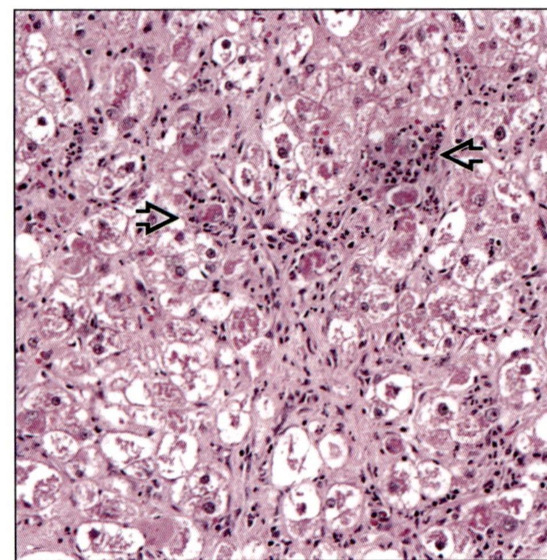

*(**Left**) Ballooned hepatocytes containing Mallory hyaline ➩ are visible in this photomicrograph of amiodarone toxicity. Fat and inflammation may not be prominent. Fibrosis is evident even on H&E ➔. (**Right**) This high-power photomicrograph illustrates abundant dark pink, irregular clumps of Mallory hyaline ➩ within ballooned hepatocytes.*

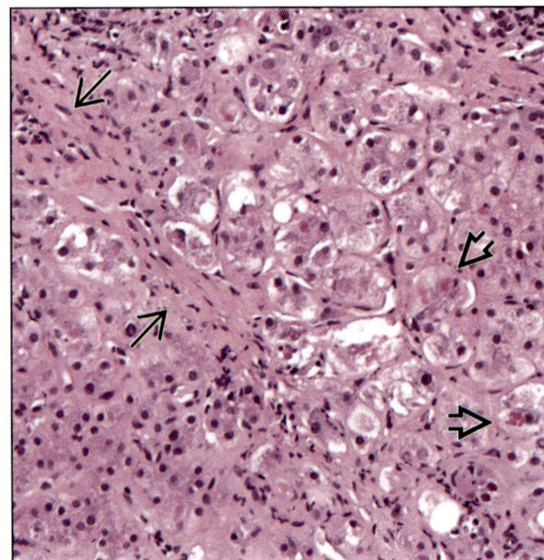

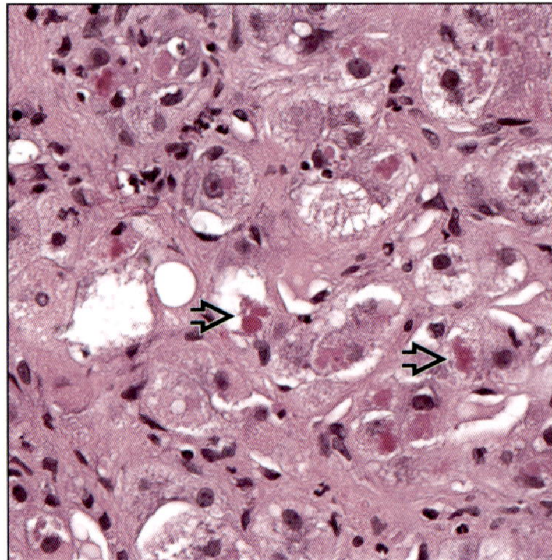

*(**Left**) This low-power view of a liver biopsy showing mild methotrexate injury features mild macrovesicular steatosis and reactive hepatocellular changes but minimal inflammation. (**Right**) Both macrovesicular and microvesicular steatosis can be seen in methotrexate injury. Inflammation may not be prominent.*

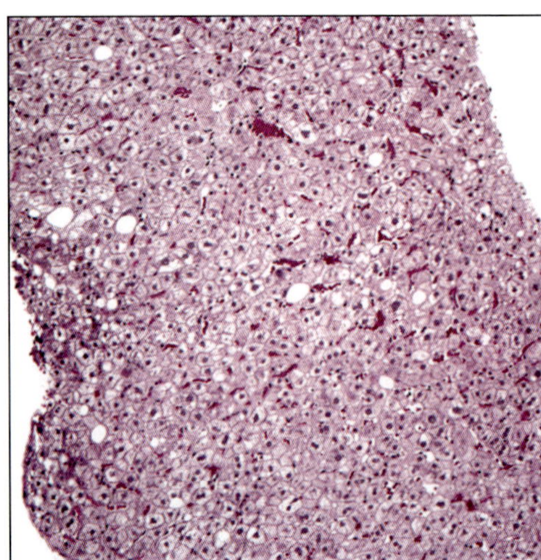

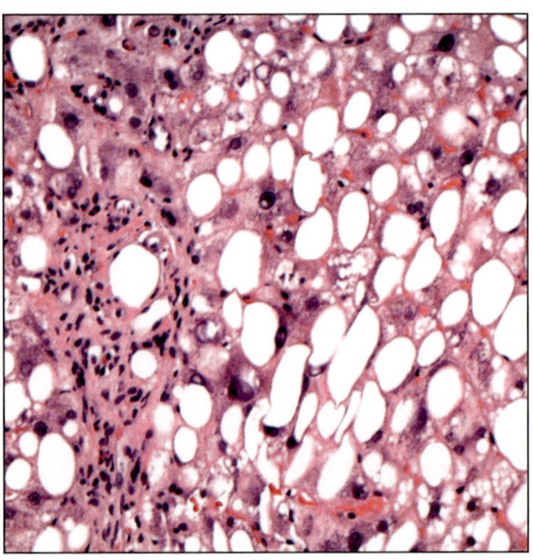

Microscopic Features

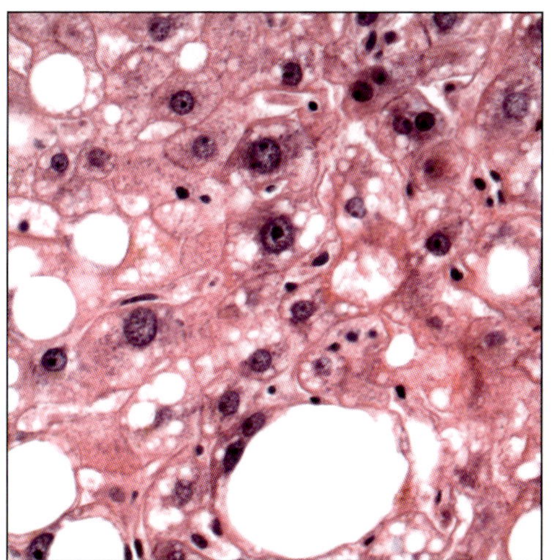
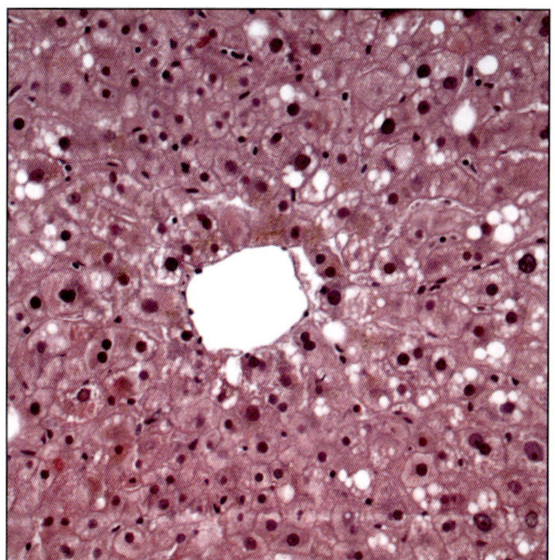

(Left) *High-power photomicrograph of methotrexate injury shows microvesicular and macrovesicular steatosis, along with nuclear anisocytosis (variation in nuclear size).* ***(Right)*** *Marked nuclear anisocytosis is a reactive change commonly seen in methotrexate toxicity.*

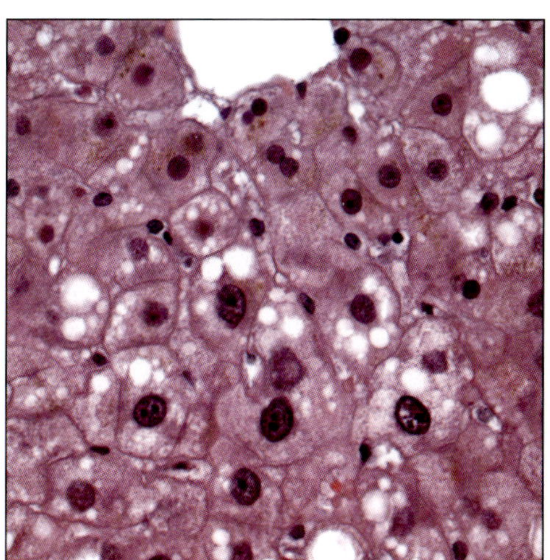
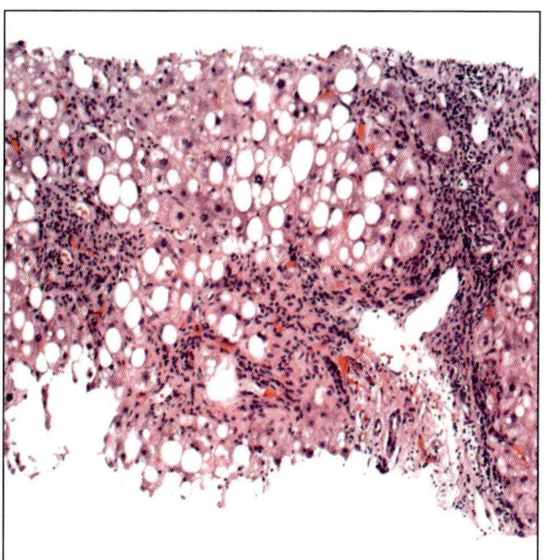

(Left) *H&E shows reactive changes in methotrexate injury including nuclear anisocytosis and double nuclei in hepatocytes. Steatosis is also present.* ***(Right)*** *Liver biopsy in methotrexate injury shows steatosis, mild portal inflammation, and expansion of portal/periportal areas by fibrosis.*

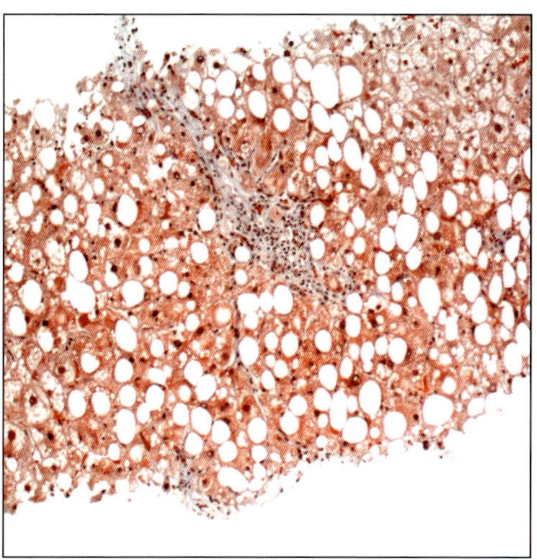
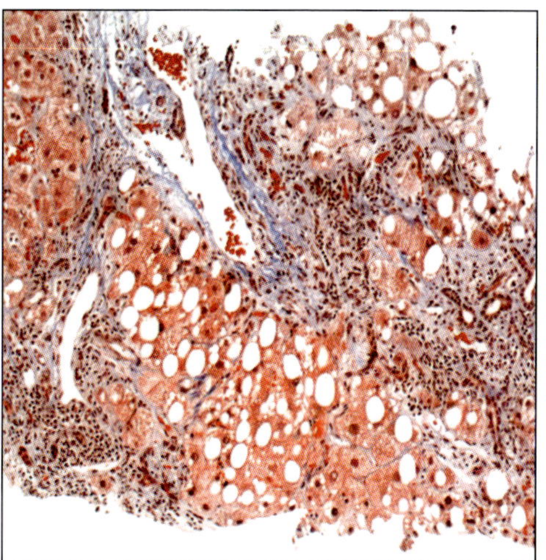

(Left) *Trichrome stain in methotrexate injury shows steatosis and delicate irregular spurs of connective tissue extending out from the portal tract.* ***(Right)*** *Trichrome stain illustrates more advanced fibrosis in methotrexate toxicity, consisting of an increase in portal/periportal fibrosis as well as established bridging fibrosis.*

REYE SYNDROME

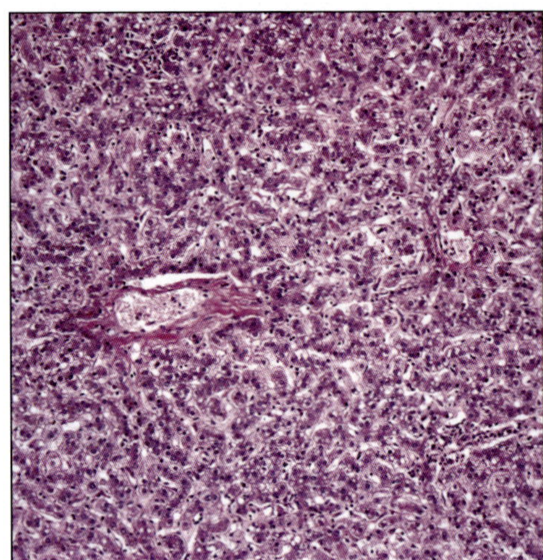

The characteristic finding in Reye Syndrome is diffuse, panlobular microvesicular steatosis without accompanying inflammation.

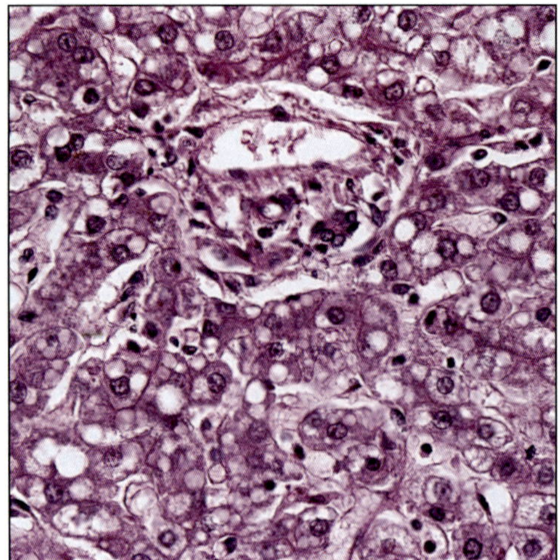

Microvesicular fat is seen within hepatocytes. A portal tract at the upper center of the field is free of inflammation.

TERMINOLOGY

Definitions

- Acute and potentially life-threatening disorder characterized by fatty liver and encephalopathy
  - Most common in infants and children under 17 years
  - Worldwide distribution
- "Classic" or "idiopathic" syndrome: Combination of resolving flu-like illness and salicylate therapy
- Reye-like syndrome: Presumed to have metabolic disorder unless clear evidence of viral illness, salicylates
  - Many children who survived acute Reye syndrome-like illness subsequently diagnosed with metabolic disorder

ETIOLOGY/PATHOGENESIS

Pathogenesis Unknown

- Probable target is mitochondria
  - Mitochondrial injury is fundamental feature
  - Failure of mitochondrial function results in carbohydrate, amino acid, and fatty acid metabolic derangement
- Initiating factors remain obscure
  - Frequent antecedent viral infection
  - Role of salicylate exposure
    - No proven causal connection
    - Reye syndrome has decreased as pediatric salicylate exposure has decreased

CLINICAL ISSUES

Presentation

- Biphasic pattern
  - Prodromal febrile illness
    - Particularly influenza B or varicella
  - Vomiting and neurologic alterations 3-5 days later
    - Lethargy and irritability initially; can progress to delirium, obtundation, seizures, coma
- Clinical evidence of liver disease often absent
- Jaundice absent
- Metabolic acidosis, respiratory alkalosis can be present

Laboratory Tests

- CSF has normal glucose and protein; minimal leukocytosis
- Increased transaminases, often marked
- Increased serum ammonia
- Normal bilirubin
- Electron microscopy
  - Enlarged, swollen, pleomorphic mitochondria
  - Disrupted, fragmented cristae
  - Lucent matrix
  - Loss of matrical dense bodies
  - Mitochondria may decrease in number as disease progresses

Treatment

- Supportive care
- Controlling increased intracranial pressure
- Correcting metabolic abnormalities

Prognosis

- Dominated by neurologic rather than hepatic manifestations
  - Death usually due to cerebral edema and complications
- Mortality approximately 30%
  - Those who survive acute illness usually recover completely
  - Small percentage have long-term neurologic sequelae
  - Diagnosis before irreversible brain damage occurs is critical

REYE SYNDROME

Key Facts

Terminology
- Acute and potentially life-threatening disorder characterized by fatty liver and encephalopathy
  - Most often seen in children
  - Classic syndrome involves combination of resolving viral illness and salicylate therapy

Clinical Issues
- Biphasic pattern: Viral prodrome followed by neurologic manifestations
  - Clinical evidence of hepatic disease may be very subtle

Microscopic Pathology
- Diffuse, panlobular microvesicular steatosis
- No significant inflammation

Top Differential Diagnoses
- Congenital metabolic conditions

MACROSCOPIC FEATURES

General Features
- Mild hepatomegaly, yellow discoloration

MICROSCOPIC PATHOLOGY

Histologic Features
- Diffuse, panlobular microvesicular steatosis
  - Most evident during 1st 3-4 days of illness
  - Droplets may be so small as to be missed
  - Lipid can be demonstrated using oil red O or Sudan black B stains in frozen sections
- Minimal or absent inflammation
- Enlarged, central hepatocyte nuclei
- Depleted glycogen
- Necrosis, cholestasis rare

DIFFERENTIAL DIAGNOSIS

Acute Fatty Liver of Pregnancy
- Different clinical scenario

Alcoholic Foamy Degeneration
- Associated with ethanol use
- Elevated bilirubin
- Other changes of alcoholic liver disease often present

Drug/Toxin-mediated Injury
- Valproic acid, IV tetracycline, salicylates

Congenital Metabolic Conditions
- Urea cycle disorders, fatty acid metabolism defects, lysosomal lipase deficiency
- Electron microscopy, extensive metabolic work-up may be needed to distinguish these from Reye Syndrome

Sepsis
- e.g., toxic shock syndrome

DIAGNOSTIC CHECKLIST

Clinically Relevant Pathologic Features
- Presumptive diagnosis can be made based on clinical and laboratory findings
  - Whether or not liver biopsy is essential to diagnosis is controversial

Pathologic Interpretation Pearls
- Microvesicular fatty change in context of neurologic alterations/encephalopathy

SELECTED REFERENCES

1. Crocker JF: Reye's syndrome. Semin Liver Dis. 2(4):340-52, 1982
2. Starko KM et al: Reye's syndrome and salicylate use. Pediatrics. 66(6):859-64, 1980
3. Reye RD et al: Encephalopathy and fatty degeneration of the viscera. A disease entity in childhood. Lancet. 2(7311):749-52, 1963

IMAGE GALLERY

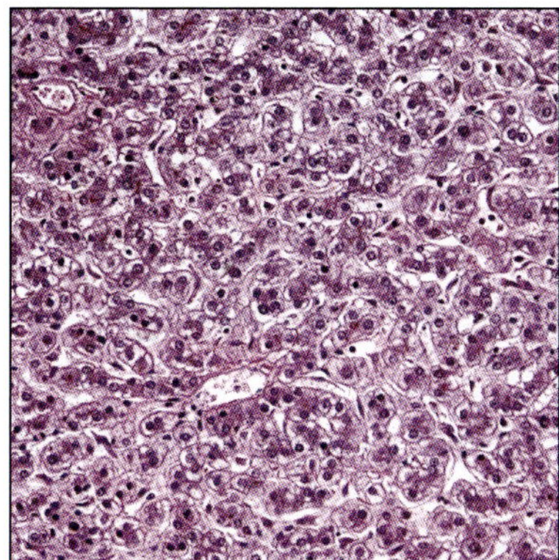

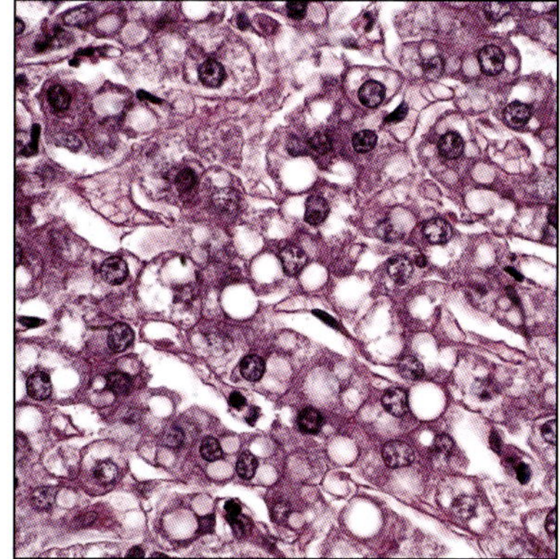

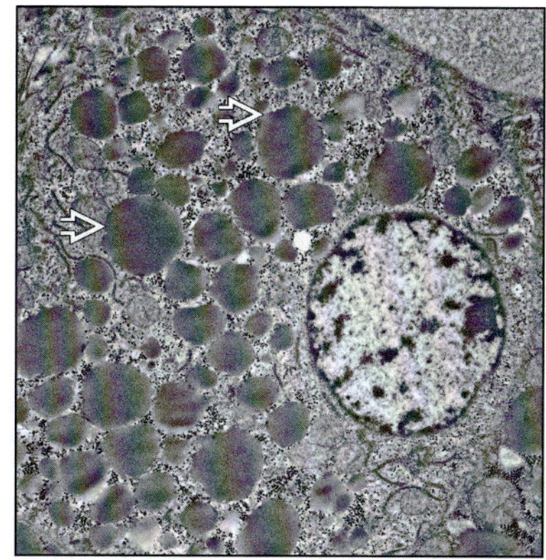

(Left) *Hepatocytes in all zones contain microvesicular fat, and there is no associated inflammation, necrosis, or hepatocyte damage.* ***(Center)*** *This H&E section demonstrates the microvesicular fat in Reye Syndrome at high power. Hepatocyte nuclei are round and centrally located. There is no hepatocyte damage.* ***(Right)*** *This electron micrograph shows numerous lipid droplets ⇒ within a hepatocyte in a patient with Reye syndrome. (Courtesy E. Sengupta, MD.)*

DRUG-RELATED CHOLANGITIS/DUCTOPENIA

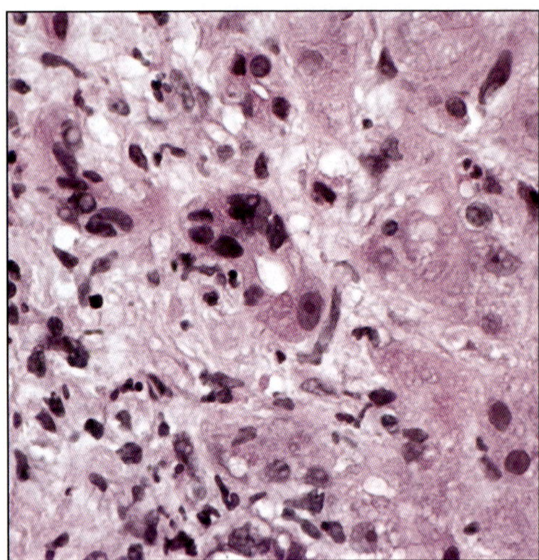

This example of drug-induced cholangitis due to an ACE inhibitor shows a damaged duct with eosinophilic cytoplasm, irregular spaces between nuclei, and variation in nuclear size and shape.

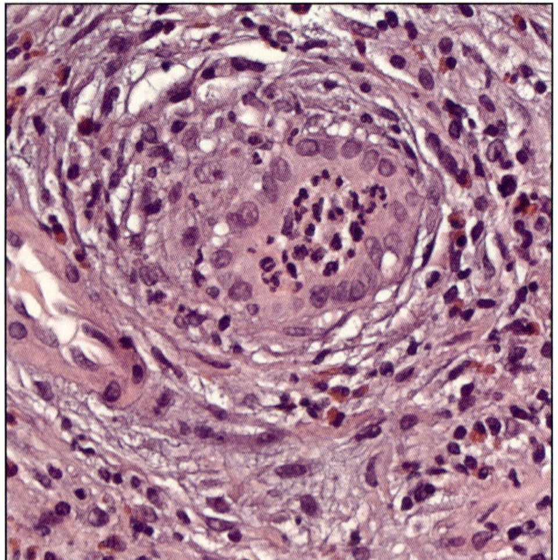

This example of drug-related cholangitis due to antibiotics shows a duct with cholangitis surrounded by portal edema and an infiltrate that is rich in eosinophils.

TERMINOLOGY

Synonyms

- Cholangiodestructive cholestasis

Definitions

- Bile duct injury, cholangitis, &/or ductopenia related to adverse drug reactions
  - Often accompanied by cholestasis
- Vanishing bile duct syndrome
  - Used to describe ductopenia related to drugs but not a specific entity
    - Also describes ductopenia occurring with graft-vs.-host disease and chronic ductopenic rejection in liver allografts
- Stevens-Johnson syndrome
  - Drug reaction associated with severe mucocutaneous manifestations and vanishing bile duct syndrome

ETIOLOGY/PATHOGENESIS

Two Categories of Injury

- Predictable
  - Dose-related, reproducible, and related to intrinsic toxicity of drug or its metabolites
- Idiosyncratic
  - Unpredictable, unrelated to dose, not reproducible in animal models
  - Allergic or autoimmune responses to drug or its metabolite may be involved

Drugs

- Many medication classes implicated
  - Anti-inflammatory: Acetaminophen, ibuprofen, phenylbutazone
  - Antibiotics: Amoxicillin-clavulanic acid, ampicillin*, clindamycin, erythromycin, tetracycline, trimethoprim-sulfa
  - Antiepileptics: Carbamazepine, phenytoin
  - Psychiatric drugs: Amytriptyline, imipramine*, Haldol
  - Tranquilizers: Chlorpromazine, prochlorperazine, phenothiazine
  - Hypoglycemics: Tolbutamide, chlorpropamide
  - Other: Cromolyn sodium (antiasthmatic), cyproheptadine (antihistamine), methyltestosterone, thiabendazole (antihelminthic)*
- *Also associated with vanishing bile duct syndrome

Herbal Preparations

- May not be considered drugs and therefore not reported by patients as part of medication and exposure history

Toxins

- Paraquat, rapeseed oil

Genetic Predisposition

- Mutations in MDR3 (phospholipid export pump involved in bile secretion) predispose to drug-related cholangitis

CLINICAL ISSUES

Presentation

- Jaundice
  - Temporal relationship between drug administration and onset of signs and symptoms
  - Usually presents within weeks of taking drug but may be delayed up to 1 year

Natural History

- Initial bile duct injury may be followed by ductopenia and prolonged cholestasis
- Effects may persist for months
- May see reduced bile duct numbers on biopsy after clinical recovery

Treatment

- Discontinue offending drug

DRUG-RELATED CHOLANGITIS/DUCTOPENIA

Key Facts

Terminology
- Bile duct injury, cholangitis, &/or ductopenia related to adverse drug reactions
  - Often accompanied by cholestasis
- Vanishing bile duct syndrome
  - Used to describe ductopenia related to drugs but not a specific term

Etiology/Pathogenesis
- Many medication classes implicated including anti-inflammatory, antiepileptic, antibiotics

Clinical Issues
- Jaundice
  - Temporal relationship between drug administration and onset of signs and symptoms
  - Most patients recover fully with discontinuation of drug
  - Few cases develop chronic cholestatic injury

Microscopic Pathology
- Generally no specific features indicating injury is drug-related
  - Cholestasis, usually zone 3
  - Bile duct epithelial cell injury, including cytoplasmic eosinophilia &/or vacuolization, nuclear pleomorphism, atrophy of ductal epithelium
  - Lymphocytic or mixed cell cholangitis
- Some cases show changes of progression/chronicity
  - Progressive ductopenia
  - Periportal hepatocyte swelling and copper accumulation

- Ursodeoxycholic acid may improve cholestasis in some patients

Prognosis
- Most patients recover fully with discontinuation of drug
- Few cases develop chronic cholestatic injury
  - Vanishing bile duct syndrome
  - Biliary cirrhosis or sclerosing cholangitis-like picture

MICROSCOPIC PATHOLOGY

Histologic Features
- **Generally no specific features indicating injury is drug-related**
- Cholestasis, usually zone 3
- Bile duct epithelial cell injury
  - Cytoplasmic eosinophilia &/or vacuolization
  - Nuclear pleomorphism
  - Uneven spacing of nuclei
  - Apoptosis
  - Flattening or atrophy of ductal epithelium
- Lymphocytic or mixed cell cholangitis
- Mild to moderate portal inflammation
  - May include large numbers of eosinophils &/or neutrophils
  - Portal edema may be present
- Variable degree of hepatocyte damage and lobular inflammation
- Bile ductular proliferation
- Changes of progression/chronicity
  - Progressive ductopenia
    - Defined as hepatic artery branches or portal tracts lacking companion bile ducts
    - Diagnosis established by 50% reduction in bile ducts
  - Periportal hepatocyte swelling and copper accumulation
  - Fibrosis
- Vanishing bile duct syndrome
  - Duct loss and cholangiolar proliferation
  - Chronic cholestasis
  - Portal inflammation and fibrosis

DIFFERENTIAL DIAGNOSIS

Primary Biliary Cirrhosis
- Positive AMA

Primary Sclerosing Cholangitis
- Characteristic ERCP findings, history of inflammatory bowel disease

Secondary Sclerosing Cholangitis
- Operative trauma, ischemia, cystic fibrosis

Infections
- Sepsis, cryptosporidiosis, microsporidiosis, Cytomegalovirus

Graft-vs.-Host Disease
- Clinical context of transplantation

Allograft Rejection
- Clinical context of liver transplantation, presence of endothelialitis

DIAGNOSTIC CHECKLIST

Clinically Relevant Pathologic Features
- Histologic features usually cannot provide definite diagnosis of drug-related injury but can assist in excluding other etiologies

SELECTED REFERENCES

1. Trauner M et al: MDR3 (ABCB4) defects: a paradigm for the genetics of adult cholestatic syndromes. Semin Liver Dis. 27(1):77-98, 2007
2. Mohi-ud-din R et al: Drug- and chemical-induced cholestasis. Clin Liver Dis. 8(1):95-132, vii, 2004
3. Velayudham LS et al: Drug-induced cholestasis. Expert Opin Drug Saf. 2(3):287-304, 2003

Microscopic Features

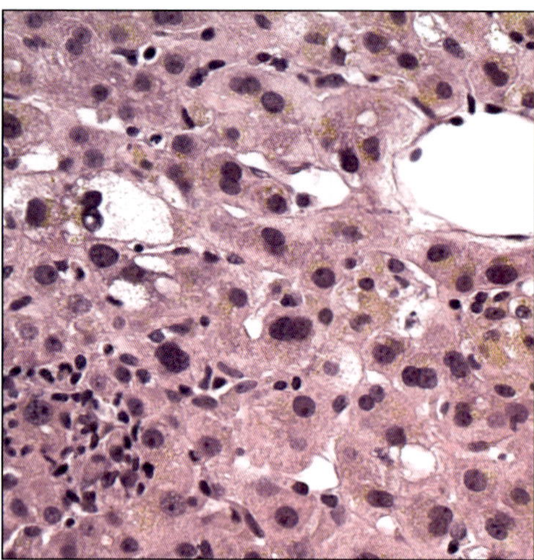

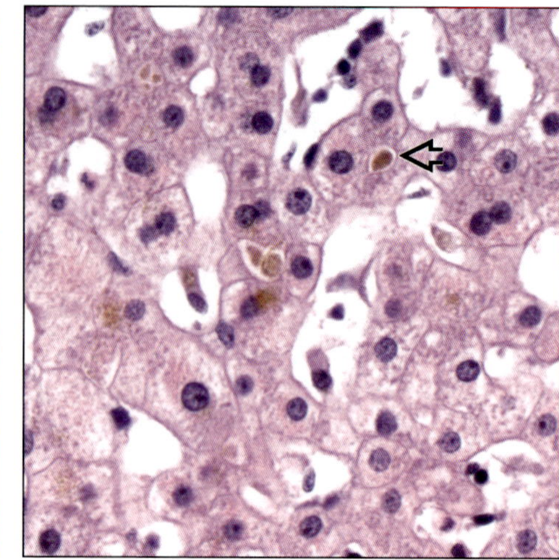

(Left) *Centrilobular cholestasis and varying degrees of lobular inflammation, hepatocyte damage, and reactive hepatocellular changes can be seen in drug-induced cholangitis. This case is due to NSAID injury.* ***(Right)*** *A high-power view shows canalicular cholestasis ⇨ in zone 3, which is a common finding in drug-associated cholangitis.*

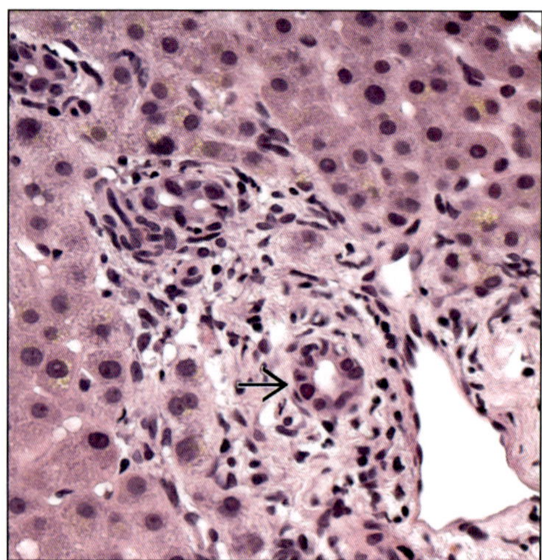

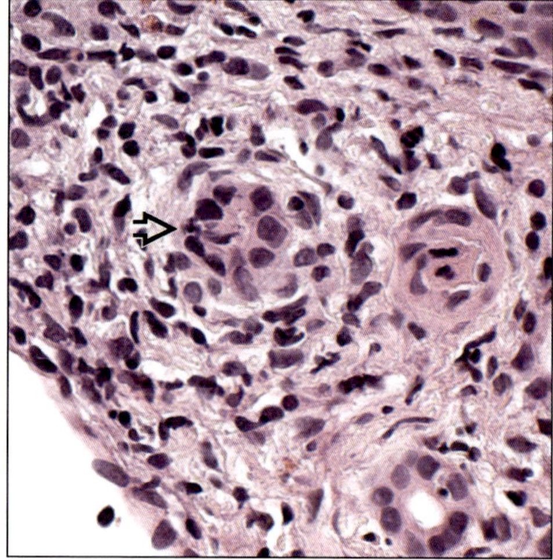

(Left) *This example of duct injury due to NSAIDs shows mild portal edema, a portal mononuclear cell infiltrate, and a damaged duct → with eosinophilic cytoplasm and variation in nuclear size.* ***(Right)*** *Portal tracts may be edematous, and the inflammatory infiltrate may be predominantly mononuclear or contain eosinophils. Note the damaged duct ⇨ with eosinophilic cytoplasm and "jumbled" nuclei.*

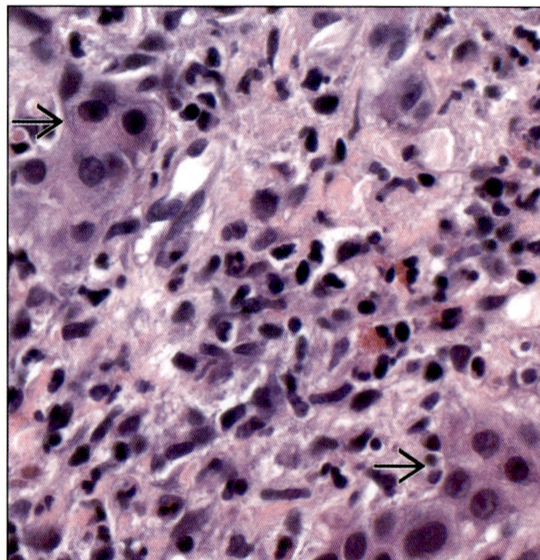

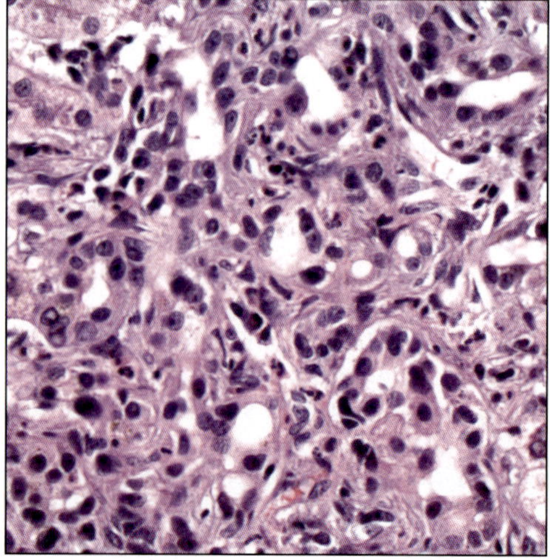

(Left) *The portal infiltrate may contain prominent eosinophils and plasma cells. Note the cholangiolar proliferation → at the edges of the portal tract.* ***(Right)*** *Patchy cholangiolar proliferation is a common finding in drug-associated cholangitis and duct injury.*

Microscopic Features

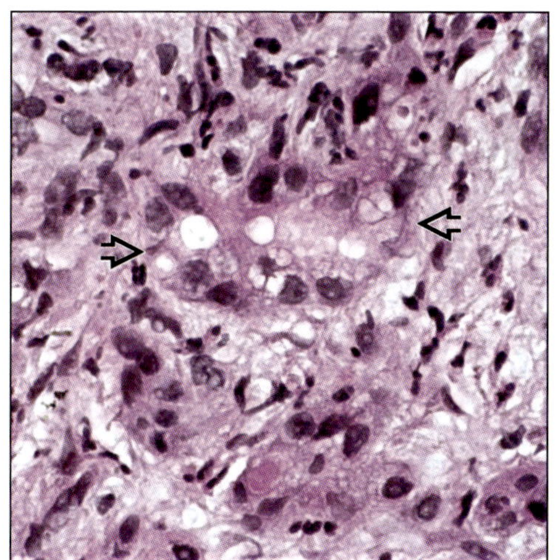

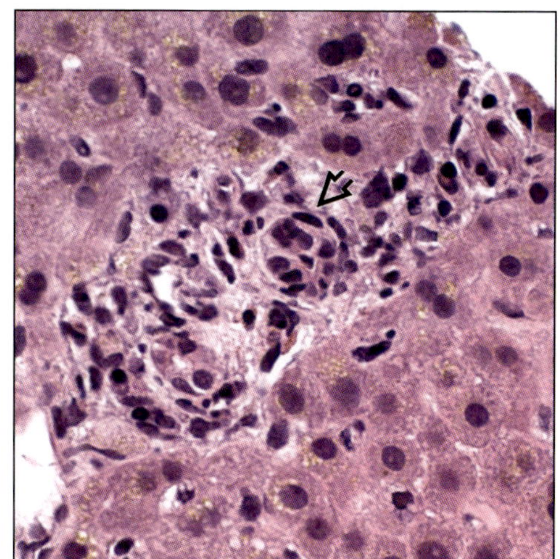

(Left) *This severely injured duct ➩ shows marked cytoplasmic vacuolization and eosinophilia as well as irregularly spaced nuclei.* ***(Right)*** *This portal tract shows an atrophic bile duct that is infiltrated by lymphocytes ➩. Note the irregularity in nuclear spacing as well as the variation in nuclear size and shape. This injury is related to NSAIDs.*

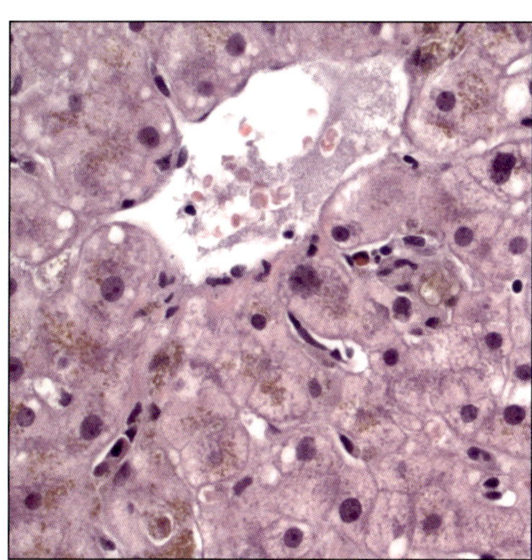

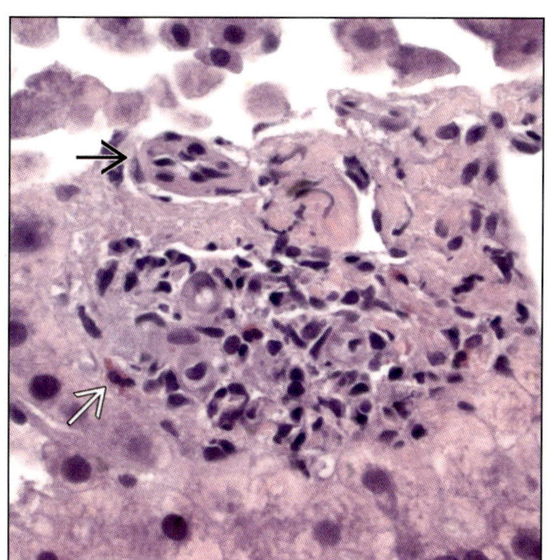

(Left) *This case of Augmentin-associated vanishing bile duct syndrome showed zone 3 cholestasis, a common finding in drug-related duct injury.* ***(Right)*** *This portal tract in vanishing bile duct syndrome lacks a duct altogether. Note the unaccompanied hepatic arteriole → and the mononuclear cell portal infiltrate with admixed eosinophils ➔.*

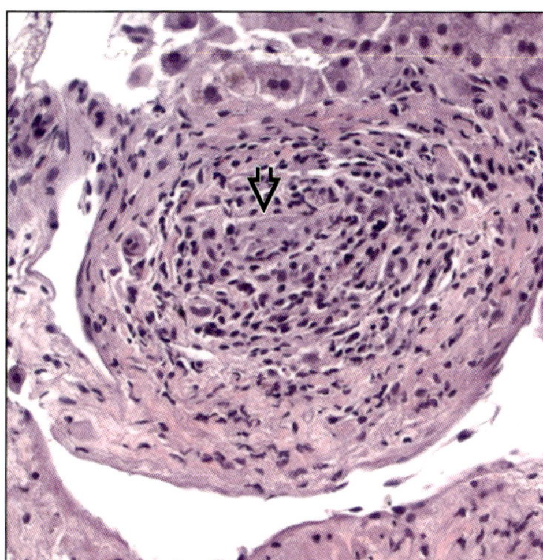

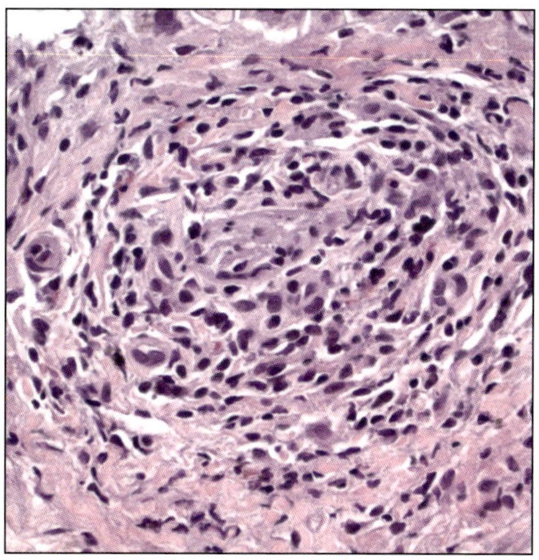

(Left) *This portal tract from a case of Augmentin-associated vanishing bile duct syndrome shows a barely discernible bile duct remnant ➩ surrounded by mononuclear cells.* ***(Right)*** *A high-power view of a portal tract from a case of Augmentin-associated vanishing bile duct syndrome shows duct destruction and a predominantly mononuclear portal inflammatory infiltrate.*

STELLATE CELL HYPERPLASIA

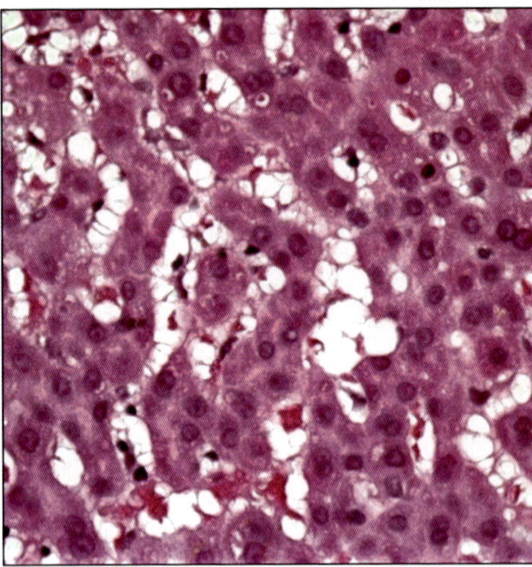

Hyperplastic, hypertrophic stellate cells are seen in the sinusoids of a patient who chronically overingested vitamin A supplements.

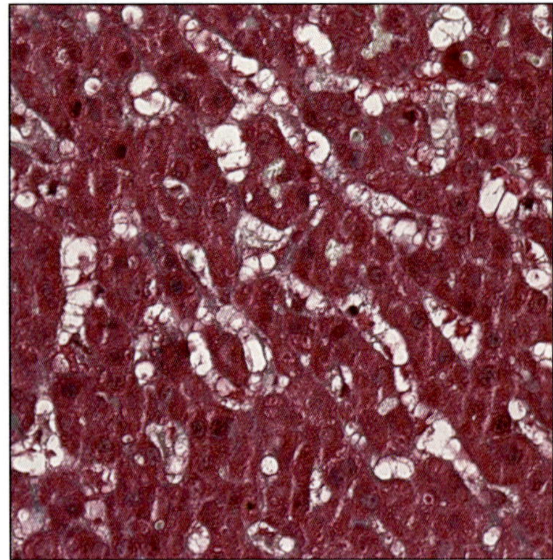

This patient does not have increased perisinusoidal fibrosis, but the contrast of the trichrome stain accentuates the bubbly cytoplasm of the stellate cells.

TERMINOLOGY

Abbreviations

- Hepatic stellate cells (HSC)

Synonyms

- Ito cell
- Perisinusoidal lipocyte

Definitions

- Phenotypic changes in stellate cells as a result of activation
  - Most commonly seen in vitamin A toxicity (hypervitaminosis A)
    - Even moderate amounts of vitamin A can cause liver disease if taken over long period of time
- Stellate cells reside in space of Disse
  - Long cytoplasmic processes surround sinusoids
  - Contain small lipid droplets that are rich in vitamin A
  - Produce extracellular proteins
  - Play a role in hepatic regeneration

ETIOLOGY/PATHOGENESIS

Environmental Exposure

- Overingestion of vitamin A
  - HSC are main site of vitamin A storage
  - Hepatotoxicity from overdose of vitamin A activates HSC
  - Activation causes sinusoidal obstruction, increased collagen synthesis

CLINICAL ISSUES

Presentation

- Very variable, many organ systems may be involved
  - Hepatomegaly
    - Varices, ascites if portal hypertension present
    - Jaundice variably present
  - Cutaneous, gastrointestinal, neuroophthalmic, musculoskeletal, renal, hematological manifestations also common
- Some patients asymptomatic
- Alcohol may potentiate toxic effects of vitamin A

Laboratory Tests

- Nonspecific elevations in transaminases, alkaline phosphatase
- Plasma vitamin A levels may be normal

Treatment

- Discontinue vitamin A ingestion

Prognosis

- Severity of liver disease depends on duration and dose of vitamin A
- Cirrhosis or noncirrhotic portal hypertension due to sinusoidal fibrosis may develop
  - Fibrosis may continue after cessation given long half-life of vitamin A in liver
- Liver failure, cirrhosis at time of diagnosis portend worse prognosis

MICROSCOPIC PATHOLOGY

Histologic Features

- Stellate cell hyperplasia and hypertrophy
  - Enlarged cells with clear cytoplasm
  - Delicate cytoplasmic processes (multivacuolated appearance)
- Hepatocellular injury, inflammation minor
- Microvesicular steatosis may be present
- Fibrosis
  - Begins as perisinusoidal fibrosis
  - Usually panlobular
  - Central vein sclerosis has been described
  - May progress to cirrhosis

STELLATE CELL HYPERPLASIA

Key Facts

Terminology
- Phenotypic changes in stellate cells as a result of activation, most commonly due to vitamin A toxicity (hypervitaminosis A)
- Severity of liver disease depends on duration and dose of vitamin A

Clinical Issues
- Hepatomegaly often present
  - Cutaneous, gastrointestinal, neuroophthalmic, musculoskeletal, renal, hematological manifestations also common

Microscopic Pathology
- Stellate cell hyperplasia and hypertrophy
- Hepatocellular injury, inflammation minor
- Fibrosis begins in perisinusoidal pattern, may progress to cirrhosis

- Peliosis, periportal sinusoidal dilatation have been described
- Immunohistochemical markers
  - Vimentin
  - Desmin
  - Smooth muscle actin
  - GFAP
  - N-CAM
  - Synaptophysin
- HSC have transient green fluorescence under ultraviolet light, particularly on frozen section

DIFFERENTIAL DIAGNOSIS

Methotrexate Therapy
- Should not have history of excessive vitamin A ingestion

Other Drugs
- Steroid use
  - Should not have history of excessive vitamin A ingestion
- IV fat emulsion administration

Post-transplant Biopsies
- Stellate cell activation has been reported in chronic viral hepatitis following transplantation
- May be marker of early fibrogenesis
- Should not have history of excessive vitamin A ingestion

DIAGNOSTIC CHECKLIST

Pathologic Interpretation Pearls
- Histologic findings are subtle and easily missed

SELECTED REFERENCES

1. Nollevaux MC et al: Hypervitaminosis A-induced liver fibrosis: stellate cell activation and daily dose consumption. Liver Int. 26(2):182-6, 2006
2. Carpino G et al: Alpha-SMA expression in hepatic stellate cells and quantitative analysis of hepatic fibrosis in cirrhosis and in recurrent chronic hepatitis after liver transplantation. Dig Liver Dis. 37(5):349-56, 2005
3. Levine PH et al: Stellate-cell lipidosis in liver biopsy specimens. Recognition and significance. Am J Clin Pathol. 119(2):254-8, 2003
4. Hautekeete ML et al: The hepatic stellate (Ito) cell: its role in human liver disease. Virchows Arch. 430(3):195-207, 1997
5. Jorens PG et al: Vitamin A abuse: development of cirrhosis despite cessation of vitamin A. A six-year clinical and histopathologic follow-up. Liver. 12(6):381-6, 1992
6. Geubel AP et al: Liver damage caused by therapeutic vitamin A administration: estimate of dose-related toxicity in 41 cases. Gastroenterology. 100(6):1701-9, 1991
7. Leo MA et al: Hypervitaminosis A: a liver lover's lament. Hepatology. 8(2):412-17, 1988

IMAGE GALLERY

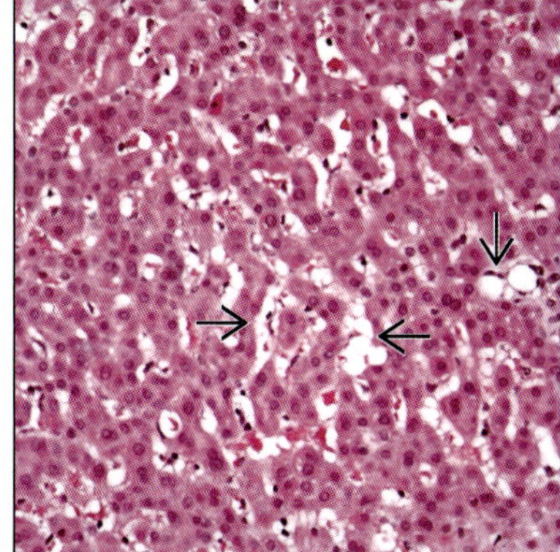

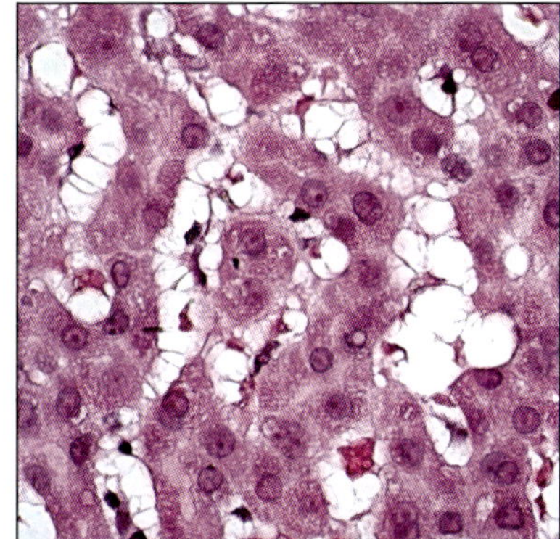

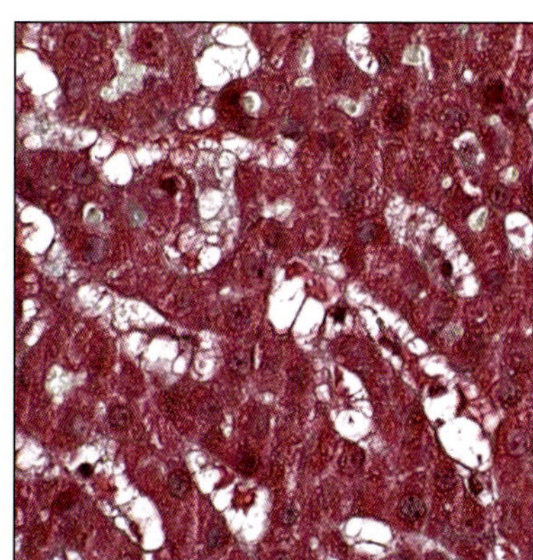

(Left) *Low-power view of stellate cell hyperplasia in hypervitaminosis A illustrates bubbly, "multivacuolated" HSC in the sinusoids ⇒. Note the lack of inflammation or hepatocyte degeneration.* ***(Center)*** *Hyperplastic, hypertrophic stellate cells reside in the sinusoids and are characterized by swollen, clear cytoplasm with delicate cytoplasmic processes.* ***(Right)*** *A trichrome stain can highlight the clear, bubbly cytoplasm of stellate cells.*

Fatty Liver Diseases

ALCOHOLIC LIVER DISEASE

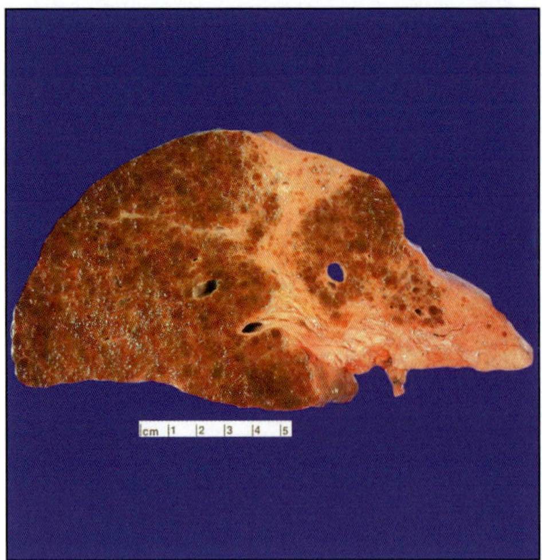

This explant from a patient with end-stage alcohol-induced cirrhosis shows a nodular cut surface.

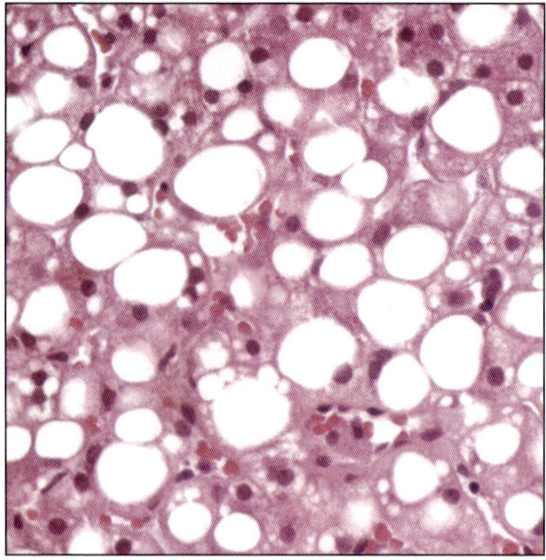

Steatosis, most often macrovesicular, is a typical finding in alcoholic liver disease.

TERMINOLOGY

Abbreviations

- Alcoholic liver disease (ALD)

Definitions

- Hepatocyte injury and inflammation that results from chronic alcohol consumption
  - Wide spectrum of clinical and pathologic disease
    - Ranges from mild/subclinical condition to end-stage cirrhosis and death

ETIOLOGY/PATHOGENESIS

Alcohol Consumption

- Alcohol is direct hepatotoxin
- Both genetic and environmental factors determine susceptibility to liver injury

CLINICAL ISSUES

Epidemiology

- Incidence
  - Approximately 20-40% of chronic alcoholics who undergo biopsy have histologic evidence of ALD

Presentation

- Very variable
  - Anorexia, nausea, vomiting
  - Abdominal pain/tenderness, hepatomegaly
  - Variably present jaundice
- Some patients are asymptomatic
- End-stage patients may have encephalopathy, ascites, coagulopathy, varices

Laboratory Tests

- Moderately elevated transaminases
  - AST/ALT ratio > 2
- Variably elevated alkaline phosphatase, bilirubin
- Hypoalbuminemia, prolonged PTT in end-stage disease

Treatment

- Abstinence
- Liver transplant

Prognosis

- Very variable course of disease
  - Leading cause of end-stage liver disease in USA

MICROSCOPIC PATHOLOGY

Histologic Features

- Combination of hepatocyte injury, inflammation, steatosis, and fibrosis
  - Hepatocyte ballooning degeneration
    - Enlarged, swollen, pale cells with granular cytoplasm
  - Acidophil bodies
  - Mallory-Denk bodies (Mallory hyaline)
    - Discrete masses of ropy eosinophilic material
    - Neither invariably present or specific
  - Megamitochondria
  - Inflammation
    - Neutrophils are principal inflammatory cell
    - Encircle Mallory body-bearing cells (satellitosis)
    - Lobular inflammation usually > portal inflammation
  - Steatosis
    - Almost always present but can be absent depending on timing of biopsy
    - Usually macrovesicular, can have mixed microvesicular
  - Fibrosis
    - Pericellular/perisinusoidal fibrosis: "Chicken wire" pattern of fibrosis that surrounds hepatocytes
    - Perivenular fibrosis around central veins
    - Eventual progression to bridging fibrosis and cirrhosis
  - Cholestasis and cholangiolitis may be seen

ALCOHOLIC LIVER DISEASE

Key Facts

Terminology
- Hepatocyte injury and inflammation that results from chronic alcohol consumption

Clinical Issues
- Very variable presentation
  - Ranges from nonspecific abdominal complaints to end-stage liver disease and death
- AST/ALT ratio > 2 favors ALD
- Some patients are asymptomatic

Microscopic Pathology
- Combination of hepatocyte injury, inflammation, steatosis, and fibrosis
  - Hepatocytic ballooning
  - Lobular inflammation with predominance of neutrophils
  - Mallory-Denk bodies (Mallory hyaline)
  - Megamitochondria
  - Steatosis
- Fibrosis is most often pericellular and perivenular, especially at first
- Cholestatic features may be seen
- Iron deposition in hepatocytes and Kupffer cells is common

Top Differential Diagnoses
- Nonalcoholic steatohepatitis (NASH)
- Chronic hepatitis C
  - Many patients have both ALD and hepatitis C infection

Comparison of Histologic Lesions in ALD and NASH

Lesions in ALD and NASH	Lesions Seen Only in ALD
Macrovesicular steatosis	Microvesicular steatosis
Ballooned hepatocytes	Sclerosing hyaline necrosis
Lobular inflammation	Satellitosis (neutrophilic aggregates in lobules)
Mallory-Denk bodies	Canalicular steatosis
Megamitochondria	Ductular reaction with neutrophilic infiltrates in portal tracts
Perivenular/pericellular ("chicken wire") fibrosis	Lymphocytic phlebitis/phlebosclerosis of terminal hepatic venules

  - Iron deposition frequent, especially in cirrhosis
  - Lymphocytic phlebitis and obliterative fibrosis of terminal hepatic venule
- Sclerosing hyaline necrosis
  - Severe alcoholic hepatitis with hepatocytic necrosis, dense perivenular/perisinusoidal fibrosis, and obliteration of terminal hepatic venules
  - May be associated with noncirrhotic portal hypertension

DIFFERENTIAL DIAGNOSIS

Nonalcoholic Steatohepatitis (NASH)
- No history of alcohol use
- Metabolic syndrome, such as diabetes, obesity, hyperlipidemia
- Cholestatic features, sclerosing hyaline necrosis, lymphocytic phlebitis uncommon in NASH
- Glycogenated nuclei uncommon in ALD

Chronic Hepatitis C
- Both ALD and HCV show steatosis, but distribution is predominantly random in HCV
- HCV usually has more portal inflammation, fewer neutrophils
- ALD and chronic hepatitis C may coexist in many patients

Drug Toxicity
- History of drug use temporally corresponding to onset of disease
- Eosinophils may be prominent

Biliary Obstruction
- Bile ductular reaction with associated neutrophilic infiltrate is common
- Abnormal ERCP or image studies

DIAGNOSTIC CHECKLIST

Pathologic Interpretation Pearls
- Histology of ALD and NASH is almost identical; favor ALD when following are seen
  - Neutrophilic aggregates in lobules (satellitosis)
  - Mallory bodies with many ballooned hepatocytes
  - Sclerosing hyaline necrosis

SELECTED REFERENCES

1. Yeh MM et al: Pathology of fatty liver: differential diagnosis of non-alcoholic fatty liver disease. Diagnostic Histopathology. 14:586-9, 2008
2. Levitsky J et al: Diagnosis and therapy of alcoholic liver disease. Semin Liver Dis. 24(3):233-47, 2004
3. Mandayam S et al: Epidemiology of alcoholic liver disease. Semin Liver Dis. 24(3):217-32, 2004
4. Brunt EM: Alcoholic and nonalcoholic steatohepatitis. Clin Liver Dis. 6(2):399-420, vii, 2002

ALCOHOLIC LIVER DISEASE

Microscopic Features

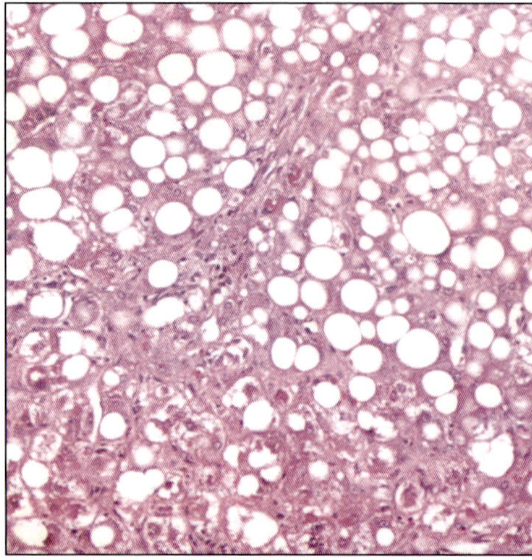

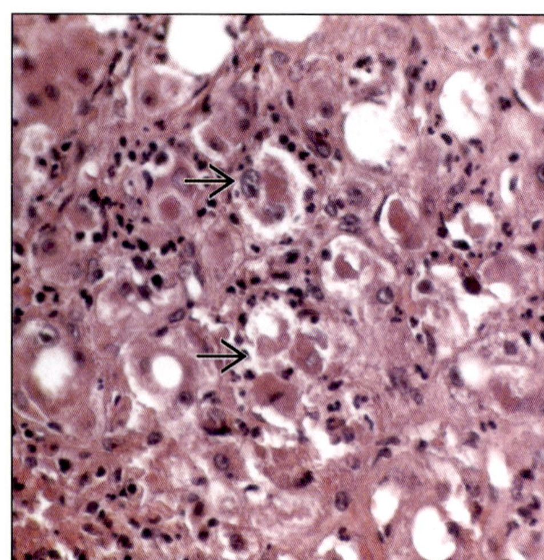

(Left) *Marked macrovesicular steatosis, lobular inflammation, and ballooned hepatocytes are common findings in alcoholic steatohepatitis.* ***(Right)*** *Ballooned hepatocytes ➔, containing many Mallory-Denk bodies, are seen in alcoholic steatohepatitis, along with lobular inflammation featuring satellitosis of neutrophils around the ballooned cells.*

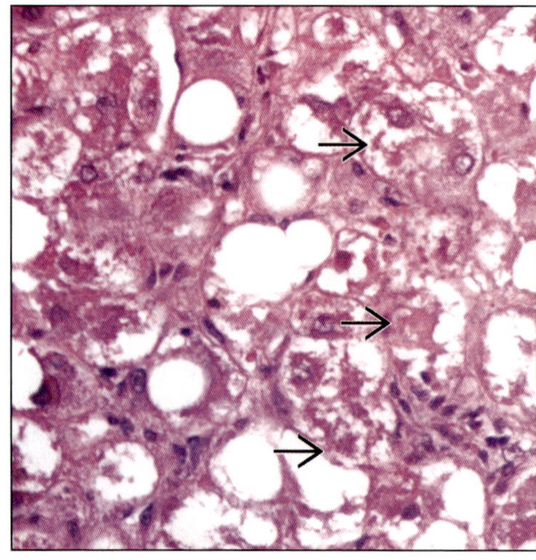

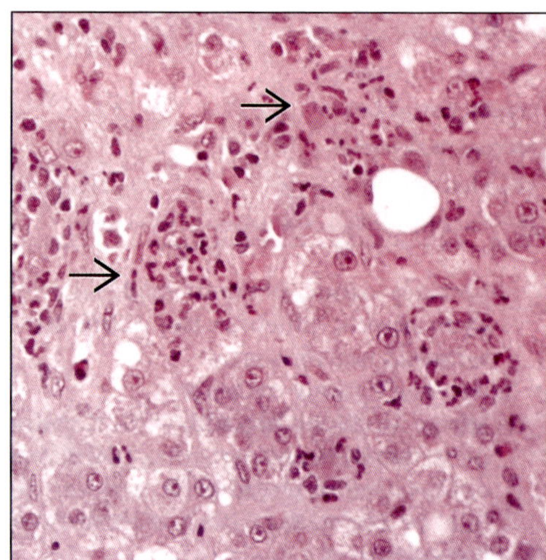

(Left) *Mallory-Denk bodies ➔ are the eosinophilic, ropy, and branching substance composed of intermediate filaments in the cytoplasm of injured hepatocytes in alcoholic steatohepatitis. Although Mallory-Denk bodies may also be seen in NASH, when abundant, ALD should be suspected.* ***(Right)*** *Aggregates of neutrophils ➔ are frequently seen in alcoholic steatohepatitis but are uncommon in NASH.*

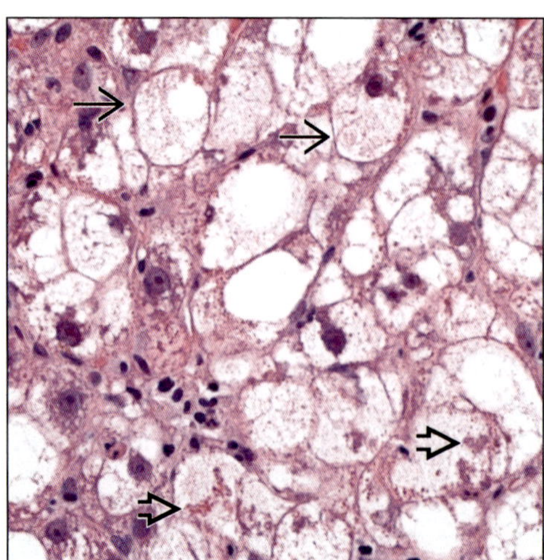

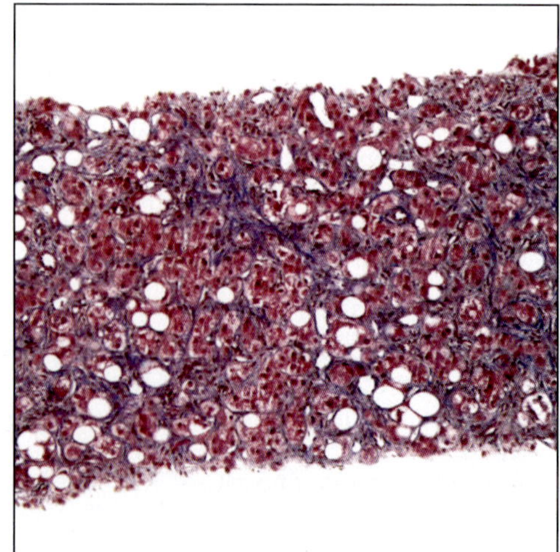

(Left) *This high-magnification photomicrograph shows ballooned hepatocytes ➔ with rarefied and clumped cytoplasm and Mallory-Denk bodies ➲ in alcoholic steatohepatitis.* ***(Right)*** *Collagen fiber deposition within the sinusoidal spaces ("chicken wire" fibrosis) is common in ALD. This pattern of fibrosis is also a feature in NASH.*

Microscopic Features

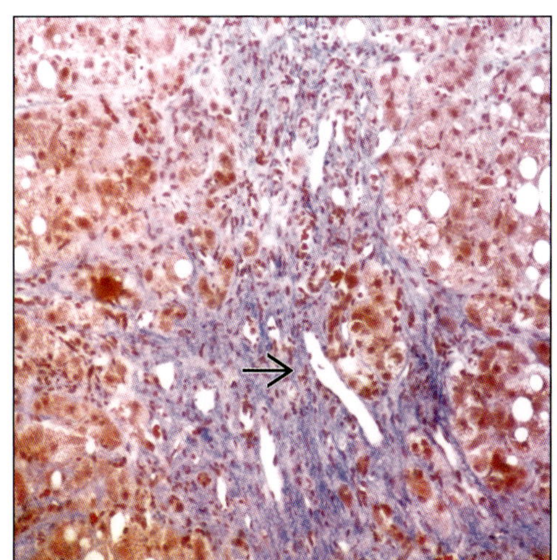
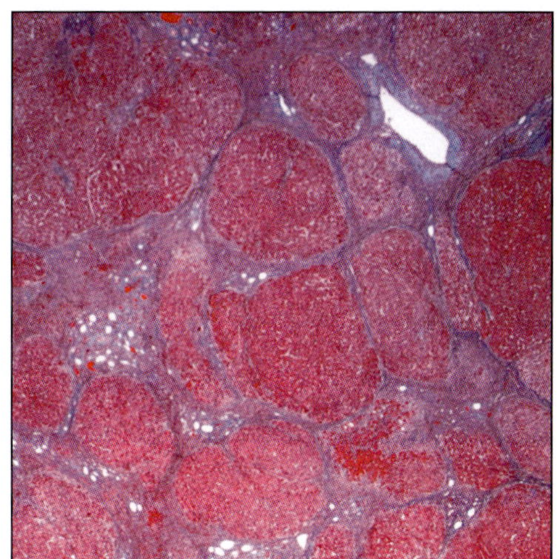

(Left) *Dense collagen fibers surround the terminal hepatic venules ⇒ and hepatocytes in ALD.* ***(Right)*** *This trichrome-stained section from an explanted liver due to ALD-induced cirrhosis shows multiple cirrhotic nodules.*

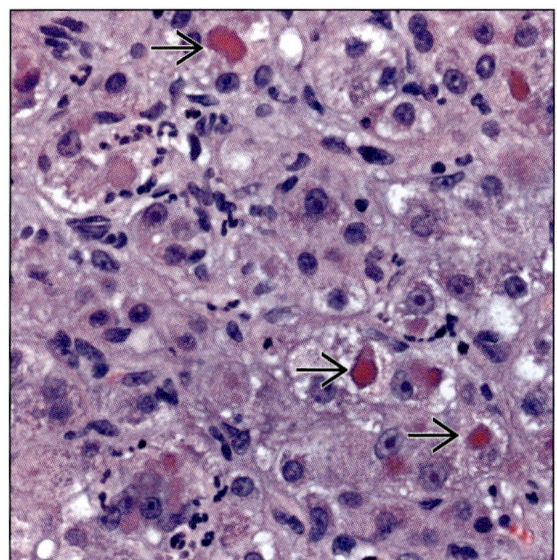
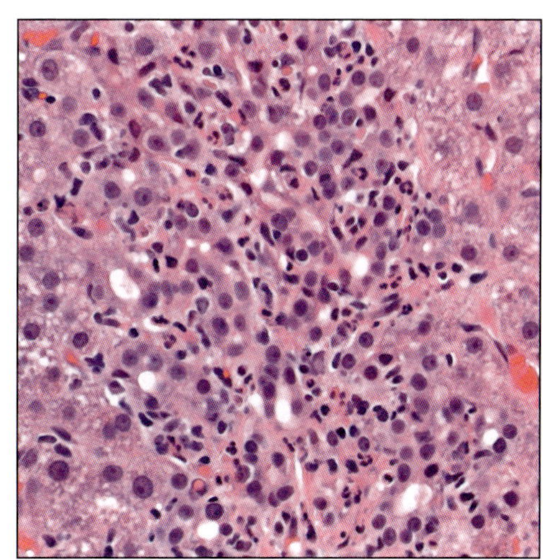

(Left) *Megamitochondria ⇒ consist of round, oblong, and eosinophilic inclusions in the hepatocytes in alcoholic liver disease.* ***(Right)*** *Some cases of ALD have bile ductular reaction with an associated neutrophilic infiltrate that can mimic large bile duct obstruction.*

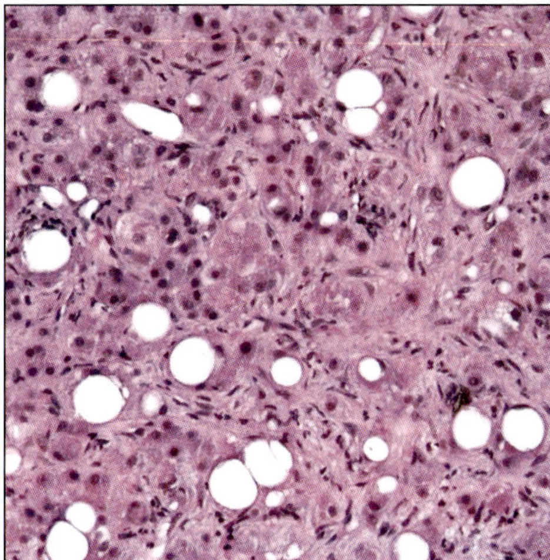
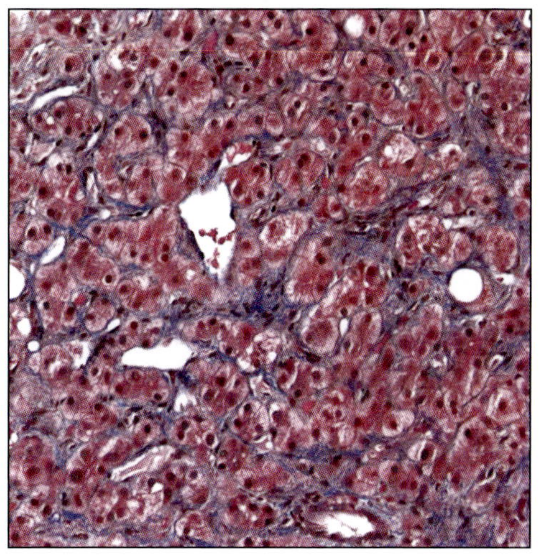

(Left) *This case of alcoholic liver disease has features of sclerosing hyaline necrosis including dense pericellular fibrosis and obliteration of central veins.* ***(Right)*** *Dense pericellular fibrosis compresses central veins in this case of alcoholic liver disease with features of sclerosing hyaline necrosis.*

NASH

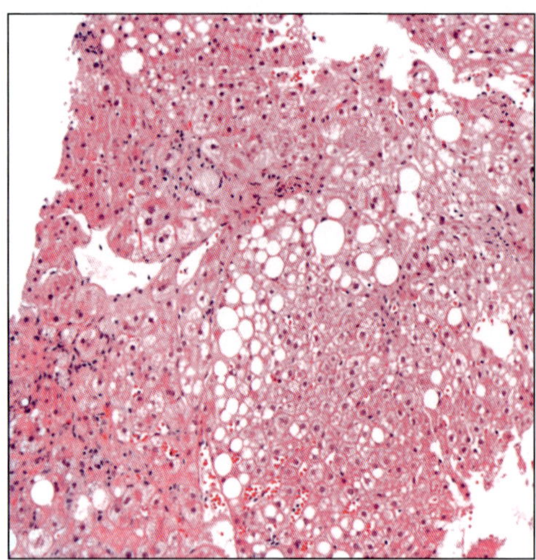

The typical features of NASH include steatosis, lobular inflammation, and ballooned hepatocytes.

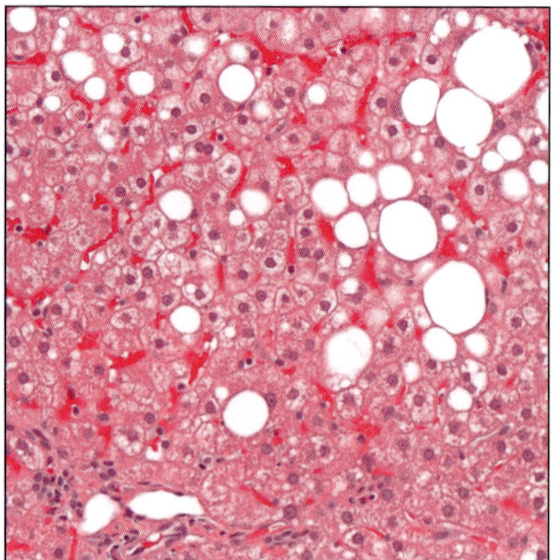

Macrovesicular steatosis is commonly seen in NASH.

TERMINOLOGY

Abbreviations

- Nonalcoholic steatohepatitis (NASH)

Definitions

- Steatosis, inflammation, and liver cell injury in absence of excessive alcohol use history

ETIOLOGY/PATHOGENESIS

Mechanism

- Abnormal accumulation of lipids in hepatocytes provide source of oxidative stress
- Leads to injury/inflammation
- Subsequent activation of TGF-β and hepatic stellate cells results in liver fibrosis

Associated Conditions

- Diabetes, obesity, hyperlipidemia, dyslipidemia, drugs, malabsorption, malnutrition

CLINICAL ISSUES

Presentation

- Hepatomegaly
- Metabolic syndrome
  - Central (visceral) obesity
  - Type 2 diabetes
  - Dyslipidemia (hypertriglyceridemia and low HDL)
  - Systemic hypertension

Laboratory Tests

- Elevated transaminases

Treatment

- Management of associated metabolic conditions (diabetes, hyperlipidemia, and dyslipidemia)
- Exercise
- Dietary control and weight reduction

Prognosis

- May lead to liver fibrosis, cirrhosis, and hepatocellular carcinoma

MICROSCOPIC PATHOLOGY

Histologic Features

- Steatosis (predominantly macrovesicular)
- Lobular inflammatory infiltrate
  - Lymphocytes, pigmented macrophages, Kupffer cells
  - Typically more severe than portal inflammation
- Liver cell injury
  - Ballooned hepatocytes
  - Apoptotic bodies
  - Hepatocyte injury predominantly zone 3
- Hepatocytes may contain Mallory-Denk bodies, megamitochondria, glycogenated nuclei
- Zone 3 perivenular/pericellular ("chicken wire") fibrosis

Variants

- Pediatric patients
  - Inflammation and fibrosis accentuated in portal (not centrilobular) region
  - Ballooning degeneration and perisinusoidal fibrosis not typically obvious
- NASH after treatment
  - Histologic improvements of steatosis, inflammation, ballooning, and fibrosis
  - Shift in proportion of lobular inflammation to portal inflammation may be seen

Grading and Staging

- Brunt scheme
  - Grade: Compilation of steatosis, ballooning, and inflammation
    - Grade 1: Mild
    - Grade 2: Moderate

Key Facts

Etiology/Pathogenesis
- Associated conditions
  - Diabetes, obesity, hyperlipidemia, dyslipidemia, drugs, malabsorption, malnutrition

Clinical Issues
- Patients often have metabolic syndrome
- Transaminases usually elevated
- May have positive ANA

Microscopic Pathology
- Zone 3 injury pattern
- Steatosis (predominantly macrovesicular)
- Lobular inflammatory infiltrate
- Ballooned hepatocytes
- Zone 3 perivenular/pericellular ("chicken wire") fibrosis
- Mallory-Denk bodies
- Megamitochondria
- Glycogenated nuclei
- NASH in pediatric population has different injury pattern
  - Inflammation, fibrosis accentuated in portal region
  - Ballooning degeneration and perisinusoidal fibrosis not obvious

Top Differential Diagnoses
- Steatosis without specific liver injury
- Alcoholic hepatitis
- Chronic hepatitis C
- Autoimmune hepatitis
- Glycogenic hepatopathy
- Microvesicular steatosis
- Wilson disease

    - Grade 3: Severe
  - Fibrosis
    - Stage 1: Zone 3 perivenular perisinusoidal/pericellular fibrosis (focal or extensive)
    - Stage 2: As above with focal or extensive periportal fibrosis
    - Stage 3: Bridging fibrosis (focal or extensive)
    - Stage 4: Cirrhosis (probable or definite)
- Nonalcoholic fatty liver disease activity (NAS) and fibrosis scoring from NIDDK NASH Clinical Research Network (CRN)
  - NAS (0-8): Summation of the following scores
    - Steatosis: 0 (< 5%); 1 (5-33%); 2 (33-66%); 3 (> 66%)
    - Lobular inflammation: Counted in 20x fields: 0, 1 (< 2 foci), 2 (2-4 foci), 3 (> 4 foci)
    - Ballooning: 0, 1 (few), 2 (many)
  - Fibrosis
    - 0: None
    - 1a: Mild, zone 3 perisinusoidal fibrosis (requires trichrome stain to see)
    - 1b: Moderate zone 3 perisinusoidal fibrosis
    - 1c: Portal fibrosis only
    - 2: Zone 3 perisinusoidal and periportal fibrosis
    - 3: Bridging fibrosis
    - 4: Probable or definite cirrhosis

DIFFERENTIAL DIAGNOSIS

Steatosis (Without Specific Liver Injury)
- Lack of ballooned hepatocytes
- Lobular inflammation usually minimal to mild

Alcoholic Hepatitis
- Almost impossible to distinguish; clinical history critical
- More abundant Mallory-Denk bodies
- Neutrophilic aggregates in lobules
- Ductular reaction and acute inflammatory infiltrate in portal regions
- Sclerosing hyaline necrosis

Chronic Hepatitis C
- Positive HCV antibody and RNA
- Portal-based chronic inflammation
- Fibrosis starting from portal regions
- Steatosis generally azonal in distribution

Autoimmune Hepatitis
- Positive ANA (antinuclear antibody) and other autoimmune serology
- 20% of cases of nonalcoholic fatty liver disease (NAFLD) have positive ANA

Glycogenic Hepatopathy
- Swollen hepatocytes may mimic ballooned hepatocytes

Microvesicular Steatosis
- May mimic ballooned hepatocytes
- Centrally located nuclei

Wilson Disease
- Positive tissue copper quantitation

SELECTED REFERENCES

1. Yeh MM et al: Pathology of nonalcoholic fatty liver disease. Am J Clin Pathol. 128(5):837-47, 2007
2. Kleiner DE et al: Design and validation of a histological scoring system for nonalcoholic fatty liver disease. Hepatology. 41(6):1313-21, 2005
3. Schwimmer JB et al: Histopathology of pediatric nonalcoholic fatty liver disease. Hepatology. 42(3):641-9, 2005
4. Brunt EM et al: Nonalcoholic steatohepatitis: a proposal for grading and staging the histological lesions. Am J Gastroenterol. 94(9):2467-74, 1999

Microscopic Features

(Left) Steatosis accentuated in zone 3 ➜ with sparing in the portal region ⇨ is a typical pattern of NASH in adults. (Right) Lobular inflammation with a mononuclear cell infiltrate in the lobule is often seen in NASH.

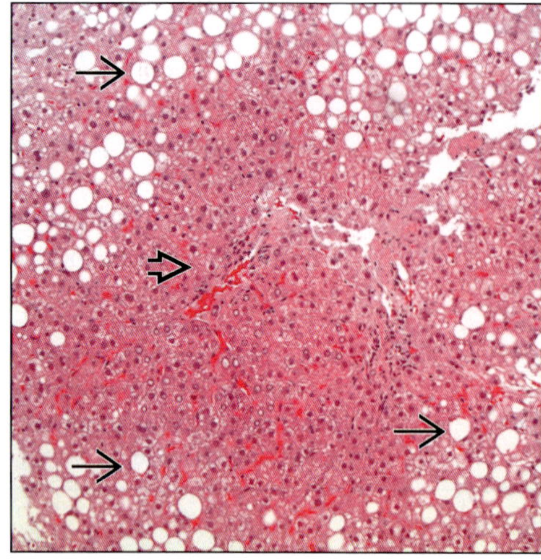

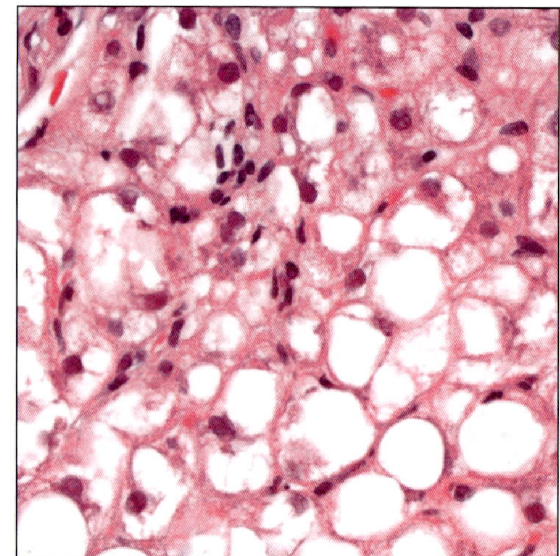

(Left) Ballooned hepatocytes ➜ are swollen and enlarged with rarefied and clumped cytoplasm. They sometimes contain Mallory-Denk bodies ↪. (Right) Mallory-Denk bodies ➜ are characterized by eosinophilic, ropy, and globular materials within ballooned hepatocytes and are commonly seen in NASH.

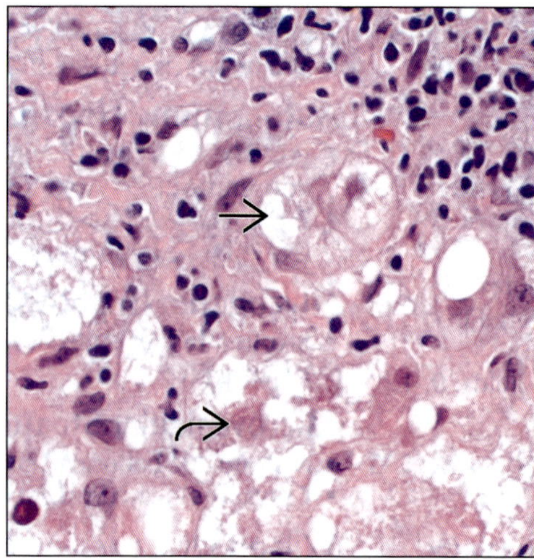

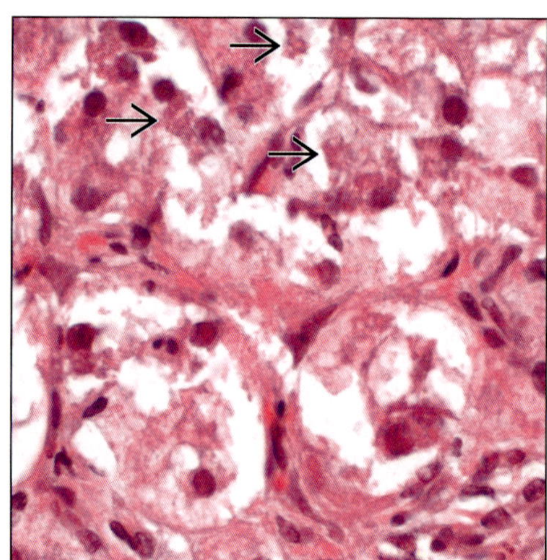

(Left) Stage 1 NASH features perivenular/pericellular fibrosis ➜. (Right) Stage 2 NASH is characterized by perivenular/pericellular fibrosis and portal fibrosis.

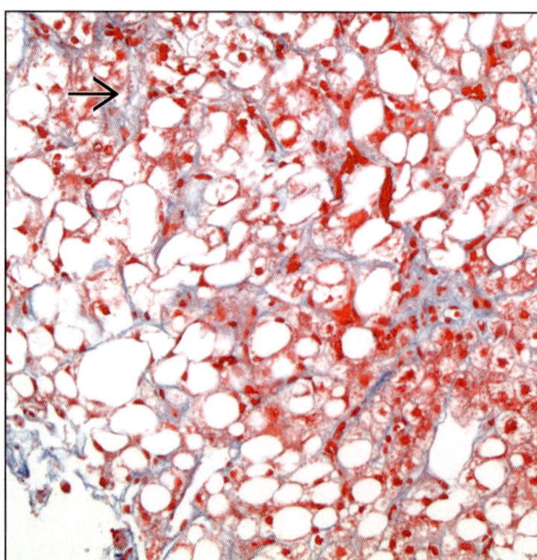

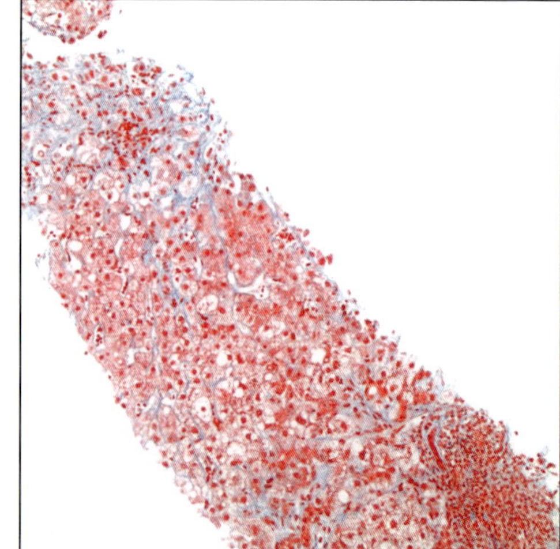

Microscopic Features

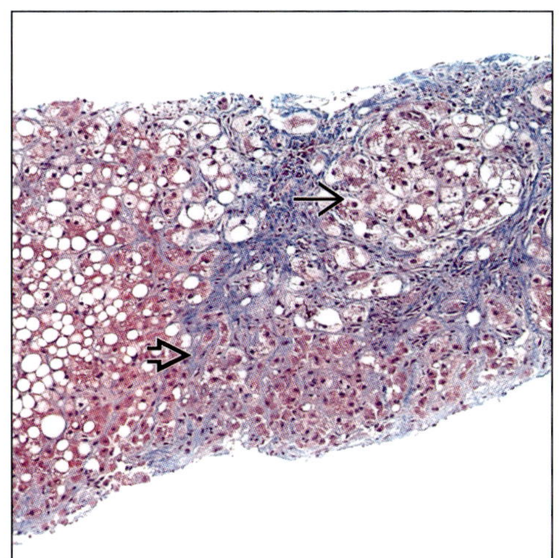

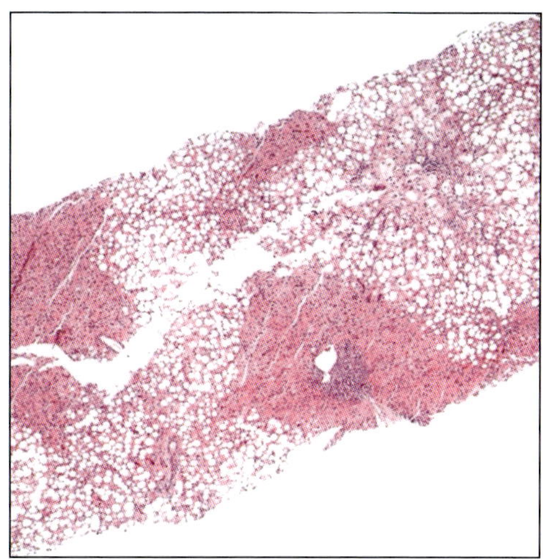

(Left) *Bridging fibrosis ⇨ and a cirrhotic nodule → are seen in late-stage NASH.* ***(Right)*** *A case of concomitant NASH and chronic hepatitis C shows zone 3 steatosis and hepatocyte injury, along with dense chronic portal inflammation and lymphoid aggregates.*

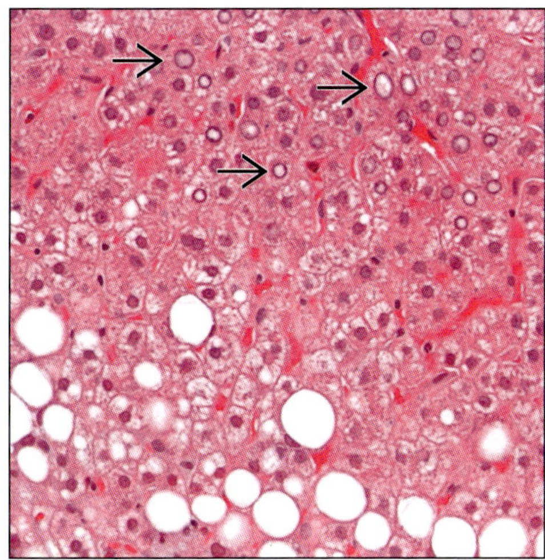

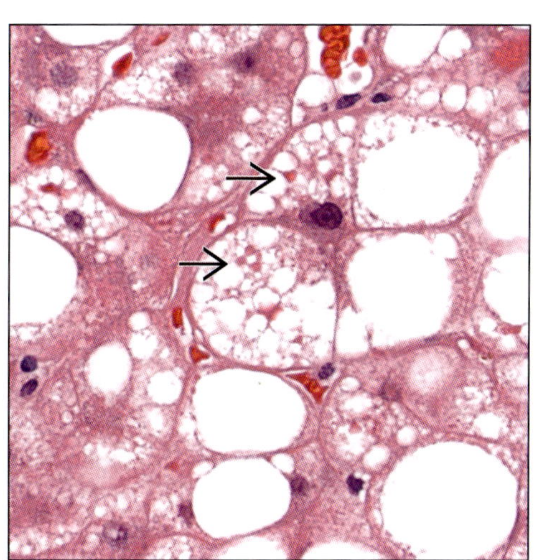

(Left) *Glycogenated nuclei → characterized by vesiculated nuclei of the hepatocytes, are common but nonspecific findings in NASH.* ***(Right)*** *Megamitochondria (i.e., "giant" mitochondria →) are often seen in NASH and are characterized by intracytoplasmic, oblong, round, and eosinophilic inclusions.*

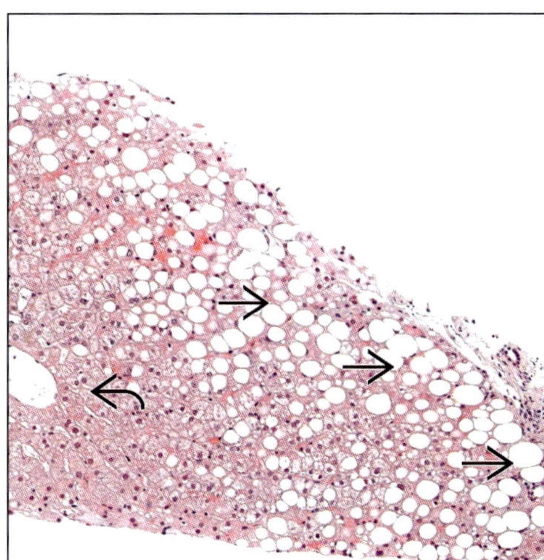

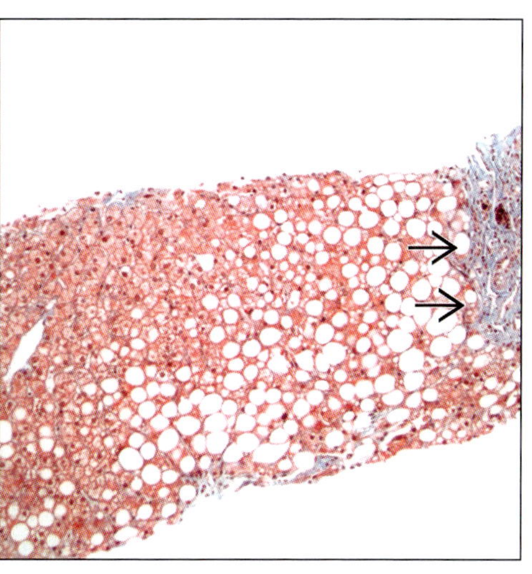

(Left) *The steatosis of NASH in pediatric patients is typically accentuated in zone 1 → with zone 3 sparing ↩.* ***(Right)*** *NASH in pediatric patients is typically characterized by portal-based fibrosis → rather than zone 3 pericellular fibrosis.*

GLYCOGENIC HEPATOPATHY

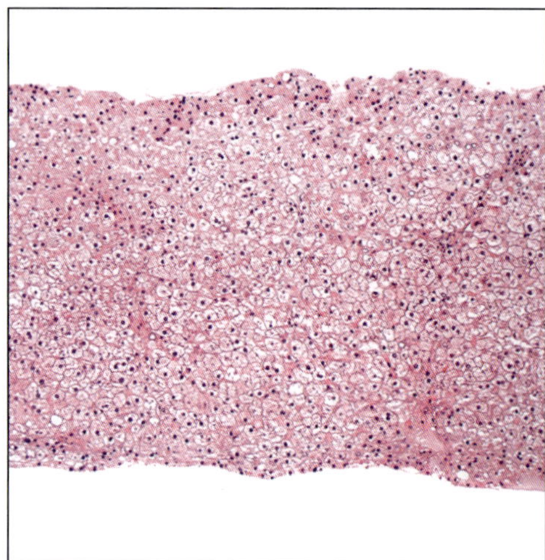

Paraffin section shows diffuse pale staining of hepatocytes. There is no inflammation or hepatocyte necrosis.

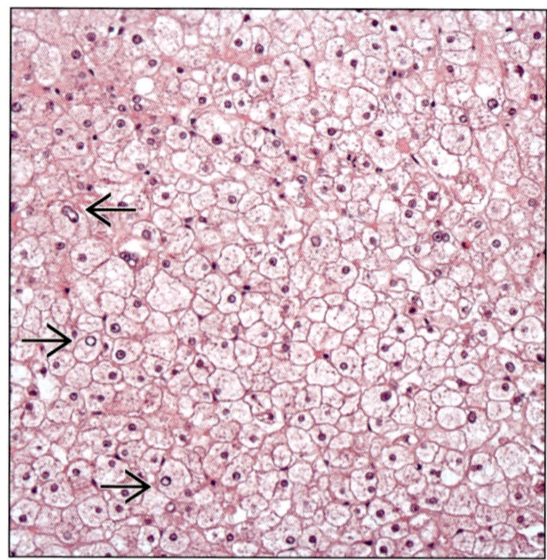

Hematoxylin & eosin demonstrates diffusely swollen and pale hepatocytes with prominent cell membranes. Occasional glycogenated hepatocyte nuclei ⇒ are seen. There is no inflammation or necrosis.

TERMINOLOGY

Synonyms

- Hepatic glycogenosis
- Liver glycogenosis
- Glycogen hepatopathy or glycogenic hepatopathy
- Diabetes mellitus-associated glycogen storage hepatomegaly
- Mauriac syndrome
  - If liver changes are accompanied by growth retardation, delayed puberty, hypercholesterolemia, and Cushingoid features

Definitions

- Excessive glycogen storage in hepatocytes secondary to poorly controlled insulin-dependent diabetes mellitus

ETIOLOGY/PATHOGENESIS

Metabolic Factors

- Chronic hyperglycemia due to poorly controlled insulin-dependent diabetes mellitus
- Longstanding high blood sugar levels lead to glycogen accumulation in hepatocytes
- Hepatomegaly and transaminase elevations attributed to this excess glycogen accumulation

CLINICAL ISSUES

Epidemiology

- Age
  - Occurs in children and adults

Presentation

- Abdominal pain
- Hepatomegaly
- Nausea
- Vomiting
- History of ketoacidosis

Laboratory Tests

- Hyperglycemia
- Elevated transaminases
- Alkaline phosphatase may also be elevated
- Elevated hemoglobin A1c (HbA1c) indicates history of poor glycemic control

Treatment

- Options, risks, complications
  - Mainstay treatment is improved management of diabetes mellitus
    - Optimization of glycemic control with insulin and diet
- Surgical approaches
  - Resolution after pancreas transplantation has been reported

Prognosis

- Excellent outcome with medical management
- Liver histology improves and transaminases normalize with optimization of glycemic control

IMAGE FINDINGS

Radiographic Findings

- Hyperdense liver on CT scan without administration of contrast material

MACROSCOPIC FEATURES

General Features

- Hepatomegaly

MICROSCOPIC PATHOLOGY

Histologic Features

- Diffuse pale-staining hepatocyte cytoplasm

GLYCOGENIC HEPATOPATHY

Key Facts

Terminology
- Hepatomegaly and elevated liver enzymes associated with poorly controlled diabetes mellitus and abundant glycogen in hepatocytes

Clinical Issues
- Abdominal pain
- Elevated transaminases
- Hepatomegaly
- Occurs in patients with history of poorly controlled insulin-dependent diabetes mellitus
- Resolves with optimization glycemic control

Microscopic Pathology
- Diffuse pale-staining hepatocytes
- Excessive glycogen storage in hepatocytes demonstrated by periodic acid-Schiff (PAS) stain
- Absence of inflammation or evidence of other liver disease

- Periodic acid-Schiff (PAS) stain confirms excessive glycogen accumulation in hepatocytes
- Rare acidophil bodies may be seen
- Glycogenated hepatocyte nuclei
- Notable absence of inflammation or other features of hepatic injury
- Fibrosis is rare

ANCILLARY TESTS

Electron Microscopy
- Marked glycogen accumulation in hepatocyte cytoplasm and nuclei

DIFFERENTIAL DIAGNOSIS

Normal Liver
- Pale, enlarged hepatocytes may be mistaken for normal or interpreted as fixation artifact

Fatty Liver Disease
- Pale, enlarged hepatocytes may be misinterpreted as ballooning hepatocyte degeneration
- Most cases of glycogenic hepatopathy show little or no steatosis

Glycogen Storage Disease
- Typically presents at younger age and without history of diabetes mellitus

DIAGNOSTIC CHECKLIST

Clinically Relevant Pathologic Features
- Marked transaminase elevation attributed to excessive glycogen accumulation in hepatocytes

Pathologic Interpretation Pearls
- Consider in patients with unexplained transaminase elevations and history of poorly controlled diabetes mellitus
- Pale, slightly swollen hepatocytes with prominent cell membranes
  - May be mistaken for normal hepatocytes, a glycogen storage disease, or fixation artifact

SELECTED REFERENCES

1. Sweetser S et al: The bright liver of glycogenic hepatopathy. Hepatology. 51(2):711-2, 2010
2. Fridell JA et al: Complete reversal of glycogen hepatopathy with pancreas transplantation: two cases. Transplantation. 83(1):84-6, 2007
3. Torbenson M et al: Glycogenic hepatopathy: an underrecognized hepatic complication of diabetes mellitus. Am J Surg Pathol. 30(4):508-13, 2006

IMAGE GALLERY

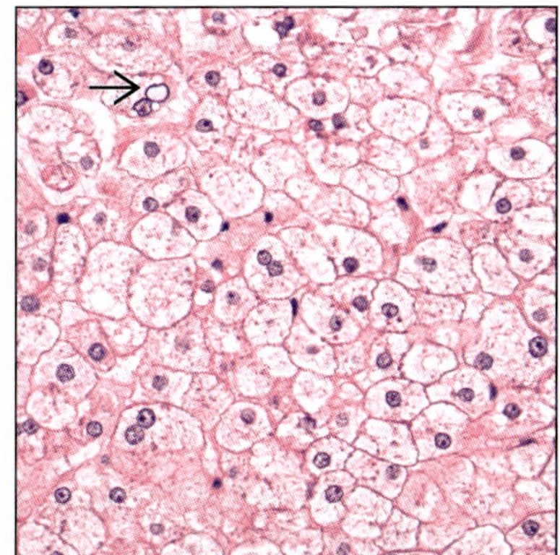

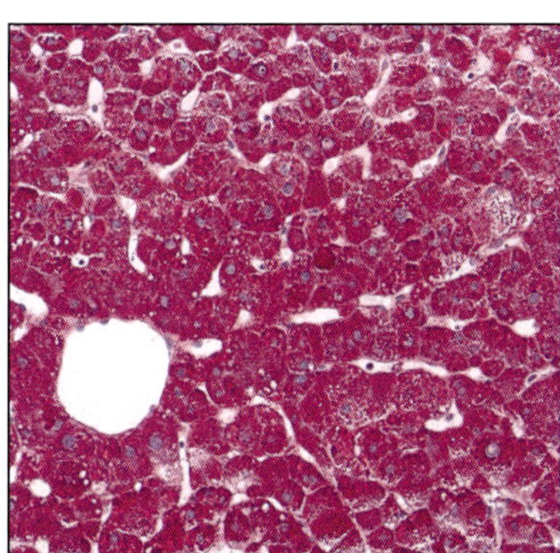

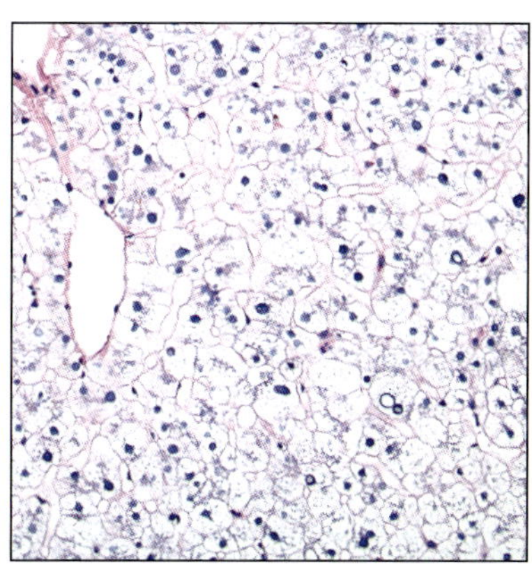

(Left) *H&E section demonstrates diffuse hepatocyte enlargement with pale cytoplasm and prominent cell membranes in a patient with poorly controlled diabetes mellitus and hepatic glycogenosis. Few glycogenated hepatocyte nuclei ⇒ are seen.* ***(Center)*** *Periodic acid-Schiff stain demonstrates abundant glycogen in hepatocytes in hepatic glycogenosis.* ***(Right)*** *Periodic acid-Schiff with diastase reveals no remaining glycogen in hepatocytes in hepatic glycogenosis.*

FATTY LIVER OF PREGNANCY

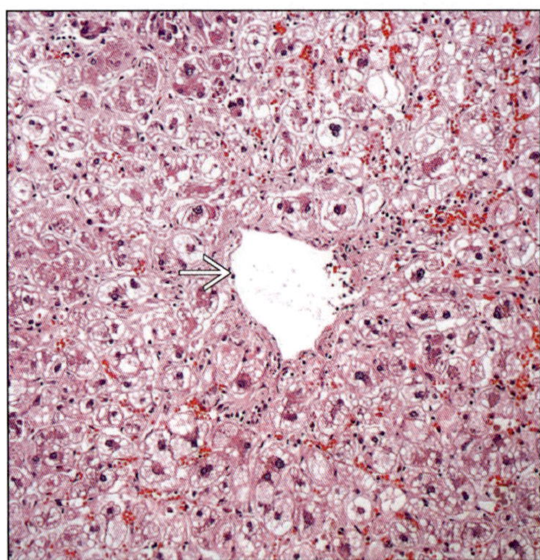

Hematoxylin and eosin section demonstrates extensive microvesicular steatosis. The centrilobular or zone 3 hepatocytes are involved. In the center of the image is a central vein ➡.

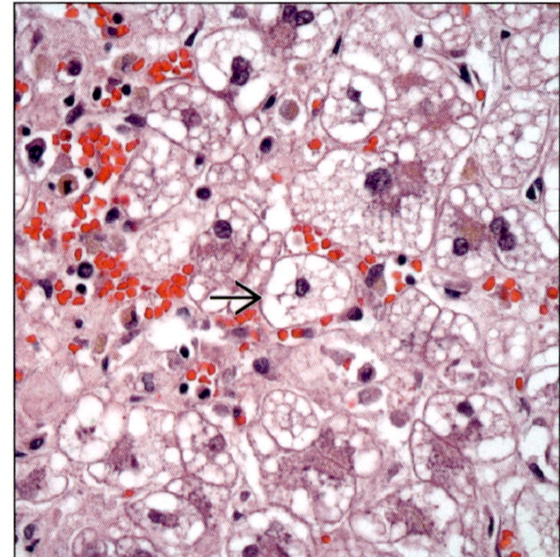

Hematoxylin and eosin section demonstrates microvesicular steatosis. Numerous small steatotic vacuoles ➡ surround and focally indent the hepatocyte nucleus.

TERMINOLOGY

Synonyms

- Acute fatty liver of pregnancy (AFLP)
- Hepatic lipidosis of pregnancy
- Sheehan syndrome

Definitions

- Acute liver failure during 2nd half of pregnancy with severe fatty infiltration of liver

ETIOLOGY/PATHOGENESIS

Etiology Unknown

- Possible mitochondrial β oxidation defect
  - Some affected mothers and infants have inherited fatty acid oxidation defects
    - Long-chain 3-hydroxyacyl-CoA dehydrogenase (LCHAD) deficiency
    - Infant and parents should be evaluated for LCHAD deficiency
  - Carnitine palmitoyltransferase I deficiency also associated with AFLP

CLINICAL ISSUES

Epidemiology

- Incidence
  - Diagnosed in 1/6,659 deliveries, although subclinical cases also exist
  - Usually occurs in late 3rd trimester but can be seen in 2nd trimester
  - More common in women who are primigravidae and have multiple gestations

Presentation

- Mild prodromal illness
- Nausea, vomiting, and abdominal pain
- Jaundice, cholestatic
- Confusion
- Rapidly progressive acute liver failure
- May also have hypertension and proteinuria
- Associated acute pancreatitis may also occur

Laboratory Tests

- Increased prothrombin time
- Low serum fibrinogen level
- Moderate hyperbilirubinemia and transaminase elevation
- Hypoglycemia
- Serum lipase and amylase elevated if acute pancreatitis also present

Natural History

- Does not progress to chronic liver disease
- Subsequent pregnancies may be unaffected or complicated by recurrent disease

Treatment

- Urgent delivery of infant
- Supportive therapy
- Transplantation in selected cases

Prognosis

- Can be fatal for mother and fetus if not diagnosed and treated early
- Early diagnosis and delivery associated with excellent outcome
  - Up to 100% maternal survival rate
  - Infant mortality 6-7% or less

IMAGE FINDINGS

Radiographic Findings

- Ultrasound and CT demonstrate fatty infiltration of liver

FATTY LIVER OF PREGNANCY

Key Facts

Terminology

- Acute liver failure during 2nd half of pregnancy associated with severe fatty infiltration of liver

Etiology/Pathogenesis

- Etiology unknown but associated with mitochondrial fatty acid oxidation defects

Clinical Issues

- Most commonly occurs in last 10 weeks and usually in last 4 weeks of pregnancy
- Rapidly progressive acute liver failure
- Early diagnosis and delivery are critical

Microscopic Pathology

- Microvesicular steatosis

MACROSCOPIC FEATURES

General Features

- Liver grossly small and pale yellow

MICROSCOPIC PATHOLOGY

Histologic Features

- Severe microvesicular steatosis, predominantly centrilobular or diffuse
  - May show small rim of periportal sparing
  - Small steatosis vacuoles may require special stains (oil red O or Sudan black), or electron microscopy
- Zone 3 perivenular canalicular cholestasis and hepatocellular cholestasis
- Hepatocyte injury and Kupffer cell hyperplasia
- Mild mononuclear infiltrates of lobules and portal tracts

DIFFERENTIAL DIAGNOSIS

Acute Hepatic Failure Unrelated to Pregnancy

- Acute viral hepatitis
- Drug-induced liver injury

Preeclampsia/Eclampsia

- Commonly also present in patients with AFLP
- Hypertension and proteinuria
- Periportal necrosis
  - In HELLP (hemolysis, elevated liver enzymes, and low platelets) syndrome, also periportal hemorrhage and fibrin deposition
- Both disorders treated by delivery

DIAGNOSTIC CHECKLIST

Pathologic Interpretation Pearls

- Microvesicular steatosis in pregnant woman

SELECTED REFERENCES

1. Gutiérrez Junquera C et al: Acute fatty liver of pregnancy and neonatal long-chain 3-hydroxyacyl-coenzyme A dehydrogenase (LCHAD) deficiency. Eur J Pediatr. 168(1):103-6, 2009
2. Lee NM et al: Liver disease in pregnancy. World J Gastroenterol. 15(8):897-906, 2009
3. Devarbhavi H et al: Pregnancy-associated acute liver disease and acute viral hepatitis: differentiation, course and outcome. J Hepatol. 49(6):930-5, 2008
4. Hay JE: Liver disease in pregnancy. Hepatology. 47(3):1067-76, 2008
5. Knight M et al: A prospective national study of acute fatty liver of pregnancy in the UK. Gut. 57(7):951-6, 2008

IMAGE GALLERY

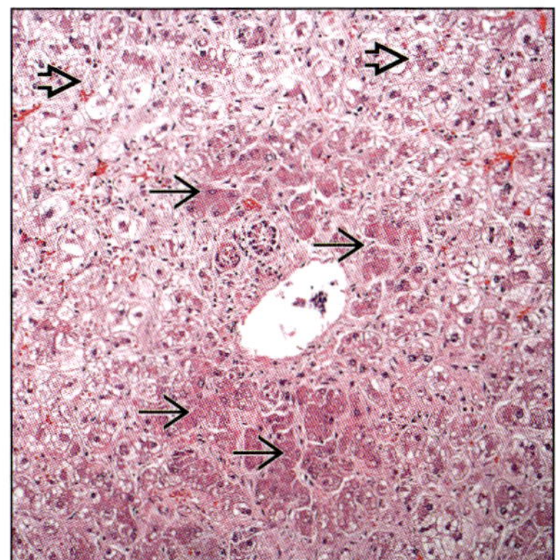

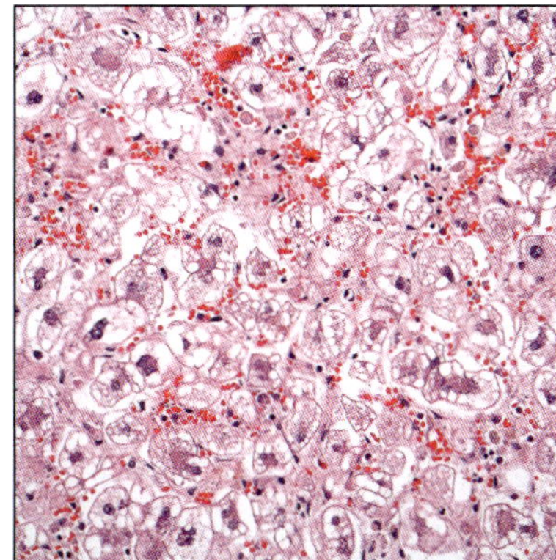

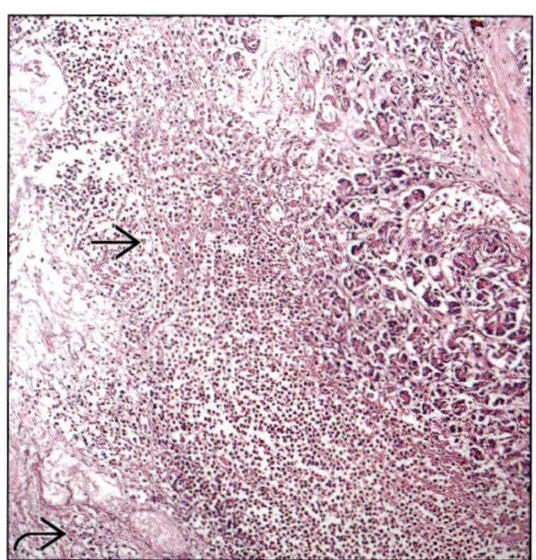

(Left) *Hematoxylin and eosin section shows a background of microvesicular steatosis ⇨ with relative sparing of a small rim of periportal hepatocytes →.* ***(Center)*** *Hematoxylin and eosin stain shows microvesicular steatosis. Small steatotic vacuoles in the hepatocyte cytoplasm surround and indent the hepatocyte nucleus.* ***(Right)*** *Hematoxylin and eosin section demonstrates acute pancreatitis → with necrosis ↗ in a patient with fatty liver of pregnancy.*

Vascular Disorders

PORTAL VENOUS OBSTRUCTION

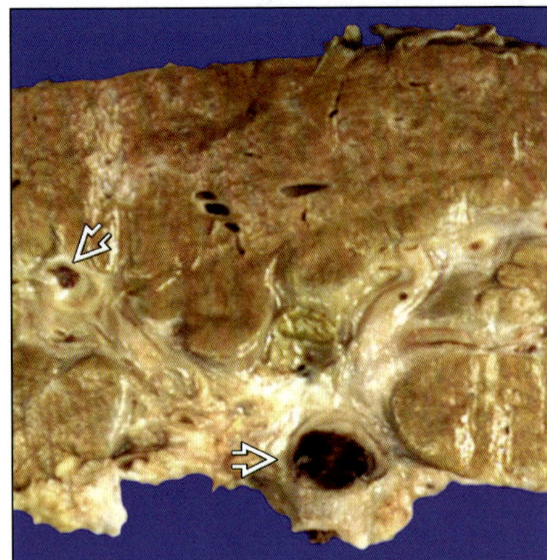
A large portal vein thrombus ➔ is seen in this liver.

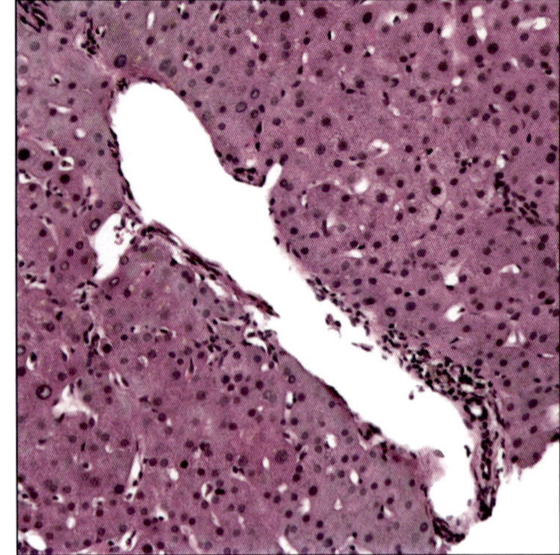
Typical changes in portal venous obstruction include dilated portal venules with "herniation" of the vessel into the surrounding parenchyma.

TERMINOLOGY

Synonyms

- Idiopathic portal hypertension
  - Many cases of idiopathic portal hypertension probably represent undetected portal vein thrombosis
- Noncirrhotic portal hypertension

Definitions

- Changes resulting from mechanical obstruction of lumen of portal vein
- Extrahepatic
  - Obstruction of portal trunk or main tributaries
    - Usually diagnosed by imaging studies
    - Inconsistent changes seen in liver biopsy
    - Many causes including tumors, thrombi, intraabdominal inflammation, congenital vascular anomalies, venous outflow obstruction, compression
- Intrahepatic
  - Obstruction of portal venules within liver
    - Lesion(s) may not be apparent on noninvasive imaging studies
    - Suggestive changes may be seen on liver biopsy
    - May result from propagation of large portal vein thrombosis or emboli
    - Specific cause often not identified
    - Can be secondary to other conditions including congenital hepatic fibrosis, sarcoidosis, schistosomiasis, and any type of cirrhosis

ETIOLOGY/PATHOGENESIS

Luminal Obstruction

- Can occur at any level of portal venous system
- Sequelae depend on location, cause, time course, and extent of blockage
  - May be well tolerated because of liver dual blood supply and development of collaterals
  - Extrahepatic: Usually caused by thrombosis
  - Intrahepatic: Specific cause usually not identified

CLINICAL ISSUES

Epidemiology

- Age
  - Both children and adults can be affected
    - Major risk factors in children: Infection, congenital cardiovascular malformations
    - Major risk factors in adults: Hypercoagulable states, cirrhosis, malignant neoplasms

Presentation

- Signs/symptoms of portal hypertension
  - Varices ± bleeding
  - Splenomegaly
  - Abdominal pain/tenderness
  - Ascites
- Patients may be asymptomatic
- Complications
  - Variceal bleeding
  - Liver failure
  - Portal biliopathy
    - Partial bile duct obstruction in patients with portal vein thrombosis, due to either compression by adjacent varices or duct ischemia

Treatment

- Managing sequelae of portal hypertension
- Must treat underlying cause of obstruction if possible

Prognosis

- Depends on underlying cause as well as location, time course, extent of obstruction

PORTAL VENOUS OBSTRUCTION

Key Facts

Etiology/Pathogenesis

- Can occur at any level of portal venous system
  - Extrahepatic: Portal trunk or large tributaries, usually caused by thrombosis
  - Intrahepatic: Intrahepatic portal venules, often no specific cause determined
- Sequelae depend on location, cause, time course, and extent of blockage

Microscopic Pathology

- Often irregularly distributed, may be missed in small biopsy specimens
  - Dilated portal venules
  - Multiple collateral venules
  - Herniation of venules into parenchyma
  - Portal fibrosis

MACROSCOPIC FEATURES

Large Vessel Findings

- Intimal plaques, intimal fibrosis, or mural calcifications
- Fresh or organizing thrombi
- Cavernous transformation (mass of collateral and recanalized vessels)

MICROSCOPIC PATHOLOGY

Histologic Features

- Often irregularly distributed, may be missed in small biopsy specimens
- Subtle alterations of portal venules
  - Dilated portal venules
  - Multiple collateral venules
  - Herniation of venules into parenchyma
  - Rarely, sclerosis of portal venules similar to hepatoportal sclerosis
- Portal fibrosis
- Infarcts of Zahn
  - Not really infarcts but rather zones of hepatocyte atrophy with sinusoidal dilatation and congestion
  - Persistent occlusion can lead to atrophy of entire segments of liver
- True infarcts rarely develop
- Venous inflammatory changes may be seen in cases complicated by pylephlebitis

DIFFERENTIAL DIAGNOSIS

Hepatoportal Sclerosis

- Has sclerotic portal venules
- May need imaging to exclude portal venous obstruction

Normal Liver

- Changes may be very subtle and easily missed
- Loss/fibrosis of small portal venules is normal finding in elderly persons

SELECTED REFERENCES

1. Chandra R et al: Portal biliopathy. J Gastroenterol Hepatol. 16(10):1086-92, 2001
2. Sahni P et al: Extrahepatic portal vein obstruction. Br J Surg. 77(11):1201-2, 1990
3. Terada T et al: Microvasculature in the small portal tracts in idiopathic portal hypertension. A morphological comparison with other hepatic diseases. Virchows Arch A Pathol Anat Histopathol. 415(1):61-7, 1989
4. Kameda H et al: Obliterative portal venopathy: a comparative study of 184 cases of extrahepatic portal obstruction and 469 cases of idiopathic portal hypertension. Hepatology. 1:139-49, 1986
5. Nakanuma Y et al: Pathological study on livers with noncirrhotic portal hypertension and portal venous thromboembolic occlusion: report of seven autopsy cases. Am J Gastroenterol. 79(10):782-9, 1984

IMAGE GALLERY

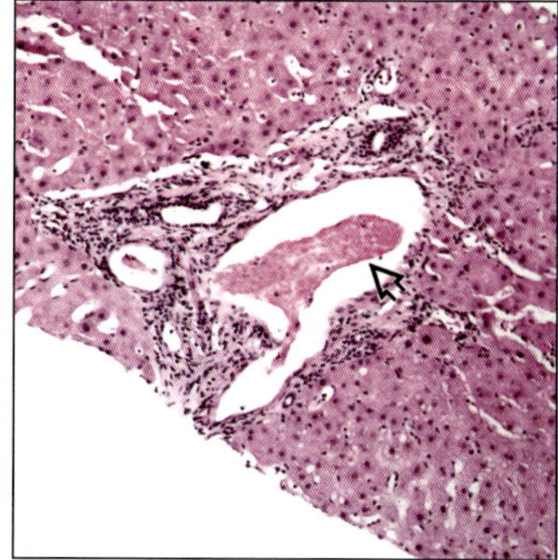

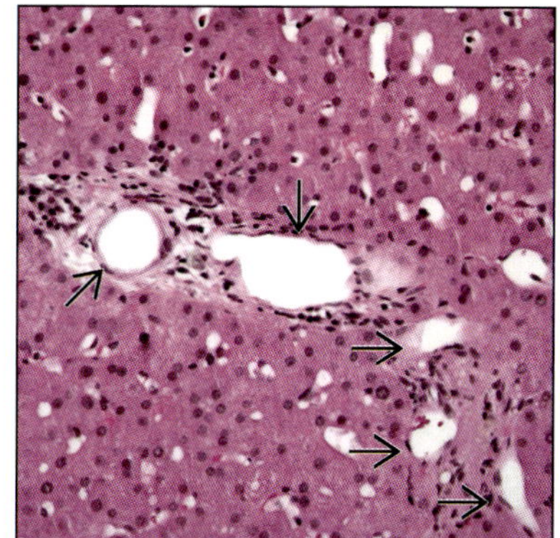

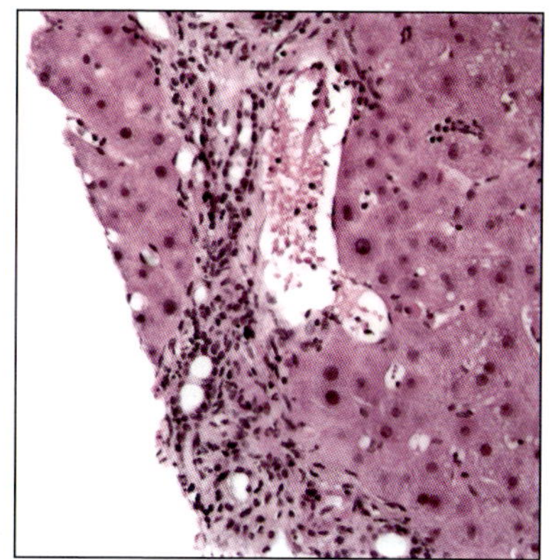

(Left) *Fibrin thrombus ⊳ is seen within a dilated portal venule in this case of intrahepatic portal vein thrombosis due to propagation of a thrombus in a larger portal vein.* ***(Center)*** *Multiple collateral venules → are present in this portal tract in a case of portal venous obstruction, indicating elevated portal pressures.* ***(Right)*** *This dilated portal venule "herniates" into the hepatic parenchyma in a case of portal venous obstruction.*

HEPATOPORTAL SCLEROSIS

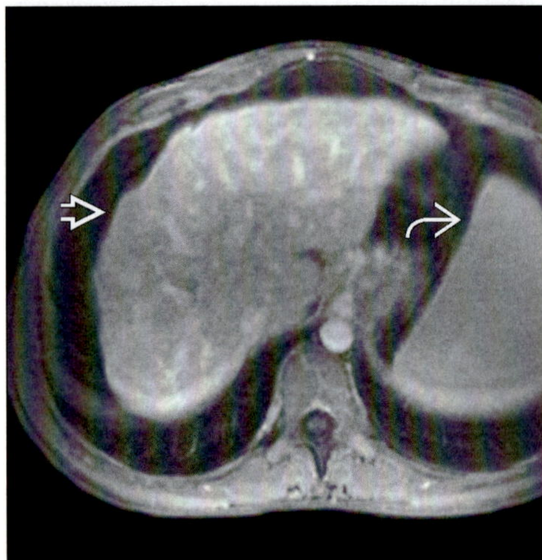

Abdominal magnetic resonance imaging shows irregular hepatic surface with a shrunken appearance ➡ and heterogeneous hepatic parenchyma. Note the presence of splenomegaly ➡.

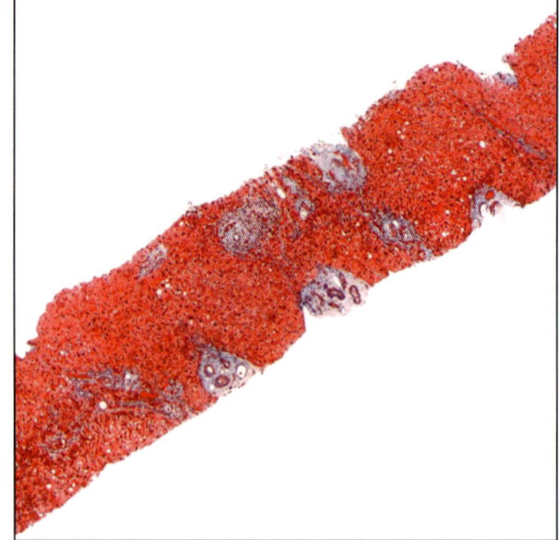

Trichrome stain highlights abnormal approximation of the portal tracts seen in a needle biopsy, resulting in an altered hepatic architecture. Portal fibrosis is evident even at low power.

TERMINOLOGY

Abbreviations

- Hepatoportal sclerosis (HPS)

Synonyms

- Idiopathic portal hypertension
- Noncirrhotic portal fibrosis
- Obliterative portal venopathy
- Intrahepatic portal venopathy
- Idiopathic presinusoidal portal hypertension
- Banti disease or Banti syndrome

Definitions

- Portal hypertension secondary to portal fibrosis and portal vein obliteration in absence of cirrhosis

ETIOLOGY/PATHOGENESIS

Mechanism Unknown

- Associated with several conditions that cause increased vascular resistance at presinusoidal level
  - Prothrombotic states
  - Infections
    - Intestinal and intraabdominal bacterial infections
    - HIV infection/antiretroviral therapy
- Chronic exposure to toxins
  - Inorganic arsenic
  - Vinyl chloride monomers
- Autoimmune disorders
- Adams-Oliver syndrome

CLINICAL ISSUES

Epidemiology

- Incidence
  - Common in India and Japan; rare in USA

Presentation

- Splenomegaly
- Upper GI bleeding
- Ascites in advanced disease

Laboratory Tests

- Usually normal or near normal liver function tests
- Anemia and thrombocytopenia
- Elevated portal venous pressure

Treatment

- Transjugular intrahepatic portosystemic shunt (TIPS)
- Endoscopic variceal sclerotherapy or band ligation
- Splenectomy
- Liver transplantation for advanced HPS

Prognosis

- Better than cirrhosis because of preserved liver function

IMAGE FINDINGS

General Features

- Sudden narrowing or paucity of intrahepatic portal vein branches
- Patent extrahepatic portal and hepatic veins, but portal vein thrombosis may be seen

MACROSCOPIC FEATURES

General Features

- Irregular, nodular, or wrinkled surface
- Dilatation and wall thickening of large portal veins
- Unusual distribution of portal tracts and vascular structures
- Shrunken in advanced disease

HEPATOPORTAL SCLEROSIS

Key Facts

Terminology

- Portal hypertension secondary to portal fibrosis and portal vein obliteration
  - Form of "noncirrhotic" portal hypertension
  - Associated with variety of conditions that lead to increased vascular resistance at presinusoidal level

Clinical Issues

- Most common in India and Japan
- Usually treated with transjugular intrahepatic portosystemic shunt (TIPS)
- Better prognosis than cirrhotic portal hypertension because of preserved liver function

Microscopic Pathology

- Lack of consistent relationship between portal tracts and central veins
- Portal fibrosis
- Narrowing or obliteration of portal veins

MICROSCOPIC PATHOLOGY

Histologic Features

- Abnormal vascular architecture
  - Distorted portal-central vein relationships (approximation or wide separation)
  - Eccentric location of central veins in lobules; multiple ectatic veins in single lobule
- Portal vein changes
  - Narrowing or obliteration of portal veins
  - Presence of numerous thin-walled vascular channels in portal tracts (angiomatoid malformation)
  - Herniation of normal caliber or dilated portal veins into lobule
- Portal fibrosis
  - Periportal and perisinusoidal fibrosis as well as slender portal-portal fibrous septa may be seen
- Marked sinusoidal dilatation (megasinusoids)
- Minimal portal inflammation
- Diffuse or localized nodular hyperplasia

DIFFERENTIAL DIAGNOSIS

Cirrhosis

- Extensive fibrous septa that divide entire liver parenchyma into regenerative nodules

Abnormal Portal Vasculature in Absence of Portal Hypertension

- Unclear clinical significance
- Correlates with increased fibrosis in HCV
- Frequently seen in allograft biopsies
- Absence of portal hypertension must be clinically documented

Portal Vein Thrombosis

- May have similar histologic features
- Demonstrate thrombus through imaging studies

Nodular Regenerative Hyperplasia

- Normal-appearing portal tracts and portal veins with no fibrosis

DIAGNOSTIC CHECKLIST

Clinically Relevant Pathologic Features

- Rule out cirrhosis or other known etiologies of portal hypertension

SELECTED REFERENCES

1. Chawla Y et al: Intrahepatic portal venopathy and related disorders of the liver. Semin Liver Dis. 28(3):270-81, 2008
2. Sarin SK et al: Noncirrhotic portal fibrosis/idiopathic portal hypertension: APASL recommendations for diagnosis and treatment. Hepatol Int. 1(3):398-413, 2007
3. Krasinskas AM et al: Abnormal intrahepatic portal vasculature in native and allograft liver biopsies: a comparative analysis. Am J Surg Pathol. 29(10):1382-8, 2005

IMAGE GALLERY

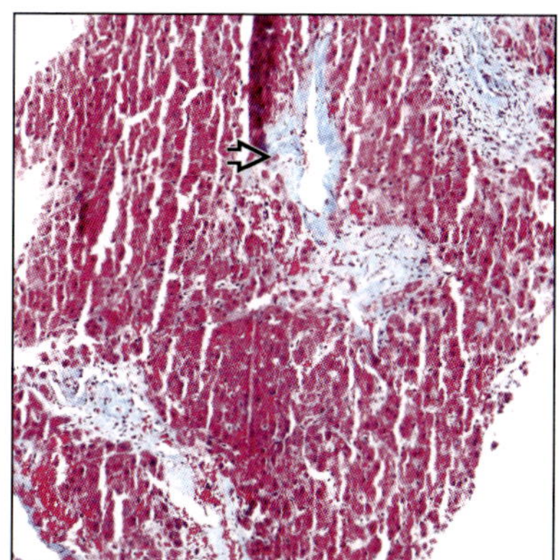
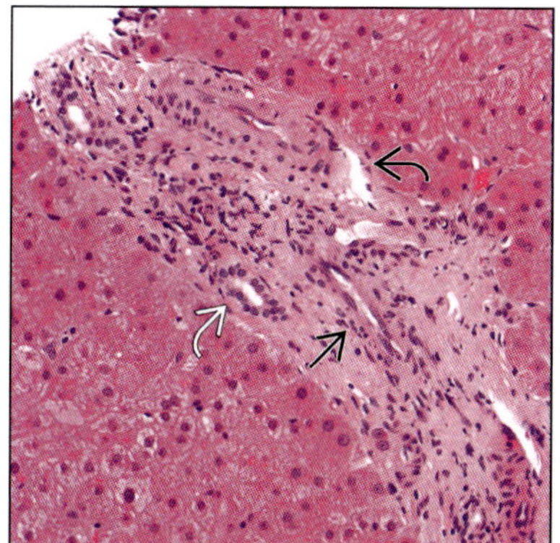
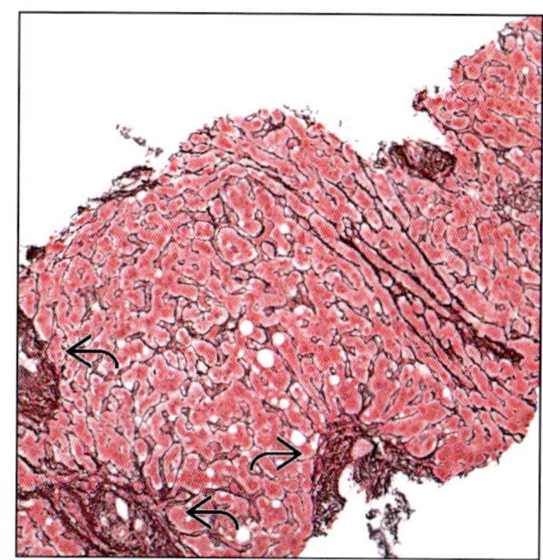

(Left) *Trichrome stain reveals portal and periportal fibrosis. Portal veins are inconspicuous. A central vein is abnormally close to a portal tract ⇨.* ***(Center)*** *The portal tract is expanded by fibrosis, with marked narrowing of the portal venule ⇨. Note the presence of normal caliber hepatic artery → and bile duct ➡.* ***(Right)*** *Reticulin stain highlights nodular hyperplasia of the hepatocytes. Note the abnormal approximation of the portal tracts ⇨.*

HEPATIC VENOUS OUTFLOW OBSTRUCTION

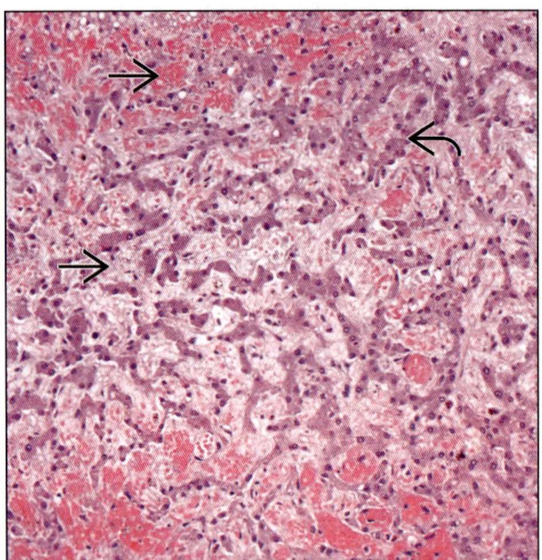

In Budd-Chiari syndrome, increased sinusoidal pressure causes sinusoidal dilatation, congestion ⇒, and hepatocellular atrophy ⇒.

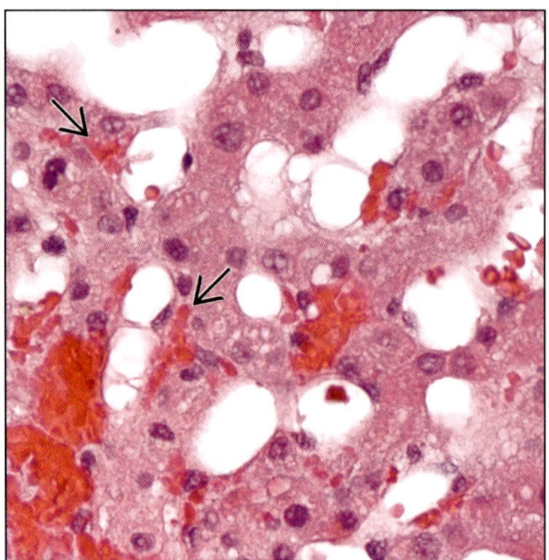

Extravasation of RBC ⇒ in the space of Disse (the potential space between the hepatocytes and sinusoidal basement membrane) is caused by increased sinusoidal pressure.

TERMINOLOGY

Abbreviations

- Hepatic venous outflow obstruction (HVOO)

ETIOLOGY/PATHOGENESIS

Venous Obstruction

- Can occur at different levels of hepatic venous outflow
  - Sinusoids or small hepatic veins: Sinusoidal obstruction syndrome (formerly veno-occlusive disease)
  - Large hepatic veins or inferior vena cava (Budd-Chiari syndrome [BCS])
  - Right heart or pericardial disease
    - Right heart failure (either isolated or result of left heart failure)
    - Tricuspid valve disease
    - Cardiac amyloidosis
    - Constrictive pericarditis

Pathogenesis

- Liver changes result from hepatic venous congestion, increased hepatic and sinusoidal pressure, and necrosis
- Secondary sinusoidal thrombosis extending into hepatic and portal veins may contribute to parenchymal damage and fibrosis

CLINICAL ISSUES

Presentation

- Subacute presentation (< 6 months) is most common with painful hepatomegaly, mild jaundice, and ascites
- Less commonly, presents as chronic liver disease or cirrhosis
- Rare cases have fulminant presentation with acute liver failure

Laboratory Tests

- Mild elevation of transaminases; marked increase in acute cases
- Alkaline phosphatase elevation is common

Treatment

- Decompression procedures in Budd-Chiari syndrome
  - Nonsurgical decompression by percutaneous transluminal angioplasty with stent: Suitable for webs or limited stenosis
  - Image-guided transjugular intrahepatic portosystemic shunt (TIPS)
  - Surgical decompression with portosystemic shunt
- For cardiac etiologies, treat underlying disease
- Liver transplant necessary in cases with advanced fibrosis
- Hematological work-up is essential to identify cause of thrombosis

Prognosis

- Budd-Chiari syndrome
  - 5-year survival after portosystemic shunt is 75-90%
  - 5-year survival after liver transplantation is 60%
- Cardiac disease
  - Depends on type and severity of underlying illness

IMAGE FINDINGS

Radiographic Findings

- For BCS, ultrasound with Doppler flow studies is initial tool of choice
- Hepatic scintigraphy, computerized tomography (CT), and magnetic resonance imaging (MR) can also contribute to diagnosis
- Hepatic venography was considered gold standard in BCS, but it is now restricted to diagnostically challenging cases
  - Normal hepatic vein flow is not seen

HEPATIC VENOUS OUTFLOW OBSTRUCTION

Key Facts

Etiology/Pathogenesis

- Sinusoids or small hepatic veins: Sinusoidal obstruction syndrome (formerly veno-occlusive disease)
- Large hepatic veins or inferior vena cava (Budd-Chiari syndrome)
- Right heart or pericardial disease

Clinical Issues

- Subacute presentation (< 6 months) is most common with painful hepatomegaly, mild jaundice, and ascites
- Less commonly, disease presents as chronic liver disease or cirrhosis
- Rare cases have fulminant presentation with acute liver failure

Microscopic Pathology

- Centrizonal-based changes: Sinusoidal dilatation and congestion, RBC extravasation, hepatic plate atrophy, necrosis
- Portal-based changes: Ductular reaction, focal bile duct damage
- Central vein-based fibrosis in chronic cases

Top Differential Diagnoses

- Biliary disease
- Other diseases that can cause sinusoidal dilatation
  - Portal vein thrombosis, systemic inflammatory conditions, some neoplasms such as renal cell carcinoma or lymphoma, artifactual sinusoidal dilatation

---

  - Collaterals attempt to decompress obstruction leading to "spider web" appearance
  - Reverse flow can be seen in portal vein
- For cardiac causes, findings depend on underlying disease

MACROSCOPIC FEATURES

General Features

- "Nutmeg liver": Alternating areas of hemorrhagic area and pale parenchyma
- Hemorrhagic areas corresponding to centrizonal areas; pale areas are relatively unaffected periportal parenchyma

MICROSCOPIC PATHOLOGY

Histologic Features

- Role of liver biopsy: Confirm diagnosis and determine degree of hepatocellular damage
  - Centrizonal-based changes
    - Sinusoidal dilatation and congestion
    - Sinusoidal dilatation compresses hepatocytes leading to hepatic plate atrophy
    - Increased sinusoidal pressure leads to RBC extravasation in space of Disse
    - Hepatocellular necrosis in acute and subacute cases
    - Pericentral and sinusoidal fibrosis in chronic cases that can progress to bridging fibrosis and cirrhosis
    - Fibrosis can be highly variable in distribution, especially in patients with heart failure
  - Portal-based changes
    - Portal expansion with bile ductular reaction with mild lymphoplasmacytic infiltrate
    - Ductular reaction is generally mild but can be florid
    - Bile duct damage can be present in form of lymphocytic cholangitis
    - Portal and periportal fibrosis can occur
- Features in certain clinical settings
  - Hyaline eosinophilic deposits in sinusoids &/or vessel walls in amyloidosis
  - Nodular regenerative hyperplasia can be seen
  - Large regenerative nodules in BCS
    - Can be multiple and range from 0.5-3.5 cm
    - Presumably result from localized increase in arterial blood flow
    - Some nodules are associated with ductular reaction resembling focal nodular hyperplasia
    - Some nodules lack bile ducts resembling hepatic adenoma
- Biopsy features can determine choice of therapy
  - Congestion without significant necrosis or fibrosis
    - Conservative management with possible repeat biopsy in 3-6 months
  - Congestion with necrosis but no significant fibrosis
    - Surgical decompression
  - Severe fibrosis or cirrhosis
    - Liver transplant

DIFFERENTIAL DIAGNOSIS

Other Causes of Sinusoidal Dilatation

- Vascular causes
  - Portal vein thrombosis
    - Obstruction of portal vein blood flow leads to hepatocyte atrophy
    - Hepatic atrophy gives appearance of dilated sinusoids
  - Nodular regenerative hyperplasia (NRH)
    - Multiple 0.1-0.2 cm nodules without fibrosis
    - Occurs in variety of clinical settings, including vascular disorders, myeloproliferative diseases, primary biliary cirrhosis
    - Nodules compress hepatic microvasculature leading to hepatocyte atrophy and resultant sinusoidal dilatation
- Systemic inflammatory conditions
  - Castleman disease, Crohn disease, rheumatoid arthritis, Still disease, polymyalgia rheumatica
  - Granulomatous conditions, such as sarcoidosis

HEPATIC VENOUS OUTFLOW OBSTRUCTION

Causes of Budd-Chiari Syndrome	
Disease Category	**Specific Etiologies**
Thrombotic diseases	
(A) Hypercoagulable states	Myeloproliferative disorders, pregnancy and oral contraceptive use, antiphospholipid antibodies, systemic lupus erythematosus, paroxysmal nocturnal hemoglobinuria, factor V Leiden
(B) Deficiencies of coagulation factors or inhibitors	Antithrombin deficiency, protein C deficiency, protein S deficiency
Mechanical causes	Membranous obstruction of inferior vena cava, obstruction by tumor, extrinsic compression by tumor or mass, post-transplant kinking of hepatic venous outflow

- Etiology of sinusoidal dilatation in inflammatory disorders is not clear
- Extrahepatic neoplasms without liver involvement
  - Sinusoidal dilatation is most commonly associated with renal cell carcinoma (RCC) and Hodgkin lymphoma
  - Other tumors: Carcinomas of stomach, uterus, and colon
- Nonspecific sinusoidal dilatation in different clinical settings
  - Artifactual sinusoidal dilatation
    - Mechanical reasons, such as rough handling or tearing of biopsy
    - Often more pronounced at biopsy edges
    - Hepatic plate atrophy or extravasation of RBC into space of Disse is not seen
  - Transplant liver biopsies
    - Commonly show sinusoidal dilatation in absence of venous outflow obstruction
    - May be related to hemodynamic changes related to vascular anastomosis
  - Regenerative nodules in cirrhosis or adjacent to mass lesions
    - Can lead to adjacent sinusoidal dilatation due to localized venous outflow obstruction
  - Intraoperative biopsies
    - Sinusoidal dilatation is common in biopsies obtained during abdominal surgeries
    - May be due to alterations in portal blood flow during abdominal surgery

Biliary Disease

- Portal changes, such as ductular reaction and lymphocytic inflammation, can occur in HVOO
- Elevation of alkaline phosphatase is also common
- Both of these features can lead to additional suspicion of biliary disease, such as bile duct obstruction or primary biliary cirrhosis
- Normal bile ducts on imaging and negative antimitochondrial antibodies do not support biliary disease

Other Causes of Parenchymal Necrosis/ Hemorrhage

- Acetaminophen toxicity
  - Centrizonal necrosis and absence of inflammation mimics venous outflow obstruction
  - Sinusoidal dilatation may be focal but is not marked
  - Drug history and acetaminophen levels point toward correct diagnosis
- Ischemic liver injury
  - Centrizonal hemorrhage, necrosis, and absence of inflammation mimics venous outflow obstruction
  - Prominent sinusoidal dilatation is usually not present
  - History of cardiogenic or noncardiogenic (septic, hypovolemic) shock, heatstroke is key to diagnosis
- Wilson disease
  - Necrosis without prominent inflammation can be seen
  - Typical features of venous outflow obstruction, such as sinusoidal dilatation and congestion, are not seen
  - Copper studies will lead to correct diagnosis
- Viral hepatitis
  - Herpes simplex and adenoviral hepatitis can lead to hemorrhagic necrosis without significant inflammation
  - Viral inclusions confirmed by immunohistochemistry establish diagnosis

SELECTED REFERENCES

1. Ibarrola C et al: Focal hyperplastic hepatocellular nodules in hepatic venous outflow obstruction: a clinicopathological study of four patients and 24 nodules. Histopathology. 44(2):172-9, 2004
2. Kakar S et al: Histologic changes mimicking biliary disease in liver biopsies with venous outflow impairment. Mod Pathol. 17(7):874-8, 2004
3. Kakar S et al: Sinusoidal dilatation and congestion in liver biopsy: is it always due to venous outflow impairment? Arch Pathol Lab Med. 128(8):901-4, 2004
4. Tanaka M et al: Pathology of the liver in Budd-Chiari syndrome: portal vein thrombosis and the histogenesis of veno-centric cirrhosis, veno-portal cirrhosis, and large regenerative nodules. Hepatology. 27(2):488-96, 1998
5. Wanless IR et al: Role of thrombosis in the pathogenesis of congestive hepatic fibrosis (cardiac cirrhosis). Hepatology. 21(5):1232-7, 1995
6. Dilawari JB et al: Hepatic outflow obstruction (Budd-Chiari syndrome). Experience with 177 patients and a review of the literature. Medicine (Baltimore). 73(1):21-36, 1994
7. Bruguera M et al: Incidence and clinical significance of sinusoidal dilatation in liver biopsies. Gastroenterology. 75(3):474-8, 1978
8. Poulsen H et al: The significance of centrilobular sinusoidal changes in liver biopsies. Scand J Gastroenterol Suppl. 7:103-9, 1970

Microscopic Features

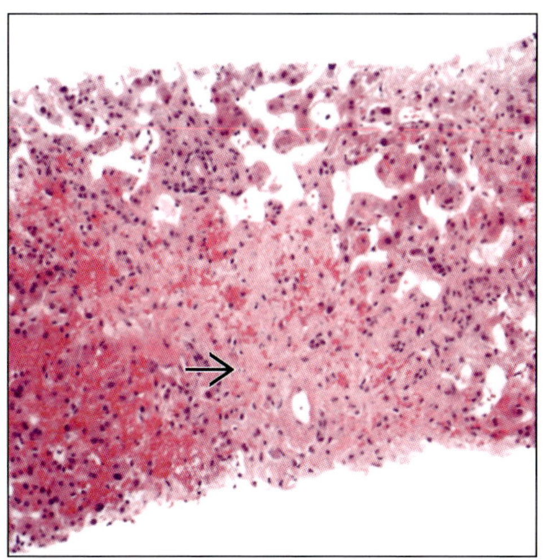

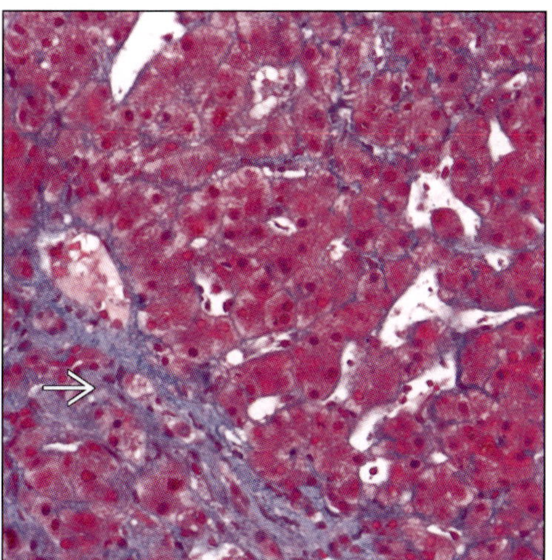

(Left) *Hepatocellular necrosis ⇨ around the central vein can be seen in hepatic venous outflow obstruction, especially in cases presenting acutely. Inflammation is typically mild or absent, unlike centrizonal necrosis seen in autoimmune hepatitis or adverse drug reaction.* ***(Right)*** *Fibrosis around the central vein ➡ can occur in a pericellular fashion in chronic cases. The fibrosis can progress to cirrhosis (cardiac cirrhosis).*

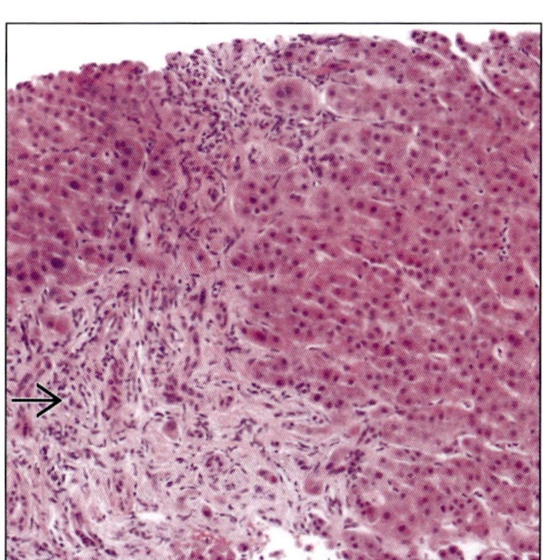

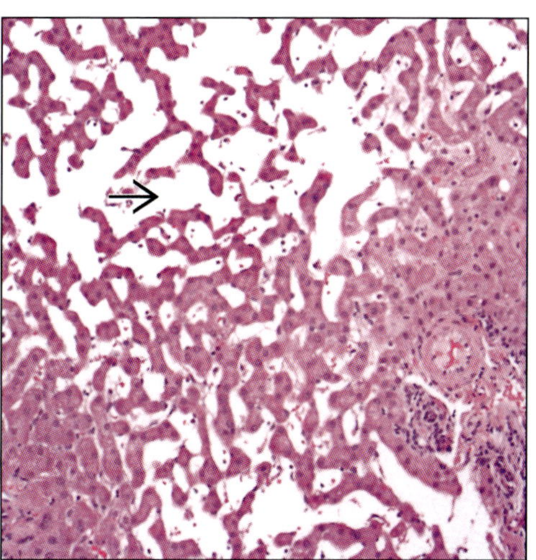

(Left) *Ductular reaction ⇨ can be seen adjacent to portal tracts. It is generally mild but can be prominent, accompanied by portal inflammation &/or focal bile duct damage. These findings can closely mimic biliary disease.* ***(Right)*** *Marked sinusoidal dilatation ⇨ and hepatic plate atrophy are seen in a case of Castleman disease. These features can occur in systemic inflammatory conditions and can mimic venous outflow obstruction.*

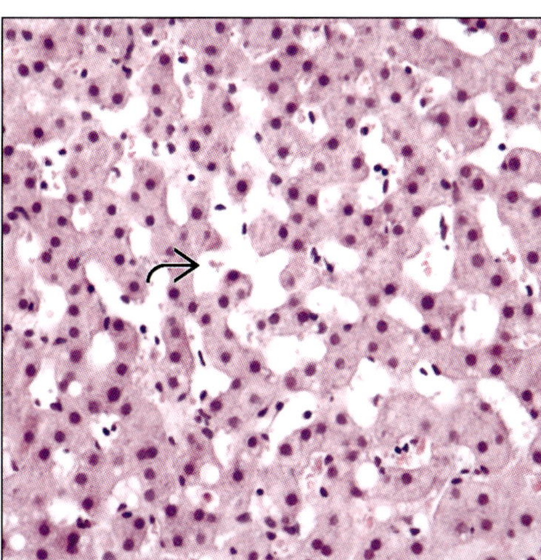

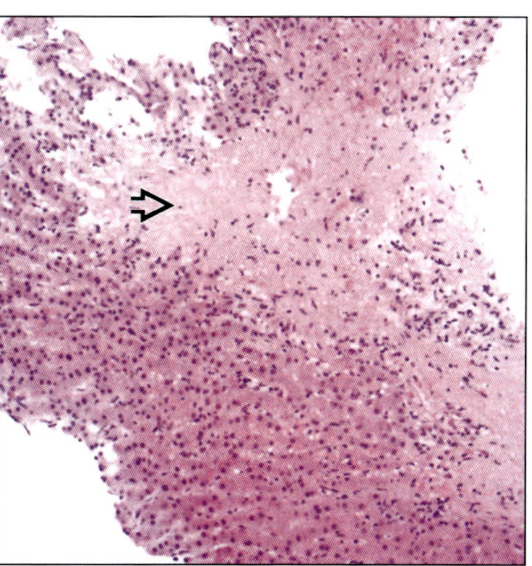

(Left) *Artifactual sinusoidal dilatation ⇨ can be distinguished from hepatic venous outflow obstruction by the lack of centrizonal distribution, hepatic plate atrophy, and RBC extravasation.* ***(Right)*** *Centrizonal necrosis ⇨ without significant inflammation is seen in a case of hepatic ischemia. The sinusoidal dilatation is not prominent. This condition can closely mimic venous outflow obstruction.*

VENO-OCCLUSIVE DISEASE

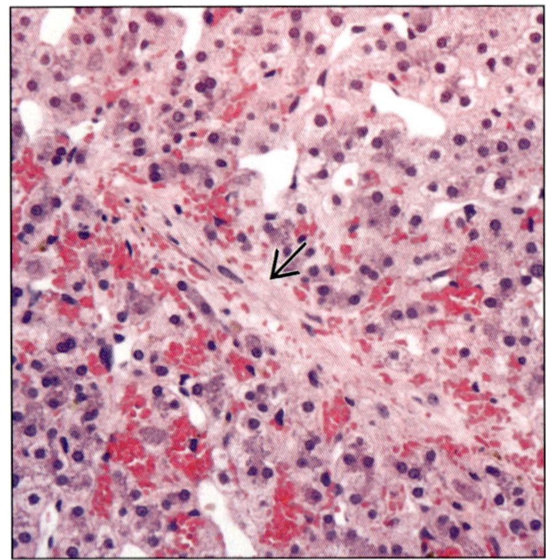

Complete obliteration of the central vein ⇒ accompanied by centrizonal sinusoidal congestion is seen in veno-occlusive disease.

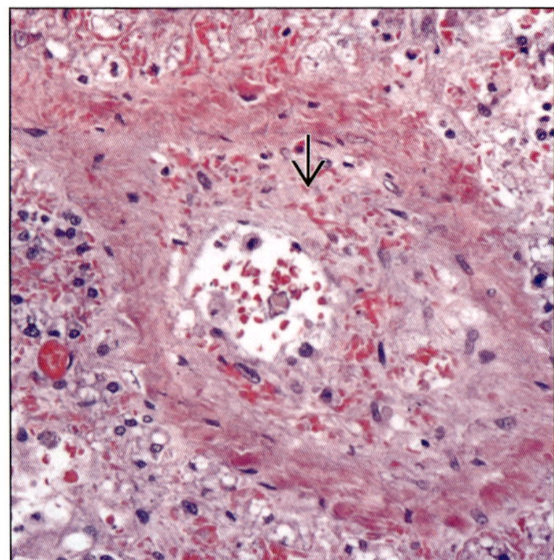

Endothelial swelling with subendothelial edema and fibrosis ⇒ lead to partial occlusion of the lumen of a small hepatic vein in veno-occlusive disease.

TERMINOLOGY

Abbreviations

- Veno-occlusive disease (VOD)

Synonyms

- Sinusoidal obstruction syndrome (SOS)

ETIOLOGY/PATHOGENESIS

Etiology

- Stem cell transplantation and high-dose chemotherapy are most common causes

Risk Factors

- Older age and poor performance status
- HLA disparity in allogeneic stem cell transplant
- Preexisting liver dysfunction
- Prior abdominal radiation
- Pretransplant use of acyclovir or vancomycin
- High-dose busulphan and cyclophosphamide therapy

Pathogenesis

- Injury to sinusoidal endothelial cells is important initial event; hence, preferred term is sinusoidal obstruction syndrome
- Major damage occurs in zone 3, which has high concentration of cytochrome P450 enzymes that metabolize many chemotherapeutic agents
- Depletion of glutathione, also predominantly present in centrizonal location, plays a role in hepatocyte necrosis

CLINICAL ISSUES

Presentation

- SOS in stem cell transplantation
  - Typically occurs in 1st 3 weeks
  - Triad of hyperbilirubinemia, weight gain, and painful hepatomegaly
  - Plasma levels of plasminogen activator inhibitor-1 are often elevated
  - Attenuated or reverse flow in portal vein on Doppler ultrasound
  - Wedged hepatic venous pressure gradient (WHVPG) > 10 mm Hg has 91% specificity and 52% sensitivity

Treatment

- Use of pharmacokinetics to monitor drug levels with intent of minimizing hepatic injury
- Fibrinolytic agents such as recombinant tissue plasminogen activator and anticoagulants like heparin
- Anti-inflammatory agents such as ursodiol and pentoxifylline
- Endothelial protective agents such as prostaglandin E1 and defibrotide
- Glutathione and N-acetyl cysteine supplementation

Prognosis

- Mild disease: No significant adverse effect from liver dysfunction with complete resolution
- Moderate disease: Requiring therapy but with eventual complete resolution
- Severe: Dismal outcome, mortality approaching 100%
- Adverse prognostic factors: Ascites, multiorgan failure, WHVPG > 20 mmHg

MICROSCOPIC PATHOLOGY

Histologic Features

- Liver biopsy is done through transjugular route; percutaneous biopsy is contraindicated given high risk for bleeding
- Changes can be patchy in early disease leading to false-negative results
- Subendothelial edema, red cell extravasation, fibrin deposition in central vein and sinusoids

VENO-OCCLUSIVE DISEASE

Key Facts

Etiology/Pathogenesis
- Stem cell transplantation and high-dose chemotherapy
- Sinusoidal endothelial cell injury is important initial event

Clinical Issues
- Hyperbilirubinemia, weight gain, and painful hepatomegaly
- Attenuated or reverse flow in portal vein on Doppler ultrasound

Microscopic Pathology
- Subendothelial edema, red cell extravasation, fibrin deposition in sinusoids and central vein
- Zone 3 sinusoidal dilatation and hepatocellular necrosis
- Venular obliteration and widespread fibrosis

Causes of Hepatic SOS

Disease Category	Specific Etiologies
Transplant-related	Stem cell or bone marrow transplant, liver transplant (rare)
Chemotherapy/radiation	Oxaliplatin (colorectal cancer metastasis), azathioprine (immunosuppressive), actinomycin D, mithramycin, dacarbazine, cytosine arabinoside, 6-thioguanine, anti-CD33 monoclonal antibody (treatment of leukemia/lymphoma)
Toxins	Pyrrolizidine alkaloids in African bush tea, herbal medications

- Narrowing of venular lumen leads to sinusoidal dilatation and hepatocyte necrosis
- Fibrosis develops in sinusoids and venular wall
- Eventually leads to venular obliteration, extensive hepatocellular necrosis, and widespread fibrosis

DIFFERENTIAL DIAGNOSIS

Acute Graft-vs.-Host Disease
- Also causes acute liver dysfunction after stem cell transplant
- Bile duct damage and apoptosis are not seen in SOS
- Centrizonal hepatocellular damage is not characteristic of GVHD
- Infections

Hepatic Venous Outflow Obstruction
- Venular luminal compromise, obliteration absent in HVOO

SELECTED REFERENCES

1. Palladino M et al: Severe veno-occlusive disease after autologous peripheral blood stem cell transplantation for high-grade non-Hodgkin lymphoma: report of a successfully managed case and a literature review of veno-occlusive disease. Clin Transplant. 22(6):837-41, 2008
2. Karoui M et al: Influence of preoperative chemotherapy on the risk of major hepatectomy for colorectal liver metastases. Ann Surg. 243(1):1-7, 2006
3. Kumar S et al: Hepatic veno-occlusive disease (sinusoidal obstruction syndrome) after hematopoietic stem cell transplantation. Mayo Clin Proc. 78(5):589-98, 2003
4. Wadleigh M et al: Hepatic veno-occlusive disease: pathogenesis, diagnosis and treatment. Curr Opin Hematol. 10(6):451-62, 2003
5. Dhillon AP et al: Hepatic venular stenosis after orthotopic liver transplantation. Hepatology. 19(1):106-11, 1994

IMAGE GALLERY

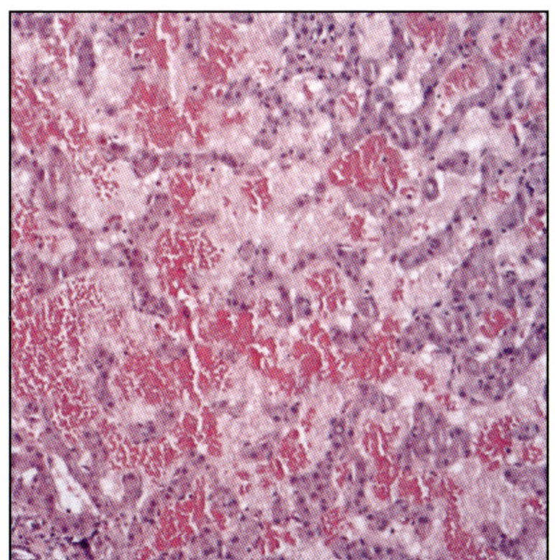
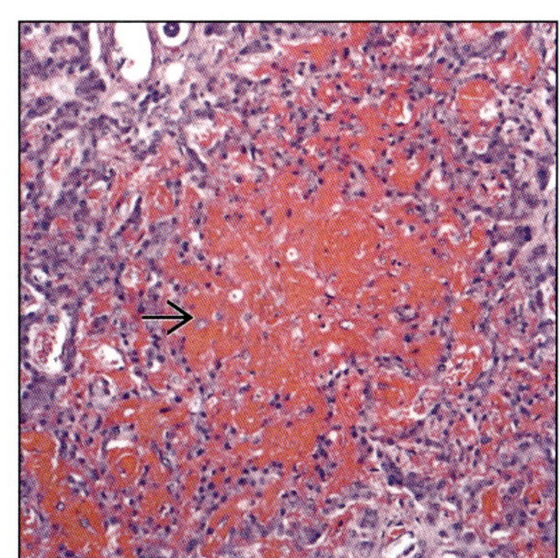
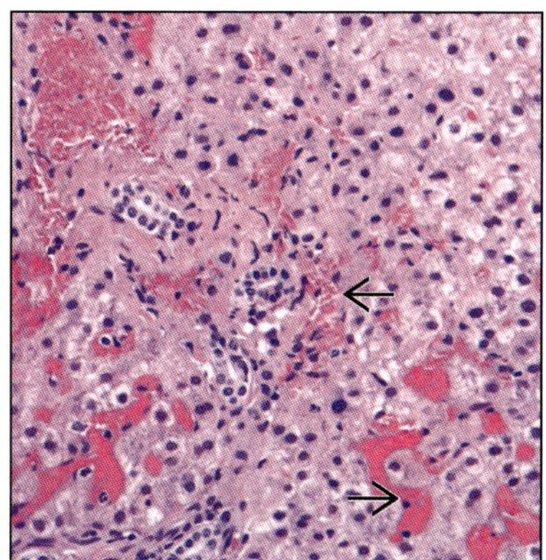

(Left) *Endothelial injury in sinusoids and small hepatic veins leads to venous outflow obstruction that manifests as sinusoidal dilatation, congestion, and hepatic plate atrophy.* ***(Center)*** *Marked congestion in the sinusoids can be accompanied by areas of hemorrhage ⇒.* ***(Right)*** *Sickled red blood cells occluding hepatic sinusoids ⇒ in hepatic sickle cell crisis can mimic SOS.*

AMYLOIDOSIS

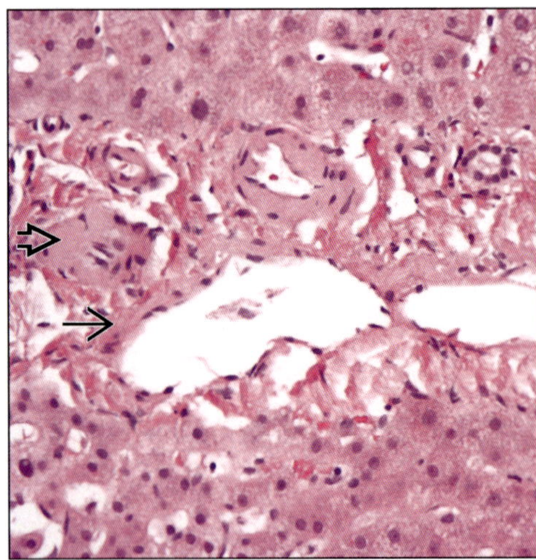

Deposits are seen in the hepatic arteriole ⇨ and portal vein → in the vascular pattern of hepatic amyloidosis. This distribution is characteristic, but not specific, for the AA form.

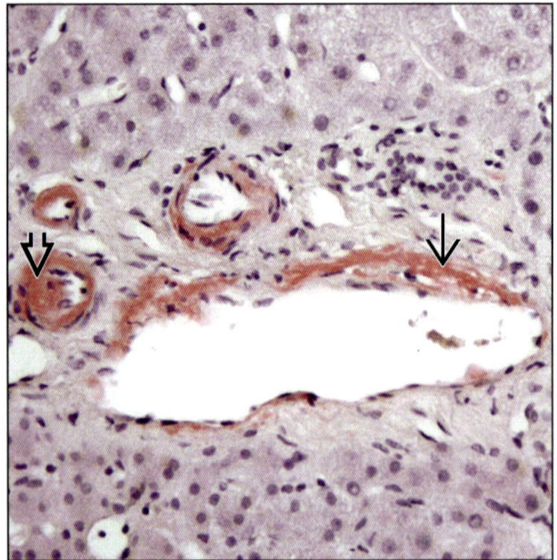

Congo red stain highlights the vascular distribution of amyloid deposits in the hepatic arteriole ⇨ and portal vein →.

TERMINOLOGY

Definitions

- Heterogeneous group of diseases characterized by deposition of glycoprotein fibrils in extracellular matrix and vessel walls
  - Deposits composed of low molecular weight subunits (5-25 KDa) derived from normal serum proteins
- Liver involvement may be seen in all 3 types
  - Primary, or AL, amyloidosis
    - Deposits are composed of fragments of monoclonal light chains
    - Occurs alone or associated with other hematologic diseases (plasmacytoma, multiple myeloma Waldenstrom macroglobulinemia)
    - Liver involved in up to 70% of cases
    - Hepatic involvement reflects advanced disease and denotes poor prognosis
  - Secondary, or AA, amyloidosis
    - Deposits are composed of fragments of serum amyloid A (SAA) protein, an acute phase reactant
    - Often secondary to chronic infections, systemic diseases such as rheumatoid arthritis
  - Hereditary amyloidosis
    - Hereditary AApoAI amyloidosis: Some mutations in apolipoprotein AI can lead to hepatic amyloidosis

CLINICAL ISSUES

Presentation

- May be asymptomatic
- More common in men; mean age: 60 years
- Common symptoms: Weight loss, fatigue, abdominal pain, anorexia, early satiety, nausea, dysgeusia
- Physical findings: Hepatomegaly, ascites, edema, purpura, splenomegaly
- Extrahepatic manifestations of amyloidosis are often present

Laboratory Tests

- Elevated alkaline phosphatase is most common laboratory abnormality (often > 500 IU/L)
- Mild elevation of liver transaminases occurs in 1/3 of cases

Treatment

- High-dose chemotherapy, autologous stem cell transplantation for AL amyloidosis
- Liver transplant for some hereditary cases

Prognosis

- Generally poor
  - Elevated bilirubin and congestive heart failure are adverse prognostic factors

MICROSCOPIC PATHOLOGY

Histologic Features

- Amyloid deposition in sinusoids or vessel walls (both involved in 20% of cases)
  - Sinusoidal pattern more common in AL amyloidosis, vascular pattern in AA
  - Distribution patterns overlap and are not reliable for definite distinction between AL and AA amyloidosis
- Macrophages, multinucleated giant cells can be seen around amyloid deposits
- Mild portal fibrosis can occur, but advanced fibrosis does not occur due to amyloidosis alone
- Congo red stain is gold standard for diagnosis
  - Amyloid deposits are congophilic and show "apple green" birefringence under polarized light
    - In practice, color varies from yellow-green to blue-green and can change with rotation of polarizer/analyzer
    - Different areas of section can demonstrate different colors

AMYLOIDOSIS

Key Facts

Etiology/Pathogenesis

- Liver involvement may be seen in AL, AA, and hereditary amyloidosis

Microscopic Pathology

- Sinusoidal pattern is more common in AL amyloidosis and vascular pattern in AA amyloidosis
- Distribution patterns show overlap and are not reliable for definite distinction between AL and AA amyloidosis
- Amyloid deposits are congophilic and show "apple green" birefringence under polarized light
- Birefringence is best demonstrated by turning light to maximum and pulling color filters out
- Immunohistochemistry for light chains and SAA help in further classification

    - Birefringence is best demonstrated by turning light to maximum and pulling color filters out
    - Thick sections (10 microns) can increase sensitivity
    - Congophilia can be reduced after prolonged fixation
  - Fluorescence microscopy using fluorescein isothiocyanate filter yields yellow fluorescence with Congo red but is not specific for amyloid
- Immunohistochemistry for glycoprotein P component, present in all amyloid deposits, can be helpful
- Immunohistochemistry for specific proteins such as immunoglobulin light chains (AL amyloid) and SAA (AA amyloid) can be done for further classification
  - Background staining can make interpretation difficult
  - Immunoglobulin deposits occasionally seen in amyloid of nonimmunological origin
- Electron microscopy shows central electron-lucent core and nonbranching fibrils of indefinite length with mean diameter of 10 nm

DIFFERENTIAL DIAGNOSIS

Monoclonal Immunoglobulin Deposit Disease (MIDD)

- Deposition of monoclonal protein (M-protein) in tissue
- AL amyloidosis is form of MIDD (distinguished from other forms by Congo red staining)
- Other forms include light chain deposition disease, heavy chain deposition disease, light and heavy chain deposition disease

DIAGNOSTIC CHECKLIST

Clinically Relevant Pathologic Features

- Diagnosis should be suspected in setting of involuntary weight loss, hepatomegaly, unexplained elevated serum alkaline phosphatase level, proteinuria, or evidence for hyposplenism

SELECTED REFERENCES

1. Howie AJ et al: Optical properties of amyloid stained by Congo red: history and mechanisms. Micron. 40(3):285-301, 2009
2. Malnick S et al: The involvement of the liver in systemic diseases. J Clin Gastroenterol. 42(1):69-80, 2008
3. Park MA et al: Primary (AL) hepatic amyloidosis: clinical features and natural history in 98 patients. Medicine (Baltimore). 82(5):291-8, 2003
4. Gertz MA et al: Hepatic amyloidosis: clinical appraisal in 77 patients. Hepatology. 25(1):118-21, 1997
5. Buck FS et al: Hepatic amyloidosis: morphologic differences between systemic AL and AA types. Hum Pathol. 22(9):904-7, 1991
6. Chopra S et al: Hepatic amyloidosis. A histopathologic analysis of primary (AL) and secondary (AA) forms. Am J Pathol. 115(2):186-93, 1984

IMAGE GALLERY

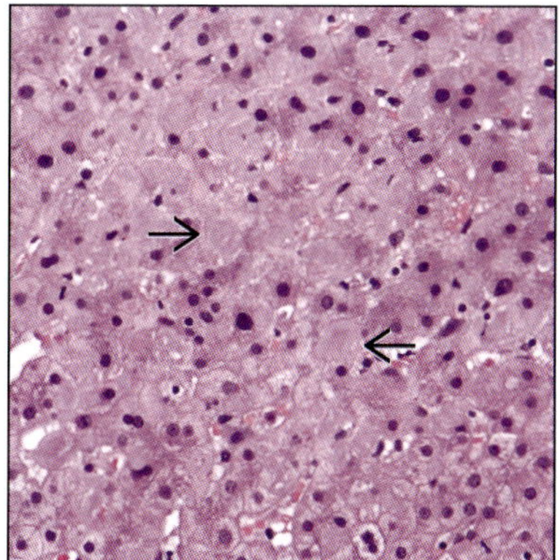

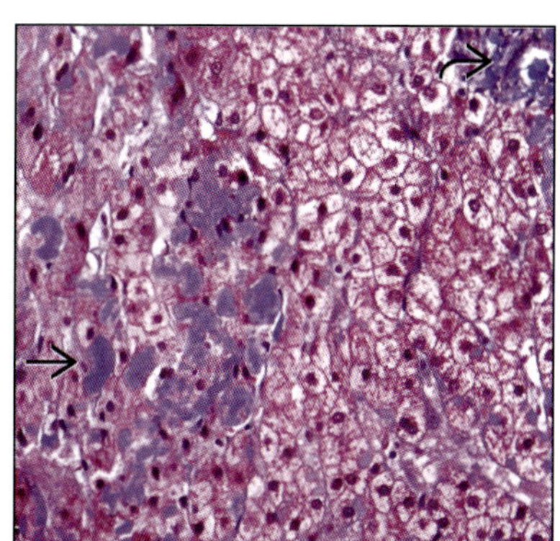

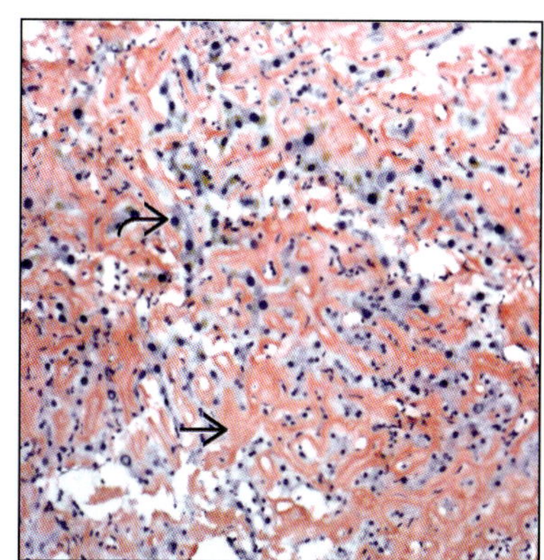

(Left) *The pale globular amyloid ⇒ deposits in the sinusoids can be overlooked on the H&E stain.* ***(Center)*** *Amyloid deposits ⇒ stain with trichrome stain, but it is often a paler staining than that seen with collagen ⇗.* ***(Right)*** *Congo red stain highlights the diffuse sinusoidal pattern ⇒ of hepatic amyloidosis. The amyloid deposits are compressing the hepatocytes ⇗, leading to hepatic plate atrophy.*

ISCHEMIA

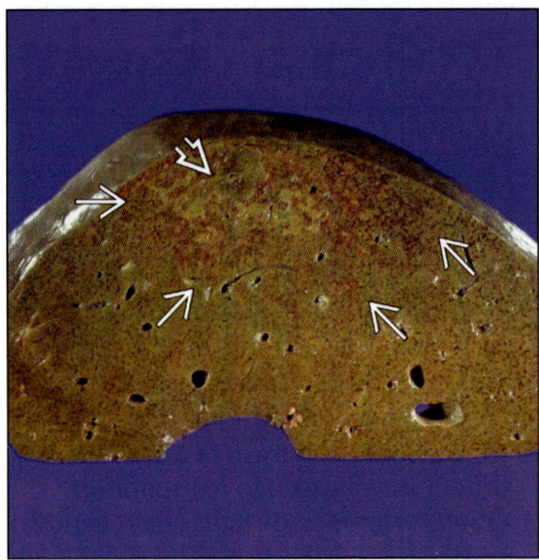

This gross photograph illustrates a subcapsular hepatic infarct. The infarcted area shows variegated red hemorrhagic areas ➡ admixed with necrosis ⇨.

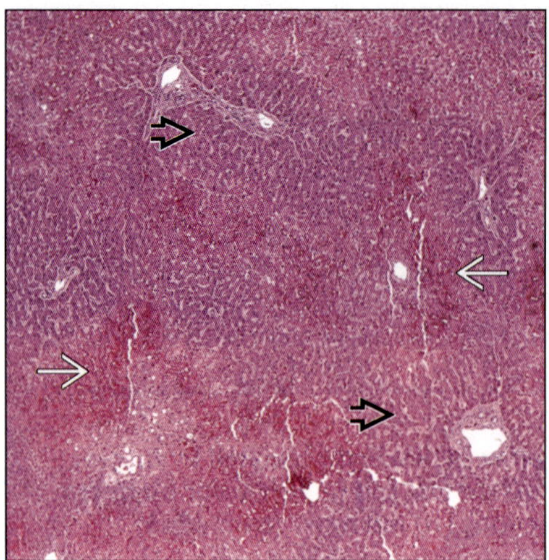

This low-power photomicrograph shows perivenular hemorrhage and necrosis ➡ in a case of hepatic ischemia. The periportal hepatocytes are well preserved ⇨.

TERMINOLOGY

Synonyms

- Ischemic hepatitis
- Shock liver
- Hypoxic hepatitis
- Hepatic infarction

Definitions

- Liver injury due to reduced blood flow

ETIOLOGY/PATHOGENESIS

Systemic Hypotension &/or Hypoxemia

- Cardiac failure
  - Acute myocardial infarction or cardiac surgery
- Circulatory shock due to sepsis, hypovolemia, severe trauma, burns, and other causes

Vascular Obstruction

- Caused by stasis, endothelial injury, and hypercoagulable state
  - 1 or more vessels may be involved
- In transplant patients, anastomotic complications lead to vascular thromboses
- In native livers, usually require obstruction of 2 vessels to result in clinically significant ischemia
  - Greater collateralization present in native livers, but allografts subject to injury with single vessel obstruction

CLINICAL ISSUES

Presentation

- Often asymptomatic
- May exhibit mild jaundice
- Severely affected patients may present with acute liver failure

Laboratory Tests

- Rapid and extreme rise in serum aminotransferases, often identified by screening laboratory tests
  - May be followed by liver failure
  - If patient survives, enzymes then normalize rapidly
- Marked elevation of lactate dehydrogenase (LDH)

Treatment

- Treat underlying cause of ischemia
- Supportive care

Prognosis

- Depends on duration and extent of liver injury
  - In severe cases, often accompanied by multisystem organ failure and poor prognosis
- Most cases are brief and followed by recovery
  - Many cases are likely subclinical
- Hepatic abscess may occur if necrotic tissue is colonized by organisms

MACROSCOPIC FEATURES

General Features

- Variably present gross abnormalities
- Infarcts evident as hyperemic areas
- "Nutmeg liver"
  - Serpiginous, red discoloration representing zones of necrosis and hemorrhage
  - Common autopsy finding

MICROSCOPIC PATHOLOGY

Histologic Features

- Range of findings, depending on location and extent of ischemic insult
  - Different regions of liver can be variably affected
  - Needle biopsies may not be representative of extent or severity of ischemic injury

ISCHEMIA

Key Facts

Terminology
- Ischemic hepatitis, hepatic infarction, and shock liver

Etiology/Pathogenesis
- Cardiac failure
- Circulatory shock due to sepsis, hypovolemia, severe trauma, burns, and other causes
- Vascular thromboses due to stasis, endothelial injury, and hypercoagulable state
- In transplant patients, anastomotic complications

Clinical Issues
- Often asymptomatic
- Characterized by rapid and extreme rise in serum aminotransferases
- Patients may develop acute liver failure

Microscopic Pathology
- Sharply demarcated zones of coagulative hepatocyte necrosis
- Minimal inflammation

- Sharply demarcated zones of coagulative hepatocyte necrosis
  - Collapse of liver cell plates seen on reticulin stain
  - Sinusoidal congestion
  - May see cholestasis at periphery of necrotic areas
  - With cardiac failure or shock, zone 3/perivenular hepatocytes most often affected
    - May extend into zone 2
  - Zone 1 necrosis more typical of diseases with intravascular fibrin deposition
    - Disseminated intravascular coagulation, toxemia of pregnancy
- Hepatic infarct
  - Ischemic necrosis of 2 or more contiguous and complete acini
- Hepatocyte swelling
- Minimal inflammation
- Aggregates of ceroid pigment-laden macrophages in hepatic lobules following resolution
- Dystrophic calcification may eventually develop

DIFFERENTIAL DIAGNOSIS

Infection
- Also causes confluent hepatocyte necrosis
- In infection, necrotic areas are nonzonal ("geographic" necrosis)
  - Herpes simplex and adenovirus hepatitis cause nonzonal confluent necrosis
  - Viral inclusions can usually be found
    - Immunohistochemical stains may be helpful

Drug-induced Liver Injury
- Acetaminophen and cocaine also cause zone 3 hepatocyte necrosis
- Distinction based on history and other clinical findings

Chronic Passive Congestion
- Causes hepatocyte atrophy and sinusoidal dilatation
- Usually lacks zonal ischemic necrosis, infarcts
- History and laboratory values may be helpful

DIAGNOSTIC CHECKLIST

Clinically Relevant Pathologic Features
- Consider in systemically ill patients or those at risk for thrombosis with rapid, extreme rise in aminotransferases

SELECTED REFERENCES

1. Ebert EC: Hypoxic liver injury. Mayo Clin Proc. 81(9):1232-6, 2006
2. Denis C et al: Acute hypoxic hepatitis ('liver shock'): still a frequently overlooked cardiological diagnosis. Eur J Heart Fail. 6(5):561-5, 2004
3. Giallourakis CC et al: The liver in heart failure. Clin Liver Dis. 6(4):947-67, viii-ix, 2002
4. Seeto RK et al: Ischemic hepatitis: clinical presentation and pathogenesis. Am J Med. 109(2):109-13, 2000

IMAGE GALLERY

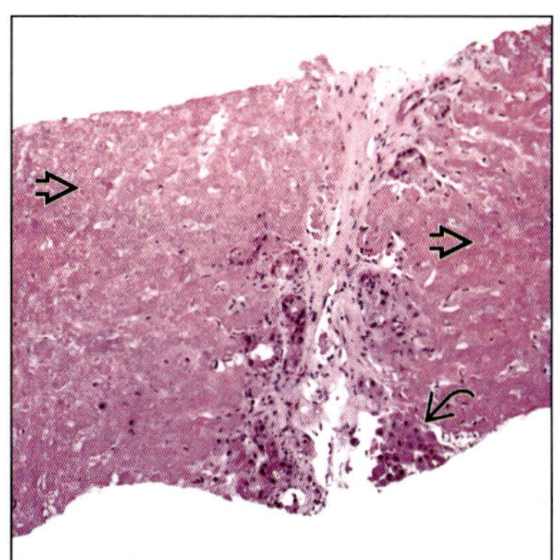

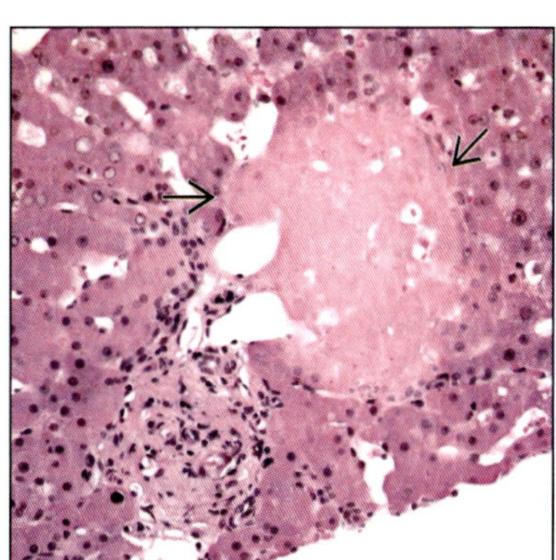

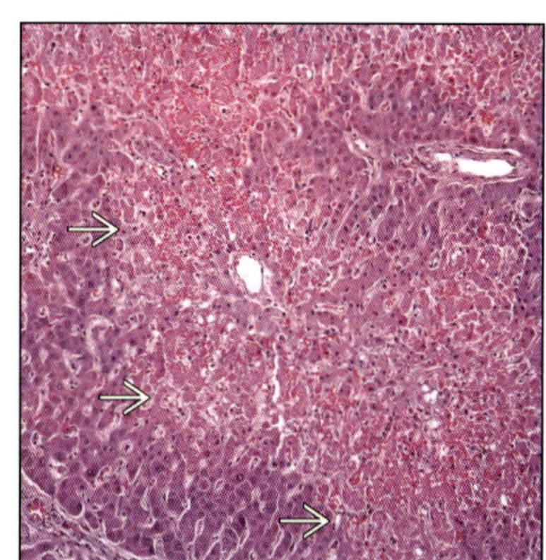

(Left) *This liver biopsy demonstrates confluent hepatocyte necrosis ⇨ involving multiple lobules. The portal tract and a few periportal hepatocytes ⇗ are preserved.* ***(Center)*** *Areas of periportal hepatocyte necrosis → secondary to ischemia are seen on a liver biopsy.* ***(Right)*** *Well-demarcated areas of hepatocyte necrosis and hemorrhage ➡ are seen in hepatic ischemia. The hemorrhage corresponds to red areas seen grossly in "nutmeg liver."*

NODULAR REGENERATIVE HYPERPLASIA

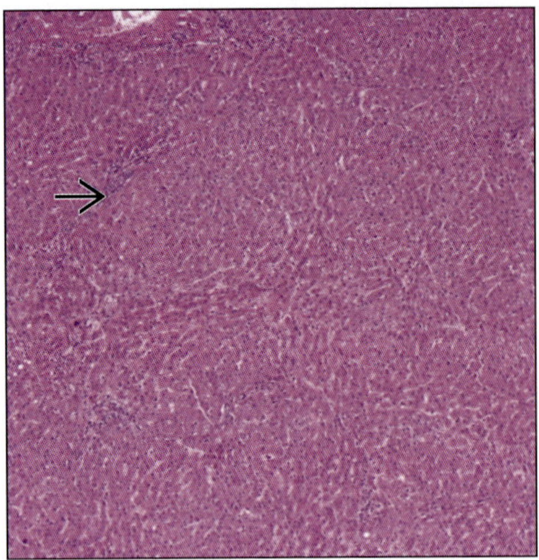

Nodular regenerative hyperplasia is characterized by diffuse replacement of liver by small nodules ➡. Nodules are typically 1-3 mm in size but can be as large as 1 cm.

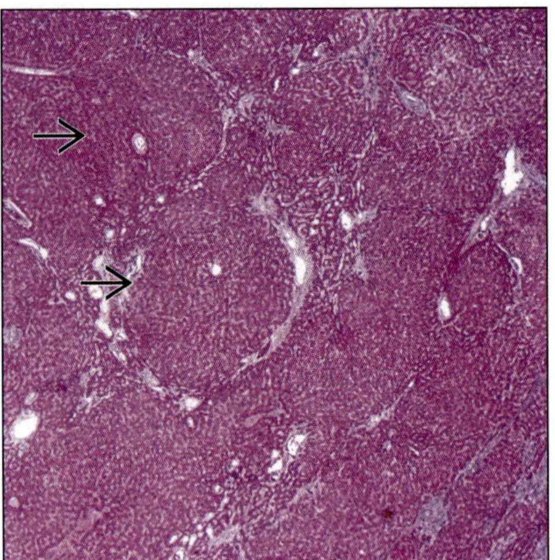

The trichrome stain highlights the nodules ➡. By definition, there are no fibrous septa between the nodules in nodular regenerative hyperplasia.

TERMINOLOGY

Abbreviations

- Nodular regenerative hyperplasia (NRH)

Definitions

- Pattern of liver injury, associated with many underlying causes, that does not represent a specific entity
  - Formation of nodules with minimal or no fibrosis
  - Believed to be related to ischemic atrophy with secondary nodular hyperplasia in areas with good blood flow

ETIOLOGY/PATHOGENESIS

Mechanism

- Results from changes in hepatic blood flow resulting from obliteration of small portal vein radicles
- Obliterative changes in some portal vein radicles lead to localized areas of decreased blood flow and atrophy
- Portal hypertension results from obliterative portal venopathy or sinusoidal compression by nodules

CLINICAL ISSUES

Presentation

- More prevalent in elderly population but can occur in children
- Underlying disease is often clinically evident long before NRH becomes symptomatic
- Symptomatic NRH manifests as portal hypertension and its sequelae: Variceal bleeding, ascites, and splenomegaly

Laboratory Tests

- Liver transaminases and serum bilirubin levels usually normal; alkaline phosphatase elevated in 25% of cases

Treatment

- Identification and treatment of underlying etiology
- Portosystemic shunt for portal hypertension

IMAGE FINDINGS

Radiographic Findings

- CT can be normal or show diffuse nodularity mimicking cirrhosis

MACROSCOPIC FEATURES

General Features

- Diffuse replacement of liver parenchyma by small nodules
  - Most nodules are 1-3 mm but can be larger

MICROSCOPIC PATHOLOGY

Histologic Features

- Diagnosis may be difficult in small biopsies
- Vague, ill-defined, diffuse parenchymal nodules
  - Hepatocytes in nodule arranged in plates that are 1-2 cells thick
  - Hepatocytes between nodules are small and atrophic; often compressed into thin, parallel plates
    - Variation in hepatocytes within and between nodules is best demonstrated on reticulin stain
  - Regenerative features (large nuclei, binucleation) may be seen
- Sinusoidal dilation in areas of hepatocellular atrophy
- There are no fibrous septa between the nodules, but focal sinusoidal or periportal fibrosis can be seen
- Occlusion of small portal vein radicals occlusion can occur; larger portal veins are generally normal
- Inflammation is absent; bile ducts and hepatic arterioles are normal

NODULAR REGENERATIVE HYPERPLASIA

Key Facts

Etiology/Pathogenesis

- NRH results from changes in hepatic blood flow resulting from obliteration of small portal vein radicles

Clinical Issues

- Symptomatic NRH clinically manifests as portal hypertension and its sequelae

Microscopic Pathology

- Diffuse replacement of liver parenchyma by small nodules without fibrous septa

Top Differential Diagnoses

- Fibrous septa around nodules in cirrhosis distinguishes it from NRH

Clinical Settings with Nodular Regenerative Hyperplasia

Disease Category	Specific Etiology
Vascular disorders	Portal vein thrombosis, Budd-Chiari syndrome
Rheumatologic diseases	Rheumatoid arthritis, systemic lupus erythematosus, antiphospholipid syndrome, polyarteritis nodosa
Hematological diseases	Lymphoma, leukemia, myeloproliferative disorders, sickle cell anemia, extramedullary hematopoiesis
Antineoplastic/immunosuppressive drugs	Azathioprine, 6-thioguanine, busulphan, doxorubicin, cyclophosphamide
Other	Primary biliary cirrhosis, cardiac failure, celiac disease

DIFFERENTIAL DIAGNOSIS

Cirrhosis

- Fibrous septa around nodules distinguishes cirrhosis from NRH

Focal Nodular Hyperplasia

- Usually solitary, < 5 cm
- Central scar and fibrous septa with aberrant arterioles and ductular reaction

Adenomatosis

- Varying sized nodules, typically larger than nodules in NRH (several cm)
- Multiple lesions but generally do not involve liver diffusely and uniformly

Partial Nodular Transformation

- Single or multiple nodules at or close to hepatic hilum
- Size of nodules larger than nodules in NRH (3-5 cm)

DIAGNOSTIC CHECKLIST

Pathologic Interpretation Pearls

- Reticulin stain should be obtained in all cases of unexplained portal hypertension

SELECTED REFERENCES

1. Wang HM et al: Nodular regenerative hyperplasia of the liver. J Chin Med Assoc. 71(10):523-7, 2008
2. Reshamwala PA et al: Nodular regenerative hyperplasia: not all nodules are created equal. Hepatology. 44(1):7-14, 2006
3. Shimamatsu K et al: Role of ischemia in causing apoptosis, atrophy, and nodular hyperplasia in human liver. Hepatology. 26(2):343-50, 1997
4. Wanless IR: Micronodular transformation (nodular regenerative hyperplasia) of the liver: a report of 64 cases among 2,500 autopsies and a new classification of benign hepatocellular nodules. Hepatology. 11(5):787-97, 1990

IMAGE GALLERY

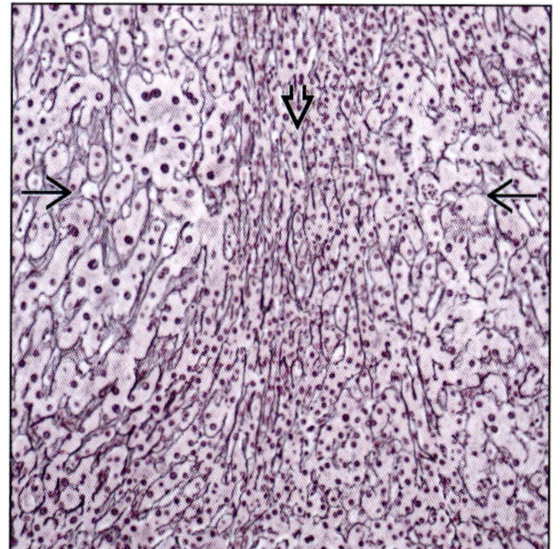

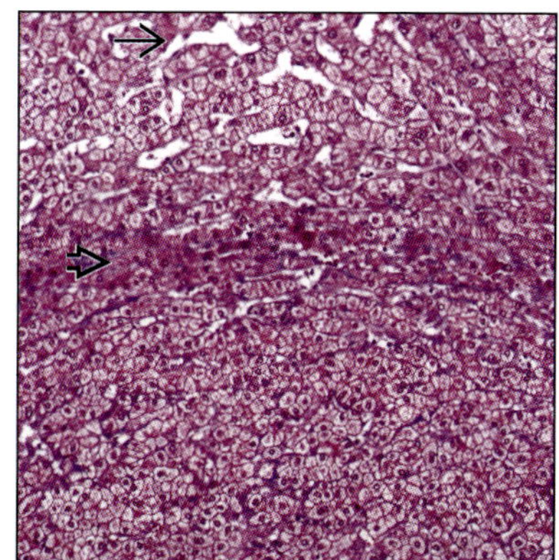

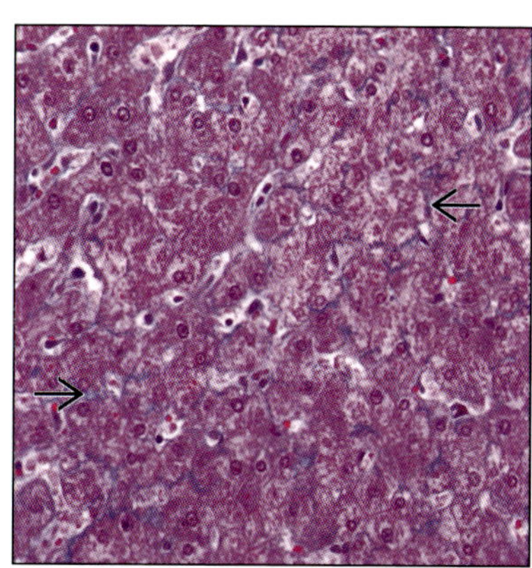

(Left) Reticulin stain highlights the nodules ➔. The reticulin network is compressed in the parenchyma between the nodules ➪. *(Center)* Focal sinusoidal dilatation can be seen in NRH ➔. The hepatocytes between the nodules are compressed and atrophic ➪. *(Right)* Fibrous septa are not present between the nodules, but focal sinusoidal fibrosis ➔ can be seen.

Transplantation Pathology

PRESERVATION INJURY

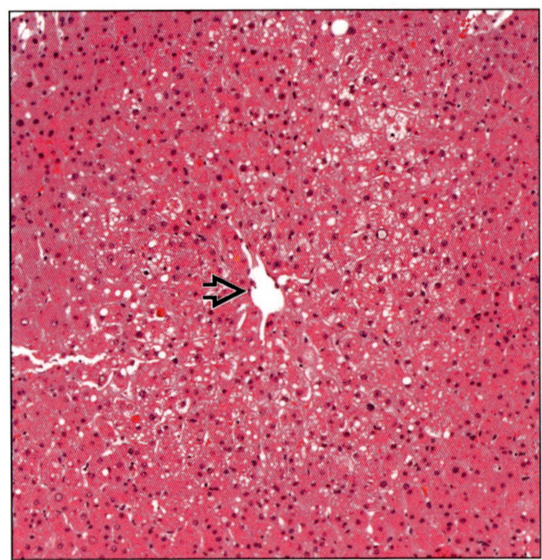

H&E section shows hepatocyte ballooning and steatosis around the terminal hepatic venule ⇨, imparting a distinctive pale appearance at zone 3 on low power.

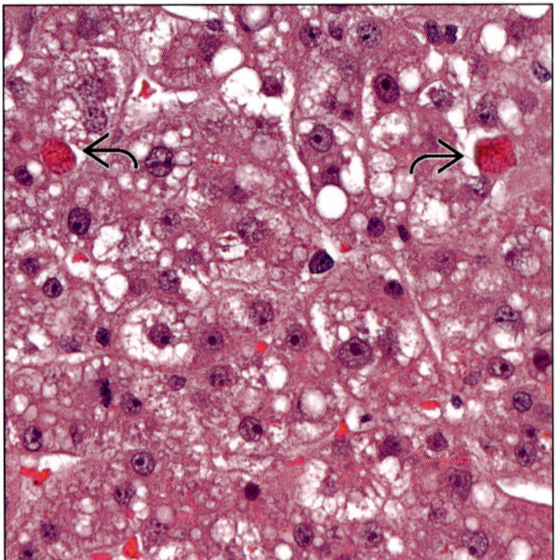

High-power view of preservation injury shows hepatocyte ballooning, microvesicular steatosis, and scattered acidophil bodies ↪ in zone 3.

TERMINOLOGY

Synonyms

- Preservation/reperfusion injury
- Harvesting injury
- Ischemia and reperfusion injury
- Functional cholestasis

Definitions

- Initial graft dysfunction secondary to tissue damage sustained during graft harvesting, preservation, transportation, and reperfusion

ETIOLOGY/PATHOGENESIS

Ischemic Injury

- Occurs in 4 stages
  - Prepreservation injury
  - Cold preservation
  - Rewarming
  - Reperfusion injury
- 2 types of ischemic injury
  - Cold ischemia
    - Prolonged storage in preservation solutions
    - Preferentially targeting sinusoidal endothelial cells
  - Warm ischemia
    - Compromised blood flow to liver at body temperature before and during harvesting
    - Resumption of blood flow after implantation
    - Primarily damaging hepatocytes
- Bile duct epithelium, Kupffer cells, and Ito cells sensitive to both cold ischemia and warm ischemia
- Preexisting donor risk factors
  - Severe macrovesicular steatosis of graft
  - Cardiovascular instability after brain death
  - Prolonged stay in intensive care unit
  - History of alcohol or drug abuse

CLINICAL ISSUES

Presentation

- Elevation of serum transaminases and poor bile production within 1st 24-48 hours after revascularization
- Severity of injury depending on type and duration of ischemic stress
- Enzyme levels typically decreasing progressively within several days if graft survives injury
- Clinical resolution usually observed within 1-4 weeks
- Abnormal liver tests may persist for as long as 3 months if injury is severe

Treatment

- No specific therapy

Prognosis

- Complete resolution in most cases
- Higher incidence of both acute and chronic rejection
- Higher incidence of biliary complications
- Increased severity of recurrent hepatitis C
- Graft failure in rare occasions (primary nonfunction)

MICROSCOPIC PATHOLOGY

Histologic Features

- Zone 3 injury
  - Hepatocyte ballooning, imparting distinctive pale appearance on low power
  - Hepatocyte necrosis and dropout
- Steatosis
  - Microvesicular
  - Pseudopeliotic steatosis, or fat released from damaged steatotic hepatocytes into extracellular spaces
- Biliary/cholestatic changes
  - Cytoplasmic and canalicular cholestasis, more pronounced in zone 3

PRESERVATION INJURY

Key Facts

Clinical Issues

- Elevation of serum transaminases and poor bile production within 24-48 hours after revascularization
- Clinical resolution usually observed within 1-4 weeks
- No specific therapy

Microscopic Pathology

- Zone 3 hepatocyte ballooning, imparting distinctive pale appearance at zone 3 on low-power view
- Zone 3 hepatocyte necrosis and dropout
- Microvesicular steatosis
- Cytoplasmic and canalicular cholestasis, more pronounced at zone 3
- No significant portal inflammation in general

Top Differential Diagnoses

- Antibody-mediated rejection
- Hepatic artery thrombosis
- Biliary obstruction

- Bile duct degeneration and detachment of duct epithelium from basement membrane
- Periportal ductular reaction, sometimes surrounded by neutrophils
- Cholangiolar cholestasis with bile plugs may be seen
- Scattered acidophil bodies
  - Periportal or confluent necrosis in severe cases
- Neutrophilic infiltration of lobules; portal inflammation rare
- Resolving preservation injury features regenerative changes of hepatocytes
  - Nuclear enlargement with frequent binucleation
  - Increased mitotic activity
  - Thickened cell plates
  - Mild ballooning, cytoplasmic cholestasis may persist for several weeks
  - Zone 3 histiocytes and other inflammatory cells

DIFFERENTIAL DIAGNOSIS

Antibody-mediated Rejection

- Preformed donor-reactive antibodies in recipient
- Low complement levels
- Hemorrhagic necrosis of graft with fibrin thrombi
- Fibrinoid necrosis of hepatic artery branches

Hepatic Artery Thrombosis

- Doppler ultrasound and angiography are diagnostic
- Massive or zone 3 coagulative necrosis
- Bile duct necrosis

Hepatic Vein Stenosis and Thrombosis

- Doppler ultrasound and venography are diagnostic
- Resembles Budd-Chiari syndrome clinically
- Zone 3 congestion, hemorrhage, and necrosis

Biliary Obstruction

- Jaundice and acholic stools
- Cholangiography is diagnostic
- Portal edema
- More prominent ductular reaction with neutrophilic infiltration (pericholangitis)

DIAGNOSTIC CHECKLIST

Pathologic Interpretation Pearls

- Zone 3 hepatocyte damage characterized by ballooning, necrosis, and cholestasis

SELECTED REFERENCES

1. Casillas-Ramírez A et al: Past and future approaches to ischemia-reperfusion lesion associated with liver transplantation. Life Sci. 79(20):1881-94, 2006
2. Husted TL et al: The role of cytokines in pharmacological modulation of hepatic ischemia/reperfusion injury. Curr Pharm Des. 12(23):2867-73, 2006
3. Fondevila C et al: Hepatic ischemia/reperfusion injury--a fresh look. Exp Mol Pathol. 74(2):86-93, 2003
4. Khettry U et al: Centrilobular histopathologic changes in liver transplant biopsies. Hum Pathol. 33(3):270-6, 2002

IMAGE GALLERY

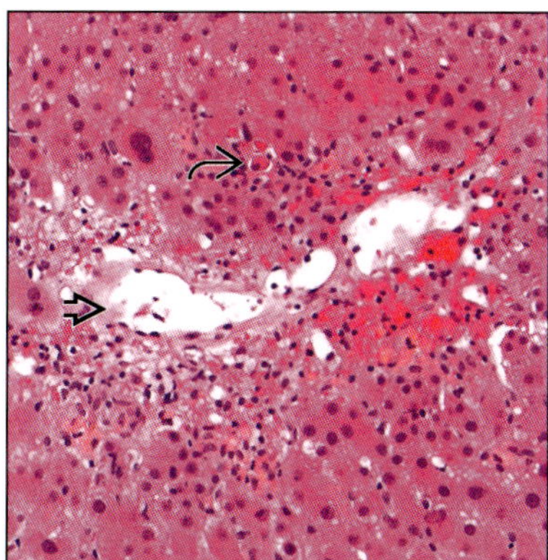

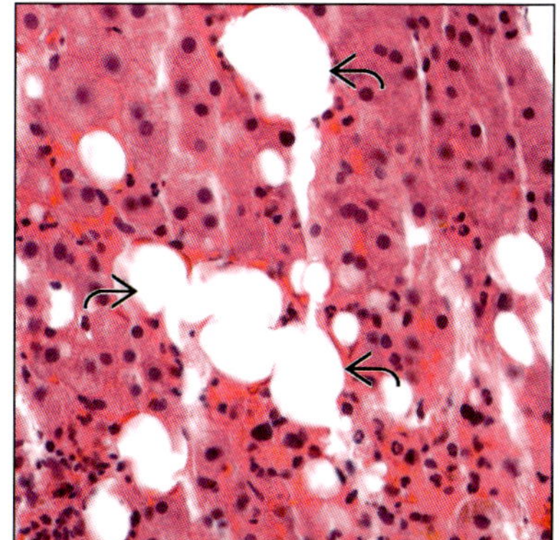

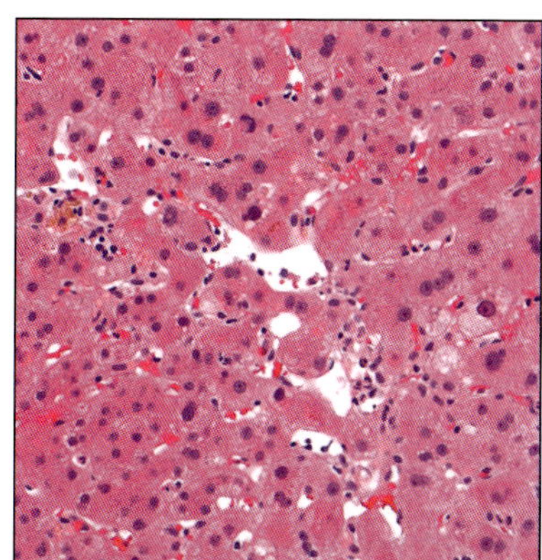

(Left) *Zone 3 necrosis is seen in a case of preservation injury. Note hepatocyte dropout around the terminal hepatic venule ⇨ and the presence of acidophil bodies ↗.* ***(Center)*** *Pseudopeliotic steatosis ↗ is caused by fat release from damaged steatotic hepatocytes.* ***(Right)*** *H&E section shows resolving preservation injury with nuclear enlargement, binucleation of hepatocytes, and mitoses. Note the persistence of hepatocyte ballooning and cholestasis.*

ANTIBODY-MEDIATED REJECTION

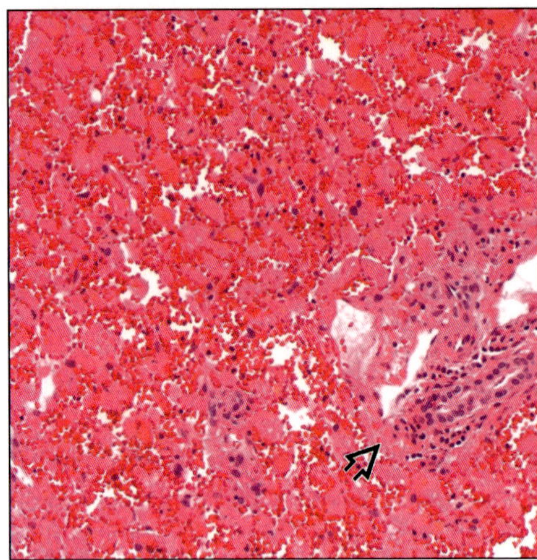

Hyperacute rejection features massive, panacinar hemorrhagic necrosis. A residual portal tract is present ⇨. Note the absence of an inflammatory response.

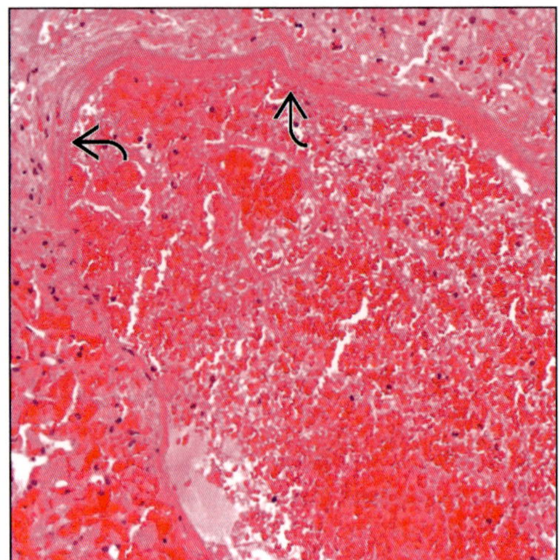

A central vein thrombus is seen in hyperacute rejection. Note the presence of circumferential fibrin deposition ⇨. The adjacent liver parenchyma shows hemorrhagic necrosis.

TERMINOLOGY

Synonyms

- Humoral rejection
- Hyperacute rejection
- Acute humoral rejection

Definitions

- Graft dysfunction and failure mediated by preformed antibodies directed against donor antigens

ETIOLOGY/PATHOGENESIS

Preformed Antibodies

- Major ABO blood group isoagglutinins
- High titer of lymphocytotoxic antibodies (especially IgG class) against MHC class I antigens
- Binding to antigens expressed on endothelial cells
- Fixation and activation of complement elements
- Initiation of clotting cascade
- Impaired blood flow and tissue damage

CLINICAL ISSUES

Epidemiology

- Incidence
  - < 1% in ABO-compatible liver transplants
  - Up to 35% in ABO-incompatible liver transplants
  - Unknown role of humoral mechanisms in conventional acute and chronic rejection

Presentation

- Severe graft dysfunction immediately (hyperacute) or during 1st week (acute) following revascularization
  - Rapid rise in serum liver enzyme and bilirubin levels
  - Consumptive coagulopathy
  - Refractory thrombocytopenia
  - Hypocomplementemia

Laboratory Tests

- Detection of preformed donor-reactive antibodies in recipient or tissue eluates from failed graft
  - Immunofluorescent detection of immunoglobulins (IgG and IgM) and complements (C1q, C3 and C4)
  - Immunohistochemical detection of C4d
    - Staining portal stroma in ABO-incompatible grafts
    - Staining endothelial cells lining sinusoids and vasculature in acute and chronic rejection
    - Specificity under further investigation

Treatment

- Vigorous immunosuppression for ABO-incompatible living donor transplantation
  - Perioperative plasmapheresis
  - Anti-CD20 antibody (rituximab) therapy
  - Splenectomy
- Retransplantation

Prognosis

- Graft failure
- Increased incidence of graft complications in recipients who survive the early insult
  - Biliary complications
  - Hepatic artery complications
  - Conventional acute and chronic rejection

IMAGE FINDINGS

Hepatic Artery Angiogram

- Segmental or diffuse luminal narrowing with poor peripheral filling, indicative of vasospasm

MACROSCOPIC FEATURES

General Features

- Graft rapidly becomes swollen, cyanotic, and mottled following initial short period of normal reperfusion
- Thrombosis in large vessels may be seen

ANTIBODY-MEDIATED REJECTION

Key Facts

Clinical Issues

- Severe graft dysfunction occurring in presensitized recipient immediately or during 1st week after transplantation
- Absence of other causes of ischemia or infarction
- Rare event in ABO-compatible liver transplants

Microscopic Pathology

- Massive hemorrhagic necrosis
- Thrombosis and fibrinoid arteritis
- Portal and periportal edema
- Demonstration of complement &/or immunoglobulin deposits in graft
- Value of C4d immunostain remains controversial

Top Differential Diagnoses

- Primary nonfunction
- Vascular thrombosis
- Preservation injury
- Biliary obstruction

MICROSCOPIC PATHOLOGY

Histologic Features

- Hyperacute rejection
  - Sinusoidal congestion and fibrin deposition
  - Fibrin thrombi in portal and central veins
  - Neutrophilic &/or fibrinoid arteritis
  - Geographic or massive hemorrhagic necrosis
  - Hemorrhage into portal tracts
- Acute humoral rejection
  - Portal and periportal edema and ductular reaction
  - Portal and lobular infiltration by neutrophils and macrophages
  - Zone 3 hepatocyte ballooning and cholestasis
  - Spotty hepatocyte necrosis
  - Lack of significant lymphocyte infiltration

Predominant Pattern/Injury Type

- Hemorrhogic necrosis

DIFFERENTIAL DIAGNOSIS

Primary Nonfunction

- Failure to produce bile and severe coagulopathy immediately following revascularization
- Lack of fibrinoid arteritis

Vascular Thrombosis

- Doppler ultrasound and angiography are diagnostic
- Zone 3 hepatocyte damage

Preservation Injury

- Zone 3 hepatocyte damage
- Progressive resolution

Biliary Obstruction

- Cholangiography is diagnostic
- More pronounced ductular reaction

DIAGNOSTIC CHECKLIST

Clinically Relevant Pathologic Features

- Severe graft dysfunction immediately or during 1st week following revascularization

Pathologic Interpretation Pearls

- Massive hemorrhagic necrosis and thrombosis

SELECTED REFERENCES

1. Bellamy CO et al: C4d immunopositivity is uncommon in ABO-compatible liver allografts, but correlates partially with lymphocytotoxic antibody status. Histopathology. 50(6):739-49, 2007
2. Sakashita H et al: Significance of C4d staining in ABO-identical/compatible liver transplantation. Mod Pathol. 20(6):676-84, 2007
3. Haga H et al: Periportal edema and necrosis as diagnostic histological features of early humoral rejection in ABO-incompatible liver transplantation. Liver Transpl. 10(1):16-27, 2004
4. Terminology for hepatic allograft rejection: International Working Party. Hepatology. 22(2):648-54, 1995

IMAGE GALLERY

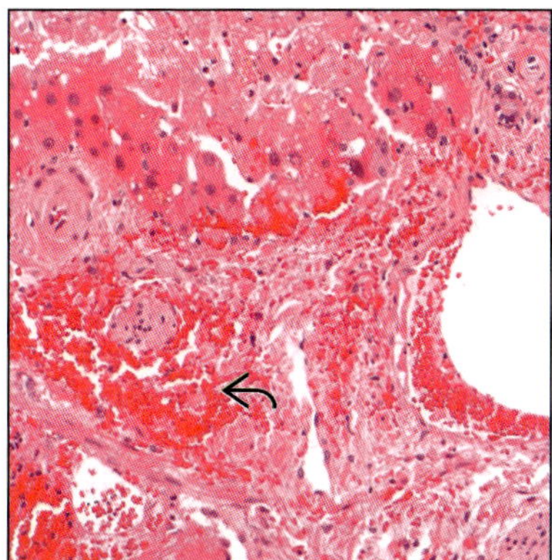

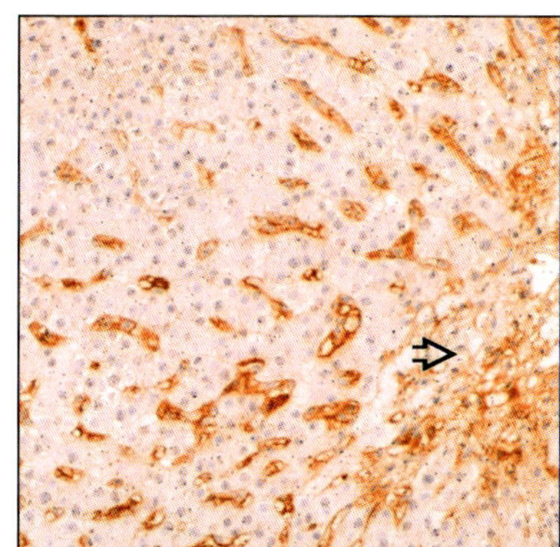

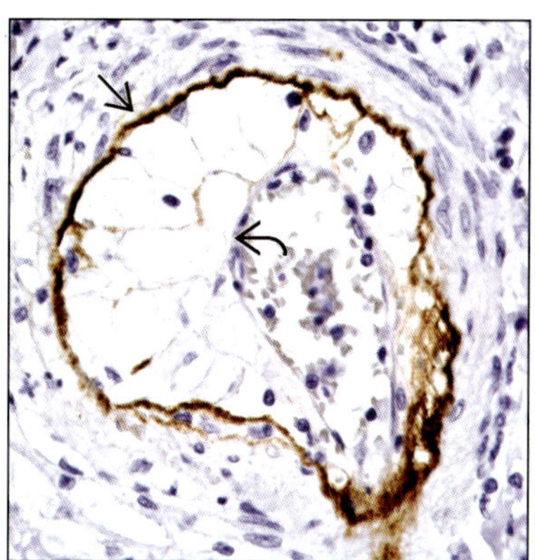

*(**Left**) A slide of hyperacute rejection shows hemorrhage into the portal tract ⮰. Note that few periportal hepatocytes remain viable. (**Center**) C4d immunostain shows sinusoidal deposition in a case of severe acute rejection with central perivenulitis ⮚, suggesting a role for humoral mechanisms. (**Right**) C4d immunostain shows circumferential deposition in an arterial branch → in a case of chronic rejection with obliterative arteriopathy and foamy macrophages ⮰.*

ACUTE CELLULAR REJECTION

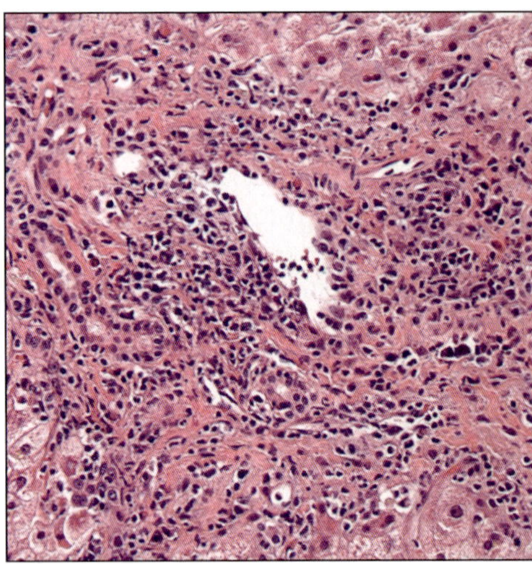

H&E section of acute rejection shows a mixed portal inflammatory cell infiltrate composed of activated-appearing lymphocytes, histiocytes, eosinophils, and other inflammatory cells.

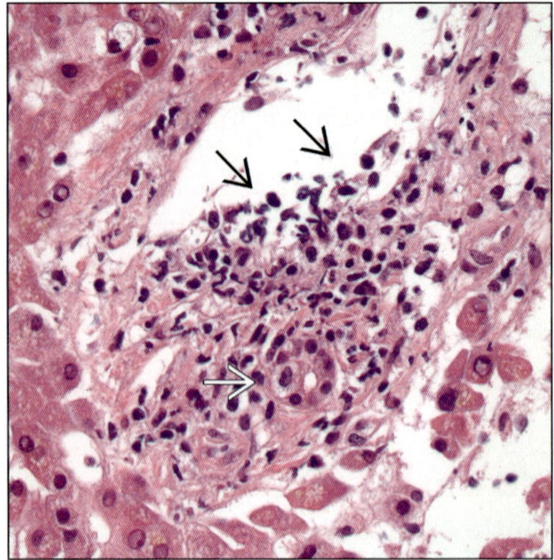

H&E stain demonstrates endotheliitis ⇨ of a portal vein branch and bile duct damage ➡. The portal tract also contains a mixed inflammatory cell infiltrate.

TERMINOLOGY

Abbreviations

- Acute cellular rejection (ACR)

Synonyms

- Acute rejection

Definitions

- Immune-mediated inflammation and injury of liver allograft due to genetic mismatch

ETIOLOGY/PATHOGENESIS

Immune-mediated Inflammatory Process

- Recipient immune system recognizes donor antigens in liver allograft as foreign
- Inflammatory cells in portal tracts and centrilobular, perivenular areas cause damage to biliary epithelium and endothelial cells

CLINICAL ISSUES

Epidemiology

- Incidence
  - Affects approximately 20-40% of liver allograft recipients
  - All liver transplant recipients susceptible, although more frequent in younger, healthier patients
    - Also more common with increased donor age, long cold ischemia time, and immune dysregulation of recipient

Presentation

- Fever
- Abdominal pain
- Hepatomegaly
- Ascites
- Often asymptomatic

Laboratory Tests

- Nonspecific elevation of transaminases, bilirubin, alkaline phosphatase, &/or γ-glutamyl transferase (GGT)

Natural History

- Rapid allograft failure or chronic rejection

Treatment

- Drugs
  - General strategy is to increase immunosuppression
  - Corticosteroids are standard therapy
  - May be managed by adjusting baseline immunosuppression

Prognosis

- Prognosis is very good for treated acute cellular rejection
- Refractory, untreated, or recurrent ACR associated with increased risk of chronic rejection

Timing

- Can occur at any time after transplantation, but most often presents within 1st month

MICROSCOPIC PATHOLOGY

Predominant Pattern/Injury Type

- Inflammatory

Histologic Features

- Mixed portal inflammatory cell infiltrates
  - Mixture of enlarged, activated, or blastic lymphocytes, eosinophils, neutrophils, and macrophages
  - Inflammation predominantly comprised of CD8(+) T lymphocytes
- Bile duct damage
  - Lymphocytic infiltration of interlobular bile ducts

ACUTE CELLULAR REJECTION

Key Facts

Terminology

- Immune-mediated inflammation and injury of liver allograft due to genetic mismatch

Etiology/Pathogenesis

- Inflammatory cells in portal tracts and centrilobular, perivenular areas cause damage to biliary epithelium and endothelial cells

Clinical Issues

- Often asymptomatic but may present with fever or abdominal pain
- Nonspecific elevation of liver function tests
- Can occur at any time after transplantation, but most often presents within 1st month

Microscopic Pathology

- Mixed portal inflammatory cell infiltrates, bile duct damage, and subendothelial venous inflammation

    - Bile duct epithelial cell injury manifests as irregular shape and spacing of nuclei, apoptosis, cytoplasmic eosinophilia, and vacuolization
  - Subendothelial venous inflammation (endotheliitis)
    - Venous inflammation with lifting and denudation of endothelial cells
    - Portal veins &/or hepatic veins may be affected
    - In severe ACR, associated with perivenular parenchymal necrosis
    - Rarely affects hepatic arterioles
    - Central vein endotheliitis may occur as isolated finding
  - At least 2 of these 3 features above required for diagnosis of ACR
  - Necrotizing arteritis is rarely sampled on needle biopsy
  - Central perivenulitis (perivenular inflammation and hepatocyte dropout) may occur with typical portal features of ACR **or** as isolated finding

DIFFERENTIAL DIAGNOSIS

Recurrent Chronic Viral Hepatitis (Hepatitis B or Hepatitis C)

- Only occurs in patients with chronic viral hepatitis
- Can be difficult to distinguish from ACR based on histology
  - Both exhibit portal inflammation and can show endotheliitis
- Features that favor chronic viral hepatitis include more mononuclear portal inflammatory cell infiltrate, interface activity, and foci of lobular inflammation
  - Late ACR can show fewer blastic lymphocytes, less endotheliitis, and more lobular inflammation

Biliary Complications

- Also exhibit portal inflammatory cell infiltrates
- Portal edema is specific feature of biliary obstruction
  - Chronic biliary strictures associated with periportal cholate stasis
- Acute cholangitis shows collections of neutrophils within bile duct lumens

Autoimmune Hepatitis

- Usually exhibits numerous plasma cells, more centrilobular perivenular inflammation, and more mononuclear portal inflammatory cell infiltrates than seen in ACR

Post-transplant Lymphoproliferative Disorders

- Vast majority are B-cell processes whereas ACR exhibits mostly T lymphocytes

SELECTED REFERENCES

1. Hübscher SG: Transplantation pathology. Semin Liver Dis. 29(1):74-90, 2009
2. Banff Working Group et al: Liver biopsy interpretation for causes of late liver allograft dysfunction. Hepatology. 44(2):489-501, 2006

IMAGE GALLERY

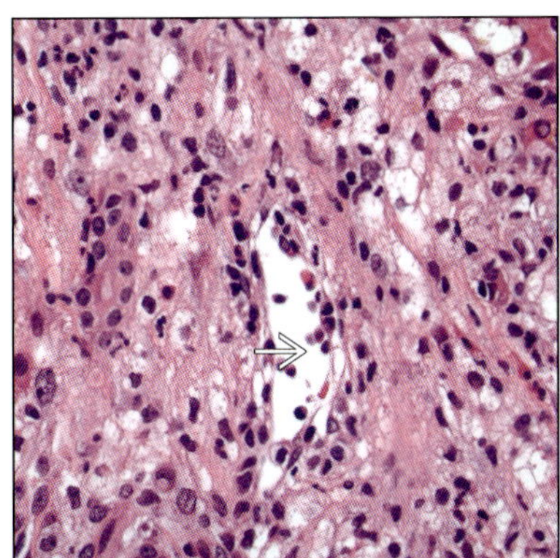

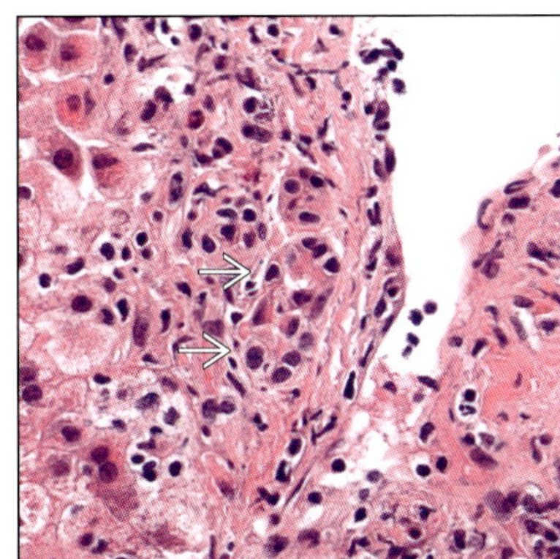

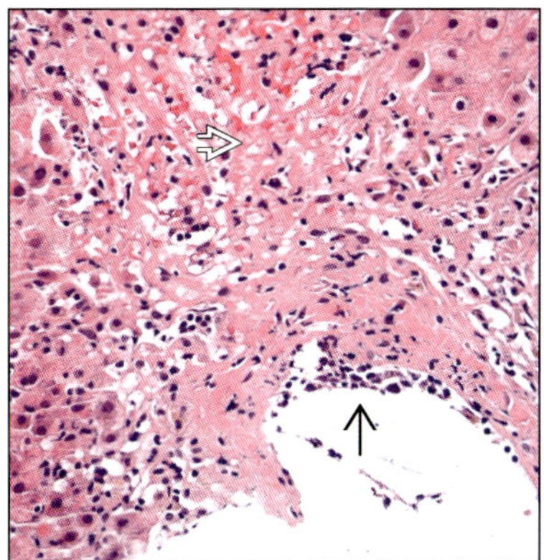

(Left) *H&E section demonstrates endotheliitis. There is inflammation of the vein wall and associated endothelial cell lifting ➡.* ***(Center)*** *H&E stain demonstrates evidence of bile duct damage ➡. The injured duct shows nuclear hyperchromasia, pleomorphism, uneven spacing, and loss of polarity.* ***(Right)*** *H&E section shows endotheliitis ⇨ affecting a terminal hepatic vein and perivenular hepatocyte necrosis ➡ in severe acute rejection.*

CHRONIC REJECTION

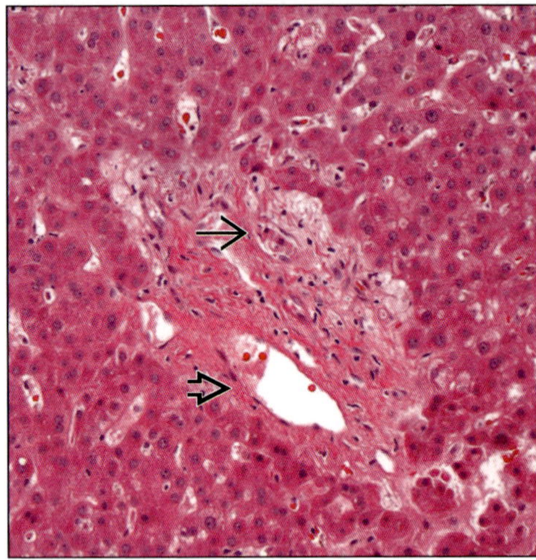

A portal tract in a case of chronic ductopenic rejection contains a hepatic artery ⇒ and portal vein ⇨ but no interlobular bile duct.

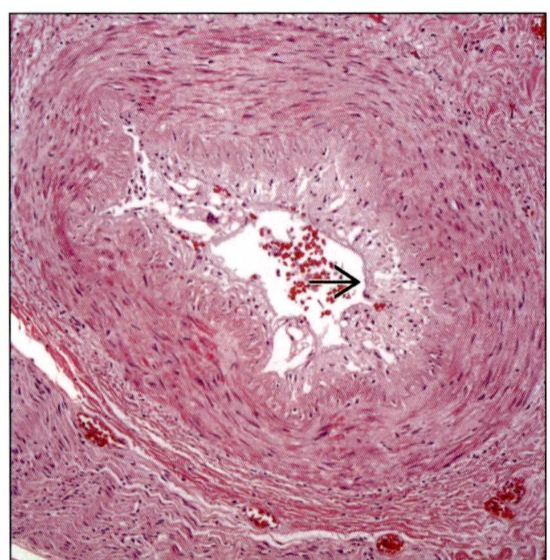

A medium-sized muscular artery shows intimal foam cell arteriopathy ⇒ in chronic rejection.

TERMINOLOGY

Abbreviations

- Chronic rejection (CR)

Synonyms

- Ductopenic rejection

Definitions

- Presents in 2 forms
    - Obliterative (foam cell) arteriopathy
        - Only seen in large- and medium-sized arteries
    - Bile duct loss
        - Most common finding in allograft biopsy

ETIOLOGY/PATHOGENESIS

Immune-mediated Damage to Allograft

- May evolve from severe or repeated acute cellular rejection and result in potentially irreversible damage to interlobular bile ducts &/or endothelium of veins and arteries
- Occurs later than acute cellular rejection

CLINICAL ISSUES

Presentation

- Progressive jaundice and elevated cholestatic enzymes

Treatment

- Early chronic rejection may respond to potent immunosuppressants such as tacrolimus, OKT3, mycophenolate, or rapamycin

Prognosis

- Usually unresponsive to immunosuppression
- Retransplantation often needed

MICROSCOPIC PATHOLOGY

Histologic Features

- Early chronic rejection
    - Lymphocytic cholangitis
    - Atypical bile duct epithelium; may resemble dysplasia
    - Centrizonal perivenular hepatocyte dropout
- Late chronic rejection
    - Loss of interlobular bile ducts
    - Loss of hepatic arteries
    - Foam cell arteriopathy with luminal narrowing by subintimal foam cells
    - Portal inflammation typically decreases over time
    - Perivenular necrosis is common
- Ductopenic rejection
    - > 50% of portal tracts do not have interlobular bile ducts
    - Ideally > 20 portal tracts need to be present in biopsy
    - Serial biopsies may be needed if sample contains fewer than 20 portal tracts
    - PAS stain with diastase digestion or CK7 or CK19 immunohistochemical stains may help identify bile ducts when ductopenia is suspected
    - Cholestasis often prominent
    - Ductular reaction, periportal fibrous expansion usually absent
    - Marked perivenular fibrosis with bridging may develop in late chronic rejection

DIFFERENTIAL DIAGNOSIS

Ischemic Cholangiopathy

- Imaging studies may help
- CR usually lacks secondary biliary features such as ductular proliferation, copper staining

CHRONIC REJECTION

Key Facts

Microscopic Pathology

- Atypical bile duct epithelium resembling dysplasia
- Centrizonal perivenular hepatocyte dropout
- Loss of interlobular bile duct
- Foam cell arteriopathy
- Luminal narrowing by subintimal foam cells
- > 50% of portal tracts do not have interlobular bile ducts in 20 portal tracts examined
- PAS stain with diastase digestion or CK7 or CK19 immunohistochemical stains may help identify bile ducts

Top Differential Diagnoses

- Ischemic cholangiopathy
- Recurrent primary biliary cirrhosis
- Recurrent primary sclerosing cholangitis
- Vanishing bile duct syndrome in drug-induced liver disease

Recurrent Primary Biliary Cirrhosis

- Has florid duct lesions, portal inflammation, and bile ductular reaction
- Positive antimitochondrial antibody (AMA)

Recurrent Primary Sclerosing Cholangitis

- Has characteristic ERCP findings
- Has sclerosing ducts
- Has portal inflammation with bile ductular reaction

Drug-induced Vanishing Bile Duct Syndrome

- History of medications known to cause ductopenia
  - Augmentin
  - Chlorpromazine
  - Phenytoin

DIAGNOSTIC CHECKLIST

Clinically Relevant Pathologic Features

- Previous episodes of severe or persistent acute cellular rejection

Pathologic Interpretation Pearls

- Centrilobular necrosis &/or cholestasis in repeated biopsy specimens should be considered warning sign of possible chronic rejection
- Foam cell arteriopathy typically occurs in medium- or large-sized arteries and is seldom seen in allograft biopsy specimens

SELECTED REFERENCES

1. Lefkowitch JH: Diagnostic issues in liver transplantation pathology. Clin Liver Dis. 6(2):555-70, ix, 2002
2. Demetris A et al: Update of the International Banff Schema for Liver Allograft Rejection: working recommendations for the histopathologic staging and reporting of chronic rejection. An International Panel. Hepatology. 31(3):792-9, 2000
3. Jones KD et al: Interpretation of biopsy findings in the transplant liver. Semin Diagn Pathol. 15(4):306-17, 1998
4. Noack KB et al: Severe ductopenic rejection with features of vanishing bile duct syndrome: clinical, biochemical, and histologic evidence for spontaneous resolution. Transplant Proc. 23(1 Pt 2):1448-51, 1991
5. van Hoek B et al: Recurrence of ductopenic rejection in liver allografts after retransplantation for vanishing bile duct syndrome. Transplant Proc. 23(1 Pt 2):1442-3, 1991
6. Ludwig J et al: Persistent centrilobular necroses in hepatic allografts. Hum Pathol. 21(6):656-61, 1990

IMAGE GALLERY

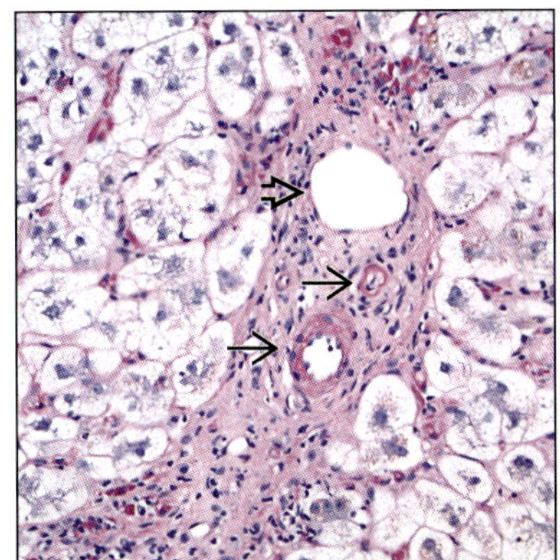

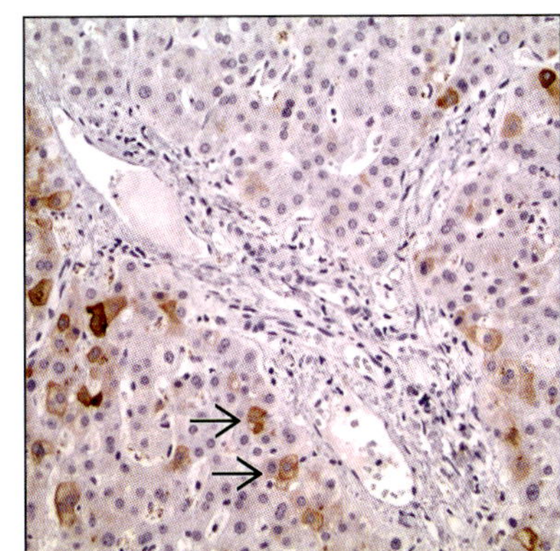

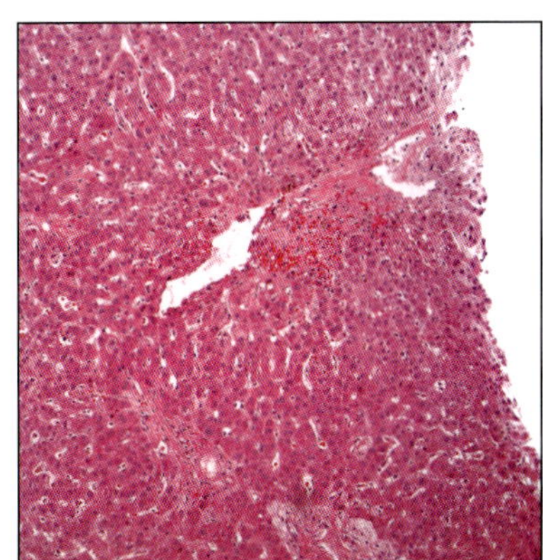

(Left) *PAS stain with diastase digestion in a case of chronic rejection shows the presence of hepatic arterioles ⇒ and portal vein ⇒ but no interlobular bile ducts.* ***(Center)*** *Immunohistochemical stain for CK7 shows cells in the hepatic progenitor cell compartment ⇒ in the periportal region but no interlobular bile ducts.* ***(Right)*** *Centrilobular hepatocellular necrosis may be an early sign of impending chronic rejection.*

HEPATIC ARTERY THROMBOSIS

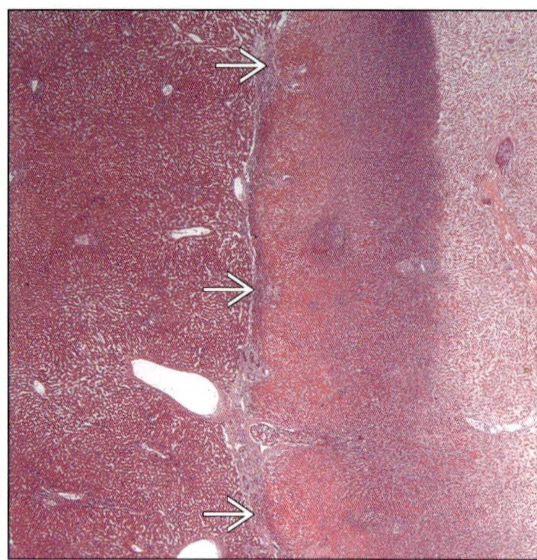

This section demonstrates a well-delineated area of hepatic parenchymal infarction ➔ following hepatic artery thrombosis.

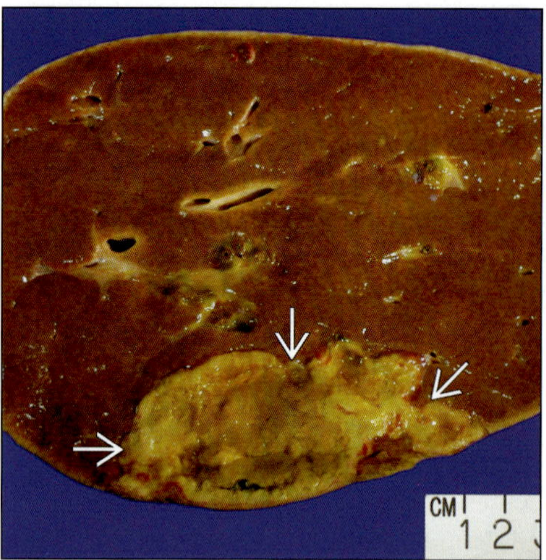

An explanted allograft liver demonstrates an area of bile duct necrosis and a bile leak ➔ in a patient who developed hepatic artery thrombosis after transplantation.

TERMINOLOGY

Abbreviations

- Hepatic artery thrombosis (HAT)

Definitions

- HAT indicates thrombotic occlusion of hepatic artery &/or its branches
- "Ischemic cholangiopathy" refers to bile duct ischemia and complications resulting from HAT or other cause

ETIOLOGY/PATHOGENESIS

Causes of Thrombosis

- Atherosclerosis
- Hypercoagulable state
- Anastomotic complication after liver transplantation
  - Greatest risk with non-heart-beating donors
- Hepatic artery infusion of chemotherapeutic agents

Bile Duct Ischemia

- Bile ducts dependent on arterial flow
  - Acute ischemia leads to biliary ulcers, duct necrosis, and bile leaks
  - Chronic ischemia leads to scarring, strictures, and duct loss

Hepatic Infarction

- Localized ischemia of hepatocytes, bile ducts, and portal connective tissue

CLINICAL ISSUES

Epidemiology

- Incidence
  - Relatively well tolerated in native livers
    - Anastomosing blood supply with good collateralization is protective against ischemic injury
  - Transplanted livers much more susceptible, especially early after transplant
    - Most frequent cause of vascular complications after liver transplant
    - Liver grafts lack anastomosing blood supply and are more dependent on arterial inflow
    - Pediatric and split-liver grafts at greatest risk due to smaller vessels and greater technical difficulty

Presentation

- Varies with clinical setting
- Symptoms related to acuity and ensuing complications
  - Fever
  - Abdominal pain
  - Jaundice
  - Bile peritonitis
  - Fulminant hepatic failure
- Cholestatic liver function abnormalities
  - Elevated bilirubin, alkaline phosphatase, γ-glutamyl transferase

Treatment

- Surgical approaches
  - Arterial thrombectomy
  - Revascularization
  - Liver transplantation/retransplantation

Prognosis

- Long-term complications include ischemic cholangiopathy with stricture and duct loss
- Can lead to fulminant hepatic failure

IMAGE FINDINGS

Radiographic Findings

- Doppler ultrasound used as screening tool
- Computed tomography-angiography used as a confirmatory test

HEPATIC ARTERY THROMBOSIS

Key Facts

Etiology/Pathogenesis

- Thrombosis may result from atherosclerosis, hypercoagulable state, complication after liver transplantation, or infusion of chemotherapeutic agents
- Bile ducts depend on arterial flow and therefore suffer ischemic injury
- Can also cause ischemia of hepatocytes, bile ducts, and portal connective tissue

Microscopic Pathology

- Bile duct necrosis with bile cast formation and bile leakage
- Necrosis of hepatocytes and portal connective tissue
- In time, chronic ischemia can lead to biliary strictures, fibrosis, and duct loss

Diagnostic Checklist

- Needle biopsy may not be representative, as ischemic features may be patchy

MACROSCOPIC FEATURES

General Features

- May appear grossly normal, especially on surface
- Mottled liver parenchyma
- Foci of parenchymal necrosis and bile leak

MICROSCOPIC PATHOLOGY

Histologic Features

- Bile duct necrosis
  - Denuded, necrotic bile duct epithelium
  - Eosinophilic bile casts comprised of sloughed, necrotic biliary epithelial cells
  - Bile leakage into periductal connective tissue
- Necrosis of hepatocytes and portal connective tissue seen in hepatic infarcts
  - May develop secondary infection and abscesses
- In time, ongoing ischemic injury can lead to biliary strictures, fibrosis, and duct loss

DIFFERENTIAL DIAGNOSIS

Primary Sclerosing Cholangitis

- May be indistinguishable from chronic ischemia based on histologic features alone
- Distinct clinical picture
  - Typically young males with history of inflammatory bowel disease

Acute or Chronic Allograft Rejection

- Acute rejection shows typical rejection-type infiltrates and endotheliitis
- Chronic rejection shows senescent duct changes; associated with refractory or untreated acute rejection

Other Biliary Complications

- Biliary obstruction

Ischemic Hepatitis

- More diffuse process with zone 3 hepatocyte injury

DIAGNOSTIC CHECKLIST

Pathologic Interpretation Pearls

- Needle biopsy may not be representative
  - Ischemic features may be patchy, and large ducts often not sampled

SELECTED REFERENCES

1. Adeyi O et al: Liver allograft pathology: approach to interpretation of needle biopsies with clinicopathological correlation. J Clin Pathol. 63(1):47-74, 2010
2. Bekker J et al: Early hepatic artery thrombosis after liver transplantation: a systematic review of the incidence, outcome and risk factors. Am J Transplant. 9(4):746-57, 2009
3. Deltenre P et al: Ischemic cholangiopathy. Semin Liver Dis. 28(3):235-46, 2008

IMAGE GALLERY

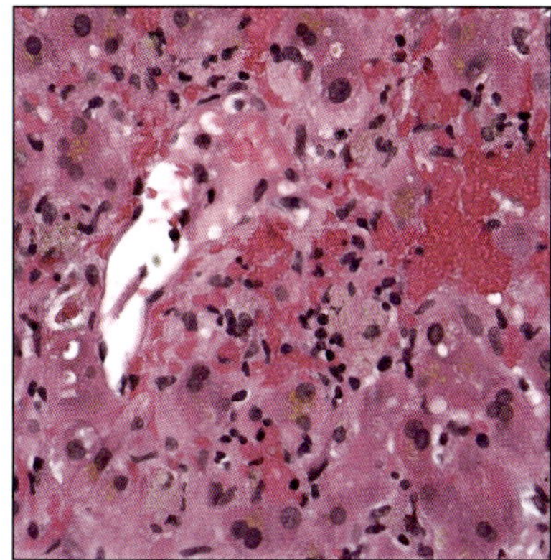

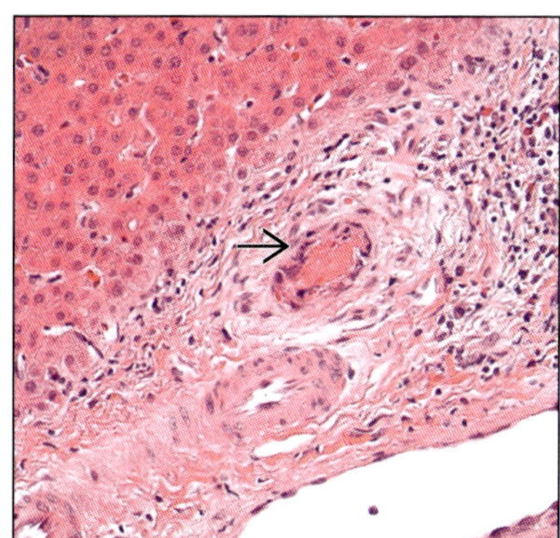

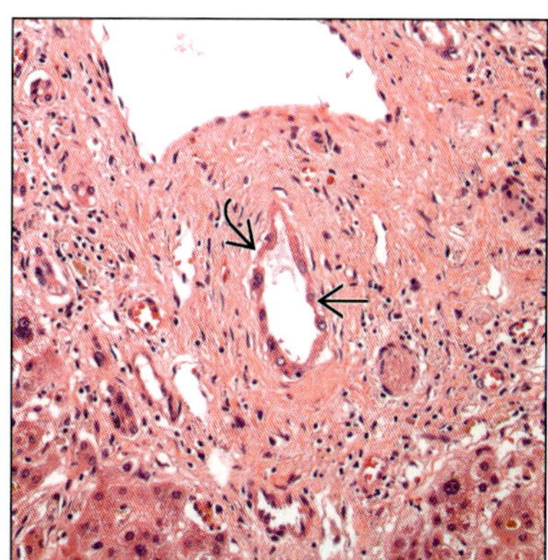

(Left) *This liver biopsy shows zone 3 hemorrhage and hepatocyte dropout in a case of post-transplant hepatic artery thrombosis.* ***(Center)*** *This example of hepatic artery thrombosis shows ischemic bile duct injury with an eosinophilic bile cast* ➔. ***(Right)*** *This example of ischemic biliary damage secondary to HAT shows flattened biliary epithelium* ➔ *and an irregular bile duct lumen* ➚.

GRAFT-VS.-HOST DISEASE

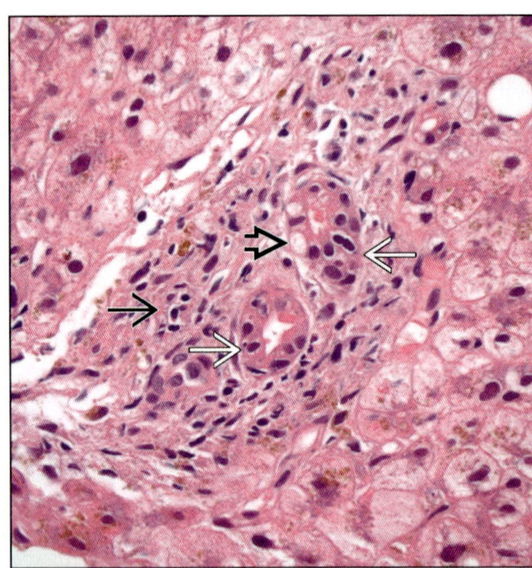

H&E stained slide shows mild portal inflammation ⇨ and bile duct damage in GVHD. The epithelial cells are irregular, unevenly spaced ➡, and show vacuolization ⇨. The duct lumen is irregular.

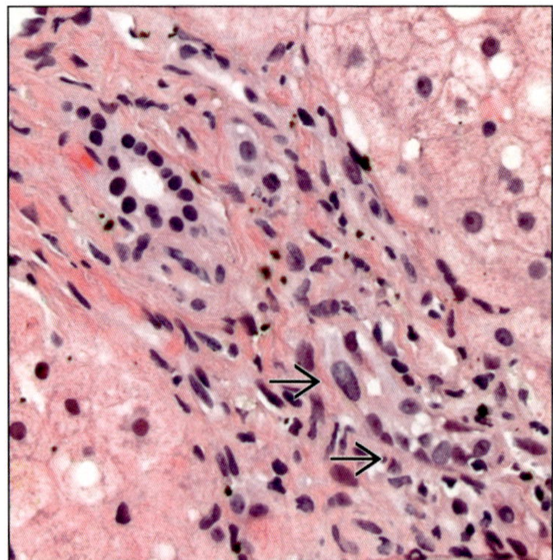

H&E stained section demonstrates portal features of GVHD. The portal inflammation is mild. Bile duct epithelial cell nuclei are pleomorphic, varying in size and polarity, and are unevenly spaced ⇨.

TERMINOLOGY

Abbreviations

- Graft-vs.-host disease (GVHD)

Synonyms

- Vanishing bile duct syndrome
  - Refers to loss of bile ducts in chronic GVHD

Definitions

- Attack of immunocompetent, donor-derived cells against recipient tissues
  - Usually occurs in bone marrow transplant or hematopoietic stem cell transplant recipients
  - Occurs infrequently after solid organ transplant
  - Rarely occurs after blood transfusion

ETIOLOGY/PATHOGENESIS

Immune-mediated

- Donor-derived T-lymphocyte response against immunocompromised host epithelium
- Usually due to graft major histocompatibility complex (MHC) incompatibility
  - Can also occur with autologous and syngeneic grafts
- Immunosuppressed recipient cannot destroy donor cells

CLINICAL ISSUES

Epidemiology

- Incidence
  - Represents major hepatic complication after stem cell transplant
  - Affects up to 70% of hematopoietic stem cell recipients at some point in their course

Presentation

- Jaundice
- Hepatomegaly
- Elevated liver function tests
  - Elevated serum alkaline phosphatase and bilirubin
  - Transaminases may also be elevated
- Acute GVHD may also be accompanied by manifestations of skin or GI tract involvement
  - Rash, diarrhea, weight loss
- Chronic GVHD often presents with widespread disease
  - Wasting disease, with salivary gland, oral, ocular, and musculoskeletal involvement
- Hepatic failure and coagulopathy with advanced disease

Natural History

- Acute and chronic forms defined clinically
  - Acute GVHD occurs < 100 days after transplant, usually between 7-50 days
  - Chronic GVHD occurs > 100 days after transplant
  - No clear dichotomy between acute and chronic GVHD with respect to liver histology

Treatment

- Drugs
  - Treatment strategy is increased immunosuppression
  - Corticosteroids are first-line therapy
  - Ursodeoxycholic acid used for prophylaxis

Prognosis

- Acute GVHD fatal in < 5% of patients
- Persistent jaundice is poor prognostic sign

MICROSCOPIC PATHOLOGY

Histologic Features

- Bile duct epithelial cell damage
  - Key feature that distinguishes GVHD from other forms of hepatic injury
    - Damage of > 50% of ducts with minimal inflammation or duct loss (< 80% of portal tracts

GRAFT-VS.-HOST DISEASE

Key Facts

Terminology

- Attack of immunocompetent, donor-derived cells against recipient tissues

Etiology/Pathogenesis

- Donor-derived T-lymphocyte response against immunocompromised host epithelium
- Immunosuppressed recipient cannot destroy donor cells

Clinical Issues

- Represents major hepatic complication after stem cell transplant

Microscopic Pathology

- Bile duct epithelial cell damage
- Portal inflammation, typically mild
- Endotheliitis in some cases

contain duct) is considered highly suggestive of GVHD
  - Lymphocytic infiltration of bile ducts
  - Epithelial cell vacuolization and attenuation
  - Withering, sloughing, and necrosis of biliary epithelial cells
  - Ductopenia with progression to chronic disease
- Endotheliitis
  - Not seen in all cases
- Other nonspecific changes
  - Portal inflammation, typically mild
  - Cholestasis
  - Hepatocyte swelling or apoptosis
  - Lobular inflammation
  - Fibrosis with chronic disease
- Histologic findings may be focal
- Acute hepatitis pattern also described in up to 25% of patients

DIFFERENTIAL DIAGNOSIS

Drug-induced Liver Injury

- Cause of elevated bilirubin but not usually biopsied
- Cyclosporine causes mild hyperbilirubinemia by inhibiting canalicular bile transport
- Tacrolimus and other drugs can cause liver dysfunction

Cholangitis Lenta

- Hyperbilirubinemia occurring in patients with neutropenia and fever
- Affected patients may also be septic or have localized infections
- Attributed to hepatocyte retention of conjugated bilirubin

Infections (Fungal, Bacterial, Viral)

- Clinical differential but usually distinct histologically

Biliary Obstruction

- Imaging studies helpful to exclude obstruction
- Portal edema, neutrophilic infiltrate, and bile infarcts favor obstruction
- Bile duct proliferation is not feature of GVHD

Post-transplant Lymphoproliferative Disorder

- More prominent lymphocytic infiltrates

SELECTED REFERENCES

1. McDonald GB: Hepatobiliary complications of hematopoietic cell transplantation, 40 years on. Hepatology. 51(4):1450-60, 2010
2. Quaglia A et al: Histopathology of graft versus host disease of the liver. Histopathology. 50(6):727-38, 2007
3. Shulman HM et al: Histopathologic diagnosis of chronic graft-versus-host disease: National Institutes of Health Consensus Development Project on Criteria for Clinical Trials in Chronic Graft-versus-Host Disease: II. Pathology Working Group Report. Biol Blood Marrow Transplant. 12(1):31-47, 2006

IMAGE GALLERY

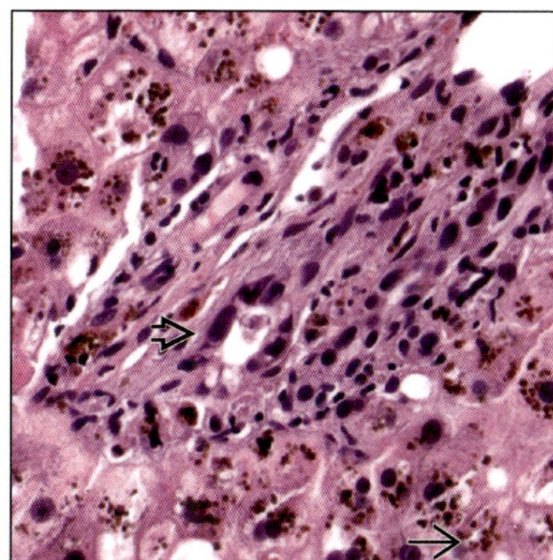
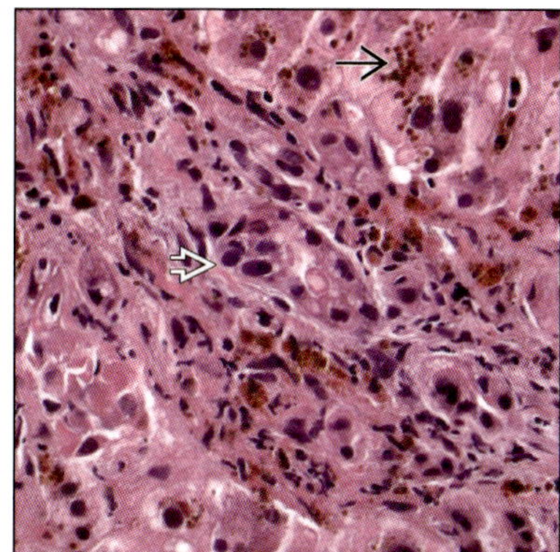
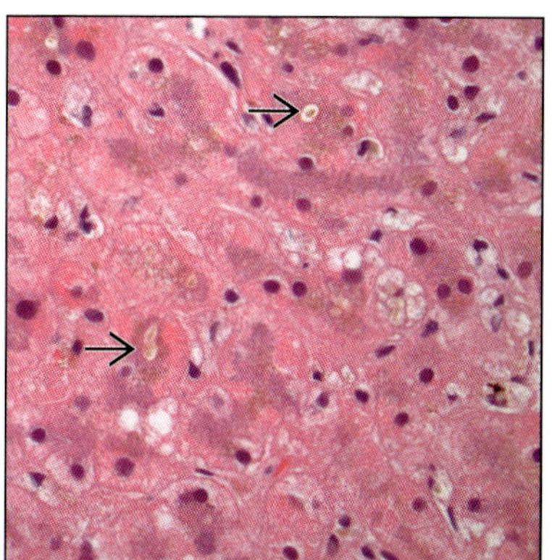

(Left) *H&E stained slide shows mild portal inflammation and biliary epithelial cell injury ⇨. Iron overload is often seen → in stem cell transplant recipients.* ***(Center)*** *H&E stained section demonstrates mild portal inflammation and marked biliary epithelial cell injury ➡ in GVHD. Also noted is iron overload →.* ***(Right)*** *H&E stained slide shows nonspecific lobular changes seen in GVHD, including cholestasis →, mild inflammation, and hepatocyte swelling.*

Tumors of the Liver

HEPATIC ADENOMA

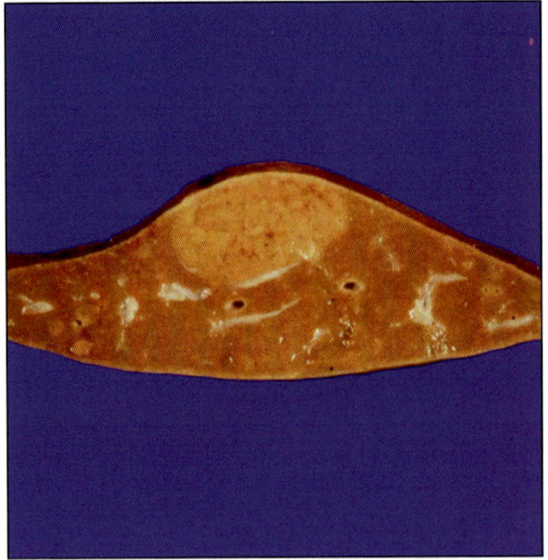

This partial hepatectomy specimen shows a well-circumscribed yellow-tan adenoma under the capsule, in a background of noncirrhotic liver.

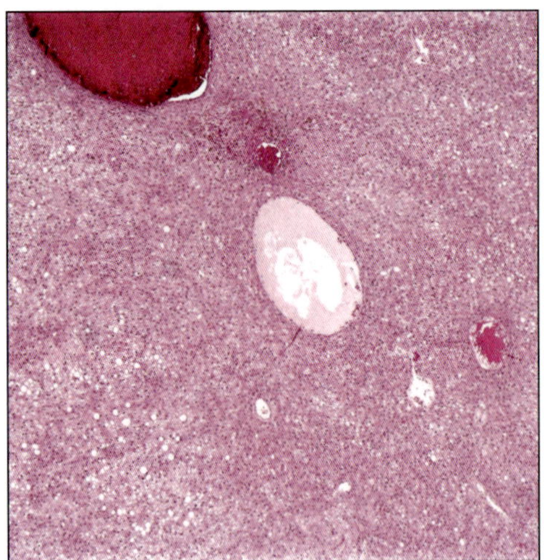

This low-power photomicrograph of hepatic adenoma shows sheets of benign tumor cells with numerous thin-walled unpaired vessels.

TERMINOLOGY

Definitions

- Benign liver neoplasm composed of cells of hepatocytic origin

ETIOLOGY/PATHOGENESIS

Definite Mechanism Unclear

- Sex hormones appear to play a role
  - Almost always associated with oral contraceptive or long-term steroid use
  - Also associated with glycogen storage disease types I and III, galactosemia, tyrosinemia

CLINICAL ISSUES

Epidemiology

- Age
  - Reproductive age
- Gender
  - Typically in women

Presentation

- Liver mass
  - Arising in noncirrhotic liver
  - Often without underlying liver disease
  - Associated with oral contraceptive use
    - May regress after withdrawal of oral contraceptives
- Symptoms
  - Abdominal pain
    - Acute, intermittent, or chronic
- May be asymptomatic; found on imaging (20% of cases)

Laboratory Tests

- Serum liver tests usually normal
- α-fetoprotein normal

Treatment

- Stop oral contraceptives
- Embolization
- Surgical resection
  - Often favored considering risks of bleeding, rupture, and malignant transformation
- Liver transplantation in unresectable cases

Prognosis

- Surgical resection may be indicated if lesion is symptomatic or increases in size
  - Complete surgical resection should be curative
- Complications
  - Bleeding
  - Rupture
    - Pregnancy is risk factor for rupture
  - Rarely, malignant transformation
    - May be associated with β-*catenin* mutation

MACROSCOPIC FEATURES

General Features

- Unencapsulated, well-demarcated mass
  - Typically solitary but may be multiple
  - Tan to brown, may have hemorrhage or necrosis
  - Often subcapsular and bulge from surface

Size

- 5-15 cm but may be up to 30 cm

MICROSCOPIC PATHOLOGY

Histologic Features

- Background of noncirrhotic liver
- Cords or sheets of benign hepatocytes
  - Low nuclear to cytoplasmic ratio
  - Regular and uniform nuclei, lack prominent nucleoli
  - Mitoses are rare
  - Fat and glycogen may be abundant in tumor cells

HEPATIC ADENOMA

Key Facts

Etiology/Pathogenesis

- Almost always associated with oral contraceptive or long-term steroid use
  - May regress after withdrawal of oral contraceptives

Clinical Issues

- Typically in women of reproductive age
  - Noncirrhotic background liver
- Symptoms
  - Abdominal pain; acute, intermittent, or chronic
- Complications
  - Bleeding
  - Rupture; pregnancy is risk factor
  - Slight chance of malignant transformation

Microscopic Pathology

- Cords or sheets of benign hepatocytes with uniform nuclei
  - Low nuclear to cytoplasmic ratio
- Portal structures lacking
- Numerous unpaired arteries
- Intact reticulin framework
- Hemorrhage &/or infarcts may be present with hemosiderin-laden macrophages or fibrotic regions

Top Differential Diagnoses

- Hepatocellular carcinoma
- Focal nodular hyperplasia
- Nodular regenerative hyperplasia

  - Pseudoacinar or pseudoglandular structures typically lacking
- Architectural features
  - Portal structures lacking
  - Increased unpaired arteries
  - Compressed sinusoidal spaces
  - Bile ducts are absent, but ductules may be present
  - Intact reticulin framework
- Hemorrhage &/or infarcts may be present with hemosiderin-laden macrophages or fibrotic regions
- Variants
  - Telangiectatic hepatic adenoma
    - Prominent sinusoidal dilatation
    - Presence of bile ductules and inflammation may mimic focal nodular hyperplasia, but recent molecular studies classify these as adenoma
  - Multiple adenoma or hepatic adenomatosis
    - Associated with glycogen storage disease and diabetes

DIFFERENTIAL DIAGNOSIS

Hepatocellular Carcinoma

- Cytologic atypia with increased nuclear to cytoplasmic ratio and prominent nucleoli
- Thickened trabecula and pseudoglandular formation
- Reticulin and immunohistochemical stains may help
  - Reticulin: Loss of reticulin suggests hepatocellular carcinoma
  - Positive glypican-3 (cytoplasmic) staining supports hepatocellular carcinoma
  - β-catenin: Positive (nuclear) staining supports hepatocellular carcinoma
  - Glutamine synthase: Extensive staining of hepatocytes in all zones supports hepatocellular carcinoma
- Often arises in background of cirrhosis &/or chronic liver disease
- More common in men and older individuals

Focal Nodular Hyperplasia

- Has thick fibrous septa
- Prominent bile ductular reaction and inflammatory infiltrate in fibrous septa
- Thick-walled arteries at periphery of septa, not in parenchyma

Nodular Regenerative Hyperplasia

- Diffuse nodular appearance throughout liver

Metastatic Carcinoma

- History of primary carcinoma elsewhere
- Usually negative for Hep-Par1 immunohistochemical stain

DIAGNOSTIC CHECKLIST

Clinically Relevant Pathologic Features

- Liver mass in woman on oral contraceptives
- Be very cautious when making this diagnosis in male patient

SELECTED REFERENCES

1. Bioulac-Sage P et al: Pathological diagnosis of liver cell adenoma and focal nodular hyperplasia: Bordeaux update. J Hepatol. 46(3):521-7, 2007
2. Zucman-Rossi J et al: Genotype-phenotype correlation in hepatocellular adenoma: new classification and relationship with HCC. Hepatology. 43(3):515-24, 2006
3. Bianchi L: Glycogen storage disease I and hepatocellular tumours. Eur J Pediatr. 152 Suppl 1:S63-70, 1993
4. Ferrell LD: Hepatocellular carcinoma arising in a focus of multilobular adenoma. A case report. Am J Surg Pathol. 17(5):525-9, 1993
5. Flejou JF et al: Liver adenomatosis. An entity distinct from liver adenoma? Gastroenterology. 89(5):1132-8, 1985
6. Edmondson HA et al: Liver-cell adenomas associated with use of oral contraceptives. N Engl J Med. 294(9):470-2, 1976

HEPATIC ADENOMA

Microscopic and Gross Features

*(**Left**) Hepatic adenomas typically show sheets of uniform tumor cells with numerous unpaired, thin-walled vessels. Note that steatosis is also present, and that there are no normal portal tracts. (**Right**) This hepatic adenoma features a thin-walled unpaired vessel surrounded by neoplastic hepatocytes with abundant steatosis.*

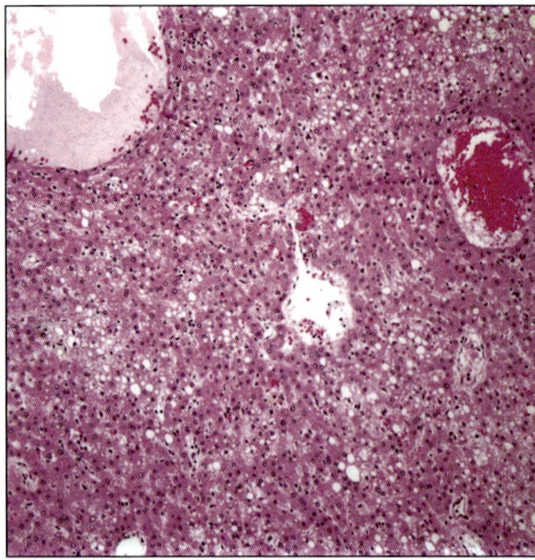

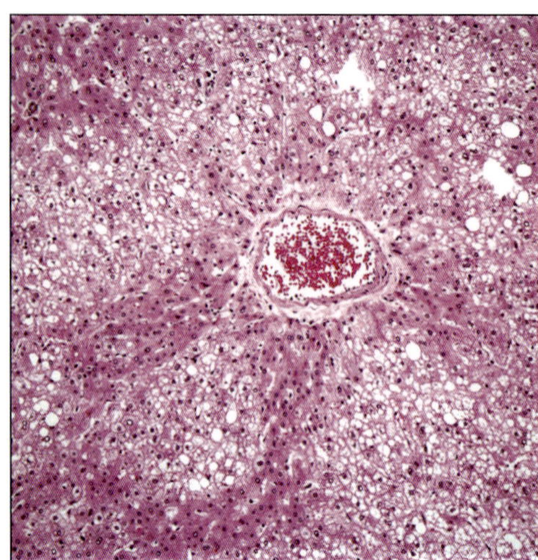

*(**Left**) This high-power view of the neoplastic hepatocytes in hepatic adenoma illustrates their uniformity and low N:C ratio. (**Right**) Hepatic adenomas have an intact, normal reticulin framework without thickened trabeculae or loss of reticulin.*

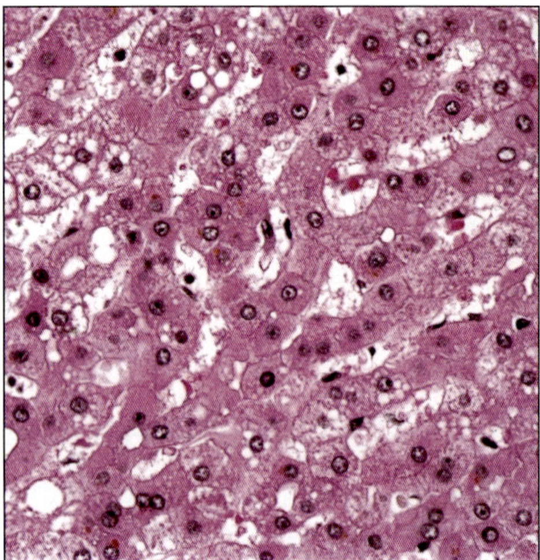

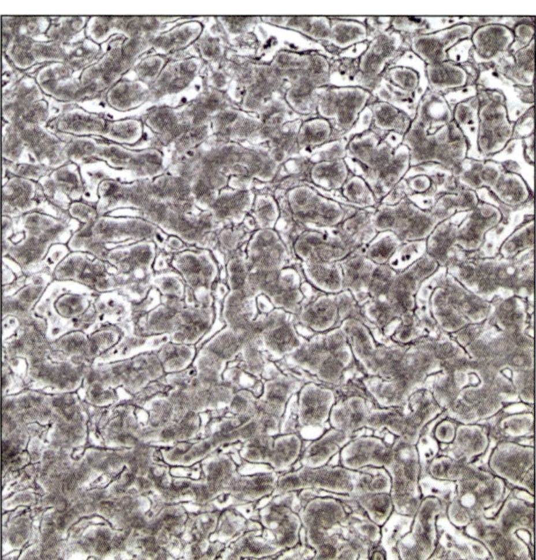

*(**Left**) This gross photograph shows multiple telangiectatic hepatic adenomas ➡. (**Right**) A low-magnification micrograph shows telangiectatic hepatic adenoma → on the left, with prominent dilated sinusoids, and nonneoplastic liver ⇨ on the right.*

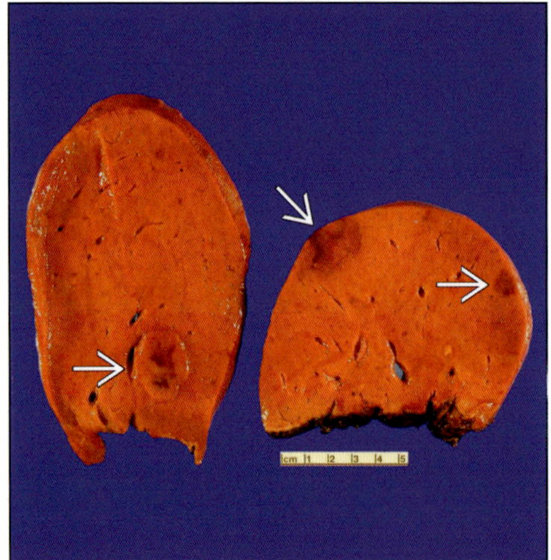

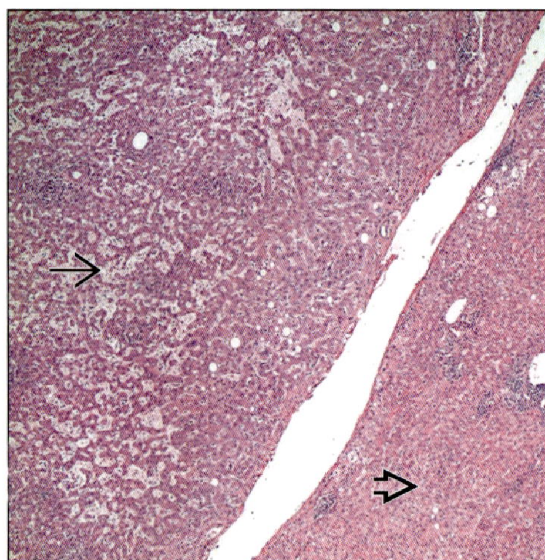

Microscopic and Gross Features

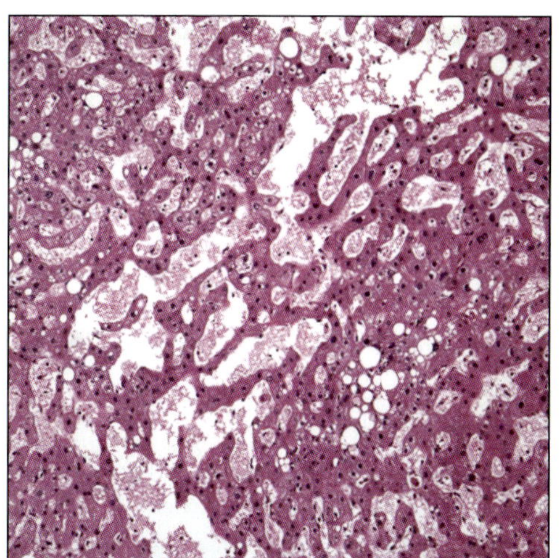

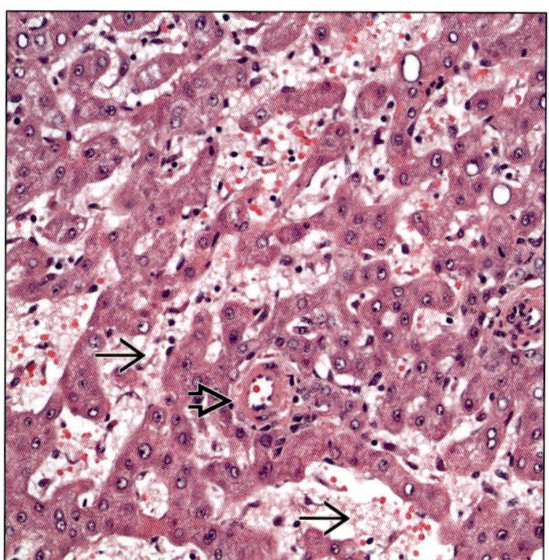

(Left) *This high-power view of a telangiectatic adenoma shows the markedly dilated sinusoids. Note the absence of portal tracts.* ***(Right)*** *Dilated sinusoids* → *and an unpaired artery* ⇨ *are seen in this telangiectatic hepatic adenoma.*

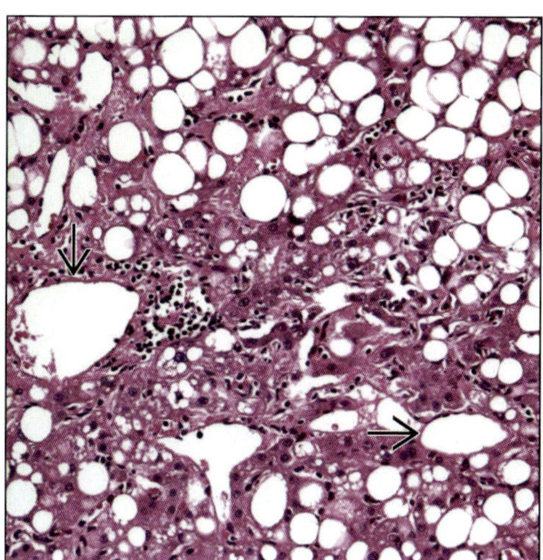

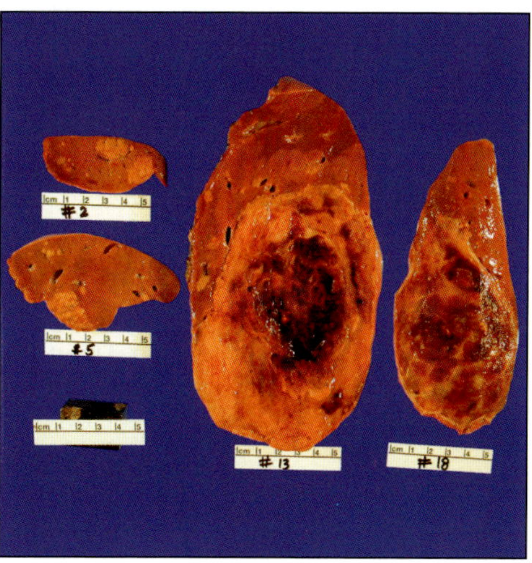

(Left) *Fat and chronic inflammation are also frequent findings in telangiectatic adenomas. Note the unpaired thin-walled vessels as well* →*.* ***(Right)*** *This case of hepatic adenomatosis features multiple adenomas with hemorrhage and necrosis.*

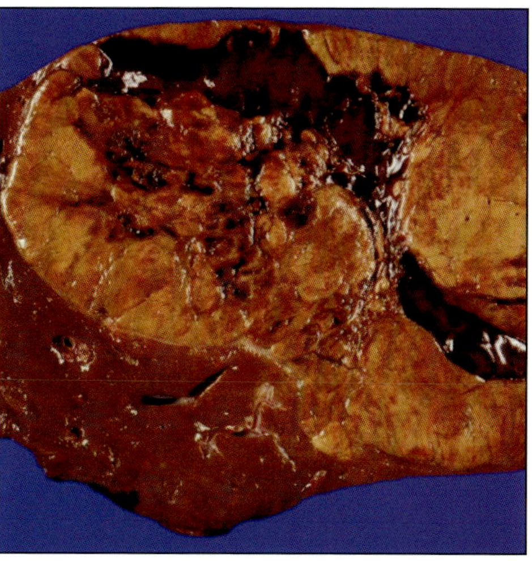

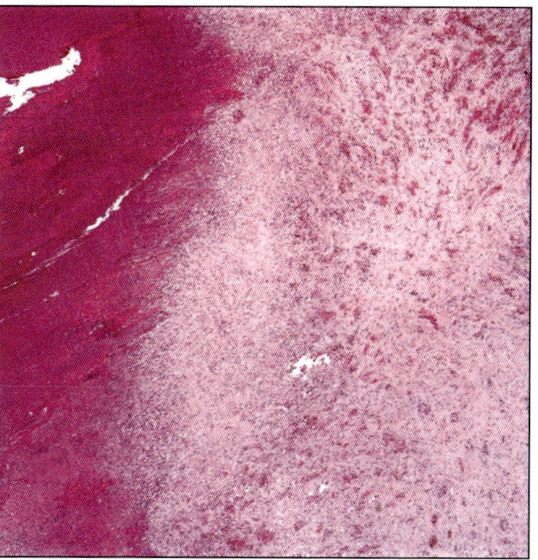

(Left) *This large adenoma has central areas of rupture and hemorrhage. The patient presented with an acute abdomen.* ***(Right)*** *This section from a ruptured hepatic adenoma shows hemorrhage on the left and areas of fibrosis and granulation tissue on the right.*

FOCAL NODULAR HYPERPLASIA

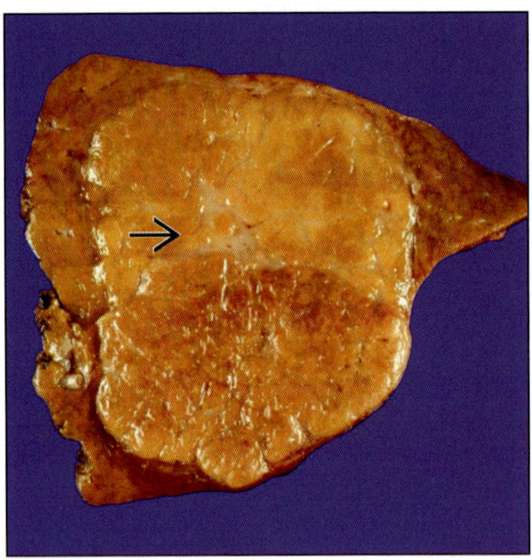

This liver wedge resection shows a well-circumscribed nodular lesion with a central stellate scar ⇒, typical of FNH.

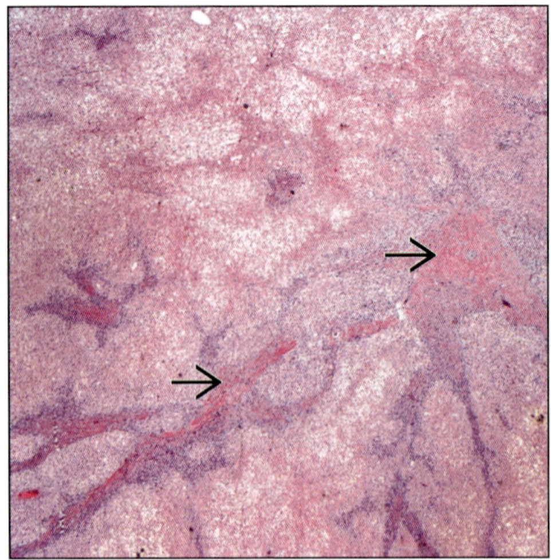

Low-power magnification illustrates the fibrous septa ⇒ in FNH, with associated ductular reaction and a mononuclear cell inflammatory infiltrate.

TERMINOLOGY

Abbreviations

- Focal nodular hyperplasia (FNH)

Synonyms

- Focal cirrhosis

Definitions

- Benign tumor-like lesion of liver caused by hyperplastic response to localized vascular abnormality

ETIOLOGY/PATHOGENESIS

Localized Abnormal Blood Flow

- Exact mechanism unclear
- Hepatocytes polyclonal, unlike hepatocytic adenomas
- Steroids are not thought to play role

CLINICAL ISSUES

Presentation

- Mostly incidental finding on imaging studies
- More common in women
- Normal liver biochemical tests

Treatment

- Surgical approaches
  - Reserved for large and symptomatic lesions

Prognosis

- Benign lesion
- Rupture, bleeding, and malignant transformation very rare

IMAGE FINDINGS

General Features

- Brightly, homogeneously enhancing mass in arterial phase CT or MR with delayed enhancement of central scar

MACROSCOPIC FEATURES

General Features

- Unencapsulated, well-circumscribed lesion
  - Approximately 20% are multiple
- Firm to rubbery cut surface that bulges from surface of liver
- Central stellate scar with radiating septa
- Noncirrhotic background liver

Size

- Most < 5 cm

MICROSCOPIC PATHOLOGY

Histologic Features

- Hyperplastic hepatocytes arranged into plates 2 cells thick
  - Subdivided into nodules by fibrous septa
  - Intact reticulin framework
- Classic triad
  - Fibrous septa, usually with large central stellate scar
    - Scar contains numerous thick-walled arteries
    - Arteries often show eccentric thickening
  - Ductular reaction (not true ducts) at junction between septa and parenchyma
  - Mononuclear inflammatory infiltrate in fibrous septa
- Periseptal hepatocytes may show positive copper staining due to cholestasis

FOCAL NODULAR HYPERPLASIA

Key Facts

Terminology
- Benign tumor-like lesion of liver caused by hyperplastic response to localized vascular abnormality

Clinical Issues
- Mostly incidental finding on imaging studies, most common in women

Macroscopic Features
- Unencapsulated, well-circumscribed lesion with bulging cut surface
  - Noncirrhotic background liver
- Central stellate scar with radiating septa

Microscopic Pathology
- Localized nodular parenchyma with fibrous septa and stellate central scar
  - Septa contain thick-walled vessels and mononuclear inflammatory infiltrate
- Ductular reaction at junction between septa and parenchyma

Top Differential Diagnoses
- Hepatocytic adenoma
- Cirrhosis
- Hepatocellular carcinoma, especially fibrolamellar variant
- Nodular regenerative hyperplasia

Cytologic Features
- Bland hepatocytes

DIFFERENTIAL DIAGNOSIS

Hepatocytic Adenoma
- Presence of unpaired arteries in parenchyma
  - Versus thick-walled arteries in fibrous septa in FNH
- Absence of portal tracts and fibrous septa
- Lack of ductular reaction
- Sinusoidal endothelial cells in adenoma are positive for CD34

Telangiectatic Hepatocytic Adenoma
- Dilated sinusoids
- Ectatic vessels
  - Vessels draining directly into sinusoids
- Absence of fibrous septa
- Immunoreactivity for serum amyloid A (SAA)

Cirrhosis
- Generalized nodules surrounded by fibrous septa
  - Imaging studies invaluable in distinguishing diffuse from focal nodular process
- Ductular reaction and inflammation may also be present in fibrous septa
- Lack thick-walled arteries
- Often underlying liver disease

Hepatocellular Carcinoma (Especially Fibrolamellar Variant)
- With or without background of cirrhosis and underlying liver disease
- Increased unpaired arteries in parenchyma
- Lack of portal structures
- Thickened hepatic trabecula or secondary structures such as pseudoacinar or pseudoglandular formation
- Cytologic atypia with increased nuclear to cytoplasmic ratio and prominent nucleoli
- Hepatocytes are positive for Glypican-3 immunohistochemistry

Nodular Regenerative Hyperplasia
- Lack of fibrous septa
- Nodularity is typically diffuse

DIAGNOSTIC CHECKLIST

Pathologic Interpretation Pearls
- Nodular liver parenchyma with fibrous septa containing thick-walled arteries at periphery, bile ductular reaction, and mixed mononuclear inflammation

SELECTED REFERENCES

1. Ahmad I et al: Diagnostic use of cytokeratins, CD34, and neuronal cell adhesion molecule staining in focal nodular hyperplasia and hepatic adenoma. Hum Pathol. 40(5):726-34, 2009
2. Bioulac-Sage P et al: Pathological diagnosis of liver cell adenoma and focal nodular hyperplasia: Bordeaux update. J Hepatol. 46(3):521-7, 2007
3. Makhlouf HR et al: Diagnosis of focal nodular hyperplasia of the liver by needle biopsy. Hum Pathol. 36(11):1210-6, 2005
4. Kondo F: Benign nodular hepatocellular lesions caused by abnormal hepatic circulation: etiological analysis and introduction of a new concept. J Gastroenterol Hepatol. 16(12):1319-28, 2001
5. Nguyen BN et al: Focal nodular hyperplasia of the liver: a comprehensive pathologic study of 305 lesions and recognition of new histologic forms. Am J Surg Pathol. 23(12):1441-54, 1999
6. Wanless IR et al: On the pathogenesis of focal nodular hyperplasia of the liver. Hepatology. 5(6):1194-200, 1985

Imaging, Gross, and Microscopic Features

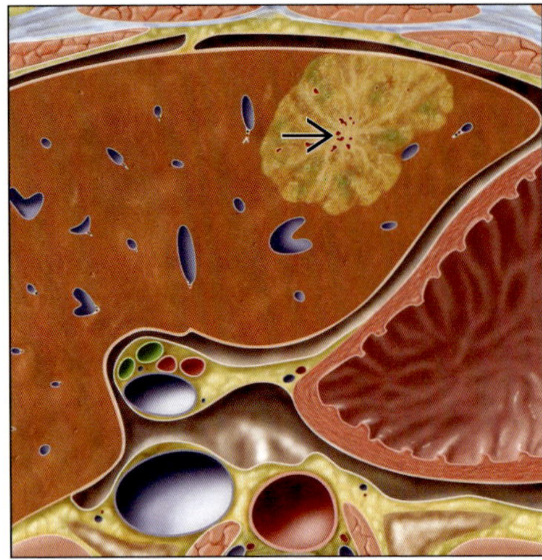

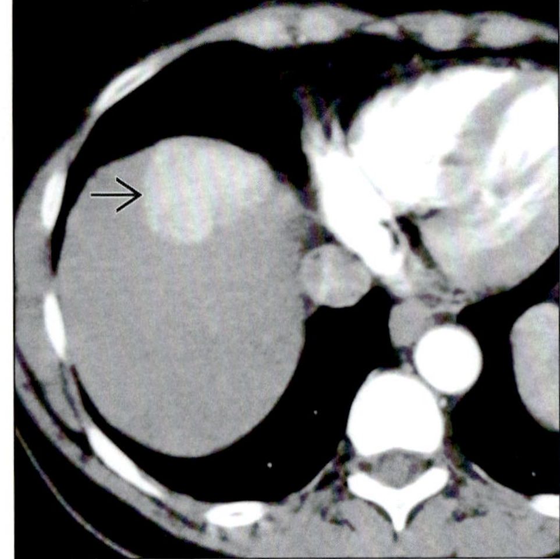

(Left) *This graphic illustrates the typical characteristics of focal nodular hyperplasia: Central vascularity* →*, radiating fibrous septae, well-defined margins, and absence of capsule.* ***(Right)*** *Axial CECT during the arterial phase shows a subcapsular enhancing hepatic mass without a central scar* →*.*

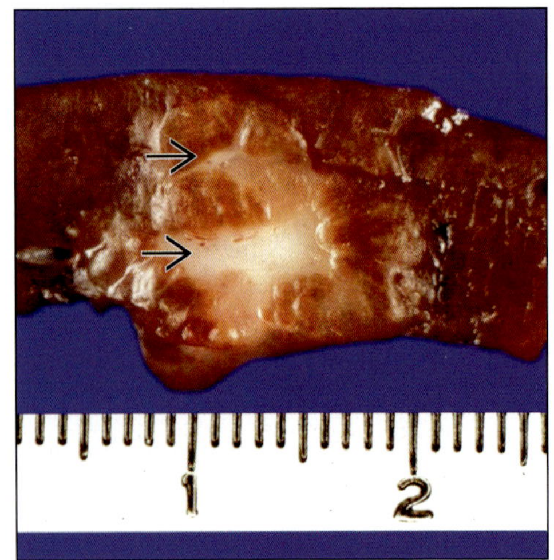

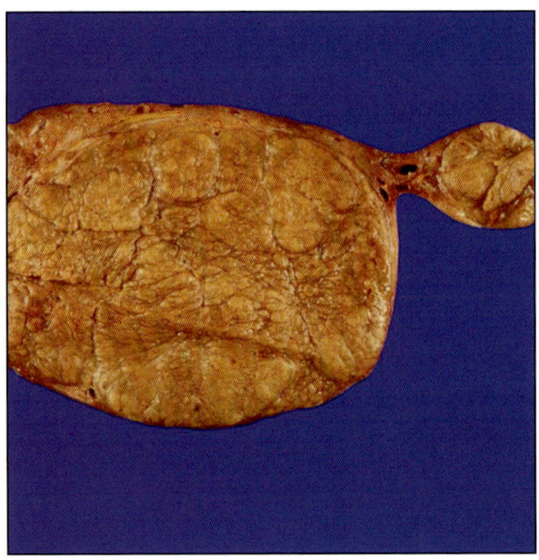

(Left) *This partial hepatectomy specimen shows a nodular brown lesion with a well-developed central scar* →*, characteristic of focal nodular hyperplasia.* ***(Right)*** *Focal nodular hyperplasia can be quite large, and occasionally they are multiple, as in this case.*

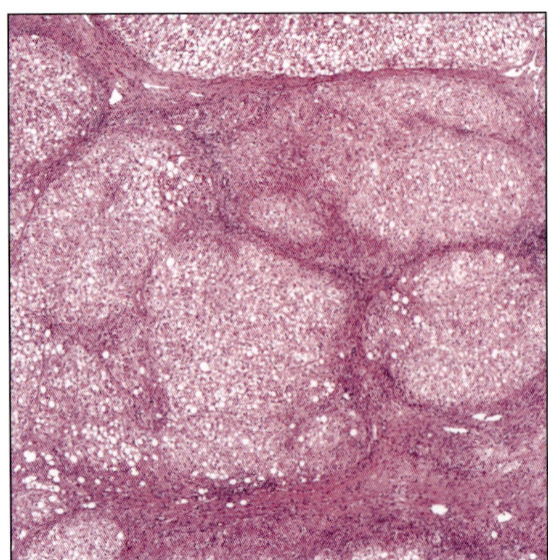

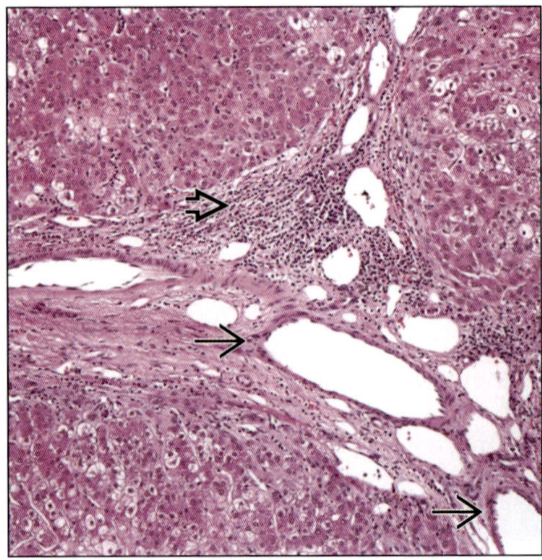

(Left) *Low-power photomicrograph of focal nodular hyperplasia shows the nodular appearance of the hepatic parenchyma. These lesions have been referred to as "focal cirrhosis."* ***(Right)*** *The fibrous septa contain a mononuclear cell infiltrate* ⇨ *and prominent vessels* →*.*

Microscopic Features

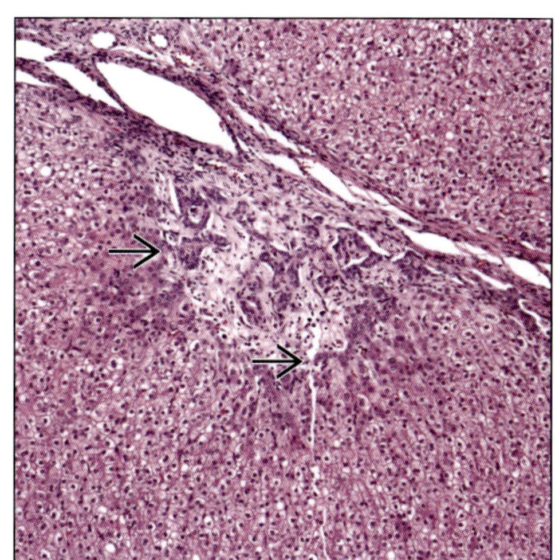

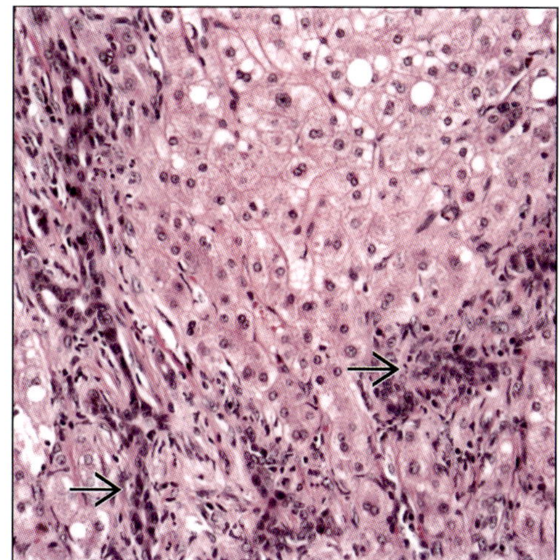

(Left) *A prominent ductular reaction* ⇒ *is often associated with the fibrous septa.* ***(Right)*** *High-power view demonstrates the ductular reaction* ⇒ *associated with the fibrous septa and the nodules of hepatic parenchyma.*

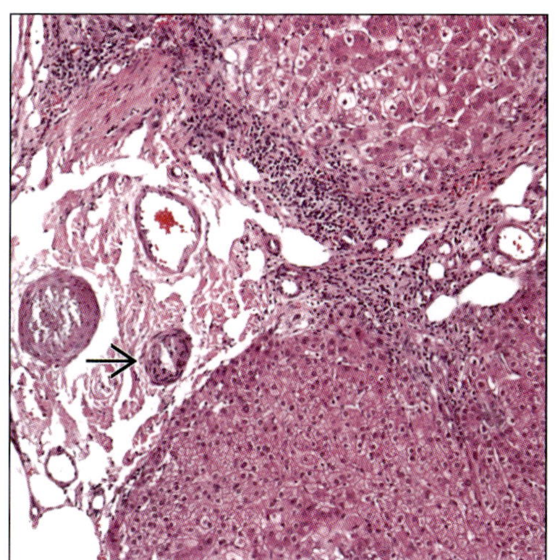

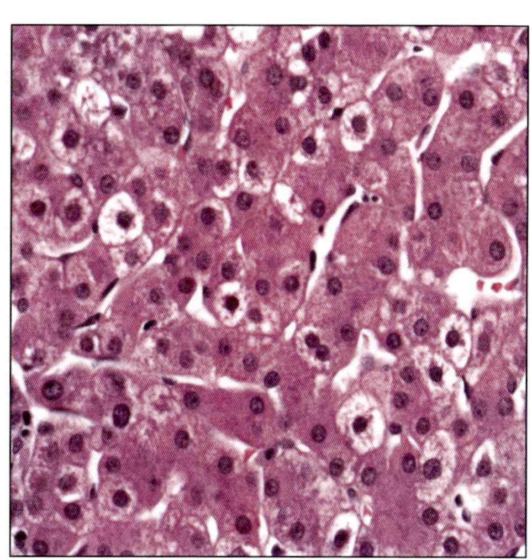

(Left) *The central scar as well as the fibrous septa may contain thick-walled vessels* ⇒. ***(Right)*** *The hepatic plates are 2 cells thick, and the reticulin framework should be intact.*

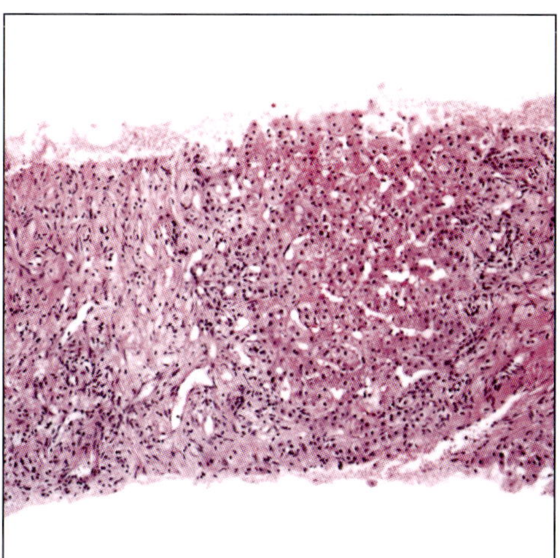

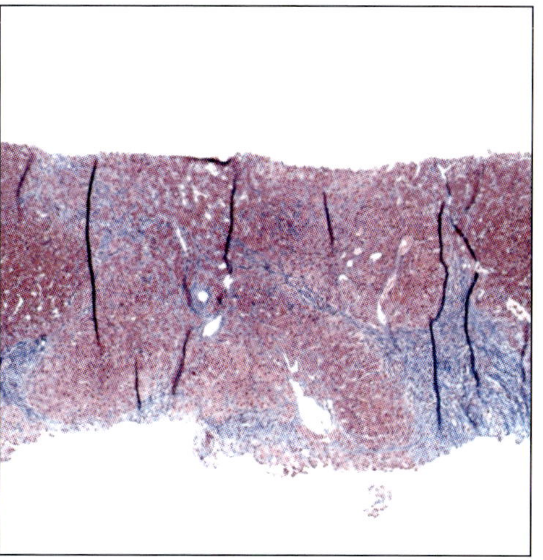

(Left) *Needle biopsy of a focal lesion shows nodular parenchyma, fibrous septa, and ductular reaction, consistent with focal nodular hyperplasia.* ***(Right)*** *Masson trichrome stain shows thick fibrous septa in a liver biopsy specimen from a focal nodular hyperplasia.*

REGENERATIVE AND DYSPLASTIC NODULES

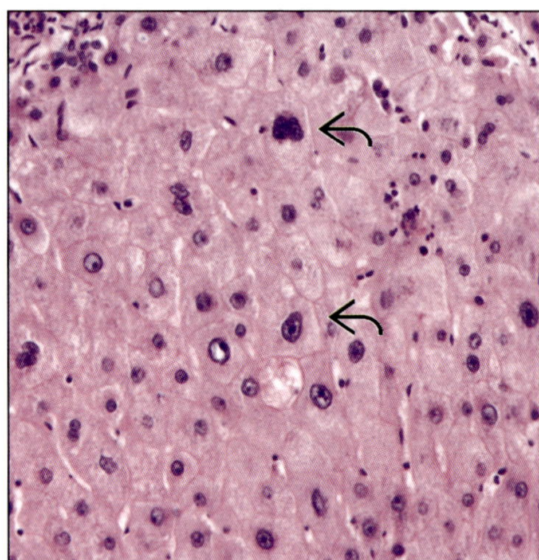

Large cell change is characterized by large hyperchromatic nuclei but preserved nuclear to cytoplasmic ratio ⇗. This change is thought to be degenerative and not preneoplastic.

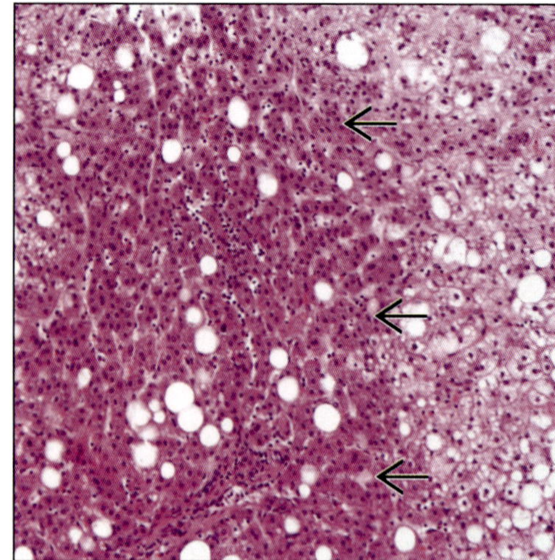

Small cell change (left 2/3 of image) ⇒ is characterized by small cells with high N:C ratio leading to increased cell density. When present in a nodule, it is the hallmark of HGDN.

TERMINOLOGY

Abbreviations

- Regenerative nodule (RN), macroregenerative nodule (MRN), low-grade dysplastic nodule (LGDN), high-grade dysplastic nodule (HGDN)

Synonyms

- RN: Large regenerative nodule, macroregenerative nodule, adenomatous hyperplasia
- HGDN: Borderline nodule, type II macroregenerative nodule, atypical adenomatous hyperplasia, atypical macroregenerative nodule

Definitions

- Dysplasia: Abnormal histologic growth that does not fulfill criteria of malignancy
  - Dysplastic focus: Cluster of dysplastic hepatocytes **less than** 1 cm in diameter
  - Dysplastic nodule: Cluster of dysplastic hepatocytes **greater than** 1 cm in diameter
- Regenerative nodule: Large (greater than 1 cm) nodule usually seen in context of cirrhosis
  - No reliable gross or histologic criteria for distinguishing RN from LGDN, thus they will be considered together here
    - LGDN thought to represent clonal proliferation of hepatocytes although likelihood of progression to carcinoma is unclear
  - Most RN are probably not preneoplastic
- HGDN: Nodule with atypical cytologic and architectural features believed to be precursor of carcinoma
- Large cell change (formerly large cell dysplasia)
  - Large hepatocytes with nuclear enlargement, hyperchromasia, prominent nucleoli, often multinucleated
    - Abundant cytoplasm and hence normal nuclear cytoplasmic ratio
  - Very common in cirrhotic liver
  - Formerly thought to be precursor of hepatocellular carcinoma (HCC)
    - No longer considered preneoplastic but rather regenerative or degenerative phenomenon
    - Low proliferation rate and absence of *P53* mutations also do not support preneoplastic process
- Small cell change (formerly small cell dysplasia)
  - Small hepatocytes with increased nuclear to cytoplasmic ratio and hyperchromatic nuclei
    - High proliferative activity and *P53* overexpression can occur
  - Likely to be preneoplastic when occurring in expansile nodules
  - Poorly defined or diffuse areas of small cell change without nodular configuration may represent regenerative phenomenon
  - Small cell regenerative foci common in biliary disease, unlikely to be preneoplastic

CLINICAL ISSUES

Presentation

- Occur in setting of cirrhosis, usually in background of hepatitis B, hepatitis C, alcoholic liver disease, hemochromatosis
  - Uncommon in chronic biliary diseases
  - Can occasionally occur in chronic liver disease without fully developed cirrhosis
  - Can occur in noncirrhotic liver in Budd-Chiari syndrome, portal vein thrombosis, or regeneration after necrosis
- May be detected at autopsy, transplantation, or by imaging
- Serum AFP is normal or mildly elevated

Treatment

- RN/LGDN: Follow-up by imaging and serological markers

REGENERATIVE AND DYSPLASTIC NODULES

Key Facts

Clinical Issues

- RN: Regenerative nodule greater than 1 cm; most believed to be nonneoplastic
  - LGDN resemble RN morphologically but are clonal
- HGDN: Preneoplastic lesion; likely precursor of HCC

Macroscopic Features

- Greater than 1 cm but usually less than 3 cm

Microscopic Pathology

- RN/LGDN: Plates 1-2 cells thick, portal tracts present, no architectural or cytologic atypia
- HGDN: Plates focally up to 3 cells thick; small cell change with increased N:C ratio
  - Unpaired arterioles and pseudoacinar architecture can be present
- Reticulin is preserved
  - May be focally lost in HGDN

Top Differential Diagnoses

- Small cell change, high N:C ratio, pseudoacinar architecture, and unpaired arterioles favor HGDN over LGDN
- Uniformly thick plates (> 3 cells) is most important feature distinguishing HCC from HGDN
  - Prominent pseudoacinar architecture, numerous unpaired arterioles and loss or fragmentation of reticulin favor HCC
- Stromal invasion distinguishes early HCC from HGDN
  - Lack of CK7(+) ductular reaction is useful in demonstrating stromal invasion

---

- HGDN: No well-defined guidelines; often ablated as they are considered preneoplastic

Prognosis

- RN: Most RN regress or remain unchanged on imaging follow-up and thus are probably not preneoplastic
  - LGDN: Unclear but probable low likelihood of progression as well
  - Difficult to ascertain prognosis since it is difficult to clearly define entity LGDN
- HGDN
  - Preneoplastic lesion, likely precursor of HCC
  - Allelic imbalance is seen in > 80% compared to 15% of regenerative nodules
  - Most remain stable or regress on follow-up; progression to HCC in 10-15%, but this data is based on limited studies

MACROSCOPIC FEATURES

Regenerative Nodules (Including LGDN)

- Larger than typical cirrhotic nodules
- By definition > 1 cm but usually < 3 cm
- May be pale yellow to tan compared to other cirrhotic nodules; some can be bile-stained
- Sharply circumscribed and bulge on cut section

High-Grade Dysplastic Nodule

- Similar gross appearance as RN/LGDN
- Some HGDN are not well circumscribed and may show irregular border

MICROSCOPIC PATHOLOGY

Histologic Features

- Regenerative nodule
  - Resemble cirrhotic nodules; cell plates are 1-2 cells thick
    - Reticulin framework is intact
  - Portal tracts are usually present within nodule, and ductular reaction may be prominent
  - Occasional unpaired arterioles may be seen, but this is not prominent finding
  - Hepatocytes typically appear normal; mild variation in cell size and scattered large cell change can be present
    - Specific morphologic features for low-grade dysplasia have not been established
    - May be indistinguishable from lesions formerly called MRN in the absence of clonality studies
  - May contain Mallory-Denk bodies, bile, clear cell changes, iron, copper, and fat
  - CD34 shows patchy sinusoidal staining at edge; occasional nodules can show more diffuse expression
  - Nodules are negative for α-fetoprotein and GPC with rare exceptions
  - No histologic criteria to distinguish RN from LGDN
- High-grade dysplastic nodule
  - HG dysplastic changes may involve entire nodule or present as one or more dysplastic foci within nodule
  - By definition, atypical features do not fulfill criteria of diagnosis of HCC
  - Focal areas with up to 3-cell thick plates may be present (normal cell plates are typically 1-2 cells thick)
    - Reticulin network is normal or focally decreased
    - Pseudoacinar architecture can be present but is usually not diffuse
  - Portal tracts are present within nodule
  - Scattered unpaired arterioles are present but not as numerous as in HCC
  - Small cell change with increased nuclear to cytoplasmic ratio is a characteristic feature
    - Results in nuclear crowding and increased nuclear density
    - Large cell change can be seen but is neither sufficient nor necessary for diagnosis
  - May contain Mallory-Denk bodies, fat, clear cell change, cytoplasmic basophilia, bile
  - Tend to lack iron (in contrast to MRN, where iron deposits are more common)

- CD34 shows patchy sinusoidal staining, usually at edge; occasional nodules can show more diffuse expression
- α-fetoprotein is negative
- Glypican-3 (GPC) expression is variable; diffuse strong expression strongly favors HCC

DIFFERENTIAL DIAGNOSIS

Other Regenerative Nodules

- By definition, size > 1 cm differentiates RN from other cirrhotic nodules

Hepatic Adenoma

- Rarely, RN may lack portal zones and resemble hepatic adenoma
- True adenomas rarely, if ever, occur in cirrhotic liver

RN/LGDN vs. HGDN

- Cytologic abnormalities like small cell change and nuclear atypia favor HGDN
- Architectural abnormalities like pseudoacinar architecture, focal reticulin loss, and unpaired arterioles favor HGDN

HGDN vs. Well-Differentiated HCC

- Cell plates more than 3 cells thick are most important feature distinguishing HCC from HGDN
- Prominent pseudoacinar architecture and numerous unpaired arterioles are typical of HCC
- Loss or fragmentation of reticulin network strongly favors HCC
- CD34 is typically diffuse in HCC and patchy in HGDN, but considerable overlap exists
- CK7(+) ductular reaction present around over 50% of circumference of HGDN in most cases; this is focal or lost in most HCC
- GPC expression favors HCC, especially if strong and diffuse
  - GPC expression described in 7-22% of HGDN also

HGDN vs. Early HCC (Early Well-Differentiated HCC or Vaguely Nodular HCC)

- Characteristic feature of early HCC is stromal invasion leading to vaguely nodular appearance
  - Stromal invasion can occur at nodule-parenchymal or nodule-septal interface within nodule or at periphery
  - Since stromal invasion can be focal, distinction from HGDN on biopsy may not be possible
  - Lack of CK7(+) ductular reaction can be useful in demonstrating stromal invasion
- Uniformly thick plates (> 3 cells), prominent pseudoglands, and loss of reticulin are typical of progressed HCC; may not be seen in early HCC
- Immunohistochemistry
  - GPC expression is more often seen in early HCC than HGDN
  - Glutamine synthetase (GS), a downstream gene in β-catenin pathway, is diffusely positive in many early HCC (up to 70%)
    - 10-15% of HGDN can be positive (usually focal)
  - Heat shock protein (HSP)-70, a cell cycle/apoptosis regulator, is overexpressed in 80% of early HCC
    - 5-10% of HGDN can be positive (usually focal)
  - When 2 of these 3 markers are positive, specificity and sensitivity for diagnosis of HCC is 100% and 72%, respectively, in **resections**
  - When 2 of these 3 markers are positive, specificity and sensitivity for diagnosis of HCC is 100% and 50%, respectively, in **biopsies**
- Most immunohistochemical stains have only been studied in limited fashion and need validation in larger studies

DIAGNOSTIC CHECKLIST

Clinically Relevant Pathologic Features

- No criteria other than clonality to distinguish LGDN from RN
  - Most RN/LGDN are probably not preneoplastic
- HGDN have significant cytologic and sometimes architectural atypia; considered precursors of HCC

SELECTED REFERENCES

1. Roskams T et al: Pathology of early hepatocellular carcinoma: conventional and molecular diagnosis. Semin Liver Dis. 30(1):17-25, 2010
2. Di Tommaso L et al: The application of markers (HSP70 GPC3 and GS) in liver biopsies is useful for detection of hepatocellular carcinoma. J Hepatol. 50(4):746-54, 2009
3. Kondo F: Histological features of early hepatocellular carcinomas and their developmental process: for daily practical clinical application : Hepatocellular carcinoma. Hepatol Int. 3(1):283-93, 2009
4. The International Consensus Group for Hepatocellular Neoplasia: Pathologic diagnosis of early hepatocellular carcinoma: a report of the international consensus group for hepatocellular neoplasia. Hepatology. 49(2):658-64, 2009. Erratum in: Hepatology. 49(3):1058, 2009
5. Shafizadeh N et al: Utility and limitations of glypican-3 expression for the diagnosis of hepatocellular carcinoma at both ends of the differentiation spectrum. Mod Pathol. 21(8):1011-8, 2008
6. Park YN et al: Ductular reaction is helpful in defining early stromal invasion, small hepatocellular carcinomas, and dysplastic nodules. Cancer. 109(5):915-23, 2007
7. Sherman M: Diagnosis of small hepatocellular carcinoma. Hepatology. 42(1):14-6, 2005
8. Seki S et al: Outcomes of dysplastic nodules in human cirrhotic liver: a clinicopathological study. Clin Cancer Res. 6(9):3469-73, 2000
9. Lee RG et al: Large cell change (liver cell dysplasia) and hepatocellular carcinoma in cirrhosis: matched case-control study, pathological analysis, and pathogenetic hypothesis. Hepatology. 26(6):1415-22, 1997
10. Nakashima O et al: Pathomorphologic characteristics of small hepatocellular carcinoma: a special reference to small hepatocellular carcinoma with indistinct margins. Hepatology. 22(1):101-5, 1995
11. Ferrell LD et al: Proposal for standardized criteria for the diagnosis of benign, borderline, and malignant hepatocellular lesions arising in chronic advanced liver disease. Am J Surg Pathol. 17(11):1113-23, 1993

Macroregenerative vs. High-Grade Dysplastic Nodule

Feature	MRN	HGDN
Morphology		
Cell plate thickness	1-2	1-2, focally up to 3
Pseudoacinar architecture	Uncommon	Often present, usually not diffuse
Unpaired arterioles	Uncommon	Often present, not in large numbers
Small cell change	Absent	Characteristic
N:C ratio	Normal	Increased
Irregular nuclear contours	Absent	Mild
Histochemical Stains		
Reticulin network	Preserved	Preserved or focally absent
Iron	Patchy or diffuse when present, usually same as surrounding liver	Can be decreased or absent compared to surrounding liver (iron free foci)
Immunohistochemistry		
CD34 sinusoidal staining	Absent or patchy at periphery, occasionally diffuse	Patchy, occasionally diffuse
AFP	Absent	Absent
Glypican-3	Absent, rare positive cases	Absent or focal, rarely strong
CK7(+) ductular reaction	Present, diffuse	Present, may be focally lost

High-Grade Dysplastic Nodule vs. Hepatocellular Carcinoma

Feature	HGDN	Well-differentiated HCC
Imaging		
Arterial phase	Usually hypovascular	Early HCC hypovascular, most progressed HCC are hypervascular
Morphology		
Cell plate thickness	1-2, focally up to 3	> 3, can be < 3 in early cases
Pseudoacinar architecture	Usually focal	Can be diffuse
Unpaired arterioles	Present, but few	Present, often numerous
Stromal invasion	Absent	Present
Small cell change	Present	Present
Nuclear to cytoplasmic ratio	Increased	Increased
Cell density	More than 1.3x normal	More than 2x normal
Abnormalities in nuclear contour	Mild	Mild to moderate
Cytoplasmic basophilia	Absent	Often present
Mitoses	Few or absent	Can be present
Histochemical Stains		
Reticulin	Present or focally absent	Fragmented or absent in most cases
Immunohistochemistry		
CD34	Patchy, occasionally diffuse	Usually diffuse
AFP	Negative	Can be positive
CK7(+) ductular reaction	Present or focally absent	Generally absent or focally present
Glypican-3	Negative or focally positive	Positive in > 50%
Glutamine synthetase	Usually negative or focally positive	Diffuse positive in most cases
HSP-70	Usually negative or focally positive	Diffuse positive in most cases
GPC, GS, HSP70: 2 of 3 positive	None	50-60%
Serum Biochemistry		
AFP > 100 μg/mL	Less common	25-30%, L3 isoform more sensitive for early HCC
Descarboxyprothrombin	Not known	15-30% early HCC

REGENERATIVE AND DYSPLASTIC NODULES

Microscopic Features

*(**Left**) Dysplastic nodules ⇒ resemble other cirrhotic nodules but are greater than 1 cm. (**Right**) This low-grade dysplastic nodule contains an intranodular portal tract with associated ductular reaction ⇒.*

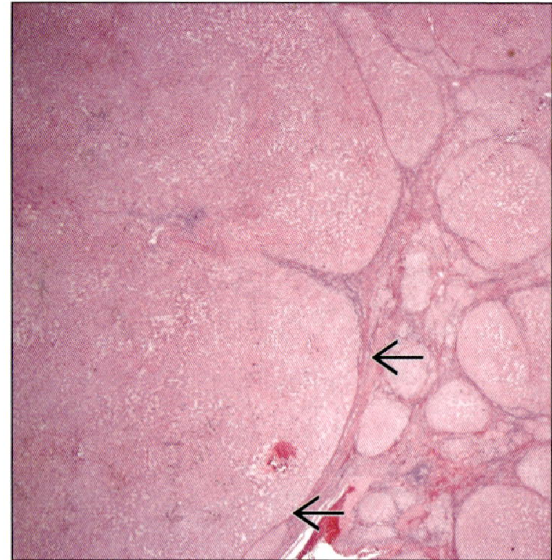

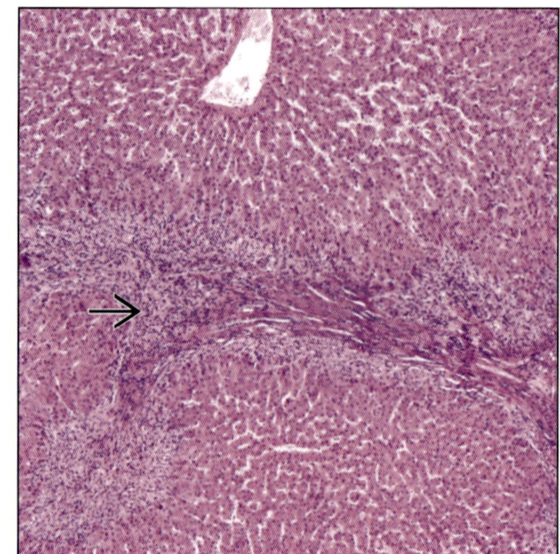

*(**Left**) Large cell change is seen in a needle biopsy of a regenerative nodule. (**Right**) This example of large cell change in a regenerative nodule features prominent glycogenated nuclei. (Courtesy E. Brunt, MD.)*

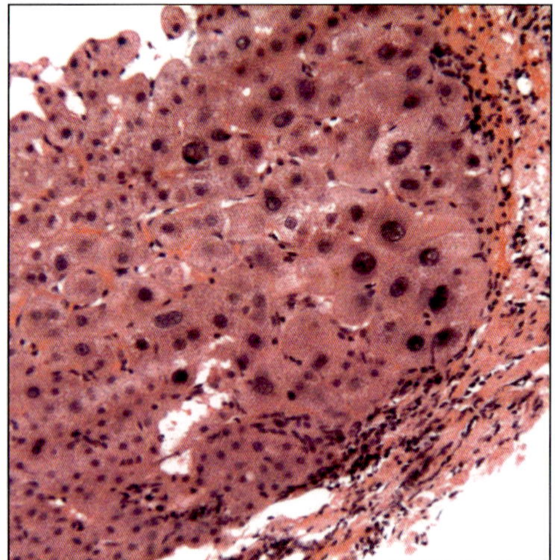

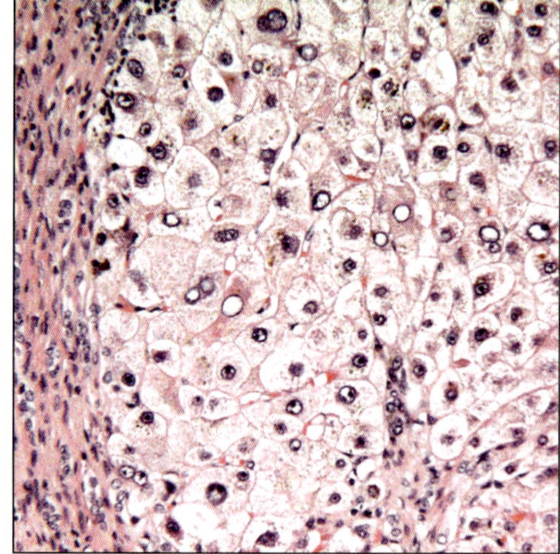

*(**Left**) This high-grade dysplastic nodule contains both small cell change ⇒ and pseudoacinar architecture ⇒, which can be seen in high-grade dysplastic nodules. (**Right**) Small cell change is characterized by increased nuclear to cytoplasmic ratio, leading to the appearance of increased cellular density in high-grade dysplastic nodules (right). A regenerative nodule is seen on the left.*

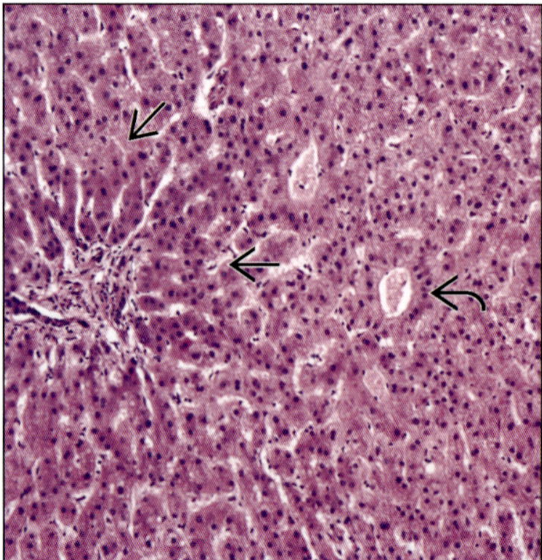

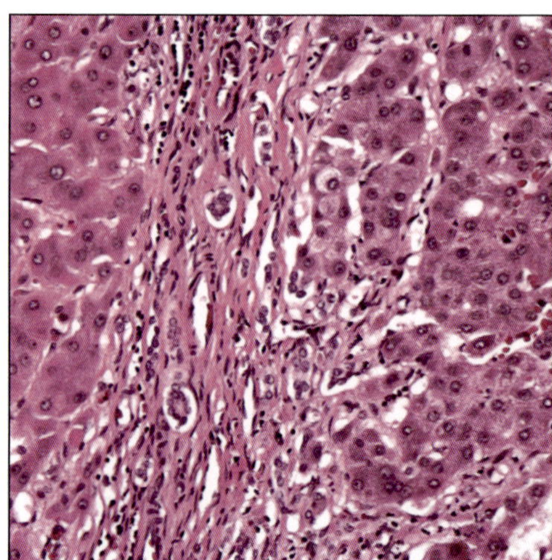

Microscopic Features

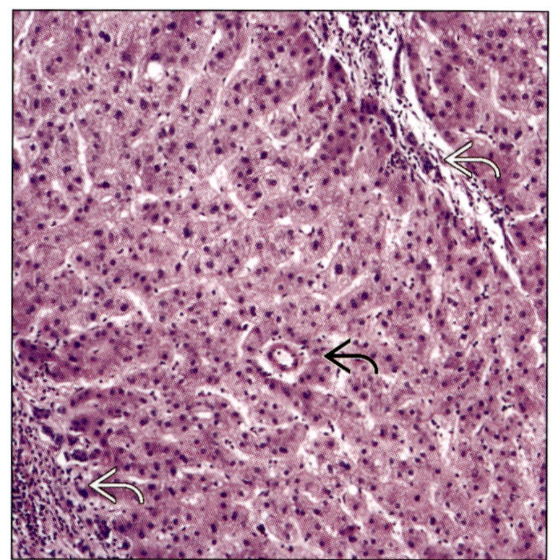

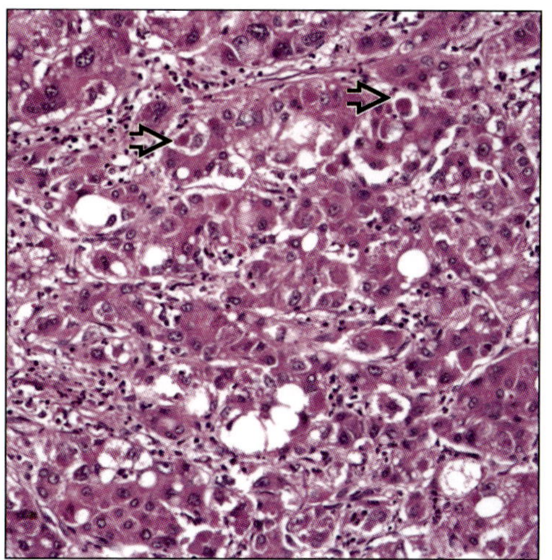

(Left) This high-grade dysplastic nodule contains an unpaired arteriole ⇨. Bile ductular reaction is seen within and at the periphery ➡. (Right) Abundant Mallory hyaline ⇨, as well as steatosis, is seen in this high-grade dysplastic nodule.

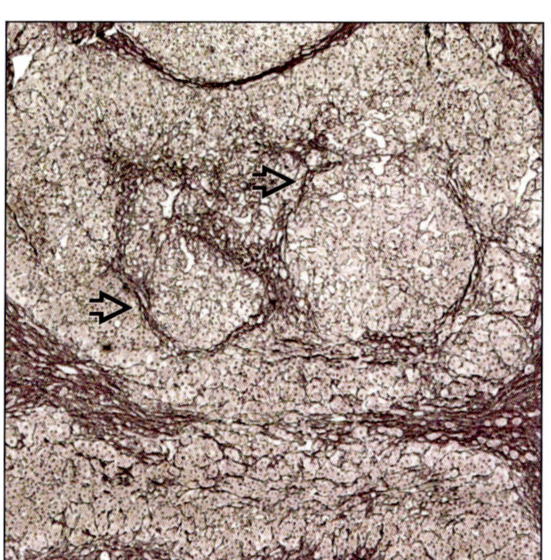

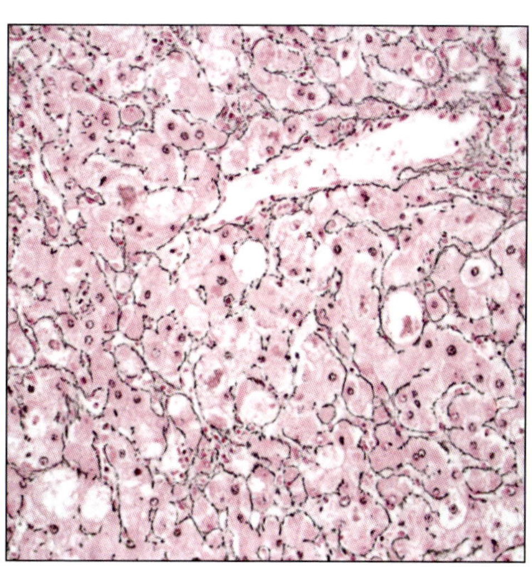

(Left) Although the reticulin framework is intact in this nodule, there is an atypical "nodule within nodule" architectural pattern ⇨ that indicates high-grade dysplasia. (Right) This high-power photograph illustrates that the reticulin network in high-grade dysplastic nodules is largely intact.

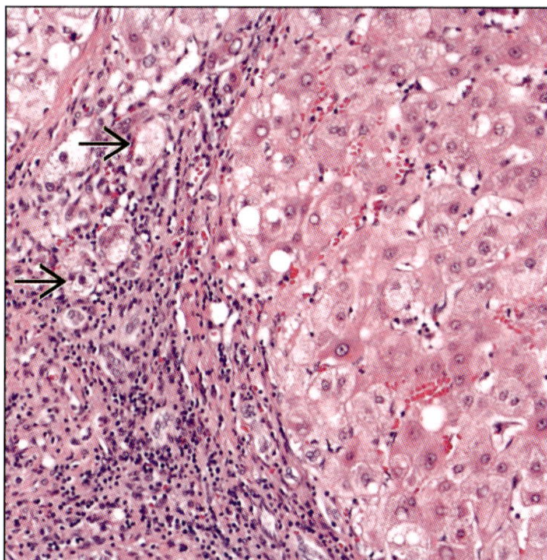

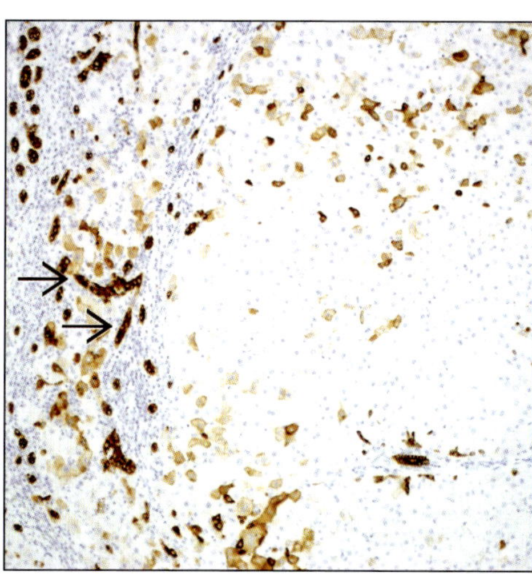

(Left) This cirrhotic nodule has an irregular extension of hepatocytes → into the fibrous septum with associated inflammation, mimicking stromal invasion. (Right) Immunohistochemistry for CK7 in a cirrhotic nodule shows CK7 positive ductules → intermingled with hepatocytes in the area of pseudoinvasion, supporting a benign diagnosis.

REGENERATIVE AND DYSPLASTIC NODULES

Microscopic Features

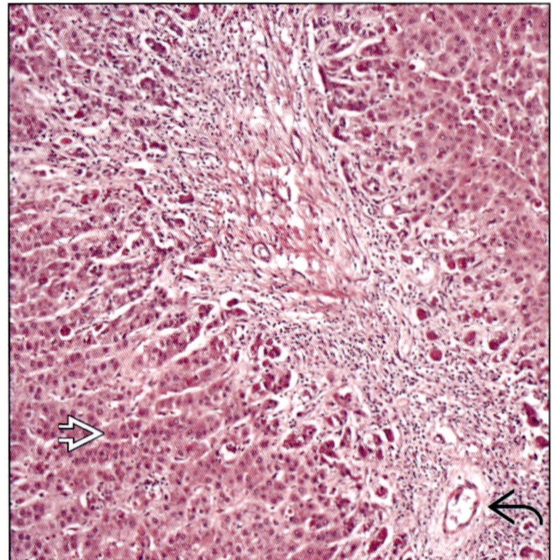

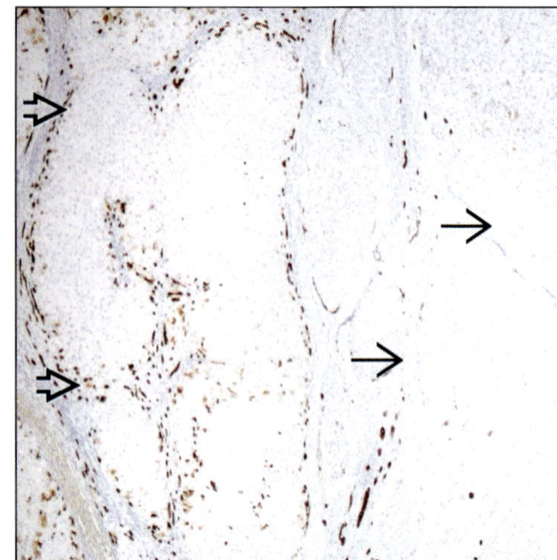

(Left) H&E illustrates the intranodular hepatocellular-stromal interface in a nodule with features of HGD including small cell change ➡ and unpaired arterioles ↷. The interface lacks bile ductular reaction, indicating that this is an early HCC. (Right) CK7 immunohistochemistry highlights the circumferential ductular reaction around regenerative nodules ➡. In contrast, the ductules are focal or absent around nodules of HCC →.

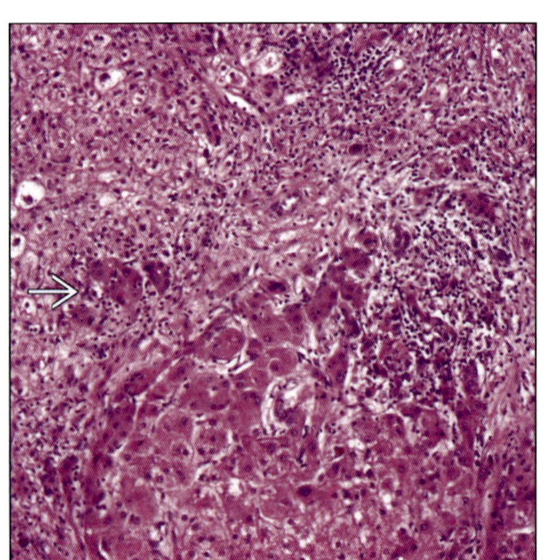

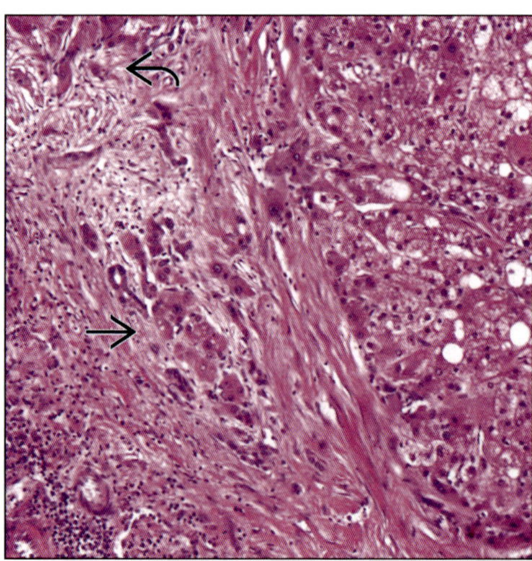

(Left) This hepatocellular nodule has features of HGD, but the infiltration of the nonneoplastic liver parenchyma at the periphery ➡ indicates this is an early HCC. Stromal invasion is key in distinguishing early HCC from high-grade dysplastic nodules. (Right) This hepatocellular nodule with high-grade dysplastic features shows infiltration of a portal tract → and fibrous septa ↷ at the periphery, supporting a diagnosis of early HCC.

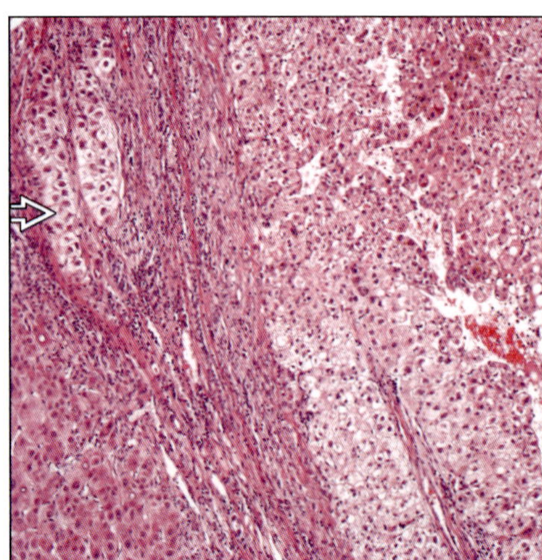

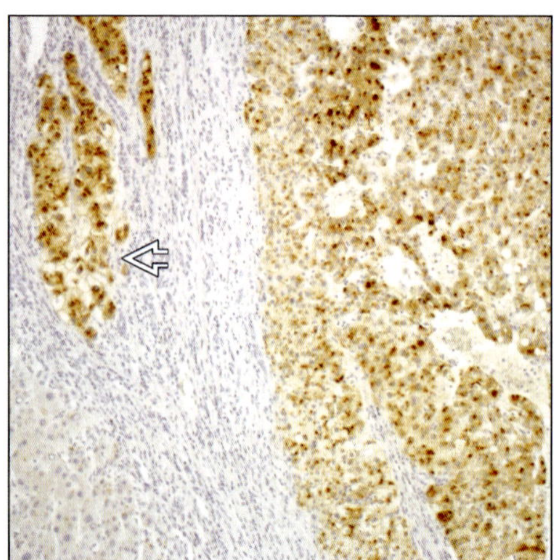

(Left) This hepatocellular nodule with high-grade dysplastic features shows stromal invasion ➡ at the periphery, supporting the diagnosis of early hepatocellular carcinoma. (Right) Glypican-3 is positive in both the high-grade dysplastic nodule and the invasive portion ➡, further supporting the diagnosis of hepatocellular carcinoma. Glypican-3 is negative or only focally positive in most high-grade dysplastic nodules.

Immunohistochemical Features

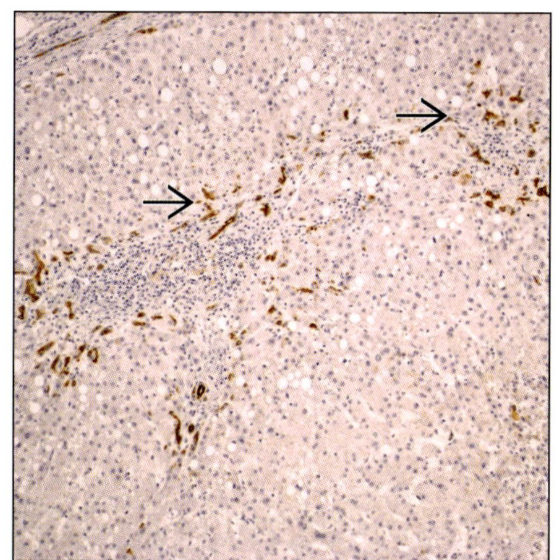

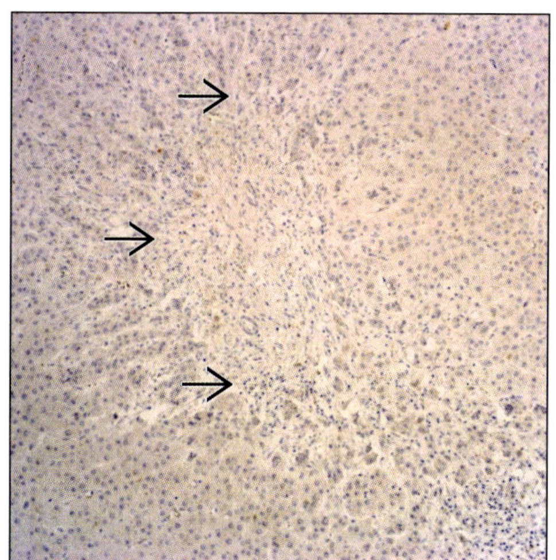

(Left) *Immunohistochemistry for CK7 demonstrates the ductular reaction ➔ at the intranodular hepatocellular-stromal interface in a regenerative nodule.* ***(Right)*** *Immunohistochemistry for CK7 demonstrates a lack of ductular reaction at the intranodular hepatocellular-stromal interface ➔, supporting a diagnosis of early hepatocellular carcinoma.*

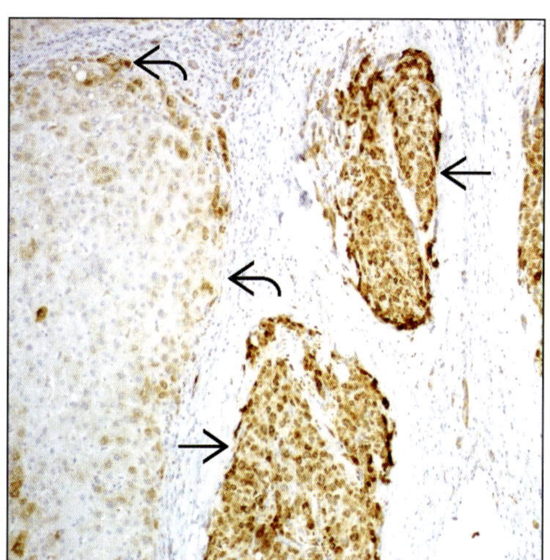

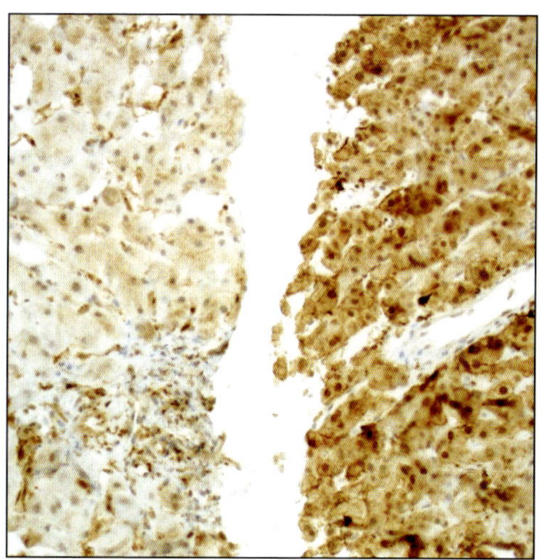

(Left) *Glutamine synthetase (GS) is helpful in the distinction of HGDN and HCC. Note the strong cytoplasmic staining in HCC ➔ vs. the adjacent HGDN that shows only weak focal staining ➚.* ***(Right)*** *HSP70 can be useful in the distinction of HGDN and HCC. Note the diffuse nuclear and patchy cytoplasmic staining in early HCC (right), as opposed to the adjacent cirrhotic liver that shows weak, focal staining (left).*

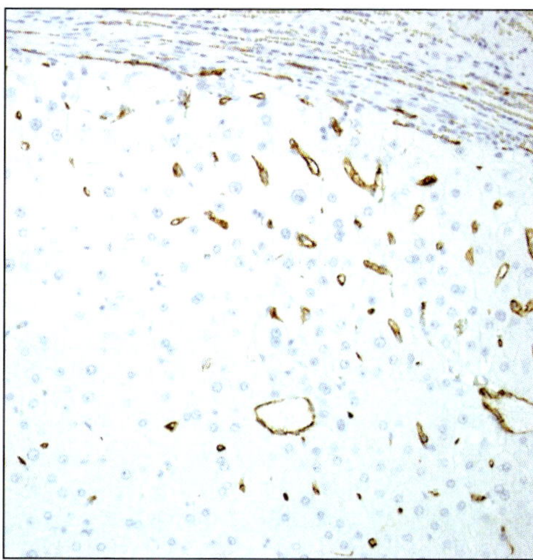

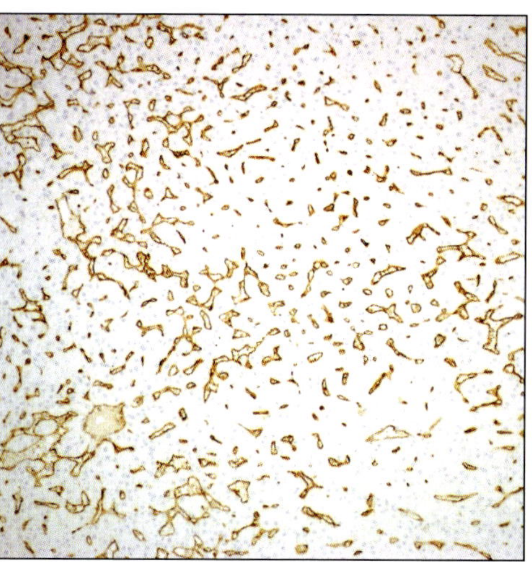

(Left) *Immunohistochemistry for CD34 typically shows either a negative or weak and patchy sinusoidal pattern of staining in regenerative and high-grade dysplastic nodules. The patchy staining is often more pronounced at the periphery of the nodule.* ***(Right)*** *Immunohistochemistry for CD34 typically shows a diffuse sinusoidal pattern of staining in HCC.*

HEPATOCELLULAR CARCINOMA AND VARIANTS

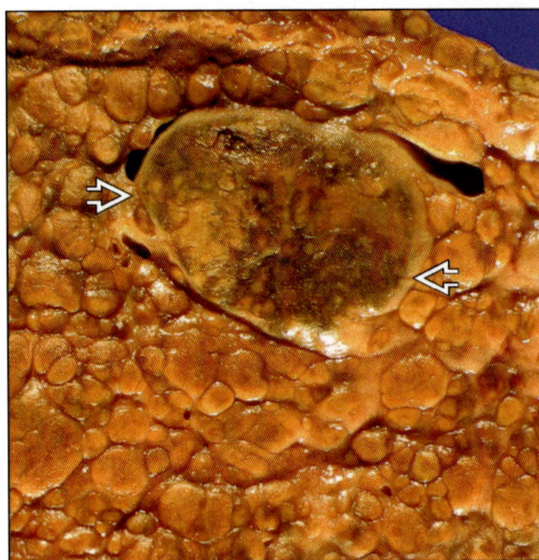

Gross photograph shows a large bile-stained tumor nodule ➡ in a background of cirrhosis. This is a classic presentation of hepatocellular carcinoma.

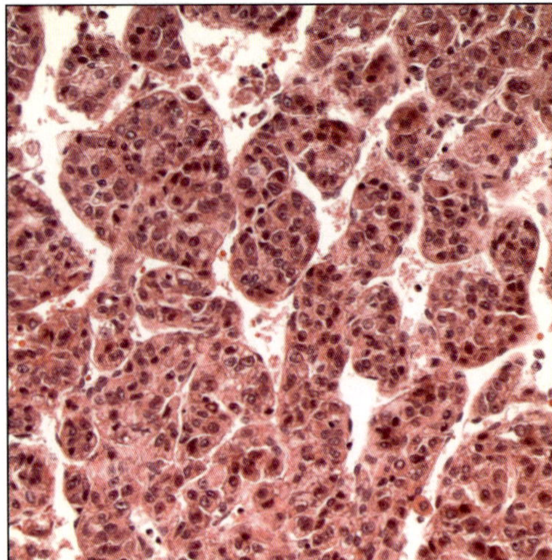

Hepatocellular carcinoma is typically composed of neoplastic cells resembling hepatocytes with a high nuclear to cytoplasmic ratio, which are organized into thick, disordered trabeculae.

TERMINOLOGY

Abbreviations

- Hepatocellular carcinoma (HCC)

Synonyms

- Hepatoma

Definitions

- Primary malignant neoplasm of liver with hepatocytic differentiation

ETIOLOGY/PATHOGENESIS

Developmental Anomaly

- HCC can occur in patients with various congenital anomalies, including Alagille syndrome, ataxia-telangiectasia, Abernethy malformation, and bile salt export protein (BSEP) deficiency

Environmental Exposure

- Aflatoxin B1, a mycotoxin produced by fungi of *Aspergillus* genus that contaminates food, is major cause of HCC in China and southern Africa
- Alcoholic cirrhosis is major cause of HCC in western populations
- Other exposures linked to HCC include anabolic steroids, Thorotrast, oral contraceptives, and smoking

Infectious Agents

- Chronic viral hepatitis (hepatitis B and hepatitis C) is leading cause of HCC worldwide

Metabolic Disorders

- Various metabolic disorders, including hemochromatosis, tyrosinemia, hypercitrullinemia, α-1-antitrypsin deficiency, and fructosemia, are associated with increased risk of HCC

Cirrhosis

- 70-90% of HCC arises in cirrhosis
- Macronodular cirrhosis is more strongly associated with HCC than micronodular

Progression of Benign Tumor

- HCC can arise in preexisting hepatocellular adenoma

CLINICAL ISSUES

Epidemiology

- Incidence
  - Varies widely depending on geography in parallel with prevalence of hepatitis B and C and aflatoxin exposure
    - East Asia and southern Africa have highest incidence worldwide, up to 150 per 100,000
    - In USA, annual incidence is approximately 4 per 100,000
- Age
  - Incidence increases with advancing age and then falls off in elderly; however, average age varies depending on geography
    - In parts of world with high incidence, average age is 35 years
    - In USA, average age is 60 years
  - Can occur in children, particularly in those with metabolic or genetic disorders
- Gender
  - More common in men

Presentation

- Abdominal pain due to stretching of Glisson capsule
- Malaise, weight loss, hepatomegaly
- Decompensation of previously stable cirrhotic patient with jaundice and rapidly accumulating ascites
- Fever, leukocytosis, and liver mass mimicking hepatic abscess

HEPATOCELLULAR CARCINOMA AND VARIANTS

Key Facts

Etiology/Pathogenesis

- Chronic viral hepatitis is leading cause of HCC worldwide
- 70-90% of HCC arises in cirrhosis

Clinical Issues

- In USA, annual incidence is approximately 4 per 100,000
- Most often presents with abdominal pain, malaise, weight loss, hepatomegaly
- AFP is elevated in 70-90% of patients
- In USA, 5-year survival is 30-40% overall, but 75% for tumors < 5 cm

Macroscopic Features

- Typically soft, bile-stained with hemorrhage and necrosis
- Can be solitary tumor, multiple discrete tumors, or small indistinct nodules throughout portion of liver
- Gross venous or bile duct invasion occurs commonly

Microscopic Pathology

- Grows as thickened hepatic plates separated by sinusoids without desmoplastic stroma
- Tumor cells resemble hepatocytes with polygonal shape, round vesicular nuclei, and prominent nucleoli
- Bile pigment in dilated canaliculi is helpful in distinguishing HCC from its mimics

Ancillary Tests

- Positive for Hep-Par1, Glypican-3, and CAM5.2 (keratins 8 and 18)

- Increasingly, small asymptomatic tumors are being found during surveillance of cirrhotic patients

Laboratory Tests

- α-fetoprotein (AFP) is elevated in 70-90% of patients

Natural History

- Metastasis occurs in 40-60% of patients
  - Most common locations are lymph nodes in porta hepatis, around pancreas, and celiac axis
- HCC has tendency for intravascular spread with involvement of hepatic and portal veins
  - Hematogenous spread most commonly occurs to lungs, but also adrenal glands, bone, stomach, heart, pancreas, kidney, spleen, and ovary
- Tumor seldom breaches Glisson capsule, and therefore dissemination throughout peritoneal cavity is rare

Treatment

- Surgical approaches
  - Resection is possible if sufficient reserve liver function
  - Transplantation is option if patient meets "Milan criteria" of single tumor < 5 cm, or fewer than 4 tumors, none > 3 cm
- Drugs
  - Sorafenib
    - Tyrosine kinase inhibitor that has proven to be at least somewhat effective in advanced cases
- Ablation therapy
  - Radiofrequency or microwave ablation or direct percutaneous ethanol injections are options for small tumors
  - Angiographic embolization of hepatic artery can infarct tumor and prolong survival

Prognosis

- Better prognosis associated with age < 50 years, female gender, resectable tumor, better differentiated tumor, low mitotic index, absence of vascular invasion, encapsulated tumor, and absence of cirrhosis
- In USA, 5-year survival is 75% for tumors < 5 cm and 30-40% overall

MACROSCOPIC FEATURES

General Features

- Soft tumor that can be bile-stained, with variable hemorrhage and necrosis
- Can be solitary tumor, solitary tumor with "satellite nodules," multiple discrete tumors, or multiple small indistinct nodules throughout portion of liver or entire liver
  - Pedunculated tumors are rare, more easily resected, and have better prognosis
  - Encapsulated tumors are rare, usually solitary tumors that arise in cirrhotic livers, and have better prognosis
- Gross venous or bile duct invasion may be seen and should be sought

MICROSCOPIC PATHOLOGY

Histologic Features

- Architectural patterns
  - Trabecular pattern: Tumor cells grow as thickened hepatic plates separated by sinusoids without desmoplastic stroma
  - Pseudoglandular or acinar pattern: Tumor cells grow in solid nests with central degenerative changes
  - Compact pattern: Trabeculae grow compressed together
  - Scirrhous pattern: Resemble trabecular HCC but with abundant stroma
  - Giant cell pattern: Multinucleate giant cells
  - Spindle cell pattern is often referred to as sarcomatoid HCC
- Tumor cell morphology
  - Tumor cells resemble hepatocytes with polygonal shape, round vesicular nuclei, and prominent nucleoli
    - Inclusions can be seen in tumor cells, including Mallory hyaline, hyaline globules, and pale bodies
    - Clear cells may be present and even numerous due to accumulation of glycogen, water, or fat

HEPATOCELLULAR CARCINOMA AND VARIANTS

- Presence of bile pigment in dilated canaliculi is helpful in distinguishing HCC from its mimics

Cytologic Features

- Neoplastic cells resemble hepatocytes but with enlarged nuclei, nuclear membrane irregularity, coarse chromatin, and prominent macronucleoli
  - May have dispersed cell pattern with numerous stripped, atypical nuclei
- Tumor cells tend to be more monotonous with less anisonucleosis and higher nuclear to cytoplasmic ratio than benign hepatocytes
- Thick, disordered plates or balls of neoplastic cells, focally lined by sinusoidal endothelial cells ("endothelial wrapping")
- Large tissue fragments traversed by blood vessels

Fibrolamellar Variant

- 5% of hepatocellular carcinomas
- Arises in noncirrhotic livers
- Affects both sexes equally, usually < 35 years of age
- Better prognosis than conventional HCC; 5-year survival rate of approximately 50%
- Grossly has lobular appearance with fibrous septa or central stellate scar
- Nests and sheets of large, eosinophilic, polygonal tumor cells with vesicular nuclei and prominent nucleoli separated by fibrous stroma

ANCILLARY TESTS

Histochemistry

- Reticulin
  - Reactivity: Not applicable
  - Staining pattern
    - Diminished or absent in sinusoids; may outline abnormally thick trabeculae as well

Immunohistochemistry

- Positive for Hep-Par1, Glypican-3, and CAM5.2 (keratins 8 and 18)
- AFP staining is highly specific but insensitive (25%)
- Polyclonal CEA and CD10 demonstrate canalicular pattern
- Sinusoidal capillarization demonstrated with CD34

DIFFERENTIAL DIAGNOSIS

Cholangiocarcinoma

- Mucicarmine(+); expresses CK7, CK19, and CA19-9
- Desmoplastic stroma
- Mixed HCC/cholangiocarcinoma may show features of both

Metastatic Neuroendocrine Tumor

- Prominent collagenous stroma; positive staining for neuroendocrine markers

Metastatic Adenocarcinoma

- Mucicarmine(+); MOC31(+), keratin profile not limited to 8 and 18

Angiomyolipoma

- Presence of adipose tissue and muscular arteries; HMB-45(+), Hep-Par1(-)

Renal Cell Carcinoma

- History of renal cell carcinoma or renal tumor, no cirrhosis
- Hep-Par1(-), pax-2(+), pax-8(+)

Hepatic Adenoma

- Patient demographics differ, cirrhosis absent, trabeculae at most 2 or 3 cells thick

Regenerative Nodule in Cirrhosis

- Cytologically benign, absence of trabecular or pseudoglandular growth pattern
- Portal tracts present in nodule
- Intact reticulin

Dysplastic Nodule in Cirrhosis

- Cytologic atypia and mild architectural abnormalities
- Contains portal tracts, lacks invasion of portal tracts by tumor
- Intact reticulin

GRADING

Edmonson and Steiner

- Grade I (well differentiated): Small hepatocytic tumor cells arranged as trabeculae
- Grade II (moderately differentiated): Larger tumor cells with abnormal nuclei and eosinophilic cytoplasm; pseudoglandular structures may be seen
- Grade III (poorly differentiated): More frequent tumor giant cells
- Grade IV (undifferentiated): Poorly differentiated tumor cells with hyperchromatic nuclei, little cytoplasm, and loss of trabecular architecture

SELECTED REFERENCES

1. Stuart KE et al: Hepatocellular carcinoma in the United States. Prognostic features, treatment outcome, and survival. Cancer. 77(11):2217-22, 1996
2. Hurlimann J et al: Immunohistochemistry in the differential diagnosis of liver carcinomas. Am J Surg Pathol. 15(3):280-8, 1991
3. Kassianides C et al: The clinical manifestations and natural history of hepatocellular carcinoma. Gastroenterol Clin North Am. 16(4):553-62, 1987
4. Craig JR et al: Fibrolamellar carcinoma of the liver: a tumor of adolescents and young adults with distinctive clinicopathologic features. Cancer. 46(2):372-9, 1980

Gross and Microscopic Features

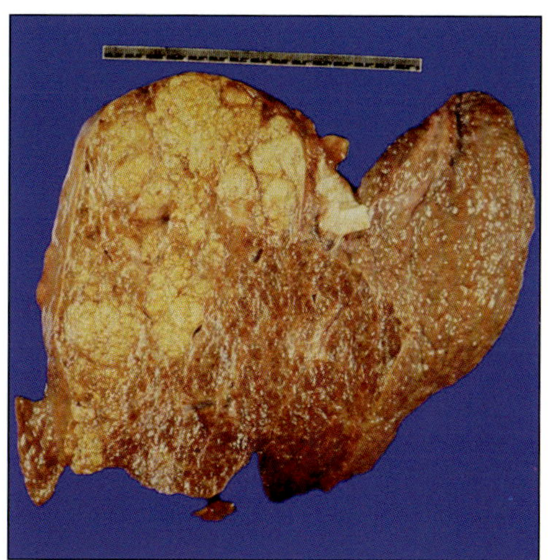

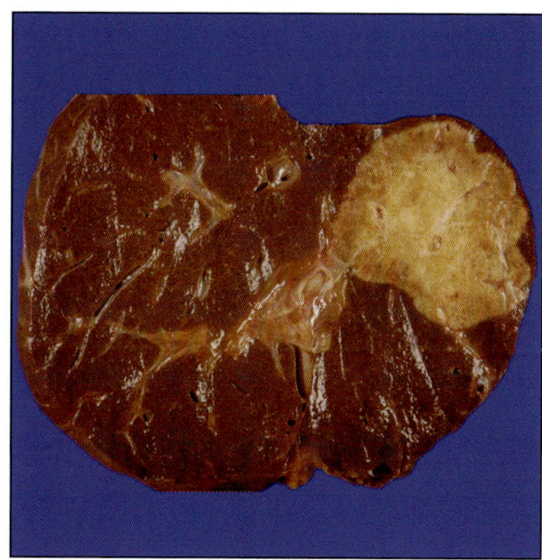

(Left) This large, multinodular hepatocellular carcinoma arises in a background of cirrhosis. **(Right)** This hepatocellular carcinoma is unifocal, yellow-tan, and well circumscribed. The background liver is not cirrhotic.

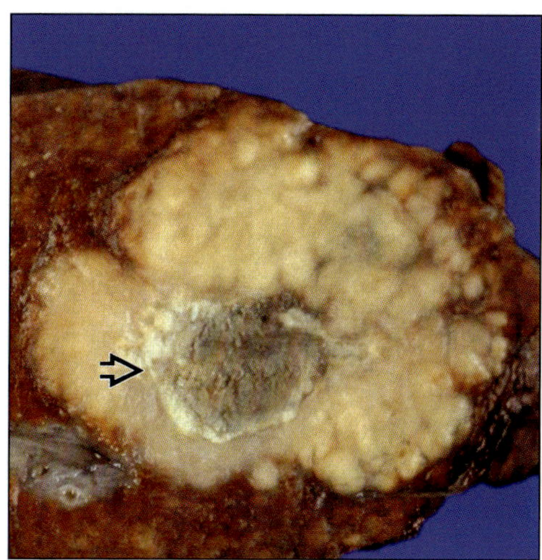

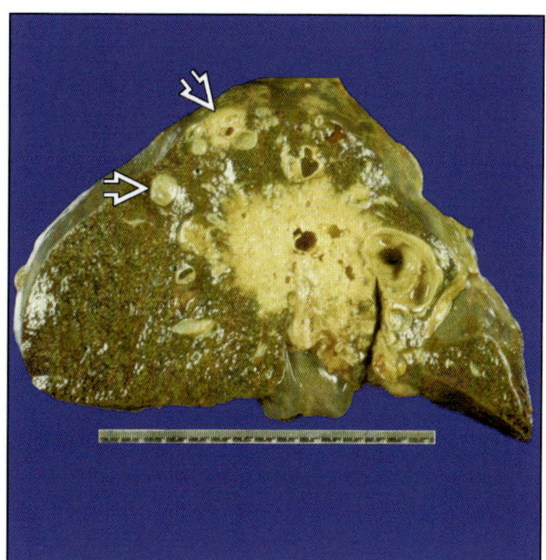

(Left) This hepatocellular carcinoma arose in a background of hereditary hemochromatosis; note the rust-colored cirrhotic liver in the background. There is also central necrosis ⇨. **(Right)** This hepatocellular carcinoma is composed of a large central mass with small satellite tumor nodules ➡. There is a background of cirrhosis.

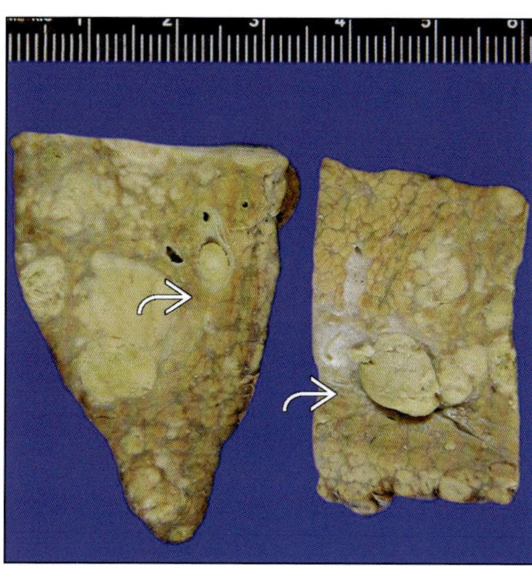

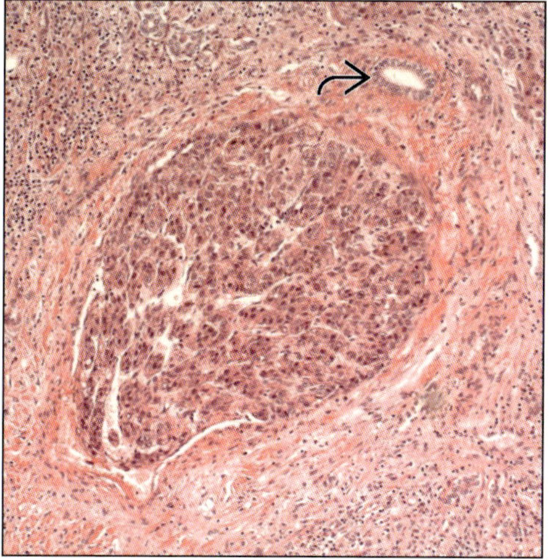

(Left) This example of the diffuse pattern of HCC shows innumerable small white-tan nodules of a tumor in a background of cirrhosis. Careful inspection shows that 2 of these nodules represent gross venous invasion ↪. **(Right)** A histologic section of a tumor shows venous invasion by HCC. A portal vein is distended and filled with trabeculae of hyperchromatic neoplastic cells. Note the adjacent accompanying bile duct ↪.

Microscopic Features

(Left) The trabecular pattern of hepatocellular carcinoma is characterized by thickened trabeculae separated by sinusoids. In this focus, the trabeculae appear to be approximately 6-8 cells thick. **(Right)** This hepatocellular carcinoma is growing in a pattern of rounded trabeculae with central degenerative changes.

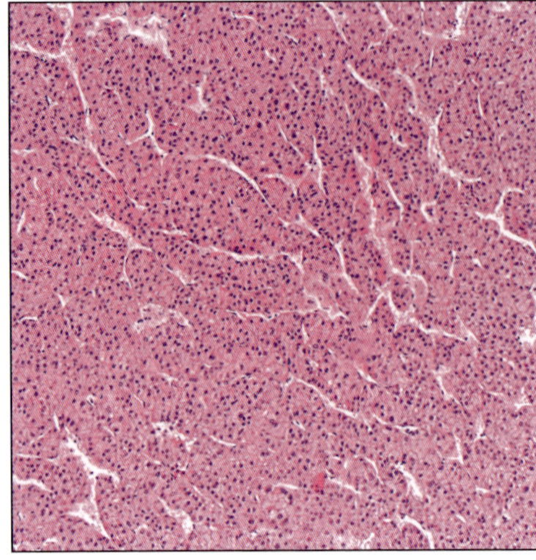

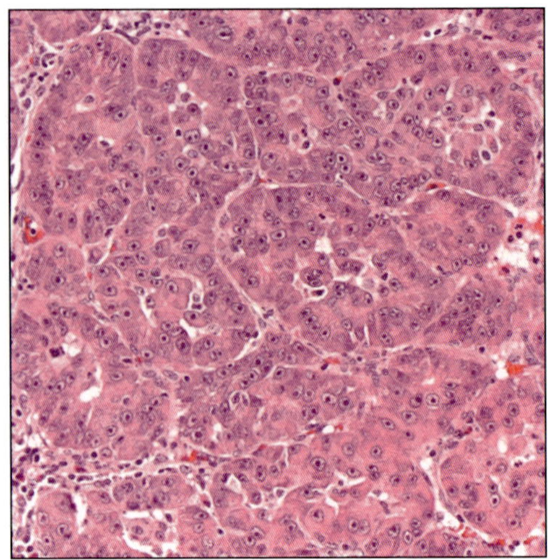

(Left) In the pseudoglandular pattern of hepatocellular carcinoma, dilated spaces in the centers of trabeculae mimic glands ➔. **(Right)** This example of sarcomatoid hepatocellular carcinoma has extensive spindle cell change. Notice the interlacing of spindle cells with more compact epithelioid tumor cells ↷.

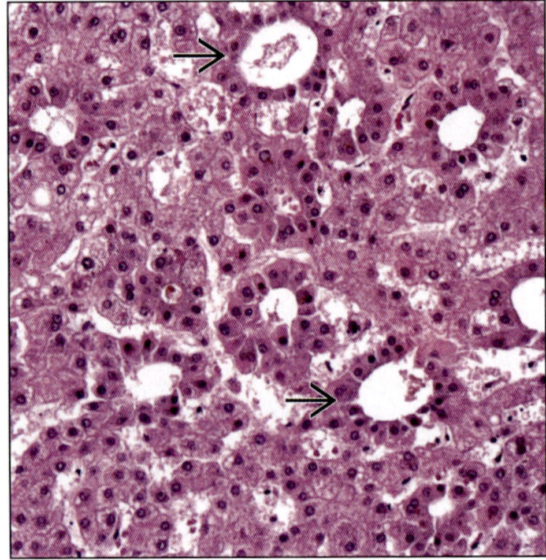

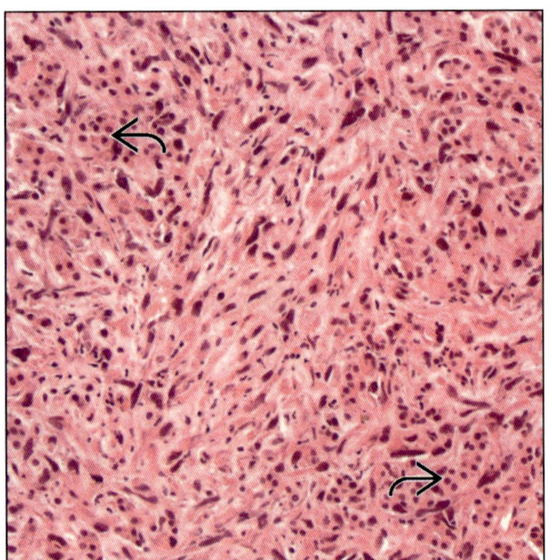

(Left) These tumor cells in HCC contain pale eosinophilic inclusions in the cytoplasm, presumably fibrinogen, known as pale bodies. **(Right)** Mallory hyaline can be seen in hepatocellular carcinoma. In this tumor, many of the tumor cells contain an oval eosinophilic inclusion ➔. Although Mallory hyaline in HCC can have the characteristic ropy appearance of alcoholic hyaline, it often is more globular and rounded.

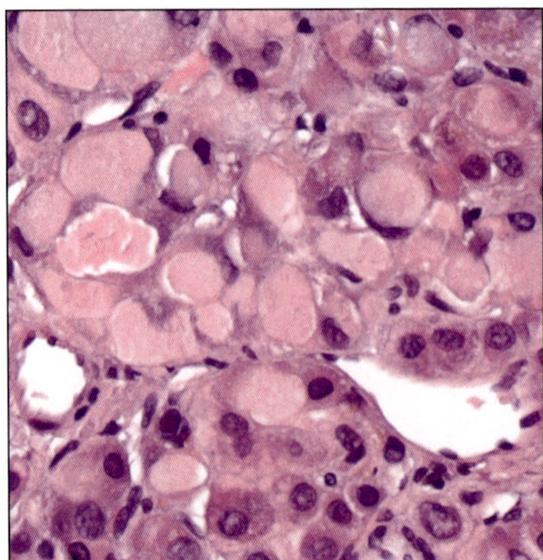

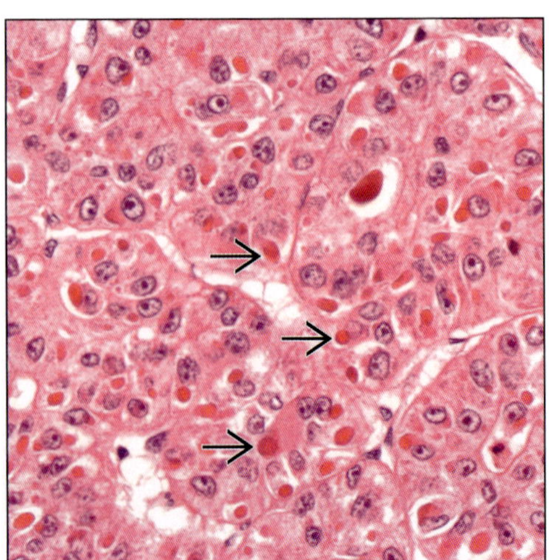

Microscopic and Gross Features and Variants

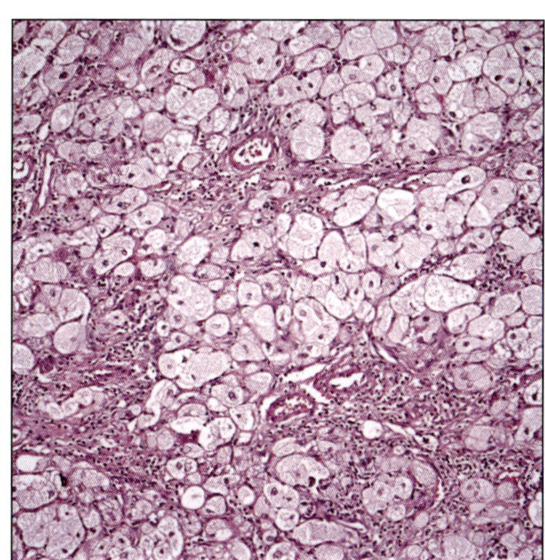

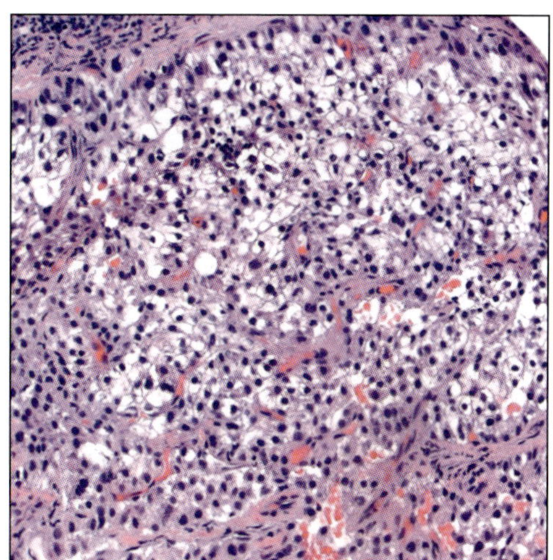

(Left) *The clear cell variant of hepatocellular carcinoma contains tumor cells with abundant glycogen in the cytoplasm, creating a clear appearance reminiscent of clear cell renal cell carcinoma.* ***(Right)*** *Metastatic renal cell carcinoma in the liver is easily mistaken for the clear cell variant of hepatocellular carcinoma. This patient had an identical renal tumor excised a few years prior to this tumor developing in the liver.*

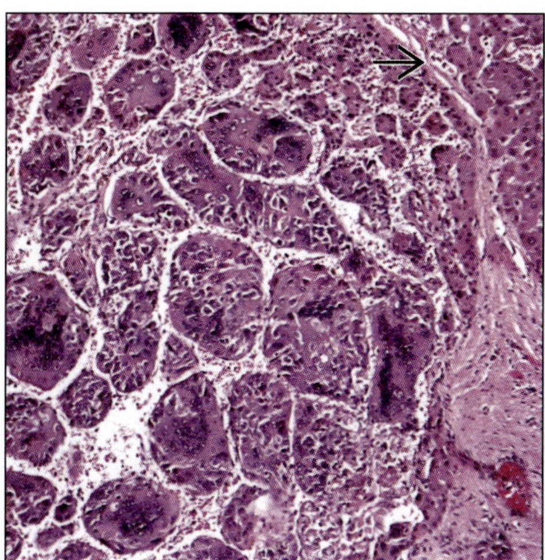

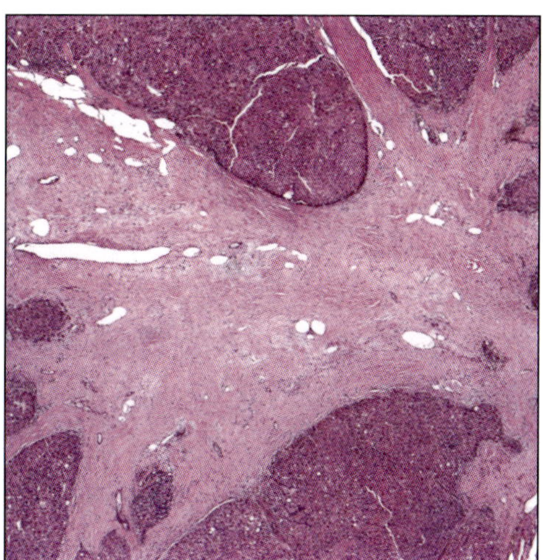

(Left) *This giant cell variant of hepatocellular carcinoma features striking multinucleated tumor giant cells. An area of more typical HCC is present at the periphery of the field →.* ***(Right)*** *The scirrhous pattern of HCC has prominent stroma and may form a large central fibrous scar that can mimic focal nodular hyperplasia or fibrolamellar variant of HCC. The other histologic features of fibrolamellar variant of HCC are absent, however.*

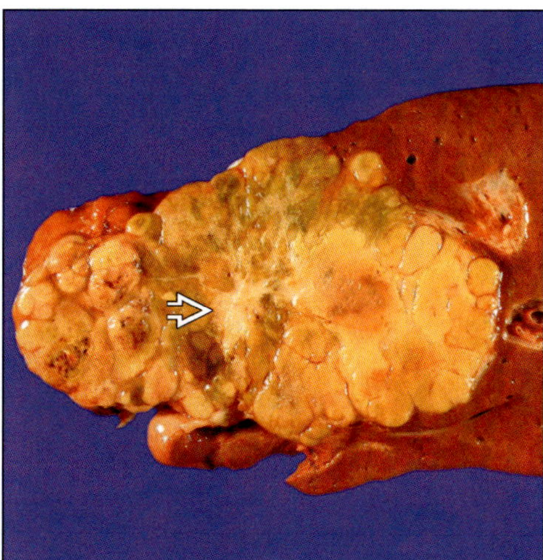

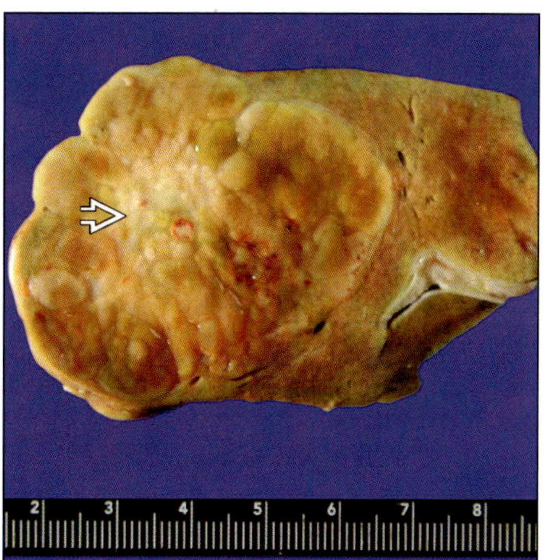

(Left) *The fibrolamellar variant of hepatocellular carcinoma typically has a lobular growth pattern and central scar ➡. Also note the absence of cirrhosis in the background liver.* ***(Right)*** *Clinically, this fibrolamellar HCC in a young woman was thought to be focal nodular hyperplasia. Note the lobular growth pattern and central scar ➡, typical of both focal nodular hyperplasia and fibrolamellar HCC.*

HEPATOCELLULAR CARCINOMA AND VARIANTS

Microscopic Features

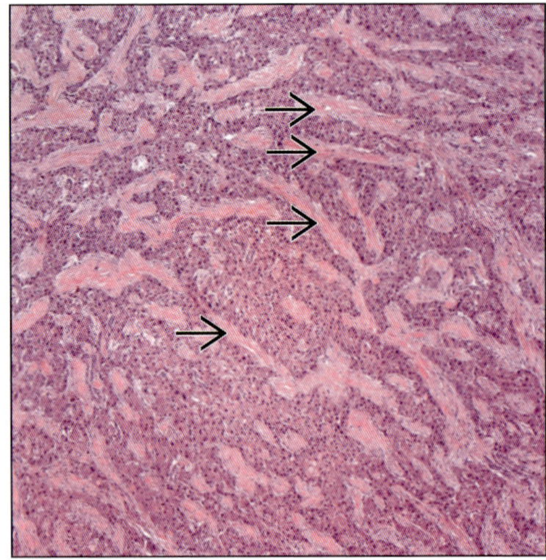

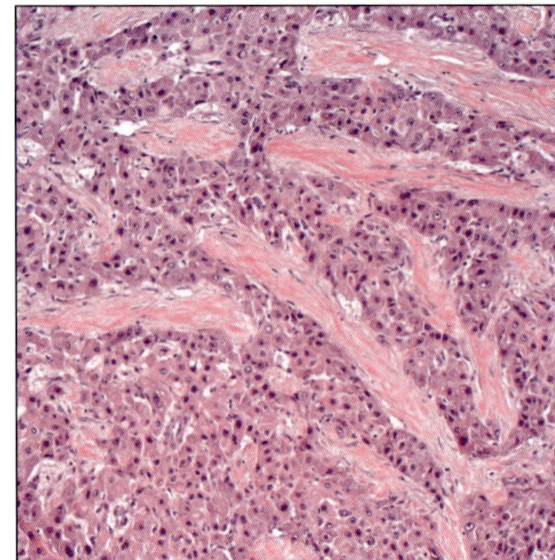

(Left) *Low-power view of fibrolamellar HCC shows cords of neoplastic hepatocytes separated by parallel arrays of collagenous stroma ⇒.* ***(Right)*** *High magnification of fibrolamellar HCC shows fibrous septae composed of parallel collagen fibers separating trabeculae of plump eosinophilic tumor cells.*

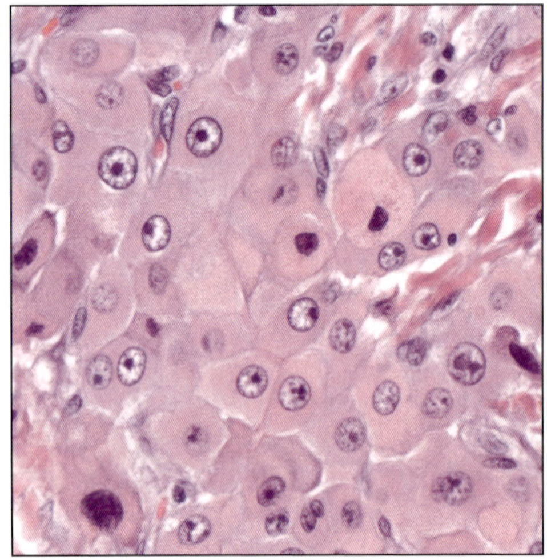

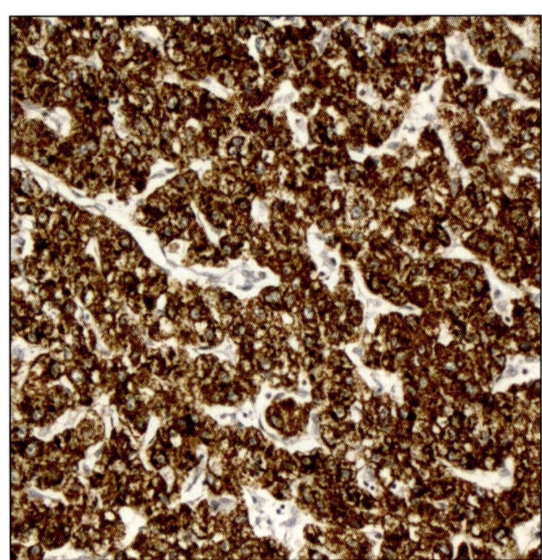

(Left) *In the fibrolamellar variant of HCC, the tumor cells are large, eosinophilic, and polygonal. They have large, vesicular nuclei with prominent nucleoli. The eosinophilic cytoplasm is due to large numbers of mitochondria.* ***(Right)*** *Hep-Par1 immunohistochemical stain in hepatocellular carcinoma shows strong positive cytoplasmic staining.*

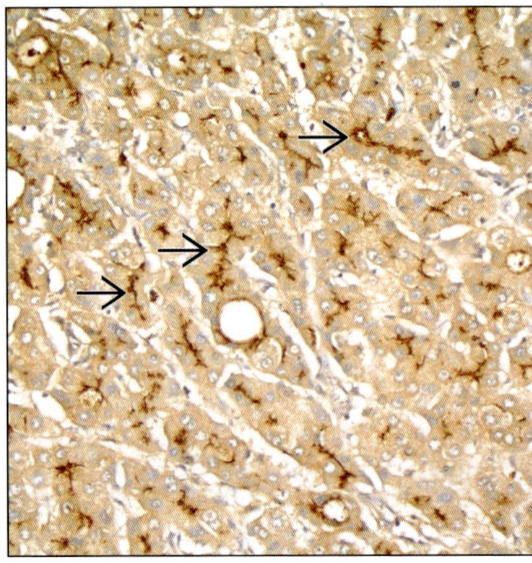

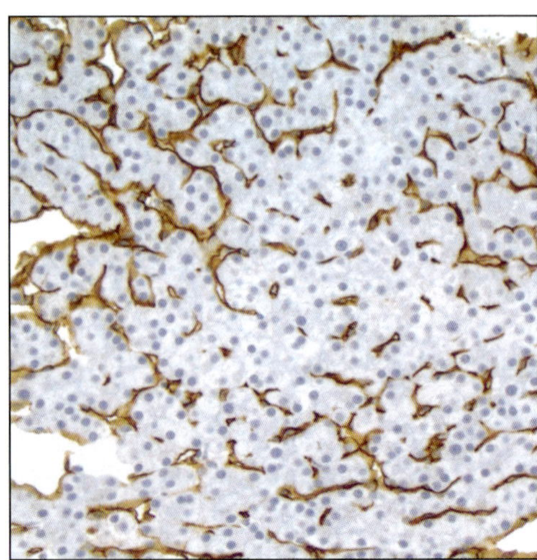

(Left) *Polyclonal CEA immunostain shows staining of bile canaliculi ⇒ in hepatocellular carcinoma, producing a so-called canalicular pattern. This is in contrast to the pattern typical of ductal adenocarcinoma in which diffuse cytoplasmic staining is seen.* ***(Right)*** *CD34 in hepatocellular carcinoma stains the sinusoidal endothelium. The sinusoids in hepatocellular carcinoma become "capillarized," and thus express antigens normally found in capillary endothelium but not in normal sinusoidal endothelium.*

Microscopic and Cytologic Features

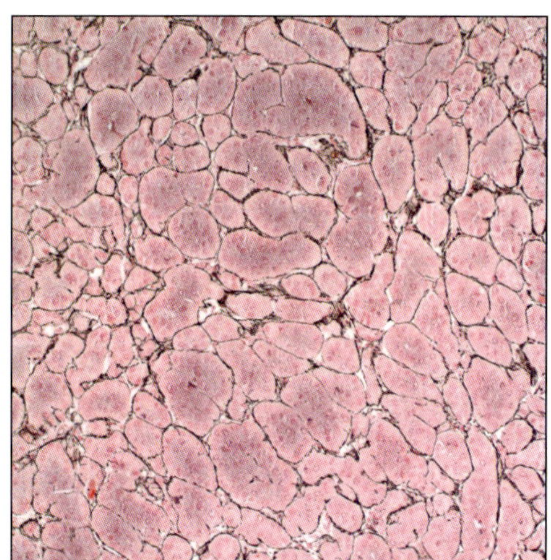

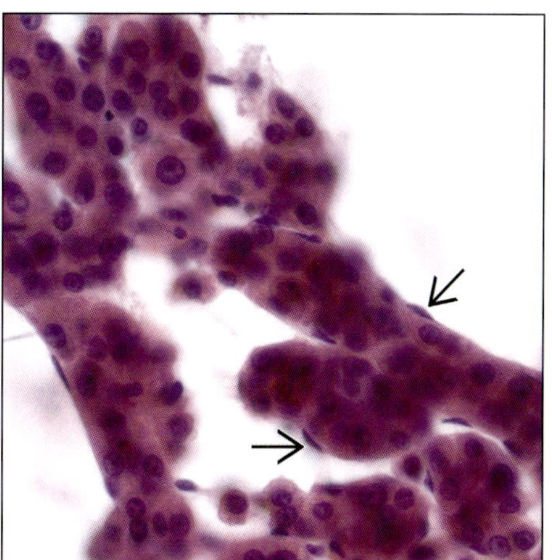

(Left) *Reticulin stain in hepatocellular carcinoma demonstrates abnormal trabecular growth pattern with thickened disorganized trabeculae. Reticulin is also frequently reduced in amount or even absent in HCC.* ***(Right)*** *Fine needle aspiration biopsy smear of HCC shows a trabecular growth pattern composed of thick trabeculae of neoplastic hepatocytes. Endothelial wrapping is present at the edges of the tumor* ⇒*.*

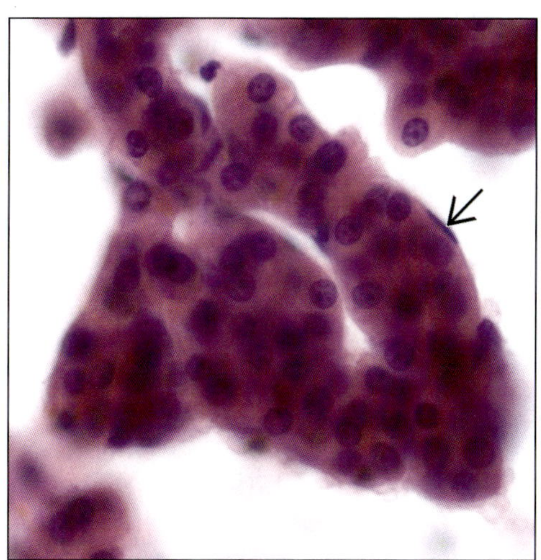

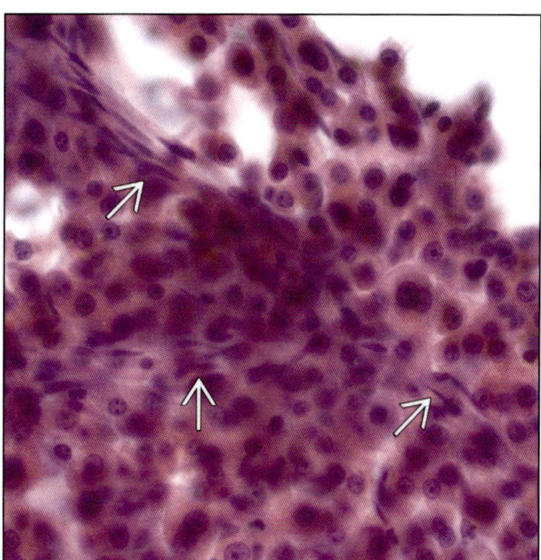

(Left) *Note the smooth contours of this group of HCC cells from an FNA created by endothelial wrapping* ⇒*. Note the increased nuclear density.* ***(Right)*** *This FNA biopsy smear of HCC shows a large cluster of neoplastic hepatocytes with traversing blood vessels* ➡ *typical of this tumor. A similar phenomenon occurs commonly in renal cell carcinoma.*

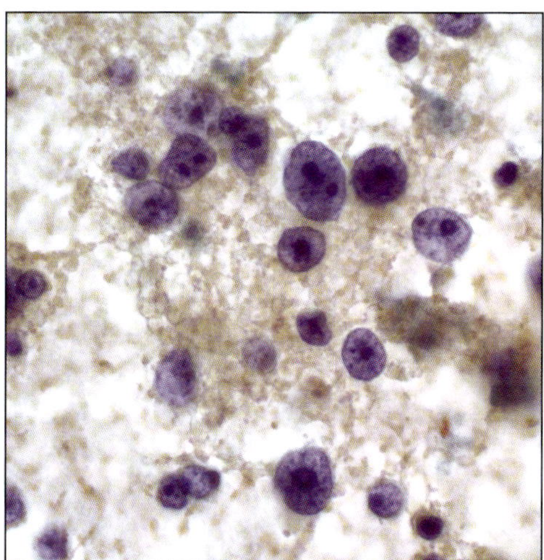

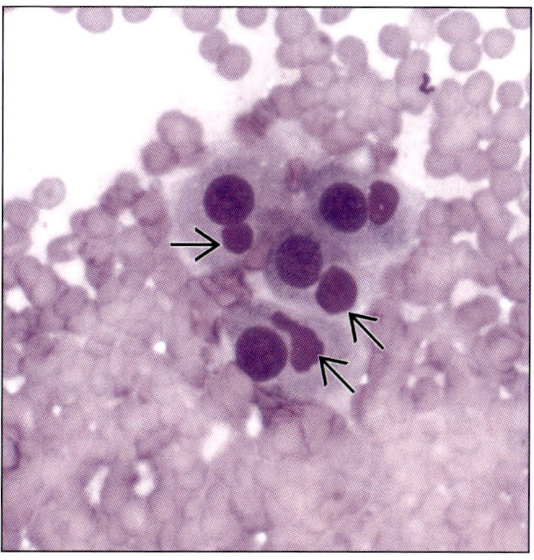

(Left) *This FNA smear of an HCC shows innumerable stripped atypical nuclei scattered throughout the slide. This pattern is not an uncommon one for HCC.* ***(Right)*** *In this air-dried preparation, the malignant hepatocytes contain cytoplasmic inclusions consistent with Mallory hyaline* ⇒*. Note that many of the inclusions are more round or oval than alcohol-related Mallory hyaline.*

HEPATOBLASTOMA

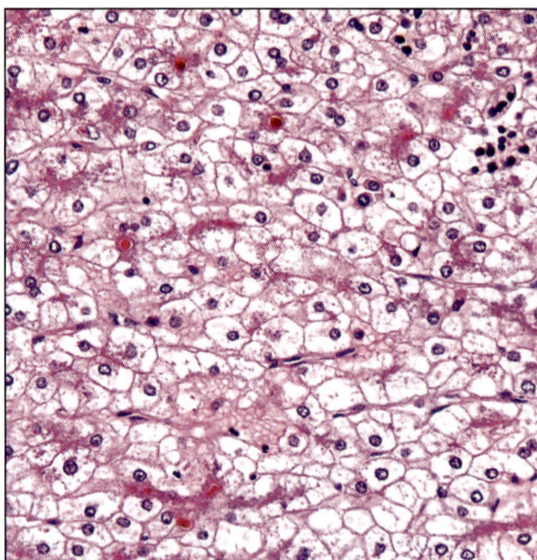

Pure fetal histology consists of uniform polygonal cells that are smaller than normal hepatocytes, have round nuclei, no nucleoli, and clear cytoplasm. This pattern is clinically significant.

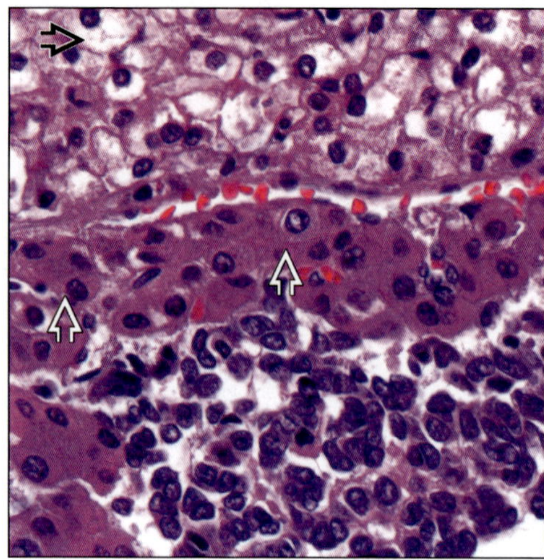

The amount of small undifferentiated cells (bottom right field) should be reported. In contrast, the fetal epithelial cells ➡ above have abundant cytoplasm with variable amounts of glycogen.

TERMINOLOGY

Abbreviations

- Hepatoblastoma (HB)

Definitions

- Predominantly pediatric liver tumor that mimics developing fetal or embryonal liver histologically

ETIOLOGY/PATHOGENESIS

Neoplasm

- β-catenin mutation-associated *Wnt* pathway activation in 70-90%

CLINICAL ISSUES

Epidemiology

- Incidence
  - Constitutes 2.1% of all pediatric cancers in 1- to 19-year-old age group
  - Increased reporting in low birth weight infants but etiology unknown
- Age
  - Most common malignant liver neoplasm in children
    - 88% in children ≤ 5 years and 3% > 15 years
    - Mean age at diagnosis is 19 months
- Gender
  - Male predominance
    - M:F = 3:2

Site

- 58% involves right lobe
- 27% involves both lobes

Presentation

- Painless abdominal mass
  - Hepatomegaly

Laboratory Tests

- Increased serum α-fetoprotein in 75-96% of patients
  - Often ≥100,000 ng/mL
    - Caveat: Neonates < 6 months of age normally have elevated α-fetoprotein
  - Useful marker of response to therapy and recurrence

Treatment

- Surgical resection
  - Only 1/3 to 1/2 have resectable disease at presentation
  - Preoperative chemotherapy converts > 50% of inoperable tumors to resectable tumors
- Orthotopic liver transplant

Children's Oncology Group Staging System (Pre-treatment Staging)

- Stage I: Completely resected tumors with negative margins
- Stage II: Grossly resected tumors with residual disease
  - Microscopic positive margin
- Stage III: Unresectable tumors
  - Biopsy diagnosis, partially resected, macroscopic residual tumor, tumor rupture
  - Positive abdominal lymph node
- Stage IV: Tumors with metastasis to lungs, other organs, or sites distant from abdomen

Prognosis

- Tumor stage is key prognostic factor in survival
  - 90% event-free survival with primary complete resection of tumor
  - < 70% event-free survival in those with nonmetastatic, unresectable tumor

Metastasis

- 10-20% of patients have metastases at presentation
- Most frequently spread to lung but can involve bone, brain, eye, or ovaries

HEPATOBLASTOMA

Key Facts

Etiology/Pathogenesis
- Aberrant Wnt/β-catenin activation

Clinical Issues
- Most common malignant liver neoplasm in children
- Typically presents with abdominal mass
- Most patients have increased serum α-fetoprotein
- Key prognostic factor of survival is tumor stage
  - May require preoperative chemotherapy before tumor is resectable

Microscopic Pathology
- Most common component is epithelial subtypes
  - Pure fetal epithelial histology is associated with favorable prognosis
  - Commonly embryonal and fetal epithelial patterns are seen together
  - Macrotrabecular is composed of fetal or embryonal type cells in wide trabeculae
  - Any amount of small undifferentiated cells often resembling neuroblasts is associated with poorer prognosis
- Mixed HB are composed of epithelial and mesenchymal components
  - Mesenchymal component can be immature spindle cells to fibrous tissue
  - Osteoid-like and even teratoid elements can be found

Top Differential Diagnoses
- Normal liver parenchyma; positive nuclear &/or cytoplasmic β-catenin staining in HB
- Hepatocellular carcinoma; presence of both fetal and embryonal cells diagnostic of HB

- 20-30% survival if there is metastatic disease at presentation

Conditions Associated with HB
- Familial adenomatous polyposis, Beckwith-Wiedemann, Li-Fraumeni, and Simpson-Golabi-Behmel syndromes
- Trisomy 18, glycogen storage disease types I-IV, and hemihypertrophy

IMAGE FINDINGS

Radiographic Findings
- Solitary or multifocal mass
  - Heterogeneous and hypervascular
  - Calcification is frequently observed

PRETEXT (Pretreatment Extent of Disease) Classification
- Assessment made prior to treatment
  - Determines number of affected liver segments and extent of venous involvement, if present
- Guides surgical approach

MACROSCOPIC FEATURES

General Features
- Solitary or multifocal, coarsely lobulated, heterogeneous mass
  - Fetal pattern areas resemble normal liver, light brown or moderately firm
  - Embryonal and small cell patterns are softer, fleshy to gelatinous, gray-tan or pale pink
  - Mesenchymal, osteoid-like areas are firm, fibrous, or calcified
  - Teratoid, melanotic component may be dark brown or black
- Carefully search for vascular invasion

Size
- Large; can be > 15 cm

MICROSCOPIC PATHOLOGY

Histologic Features
- Epithelial patterns
  - Fetal
    - Uniform cells arranged in slender cords (2-3 cells thick) and thin trabeculae
    - Fetal epithelial cells are smaller than normal hepatocytes
    - Central round to oval nuclei, inconspicuous nucleolus, and abundant clear to pink cytoplasm with distinct membrane
    - Alternating light and dark areas based on cytoplasmic glycogen content; may have fat
    - Low mitotic index (≤ 2 mitoses/10 high-power fields)
  - Crowded fetal (fetal with mitoses)
    - Similarities to pure fetal pattern but cells are closely packed and have higher mitotic count (≥ 2 mitoses/10 high-power fields)
    - Slightly increased nuclear to cytoplasmic ratio, round nuclei, and eosinophilic cytoplasm
    - Intermixed with pure fetal pattern and merged into embryonal pattern; can be difficult to differentiate
  - Embryonal
    - Primitive cells in sheets, pseudorosettes, acini, or tubules
    - Small, angulated nuclei (larger than fetal nuclei) with coarse nuclear chromatin, prominent nucleoli, scant cytoplasm, indistinct membranes
    - Mitotic figures more frequent
  - Small undifferentiated
    - Can be difficult to recognize and diagnose
    - Resembles neuroblast, blastemal cells, or cells found in "small round blue cell" neoplasms
    - Grows in sheets, lacks cohesiveness, and infiltrative
    - High nuclear to cytoplasmic ratio with almost no cytoplasm, hyperchromatic nuclei, inconspicuous nucleoli

HEPATOBLASTOMA

- Can have rhabdoid-like cells with eccentric cytoplasm
- Variable mitotic rate
- Extramedullary hematopoiesis occurs in fetal and embryonal patterns
  - Not useful to distinguish these epithelial patterns based on this finding alone
- Mesenchymal component
  - Highly cellular primitive mesenchymal cells (immature spindle cells) with scant cytoplasm and elongated, plump nuclei
  - Collagenous stroma with loose fibrosis &/or mature fibrous tissue
  - Osteoid-like areas
    - Immunoreactive for cytokeratin and epithelial membrane antigen; a metaplastic phenomenon
  - Bone, cartilage, and rhabdomyoblasts
- Teratoid component
  - Primitive neuroglia, ganglion cells, or melanin pigment
  - Can also show bone, cartilage, rhabdomyoblasts, squamous cells, and mucinous glands

Morphologic Classification

- Epithelial HB (majority of HBs)
  - Epithelial patterns can occur alone or in combination with other epithelial patterns
    - Embryonal subtype alone or with fetal component
    - Squamous epithelium and mucinous glands can be part of an epithelial HB
  - Pure fetal histology HB
    - 100% composed of fetal epithelial cells, not crowded fetal
    - Low mitotic index (≤ 2 mitoses/10 high-power fields)
  - Macrotrabecular HB
    - Fetal &/or embryonal cells in wide trabeculae, > 10 cells thick
  - Small undifferentiated or small cell anaplastic HB
    - For a diagnosis of pure small undifferentiated HB, > 70% of tumor is composed of small undifferentiated cells
    - Any amount of small undifferentiated cells should be reported; provide percentage of small undifferentiated cells
    - May be located toward center of an embryonal region
- Mixed HB
  - Both epithelial and mesenchymal elements
- Mixed HB with teratoid (heterologous) features

Prognostic Factors

- Stage
  - Stage IV associated with uniform poor prognosis (39% 5-year, event-free survival)
- Histology
  - Pure fetal epithelial HB is associated with excellent prognosis (100% 5-year, event-free survival)
  - Significantly poorer than pure fetal HB
    - HB with any amount of small cell undifferentiated cells
    - Potentially macrotrabecular HB
- α-fetoprotein < 100 confers worse prognosis

ANCILLARY TESTS

Immunohistochemistry

- Nuclear β-catenin staining in epithelial and mesenchymal components (70% of HB)
  - Positive in small undifferentiated cells
- Positive glypican-3 and Hep-Par1 staining in fetal and embryonal epithelial cells
- Positive glutamine synthetase staining in fetal and variably in embryonal cells
- INI1/BAF47 loss in some small undifferentiated cells, especially if rhabdoid phenotype

DIFFERENTIAL DIAGNOSIS

Normal Liver Parenchyma

- Must distinguish fetal epithelial cells of hepatoblastoma from normal hepatocytes, particularly near a margin
  - HB has nuclear &/or cytoplasmic immunoreactivity for β-catenin
  - Fetal cells are smaller than normal hepatocytes

Hepatocellular Carcinoma

- May be indistinguishable from macrotrabecular variant of HB
  - Biphasic pattern with both fetal and embryonal cells points to HB
  - Nuclear β-catenin and glypican-3 more consistently positive in HB

DIAGNOSTIC CHECKLIST

Clinically Relevant Pathologic Features

- Stage 1 pure fetal HB cured by surgical resection alone
- Important to report any amount of small undifferentiated cells; confers worse prognosis

SELECTED REFERENCES

1. Wang LL et al: Effects of neoadjuvant chemotherapy on hepatoblastoma: a morphologic and immunohistochemical study. Am J Surg Pathol. 34(3):287-99, 2010
2. Meyers RL et al: Predictive power of pretreatment prognostic factors in children with hepatoblastoma: a report from the Children's Oncology Group. Pediatr Blood Cancer. 53(6):1016-22, 2009
3. Finegold MJ et al: Protocol for the examination of specimens from pediatric patients with hepatoblastoma. Arch Pathol Lab Med. 131(4):520-9, 2007
4. Rowland JM: Hepatoblastoma: assessment of criteria for histologic classification. Med Pediatr Oncol. 39(5):478-83, 2002
5. Stocker JT: Hepatic tumors in children. Clin Liver Dis. 5(1):259-81, viii-ix, 2001

Microscopic Features

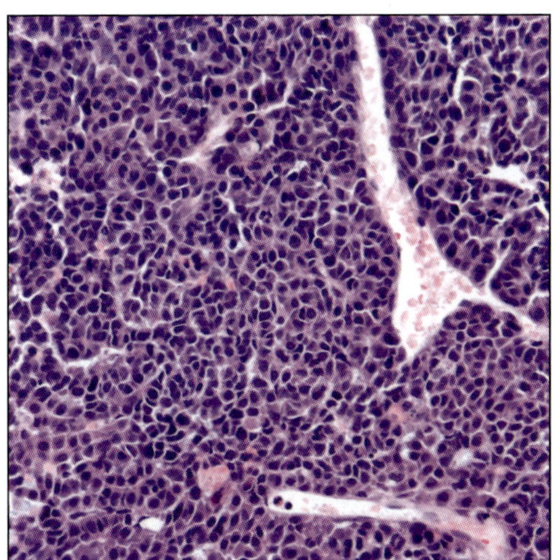

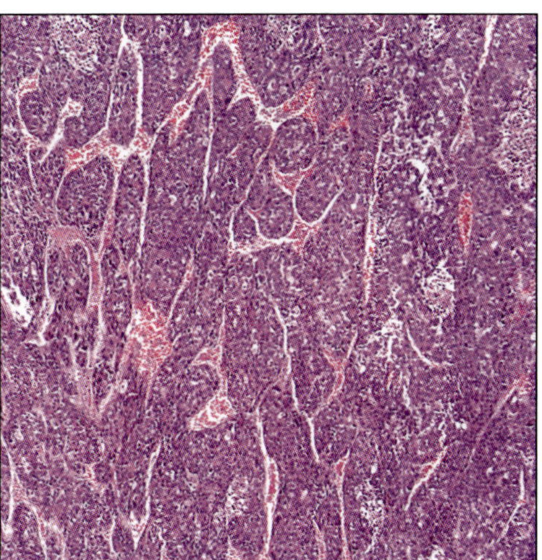

(Left) *Sheets and poorly formed nests of embryonal epithelial cells have angulated nuclei and less cytoplasm than fetal epithelial cells, which can often coexist within the same tumor. Embryonal cells have nuclear or cytoplasmic reactivity to β-catenin and are diffusely positive for glypican-3.* ***(Right)*** *Macrotrabecular HB can mimic hepatocellular carcinoma at low power. Look for mesenchymal components or fetal epithelial pattern to assist in the diagnosis.*

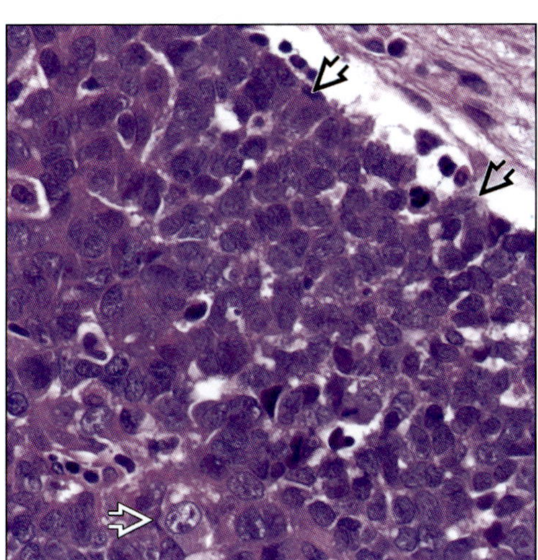

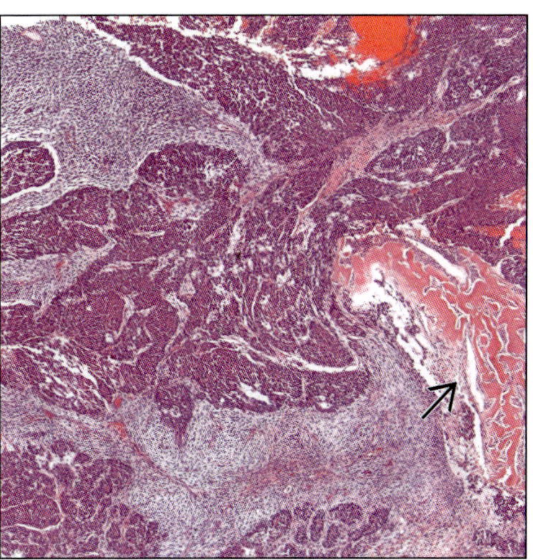

(Left) *This HB shows embryonal epithelial cells ➡ merging into a focus of small undifferentiated cells ⇨. The latter have even less cytoplasm and are often discohesive. These cells look like neuroblasts or blastemal cells but have positive nuclear stain for β-catenin. Even a microscopic focus of small undifferentiated cells confers a poorer prognosis.* ***(Right)*** *This mixed HB has embryonal epithelial cells, spindled mesenchymal component, and a focus of osteoid-like tissue →.*

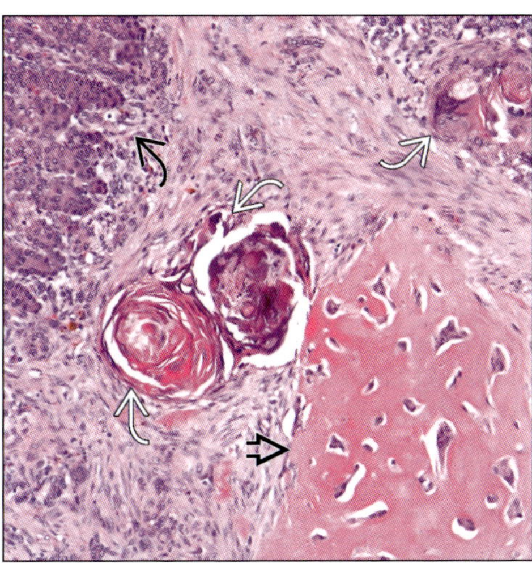

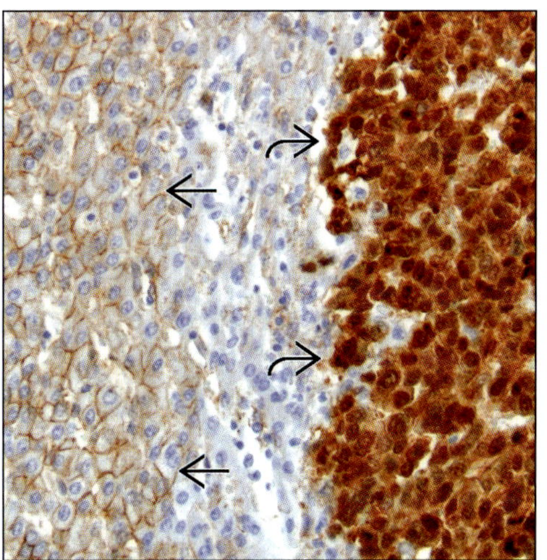

(Left) *This mixed HB has neoplastic epithelial cells ↪ in cords, squamoid nests ↪ within dense fibrous stroma, and an osteoid-like ➡ focus. This is not considered a mixed HB with teratoid features because there is no neural or neuroectodermal differentiation.* ***(Right)*** *Immunohistochemical staining for β-catenin can be useful. The liver parenchyma → shows membranous staining of normal hepatocytes, while the hepatoblastoma ↪ has nuclear staining in neoplastic cells.*

PERIBILIARY HAMARTOMA (BILE DUCT ADENOMA)

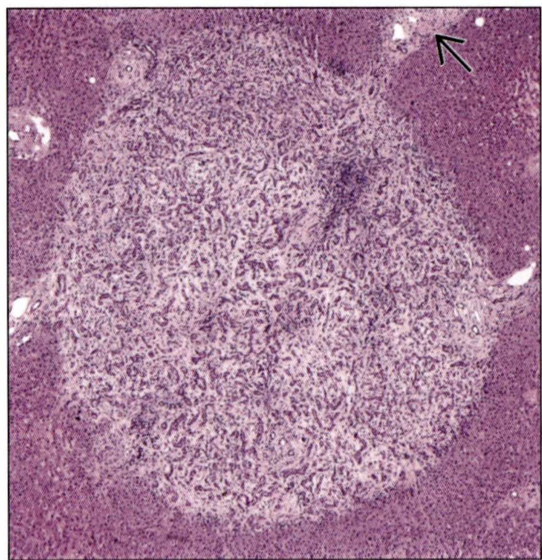

Peribiliary gland hamartomas are well circumscribed but unencapsulated. Note the obvious fibrous stroma and the adjacent portal tract ➔.

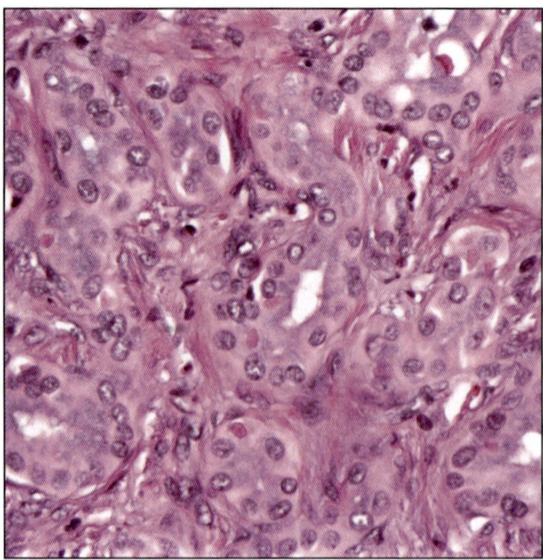

The glands in PGH are rounded and closely packed, with a single layer of cuboidal epithelium. Lumens are small or inapparent. Note the lack of nuclear atypia and mitoses.

TERMINOLOGY

Abbreviations

- Bile duct adenoma (BDA)
- Peribiliary gland hamartoma (PGH)

Synonyms

- Bile duct adenoma
- Cholangioma
- Cholangioadenoma

Definitions

- Small, benign epithelial tumor composed of glands that resemble bile ducts
  - Historically called "bile duct adenoma"
  - Recently shown that cells have phenotype of peribiliary glands rather than bile ducts

CLINICAL ISSUES

Epidemiology

- Age
  - Adults older than 40 years
- Gender
  - Equal gender distribution

Presentation

- Almost always incidental findings during surgery for another reason
  - Often submitted for frozen section during intraabdominal surgery to exclude metastasis

Prognosis

- Excellent
  - Malignant degeneration has not been well documented

MACROSCOPIC FEATURES

General Features

- Typically small (< 1 cm)
  - Rare lesions up to 4 cm
- Usually single but can be multiple
- Well circumscribed but not encapsulated
- Often subcapsular
- Firm and gray-white

MICROSCOPIC PATHOLOGY

Histologic Features

- Uniformly sized tubules and acini
  - Single layer of cuboidal to columnar cells
    - Basal nuclei without atypia
    - No hyperchromasia
    - No mitoses
  - Small or inapparent lumens
  - Rounded outlines
- Fibrous stroma either scant or dense and hyalinized
  - More abundant centrally than peripherally
- Variable amount of inflammation present
- Normal portal tracts &/or large bile ducts often associated with BDA
- Bile is not present
  - Ducts do not communicate with biliary tree
- Acidic mucin is usually present
- Variant features
  - Mucinous metaplasia
  - Neuroendocrine differentiation
  - α-1-antitrypsin globules
    - Rare cases associated with α-1-antitrypsin deficiency also contain α-1-antitrypsin globules
  - Rare variant with clear cells can be mistaken for primary or metastatic clear cell carcinoma

PERIBILIARY HAMARTOMA (BILE DUCT ADENOMA)

Key Facts

Terminology

- Historically called "bile duct adenoma" but shown to have phenotype of peribiliary glands rather than bile ducts

Clinical Issues

- Almost always incidental findings during surgery for another reason
  - Submitted for frozen section to rule out metastasis

Microscopic Pathology

- Uniformly sized tubules and acini with rounded outlines
- Single layer of cuboidal to columnar cells that lack atypia, hyperchromasia, mitoses
- Fibrous stroma either scant or dense and hyalinized
- Bile is not present, and ducts do not communicate with biliary tree

DIFFERENTIAL DIAGNOSIS

Biliary Micro-Hamartoma (von Meyenburg Complex)

- Curvilinear and angular rather than round ducts
- More abundant stroma
- Often contain bile
- Associated with polycystic liver disease

Cholangiocarcinoma/Metastatic Adenocarcinoma

- Nuclear atypia
- Poorly circumscribed
  - Infiltrative or destructive growth pattern
- Lymphovascular or perineural invasion
- Mitoses
- Bile duct adenomas are small (usually < 1 cm) and almost always found incidentally in asymptomatic patients

Neuroendocrine Tumor

- Endocrine cell clusters in some bile duct adenomas can be confused with metastatic neuroendocrine tumors

DIAGNOSTIC CHECKLIST

Clinically Relevant Pathologic Features

- Almost always incidental findings at time of surgery for another intraabdominal process
  - This lesion is most noteworthy for being mistaken for metastatic adenocarcinoma

SELECTED REFERENCES

1. Hornick JL et al: Immunohistochemistry can help distinguish metastatic pancreatic adenocarcinomas from bile duct adenomas and hamartomas of the liver. Am J Surg Pathol. 29(3):381-9, 2005
2. Albores-Saavedra J et al: Atypical bile duct adenoma, clear cell type: a previously undescribed tumor of the liver. Am J Surg Pathol. 25(7):956-60, 2001
3. Bhathal PS et al: The so-called bile duct adenoma is a peribiliary gland hamartoma. Am J Surg Pathol. 20(7):858-64, 1996
4. O'Hara BJ et al: Bile duct adenomas with endocrine component. Immunohistochemical study and comparison with conventional bile duct adenomas. Am J Surg Pathol. 16(1):21-5, 1992
5. Allaire GS et al: Bile duct adenoma. A study of 152 cases. Am J Surg Pathol. 12(9):708-15, 1988
6. Govindarajan S et al: The bile duct adenoma. A lesion distinct from Meyenburg complex. Arch Pathol Lab Med. 108(11):922-4, 1984

IMAGE GALLERY

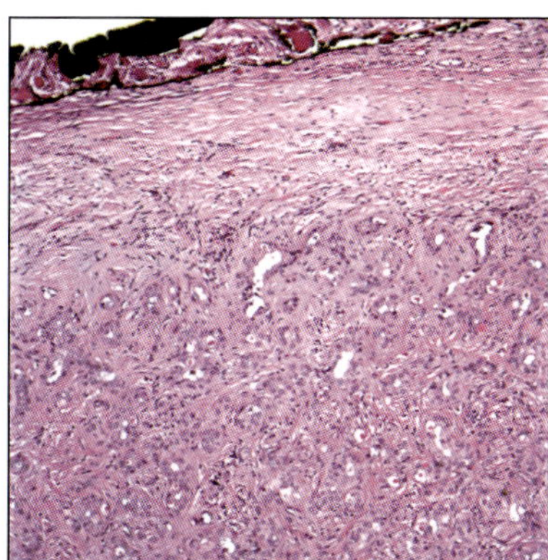

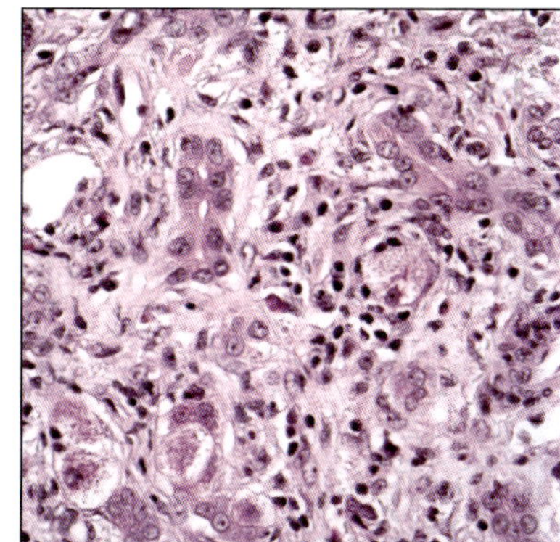

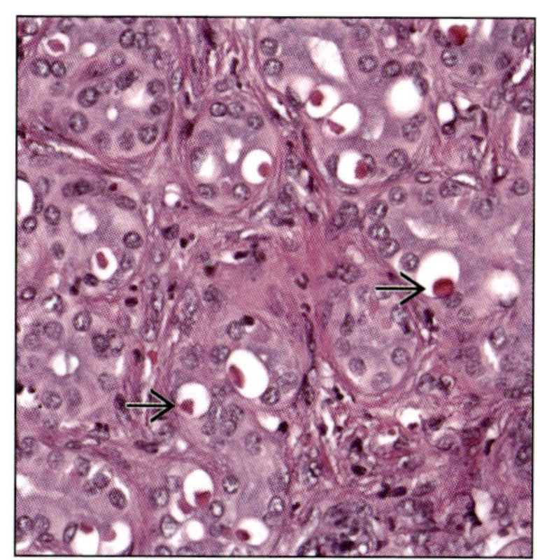

(Left) *Peribiliary gland hamartomas are often subcapsular, as seen in this case.* ***(Center)*** *This peribiliary gland hamartoma has abundant loose fibrous stroma with admixed chronic inflammation. The tubular glands are lined by a single layer of cuboidal epithelium with uniform nuclei.* ***(Right)*** *Some peribiliary gland hamartomas contain α-1-antitrypsin globules ⇒. Note the lack of nuclear atypia, mitoses, or nuclear hyperchromasia within the small rounded glands.*

VON MEYENBURG COMPLEX (BILIARY MICROHAMARTOMA)

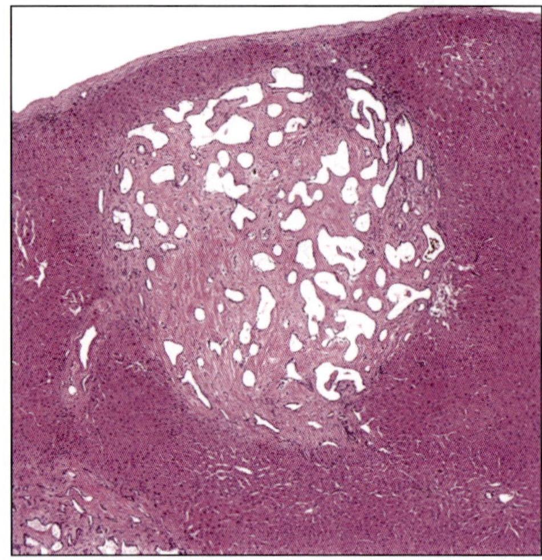
This small, subcapsular VMC features branching, irregular, angulated glands embedded in a dense fibrous stroma.

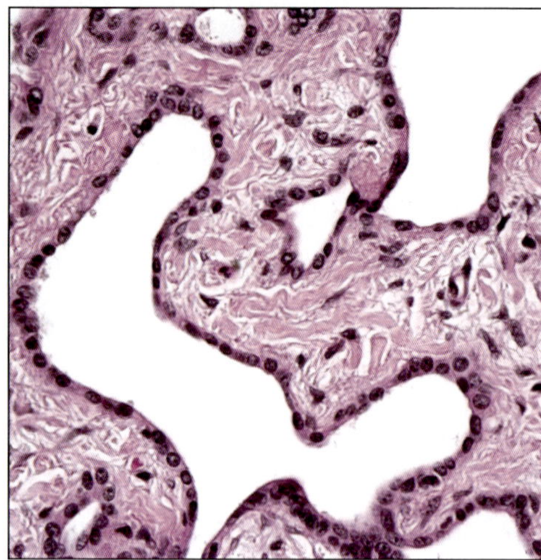
The branching, angulated glands in VMC are lined by a single layer of flattened cuboidal epithelium. There is no nuclear atypia.

TERMINOLOGY

Abbreviations

- von Meyenburg complex (VMC)

Synonyms

- Biliary microhamartoma
- Ductal plate malformation

Definitions

- Developmental malformation resulting from aberrant construction/remodeling of embryonic bile ducts

ETIOLOGY/PATHOGENESIS

Developmental Anomaly

- Within spectrum of fibropolycystic diseases of liver
  - Most often sporadic
  - Also associated with numerous fibropolycystic diseases including congenital hepatic fibrosis, Caroli disease, autosomal dominant polycystic disease
    - Considered precursor lesion of autosomal dominant polycystic liver disease
    - Basic lesion of congenital hepatic fibrosis

CLINICAL ISSUES

Epidemiology

- Incidence
  - Not precisely known
  - Occur in approximately 3% of autopsied patients

Presentation

- Often incidental findings at surgery or autopsy
  - May be submitted for frozen section during abdominal surgery to exclude metastasis

Treatment

- None for sporadic lesions
- Treat underlying disease if part of fibropolycystic disease

Prognosis

- Not considered premalignant
  - Rare cases of cholangiocarcinoma arising in VMC have been reported

MACROSCOPIC FEATURES

General Features

- Most are small (usually < 0.5 cm), gray-white, irregular, and commonly multifocal
- Most often multiple
  - Can be solitary
  - Presence of numerous, widely scattered VMC raises possibility of fibropolycystic disease or congenital hepatic fibrosis
- Gray-white or green
- Often subcapsular

MICROSCOPIC PATHOLOGY

Histologic Features

- Located within and at edge of portal tracts
- Dense fibrous stroma
- Small to medium-sized ducts embedded in dense fibrous stroma
  - Many ducts are irregularly shaped, angulated, or branching and dilated
    - Ducts are lined by cuboidal to flattened epithelium
    - No atypia
    - No mitotic activity
    - Ducts may contain eosinophilic proteinaceous debris or inspissated bile
  - Varying degrees of dilatation that may eventually lead to cyst formation
  - Not connected to normal biliary tree

VON MEYENBURG COMPLEX (BILIARY MICROHAMARTOMA)

Key Facts

Terminology

- Developmental malformation resulting from aberrant construction/remodeling of embryonic bile ducts

Etiology/Pathogenesis

- Most often sporadic; also associated with several fibropolycystic liver diseases

Macroscopic Features

- Usually multifocal and < 0.5 cm

Microscopic Pathology

- Angulated, branching, irregular ducts embedded in dense fibrous stroma
- Usually within or at edge of portal tracts

Diagnostic Checklist

- Multiple widely scattered VMC raise possibility of associated fibropolycystic disease

---

- Transition to hyperplasia, dysplasia, and cholangiocarcinoma has been very rarely noted

DIFFERENTIAL DIAGNOSIS

Bile Duct Adenoma (BDA)

- Glands have uniform round outlines
- Bile is absent
- Absence of cystic changes
- Not associated with fibropolycystic liver diseases
- Immunohistochemistry
  - BDA expresses 1F6 and D10, similar to bile ductules and canals of Hering
  - VMC expresses D10 but not 1F6

Cholangiocarcinoma/Metastatic Adenocarcinoma

- Nuclear atypia, infiltrative or destructive growth pattern, mitoses
- Lymphovascular or perineural invasion

Biliary Adenofibroma

- Rare entity with few reported cases
- Tortuous and branching ductular elements with
  - Microcystic dilatation
  - Cuboidal to flattened lining epithelium
  - Prominent fibroblastic stroma
- Immunophenotype same as VMC
- Bears marked resemblance to biliary hamartoma but is larger, not associated with any typical VMC

DIAGNOSTIC CHECKLIST

Clinically Relevant Pathologic Features

- Multiple widely scattered VMC raise possibility of associated congenital hepatic fibrosis or polycystic liver disease

SELECTED REFERENCES

1. Hornick JL et al: Immunohistochemistry can help distinguish metastatic pancreatic adenocarcinomas from bile duct adenomas and hamartomas of the liver. Am J Surg Pathol. 29(3):381-9, 2005
2. Jain D et al: Evidence for the neoplastic transformation of Von-Meyenburg complexes. Am J Surg Pathol. 24(8):1131-9, 2000
3. Desmet VJ: Congenital diseases of intrahepatic bile ducts: variations on the theme "ductal plate malformation". Hepatology. 16(4):1069-83, 1992
4. Karhunen PJ: Adult polycystic liver disease and biliary microhamartomas (von Meyenburg's complexes). Acta Pathol Microbiol Immunol Scand A. 94(6):397-400, 1986

IMAGE GALLERY

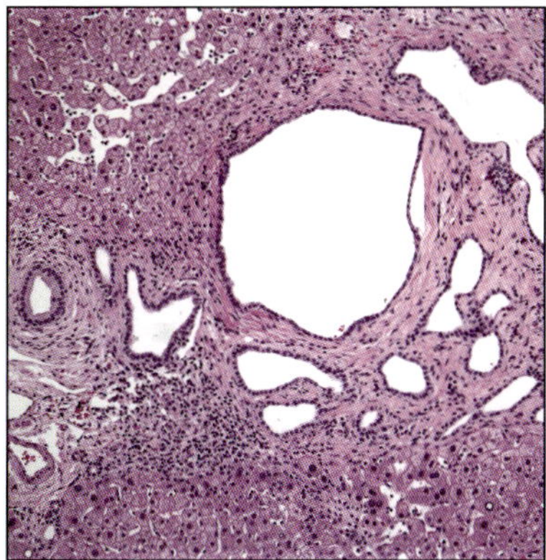

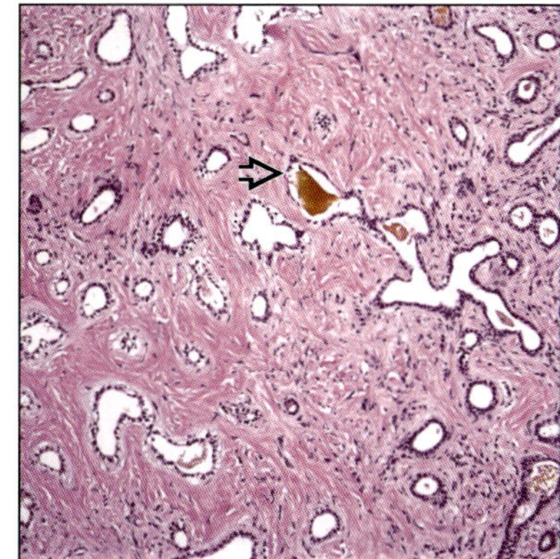

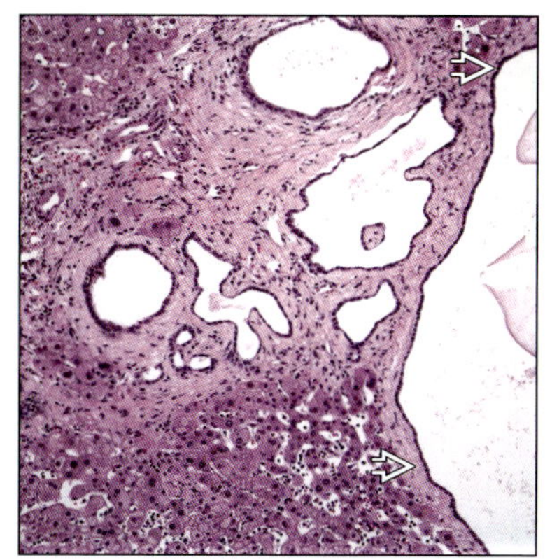

(Left) *von Meyenburg complex are located within or at the edge of portal tracts.* ***(Center)*** *VMC is characterized by angulated, branching glands within dense fibrous stroma. Note the inspissated bile ⇨. There is no nuclear atypia and no mitoses.* ***(Right)*** *Some of the glands within the von Meyenburg complex have dilated to produce a cyst ➡, which is filled with eosinophilic proteinaceous material. This patient has autosomal dominant polycystic disease.*

BILIARY CYSTADENOMA AND CYSTADENOCARCINOMA

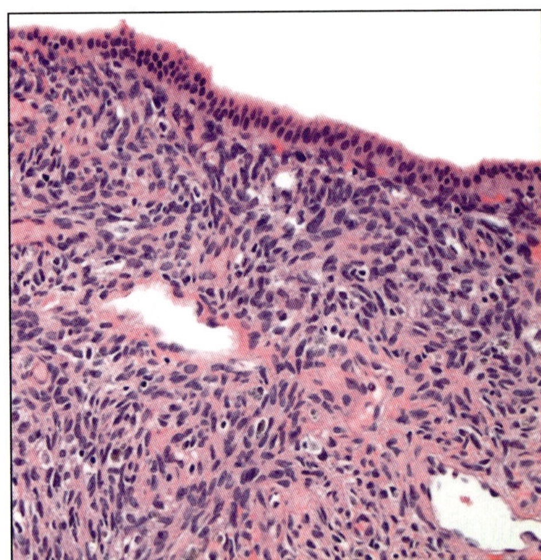

The classic spindled and cellular ovarian-type stroma is seen underneath the cyst lining of a biliary cystadenoma.

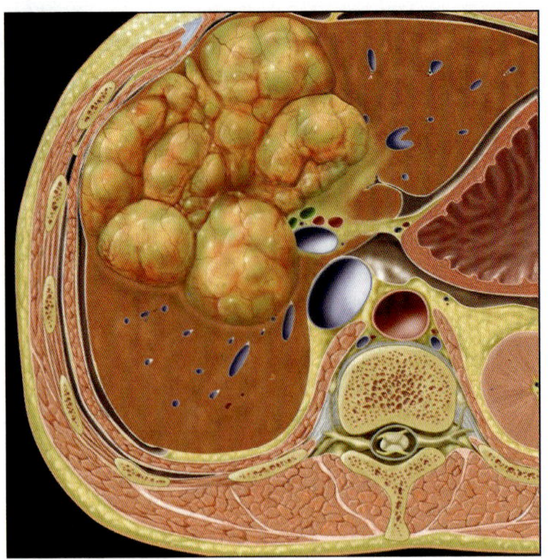

This graphic shows a lobulated complex cystic mass with a vascularized wall, areas of solid growth, and well-defined septa typical of biliary cystadenocarcinoma.

TERMINOLOGY

Definitions

- Cystic biliary neoplasm arising within liver
  - May arise in extrahepatic biliary tree, including gallbladder

ETIOLOGY/PATHOGENESIS

Unknown

- May arise from gallbladder precursor elements or peribiliary glands
- Most cystadenocarcinomas arise from preexisting biliary cystadenoma
  - Some may represent cystic variant of cholangiocarcinoma
  - Occasionally may arise in biliary cysts

CLINICAL ISSUES

Epidemiology

- Incidence
  - Rare; < 5% of cystic lesions of liver
- Age
  - Average is 40-50 years
- Gender
  - Biliary cystadenoma almost exclusively occurs in women
  - Biliary cystadenocarcinoma may be seen in men, given varied pathogenesis

Presentation

- Pain, mass, and occasionally jaundice
  - Some patients are asymptomatic

Laboratory Tests

- CA19-9 and CEA in cyst fluid helps differentiate between simple cyst and biliary cystic neoplasm

Treatment

- Surgical approaches
  - Complete resection

Prognosis

- Surgical resection should be curative
  - Incompletely resected tumor may recur or undergo malignant transformation

IMAGE FINDINGS

Ultrasonographic Findings

- Large, well-defined, multiloculated, anechoic mass with highly echogenic septations
- Mural or septal calcifications or fluid levels

CT Findings

- Nonenhancing CT
  - Large, well-defined, homogeneous, hypodense heterogeneous mass (cystic & hemorrhagic areas)
  - Cystadenoma: Septations without nodularity
  - Cystadenocarcinoma: Septations and nodularity
  - Fine mural or septal calcifications
  - Biliary dilatation
- Contrast-enhancing CT
  - Nonenhancing cystic spaces
  - Enhancement of internal septa, capsule, and papillary excrescences or nodules
  - Fine mural or septal calcifications

MACROSCOPIC FEATURES

General Features

- Solitary, multiloculated cystic neoplasm
  - Typically large, with variable numbers of internal septations
  - Clear, straw-colored, mucinous, or opalescent cystic fluid
    - Rarely hemorrhagic or purulent

BILIARY CYSTADENOMA AND CYSTADENOCARCINOMA

Key Facts

Clinical Issues

- Biliary cystadenoma almost exclusively occurs in women
- CA19-9 and CEA in cyst fluid helps differentiate between simple cyst and biliary cystic neoplasm

Macroscopic Features

- Solitary, multiloculated cystic neoplasm
- Clear, mucinous, or opalescent cystic fluid
- Cyst lining may be smooth, trabeculated, or have papillary excrescences
- Thickened, nodular areas suggest malignancy

Microscopic Pathology

- Similar to mucinous cystic neoplasm of pancreas
- Cystadenoma
  - Lined by mucinous columnar epithelium with focal cuboidal, flattened, or papillary areas
  - May have gastric or intestinal metaplasia
  - Varying degrees of dysplasia may be present
  - Densely cellular ovarian-like stroma positive for estrogen and progesterone receptors and inhibin
- Cystadenocarcinoma
  - Most arise from preexisting cystadenoma
  - Invasion of underlying stroma by malignant glands or single cells

Top Differential Diagnoses

- Cystic variant of biliary intraductal papillary neoplasm
- Solitary bile duct cysts
- Ciliated hepatic foregut cyst

- Cyst lining may be smooth, trabeculated, or have papillary excrescences
  - Thickened areas suggest malignancy, and extensive sampling is warranted

Size

- Ranges from several cm to > 20 cm

MICROSCOPIC PATHOLOGY

Histologic Features

- Cystadenoma
  - Cystic spaces are lined by benign columnar epithelium
    - Focally may be cuboidal, flattened, or papillary
    - Epithelial cells almost always contain cytoplasmic mucin that stains positive with Alcian blue or mucicarmine
    - Gastric-type or intestinal metaplasia may be present
    - Epithelial cells are immunoreactive to CK8, CK18, CK7, and CK19
  - Densely cellular ovarian-type stroma
    - Only present in women
    - Immunoreactive to estrogen and progesterone receptors and inhibin
  - Varying degrees of dysplasia may be present
- Cystadenocarcinoma
  - Cytological atypia present in epithelial lining
  - Invasion of underlying stroma by malignant glands or single cells
  - Mitoses
  - Ovarian-type stroma present in female patients

DIFFERENTIAL DIAGNOSIS

Cystic Variant of Biliary Intraductal Papillary Neoplasm

- No gender predilection
- Lack of ovarian-type stroma
- Has prominent papillary proliferation with fibrovascular cores
- Communication with prominent, cystically dilated bile duct

Solitary Biliary Cyst

- Asymptomatic, often incidental findings
- Usually unilocular
- No gender predilection
- Lack of ovarian-type stroma

Ciliated Hepatic Foregut Cyst

- Ciliated epithelium
- Usually small, asymptomatic, incidental findings
- No gender predilection
- Lack of ovarian-type stroma

DIAGNOSTIC CHECKLIST

Pathologic Interpretation Pearls

- Multilocular cystic neoplasm lined by mucinous epithelial cells with underlying ovarian-type stroma

SELECTED REFERENCES

1. Zen Y et al: Biliary cystic tumors with bile duct communication: a cystic variant of intraductal papillary neoplasm of the bile duct. Mod Pathol. 19(9):1243-54, 2006
2. Weihing RR et al: Hepatobiliary and pancreatic mucinous cystadenocarcinomas with mesenchymal stroma: analysis of estrogen receptors/progesterone receptors and expression of tumor-associated antigens. Mod Pathol. 10(4):372-9, 1997
3. Devaney K et al: Hepatobiliary cystadenoma and cystadenocarcinoma. A light microscopic and immunohistochemical study of 70 patients. Am J Surg Pathol. 18(11):1078-91, 1994
4. Wheeler DA et al: Cystadenoma with mesenchymal stroma (CMS) in the liver and bile ducts. A clinicopathologic study of 17 cases, 4 with malignant change. Cancer. 56(6):1434-45, 1985

BILIARY CYSTADENOMA AND CYSTADENOCARCINOMA

Gross, Radiographic, and Microscopic Features

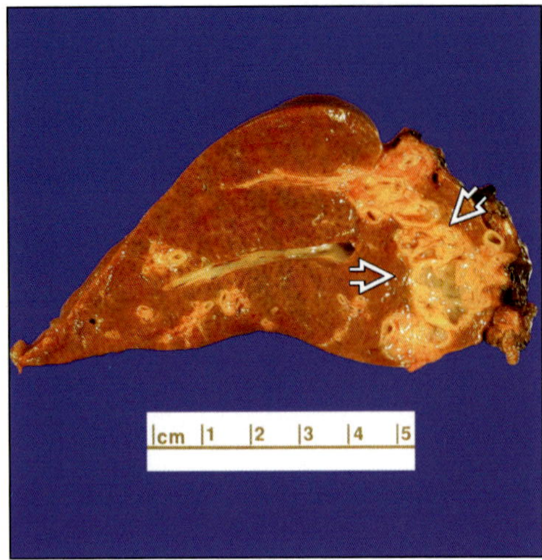

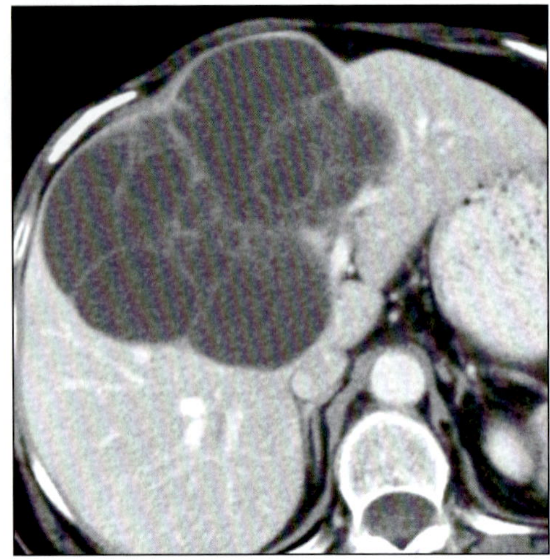

(Left) *This biliary cystadenoma consists of a multiloculated cystic tumor that is visible on the cut surface of the specimen* ➪. **(Right)** *An axial CECT shows a complex multiloculated cystic mass in the liver, with lobulated margins and an enhancing wall and septa, typical of biliary cystadenoma.*

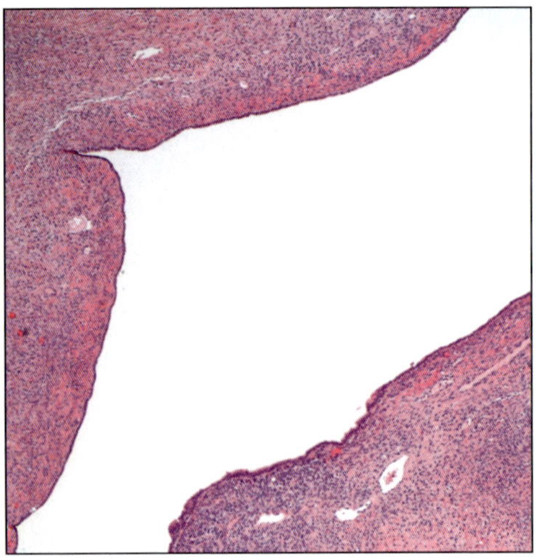

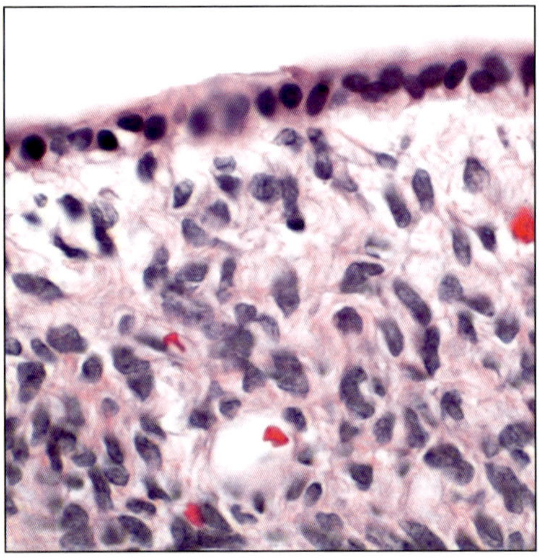

(Left) *Biliary cystadenomas are composed of cystic spaces lined by cuboidal or low columnar biliary epithelium. The ovarian-type stroma, composed of abundant spindly cells, is visible even at low power.* **(Right)** *The lining epithelial cells of biliary cystadenomas are typically simple columnar cells without cytologic atypia. Note the underlying cellular stroma composed of spindly cells.*

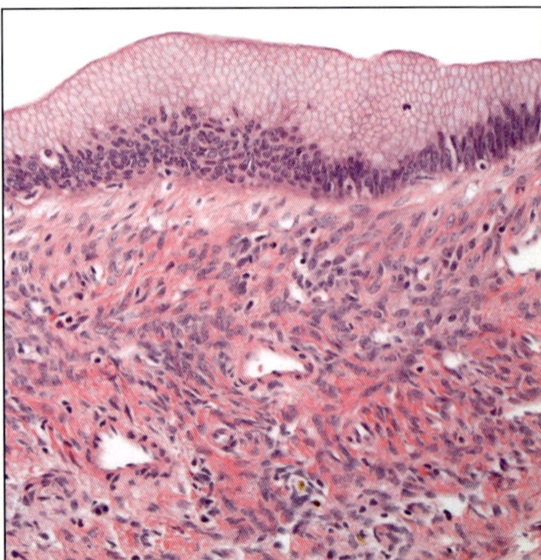

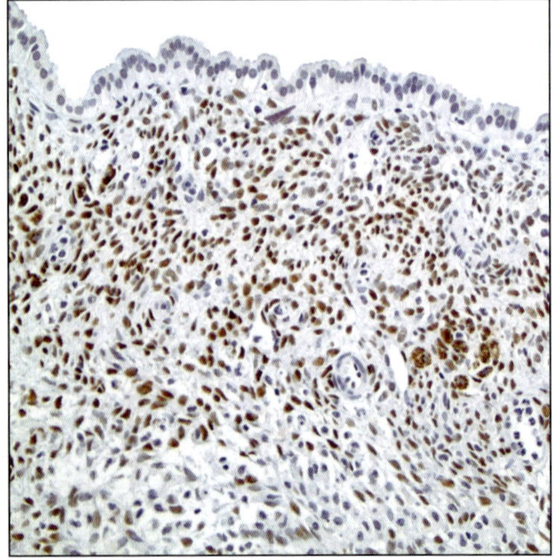

(Left) *The lining epithelial cells in biliary cystadenomas may show gastric-type metaplasia with cytoplasmic mucin.* **(Right)** *The stromal cells in biliary cystadenomas are positive for progesterone receptor (PR) upon immunohistochemical staining.*

Microscopic and Radiographic Features

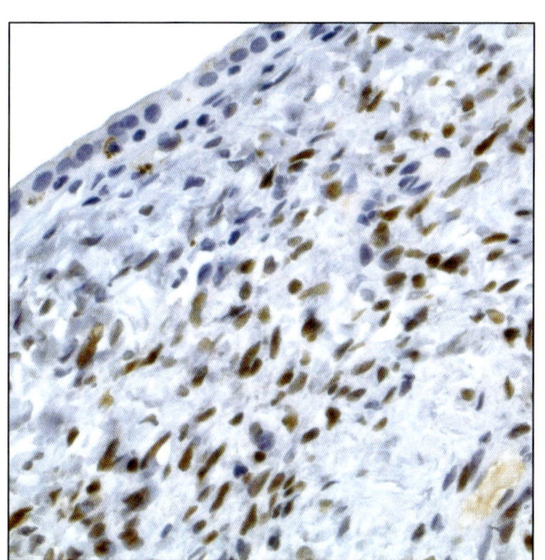

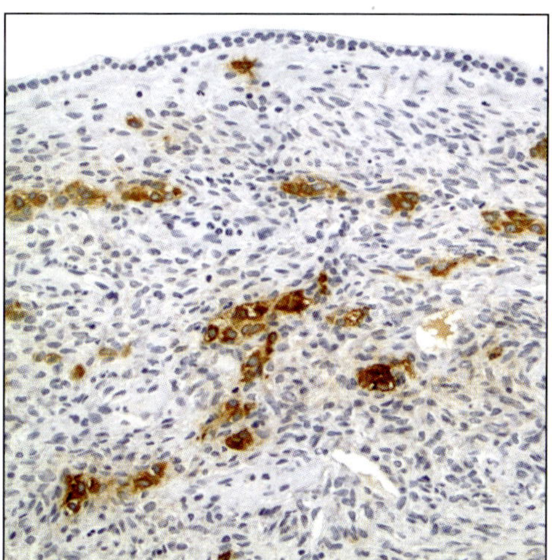

(Left) *The stromal cells in biliary cystadenomas are positive for estrogen receptor (ER) upon immunohistochemical staining.* ***(Right)*** *The stromal cells in biliary cystadenomas can be focally positive for inhibin on immunohistochemical staining.*

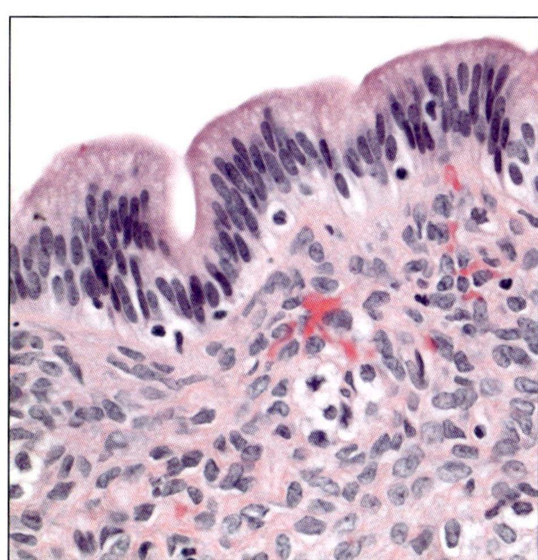

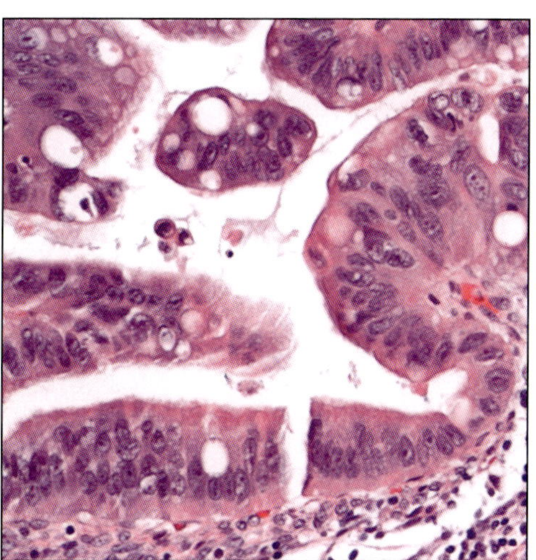

(Left) *This biliary cystadenoma shows low-grade dysplasia with enlarged, hyperchromatic, and crowded nuclei in the biliary-type epithelial cells lining the cysts. The dysplastic nuclei still maintain the polarity with the axis perpendicular to the basement membrane* ***(Right)*** *This biliary cystadenoma shows high-grade dysplasia in the lining epithelial cells, which are characterized by crowded and hyperchromatic nuclei with loss of polarity.*

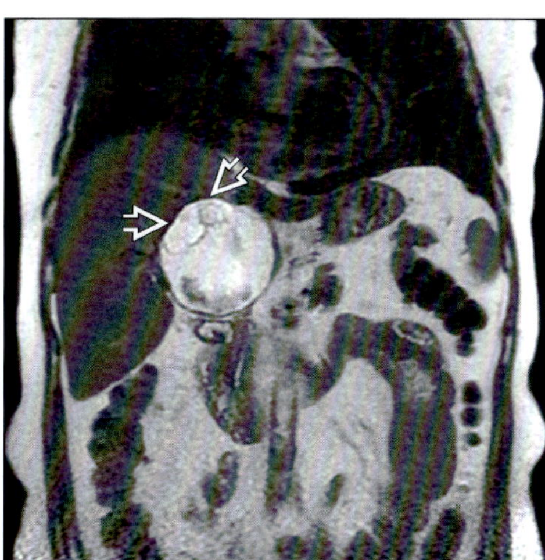

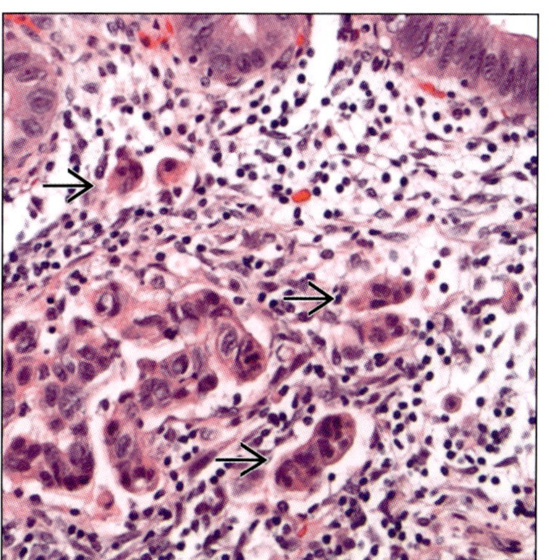

(Left) *This MR of a biliary cystadenocarcinoma shows a complex cystic mass in the liver with areas of nodular thickening of the wall* ➪*. (Courtesy R. Bentley, MD.)* ***(Right)*** *This biliary cystadenocarcinoma, arising in a biliary cystadenoma, shows focal invasion of the underlying stroma* →*.*

INTRAHEPATIC CHOLANGIOCARCINOMA

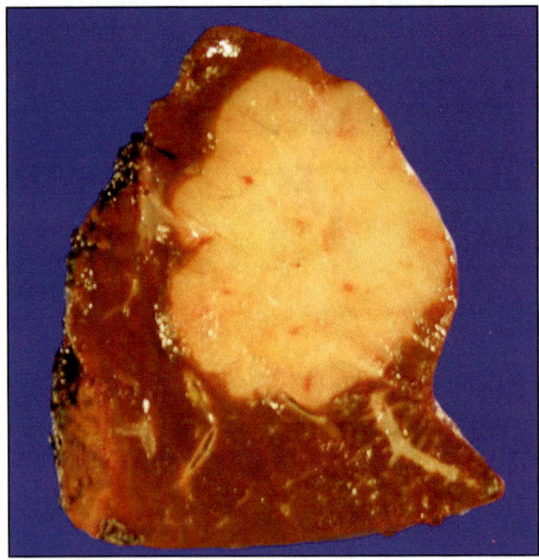

Intrahepatic cholangiocarcinomas generally arise in noncirrhotic livers. This gross photograph shows a white-tan, firm, and distinct mass in a background of noncirrhotic liver.

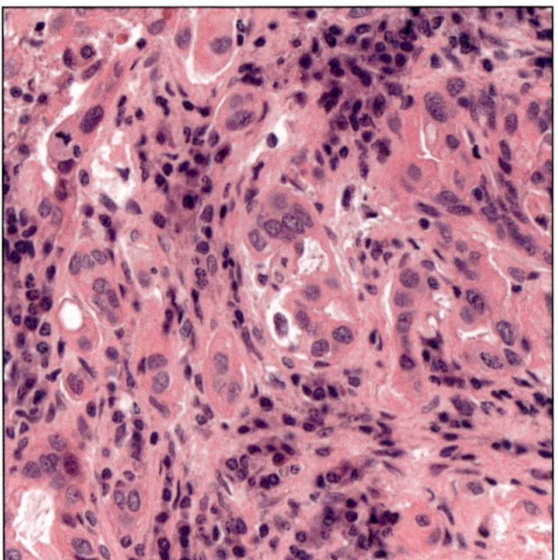

Intrahepatic cholangiocarcinomas form irregular glandular structures with an infiltrative appearance, surrounded by a prominent stroma. The nuclei are hyperchromatic and pleomorphic.

TERMINOLOGY

Definitions

- Malignant adenocarcinoma arising from bile duct epithelium within liver

ETIOLOGY/PATHOGENESIS

Multistep Carcinogenesis

- Chronic inflammation may be common pathogenic pathway

CLINICAL ISSUES

Epidemiology

- Age
  - Average age at presentation is 60 years old
- Gender
  - Equal frequency in men and women
- Ethnicity
  - Very prevalent in Asia, particularly in northeastern Thailand (associated with liver fluke infestation)

Presentation

- 10-20% of primary liver malignancies
  - Incidence and mortality rates have been increasing in several regions around world
  - Incidence has also increased 3x in past few decades in USA
- Most patients are diagnosed with advanced stages of disease
- Symptoms
  - Abdominal pain
  - Weight loss
  - Malaise
  - Jaundice

Laboratory Tests

- Serum level of CA19-9 is currently most important tumor marker
- Alkaline phosphatase and bilirubin variably elevated

Prognosis

- Long-term survival is dismal

Risk Factors

- Liver fluke infection
  - *Clonorchis sinensis*
  - *Opisthorchis viverrini*
- Primary sclerosing cholangitis
- Hepatolithiasis
- Thorotrast exposure (radiographic contrast medium widely used from 1930-1955)
- Congenital anomalies of bile ducts
  - Choledochal cysts
- Hepatitis B and C infection, alcohol use, and cirrhosis have recently been suggested as potential risk factors

MACROSCOPIC FEATURES

General Features

- Firm, irregular, white-tan scirrhous mass with infiltrative borders
  - May be single or multiple
- Peripheral type: Arise from smaller intrahepatic bile ducts (50-70% of total)
- Hilar type: Arise from major bile ducts at hepatic hilum, including right and left hepatic ducts (Klatskin tumor)

MICROSCOPIC PATHOLOGY

Histologic Features

- Usually well to moderately differentiated adenocarcinoma

INTRAHEPATIC CHOLANGIOCARCINOMA

Key Facts

Clinical Issues

- Incidence has been increasing around world, including USA
  - Very prevalent in Asia, particularly in northeastern Thailand
- Well-known risk factors include liver fluke infection, primary sclerosing cholangitis, hepatolithiasis, Thorotrast exposure, congenital anomalies of bile ducts
- Serum level of CA19-9 is commonly elevated
- Most patients are diagnosed with advanced stages of disease
  - Dismal prognosis

Macroscopic Features

- Can be peripheral or hilar (Klatskin tumor)

Microscopic Pathology

- Well to moderately differentiated adenocarcinoma
  - Desmoplastic stroma
  - Frequently shows perineural invasion
  - Mucin typically present
  - CK19, CK7 positive
- Neoplastic cells can form glands, solid nests, cords, or papillary structures

Top Differential Diagnoses

- Hepatocellular carcinoma
- Metastatic adenocarcinoma
- Epithelioid hemangioendothelioma
- Bile ductular reaction or atypical biliary epithelium due to inflammation
- Benign hamartoma

  - Neoplastic cells can form glands, solid nests, cords, or papillary structures
  - Tumor cells are columnar to cuboidal with eosinophilic and granular cytoplasm
- Desmoplastic stroma surrounding carcinoma cells is typical
- Mucin is typically present, either intracytoplasmic or extracellular, and may be demonstrated by mucicarmine, PAS with diastase, or Alcian blue
- Immunopositive for CK7 and CK19
- Uncommon variants include adenosquamous, squamous, mucinous, clear cell, and sarcomatous
- Perineural invasion is common

Precursor Lesions

- Flat- or low-papillary dysplastic epithelium
- Biliary papillomatosis
  - Macroscopic lesion with characteristic papillary proliferation of dysplastic epithelium

DIFFERENTIAL DIAGNOSIS

Hepatocellular Carcinoma

- Positive for Hep Par 1, glypican-3, and polyclonal CEA and CD10 (canalicular staining pattern)
- CD34 positive for sinusoidal endothelial cells
- Bile production and negative mucin staining

Metastatic Adenocarcinoma

- Much more common in western world
- Clinical history of primary carcinoma in other sites
- Immunoprofile may be helpful

Epithelioid Hemangioendothelioma

- Intracytoplasmic lumens, may contain red blood cells
- Positive for CD34, CD31, and factor VIII

Combined Hepatocellular/ Cholangiocarcinoma

- Has hepatocellular carcinoma component

Bile Ductular Reaction

- Abundant inflammation in clinical setting of biliary obstruction

Peribiliary Gland Hamartoma/Bile Duct Hamartoma (von Meyenburg complex)

- Smaller and more well circumscribed
- Lack of cytologic atypia
- May have angulated bile ducts

Atypical Reactive Bile Duct Epithelium

- Presence of marked background inflammation
- Lack of lymphovascular or perineural invasion
- Respects normal architecture of portal tracts

DIAGNOSTIC CHECKLIST

Pathologic Interpretation Pearls

- Immunophenotypic profiles of cholangiocarcinoma and pancreatic adenocarcinoma are virtually identical, and final distinction relies on clinical and imaging correlation

SELECTED REFERENCES

1. Pritchard CC et al: Pathology and Diagnostic Pitfalls of Cholangiocarcinoma: Rising Incidence of an Old Cancer. Pathology Case Reviews. 14:28-33, 2009
2. Zen Y et al: Biliary intraepithelial neoplasia: an international interobserver agreement study and proposal for diagnostic criteria. Mod Pathol. 20(6):701-9, 2007
3. Shaib Y et al: The epidemiology of cholangiocarcinoma. Semin Liver Dis. 24(2):115-25, 2004
4. Tan G et al: Immunohistochemical analysis of biliary tract lesions. Appl Immunohistochem Mol Morphol. 12(3):193-7, 2004
5. Lau SK et al: Comparative immunohistochemical profile of hepatocellular carcinoma, cholangiocarcinoma, and metastatic adenocarcinoma. Hum Pathol. 33(12):1175-81, 2002

INTRAHEPATIC CHOLANGIOCARCINOMA

Gross and Microscopic Features

(Left) *Intrahepatic cholangiocarcinomas can occasionally arise in cirrhotic livers. This gross photograph shows a white, green to tan, irregular and firm mass ⇨ in a background of hepatitis C-associated cirrhosis.* ***(Right)*** *Dysplastic epithelium of the intrahepatic bile ducts is considered to be a precursor lesion of intrahepatic cholangiocarcinoma. This image shows low-grade dysplasia with the nuclear axis perpendicular to the basement membrane.*

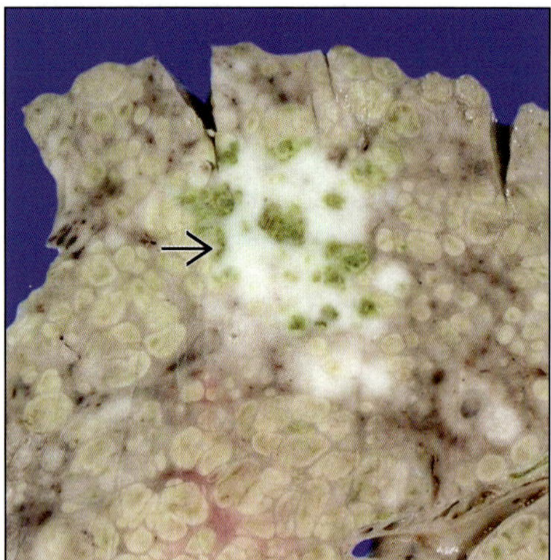

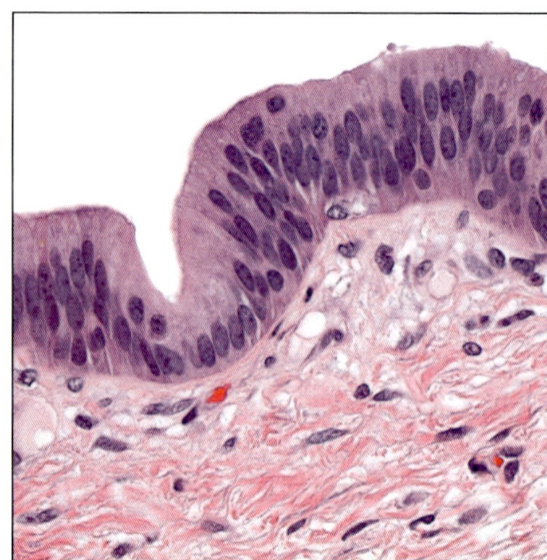

(Left) *High-grade dysplasia in an intrahepatic bile duct found adjacent to an intrahepatic cholangiocarcinoma is shown. The dysplastic epithelium shows loss of polarity of the nuclei.* ***(Right)*** *This well-differentiated intrahepatic cholangiocarcinoma has a prominent fibrous stroma surrounding infiltrative glands with minimal nuclear atypia.*

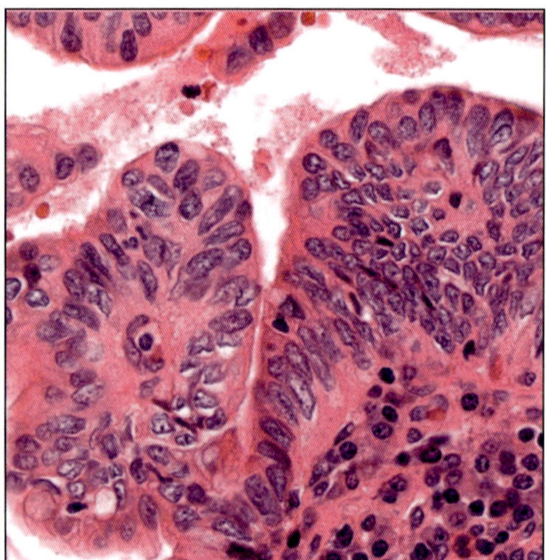

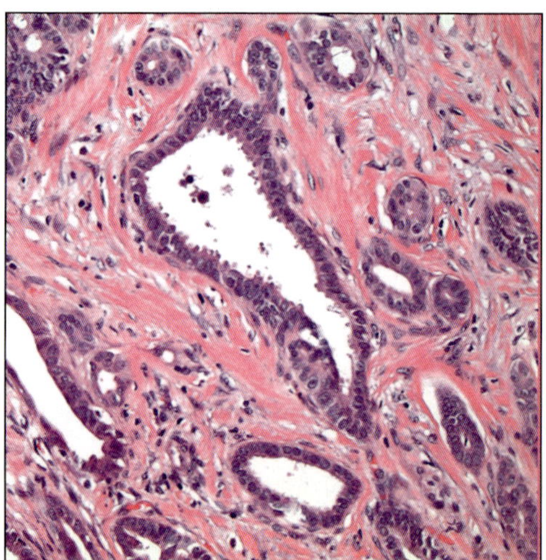

(Left) *This moderately differentiated intrahepatic cholangiocarcinoma is composed of back-to-back small glands with relatively uniform nuclei.* ***(Right)*** *Poorly differentiated intrahepatic cholangiocarcinoma, as seen here forming solid sheets, can be difficult to distinguish from hepatocellular carcinoma without immunostains.*

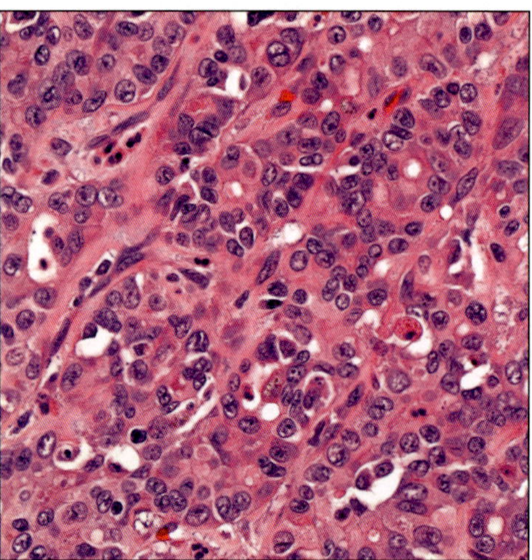

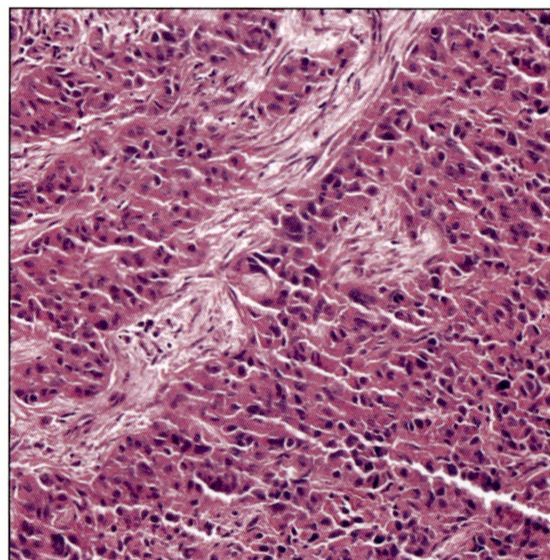

Microscopic Features

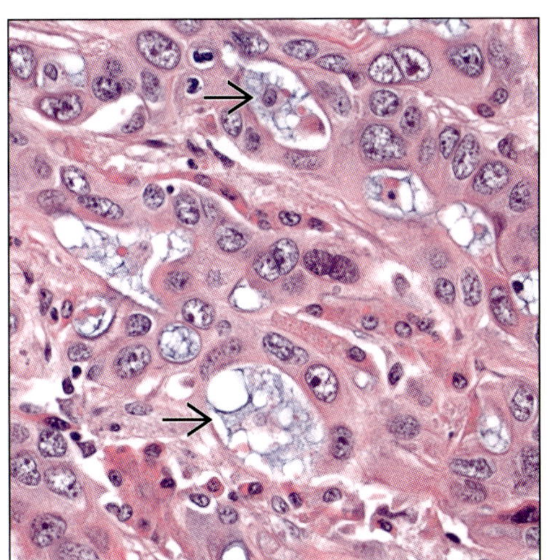

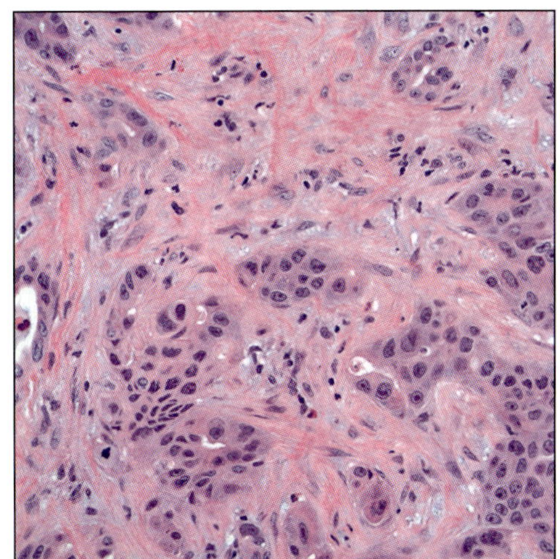

(Left) *Mucin production ⇒ is typically present in intrahepatic cholangiocarcinomas.* ***(Right)*** *Desmoplastic stroma is a common finding in intrahepatic cholangiocarcinoma.*

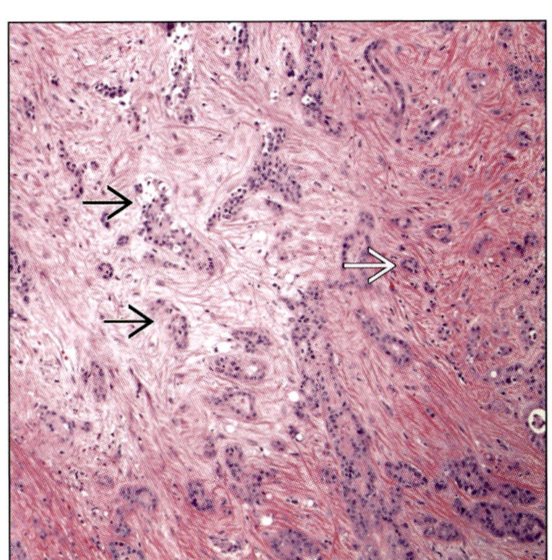

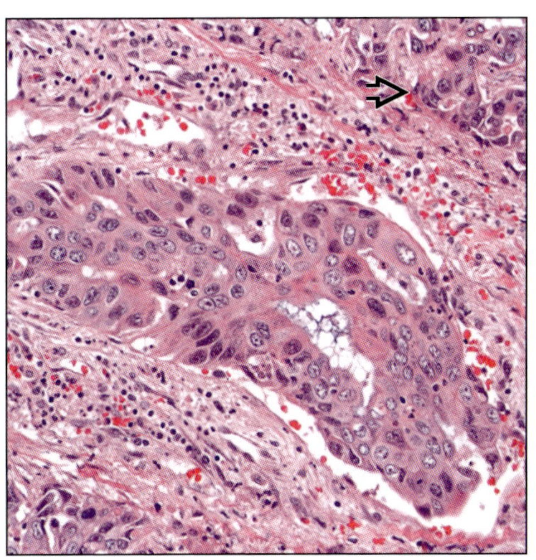

(Left) *Intrahepatic cholangiocarcinoma ⇒ must be distinguished from benign bile ducts ➡, which respect the normal lobular architecture and lack the desmoplastic stroma.* ***(Right)*** *In situ carcinoma within a large intrahepatic bile duct was found adjacent to invasive intrahepatic cholangiocarcinoma ⊳.*

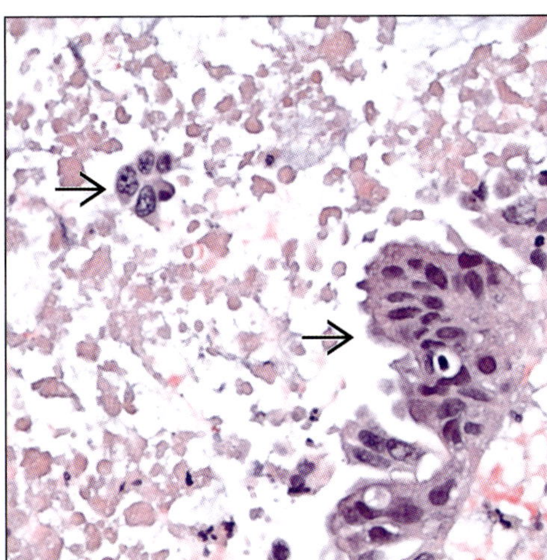

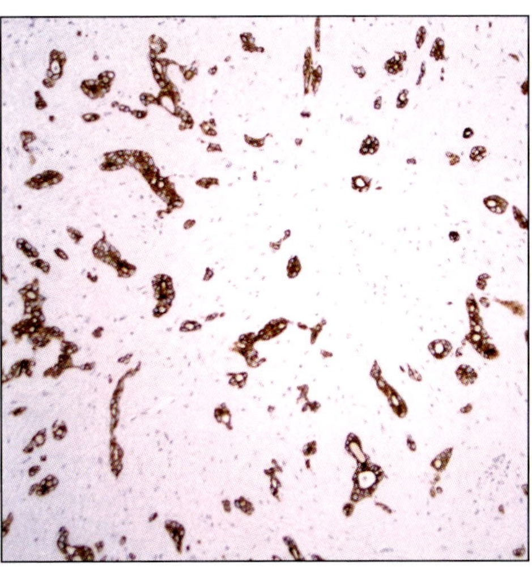

(Left) *This intrahepatic cholangiocarcinoma ⇒ was diagnosed from a fine needle aspiration of a liver mass.* ***(Right)*** *CK7 immunostaining highlights the carcinoma cells in intrahepatic cholangiocarcinoma.*

HEMANGIOMA

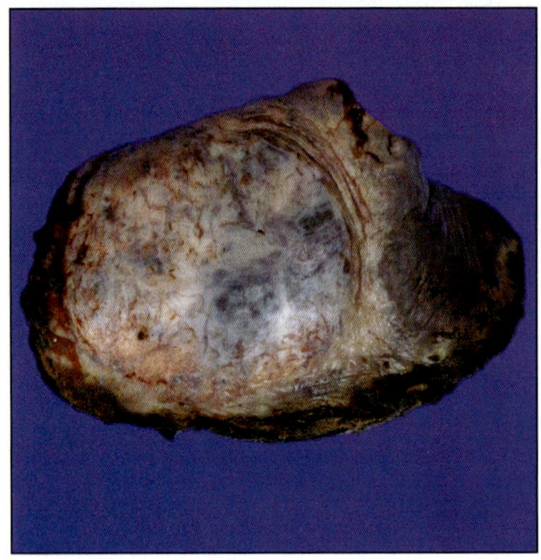

Gross photograph illustrates a subcapsular hemangioma with extensive fibrosis and hemorrhage on the cut surface. (Courtesy S. Sharma, MD.)

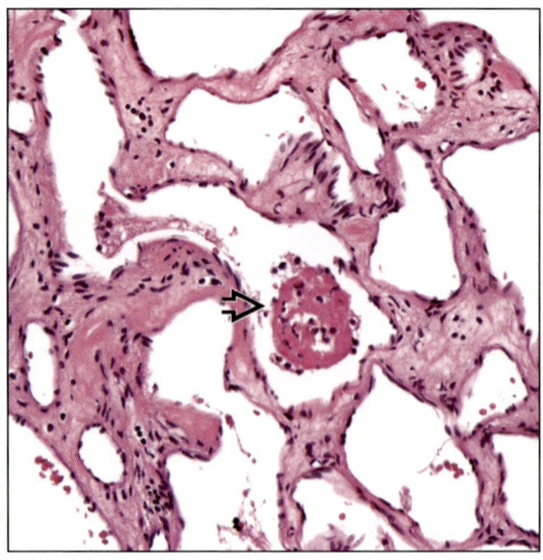

Hemangiomas are composed of dilated vascular spaces with a bland, flat endothelial lining. Note the organizing thrombus in 1 vascular space ➡.

TERMINOLOGY

Synonyms

- Cavernous hemangioma
- Sclerosing hemangioma
- Solitary necrotic nodule

Definitions

- Benign vascular tumor
    - Most common primary tumor of liver

ETIOLOGY/PATHOGENESIS

Unknown

- Postulated but unproven role of sex hormones

CLINICAL ISSUES

Epidemiology

- Incidence
    - Ranges from 1-20% in autopsy studies
- Age
    - All ages
        - More frequent in older patients
- Gender
    - More common in women
        - May be that hemangiomas are larger and more often symptomatic in women, so more likely to be diagnosed

Presentation

- Majority clinically silent, discovered incidentally
    - Tumors under 4 cm rarely symptomatic
    - Larger tumors may be symptomatic
        - Vague abdominal pain
        - Hepatomegaly
        - Palpable mass
- Complications rare
    - Spontaneous rupture
    - Consumptive coagulopathy

Treatment

- Surgical resection or ablative therapy if symptomatic

Prognosis

- Excellent

IMAGE FINDINGS

MR Findings

- Heterogeneous appearance that is virtually diagnostic

MACROSCOPIC FEATURES

General Features

- Usually solitary
    - 10% or less are multiple
- Usually subcapsular
    - May appear as red or purple capsular blotches
- Cut surface shows dark red, spongy mass composed of blood-filled cavities
    - Variably present scarring, calcification
- Occurs anywhere in liver
- Involuted lesions may consist mostly of fibrosis, calcification, &/or necrosis

Size

- Most < 4 cm
    - Tumors up to 30 cm have been described

MICROSCOPIC PATHOLOGY

Histologic Features

- Well-demarcated from surrounding liver
    - Occasional irregular borders
- Dilated, variably sized vascular spaces
    - Spaces lined by flat, bland endothelial cells
        - No atypia

ANGIOMYOLIPOMA

Key Facts

Terminology
- Rare benign mesenchymal neoplasm composed of smooth muscle, adipose tissue, and vessels

Clinical Issues
- Infrequently associated with tuberous sclerosis (6-10%)
- Benign behavior in nearly all cases

Microscopic Pathology
- Diagnostic component is smooth muscle cells that can be spindle or epithelioid
- Epithelioid smooth muscle cells are typically large, with round to oval nuclei, a single nucleolus, and eosinophilic to fibrillar or vacuolated cytoplasm
- Features that predict malignant behavior are not well defined but include large size (> 10 cm), coagulative necrosis, and clinical evidence of metastasis
  - Nuclear atypia and infiltrative margins can be seen in benign tumors

Ancillary Tests
- Smooth muscle cells stain with antibodies to HMB-45, mart-1, but not keratin or Hep-Par1

Top Differential Diagnoses
- Hepatocellular neoplasm, particularly hepatocellular carcinoma
- Metastatic malignant tumor, either carcinoma or sarcoma
- Malignant melanoma

Size
- 0.1-36 cm

MICROSCOPIC PATHOLOGY

Histologic Features
- Tumor consists of 3 major elements in varying proportions: Adipose tissue, vessels, and smooth muscle cells
- Smooth muscle cells can be epithelioid, intermediate (ovoid or short spindle), or spindled
  - Epithelioid smooth muscle cells
    - Large, polygonal, or spheroid
    - Cytoplasm characteristically described as clear, reticulated, vacuolated, or spider-web-like at periphery of cell and eosinophilic and granular in center of cell
    - Cytoplasmic clearing is due to glycogen and occasionally small fat vacuoles in periphery of smooth muscle cells
    - Round to oval eccentric nuclei that may be highly atypical
    - Mitoses rare or absent
    - Single eosinophilic nucleolus
  - Spindled smooth muscle cells
    - Plump
    - Round to oval pale nuclei
    - Rim of eosinophilic cytoplasm
- Variable features
  - Intracytoplasmic hyaline globules, erythropoietic elements, hemorrhage/hemosiderin, peliosis, foamy macrophages, cholesterol clefts, lymphocytic infiltrates, melanin
- Tumor margins may show infiltration of surrounding liver sinusoids or even "invasion" into adjacent liver tissue
  - This does not reflect biologic behavior
- Features that predict malignant behavior are not well defined
  - Large size (> 10 cm)
  - Coagulative necrosis
  - Clinical evidence of metastasis

Cytologic Features
- Clusters of plump smooth muscle cells with arborizing traversing capillaries but no peripherally wrapping endothelium admixed with adipocytes
- Smooth muscle cells show fibrillar cytoplasm, indistinct cytoplasmic borders, and spindle and elongate or oval nuclei with nucleoli and occasional intranuclear inclusions

Variants
- Myomatous, lipomatous, or angiomatous: Tumors composed predominantly of smooth muscle cells, adipose tissue, or vessels, respectively
- Tumors with predominantly or purely sinusoidal trabecular growth pattern frequently have little or no adipose tissue and are likely to be misdiagnosed as hepatocellular carcinoma
- Oncocytic AML shows relatively homogeneous cytologic features with little or no adipose tissue and prominent degenerative-type cytologic atypia
- Histologic variants have no bearing on prognosis, specific symptoms, or gross tumor characteristics

ANCILLARY TESTS

Histochemistry
- PAS-diastase
  - Reactivity: Positive
  - Staining pattern
    - Hyaline globules
- Iron
  - Reactivity: Positive
  - Staining pattern
    - Stains hemosiderin in some tumors
- Fontana-Masson
  - Reactivity: Positive
  - Staining pattern
    - Stains melanin pigment in some tumors

ANGIOMYOLIPOMA

Immunohistochemistry

- Smooth muscle cells stain with antibodies to HMB-45, mart-1, actin-sm, and vimentin but not keratin or Hep-Par1
  - Epithelioid smooth muscle cells stain most intensely with HMB-45 and are less likely to stain with usual smooth muscle markers
  - Spindle smooth muscle cells stain most intensely with actin-sm, myosin, desmin, and vimentin, and less intensely with HMB-45
- Other melanoma markers such as tyrosinase, MITF, HMSA-5, mart-1, HMB-50, and CD63 can be positive in some cases
- Smooth muscle cells are occasionally positive for S100 and NSE
- Mature adipocytes frequently stain with antibodies to S100 and vessels stain with CD34 and other vascular markers
- Although 1 study reported CD117 positivity in hepatic AML, other studies report low frequency of positivity

Flow Cytometry

- Diploid DNA pattern, favoring benign nature

Electron Microscopy

- Transmission
  - Cytoplasmic-bound granules consistent with premelanosomes and intracytoplasmic filaments that aggregate to produce dense bodies

DIFFERENTIAL DIAGNOSIS

Hepatocellular Neoplasm

- Hepatocellular adenoma
- Hepatocellular carcinoma (HCC)
  - Clear cell variant
- Fat may be within cells as steatosis but not as adipocytes
- Stains with antibodies to keratin and Hep-Par1
- HMB-45 and actin-sm should be negative

Metastatic Malignant Tumor

- Sarcoma
- Carcinoma
  - Renal cell carcinoma
- Absence of adipose tissue component or abnormal vessels
- Numerous mitoses may be present
- Immunohistochemistry for various antigens distinguishes AML from other neoplasms

Malignant Melanoma

- Absence of adipose tissue component or abnormal vessels
- Immunohistochemical staining shows S100 staining in spindle or epithelioid cells

Gastrointestinal Stromal Tumor (GIST)

- Absence of adipose tissue
- Positive staining with CD117 and CD34
- HMB-45 negative

Smooth Muscle Tumor

- Leiomyoma
- Leiomyosarcoma
- Absence of adipose tissue
- Negative staining for HMB-45

Lipoma, Focal Fatty Change, or Myelolipoma

- Absence of spindle or epithelioid cell component that stains with HMB-45

DIAGNOSTIC CHECKLIST

Clinically Relevant Pathologic Features

- Fat component may be noted on radiologic studies

Pathologic Interpretation Pearls

- Heterogeneous tumor that contains mixture of plump eosinophilic cells and fat should raise suspicion for angiomyolipoma
- Any unusual presumed carcinomas or sarcomas of liver should be tested for reactivity to HMB-45

SELECTED REFERENCES

1. Li T et al: Hepatic angiomyolipoma: a retrospective study of 25 cases. Surg Today. 38(6):529-35, 2008
2. Nguyen TT et al: Malignant hepatic angiomyolipoma: report of a case and review of literature. Am J Surg Pathol. 32(5):793-8, 2008
3. Petrolla AA et al: Hepatic angiomyolipoma. Arch Pathol Lab Med. 132(10):1679-82, 2008
4. Hornick JL et al: PEComa: what do we know so far? Histopathology. 48(1):75-82, 2006
5. Xu AM et al: Pathological and molecular analysis of sporadic hepatic angiomyolipoma. Hum Pathol. 37(6):735-41, 2006
6. Lin KJ et al: Hepatic angiomyolipoma: report of two cases with emphasis on smear cytomorphology and the use of cell block with immunohistochemical stains. Diagn Cytopathol. 31(4):263-6, 2004
7. Makhlouf HR et al: Expression of KIT (CD117) in angiomyolipoma. Am J Surg Pathol. 26(4):493-7, 2002
8. Ji Y et al: Hepatic angiomyolipoma: a clinicopathologic study of 10 cases. Chin Med J (Engl). 114(3):280-5, 2001
9. Tsui WM et al: Hepatic angiomyolipoma: a clinicopathologic study of 30 cases and delineation of unusual morphologic variants. Am J Surg Pathol. 23(1):34-48, 1999
10. Nonomura A et al: Angiomyolipoma predominantly composed of smooth muscle cells: problems in histological diagnosis. Histopathology. 33(1):20-7, 1998
11. Sawai H et al: Angiomyolipoma of the liver: case report and collective review of cases diagnosed from fine needle aspiration biopsy specimens. J Hepatobiliary Pancreat Surg. 5(3):333-8, 1998
12. Nonomura A et al: Immunohistochemical study of hepatic angiomyolipoma. Pathol Int. 46(1):24-32, 1996

ANGIOMYOLIPOMA

Microscopic Features

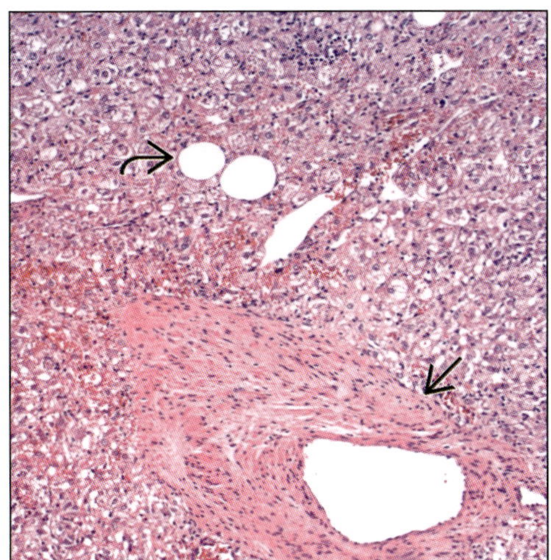
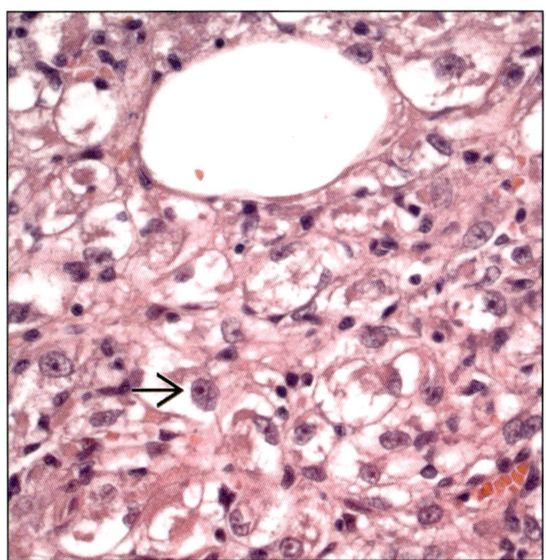

(Left) *Hematoxylin & eosin stained section shows a tumor composed largely of plump spindle and epithelioid cells, with scant adipose tissue ⮣ and abnormal thickened vessels →.* ***(Right)*** *Hematoxylin & eosin stained section shows epithelioid smooth muscle cells with a rarefied cytoplasm that resembles "spider webs." Note the enlarged oval nuclei and distinct nucleoli →.*

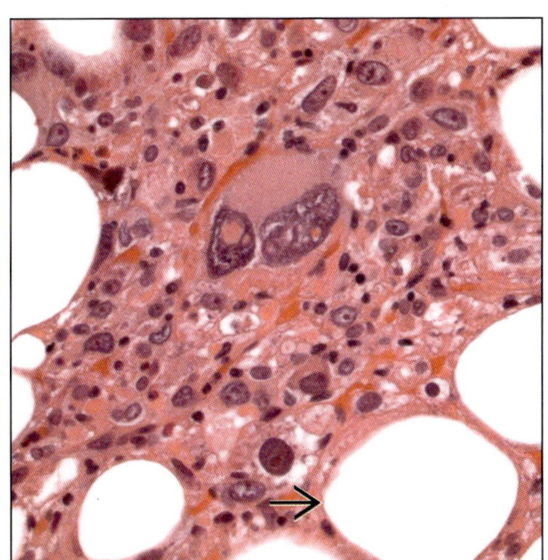
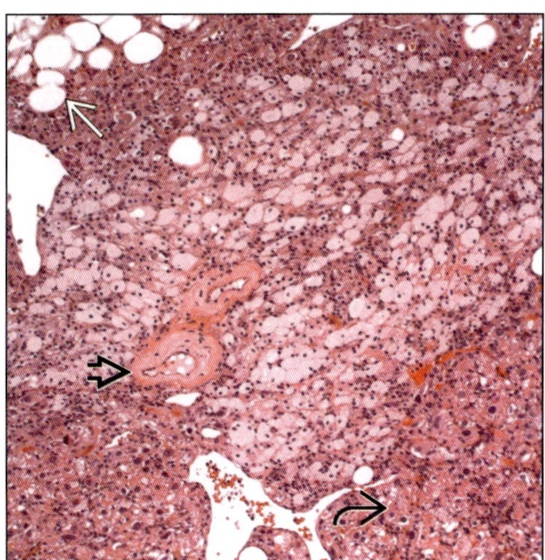

(Left) *Hematoxylin & eosin section shows highly atypical epithelioid cells with markedly enlarged nuclei, binucleation, intranuclear inclusions, and coarse chromatin admixed with adipocytes →. Mitoses are absent.* ***(Right)*** *Hematoxylin & eosin section shows aggregates of foamy macrophages and lymphocytes within this angiomyolipoma. The smooth muscle cells ⮣, adipocytes →, and abnormal vessels ⇨ typical of AML are present as well.*

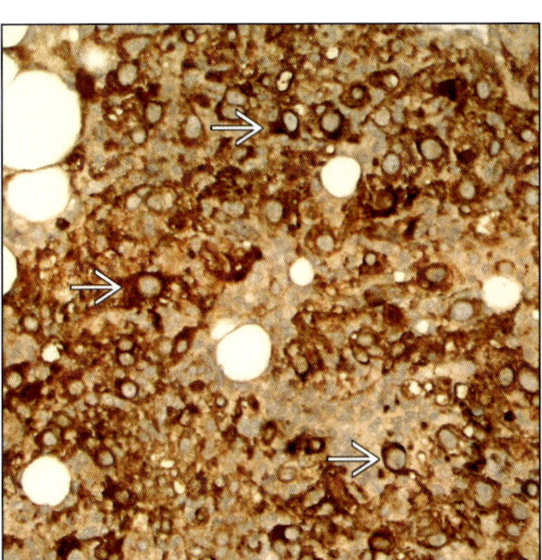
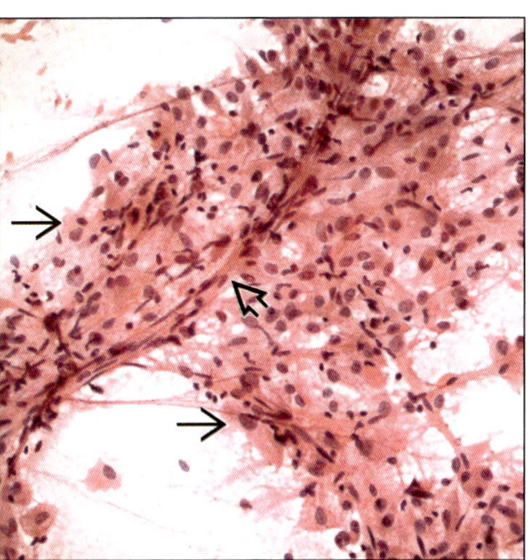

(Left) *HMB-45 immunostain shows strong positive staining (brown staining →) in the epithelioid smooth muscle cells.* ***(Right)*** *Hematoxylin & eosin intraoperative tumor smear shows loosely cohesive epithelioid smooth muscle cells → with oval nuclei adherent to traversing vessels ⇨.*

EPITHELIOID HEMANGIOENDOTHELIOMA

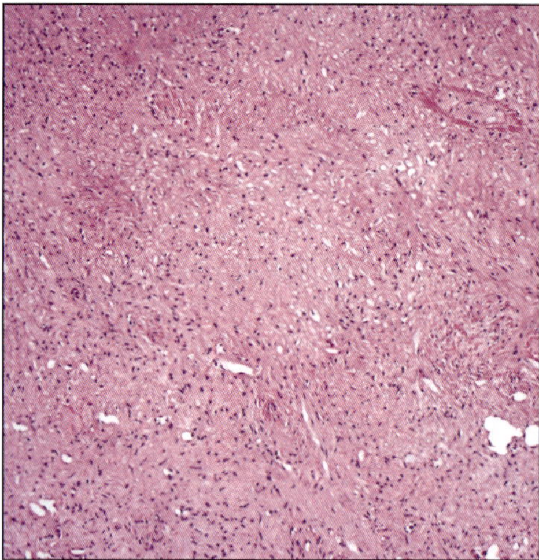

Central portion of epithelioid hemangioendothelioma (EHE) typically is hypocellular with loosely arranged spindle cells in a fibromyxoid or sclerotic stroma. The findings can simulate a scar or sclerosed hemangioma.

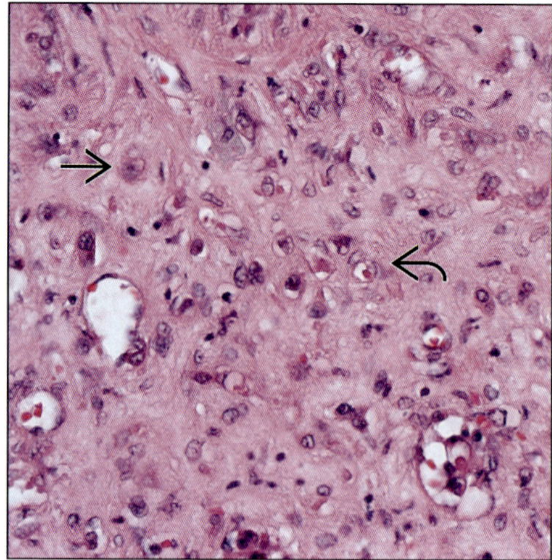

Cellular area with epithelioid tumor cells ⇒ in a fibromyxoid stroma demonstrates mild nuclear atypia with no mitoses. Vascular differentiation is seen in the form of intracytoplasmic lumina with RBCs ⇗.

TERMINOLOGY

Abbreviations

- Epithelioid hemangioendothelioma (EHE)

Definitions

- Uncommon vascular tumor, considered low-grade malignancy

ETIOLOGY/PATHOGENESIS

Unknown

- No known risk factors

CLINICAL ISSUES

Presentation

- Primarily affects adults (30-40 years)
  - Rare in children
- Slightly more common in women
- Upper abdominal mass or discomfort and elevated alkaline phosphatase may be present
  - Often discovered as incidental finding

Treatment

- Primary treatment is hepatic resection
- Liver transplantation has been successful in unresectable cases
  - Extrahepatic disease is not contraindication for transplantation
- Radiotherapy or chemotherapy are generally ineffective

Prognosis

- Natural history is extremely variable
  - Long survival despite no treatment or incomplete resection in some cases
  - Adverse outcome in others despite adequate resection and adjuvant therapy
- Prognosis better than that of angiosarcoma, even with incomplete excision or extrahepatic metastases

MACROSCOPIC FEATURES

General Features

- Firm, white to yellow with ill-defined borders
- Focal calcification can cause gritty consistency
- Can be multifocal with involvement of both right and left liver lobes
- 2 different types, depending on distribution in liver
  - Nodular type, representing early stage of disease; observed in around 10% of cases
  - Diffuse type, considered advanced stage due to coalescence of multiple lesions

MICROSCOPIC PATHOLOGY

Histologic Features

- Infiltrative tumor grows around preexisting structures and leaves portal zones and terminal hepatic venules intact
  - Periphery has higher cellularity
  - Center of tumor is often fibrotic and paucicellular
- Myxoid to fibrous stroma
  - Calcification may be present in dense areas of stroma
- Intravascular small papillary projections or tufts can occur within thin-walled vascular spaces
- Tumor cells can be dendritic or epithelioid in appearance
  - Dendritic cells are irregular, elongated, or stellate with branching processes
  - Epithelioid tumor cells are round with more abundant cytoplasm
  - Cytoplasm may contain vacuole, which represents intracellular lumina and may contain erythrocytes
  - Nuclear atypia and mitoses can be seen but are not prominent

EPITHELIOID HEMANGIOENDOTHELIOMA

Key Facts

Clinical Issues

- Rare low-grade malignant vascular neoplasm
- Prognosis better than angiosarcoma

Macroscopic Features

- Firm, white to yellow with ill-defined borders

Microscopic Pathology

- Central portion is fibrotic and paucicellular
- Dendritic or epithelioid tumor cells, often with intracytoplasmic vacuoles, in fibrous stroma
- Tumor cells express vascular markers like CD31

Top Differential Diagnoses

- Dense myxoid stroma and intracytoplasmic vacuoles can mimic adenocarcinoma
- Greater nuclear atypia, mitotic activity, and destructive growth pattern distinguish angiosarcoma from EHE

- Scattered inflammatory cells such as lymphocytes and neutrophils often present
- Residual hepatocytes or bile ducts can be present within tumor
- Tumor can invade vascular structures, such as portal and central veins, mimicking vascular thrombosis
- Immunohistochemical features
  - Vascular markers like CD31, CD34, &/or FVIIIRAg are positive in tumor cells
  - FLI-1, endothelial transcription factor, is expressed in nuclei of tumor cells
  - Podoplanin (recognized by antibody D2-40), lymphatic endothelial marker, is expressed in most EHE
    - D2-40 is not expressed in angiosarcoma although experience with this is limited

DIFFERENTIAL DIAGNOSIS

Adenocarcinoma (Including Cholangiocarcinoma)

- Intracytoplasmic lumina and dense sclerotic stroma in EHE can be mistaken for adenocarcinoma
- Focal keratin positivity in EHE due to entrapped hepatocytes, bile ducts, and possibly also in tumor cells can mimic carcinoma
- Young age, multifocal involvement, characteristic pattern of tumor infiltration at periphery and occasional calcification favor EHE
- Immunohistochemical expression of endothelial markers in tumor cells required to confirm diagnosis

Angiosarcoma

- Both EHE and angiosarcoma express endothelial markers
- Angiosarcomas tend to be large and hemorrhagic
- Angiosarcoma has greater degree of nuclear atypia, mitotic activity, and destructive growth pattern

SELECTED REFERENCES

1. Lin J et al: CT and MRI diagnosis of hepatic epithelioid hemangioendothelioma. Hepatobiliary Pancreat Dis Int. 9(2):154-8, 2010
2. Weinreb I et al: CD10 is expressed in most epithelioid hemangioendotheliomas: a potential diagnostic pitfall. Arch Pathol Lab Med. 133(12):1965-8, 2009
3. Fujii T et al: Podoplanin is a useful diagnostic marker for epithelioid hemangioendothelioma of the liver. Mod Pathol. 21(2):125-30, 2008
4. Mehrabi A et al: Primary malignant hepatic epithelioid hemangioendothelioma: a comprehensive review of the literature with emphasis on the surgical therapy. Cancer. 107(9):2108-21, 2006
5. Uchimura K et al: Hepatic epithelioid hemangioendothelioma. J Clin Gastroenterol. 32(5):431-4, 2001

IMAGE GALLERY

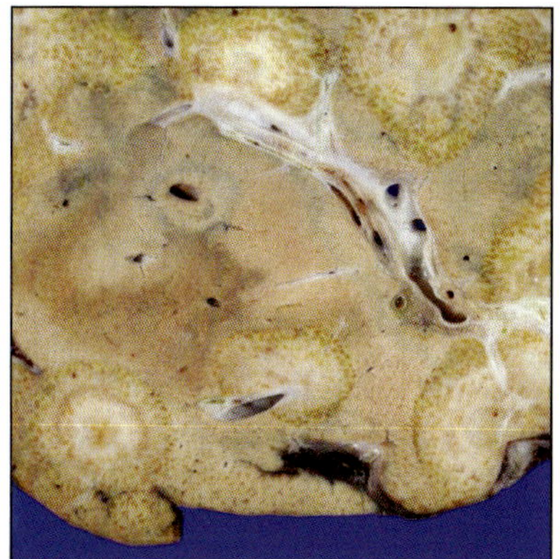

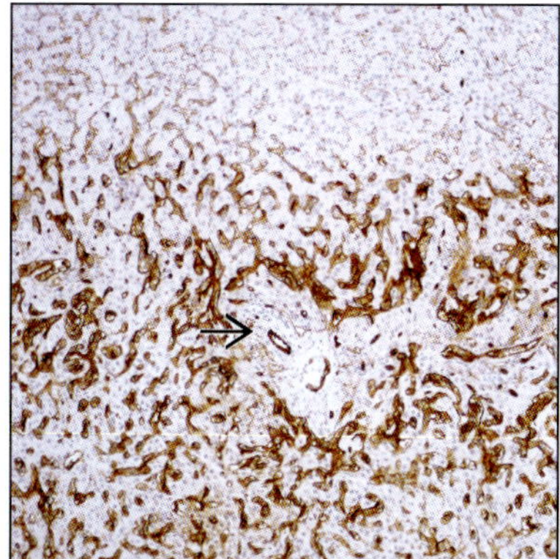

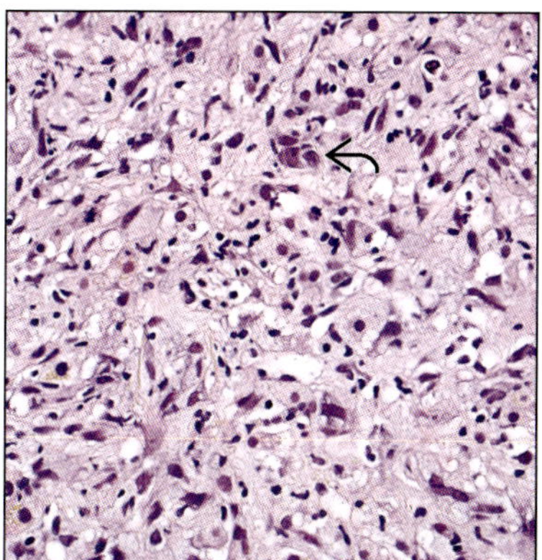

(Left) *This gross photograph illustrates the diffuse and infiltrative growth pattern of EHE.* ***(Center)*** *CD31 is strongly expressed in EHE tumor cells, highlighting the characteristic infiltrative pattern with entrapment of portal tracts* ➔ *and extension along the sinusoids in adjacent liver.* ***(Right)*** *Epithelioid angiosarcoma can mimic EHE, but it is distinguished by prominent nuclear atypia* ➔*, frequent mitoses, and lack of zonation.*

INFANTILE HEMANGIOENDOTHELIOMA

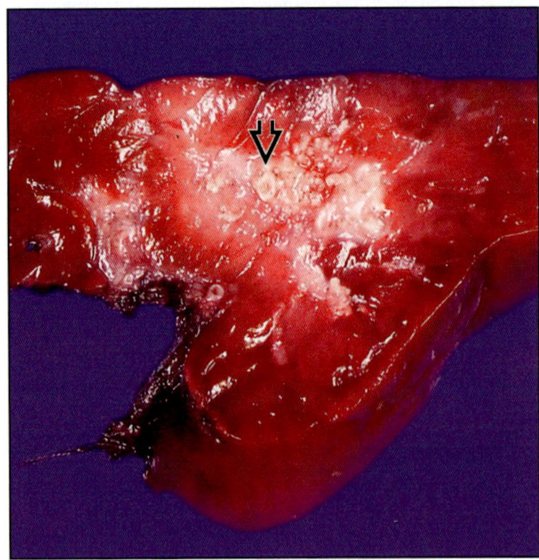

This partial hepatectomy specimen contains a poorly circumscribed, white-tan mass ⊳ with central calcification.

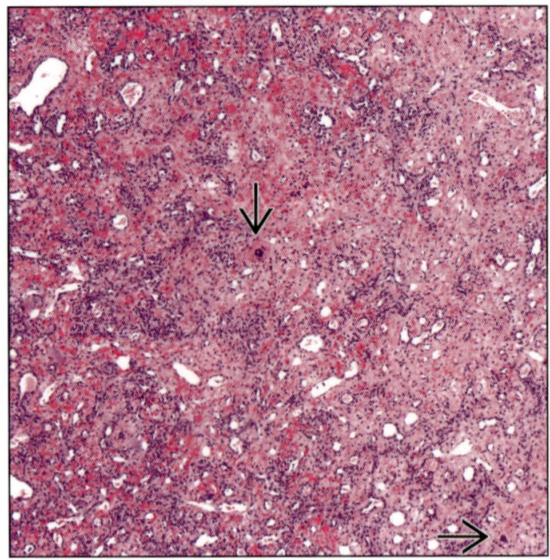

A proliferation of small, thin-walled vascular channels is present within a fibrous stroma containing entrapped bile ducts →.

TERMINOLOGY

Synonyms

- Originally described by Dehner and Ishak as infantile hemangioendothelioma type 1

Definitions

- Hepatic vascular neoplasm
  - Most common hepatic neoplasm during 1st year of life
  - Accounts for 15% of primary liver tumors in pediatric population

CLINICAL ISSUES

Epidemiology

- Age
  - Most present before age of 6 months
  - Rare in adults
- Gender
  - Female predominance

Presentation

- Hepatomegaly, abdominal enlargement, palpable mass
  - Small tumors may be asymptomatic
- Frequently have cutaneous hemangiomas
- Complications
  - High-output cardiac failure due to shunting through tumor
  - Kasabach-Merritt syndrome
    - Thrombocytopenia, hypofibrinogenemia

Natural History

- Spontaneous regression (5-10%)
- Malignant transformation has been reported

Treatment

- Intravenous steroids
- Chemotherapy
- Hepatic artery ligation
- Embolization of feeding vessels
- Surgical resection
- Orthotopic liver transplantation

Prognosis

- Survival rate of 70% with treatment

MACROSCOPIC FEATURES

General Features

- Solitary or multifocal
- Size ranges from 0.3-13 cm
- Nonencapsulated

MICROSCOPIC PATHOLOGY

Histologic Features

- Proliferation of vascular channels
  - Small capillary-like and thin-walled
  - Slightly dilated and irregular
  - In background of loose fibrous stroma
  - Some ectatic (cavernous) vessels
- Entrapped hepatocytes and bile ducts near periphery
- Secondary involutional changes more centrally
  - Myxoid change
  - Necrosis
  - Fibrosis
  - Thrombosis
  - Calcification

Cytologic Features

- Single layer of bland endothelial cells
  - Elongated plump cells with scant cytoplasm
  - Round to oval nuclei with finely granular nuclear chromatin

INFANTILE HEMANGIOENDOTHELIOMA

Key Facts

Clinical Issues

- Most common hepatic neoplasm in 1st year of life
- > 90% present before age of 6 months

Microscopic Pathology

- Vascular proliferation resembling small capillaries
  - Slightly dilated and irregular in shape
  - Lined by single layer of bland endothelial cells

Top Differential Diagnoses

- Angiosarcoma
  - Previously termed infantile hemangioendothelioma type 2
  - Key distinguishing feature is nuclear atypia of endothelial cells

ANCILLARY TESTS

Immunohistochemistry

- Tumor cells positive for vascular markers
  - Factor VIII
  - CD31
  - CD34
  - Fli-1
- Endothelial cells are surrounded by smooth muscle actin immunoreactivity
  - Negative for desmin

DIFFERENTIAL DIAGNOSIS

Angiosarcoma

- Previously termed infantile hemangioendothelioma type 2 by Dehner and Ishak
- Poorly formed, irregular, branching, and budding vascular spaces
  - Lined by stratified and atypical endothelial cells
    - Pleomorphic, large, and hyperchromatic nuclei
- Peripheral region of sinusoidal growth pattern
  - Dilated sinusoids lined by enlarged atypical cells
- Kaposiform spindle cell areas
- Absence of bile ducts within mass

Cavernous Hemangioma

- Contains mostly larger and dilated thin-walled, blood-filled spaces
  - Lined by flattened endothelium

Lymphangioma

- Similar to cavernous hemangioma, with large vascular spaces
  - Lined by attenuated endothelium
  - Spaces filled with proteinaceous fluid
  - Small lymphoid aggregates in stroma
- Immunoreactive for D2-40

Mesenchymal Hamartoma

- Overlapping age and clinical presentation
- Contains mixture of epithelial and stromal component
- Cystic spaces are not lined by endothelial cells
- Vessels are thick walled with round lumens

SELECTED REFERENCES

1. Mo JQ et al: GLUT1 endothelial reactivity distinguishes hepatic infantile hemangioma from congenital hepatic vascular malformation with associated capillary proliferation. Hum Pathol. 35(2):200-9, 2004
2. Awan S et al: Angiosarcoma of the liver in children. J Pediatr Surg. 31(12):1729-32, 1996
3. Selby DM et al: Infantile hemangioendothelioma of the liver. Hepatology. 20(1 Pt 1):39-45, 1994
4. Kirchner SG et al: Infantile hepatic hemangioendothelioma with subsequent malignant degeneration. Pediatr Radiol. 11(1):42-5, 1981
5. Dehner LP et al: Vascular tumors of the liver in infants and children. A study of 30 cases and review of the literature. Arch Pathol. 92(2):101-11, 1971

IMAGE GALLERY

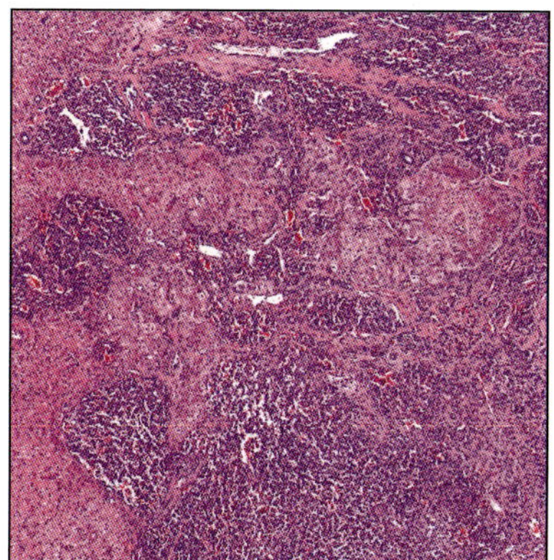

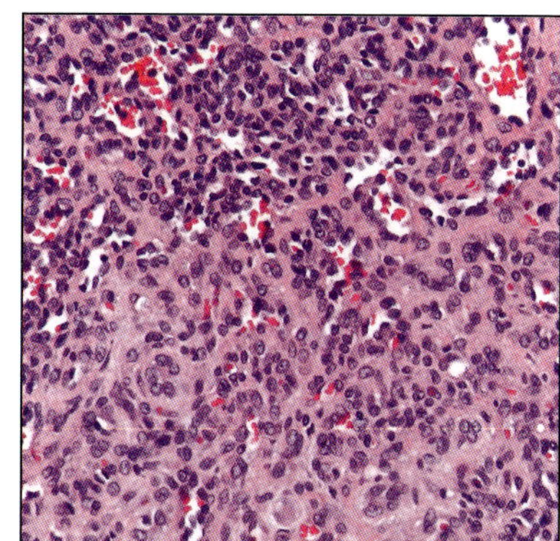

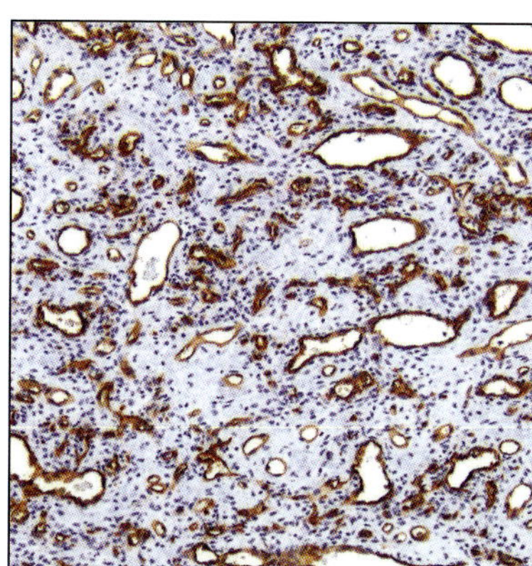

(Left) *This photograph demonstrates the irregular interface of an infantile hemangioendothelioma, more toward the right side, and adjacent hepatic parenchyma on the left side.* ***(Center)*** *Closely packed vascular channels are lined by a single layer of plump, bland endothelial cells.* ***(Right)*** *The slightly dilated, irregular capillary-like vascular channels are immunoreactive for the endothelial marker CD34.*

ANGIOSARCOMA

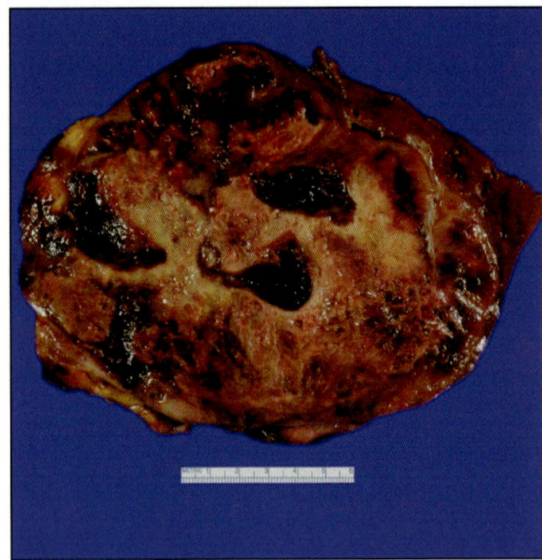

This cross section from a partial hepatectomy for angiosarcoma shows numerous cystic, blood-filled spaces. (Courtesy C. Trower, PA (ASCP) and A. Folpe, MD.)

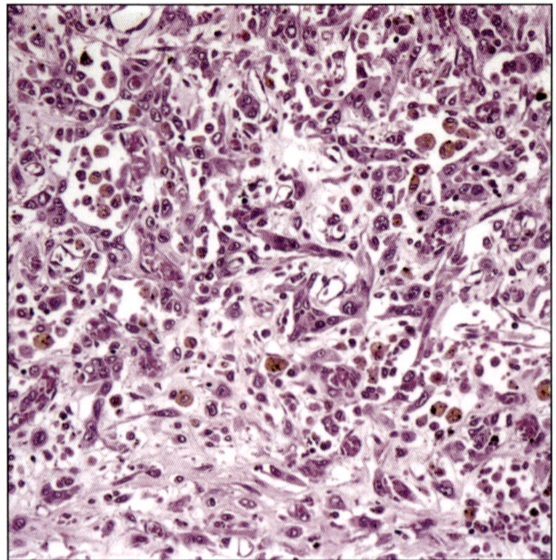

Markedly atypical neoplastic endothelial cells line vascular spaces. Note that the normal hepatic architecture has been destroyed.

TERMINOLOGY

Definitions

- Rare malignant vascular tumor of liver
  - Most common primary hepatic sarcoma
  - Approximately 2% of malignant liver tumors

ETIOLOGY/PATHOGENESIS

Environmental Exposure

- Drugs/toxins
  - Vinyl chloride
  - Arsenic
  - Thorotrast
  - Androgens
  - Contraceptive steroids
  - Copper sulfate
  - Diethylstilbestrol
  - Phenelzine
- About 25-40% of cases associated with vinyl chloride, Thorotrast, arsenic, or steroids
  - Many of these agents no longer used or strictly controlled, but they have very long latency period of up to several decades after exposure

CLINICAL ISSUES

Epidemiology

- Age
  - Predominantly older patients
    - Peak incidence in 6th-7th decades
    - Rare cases in children, often associated with infantile hemangioendothelioma
- Gender
  - Male:female ratio = 3:1

Presentation

- Signs and symptoms are nonspecific
  - Abdominal pain &/or distension
  - Hepatomegaly or palpable mass
  - Ascites
  - Jaundice
  - Weakness
  - Fatigue
  - Weight loss

Laboratory Tests

- Most patients have abnormal liver tests
  - Mildly elevated alkaline phosphatase, transaminases, bilirubin
  - Decreased albumin
  - Increased PT
  - α-fetoprotein and CEA are not elevated
- Anemia, leukocytosis, thrombocytopenia common

Treatment

- Surgery
  - Many cases inoperable at presentation
- Chemotherapy

Prognosis

- Most patients die of liver failure within 1 year
- Numerous complications related to vascular nature of tumor
  - GI and intraabdominal bleeding
  - Vascular shunts involving tumor
- Metastases common to lung, bone, lymph nodes, and spleen

MACROSCOPIC FEATURES

General Features

- Liver often markedly enlarged
- Usually multicentric
  - Both lobes involved
  - Tumor nodules range from barely visible to many centimeters
- Cut surface is red-brown, spongy, and hemorrhagic

ANGIOSARCOMA

Key Facts

Terminology
- Most common primary hepatic sarcoma

Etiology/Pathogenesis
- 25-40% of cases associated with vinyl chloride, Thorotrast, arsenic, or steroids

Clinical Issues
- Predominantly older patients, strong male predominance
- Liver biopsy may result in bleeding and death

Microscopic Pathology
- Proliferation of malignant endothelial cells in vascular structures
  - Eventually destroys hepatic parenchyma
  - Solid, epithelioid, and spindled areas may be present
- Immunopositive for vascular markers

MICROSCOPIC PATHOLOGY

Histologic Features
- Proliferation of malignant endothelial cells
  - Enlarged, pleomorphic, hyperchromatic nuclei
  - Pale ill-defined cytoplasm
  - Solid, epithelioid, and spindled areas may be present
  - Mitoses frequent
- Tumor infiltrates preexisting vascular structures
  - As tumor progresses, sinusoids dilate further and are filled with malignant endothelial cells
    - Papillary cell clusters, blood, necrotic debris may be seen
  - Eventually involves liver parenchyma, which atrophies, and then entirely disappears
  - Tumor may invade and occlude central veins or portal venules

ANCILLARY TESTS

Immunohistochemistry
- Positive for CD31, CD34, factor VIII
- Staining may be weak or absent in poorly differentiated tumors

DIFFERENTIAL DIAGNOSIS

Epithelioid Hemangioendothelioma
- Less nuclear atypia, prominent stroma
- Characteristic infiltrative growth pattern

Carcinoma
- Keratin immunostaining may be needed to distinguish from epithelioid angiosarcomas

Other Sarcomas
- Angiosarcoma positive for vascular markers

Bacillary Angiomatosis
- Abundant inflammation
- Associated with *Bartonella* infection

DIAGNOSTIC CHECKLIST

Clinically Relevant Pathologic Features
- Historically, 25-40% are associated with drug/toxin exposure
- Liver biopsy may result in bleeding and death

SELECTED REFERENCES

1. Neshiwat LF et al: Hepatic angiosarcoma. Am J Med. 93(2):219-22, 1992
2. Popper H et al: Development of hepatic angiosarcoma in man induced by vinyl chloride, thorotrast, and arsenic. Comparison with cases of unknown etiology. Am J Pathol. 92(2):349-76, 1978
3. Mark L et al: Clinical and morphologic features of hepatic angiosarcoma in vinyl chloride workers. Cancer. 37(1):149-63, 1976

IMAGE GALLERY

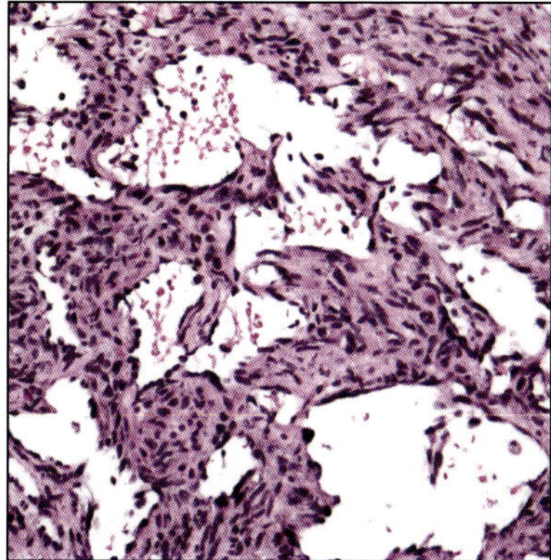

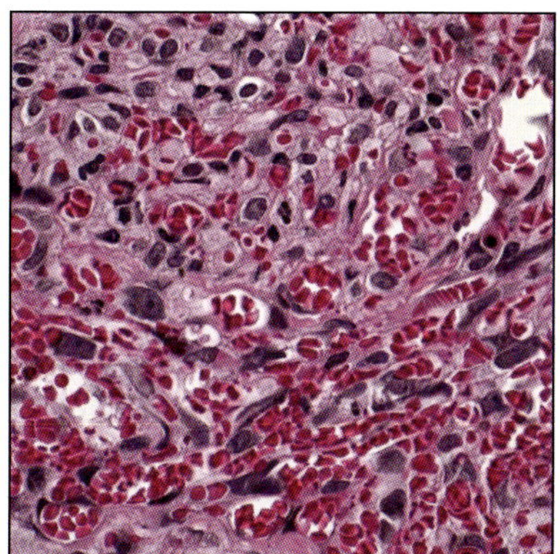

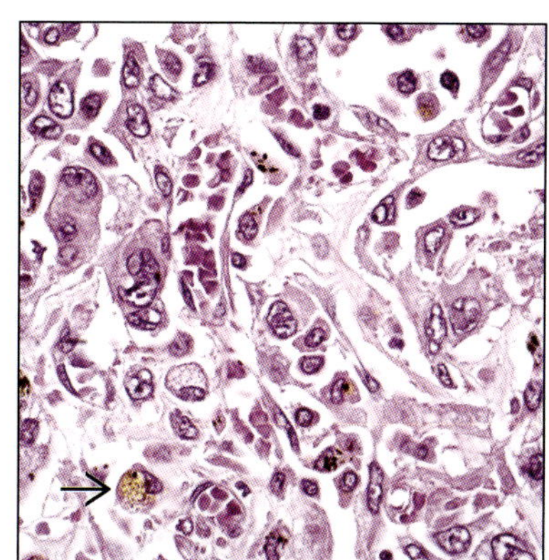

*(**Left**) This angiosarcoma is characterized by dilated sinusoids lined by malignant endothelial cells. The growth pattern is somewhat "tufted." (**Center**) This angiosarcoma has a spindled growth pattern with admixed red blood cells. The normal hepatic architecture is no longer apparent. (**Right**) This angiosarcoma shows markedly atypical endothelial cells with enlarged, bizarre nuclei. Note the admixed red blood cells and hemosiderin-laden macrophages ⇒.*

MESENCHYMAL HAMARTOMA

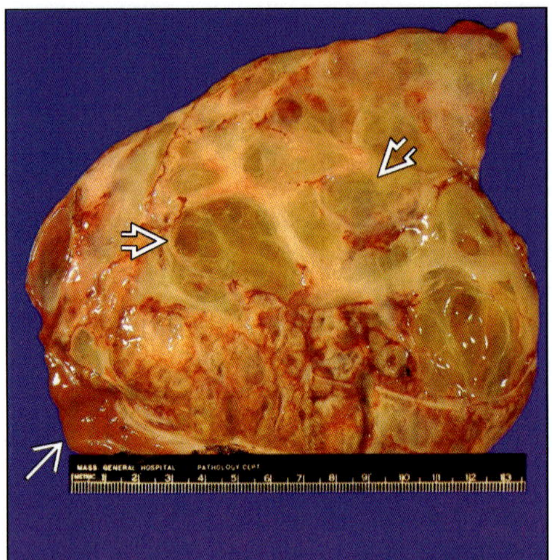

The cut surface of a large mesenchymal hamartoma shows numerous variably sized cystic spaces admixed with solid areas. Minimal uninvolved liver tissue is present at the resection margin.

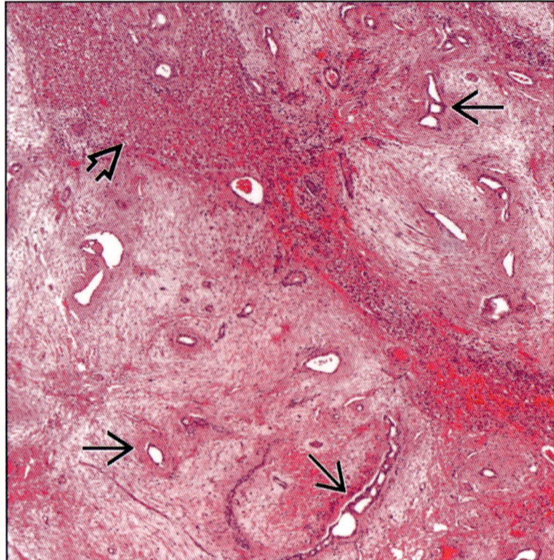

Low-power view shows numerous bile ducts in a loose, myxoid mesenchymal stroma. Note the presence of a large island of normal-appearing hepatocytes within the tumor.

TERMINOLOGY

Definitions

- Benign mass lesion of liver primarily occurring in young children

ETIOLOGY/PATHOGENESIS

Unknown

- Presumed developmental malformation of primitive hepatic mesenchyme
  - Occurs late in embryogenesis
  - Postnatal growth largely due to cystic degeneration
- Some evidence for neoplasia
  - Balanced translocation involving same breakpoint at chromosome band 19q13.4 or 19q13.3

CLINICAL ISSUES

Epidemiology

- Incidence
  - Approximately 5% of pediatric liver tumors
- Age
  - Usually seen in 1st 2 years of life
  - < 5% of cases occur after age of 5 years
  - Rarely seen in adults
- Gender
  - Male predominance in pediatric cases
  - Female predominance in adult cases

Presentation

- Painless abdominal mass
- Sudden abdominal distention due to rapid fluid accumulation in tumor

Laboratory Tests

- Normal or mildly elevated liver tests
- Moderately elevated serum α-fetoprotein level

Treatment

- Surgical resection

Prognosis

- Excellent after complete excision
- Occasional spontaneous regression without treatment
- Malignant transformation into undifferentiated embryonal sarcoma in rare case reports

IMAGE FINDINGS

General Features

- Hypodense, hypovascular, solid or multicystic lesion
- Can be detected prenatally by ultrasound and MR

MACROSCOPIC FEATURES

General Features

- Typically solitary, rarely multifocal
- Pedunculated in up to 20% of cases, usually attached to inferior surface of liver
  - 75% of cases involve right lobe of liver
- Few centimeters to > 30 cm in size
- Solid &/or cystic
  - Solid areas: White, yellow, or tan
  - Cystic spaces
    - Few millimeters to 14 cm in diameter
    - Clear to yellow fluid, or gelatinous material

MICROSCOPIC PATHOLOGY

Histologic Features

- Mixture of varying components of mesenchymal cells, bile ducts, hepatocytes, blood vessels, and cystic spaces
- Mesenchymal cells
  - Spindled or stellate fibroblasts and myofibroblasts
  - Loosely distributed in edematous, myxoid, collagenous, or hyalinized stroma

MESENCHYMAL HAMARTOMA

Key Facts

Etiology/Pathogenesis
- Developmental anomaly vs. neoplasm
- Recurrent balanced translocation involving chromosome band 19q13.4 or 19q13.3

Clinical Issues
- Typically occurring in 1st 2 years of life, rarely seen in adults
- Excellent prognosis after complete excision
- Malignant transformation only in rare case reports

Macroscopic Features
- Large, solid, &/or cystic hepatic lesion

Microscopic Pathology
- Mixture of varying portions of mesenchymal cells, bile ducts, hepatocytes, blood vessels, and cystic spaces

Top Differential Diagnoses
- Hepatoblastoma

  - Lack of nuclear pleomorphism
  - Lack of mitotic activity
  - Lack of necrosis
- Bile ducts
  - May be dilated, tortuous, compressed, branching, or arranged in ductal-plate-malformation pattern
  - Lined by cuboidal or atrophic biliary epithelium
  - Neutrophil infiltration may be seen
  - Surrounded by loose mesenchyme or dense collagen
- Hepatocytes
  - Present as large islands, small clusters, or thin compressed strips
  - More abundant at periphery of tumor
  - Cytologically normal-appearing but may show reactive changes
  - Preserved cell plate structure but lacking normal acinar architecture
- Blood vessels
  - Numerous arteries, veins, and capillaries throughout
  - Thick-walled vessels may be prominent at periphery of tumor
- Cystic spaces
  - Lymphangioma-like but lacking endothelial lining
  - Likely representing cystic degeneration of loose, primitive mesenchyme
- Absence of normal portal tracts
- Foci of extramedullary hematopoiesis may be seen
- Irregular tumor border without true capsule

ANCILLARY TESTS

Immunohistochemistry
- Mesenchyme positive for vimentin, smooth muscle actin, and desmin
- Bile ducts positive for cytokeratins 7 and 19
- Hepatocytes positive for Hep Par 1

DIFFERENTIAL DIAGNOSIS

Hepatoblastoma
- Fetal &/or embryonal liver cells with alternating light-and-dark pattern
- Much higher cellularity
- Mesenchymal elements usually include cartilaginous and osteoid-like tissues

Infantile Hemangioendothelioma
- Small intercommunicating vascular channels lined by plump endothelial cells
- Immunohistochemical stains are helpful

SELECTED REFERENCES

1. Sugito K et al: Mesenchymal hamartoma of the liver originating in the caudate lobe with t(11;19)(q13;q13.4): report of a case. Surg Today. 40(1):83-7, 2010
2. Stringer MD et al: Mesenchymal hamartoma of the liver: a systematic review. J Pediatr Surg. 40(11):1681-90, 2005

IMAGE GALLERY

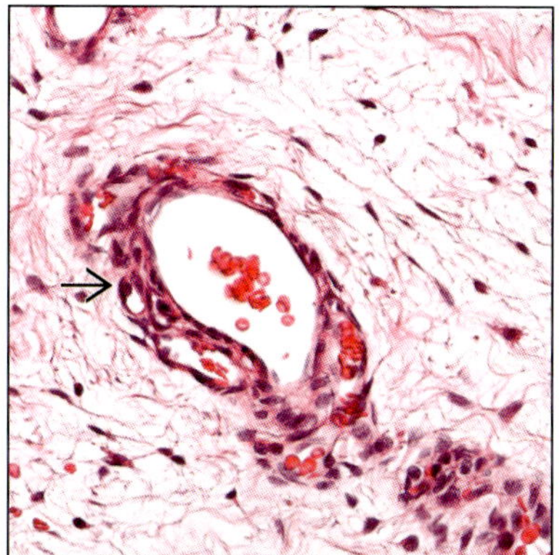

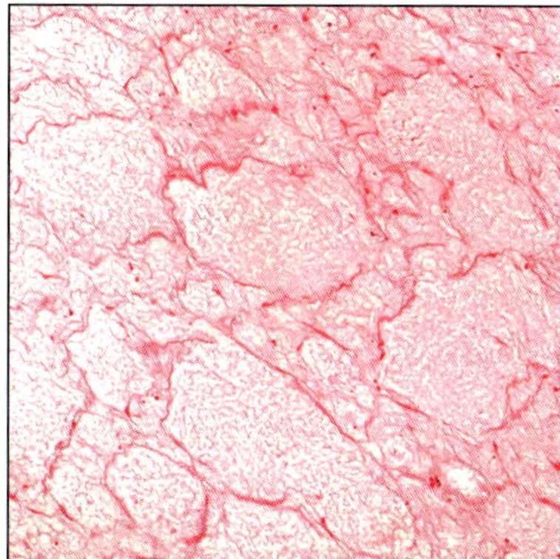

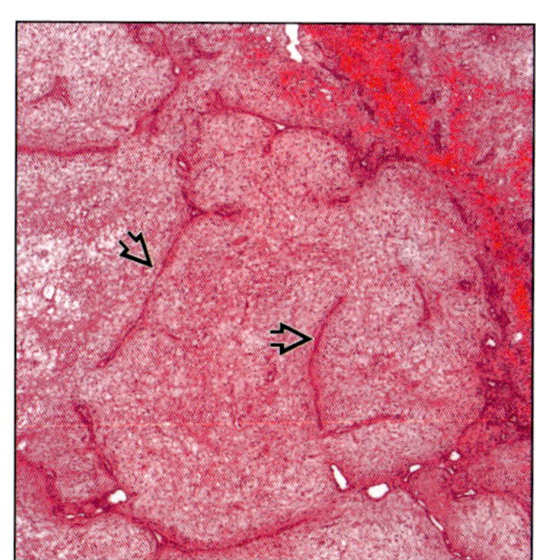

(Left) *High-power view shows scattered stellate mesenchymal cells loosely embedded in an edematous stroma. Note the presence of blood vessels ⇒.* ***(Center)*** *Accumulation of proteinaceous fluid is seen in fully developed cystic spaces, mimicking lymphangioma. However, there is no endothelial lining.* ***(Right)*** *Compressed and branching bile ducts within collagenous stroma have a ductal plate malformation-like pattern ⇒.*

UNDIFFERENTIATED EMBRYONAL SARCOMA

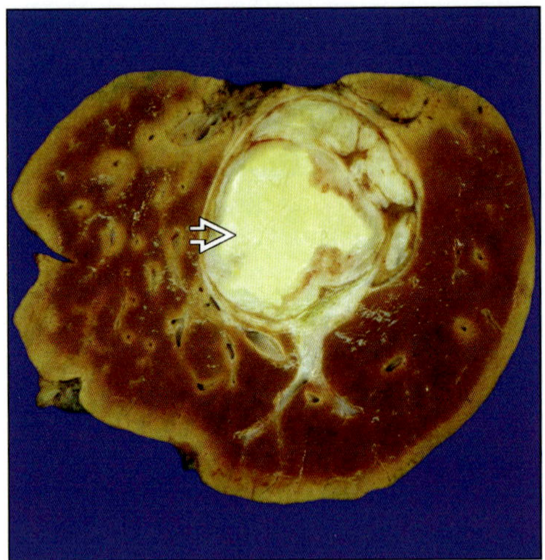

Gross photograph shows a well-demarcated liver mass with a compressed pseudocapsule. The cut surface is variegated with admixed solid areas and a large area of yellow necrosis ⇨.

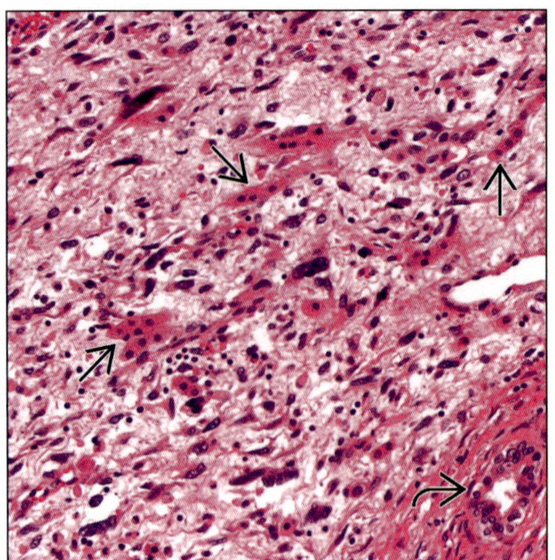

UES contains scattered pleomorphic and multinucleated tumor cells loosely distributed in a myxoid matrix. Note the presence of entrapped hepatocytes → and a bile duct ↪.

TERMINOLOGY

Abbreviations

- Undifferentiated embryonal sarcoma (UES)

Synonyms

- Embryonal sarcoma
- Undifferentiated sarcoma
- Malignant mesenchymoma

Definitions

- Malignant tumor of liver composed of primitive mesenchymal cells with partial, divergent differentiation

ETIOLOGY/PATHOGENESIS

Unknown

- Rare case reports showing association with mesenchymal hamartoma
  - UES arising in mesenchymal hamartoma
  - Share same chromosome translocation involving 19q13.4 breakpoint

CLINICAL ISSUES

Epidemiology

- Incidence
  - 6-13% of all primary hepatic tumors in childhood
- Age
  - Usually occurring from 5-20 years of age
    - > 50% occurring from 6-10 years of age
  - Rarely seen in middle-aged and elderly patients
- Gender
  - Equal gender distribution

Presentation

- Abdominal distention and pain
- Palpable mass
- Weight loss, fever

Laboratory Tests

- Normal or mildly elevated liver tests
  - Usually slightly increased alkaline phosphatase activity
- Normal serum α-fetoprotein level

Treatment

- Surgical resection
- Neoadjuvant and adjuvant chemotherapy
- Radiotherapy

Prognosis

- Markedly improved survival in recent years with combined modality therapy
  - Survival of ≥ 5 years in some patients (median survival < 1 year until 1980s)
- Local recurrence is common even with complete excision and adjuvant chemotherapy
- Distant metastasis is infrequent
  - If metastases occur, usually in lungs, pleura, peritoneal cavity

IMAGE FINDINGS

General Features

- Heterogeneous mass with solid and cystic components
- Difficult to distinguish from mesenchymal hamartoma

MACROSCOPIC FEATURES

General Features

- Predilection for right lobe
- 9-30 cm in size
- Solitary, well-demarcated, typically nonencapsulated
- Variegated cut surface with solid areas alternating with gelatinous cystic areas and foci of necrosis and hemorrhage

UNDIFFERENTIATED EMBRYONAL SARCOMA

Key Facts

Clinical Issues
- 6-13% of all primary hepatic tumors in childhood
- > 50% occurring from 6-10 years of age
- Rarely seen in middle-aged and elderly patients
- Improved survival in recent years with combined modality therapy

Microscopic Pathology
- Spindled, oval, or stellate tumor cells loosely or compactly distributed in myxoid or fibrous stroma
- Marked nuclear pleomorphism and hyperchromasia with frequent multinucleated or bizarre giant cells and brisk mitotic activity
- Characteristic PAS-positive, diastase-resistant cytoplasmic and extracellular eosinophilic globules
- Immunohistochemical evidence of partial divergent differentiation

Top Differential Diagnoses
- Embryonal rhabdomyosarcoma

MICROSCOPIC PATHOLOGY

Histologic Features
- Spindled, oval, or stellate tumor cells loosely or compactly distributed in myxoid or fibrous stroma
- Marked nuclear pleomorphism and hyperchromasia with frequent multinucleated or bizarre giant cells
- Brisk mitotic activity
- Varying amounts of pink granular cytoplasm with ill-defined cell borders
- Multiple varying-sized, PAS-positive, diastase-resistant cytoplasmic eosinophilic globules may be seen, which can also be extracellular
- Tumor necrosis can be extensive
- Intratumoral hemorrhage is common
- Foci of extramedullary hematopoiesis may be seen
- Entrapped hepatocytes and bile ducts often present at periphery of tumor

ANCILLARY TESTS

Immunohistochemistry
- Tumor cells diffusely positive for vimentin, α-1-antitrypsin, and α-1-antichymotrypsin
  - Focally positive for glypican-3, smooth muscle actin, muscle specific actin, desmin, calponin, pancytokeratin, cytokeratins 18 and 19, CD10, CD68, Bcl-2, p53
- Ki-67 proliferation index: 30-95%
- Eosinophilic globules stain with α-1-antitrypsin, α-1-antichymotrypsin, vimentin, immunoglobulins, and albumin

DIFFERENTIAL DIAGNOSIS

Embryonal Rhabdomyosarcoma
- Usually arises in extrahepatic biliary tree
- Rhabdomyoblasts with cross striations
- Immunostains for muscle markers are positive

Metastatic Gastrointestinal Stromal Tumor
- Clinical history of gastrointestinal primary
- Usually not in children
- Positive for c-kit, DOG-1

Sarcomatoid Carcinoma
- Immunostains that mark hepatocellular carcinoma or cholangiocarcinoma are helpful
- Usually not in children

SELECTED REFERENCES

1. Lenze F et al: Undifferentiated embryonal sarcoma of the liver in adults. Cancer. 112(10):2274-82, 2008
2. Pachera S et al: Undifferentiated embryonal sarcoma of the liver: case report and literature survey. J Hepatobiliary Pancreat Surg. 15(5):536-44, 2008
3. Zheng JM et al: Primary and recurrent embryonal sarcoma of the liver: clinicopathological and immunohistochemical analysis. Histopathology. 51(2):195-203, 2007

IMAGE GALLERY

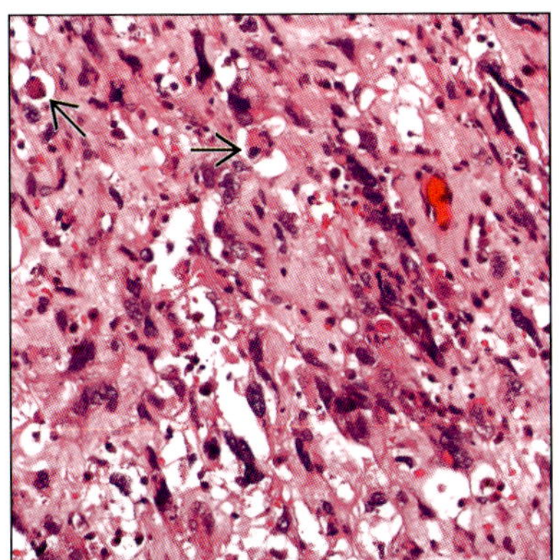
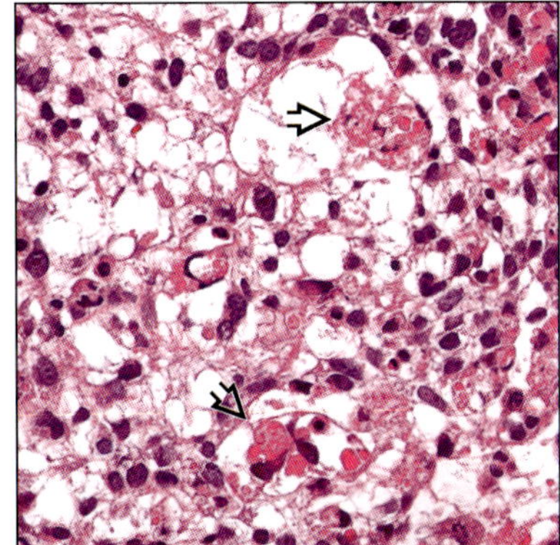
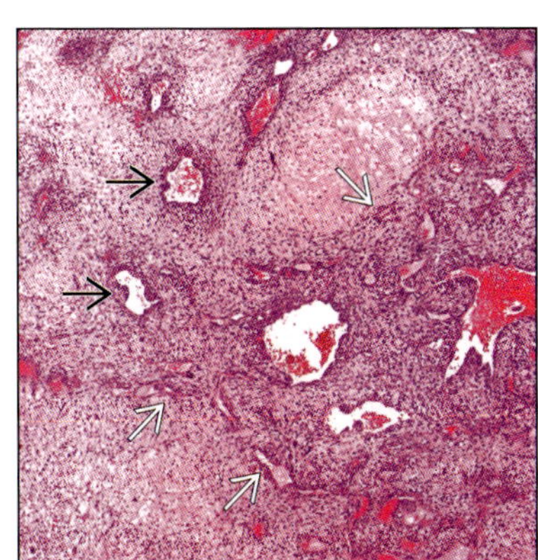

(Left) *High-power view shows markedly pleomorphic tumor cells separated by a fibrous stroma. Note the presence of apoptotic tumor cells* →. ***(Center)*** *High-power view shows ovoid tumor cells with minimal intervening stroma. Numerous cytoplasmic and extracellular eosinophilic globules are seen* ⇨. ***(Right)*** *A case of UES arising in mesenchymal hamartoma shows the presence of numerous bile ducts* →*, some arranged in a ductal plate malformation-like pattern* ➔.

HEPATECTOMY SPECIMEN HANDLING

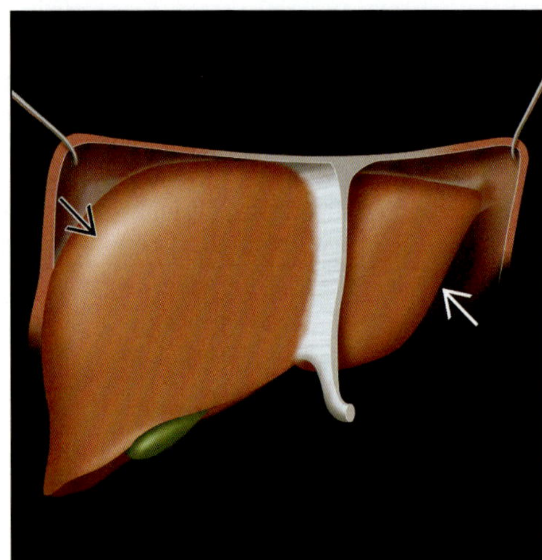

In order to orient the liver, it is important to identify the right lobe ➔ lateral to the falciform ligament and the left lobe medial to the falciform ligament ➔.

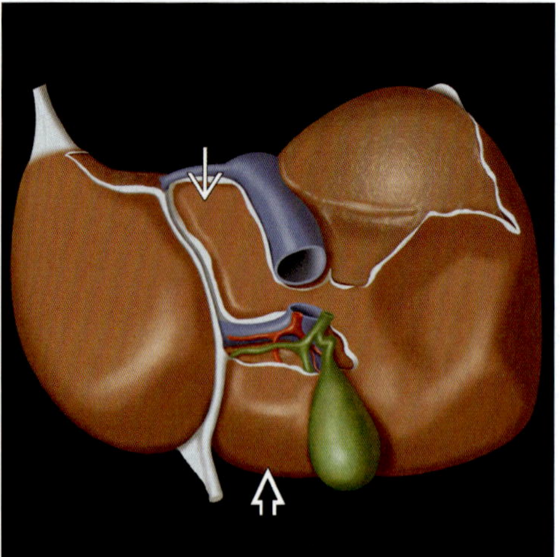

Viewed from below, the quadrate lobe is between the gallbladder fossa and the ligamentum teres ➔, and the caudate lobe ➔ is between the portal vein and the inferior vena cava.

TERMINOLOGY

Partial Hepatectomy

- Ranges from removal of a small wedge to a lobe or more
- Typically consists of lesion plus a variably sized rim of nonneoplastic liver parenchyma

Liver Explant

- Result of liver transplantation
  - Tumors
    - Goals of evaluation are to assess margins and stage tumor
  - Medical liver disease
    - Goal of evaluation is to determine or confirm cause of liver disease &/or liver failure

MACROSCOPIC FINDINGS

Specimen Handling

- Partial hepatectomy
  - Determine what procedure was performed
    - Including exactly what structures/organs are present
  - Orient specimen
    - May require surgeon's assistance
  - Identify surgical margin (exposed, cauterized, cut surface of hepatic parenchyma) and ink it
  - Weigh specimen, and measure it in each dimension
  - Examine external surface
    - Bulges and areas of serosal retraction may indicate tumors
    - Resection for trauma may have capsular lacerations, similar to spleen
  - Make initial slice through center of tumor, perpendicular to resection margin
  - Continue to thinly serially section specimen perpendicular to margin, parallel to the initial slice
    - Identify closest approach of tumor(s) to margin, and take these sections
    - Examine all cut surfaces for additional lesions
  - Document all lesions
    - Location
    - Size
    - Circumscription
    - Color
    - Consistency
    - Note necrosis, scarring, or hemorrhage
    - Sections of tumor(s) should demonstrate relationship of tumor to surrounding liver and margin
    - Interface between nonneoplastic liver and tumor are important and often less necrotic
    - Primary tumors should be sampled more extensively than known metastases
  - Search for vascular invasion
    - Document and sample if present grossly
    - Document tumor thrombi
  - Examine and describe nonneoplastic hepatic parenchyma, and take sections
    - Note especially if there is a background of cirrhosis
    - Take sections of nonneoplastic liver away from tumor mass
  - Examine lymph nodes if applicable
- Liver explant
  - Determine what procedure was performed
    - Note exactly what structures/organs are present
  - Orient liver
    - Identify right and left lobes (best viewed from above)
    - Caudate lobe is between portal vein and inferior vena cava; best viewed from below
    - Quadrate lobe is between gallbladder fossa and ligamentum teres, separated from caudate lobe by inferior vena cava; best viewed from below
    - Porta hepatis contains bile duct, hepatic artery, portal vein, nerves, lymphatics

HEPATECTOMY SPECIMEN HANDLING

- Weigh specimen, and measure it in each dimension
  - Measure gallbladder too, if present
- Examine external surface
  - Document any abnormalities/lesions
- Identify porta hepatis first
  - Document if tumor involves structures at portal hepatis and if tumor is at margin of these structures
  - Look for thrombi in vessels
  - Submit complete cross section of all structures including portal vein, bile duct, hepatic artery
  - Identify hepatic veins and submit section
  - In cases of biliary disease, extrahepatic bile duct may be hard to find; can insert probe into an intrahepatic duct near hilum and work backward
  - Look for hilar lymph nodes
- Submit section of soft tissue and liver perpendicular to hilum
  - Allows evaluation of larger bile ducts and peribiliary glands
- Dissect gallbladder
  - Describe and section as per routine cholecystectomy
- Section liver perpendicular to its long axis with long, sharp knife
  - Record color and consistency of liver parenchyma
  - Describe any focal lesions
  - Submit sections of right lobe (3), left lobe (3), caudate lobe (1), quadrate lobe (1), any other areas with distinct appearance, and any focal lesions

Anatomic Features

- Liver has dual blood supply
  - Portal vein carries blood away from intestines and pancreas
    - Enters liver at porta hepatis
  - Hepatic artery supplies oxygen-rich blood from celiac axis
    - Enters liver at porta hepatis
- Right, middle, and left hepatic veins drain liver and enter vena cava
- Bile ducts follow courses of hepatic artery and portal vein through liver
  - Nourished by hepatic arteries via peribiliary plexus
  - Bile is formed in hepatocytes, secreted into canaliculi and eventually into bile ducts
- Capsule and stroma of liver are rich in lymphatics
  - Hepatic lymphatics exit at porta hepatis
  - Drain primarily to hepatic nodes along hepatic artery and celiac nodes
- Anatomic divisions
  - Right lobe lateral to falciform ligament
  - Left lobe medial to falciform ligament
  - Caudate and quadrate lobes
  - 8 functional segments are served by their own vascular pedicles and branches of biliary tree
    - More important anatomy in terms of surgical approaches
- Superior, anterior, and lateral surfaces are smooth and covered by peritoneum
  - Except for "bare area" below diaphragm
- Falciform and round ligaments connect liver to abdominal wall

SELECTED REFERENCES

1. Torbenson M. Liver. Westra WH et al: Surgical Pathology Dissection: An Illustrated Guide. 2nd ed. New York: Springer. 76-81, 2003
2. Qin LX et al: The prognostic significance of clinical and pathological features in hepatocellular carcinoma. World J Gastroenterol. 8(2):193-9, 2002
3. Shirabe K et al: Intrahepatic cholangiocarcinoma: its mode of spreading and therapeutic modalities. Surgery. 131(1 Suppl):S159-64, 2002
4. Emond JC et al: Surgical anatomy of the liver and its application to hepatobiliary surgery and transplantation. Semin Liver Dis. 14(2):158-68, 1994
5. Bismuth H: Surgical anatomy and anatomical surgery of the liver. World J Surg. 6(1):3-9, 1982

IMAGE GALLERY

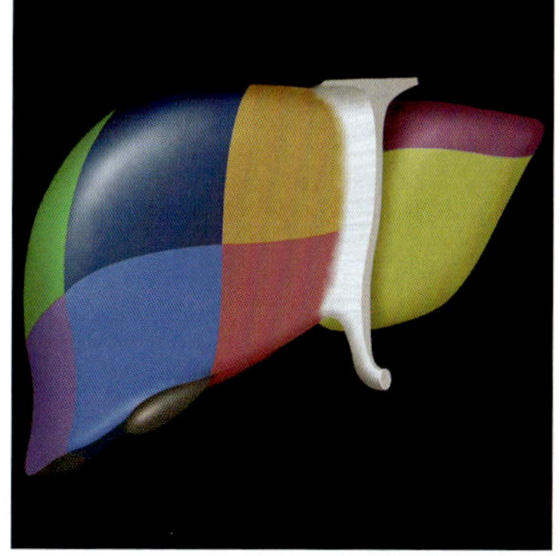

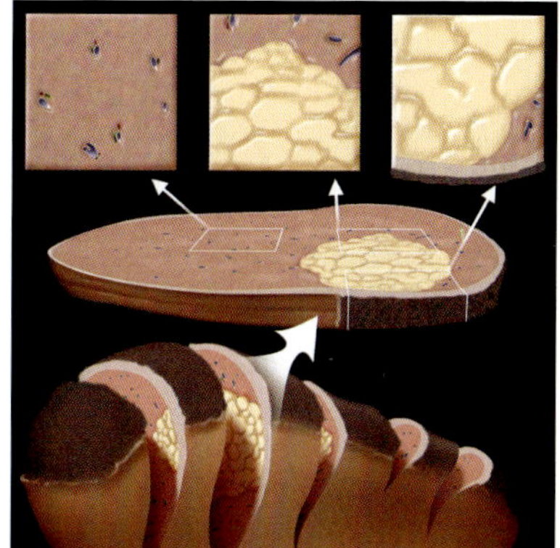

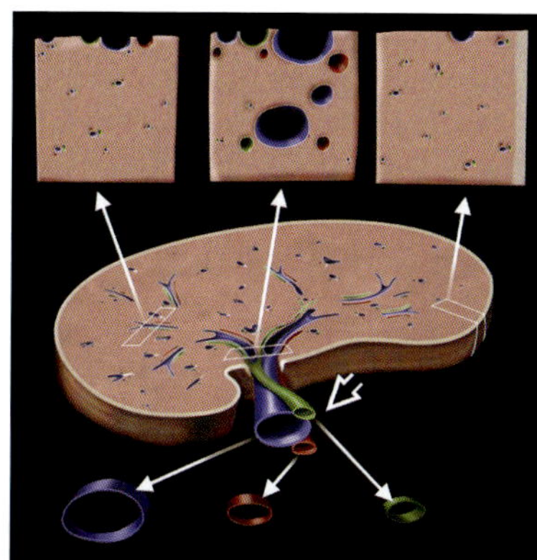

(Left) *Functionally, the liver is divided into 8 segments. These segments, more than the lobar anatomy, are relevant to the planning of surgical resections.* ***(Center)*** *Important sections from a partial hepatectomy include tumor and margin (right), tumor/nonneoplastic liver interface (center), and nonneoplastic liver (left).* ***(Right)*** *Important sections from an explant include a shave margin of the porta hepatis ⮕, a section of hilum (center), and sections of parenchyma (left and right).*

HEPATOCELLULAR CARCINOMA CANCER PROTOCOL

Hepatocellular Carcinoma: Hepatic Resection

Surgical Pathology Cancer Case Summary (Checklist)

Specimen (select all that apply)

- ___ Liver
- ___ Gallbladder
- ___ Other (specify): ______________________
- ___ Not specified

Procedure (select all that apply)

- ___ Wedge resection
- ___ Partial hepatectomy
  - *___ Major hepatectomy (3 segments or more)
  - *___ Minor hepatectomy (< 3 segments)
- ___ Other (specify): ______________________
- ___ Not specified

Tumor Size

Greatest dimension: ________ cm

*Additional dimensions: ________ x ________ cm

___ Cannot be determined

Tumor Focality

- ___ Solitary (specify location): ______________________
- ___ Multiple (specify location: ______________________

Histologic Type

- ___ Hepatocellular carcinoma
- ___ Fibrolamellar hepatocellular carcinoma
- ___ Undifferentiated carcinoma
- ___ Other (specify): ______________________
- ___ Carcinoma, type cannot be determined

Histologic Grade

- ___ Not applicable
- ___ GX: Cannot be assessed
- ___ GI: Well differentiated
- ___ GII: Moderately differentiated
- ___ GIII: Poorly differentiated
- ___ GIV: Undifferentiated/anaplastic
- ___ Other (specify): ______________________

Tumor Extension (select all that apply)

- ___ Tumor confined to liver
- ___ Tumor involves a major branch of portal vein
- ___ Tumor involves 1 or more hepatic vein(s)
- ___ Tumor involves visceral peritoneum
- ___ Tumor directly invades gallbladder
- ___ Tumor directly invades other adjacent organs (specify): ______________________

Margins (select all that apply)

Parenchymal margin

- ___ Cannot be assessed
- ___ Uninvolved by invasive carcinoma
  - Distance of invasive carcinoma from closest margin: ________ mm
  - Specify margin: ______________________
- ___ Involved by invasive carcinoma

Other margin

Specify margin: ______________________

____ Cannot be assessed

____ Uninvolved by invasive carcinoma

____ Involved by invasive carcinoma

Lymph-Vascular Invasion

Macroscopic venous (large vessel) invasion (V)

____ Not identified

____ Present

____ Indeterminate

Microscopic (small vessel) invasion (L)

____ Not identified

____ Present

____ Indeterminate

**Perineural Invasion*

*____ Not identified

*____ Present

*____ Indeterminate

Pathologic Staging (pTNM)

TNM descriptors (required only if applicable) (select all that apply)

____ m (multiple primary tumors)

____ r (recurrent)

____ y (post-treatment)

Primary tumor (pT)

____ pTX: Cannot be assessed

____ pT0: No evidence of primary tumor

____ pT1: Solitary tumor without vascular invasion

____ pT2: Solitary tumor with vascular invasion or multiple tumors, none > 5 cm

____ pT3a: Multiple tumors > 5 cm

____ pT3b: Single tumor or multiple tumors of any size involving a major branch of portal vein or hepatic veins

____ pT4: Tumor(s) with direct invasion of adjacent organs other than gallbladder or with perforation of visceral peritoneum

Regional lymph nodes (pN)

____ pNX: Cannot be assessed

____ pN0: No regional lymph node metastasis

____ pN1: Regional lymph node metastasis

Specify: Number examined: ________

Number involved: ________

Distant metastasis (pM)

____ Not applicable

____ pM1: Distant metastasis

*Specify site(s), if known: ________________________

**Additional Pathologic Findings (select all that apply)*

*Fibrosis score:

*____ Cirrhosis/severe fibrosis (Ishak score 5-6) (F1)

*____ None to moderate fibrosis (Ishak score 0-4) (F2)

*____ Hepatocellular dysplasia

*____ Low-grade dysplastic nodule

*____ High-grade dysplastic nodule

*____ Steatosis

*____ Iron overload

*____ Chronic hepatitis (specify etiology): ________________________

*____ Other (specify): ________________________

*____ None identified

**Ancillary Studies*

*Specify: ________________________

HEPATOCELLULAR CARCINOMA CANCER PROTOCOL

Clinical History (select all that apply)

*____ Cirrhosis

*____ Hepatitis C infection

*____ Hepatitis B infection

*____ Alcoholic liver disease

*____ Obesity

*____ Hereditary hemochromatosis

*____ Other (specify): ____________________________

*____ Not known

**Data elements with asterisks are not required. However, these elements may be clinically important but they are not yet validated or regularly used in patient management. Adapted with permission from College of American Pathologists, "Protocol for the Examination of Specimens from Patients with Hepatocellular Carcinoma." Web posting date October 2009, www.cap.org.*

Stage Groupings

Stage	Tumor	Node	Metastasis
I	T1	N0	M0
II	T2	N0	M0
IIIA	T3a	N0	M0
IIIB	T3b	N0	M0
IIIC	T4	N0	M0
IVA	Any T	N1	M0
IVB	Any T	Any N	M1

Adapted from 7th edition AJCC Staging Forms.

HEPATOCELLULAR CARCINOMA CANCER PROTOCOL

GENERAL PREDICTORS OF OUTCOME

Resectability for Cure

- Multiple tumors with any tumor > 5 cm associated with decreased survival
- Positive surgical margin associated with decreased survival

Extent of Vascular Invasion

- Major vessel invasion associated with decreased survival

Adverse Clinical Indicators

- Elevated serum AFP
- Cirrhosis with Child-Pugh class B or C disease

PRIMARY TUMOR CLASSIFICATION

Vascular Invasion

- For pathologic staging, vascular invasion includes gross and microscopic involvement
- Major vascular invasion is defined as invasion of branches of main portal vein or invasion of 1 or more of the 3 branches of hepatic vein
- For clinical staging, vascular invasion may be assessed pathologically &/or radiographically
- If tumor is solitary and lacks vascular invasion, size does not affect prognosis (T1 disease)

Number/Size of Tumor Nodules

- Single vs. multiple
- Size of largest tumor nodule (< 5 cm vs. > 5 cm)
- "Multiple tumors" includes tumor satellitosis, multifocal tumor nodules, and intrahepatic metastases
- Invasion of adjacent structures other than gallbladder is considered T4 disease
- Perforation of visceral peritoneum is considered T4 disease

OTHER HISTOLOGIC VARIABLES

Grade

- Edmondson and Steiner grading scheme recommended
  - Based on nuclear pleomorphism
    - Well differentiated
    - Moderately differentiated
    - Poorly differentiated
    - Undifferentiated

Status of Adjacent Liver

- Presence of cirrhosis
- Presence of chronic liver disease

REGIONAL LYMPH NODE INVOLVEMENT

Regional Nodes

- Hilar, hepatoduodenal ligament, caval, inferior phrenic comprise the regional nodes
  - Regional node involvement is rare (approximately 5%) except in fibrolamellar HCC
- Any nodal involvement considered N1, but stage IV disease (carry same prognosis as distant metastases)

METASTASES

Route of Dissemination

- Main route of dissemination is vascular (via intrahepatic portal and hepatic veins)

Common Sites

- Most common sites of distant metastasis are lung, bones

Intrahepatic

- Intrahepatic venous dissemination considered same as satellitosis or multifocal tumors

SELECTED REFERENCES

1. American Joint Committee on Cancer: AJCC Cancer Staging Manual. 7th ed. New York: Springer. 191-5, 2010
2. Pawlik TM et al: Hepatectomy for hepatocellular carcinoma with major portal or hepatic vein invasion: results of a multicenter study. Surgery. 137(4):403-10, 2005
3. Varotti G et al: Comparison between the fifth and sixth editions of the AJCC/UICC TNM staging systems for hepatocellular carcinoma: multicentric study on 393 cirrhotic resected patients. Eur J Surg Oncol. 31(7):760-7, 2005
4. Mino M et al: Pathologic spectrum and prognostic significance of underlying liver disease in hepatocellular carcinoma. Surg Oncol Clin N Am. 12(1):13-24, 2003
5. Lauwers GY et al: Prognostic histologic indicators of curatively resected hepatocellular carcinomas: a multi-institutional analysis of 425 patients with definition of a histologic prognostic index. Am J Surg Pathol. 26(1):25-34, 2002
6. Vauthey JN et al: Simplified staging for hepatocellular carcinoma. J Clin Oncol. 20(6):1527-36, 2002
7. Poon RT et al: Significance of resection margin in hepatectomy for hepatocellular carcinoma: A critical reappraisal. Ann Surg. 231(4):544-51, 2000
8. Nzeako UC et al: Hepatocellular carcinoma in cirrhotic and noncirrhotic livers. A clinico-histopathologic study of 804 North American patients. Am J Clin Pathol. 105(1):65-75, 1996
9. Vauthey JN et al: A simplified staging system for hepatocellular carcinomas. Gastroenterology. 108(2):617-8, 1995

HEPATOCELLULAR CARCINOMA CANCER PROTOCOL

Staging Parameters

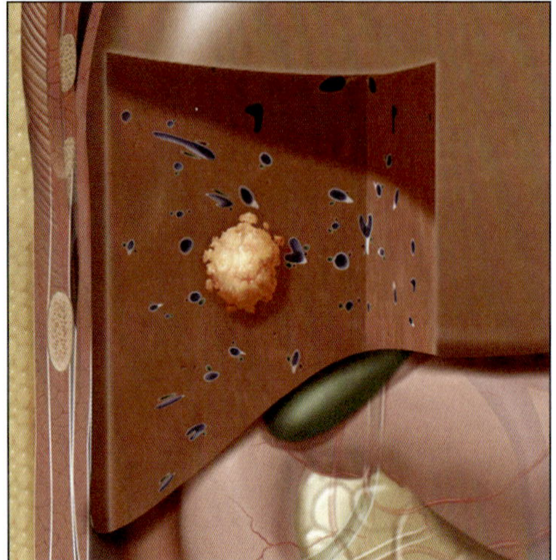

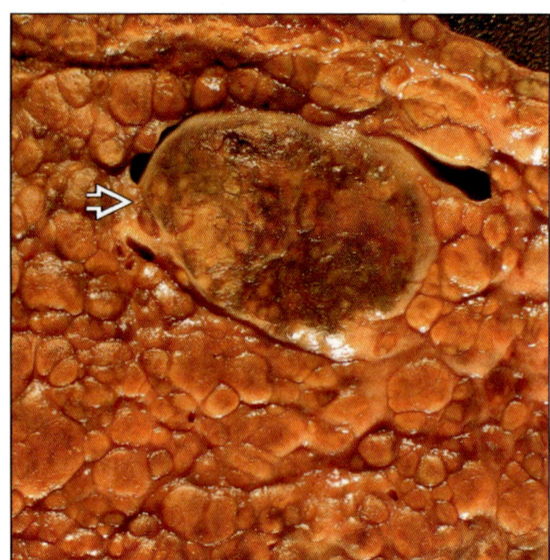

(Left) *Graphic illustrates a T1 tumor, defined as a solitary tumor without vascular invasion.* ***(Right)*** *Gross photograph shows a solitary nodule of hepatocellular carcinoma without vascular invasion (T1 disease) ➔ in a background of cirrhosis.*

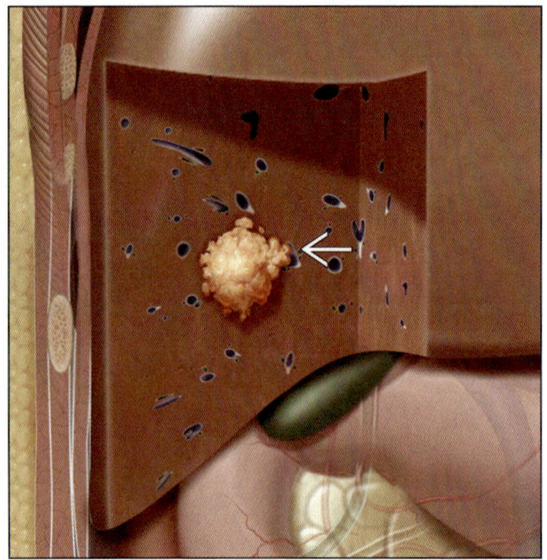

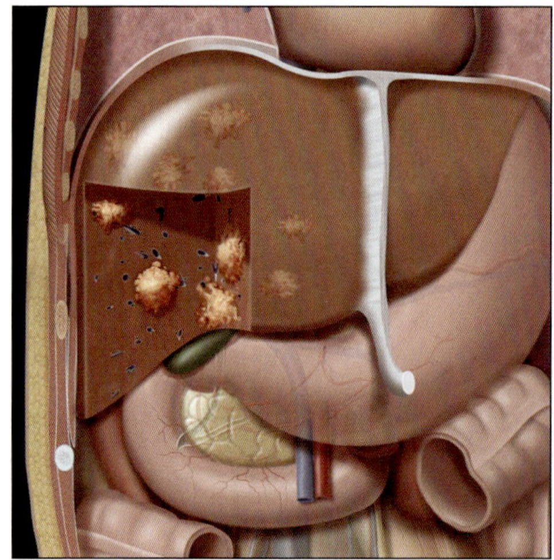

(Left) *Graphic illustrates a solitary tumor nodule with vascular invasion, consistent with T2 disease ➔.* ***(Right)*** *The presence of multiple tumor nodules, none of which are more than 5.0 cm in greatest dimension, is also classified as T2 disease.*

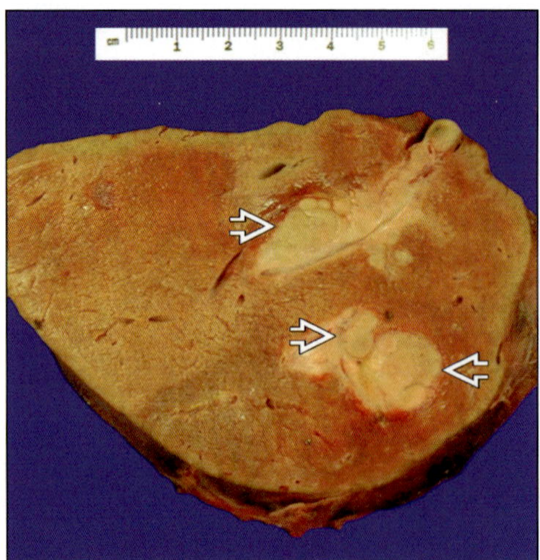

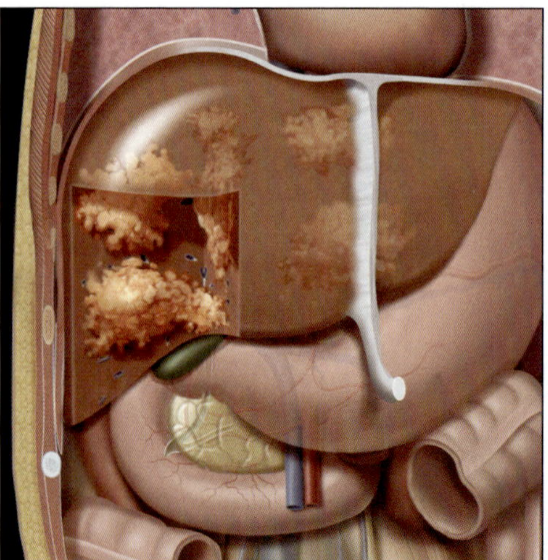

(Left) *Gross photograph shows a hepatectomy specimen with multiple tumor nodules ➔, none of which are greater than 5.0 cm (T2 disease).* ***(Right)*** *Graphic illustrates T3a disease, defined as multiple tumors with some measuring more than 5.0 cm.*

Staging Parameters

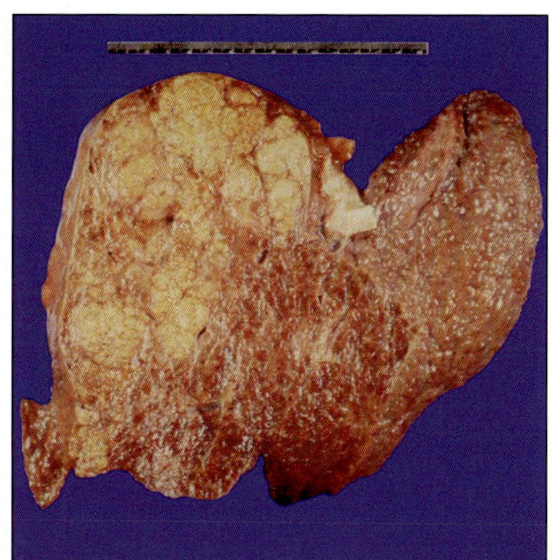

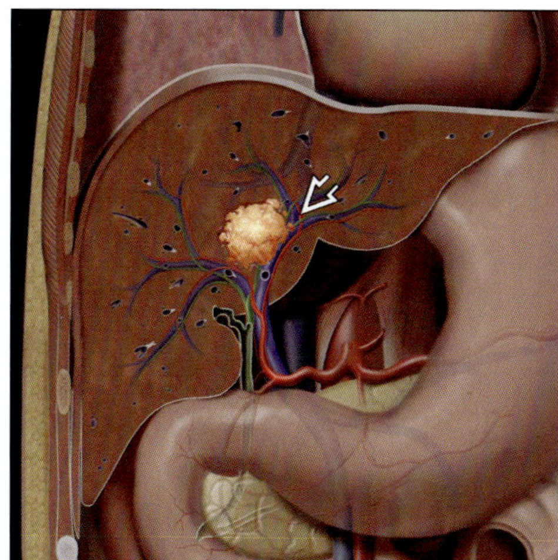

(Left) *This explant shows multiple tumor nodules, some of which are more than 5.0 cm in maximum dimension (T3a disease). Note the background of cirrhosis.* ***(Right)*** *Graphic illustrates T3b disease in which a single tumor invades a major branch of the portal vein ➡.*

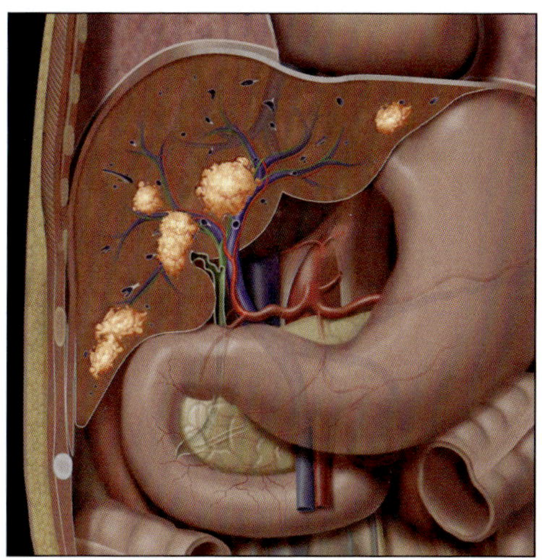

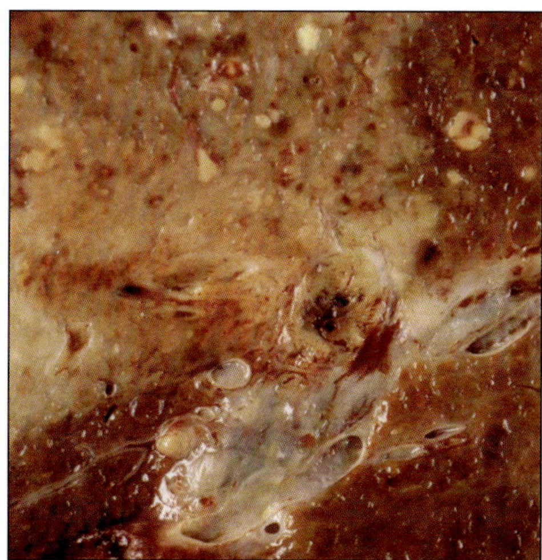

(Left) *Graphic shows multiple tumor nodules throughout the liver with portal venous invasion. T3b disease is defined as single or multiple tumors of any size involving a major branch of the portal or hepatic vein.* ***(Right)*** *Gross photograph shows vascular invasion involving a major vein (T3b disease).*

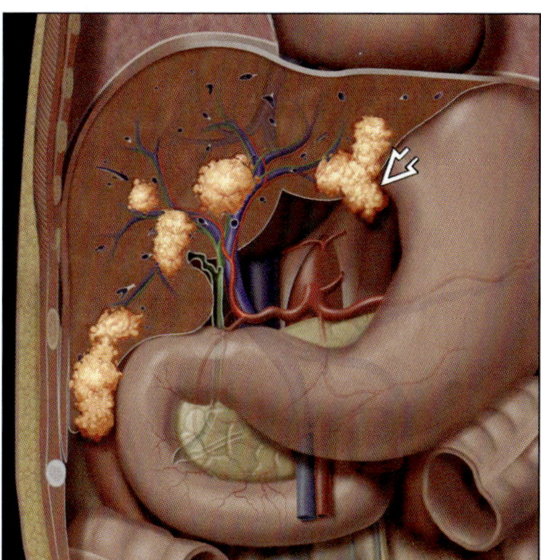

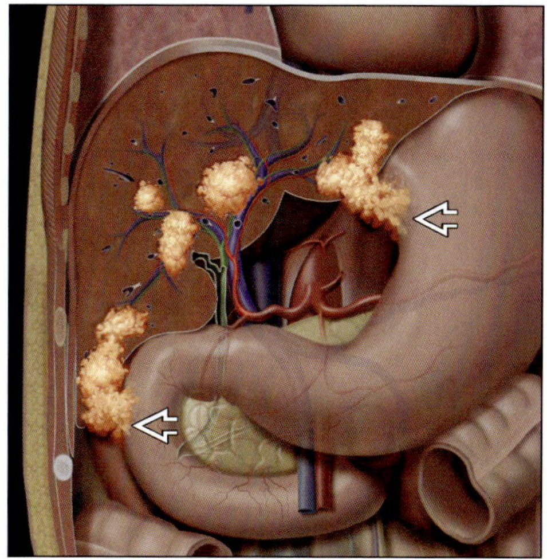

(Left) *Graphic illustrates multiple tumors throughout the liver, some of which extend through the capsule of the liver ➡ (T4 disease). Extracapsular tumoral extension with perforation of the visceral peritoneum is classified as T4.* ***(Right)*** *Direct invasion of adjacent organs other than the gallbladder, including duodenum and stomach as illustrated in this graphic ➡, is also considered T4 disease.*

INTRAHEPATIC BILE DUCT CANCER PROTOCOL

Intrahepatic Bile Ducts

Surgical Pathology Cancer Case Summary (Checklist)

Specimen

___ Liver

___ Gallbladder

___ Other (specify): ___________________________

Procedure (select all that apply)

___ Wedge resection

___ Partial hepatectomy

  *___ Major hepatectomy (3 segments or more)

  *___ Minor hepatectomy (< 3 segments)

___ Total hepatectomy

___ Other (specify): ___________________________

___ Not specified

Tumor Size

Greatest dimension: ___ cm

*Additional dimensions: ___ x ___ cm

___ Cannot be determined

Tumor Focality

___ Solitary (specify location): ___________________________

___ Multiple (specify location): ___________________________

Histologic Type

___ Cholangiocarcinoma

___ Combined hepatocellular and cholangiocarcinoma

___ Bile duct cystadenocarcinoma

___ Other (specify): ___________________________

Histologic Grade

___ Not applicable

___ GX: Cannot be assessed

___ GI: Well differentiated

___ GII: Moderately differentiated

___ GIII: Poorly differentiated

___ GIV: Undifferentiated

___ Other (specify): ___________________________

Tumor Growth Pattern

___ Mass forming

___ Periductal infiltrating

___ Mixed mass-forming and periductal infiltrating

___ Cannot be determined

Microscopic Tumor Extension (select all that apply)

___ Cannot be assessed

___ No evidence of primary tumor

___ Tumor confined to intrahepatic bile ducts histologically (carcinoma in situ)

___ Tumor confined to hepatic parenchyma

___ Tumor involves visceral peritoneal surface

___ Tumor directly invades adjacent organs other than gallbladder
  (specify): ___________________________

Margins (select all that apply)

Hepatic parenchymal margin

  ___ Cannot be assessed

  ___ Uninvolved by invasive carcinoma

Distance of invasive carcinoma from closest margin: ________ mm

Specify margin: ____________________________

____ Involved by invasive carcinoma

Bile duct margin

____ Cannot be assessed

____ Uninvolved by invasive carcinoma

*____ Dysplasia/carcinoma in situ not identified

*____ Dysplasia/carcinoma in situ present

____ Involved by invasive carcinoma

Other margin

Specify margin: ____________________________

____ Cannot be assessed

____ Uninvolved by invasive carcinoma

____ Involved by invasive carcinoma

Lymph-Vascular Invasion

Venous (major vessel) invasion (V)

(invasion of right or left portal vein, 1 or more hepatic veins)

____ Not identified

____ Present

____ Indeterminate

**Perineural Invasion*

*____ Not identified

*____ Present

*____ Indeterminate

Pathologic Staging (pTNM)

TNM descriptors (required only if applicable) (select all that apply)

____ m (multiple primary tumors)

____ r (recurrent)

____ y (post-treatment)

Primary tumor (pT)

____ pTX: Cannot be assessed

____ pT0: No evidence of primary tumor

____ pTis: Carcinoma in situ (intraductal tumor)

____ pT1: Solitary tumor without vascular invasion

____ pT2a: Solitary tumor with vascular invasion

____ pT2b: Multiple tumors, ± vascular invasion

____ pT3: Tumor perforating visceral peritoneum or involving local extrahepatic structures by direct invasion

____ pT4: Tumor with periductal invasion

Regional lymph nodes (pN)

____ pNX: Cannot be assessed

____ pN0: No regional lymph node metastasis

____ pN1: Regional lymph node metastasis

Specify: Number examined: ________

Number involved: ________

Distant metastasis (pM)

____ Not applicable

____ pM1: Distant metastasis

*Specify site(s), if known: ____________________________

**Additional Pathologic Findings (select all that apply)*

*____ Cirrhosis/severe fibrosis (Ishak fibrosis score 5-6)

*____ Primary sclerosing cholangitis

*____ Biliary stones

*____ Chronic hepatitis (specify type): ____________________________

INTRAHEPATIC BILE DUCT CANCER PROTOCOL

*____ Other (specify): ____________________________

*____ None identified

*Ancillary Studies

*Specify: ____________________________

*Clinical History (select all that apply)

*____ Cirrhosis

*____ Primary sclerosing cholangitis

*____ Inflammatory bowel disease

*____ Hepatitis C infection

*____ Other (specify): ____________________________

*____ Not known

**Data elements with asterisks are not required. However, these elements may be clinically important but are not yet validated or regularly used in patient management. Adapted with permission from College of American Pathologists, "Protocol for the Examination of Specimens from Patients with Carcinoma of the Intrahepatic Bile Ducts." Web posting date October 2009, www.cap.org.*

Stage Groupings

Stage	Tumor	Node	Metastasis
0	Tis	N0	M0
I	T1	N0	M0
II	T2	N0	M0
III	T3	N0	M0
IVA	T4	N0	M0
	Any T	N1	M0
IVB	Any T	Any N	M1

Adapted from 7th edition AJCC Staging Forms.

INTRAHEPATIC BILE DUCT CANCER PROTOCOL

INTRAHEPATIC CHOLANGIOCARCINOMA

General

- 15-20% of primary hepatic malignancies
- 20% of bile duct cholangiocarcinomas are intrahepatic
- Currently staged differently than hepatocellular carcinoma
  - Differences in
    - Prognosis
    - Clinical behavior
    - Epidemiology
    - Treatment
  - Size not prognostic factor for IHBDC

PRIMARY TUMOR

Growth Patterns and Staging

- Mass-forming lesion (60%)
- Periductal infiltrating pattern (20%)
  - Defined as diffuse longitudinal growth pattern along intrahepatic bile ducts on gross &/or microscopic evaluation
  - T4 by definition
  - Associated with poor prognosis, although analysis limited
- Mixed mass-forming and periductal patterns (20%)
  - Also staged as T4 disease
- Intraductal papillary cholangiocarcinomas defined as Tis
- Solitary vs. multiple tumors helps determines T1 vs. T2 disease
  - Multiple tumors include
    - Satellitosis
    - Multifocal tumor nodules
    - Intrahepatic metastases
- Perforation of visceral peritoneum &/or directly invading adjacent structures is T3 disease

VASCULAR INVASION

Location

- Includes both major vessel and microscopic vessel invasion

LYMPH NODES

Right Liver

- Regional nodes include hilar, periduodenal, peripancreatic nodes

Left Liver

- Regional nodes include hilar and gastrohepatic

Other

- Inferior phrenic nodes considered regional
- Spread to celiac &/or periaortic and caval nodes is considered distant metastatic disease (M1)

METASTASES

Intrahepatic

- Intrahepatic metastases classified as multiple tumors

Distant

- Distant metastases usually to peritoneum, lungs, pleura

PROGNOSTIC FEATURES

Adverse Indicators

- Elevated CA19-9
- Underlying liver disease
  - Including primary sclerosing cholangitis
- Lymph node involvement
- Incomplete resection

SELECTED REFERENCES

1. American Joint Committee on Cancer: AJCC Cancer Staging Manual. 7th ed. New York: Springer. 201-5, 2010
2. Ercolani G et al: Intrahepatic cholangiocarcinoma: primary liver resection and aggressive multimodal treatment of recurrence significantly prolong survival. Ann Surg. 252(1):107-14, 2010
3. Hatzaras I et al: Elevated CA 19-9 portends poor prognosis in patients undergoing resection of biliary malignancies. HPB (Oxford). 12(2):134-8, 2010
4. Nathan H et al: Staging of intrahepatic cholangiocarcinoma. Curr Opin Gastroenterol. 26(3):269-73, 2010
5. Choi SB et al: The prognosis and survival outcome of intrahepatic cholangiocarcinoma following surgical resection: association of lymph node metastasis and lymph node dissection with survival. Ann Surg Oncol. 16(11):3048-56, 2009
6. Yamamoto Y et al: Clinicopathological characteristics of intrahepatic cholangiocellular carcinoma presenting intrahepatic bile duct growth. J Surg Oncol. 99(3):161-5, 2009
7. Yamasaki S: Intrahepatic cholangiocarcinoma: macroscopic type and stage classification. J Hepatobiliary Pancreat Surg. 10(4):288-91, 2003
8. Isa T et al: Predictive factors for long-term survival in patients with intrahepatic cholangiocarcinoma. Am J Surg. 181(6):507-11, 2001

INTRAHEPATIC BILE DUCT CANCER PROTOCOL

Staging Parameters

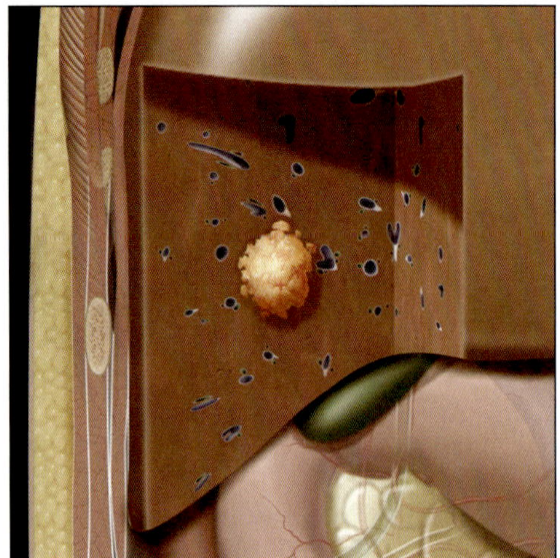

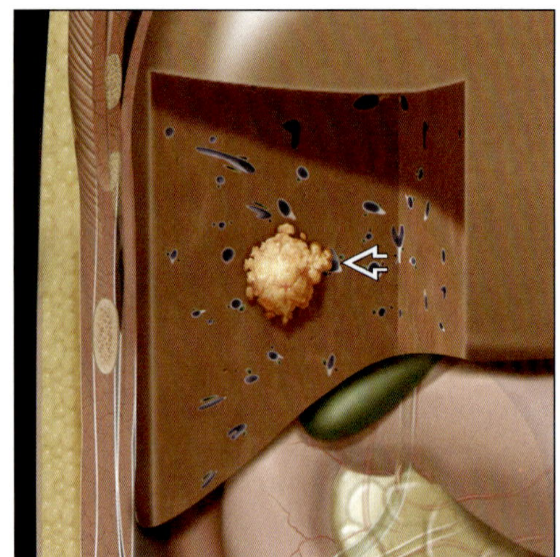

(Left) *T1 disease is defined as a solitary tumor of the intrahepatic bile ducts without vascular invasion.* ***(Right)*** *T2a disease is defined as a solitary tumor with vascular invasion ➡.*

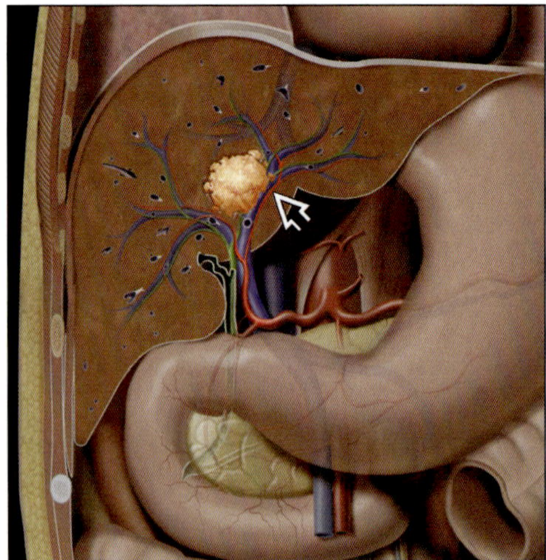

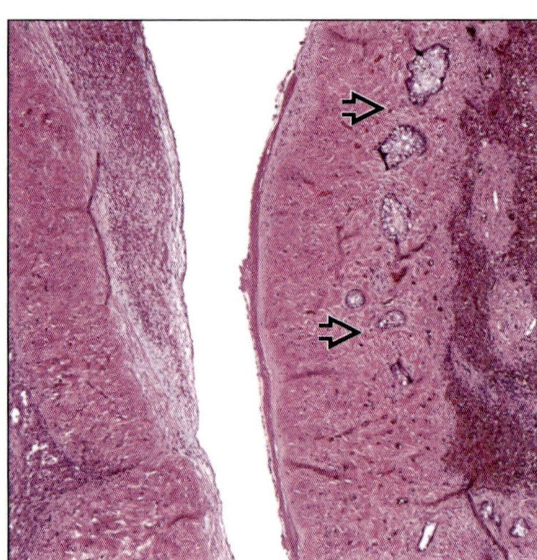

(Left) *This tumor, a solitary tumor of the intrahepatic bile ducts with major vessel invasion ➡, is also classified as T2a. T2a tumors can have either small or large vessel invasion.* ***(Right)*** *This cholangiocarcinoma invaded large veins, as seen here. The tumor is present within the wall of the vein in this longitudinal section ➡.*

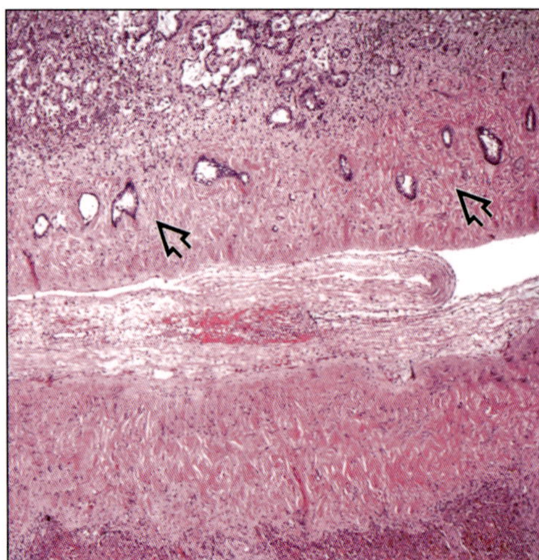

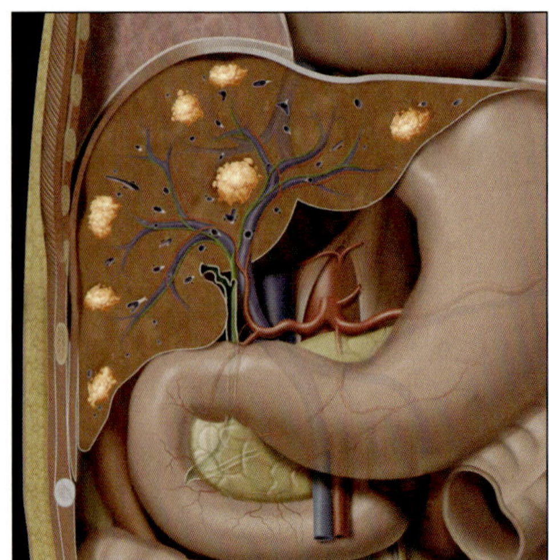

(Left) *High-power view shows large vein invasion by cholangiocarcinoma ➡. Invasion of either large or small vessels is classified as T2a.* ***(Right)*** *The presence of multiple tumors, with or without vascular invasion, defines T2b disease.*

Staging Parameters

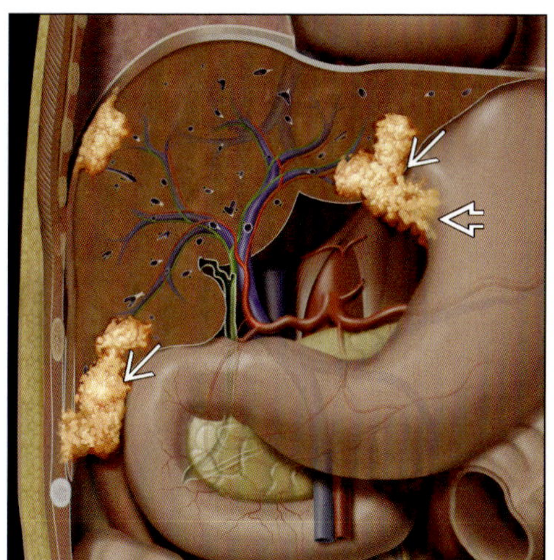

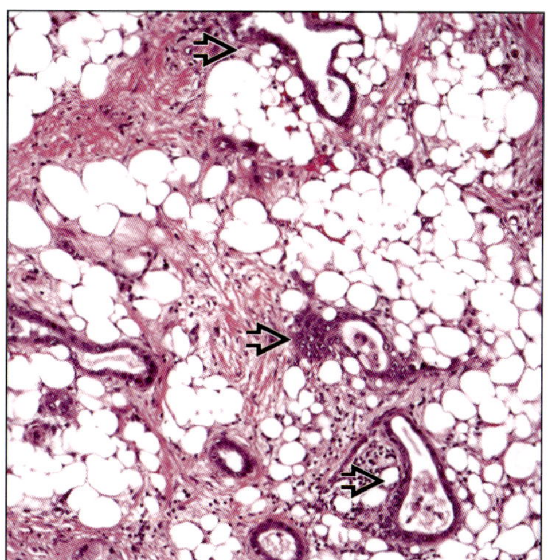

(Left) T3 disease is defined as tumor perforating the visceral peritoneum or invading local extrahepatic structures by direct extension. This graphic illustrates penetration of the visceral peritoneum ➔ and involvement of the stomach ➲. (Right) This cholangiocarcinoma of the intrahepatic bile ducts extended into the perihepatic fat by direct extension ➲.

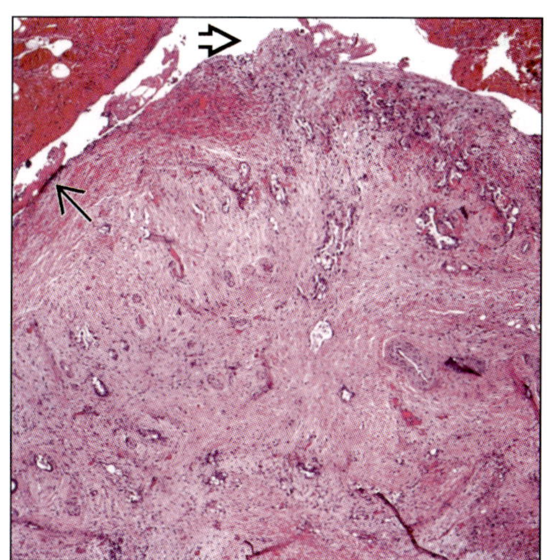

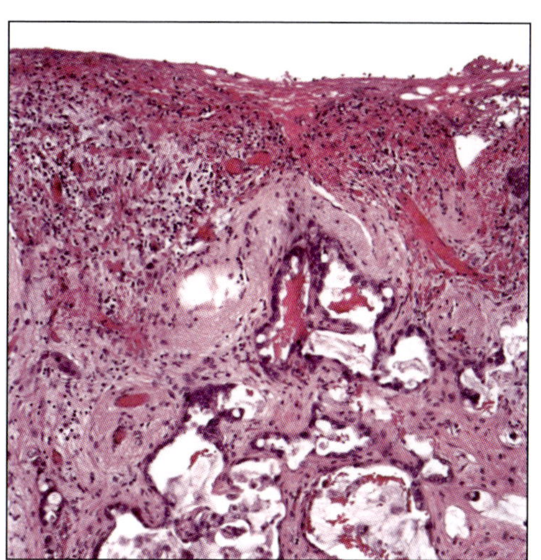

(Left) The same cholangiocarcinoma also penetrated the visceral peritoneum ➲ (T3 disease). There is a thin rim of intact mesothelial cells ➔ to the left of the area of penetration. (Right) High-power view shows penetration of the visceral peritoneum by cholangiocarcinoma. The peritoneal surface has been obliterated by tumor, fibrosis, and inflammation.

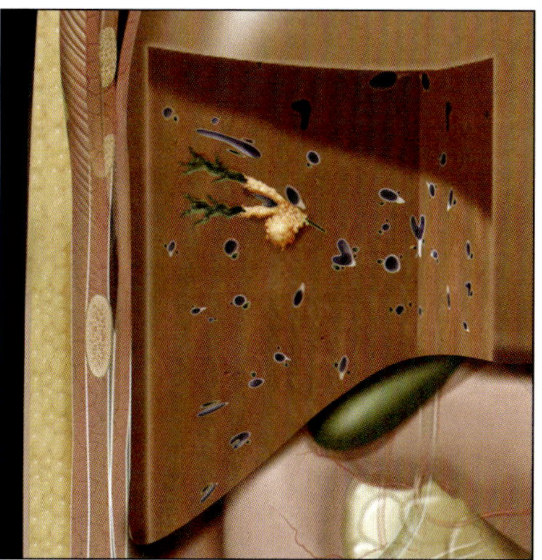

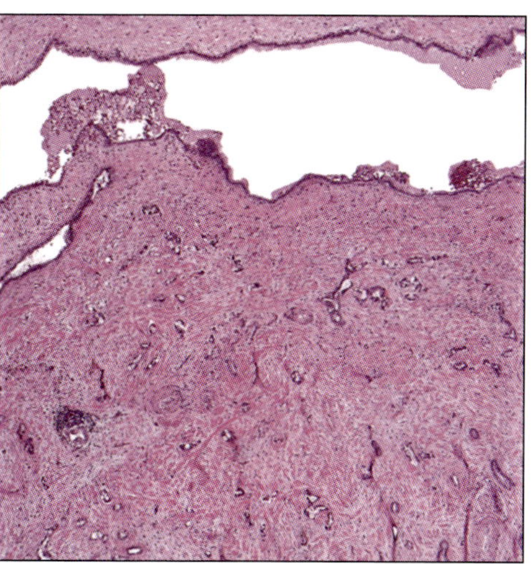

(Left) Periductal invasion, defined as diffuse longitudinal growth along the intrahepatic bile ducts, typifies T4 disease. There may or may not be a discrete tumor mass. (Right) This intrahepatic bile duct contains diffuse longitudinal tumor within the wall, consistent with T4 disease. Note the benign epithelial lining of the duct above the infiltrating tumor.

Miscellaneous Hepatic Disorders

LANGERHANS CELL HISTIOCYTOSIS

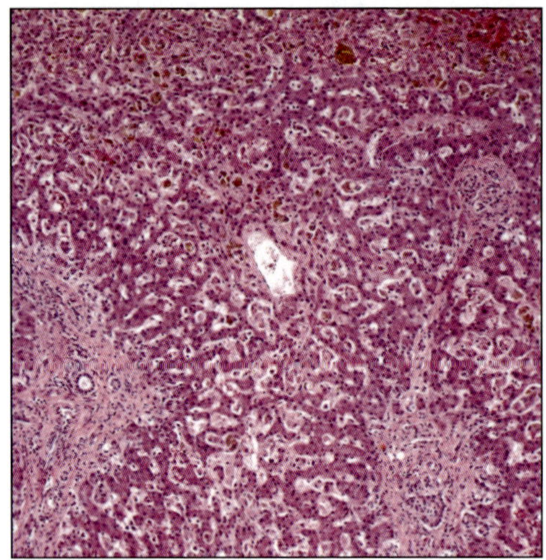

Langerhans cell histiocytosis in the liver features infiltration of the hepatic sinusoids by a mixture of Langerhans and non-Langerhans cells, with portal expansion and fibrosis.

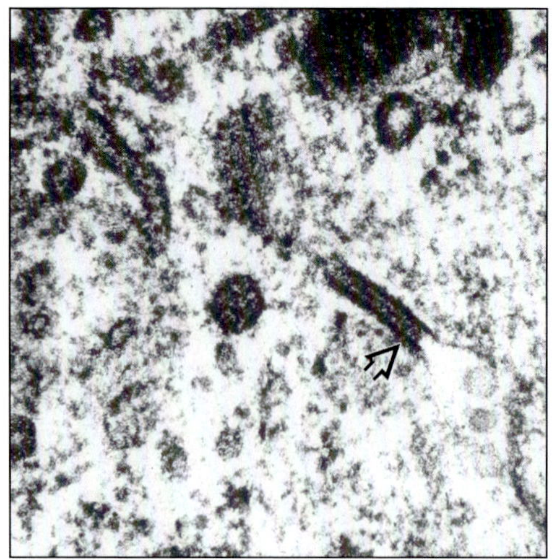

Transmission electron microscopy demonstrates a Birbeck granule ⇒, which is a trilamellar, striated tennis racket-shaped structure.

TERMINOLOGY

Abbreviations

- Langerhans cell histiocytosis (LCH)

Synonyms

- Histiocytosis X
- Eosinophilic granuloma
- Hans-Schüller-Christian disease
- Letterer-Siwe disease

Definitions

- Group of disorders characterized by clonal proliferation of Langerhans dendritic cells

ETIOLOGY/PATHOGENESIS

Clonal Disorder

- Evidence of genetic aberrations favors neoplastic process
  - Loss of heterozygosity, chromosomal instability, elevated expression of cell-cycle-related proteins and oncogene products

CLINICAL ISSUES

Epidemiology

- Incidence
  - Occurs in 4 per 1,000,000 children in United Kingdom of whom < 20% have hepatic involvement
- Age
  - Infants and children, rarely adults

Site

- LCH can involve single organ or multiple organs
  - Single-organ disease is most often bone or skin
- Multisystem disease is subtyped according to involvement of "risk" organs
  - "Risk LCH" indicates involvement of liver, spleen, hematopoietic system

Presentation

- Hepatosplenomegaly
- Jaundice, cholestatic
- Ascites
- Hepatic dysfunction

Natural History

- Permanent fibrosis of liver and lungs may occur, possibly due to "cytokine storm" produced by Langerhans cells
  - Results in pattern of sclerosing cholangitis
  - May progress to liver failure requiring transplantation

Treatment

- Drugs
  - Etoposide, vinblastine, methotrexate

Prognosis

- "Risk LCH" has 80% survival
  - Early therapy with nontoxic chemotherapy improves survival
  - Lack of response to chemotherapy at 6 weeks predicts poor survival
- Reactivation usually occurs in nonrisk organs and is rarely fatal

IMAGE FINDINGS

Radiographic Findings

- Endoscopic retrograde cholangiopancreatography (ERCP) shows strictures and beading of large intrahepatic and extrahepatic bile ducts, similar to primary sclerosing cholangitis

LANGERHANS CELL HISTIOCYTOSIS

Key Facts

Etiology/Pathogenesis
- Clonal proliferation of Langerhans dendritic cells

Clinical Issues
- Affects infants and children
- Multisystem LCH can involve "risk" organs: Liver, spleen, hematopoietic system
- Permanent fibrosis of liver and lungs may occur, possibly due to "cytokine storm" produced by Langerhans cells
  - Results in secondary sclerosing cholangitis

Microscopic Pathology
- Infiltration of liver by Langerhans cells, in small clusters or as a mass
- Small duct infiltration and destruction, with features of chronic cholestasis and biliary fibrosis
- Destructive cholangitis of large bile ducts with cystic dilatation and bile extravasation
- Langerhans cells show abundant pink cytoplasm and lobulated nuclei, with fine chromatin
- Langerhans cells often associated with eosinophils and other inflammatory cells, including non-Langerhans histiocytes

Ancillary Tests
- Langerhans cells positive for S100, CD1a, and langerin
- Electron microscopy shows Birbeck granules

Diagnostic Checklist
- LCH should be excluded in children with sclerosing cholangitis by staining for S100, CD1a, and langerin

MACROSCOPIC FEATURES

General Features
- Involvement of larger ducts may lead to cystic dilatation of intrahepatic bile ducts
- Masses of Langerhans cells may form tumor-like mass

MICROSCOPIC PATHOLOGY

Histologic Features
- Infiltration of liver by Langerhans cells
  - Ranges from small, granulomatoid foci to large tumor-like masses
  - Langerhans cells show abundant pink cytoplasm and lobulated, coffee-bean-shaped, or contorted nuclei, with fine chromatin and no nucleoli
    - Often accompanied by eosinophils, lymphocytes, neutrophils, plasma cells, non-Langerhans histiocytes, and multinucleated giant cells
    - Accompanying macrophage activation syndrome, with infiltration by non-Langerhans macrophages, can cause hypoalbuminemia and hepatomegaly
- Small bile duct infiltration and destruction
  - Small duct epithelial cells can be replaced by Langerhans cells within basement membrane
  - Changes of sclerosing cholangitis with periductal fibrosis, duct destruction, ductopenia, periportal ductular reaction, pseudoxanthomatous transformation, and copper deposition in periportal hepatocytes
    - Sclerosing cholangitis may be due to cytokines produced by Langerhans cells, and Langerhans cell may be absent in biopsy material or explant
    - May not resolve or might even progress after LCH is successfully treated
    - May evolve to biliary fibrosis and micronodular cirrhosis
- Destructive cholangitis of large bile ducts
  - Cystic dilatation of large ducts with bile extravasation and xanthogranulomatous reaction

ANCILLARY TESTS

Immunohistochemistry
- Langerhans cells stain with antibodies to S100 protein, CD1a, and langerin (CD207)

Electron Microscopy
- Transmission
  - Langerhans cells contain Birbeck granules: Tennis racket-shaped structures with striated appearance

DIFFERENTIAL DIAGNOSIS

Primary Sclerosing Cholangitis
- Rare in children
- Association with inflammatory bowel disease

Extrahepatic Biliary Atresia
- Absence of extrahepatic bile ducts and gallbladder on cholangiogram
- Biopsy shows bile duct proliferation and inspissated bile in cholangioles

DIAGNOSTIC CHECKLIST

Pathologic Interpretation Pearls
- Liver biopsies from children with features of sclerosing cholangitis should be stained with antibodies to S100, CD1a, and langerin to exclude LCH

SELECTED REFERENCES

1. Weitzman S et al: Langerhans cell histiocytosis: update for the pediatrician. Curr Opin Pediatr. 20(1):23-9, 2008
2. Braier J et al: Cholestasis, sclerosing cholangitis, and liver transplantation in Langerhans cell Histiocytosis. Med Pediatr Oncol. 38(3):178-82, 2002
3. Kaplan KJ et al: Liver involvement in Langerhans' cell histiocytosis: a study of nine cases. Mod Pathol. 12(4):370-8, 1999
4. Debray D et al: Sclerosing cholangitis in children. J Pediatr. 124(1):49-56, 1994

LANGERHANS CELL HISTIOCYTOSIS

Infiltration of Liver by LCH

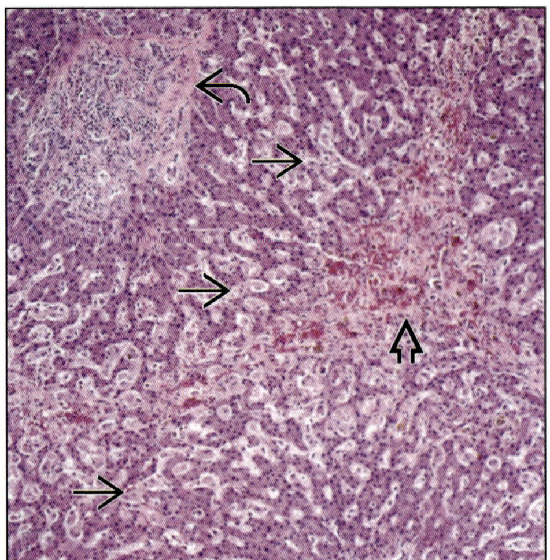

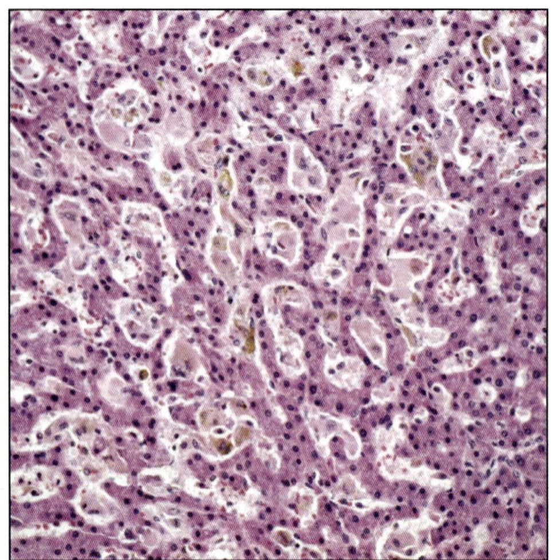

(Left) *Langerhans cell histiocytosis in the liver shows extensive infiltration of the sinusoids by histiocytes →, perivenular collapse and hemorrhage ⇨, and portal expansion with fibrosis and a mononuclear cell infiltrate ↪.* ***(Right)*** *Medium-power view of liver in LCH shows extensive infiltration of sinusoids by a mixture of Langerhans cells and non-Langerhans histiocytes.*

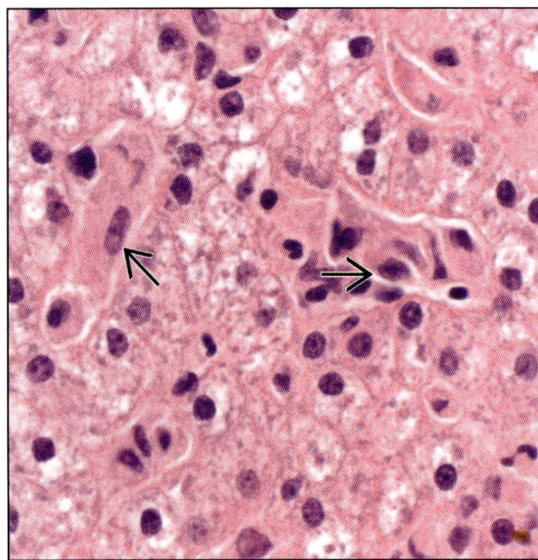

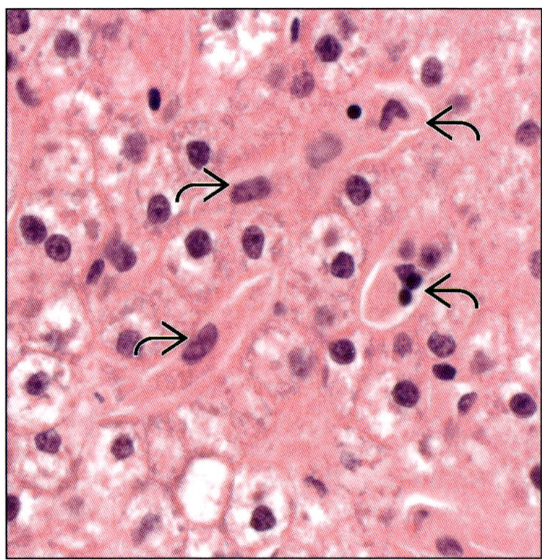

(Left) *High-power view of hepatic LCH shows histiocytic cells within sinusoids →, some of which are Langerhans cells and others that are part of the macrophage activation syndrome. Immunohistochemical stains for CD1a and langerin would identify the Langerhans cells.* ***(Right)*** *Hepatic involvement in LCH features sinusoidal histiocytic cells ↪, some of which are Langerhans cells and some of which are part of the inflammatory reaction accompanying the Langerhans cells.*

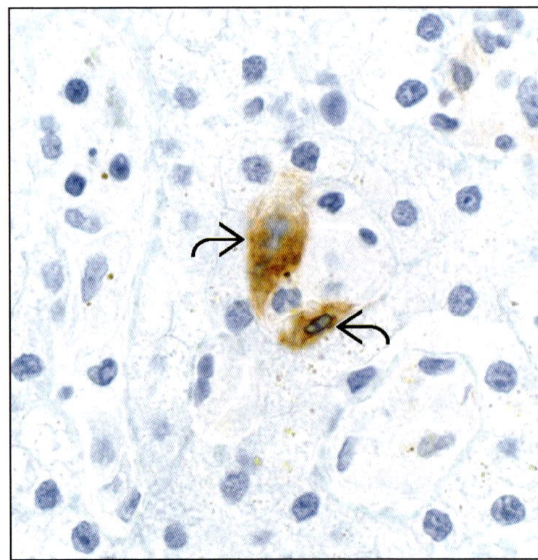

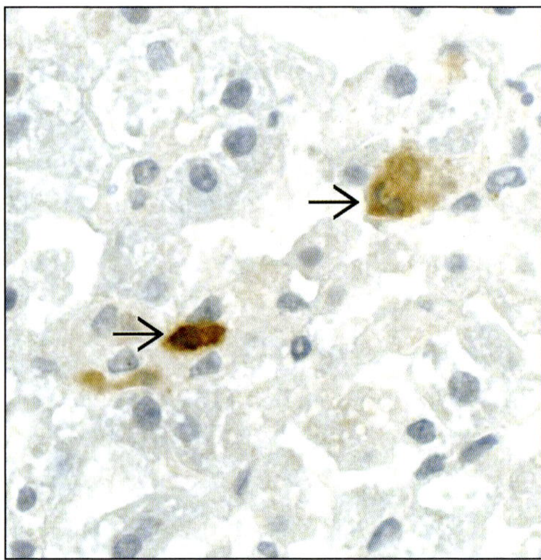

(Left) *CD1a immunohistochemical stain highlights 2 Langerhans cells ↪ within the hepatic sinusoids in hepatic involvement by LCH.* ***(Right)*** *Immunohistochemical stain for S100 protein highlights Langerhans cells within the hepatic sinusoids → in hepatic LCH.*

Microscopic Features of Sclerosing Cholangitis in LCH

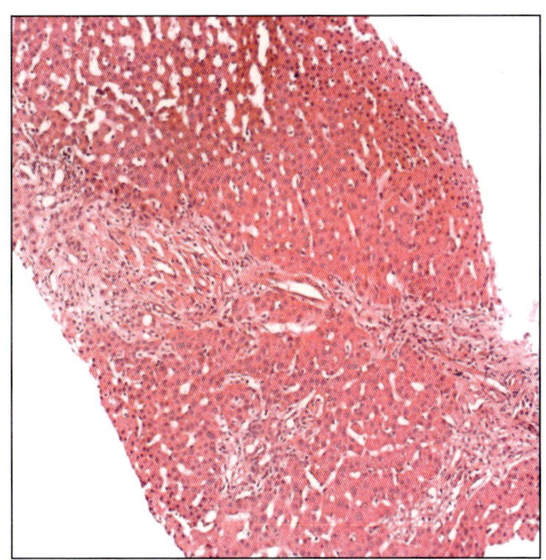

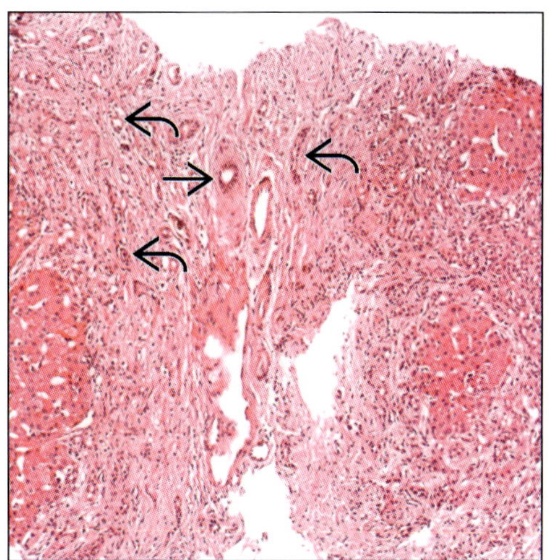

(Left) *Liver biopsy in a child with LCH shows portal-portal bridging fibrosis with a mild mononuclear infiltrate in portal areas.* ***(Right)*** *Liver biopsy in a child with LCH shows marked portal expansion with ductular proliferation ⇗, reminiscent of sclerosing cholangitis. The native bile duct is in the center of the field ⇒.*

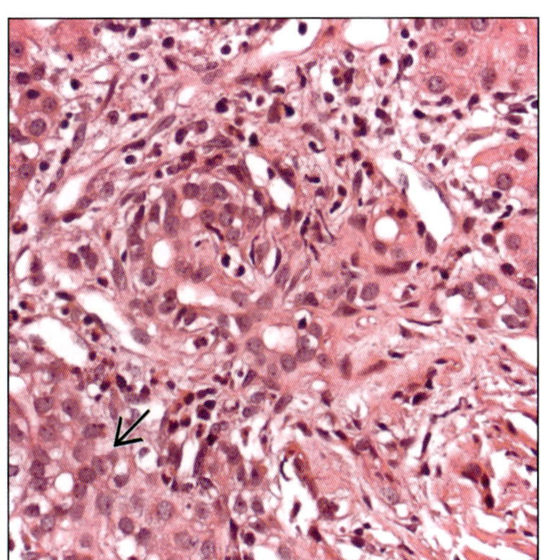

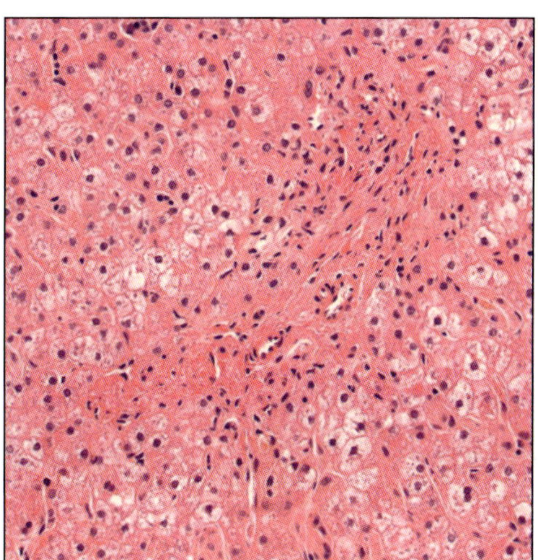

(Left) *Closer view of a liver biopsy in a child with LCH shows marked ductular reaction with cholate stasis ⇒ in periportal hepatocytes and a mild inflammatory infiltrate in the portal tract, indicative of sclerosing cholangitis secondary to LCH.* ***(Right)*** *Liver section in a child with LCH and cholangiographic evidence of sclerosing cholangitis shows irregular expansion and fibrosis of the portal tract with indistinct bile ducts.*

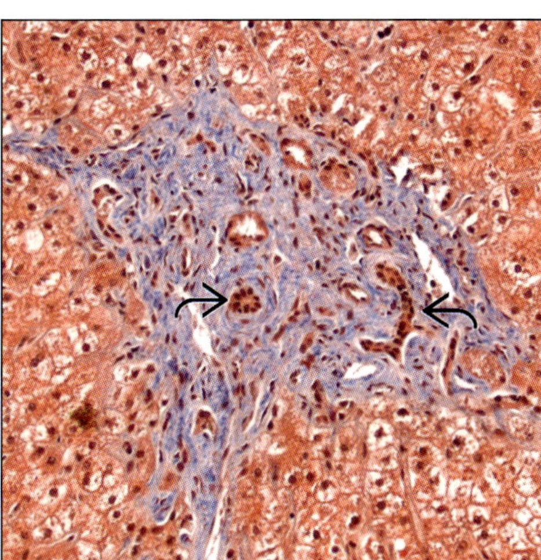

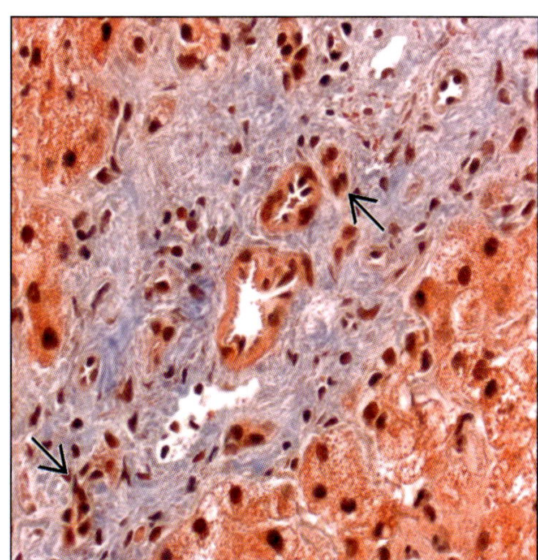

(Left) *Trichrome stain of the liver section in a child with LCH and sclerosing cholangitis shows irregular portal expansion and fibrosis with injured, distorted, and squeezed bile ducts ⇗.* ***(Right)*** *Trichrome stain of another portal tract in a child with LCH and secondary sclerosing cholangitis shows portal fibrosis and small remnants of bile ducts ⇒.*

HEMOPHAGOCYTIC SYNDROMES

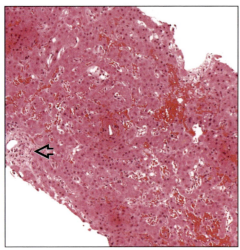

Sinusoidal dilatation and congestion are seen on low power in a case of reactive hemophagocytic syndrome. The hepatocytes and portal tracts ⇨ are otherwise unremarkable.

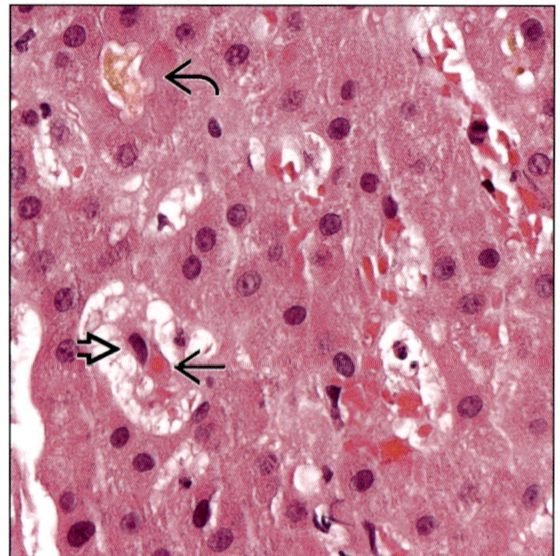

Hypertrophic Kupffer cells ⇨ in dilated sinusoids contain engulfed red cells in the cytoplasm →, which can be easily overlooked. Focal cholestasis ↷ is noted in this case.

TERMINOLOGY

Abbreviations

- Hemophagocytic lymphohistiocytosis (HLH)

Synonyms

- Hemophagocytic lymphohistiocytosis

Definitions

- Proliferation and activation of macrophages with hemophagocytosis in reticuloendothelial system

ETIOLOGY/PATHOGENESIS

Primary or Familial HLH (FHL)

- Autosomal recessive inheritance
- 4 subtypes based on causative genes
  - FHL1: Mutations in *HPLH1* gene
  - FHL2: Mutations in *PRF1* gene (encoding perforin)
  - FHL3: Mutations in *UNC13D* gene
  - FHL4: Mutations in *STX11* gene

Secondary or Reactive HLH

- Infections
  - Viruses (EBV, HIV, other herpes viruses, etc.)
  - Bacteria
  - Fungi
  - Parasites
- Malignancies
  - Lymphomas
  - Carcinomas
- Autoimmune diseases
  - Rheumatologic disorders

Pathogenesis

- T-cell dysregulation
- Hyperproduction of cytokines and chemokines (interferon-γ, TNF-α, etc.)
- Proliferation and activation of T lymphocytes and macrophages

CLINICAL ISSUES

Epidemiology

- Incidence
  - 1 in 50,000 live births for FHL
  - Unknown for secondary HLH
- Age
  - Typically seen in infants and young children for FHL
  - Typically seen in adolescents and adults for secondary HLH

Presentation

- Fever
- Hepatosplenomegaly
- Lymphadenopathy
- Jaundice
- Acute liver failure
- Neurologic abnormalities
- Skin rash

Laboratory Tests

- Molecular genetic testing
- Pancytopenia
- Hypertriglyceridemia
- Hypofibrinogenemia
- Hyperferritinemia
- Low or absent natural killer cell activity
- Bone marrow biopsy and aspirate

Treatment

- Combined cytotoxic chemotherapy and immunotherapy
- Antibiotics &/or antiviral agents
- Hematopoietic stem cell transplantation
- Treatment of underlying diseases

Prognosis

- Invariably fatal for FHL if untreated, with median survival of 2-6 months after diagnosis
- 20-25% 5-year survival even with treatment for FHL

HEMOPHAGOCYTIC SYNDROMES

Key Facts

Etiology/Pathogenesis
- Familial hemophagocytic syndrome
  - Autosomal recessive inheritance
- Reactive hemophagocytic syndrome
  - Infections, malignancies, and autoimmune diseases
- Abnormal activation of benign macrophages due to T-cell dysregulation

Clinical Issues
- Invariably fatal for familial form if untreated

Microscopic Pathology
- Cytoplasmic engulfment of erythrocytes, leukocytes, and platelets by hypertrophic Kupffer cells

Ancillary Tests
- Molecular genetic testing

Top Differential Diagnoses
- Familial vs. reactive hemophagocytic syndrome
- Hepatic Rosai-Dorfman disease

- Varied outcomes for secondary HLH, but full recovery can be achieved

MICROSCOPIC PATHOLOGY

Histologic Features
- Sinusoidal dilatation and congestion
- Kupffer cell hyperplasia and hypertrophy
  - Cytoplasmic engulfment of erythrocytes, leukocytes, and platelets by Kupffer cells
  - Stainable iron in Kupffer cells
- Mild portal lymphohistiocytic infiltrates
- Features of underlying diseases

Predominant Pattern/Injury Type
- Hemophagocytosis

DIFFERENTIAL DIAGNOSIS

FHL vs. Secondary HLH
- Age of onset
- Family history
- Molecular genetic testing

Hepatic Rosai-Dorfman Disease
- Usually seen as multiple small granuloma-like histiocytic infiltrates or larger nodules
- Portal and sinusoidal infiltration may be seen
- Characteristic phagocytosis of intact lymphocytes and red cells by large histiocytes (emperipolesis)
- Positive S100 immunostain

Involvement by Leukemia or Lymphoma
- Infiltration by monotonous or atypical cells
- Flow cytometry and immunostains are helpful

DIAGNOSTIC CHECKLIST

Clinically Relevant Pathologic Features
- Abnormal activation of benign macrophages by genetic or reactive mechanisms

Pathologic Interpretation Pearls
- Kupffer cell hyperplasia with phagocytosed hematopoietic cells, which can be easily overlooked

SELECTED REFERENCES

1. Gupta S et al: Primary and secondary hemophagocytic lymphohistiocytosis: clinical features, pathogenesis and therapy. Expert Rev Clin Immunol. 6(1):137-54, 2010
2. Rouphael NG et al: Infections associated with haemophagocytic syndrome. Lancet Infect Dis. 7(12):814-22, 2007
3. Zhang K, Filipovich AH, Johnson J, Marsh RA, Villanueva J. Hemophagocytic Lymphohistiocytosis, Familial. 1993-, 2006
4. de Kerguenec C et al: Hepatic manifestations of hemophagocytic syndrome: a study of 30 cases. Am J Gastroenterol. 96(3):852-7, 2001

IMAGE GALLERY

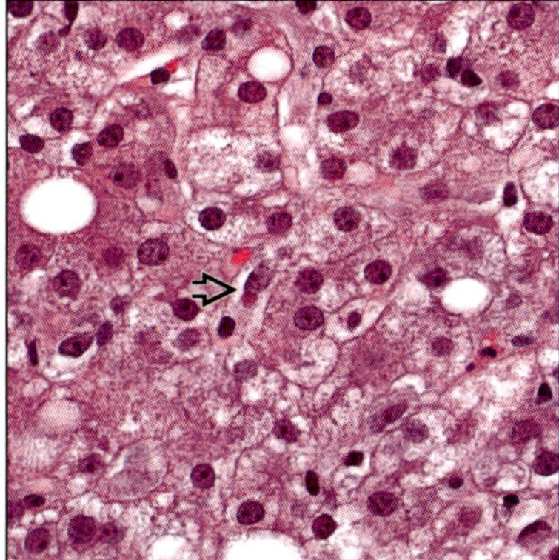

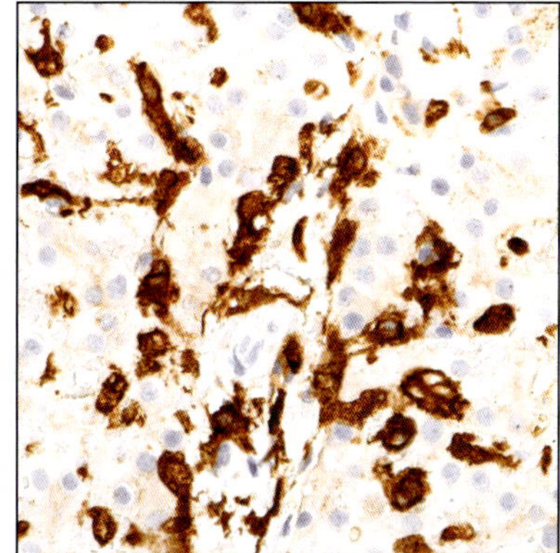

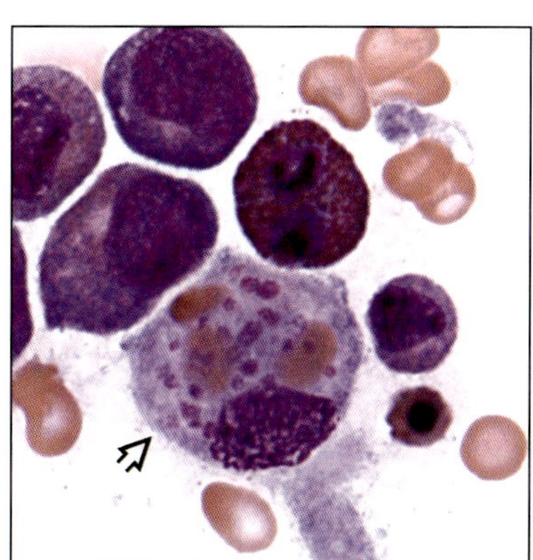

(Left) *Erythrophagocytosis by a Kupffer cell ⇨ is seen in a case of EBV-induced infectious mononucleosis.* ***(Center)*** *CD163 immunohistochemical stain highlights hyperplastic and hypertrophic Kupffer cells but does not help identify hemophagocytosis.* ***(Right)*** *Compared to that in liver biopsy, hemophagocytosis is easier to recognize on a Wright-Giemsa stained bone marrow smear, which shows a macrophage ⇨ containing phagocytosed red cells, platelets, and leukocyte debris.*

Developmental/Congenital

CONGENITAL PANCREATIC CYST

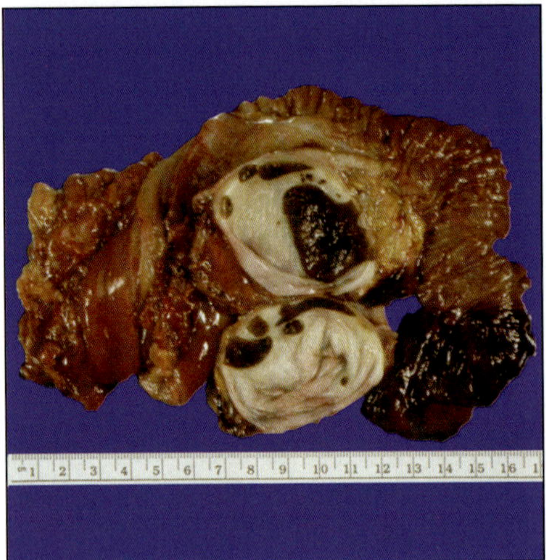

The enlarged pancreatic head mass was bisected to reveal a uniloculate cyst that did not communicate with the pancreatic duct. The thin fibrous cyst wall is smooth with focal areas of hemorrhage.

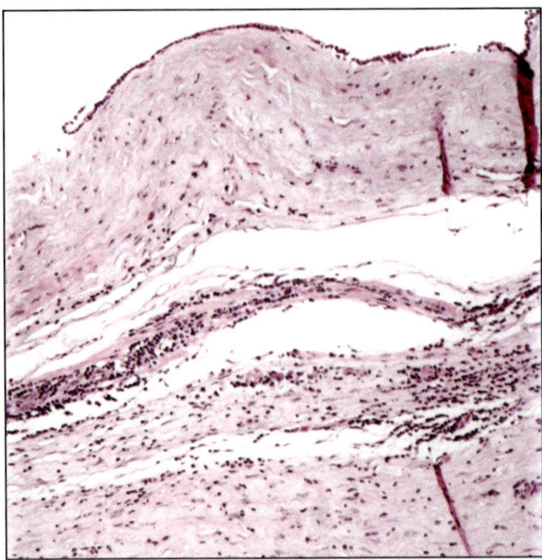

This low-power view of a congenital cyst shows a benign unilocular cyst with a fibrous wall and a partially denuded epithelial lining.

TERMINOLOGY

Synonyms

- Dysgenetic cyst

Definitions

- Rare benign congenital epithelial-lined cyst that does not communicate with ductal system

ETIOLOGY/PATHOGENESIS

Developmental Anomaly

- Thought to be caused by anomalous development of pancreatic ductal system
  - Not associated with ductal obstruction or other pancreatic abnormalities

CLINICAL ISSUES

Epidemiology

- Incidence
  - Exceedingly rare
- Age
  - May be found at any age but usually in children
    - Most present before 2 years of age
- Gender
  - Female predominance

Site

- Any location within pancreas
  - More frequently in body or tail

Presentation

- Abdominal mass or distention
  - Usually not tender
- Often incidental findings
  - May be detected on antenatal ultrasound

Laboratory Tests

- Serum amylase usually normal

Treatment

- Complete excision is treatment of choice
  - Feasible when located in pancreatic body or tail
- Internal drainage or cystenterostomy
  - For those arising from pancreatic head

Prognosis

- Good

MACROSCOPIC FEATURES

General Features

- Usually single, unilocular, thin-walled cystic lesion
  - Occasionally multilocular
- Does not communicate with pancreatic ductal system
- Contains serous fluid
  - Aspirated fluid may have elevated amylase level

Size

- 1-2 cm

MICROSCOPIC PATHOLOGY

Histologic Features

- Lined by flattened cuboidal to columnar epithelium
  - Fibroinflammatory changes of cyst wall can obscure epithelial lining

DIFFERENTIAL DIAGNOSIS

Pancreatic Cysts Associated with Hereditary Disorders or Congenital Syndromes

- Entities with multiple pancreatic cysts or polycystic pancreas
  - von Hippel-Lindau disease

CONGENITAL PANCREATIC CYST

Key Facts

Terminology
- Rare benign congenital epithelial-lined cyst that is not associated with ductal obstruction or other pancreatic anomalies
  - Does not communicate with ductal system

Clinical Issues
- Exceedingly rare
- Most present before 2 years of age
- Often incidental finding

Macroscopic Features
- Thin-walled unilocular or multilocular cyst
- Occurs anywhere in pancreas
- Generally 1-2 cm in size

Microscopic Pathology
- Lined by flattened cuboidal to columnar epithelium
- Fibroinflammatory changes can obscure epithelial lining

    - Epithelial lining identical to serous cystadenoma
  - Polycystic kidney disease
  - Jeune syndrome
  - Oral-facial-digital syndrome type 1
  - Meckel-Gruber syndrome
  - Trisomy 13

Intrapancreatic Enteric Cyst/Enteric Duplication Cyst of Pancreas
- Diagnostic consideration on imaging
- Histologic features recapitulate gut
  - Gastric mucosal epithelial lining or, rarely, ciliated epithelium surrounded by smooth muscle

Retention Cyst
- May be indistinguishable from congenital cyst in adults
- Usually found in context of pancreatitis or mass lesion
- Communicates with ductal system

Congenital Pancreatic Pseudocyst
- No epithelial lining
- Entire cyst wall may need to be sampled to confirm this diagnosis

Serous Cystadenoma, Oligocystic (Macrocystic) Variant
- Lined by single layer of bland cuboidal to flattened epithelium associated with rich capillary network
- Positive for periodic acid-Schiff stain, α-inhibin, calponin, &/or GLUT1

Cystic Fibrosis
- Pancreatic cysts are not congenital but develop in 1st few months of life
- Dilatation of acini and ductules with eosinophilic secretions
- Acinar and lobular atrophy
- Pancreas replaced by adipose tissue

SELECTED REFERENCES

1. Castellani C et al: Neonatal congenital pancreatic cyst: diagnosis and management. J Pediatr Surg. 44(2):e1-4, 2009
2. Hunter CJ et al: Enteric duplication cysts of the pancreas: a report of two cases and review of the literature. Pediatr Surg Int. 24(2):227-33, 2008
3. Chung JH et al: Congenital true pancreatic cyst detected prenatally in neonate: a case report. J Pediatr Surg. 42(9):E27-9, 2007
4. Kazez A et al: Congenital true pancreatic cyst: a rare case. Diagn Interv Radiol. 12(1):31-3, 2006
5. Boulanger SC et al: Congenital pancreatic cysts in children. J Pediatr Surg. 38(7):1080-2, 2003
6. Kurrer MO et al: Congenital pancreatic pseudocyst: report of two cases. J Pediatr Surg. 31(11):1581-3, 1996
7. Auringer ST et al: Congenital cyst of the pancreas. J Pediatr Surg. 28(12):1570-1, 1993
8. Mares AJ et al: Congenital cysts of the head of the pancreas. J Pediatr Surg. 12(4):547-52, 1977

IMAGE GALLERY

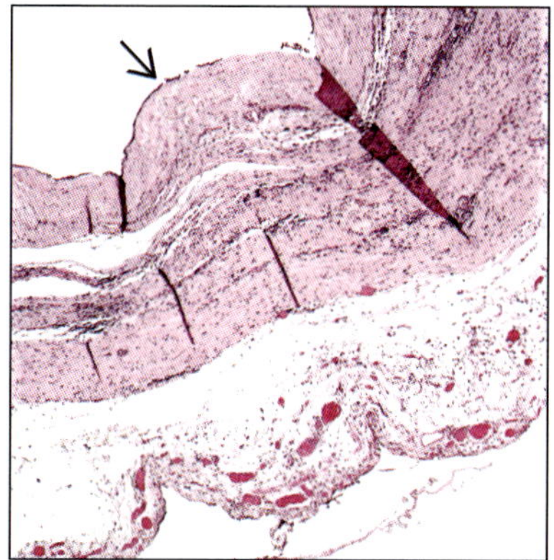

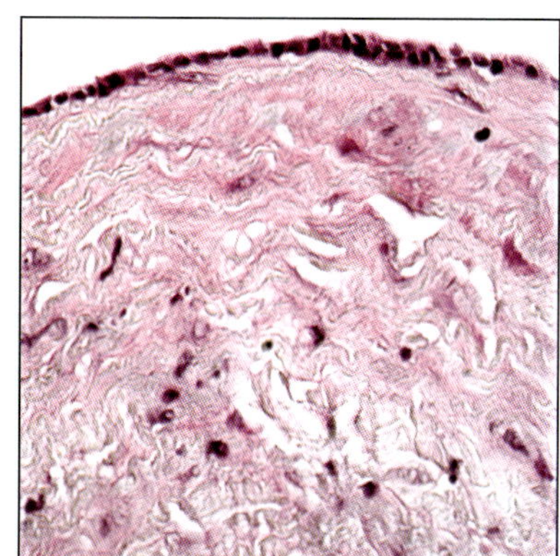

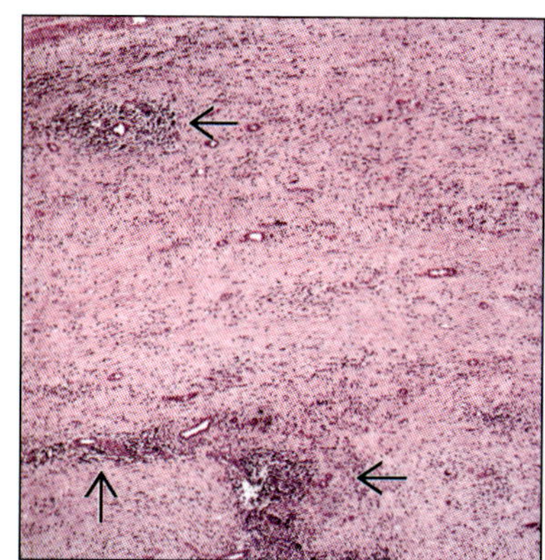

(Left) *This low-power view of a congenital pancreatic cyst shows a unilocular cyst with a fibrous wall, chronic inflammation, and lined by a single layer of nonmucinous epithelium ➔.* ***(Center)*** *The epithelial lining in a congenital pancreatic cyst is typically nonmucinous cuboidal or flattened columnar epithelium similar to that in normal ducts.* ***(Right)*** *The wall of a congenital cyst can contain varying amounts of inflammation; this one has clusters of lymphocytes ➔.*

CYSTIC FIBROSIS, PANCREAS

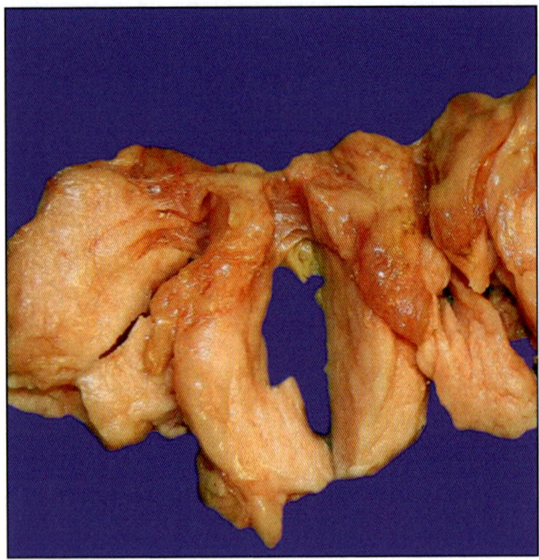

This pancreas from a 32-year-old CF patient demonstrates complete replacement of the parenchyma by fat. Note the overall architecture of the pancreas is well-maintained.

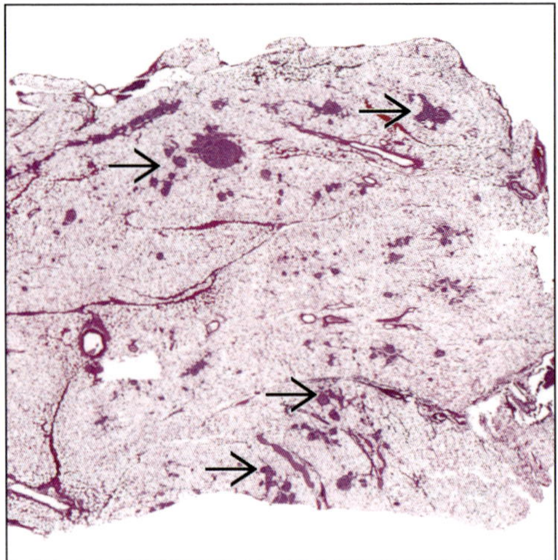

At the advanced stage, total atrophy of the exocrine portion of the pancreas may occur, leaving only the islets ⇒ within a fibrofatty stroma.

TERMINOLOGY

Abbreviations

- Cystic fibrosis (CF)

Synonyms

- Mucoviscidosis

Definitions

- Autosomal recessive disease affecting fluid secretion in exocrine glands and epithelial lining of respiratory, gastrointestinal, and reproductive tracts

ETIOLOGY/PATHOGENESIS

Cystic Fibrosis Gene

- Cystic fibrosis transmembrane conductance regulator (*CFTR*) gene on chromosome 7q31.2
  - Encodes an epithelial chloride channel protein and regulates multiple additional ion channels and cellular processes
  - More than 800 disease-causing mutations have been identified and can be grouped into 6 classes
- Most common mutation is ΔF508
  - Deletion of 3 nucleotides coding for phenylalanine at amino acid position 508
  - Results in complete lack of CFTR protein at apical surface of epithelial cells due to abnormal protein folding, processing, and trafficking
  - Found in approximately 70% of CF patients worldwide

CLINICAL ISSUES

Epidemiology

- Incidence
  - Most common inherited lethal disease in Caucasian population
    - 1 out of 3,200 live births in USA
  - Uncommon among Asians (1 in 31,000 live births) and African-Americans (1 in 15,000 live births)
  - Exocrine pancreatic insufficiency occurs in majority (85-90%) of CF patients and is associated with severe *CTFR* mutations on both alleles
- Age
  - Pathologic abnormalities of pancreas can be seen as early as 32-38 weeks gestation and progressively worsen with age
  - Onset of pancreatic insufficiency varies and may occur in patients older than 6 months
- Gender
  - Male patients appear to be less affected than female patients with CF

Presentation

- Large, foul-smelling stools
- Abdominal distention
- Poor weight gain
- Avitaminosis A, D, or K

Treatment

- Enzyme supplements, multivitamin and mineral supplements
- Pancreas or liver-pancreas transplantation
- Possible gene therapy (transfer of *CFTR* gene)

Prognosis

- Currently, median age of overall survival is 36.9 years and continues to increase

IMAGE FINDINGS

Ultrasonographic Findings

- Hyperechoic and atrophic pancreatic parenchyma

MR Findings

- Fibrosis and fatty replacement
- Pancreatic cysts are relatively common in CF patients

CYSTIC FIBROSIS, PANCREAS

Key Facts

Etiology/Pathogenesis

- Cystic fibrosis transmembrane conductance regulator (CFTR) gene on chromosome 7q31.2

Clinical Issues

- Exocrine pancreatic insufficiency occurs in majority of patients

Macroscopic Features

- Granular pancreatic parenchyma secondary to extensive fibrosis, often with cystic spaces
- Complete replacement of pancreas by fat, usually with well-preserved architecture

Microscopic Pathology

- Multiple ducts totally plugged with concrete mucous resulting in atrophy of exocrine gland, progressive fibrosis, and cyst formation

CT Findings

- Complete fatty replacement is most common finding in adult CF patients

MACROSCOPIC FEATURES

General Features

- Granular pancreatic parenchyma secondary to extensive fibrosis, often with cystic spaces
- Complete replacement of pancreas by fat, usually with well-preserved architecture, is seen in older children or adolescents

MICROSCOPIC PATHOLOGY

Histologic Features

- Milder form
  - Accumulations of mucous in small ducts with some dilatation of exocrine glands
- Advanced form
  - Usually seen in older children or adolescents
  - Multiple ducts totally plugged with concrete mucous
  - Atrophy of exocrine glands, progressive fibrosis, and fatty replacement
  - Small cysts measuring 1-3 mm (secondary to obstruction of pancreatic ducts associated with lobular atrophy)
- Lipomatous hypertrophy of pancreas
  - Total atrophy of exocrine glands resulting in markedly enlarged parenchyma with fatty replacement
  - Only islets are seen within fibrofatty stroma
- Pancreatic cystosis
  - Aggregates of epithelium-lined cysts completely replacing pancreatic parenchyma

DIFFERENTIAL DIAGNOSIS

Other Forms of Chronic Pancreatitis

- Age of onset is much older than CF
- Multiple small ducts plugged with concrete mucous are characteristic of (early-stage) CF but not other forms of chronic pancreatitis

Cystic Pancreatic Neoplasms

- Lack of characteristic signs and symptoms of CF
- Cysts are usually larger than those seen in CF

SELECTED REFERENCES

1. Robertson MB et al: Review of the abdominal manifestations of cystic fibrosis in the adult patient. Radiographics. 26(3):679-90, 2006
2. Witt H: Chronic pancreatitis and cystic fibrosis. Gut. 52 Suppl 2:ii31-41, 2003

IMAGE GALLERY

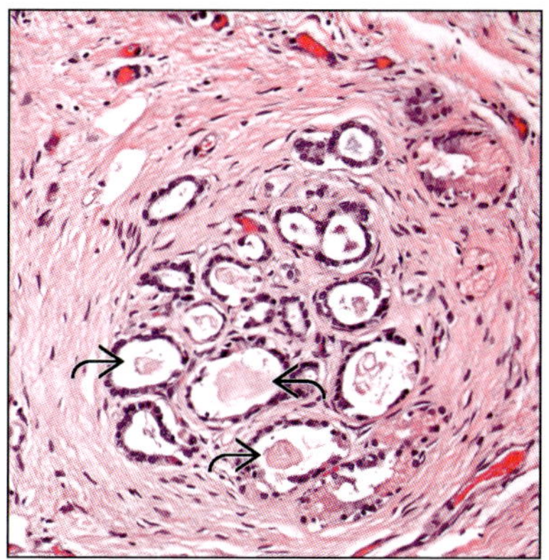

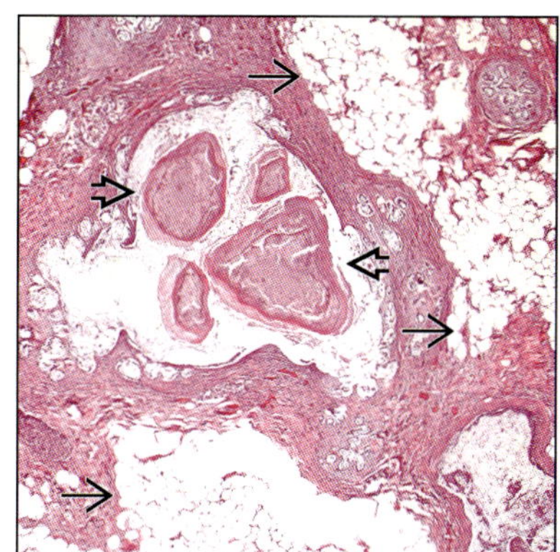

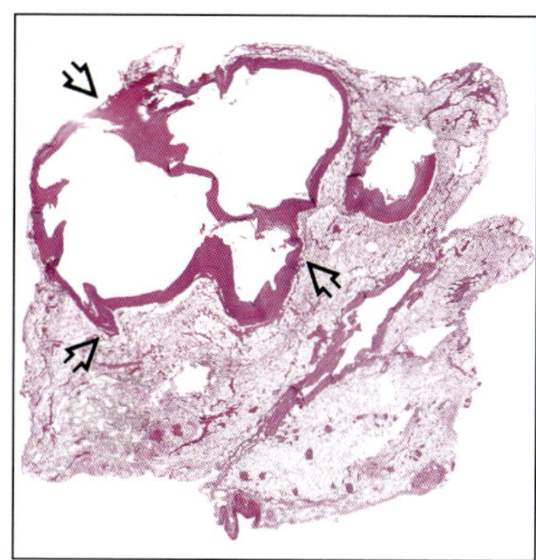

(Left) *Dilatation of ducts, which contain eosinophilic concrete mucous secretions ➚, is common in CF.* ***(Center)*** *Continued involution of the exocrine portion of the pancreas occurs during childhood, initially with a proliferation of fibroblasts but subsequently by fatty replacement →. Cystically dilated ducts are plugged with concentric concretions ⇨.* ***(Right)*** *This case shows cyst formation ⇨ in the background of fatty replacement of the pancreatic parenchyma.*

NESIDIOBLASTOSIS

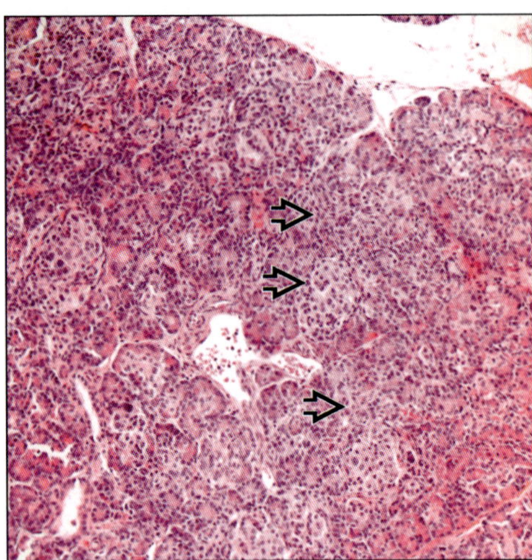

This image shows predominantly unremarkable pancreatic acinar tissue. Large and back to back islet cell-like structures ➪ are present, a finding that suggests focal nesidioblastosis.

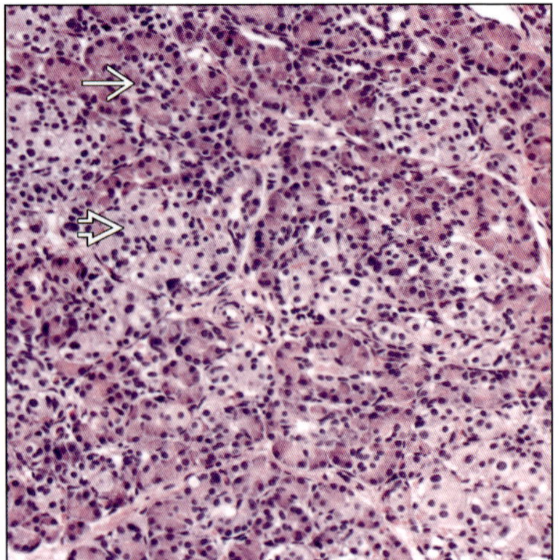

Focal nesidioblastosis features confluent growth of endocrine cells ➪. The endocrine cells are very similar to those seen in normal pancreatic islets. Note the intervening normal acinar cells ➡.

TERMINOLOGY

Abbreviations

- Nesidioblastosis (NB)

Definitions

- Morphologic findings associated with functional disorders of β cells (hyperinsulinemic hypoglycemia) in absence of insulinoma

ETIOLOGY/PATHOGENESIS

Potassium Channel Abnormalities

- *ACCC8* (formerly *SUR1*)
- *KCNJ11* (formerly *Kir6.2*)
- Diffuse NB-homozygous or compound heterozygous for *ABCC8/KCNJ11* mutations
- Focal NB: Paternally inherited mutation of potassium channel gene and somatic loss of maternal gene

Gain of Function Mutations

- Glucokinase
- Glutamate dehydrogenase

Adult Nesidioblastosis

- Some cases secondary to gastric bypass surgery

CLINICAL ISSUES

Presentation

- Neonates
  - Persistent hypoglycemia
  - Seizures, cyanosis, hypotonia, somnolence
- Adults
  - Very rare
  - Hyperinsulinemic hypoglycemia

Laboratory Tests

- Inappropriate elevations in serum insulin in the presence of hypoglycemia

Treatment

- Surgical approaches
  - Focal NB
    - Limited resection of pancreas
    - Surgical resection is curative
  - Diffuse NB
    - Near total pancreatectomy
    - Results in diabetes
- Drugs
  - Diazoxide
    - Neonates with potassium channel mutations fail medical therapy

MACROSCOPIC FEATURES

General Features

- Focal NB may be grossly inapparent or may produce firm nodule
- Diffuse NB lacks macroscopic abnormalities

MICROSCOPIC PATHOLOGY

Histologic Features

- Neonatal focal NB
  - Confluent or partially confluent clusters of endocrine cells (islet cell adenomatosis)
    - Ductuloinsular complexes
    - Giant endocrine cells (3x larger than normal endocrine cells)
  - Islets away from lesion are unremarkable
  - Rarely multifocal
- Neonatal diffuse NB
  - Islet cell abnormalities throughout gland

NESIDIOBLASTOSIS

Key Facts

Terminology

- Morphologic findings associated with functional disorders of β cells (hyperinsulinemic hypoglycemia) in absence of insulinoma

Etiology/Pathogenesis

- Abnormalities in potassium channels

Clinical Issues

- Persistent neonatal hypoglycemia
- Adult NB very rare

Microscopic Pathology

- Neonatal focal NB
  - Confluent or partially confluent clusters of endocrine cells
- Neonatal diffuse NB
  - Giant endocrine cells (3x larger than normal endocrine cells)
    - Markedly enlarged, hyperchromatic β-cell nuclei (40% increase in nuclear volume compared to normal)
  - Ductuloinsular complexes
- Adult NB
  - Multiple β cells with enlarged hyperchromatic nuclei
  - Normal distribution of various islet cell types
  - No proliferative activity in endocrine cells

ANCILLARY TESTS

Immunohistochemistry

- Chromogranin highlights confluent islets in focal NB
- Focal and diffuse NB have all 4 endocrine cell types; insulin cells often predominate

DIFFERENTIAL DIAGNOSIS

Insulinoma

- Well-circumscribed endocrine neoplasm, positive for insulin
  - Focal NB shows admixture of insulin, glucagon, pancreatic polypeptide-producing cells

Conditions with Islet Hypertrophy and Hyperplasia

- Infants of diabetic mothers
- Beckwith-Wiedemann syndrome
- Multiple endocrine neoplasia type 1

DIAGNOSTIC CHECKLIST

Clinically Relevant Pathologic Features

- Frozen section perfomed to guide extent of resection
  - Examine multiple random pancreatic sections
    - Presence of giant endocrine cell nuclei indicates diffuse NB
    - Absence of giant endocrine nuclei suggests focal NB
- Diagnosis of adult NB requires absence of insulinoma

SELECTED REFERENCES

1. Anlauf M et al: Persistent hyperinsulinemic hypoglycemia in 15 adults with diffuse nesidioblastosis: diagnostic criteria, incidence, and characterization of beta-cell changes. Am J Surg Pathol. 29(4):524-33, 2005
2. Service GJ et al: Hyperinsulinemic hypoglycemia with nesidioblastosis after gastric-bypass surgery. N Engl J Med. 353(3):249-54, 2005
3. Suchi M et al: Congenital hyperinsulinism: intraoperative biopsy interpretation can direct the extent of pancreatectomy. Am J Surg Pathol. 28(10):1326-35, 2004
4. Sadeghi-Nejad A et al: Case records of the Massachusetts General Hospital. Weekly clinicopathological exercises. Case 39-2001. A newborn girl with seizures and persistent hypoglycemia. N Engl J Med. 345(25):1833-9, 2001
5. Goossens A et al: Diffuse and focal nesidioblastosis. A clinicopathological study of 24 patients with persistent neonatal hyperinsulinemic hypoglycemia. Am J Surg Pathol. 13(9):766-75, 1989

IMAGE GALLERY

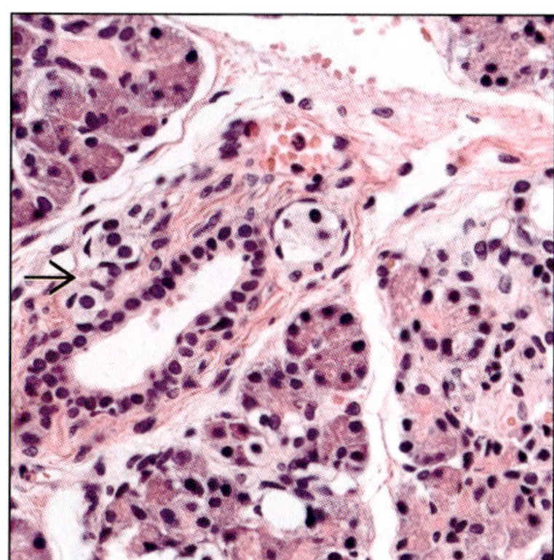

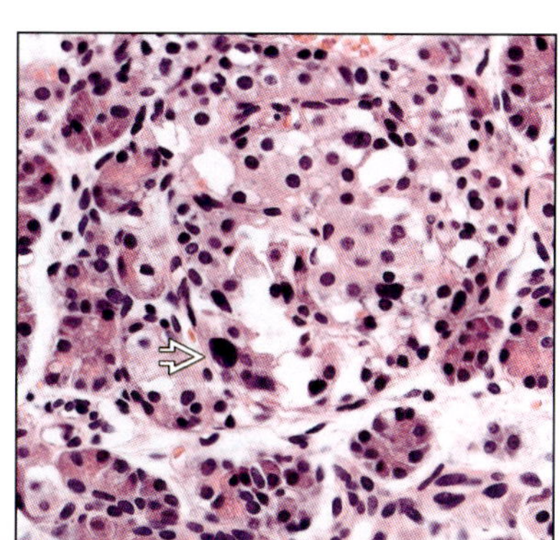

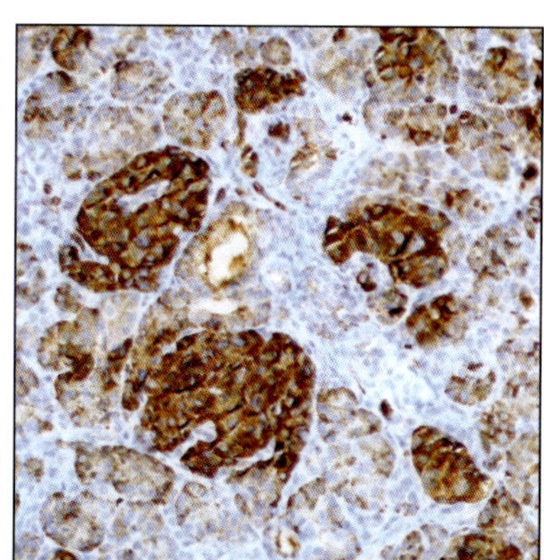

*(**Left**) The term nesidioblastosis refers to the budding off of endocrine cells from pancreatic ducts ⇒. This phenomenon is normally seen in fetal and neonatal pancreata. (**Center**) A case of diffuse nesidioblastosis features enlarged hyperchromatic endocrine cells ➡ that were seen on multiple random sections of the pancreas. This finding excludes the diagnosis of focal NB. (**Right**) Chromogranin highlights the semiconfluent growth of endocrine cells in a case of focal nesidioblastosis.*

CHOLEDOCHAL CYST

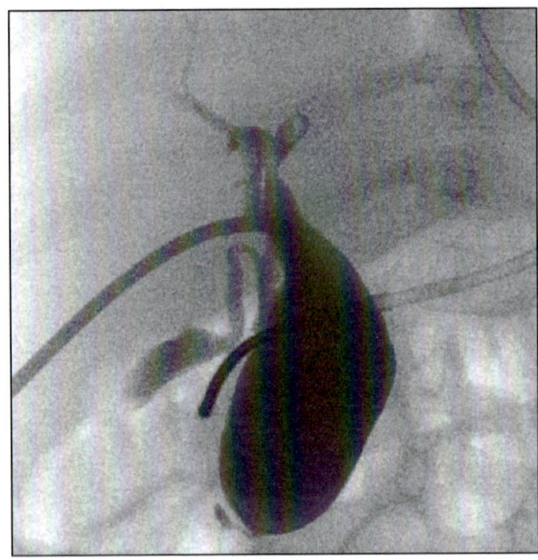

Anteroposterior radiograph during percutaneous cholangiogram shows fusiform dilatation of the common bile duct with rapid change in caliber at the sphincter of Oddi, confirming type I choledochal cyst.

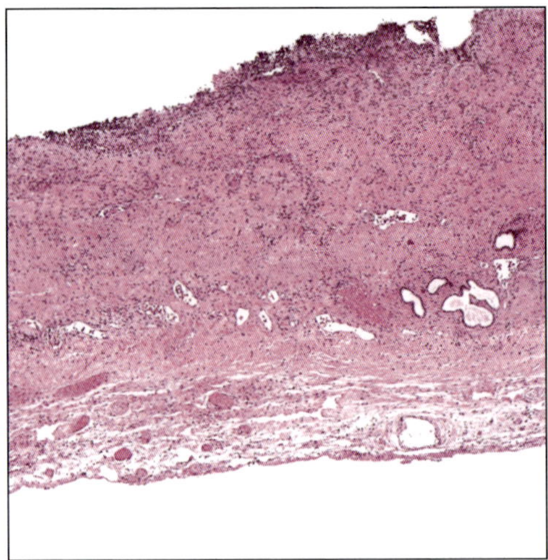

This section of choledochal cyst from a resection specimen shows a thickened fibrotic wall with chronic inflammation and ulcerated overlying epithelium.

TERMINOLOGY

Definitions

- Cystic dilatation of biliary tract, usually extrahepatic

ETIOLOGY/PATHOGENESIS

Unknown

- Possible congenital malformation
  - Majority of patients have abnormal pancreaticobiliary junction
    - Long common channel between distal common bile duct and pancreatic duct
    - May allow pancreatic secretions to reflux into bile ducts, possibly causing damage and eventual dilatation
- No specific inheritance pattern
- Occasionally coexists with congenital hepatic fibrosis, biliary dysgenesis, extrahepatic cystic disease

CLINICAL ISSUES

Epidemiology

- Age
  - Usually presents before age 10
    - Can manifest at any age, however
- Gender
  - 75% of patients are female
- Ethnicity
  - Rare in United States (1 in 13,000 live births)
  - Very common in Asian populations, particularly in Japan

Presentation

- Classic presentation is right upper quadrant mass with intermittent abdominal pain, jaundice
  - Seen only in a minority of cases
- Infants usually present with jaundice
  - Acholic stools, hepatomegaly may be present
- Some cases are asymptomatic

Treatment

- Complete excision

Prognosis

- Variable clinical course depending on complications
  - Infants at particular risk for chronic low-grade biliary obstruction leading to cirrhosis
  - Other complications
    - Bile duct perforation
    - Choledocholithiasis
    - Bacterial cholangitis
- Increased risk of carcinoma (usually adenocarcinoma)
  - Up to 20x increased risk over general population
    - 30% of patients with biliary cysts develop carcinoma
  - Risk increases with age
  - Cyst itself is most common site for carcinoma to develop (usually posterior wall), but other portions of biliary tree may also be at increased risk

IMAGE FINDINGS

General Features

- Ultrasonography, CT scan may be useful
- Cholangiography is definitive diagnostic procedure

MACROSCOPIC FEATURES

General Features

- Thickened, fibrotic cyst wall
  - Stones, calcifications variably present

Size

- Range from a few centimeters to > 15 cm
- Contain from 30-5,000 mL of bile

CHOLEDOCHAL CYST

Key Facts

Terminology
- Cystic dilatation of biliary tract, usually extrahepatic

Clinical Issues
- Usually presents in childhood; most patients female
- Most common in Japan
- Jaundice, abdominal pain, mass are common findings
- Markedly increased risk of carcinoma

Macroscopic Features
- Type I (segmental or diffuse fusiform dilatation of common bile duct) is most common

Microscopic Pathology
- Thickened, fibrotic cyst wall most commonly lined by biliary epithelium
- Liver biopsy specimen shows nonspecific changes of acute or chronic biliary obstruction

Anatomic (Todani) Classification
- Type I: Segmental or diffuse fusiform dilatation of common bile duct
  - Most common
  - 75-95% of cases
- Type II: Supraduodenal diverticulum of common bile duct, usually lateral wall; rest of biliary tree normal
- Type III: Choledochocele that usually occurs within duodenal wall
- Type IV: Multiple extrahepatic bile duct cysts
  - IVa: Associated with Caroli disease-like cystic dilatation of intrahepatic bile ducts
  - IVb: Cysts exclusively extrahepatic
- Type V: Intrahepatic cystic dilatation equivalent to Caroli disease

MICROSCOPIC PATHOLOGY

Histologic Features
- Thickened, fibrotic cyst wall
  - Chronic inflammation often present
  - Elastic and smooth muscle fibers variably present
- Biliary epithelial lining may be intact or damaged, attenuated, or absent altogether
  - Intestinal metaplasia well described
  - Dysplasia can occur
  - Type III cyst (choledochocele) often lined by duodenal epithelium
- Liver biopsy specimen shows changes of acute or chronic biliary obstruction, including biliary cirrhosis

DIFFERENTIAL DIAGNOSIS

Biliary Atresia
- May be clinically and histologically (on liver biopsy) difficult to distinguish from choledochal cyst in infants
- Radiographic studies required

Other Causes of Biliary Obstruction
- Changes on liver biopsy often similar
- Imaging required to detect choledochal cyst

SELECTED REFERENCES

1. Chaudhary A et al: Choledochal cysts--differences in children and adults. Br J Surg. 83(2):186-8, 1996
2. Katyal D et al: Choledochal cysts: a retrospective review of 28 patients and a review of the literature. Can J Surg. 35(6):584-8, 1992
3. O'Neill JA Jr: Choledochal cyst. Curr Probl Surg. 29(6):361-410, 1992
4. Rossi RL et al: Carcinomas arising in cystic conditions of the bile ducts. A clinical and pathologic study. Ann Surg. 205(4):377-84, 1987
5. Cheney M et al: Choledochal cyst. World J Surg. 9(2):244-9, 1985
6. Yamaguchi M: Congenital choledochal cyst. Analysis of 1,433 patients in the Japanese literature. Am J Surg. 140(5):653-7, 1980
7. Todani T et al: Congenital bile duct cysts: Classification, operative procedures, and review of thirty-seven cases including cancer arising from choledochal cyst. Am J Surg. 134(2):263-9, 1977

IMAGE GALLERY

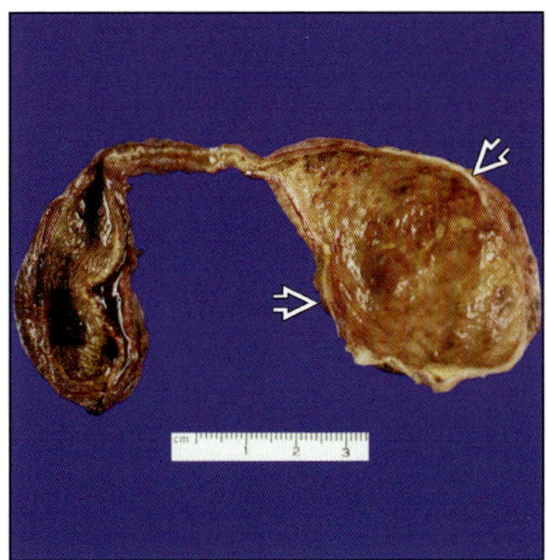

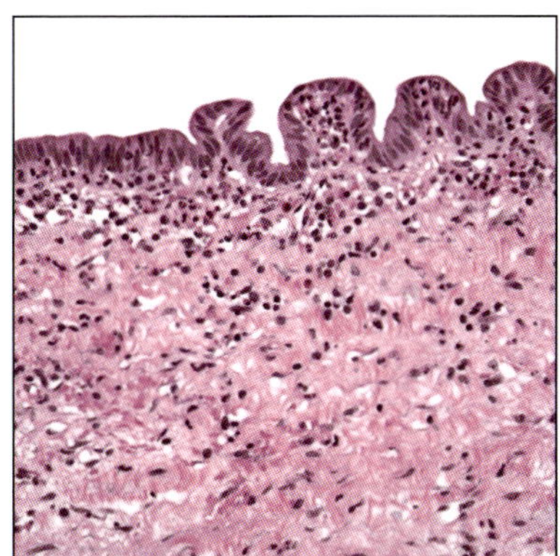

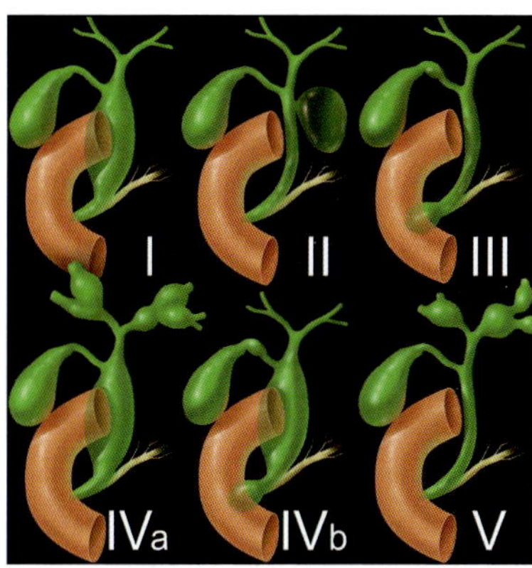

(Left) *This resection shows a large saccular choledochal cyst ➡ on the right.* ***(Center)*** *This section of a choledochal cyst shows a fibrotic wall with chronic inflammation and intact overlying biliary epithelium.* ***(Right)*** *The Todani classification includes types I (dilated common duct), II (diverticulum), III (choledochocele), IVa (extrahepatic cysts and cystic dilatation of intrahepatic ducts), IVb (multiple extrahepatic cysts), and V (multiple intrahepatic cysts).*

Inflammatory Disorders of the Gallbladder and Extrahepatic Biliary Tree

CHOLELITHIASIS

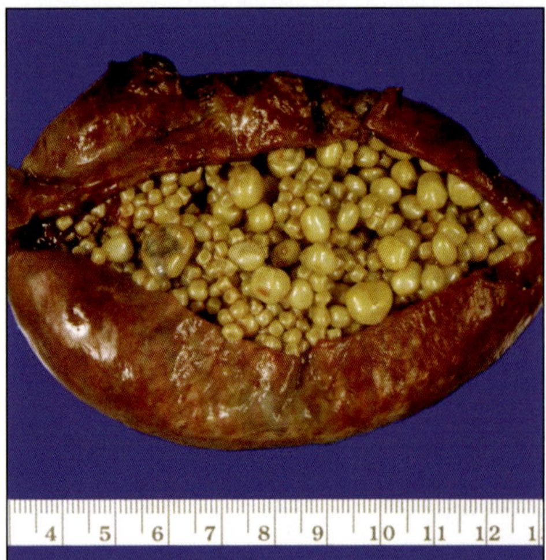

Gross photograph shows a gallbladder filled with numerous smooth yellow cholesterol stones. The gallbladder wall is mildly thickened and hyperemic. (Courtesy G. F. Gray, MD.)

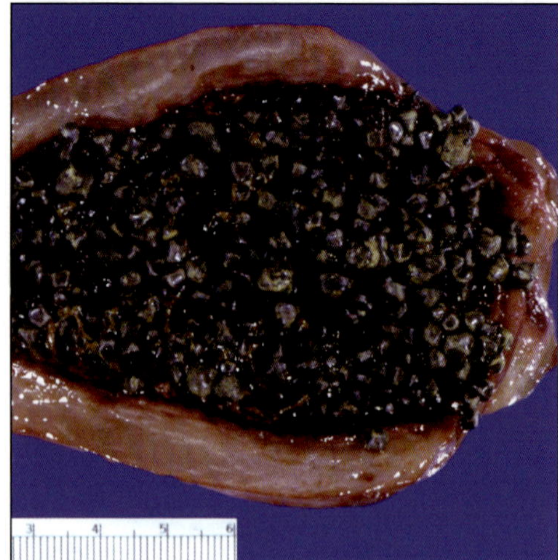

Gross photograph shows numerous faceted black pigment stones distending the gallbladder lumen. The gallbladder wall is thickened and edematous. (Courtesy G. F. Gray, MD.)

TERMINOLOGY

Definitions

- Stones in gallbladder or common bile duct
  - Classified by chemical composition into 2 main types: Cholesterol stones and pigment stones

ETIOLOGY/PATHOGENESIS

Cholesterol Stone Formation

- Bile, supersaturated with cholesterol, is secreted by liver
- Nucleation or initiation of stone formation
- Growth to detectable size

Pigment Stone Formation

- Increase in bile concentration of unconjugated bilirubin, which combines with calcium

CLINICAL ISSUES

Epidemiology

- Incidence
  - Variable in different parts of world
  - In United States, estimated 10-20% of population have gallstones
  - Majority of stones are cholesterol stones (> 80%)
    - Associated with obesity, multiparity, rapid weight loss, estrogen replacement therapy, oral contraceptive use, hypertriglyceridemia, Crohn disease, and total parenteral nutrition (TPN)
  - Black stones
    - Commonly found in individuals with hemolytic disorders, cirrhosis, alcoholism, and sclerosing cholangitis
  - Brown pigment stones
    - Strongly associated with ascending cholangitis and biliary inflammation, especially due to *E. coli*
- Age
  - Overall, increased incidence with age; quite uncommon in children
- Gender
  - More common in women
- Ethnicity
  - Cholesterol stones
    - Higher rates in Latin American women (Hispanic Americans) and Native Americans in both North and South America
    - Lower rates in women from Asia, sub-Saharan Africa, and black women living in United States
  - Pigment stones are much more common in Asian populations

Presentation

- Majority of gallstones are clinically silent
- Symptoms usually consist of right upper quadrant pain, flatulence, and intolerance of fatty food
- Complications include acute and chronic cholecystitis, choledocholithiasis, acute pancreatitis, and gallbladder cancer

Treatment

- Laparoscopic or open cholecystectomy most common treatment
- Recently developed therapies are shock wave lithotripsy and pharmacologic dissolution

IMAGE FINDINGS

Radiographic Findings

- 70-90% of gallstones are radiolucent; at least 80% of these are cholesterol stones
- Black stones may be radiopaque
- Ultrasound can detect stones > 3 mm in diameter

CHOLELITHIASIS

Key Facts

Terminology

- Stones in gallbladder or common bile duct
- Classified by chemical composition into 2 main types: Cholesterol stones and pigment stones

Clinical Issues

- Majority of stones are cholesterol stones (> 80%)
- Most gallstones are clinically silent
- Symptoms usually consist of right upper quadrant pain, flatulence, and intolerance of fatty food

Macroscopic Features

- Cholesterol stones contain > 75% cholesterol with smaller amounts of calcium bilirubinate
- Pigment stones consist predominantly of calcium bilirubinate, with smaller amounts (< 25%) of cholesterol

MACROSCOPIC FEATURES

Cholesterol Stones

- Contain > 75% cholesterol with smaller amounts of calcium bilirubinate
- Rarely measure > 2 cm in diameter
- Commonly multifaceted and have smooth contour
- Cut surface is laminated with alternating layers having variegated appearance depending on how much pigment is present
- Stones with > 90% cholesterol are referred to as pure cholesterol stones
    - Larger, usually between 2-4 cm in diameter
    - Round or ovoid
    - Cut surface shows radial arrangement of crystals; pigment is either absent or present only in scanty amounts

Pigment Stones

- Consist predominantly of calcium bilirubinate, with smaller amounts (< 25%) of cholesterol
- 2 major subtypes
    - **Black pigment stones**
        - Contain calcium bilirubinate, calcium phosphate, and calcium carbonate
        - 2-5 mm shiny, irregular, multifaceted
    - **Brown pigment stones**
        - Contain calcium bilirubinate, calcium palmitate, and cholesterol
        - Similar size to black stones but have softer texture and flaky appearance

Unusual Types of Gallstones

- Disappearing gallstones
    - Possible spontaneous passage via common bile duct, passage through cholecystoenteric fistula, and spontaneous dissolution
- Intramural gallstones
    - Stones become adherent to wall, leading to ulceration and erosion into muscularis
    - May form within preexisting diverticula or Rokitansky-Aschoff sinuses
- Floating gallstones
    - Usually result of high cholesterol content
    - Radiologic interest only
- Gas-containing gallstones
    - Gas predominantly nitrogen with smaller amounts of carbon dioxide and traces of oxygen
    - Makes stones more susceptible to effects of ultrasonic lithotripsy

SELECTED REFERENCES

1. Dowling RH: Review: pathogenesis of gallstones. Aliment Pharmacol Ther. 14 Suppl 2:39-47, 2000
2. Moser AJ et al: The pathogenesis of gallstone formation. Adv Surg. 26:357-86, 1993
3. Bowen JC et al: Gallstone disease. Pathophysiology, epidemiology, natural history, and treatment options. Med Clin North Am. 76(5):1143-57, 1992
4. Paumgartner G et al: Gallstones: pathogenesis. Lancet. 338(8775):1117-21, 1991

IMAGE GALLERY

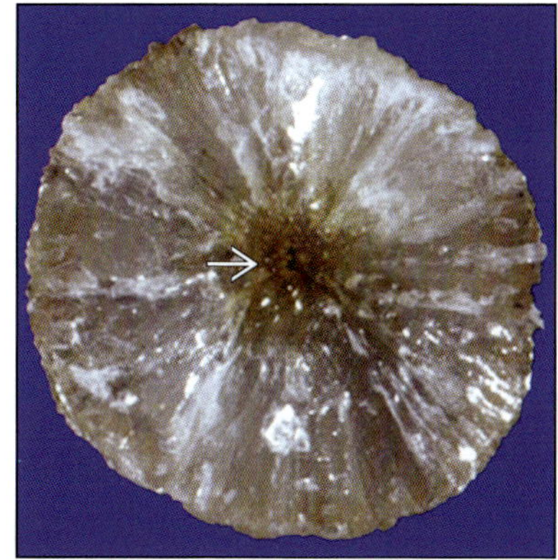

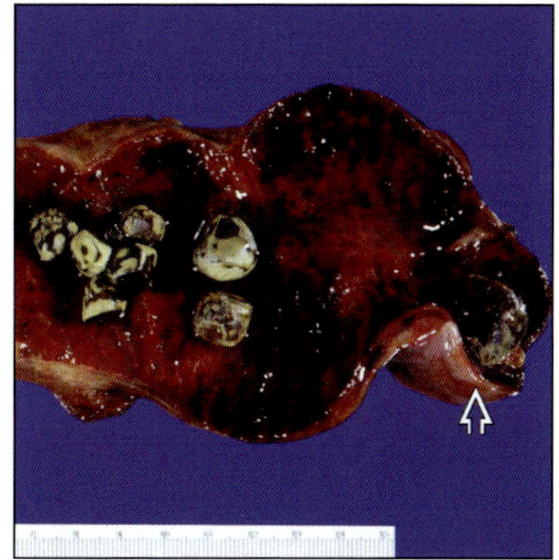

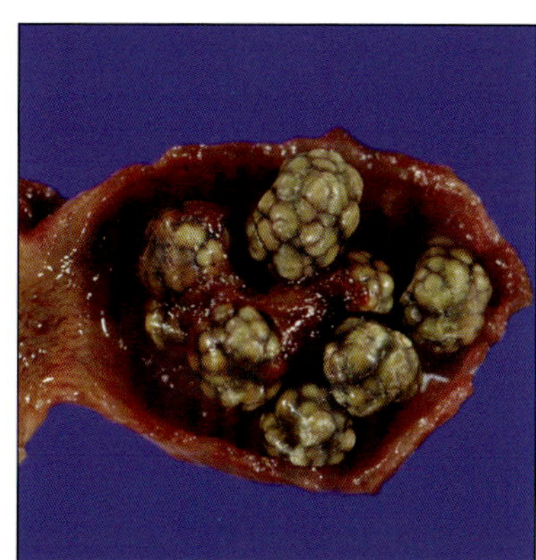

*(**Left**) The cut surface of this large gallstone shows a radial arrangement of cholesterol crystals around a central pigmented core ➡. (**Center**) This gross photograph shows mixed cholesterol-pigment stones within the gallbladder lumen and within a dilated cystic duct ⇨. The gallbladder wall is thickened and hemorrhagic. (**Right**) Gross photograph shows lobulated cholesterol stones, some of which appear partially intramural. (Courtesy G. F. Gray, MD.)*

ACUTE CHOLECYSTITIS

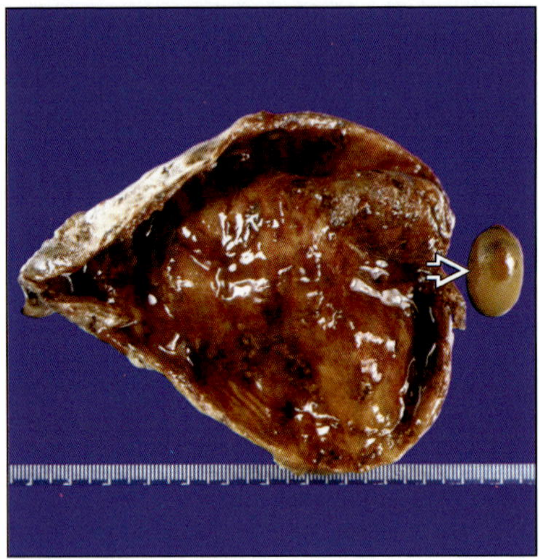

The thickened wall and congested mucosa suggest acute cholecystitis in this gallbladder. The gallstone ➡ was impacted in the neck of the gallbladder.

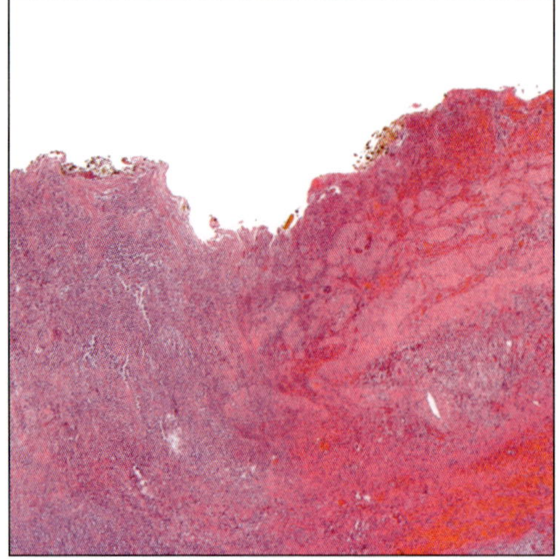

Diffuse ulceration, fresh hemorrhage, and full thickness necrosis of the muscularis propria are characteristic of acute cholecystitis.

TERMINOLOGY

Definitions

- Acute inflammation of gallbladder

ETIOLOGY/PATHOGENESIS

Acute Calculous Cholecystitis

- Key elements are obstruction of cystic duct by stones and bile supersaturated with cholesterol
- Trauma to mucosa releases phospholipase from lysosomes
  - Phospholipase converts lecithin in bile to lysolecithin, which damages gallbladder epithelium
- Secondary bacterial infection with enteric organisms occurs in 20% of cases
- Overgrowth by gas-producing organisms leads to emphysematous cholecystitis

Acute Acalculous Cholecystitis

- Accounts for 5% of cases
- Risk factors
  - Critical illness, burns, trauma, major surgical procedures, diabetes, immunosuppression
    - Key common elements in this diverse group of disorders include biliary sludge formation and mucosal ischemia

CLINICAL ISSUES

Epidemiology

- Age
  - Commonly seen between 40-80 years
- Gender
  - Female predominance

Presentation

- Right upper quadrant pain, tenderness, and guarding
- Fever, leukocytosis
- Murphy sign: Arrest of inspiration while palpating gallbladder during deep inspiration

Treatment

- Surgical approaches
  - Early laparoscopic cholecystectomy is considered treatment of choice for most patients
  - Conservative measures reserved for poor surgical candidates
    - Percutaneous cholecystostomy may be performed

Prognosis

- Acute acalculous cholecystitis, unlike acute calculous cholecystitis, is associated with high mortality

Complications

- Gangrenous cholecystitis
- Perforation
- Emphysematous cholecystitis
  - Caused by overgrowth by gas-producing organisms
- Empyema of gallbladder

IMAGE FINDINGS

Ultrasonographic Findings

- Gallstones in 95% of cases
- Thickening of gallbladder (5 mm or more), pericholecystic fluid, ultrasonographic Murphy sign

Hepatobiliary Scintigraphy

- Absence of gallbladder filling within 60 minutes after tracer administration indicates acute cholecystitis

MACROSCOPIC FEATURES

General Features

- Gallbladder wall thickened, congested, and may appear necrotic
- Serosa dull, occasionally with fibrinopurulent exudates

ACUTE CHOLECYSTITIS

Key Facts

Etiology/Pathogenesis
- Acute **calculous** cholecystitis: 95% of cases
- Acute **acalculous** cholecystitis: 5% of cases

Clinical Issues
- Right upper quadrant pain, tenderness, and guarding
- Fever, leukocytosis
- Laparoscopic cholecystectomy is procedure of choice

Macroscopic Features
- Mural thickening, congestion, purulent exudate, adhesions

Microscopic Pathology
- Changes depend on duration of disease
  - Inflammation may be sparse in early disease
- Congestion, edema, variable necrosis
- Widespread fibroblastic proliferation

- Mucosal changes range from edema to widespread ulceration; pus may be present
- 95% have stones
- Serosal adhesions

MICROSCOPIC PATHOLOGY

Histologic Features
- Changes depend on duration of disease
  - Early uncomplicated acute cholecystitis may show only edema, congestion, and hemorrhage
    - May lack inflammation altogether
- Inflammatory infiltrate
  - Acute inflammation with neutrophil cell predominance
    - Inflammation may be sparse, especially early in disease course
  - Eosinophils, macrophages, and lymphocytes appear as disease evolves
  - Eventually transmural inflammation, secondary vasculitis, and mural necrosis develop
- Widespread fibroblastic proliferation with tissue culture-like look
- Mucosal ulceration
- Transmural fibrosis and Rokitansky-Aschoff sinuses, stigmata of chronic cholecystitis, may be present
- No histologic differences between acute calculous and noncalculous cholecystitis
- Acute emphysematous cholecystitis shows necrotic wall with gas bubbles and often contains gram-positive bacilli

DIFFERENTIAL DIAGNOSIS

Chronic Cholecystitis
- Lacks acute inflammation, fibroblastic proliferation, edema/congestion

Gallbladder Dysplasia and Carcinoma
- Regenerative mucosal changes may mimic dysplasia and, infrequently, carcinoma
- Regenerative mucosal changes are diffuse and arise in background of ulcerated and inflamed mucosa

SELECTED REFERENCES

1. Elwood DR: Cholecystitis. Surg Clin North Am. 88(6):1241-52, viii, 2008
2. Strasberg SM: Clinical practice. Acute calculous cholecystitis. N Engl J Med. 2008 Jun 26;358(26):2804-11. Review. Erratum in: N Engl J Med. 359(3):325, 2008
3. Laurila JJ et al: Histopathology of acute acalculous cholecystitis in critically ill patients. Histopathology. 47(5):485-92, 2005
4. Babb RR: Acute acalculous cholecystitis. A review. J Clin Gastroenterol. 15(3):238-41, 1992

IMAGE GALLERY

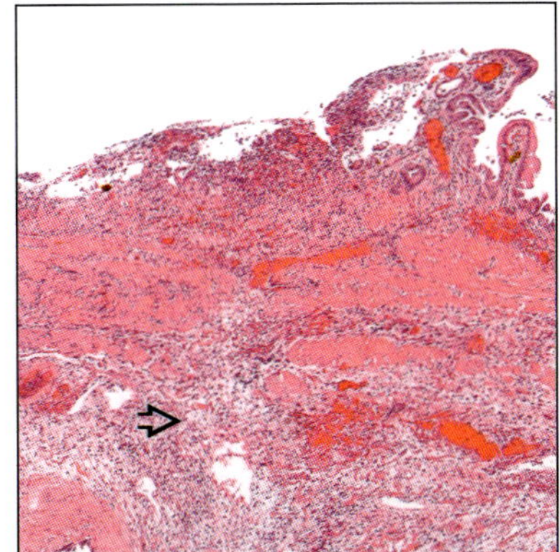

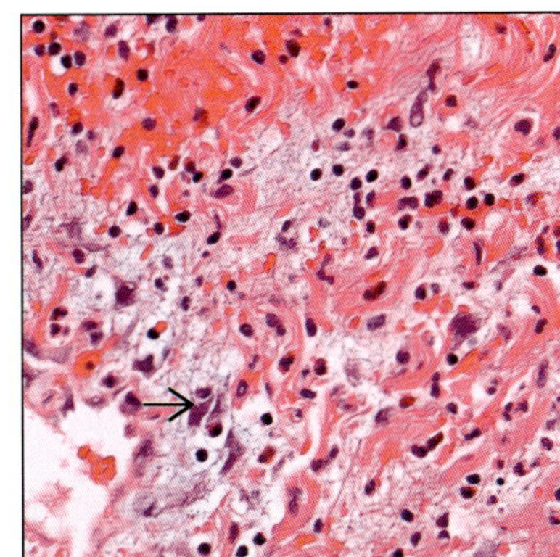

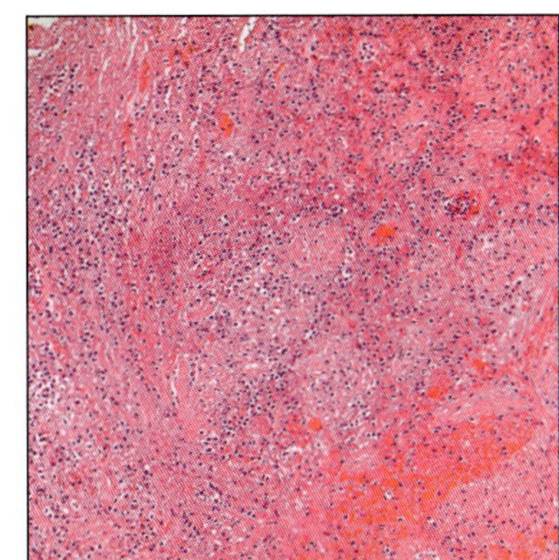

*(**Left**) This case of acute cholecystitis shows focal ulceration and edema ⇨ in the muscularis propria and subserosal tissue. (**Center**) Early acute cholecystitis may show marked edema and hemorrhage but minimal inflammation. Also note the reactive fibroblasts →. (**Right**) A case of severe acute cholecystitis shows mural necrosis, fresh hemorrhage, and neutrophilic exudate.*

CHRONIC CHOLECYSTITIS

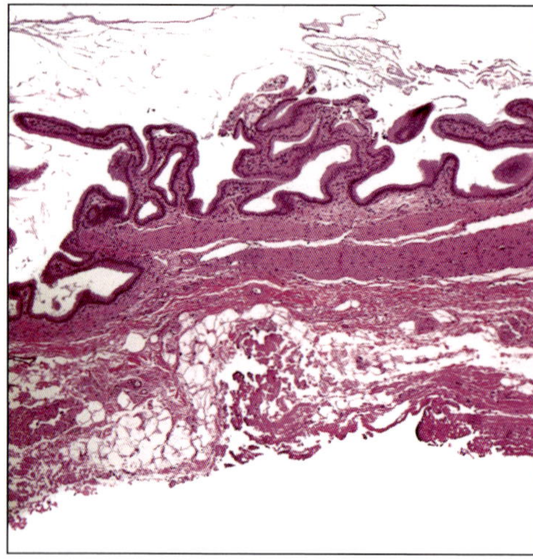

This section illustrates a normal gallbladder with typical wall thickness and a normal complement of chronic inflammatory cells.

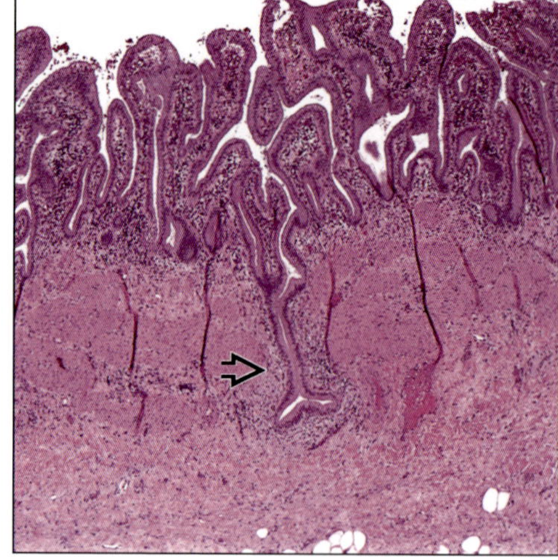

This example of chronic cholecystitis shows an increase in chronic inflammation within the lamina propria and the submucosa. A Rokitansky-Aschoff sinus ⇨ is present as well.

TERMINOLOGY

Definitions

- Chronic inflammation of gallbladder

ETIOLOGY/PATHOGENESIS

Pathogenesis

- Poorly understood
- Almost always associated with gallstones
- Possible association with trauma induced by gallstones, prior episodes of acute cholecystitis, or abnormal composition of bile

CLINICAL ISSUES

Epidemiology

- Age
  - Patients in their 40s or 50s
- Gender
  - More common in women (3:1)

Presentation

- Episodic, steady, abdominal pain ("biliary colic")
  - Usually located in epigastrium or right upper quadrant
  - May be precipitated by ingestion of food

Treatment

- Cholecystectomy is curative

IMAGE FINDINGS

Ultrasonographic Findings

- Method of choice to demonstrate stones and abnormalities in gallbladder wall

MACROSCOPIC FEATURES

General Features

- Variable, depending on degree of inflammation and fibrosis
- May appear normal or show mild wall thickening and serosal adhesions
- Some gallbladders are shrunken with marked wall thickening and scarring
- Mucosa may be
  - Flattened
  - Granular
  - Ulcerated
  - Polypoid

MICROSCOPIC PATHOLOGY

Histologic Features

- Inflammation
  - Predominantly mononuclear infiltrate predominantly composed of lymphocytes
  - Distribution focal or diffuse in lamina propria with or without extension into muscularis and pericholecystic tissues
  - Minor component of eosinophils and neutrophils may be present
- Wall thickening
  - Secondary to muscular hypertrophy and fibrosis
  - Adventitia is frequently thickened with diffuse scarring
- Metaplastic changes
  - Most common type is pyloric (antral) type
  - Surface epithelium may show mucinous columnar metaplasia of gastric type
  - Less frequently, intestinal metaplasia may occur
- Rokitansky-Aschoff sinuses
  - Herniation of mucosa into or through muscularis

CHRONIC CHOLECYSTITIS

Key Facts

Etiology/Pathogenesis
- Almost always associated with gallstones

Clinical Issues
- More common in women; approximately 3:1

Microscopic Pathology
- Predominantly mononuclear inflammatory infiltrate with lymphocytes dominating over plasma cells and histiocytes
- Minor component of eosinophils and neutrophils may be present
- Wall thickening secondary to muscular hypertrophy and fibrosis
- Metaplastic changes; most common is antral type
- Rokitansky-Aschoff sinuses

Diagnostic Checklist
- Presence of gallstones is neither necessary nor sufficient for diagnosis of chronic cholecystitis

---

    - Indicative of increased intraluminal pressure or outflow obstruction, commonly associated with hypertrophic muscularis
    - Sole occurrence is not sufficient for diagnosis of chronic cholecystitis
- Variants
    - Follicular cholecystitis
        - Numerous mucosal lymphoid follicles with hyperplastic germinal centers
        - Large follicles may cause polyps
        - May occur with infections (especially gram-negative) and primary sclerosing cholangitis
    - Chronic acalculous cholecystitis
        - No gallstones
        - Variant with diffuse lymphoplasmacytic infiltrate confined to lamina propria may be associated with extrahepatic bile duct obstruction
    - Porcelain gallbladder
        - Multiple areas of dystrophic calcification imparting "eggshell" gross appearance
        - Associated with higher risk of carcinoma

DIFFERENTIAL DIAGNOSIS

Normal Gallbladder
- Sparse, focally distributed lymphoid cells
- Lack fibrosis, Rokitansky-Aschoff sinuses

Acute Cholecystitis
- Has acute inflammation, edema, hemorrhage

Eosinophilic Cholecystitis
- More than 50% of infiltrate is composed of eosinophils

DIAGNOSTIC CHECKLIST

Pathologic Interpretation Pearls
- Presence of gallstones is neither necessary nor sufficient for diagnosis of chronic cholecystitis
- Normal gallbladders contain some chronic inflammatory cells
- It is possible to encounter histologically normal gallbladders with symptomatic calculi

SELECTED REFERENCES

1. Elwood DR: Cholecystitis. Surg Clin North Am. 88(6):1241-52, viii, 2008
2. Halpert B: Significance of the Rokitansky-Aschoff sinuses. Am J Gastroenterol. 36:534-9, 1961
3. Edulund Y et al: Histopathology of the gallbladder in gallstone disease related to clinical data; with a proposal for uniform surgical and clinical terminology. Acta Chir Scand. 116(5-6):450-60, 1959

IMAGE GALLERY

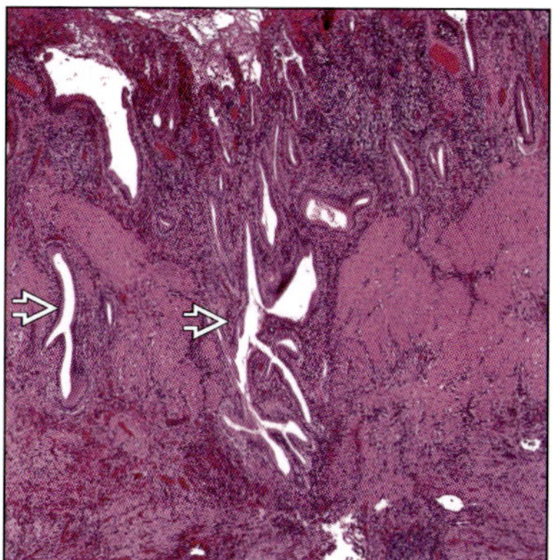

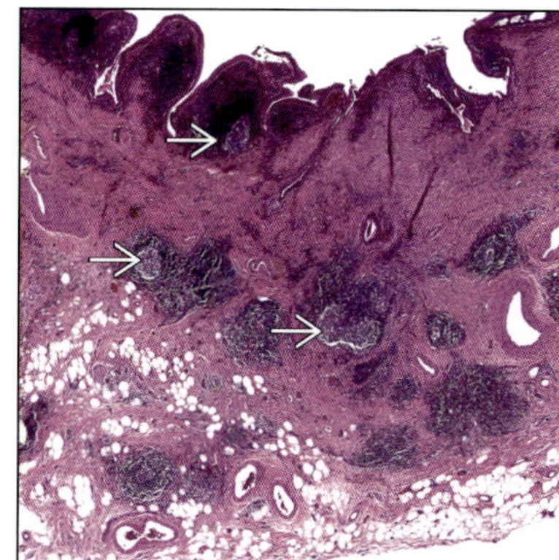

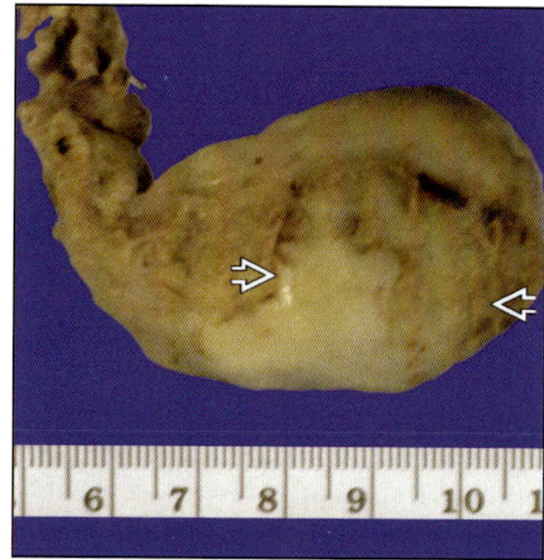

(Left) *Rokitansky-Aschoff sinuses ➡ occur when the mucosa herniates through the muscle bundles of the muscularis of the gallbladder.* ***(Center)*** *This low-power view of chronic follicular cholecystitis is characterized by reactive lymphoid follicles within the gallbladder mucosa and wall ➡.* ***(Right)*** *This porcelain gallbladder shows a thick, fibrotic gallbladder with areas of dystrophic calcification ➡ reminiscent of porcelain.*

XANTHOGRANULOMATOUS CHOLECYSTITIS

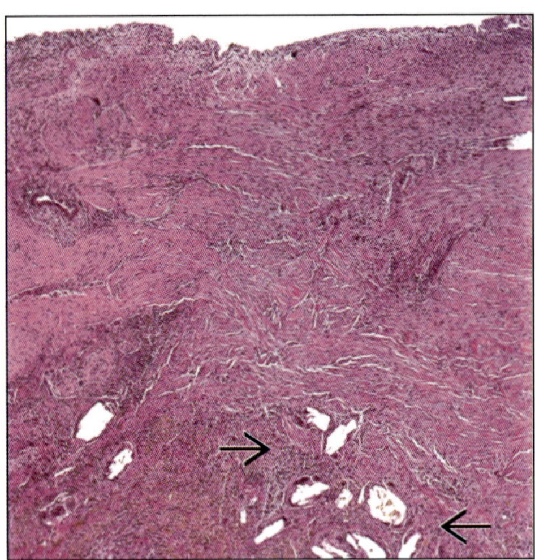

Xanthogranulomatous cholecystitis often features a markedly thickened wall with overlying mucosal ulceration. Note the associated cholesterol clefts ⇒ in the granulomatous inflammation.

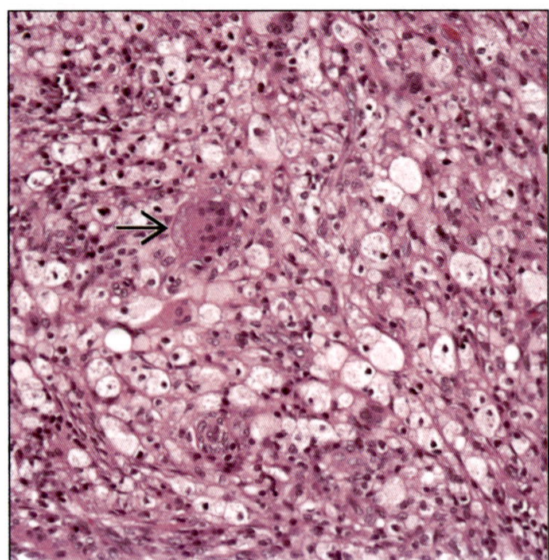

Xanthogranulomatous cholecystitis is often characterized by a dense infiltrate of foamy histiocytes, many of which contain ceroid pigment. Multinucleated giant cells are also common ⇒.

TERMINOLOGY

Abbreviations

- Xanthogranulomatous cholecystitis (XGC)

Synonyms

- Cholegranulomas
- Ceroid granulomas

Definitions

- Variant of chronic cholecystitis featuring florid proliferation of foamy macrophages and granulomatous reaction to bile

ETIOLOGY/PATHOGENESIS

Reaction to Bile

- Usually preceded by rupture of Rokitansky-Aschoff sinus
- Bile and lipid extruded into gallbladder wall produces granulomatous reaction

CLINICAL ISSUES

Epidemiology

- Incidence
  - 4-9% of cholecystectomy specimens

Presentation

- Similar to chronic cholecystitis
- Majority of cases associated with gallstones

Treatment

- Cholecystectomy

Prognosis

- Surgery is generally curative
- Rarely, inflammation extends from gallbladder to other organs to form adhesions or fistulas
  - Some reports of higher complication rates in xanthogranulomatous cholecystitis
- No established association with cholangiocarcinoma
  - Rare reports of elevated CA19-9 associated with XGC

IMAGE FINDINGS

Ultrasonographic Findings

- Thickened wall with echogenic, isoechoic, or hyperechoic nodules

MACROSCOPIC FEATURES

General Features

- Tumor-like masses, nodules, or plaques often can be seen grossly
  - Often multiple
  - Usually intramural
    - Can produce mucosal masses as well
  - Cream to brown color
  - Poorly circumscribed and soft
- Gallbladder wall often markedly thickened (up to 2 cm)

Size

- Few millimeters to 3 cm

MICROSCOPIC PATHOLOGY

Histologic Features

- Spectrum of granulomatous lesions
  - Usually centered on ruptured Rokitansky-Aschoff sinuses
  - Granulomatous inflammation forms mural nodules
    - Mucosal surface may ulcerate as nodules expand
  - Foamy histiocyte infiltrate
    - Histiocytes may contain light brown ceroid granules

XANTHOGRANULOMATOUS CHOLECYSTITIS

Key Facts

Terminology
- Variant of chronic cholecystitis characterized by granulomatous reaction to bile

Macroscopic Features
- Cream to brown tumor-like masses, nodules, or plaques
  - Usually intramural
- Gallbladder wall often markedly thickened (up to 2 cm)

Microscopic Pathology
- Spectrum of granulomatous lesions centered on ruptured Rokitansky-Aschoff sinuses
  - Range of lesions from foamy histiocytes to granulomas
  - Associated ceroid pigment, bile, cholesterol clefts
- Pools of extravasated bile may be present in wall of gallbladder

    - Occasionally histiocytes are spindled
  - Well- or loosely formed granulomas
    - Bile may be present in center
    - Multinucleated giant cells common, often containing cholesterol clefts
  - Mixture of other inflammatory cells, especially lymphocytes
- Pools of extravasated bile may be present in wall of gallbladder
- Over time, organization occurs, and fibrosis may predominate
- Calcifications also seen in older lesions

DIFFERENTIAL DIAGNOSIS

Carcinoma
- Nodules and markedly thickened wall of xanthogranulomatous cholecystitis can mimic malignancy grossly and radiographically
  - Surgeons may submit frozen section of XGC to rule out malignancy

Malakoplakia
- Has Michaelis-Gutmann bodies
- Lacks ceroid-laden histiocytes, cholesterol clefts, and bile

DIAGNOSTIC CHECKLIST

Clinically Relevant Pathologic Features
- Markedly thickened gallbladder wall may mimic malignancy grossly and radiographically

Pathologic Interpretation Pearls
- Spectrum of granulomatous inflammation associated with
  - Ruptured Rokitansky-Aschoff sinuses
  - Ceroid pigment
  - Bile
  - Cholesterol clefts

SELECTED REFERENCES

1. Houston JP et al: Xanthogranulomatous cholecystitis. Br J Surg. 81(7):1030-2, 1994
2. Roberts KM et al: Xanthogranulomatous cholecystitis: clinicopathological study of 13 cases. J Clin Pathol. 40(4):412-7, 1987
3. Fligiel S et al: Xanthogranulomatous cholecystitis: case report and review of the literature. Arch Pathol Lab Med. 106(6):302-4, 1982
4. Goodman ZD et al: Xanthogranulomatous cholecystitis. Am J Surg Pathol. 5(7):653-9, 1981

IMAGE GALLERY

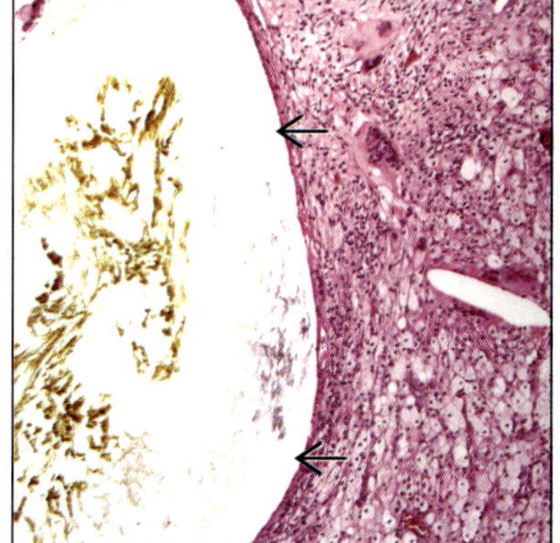

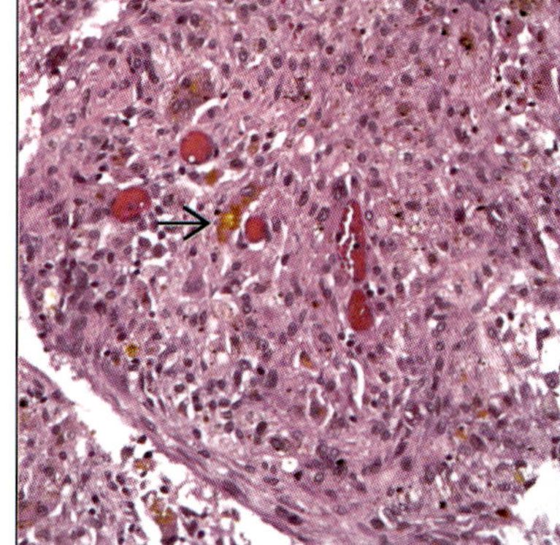

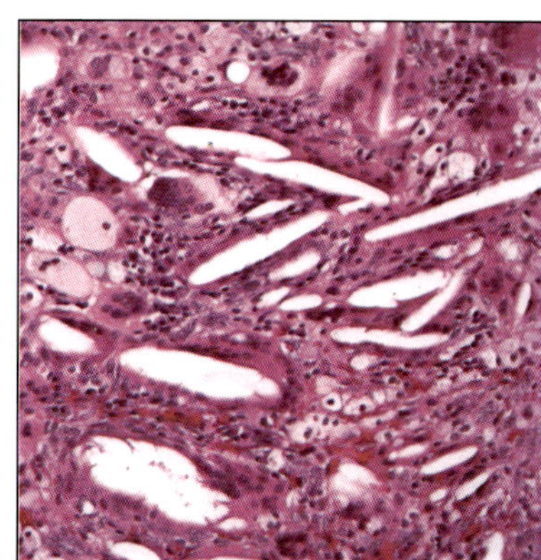

__(Left)__ The granulomatous inflammation is often centered on a Rokitansky-Aschoff sinus. The one seen here ⇨ is dilated and filled with bile. Note the foamy histiocytes, cholesterol clefts, and giant cells to the right. __(Center)__ This granuloma in the wall of the gallbladder contains bile ⇨ and ceroid-laden histiocytes. __(Right)__ This high-power view of a cholegranuloma shows foamy histiocytes, cholesterol clefts, and multinucleated giant cells.

EOSINOPHILIC CHOLECYSTITIS

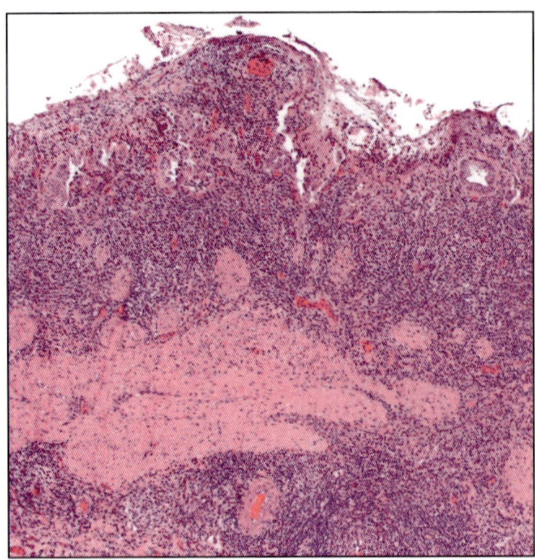

This case of eosinophilic cholecystitis shows a transmural infiltrate consisting of both lymphocytes and eosinophils.

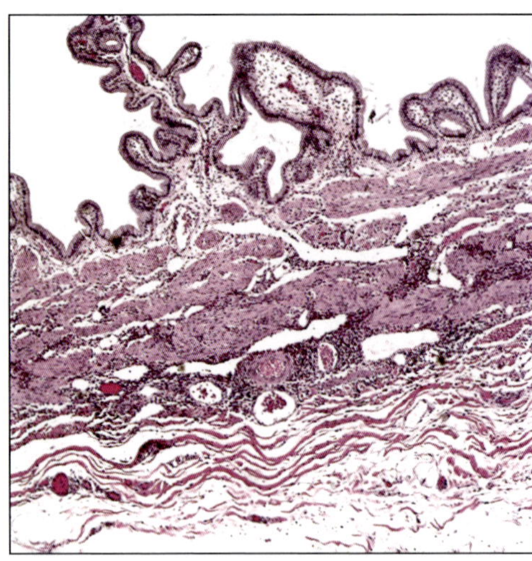

This case of "pure" eosinophilic cholecystitis shows an infiltrate composed entirely of eosinophils extending into the wall of the gallbladder.

TERMINOLOGY

Abbreviations

- Eosinophilic cholecystitis (EC)

Definitions

- Inflammatory disease of gallbladder in which inflammatory infiltrate is composed predominantly of eosinophils

ETIOLOGY/PATHOGENESIS

Hypersensitivity Reaction

- Hypersensitivity reaction to drugs, infections (*Echinococcus*, *Clonorchis sinensis*)
- Hypersensitive reaction to bile and bile stones has been hypothesized but never proven

Other Eosinophilic Diseases

- Eosinophilic cholangitis
  - Occasionally, biliary tree may be involved, leading to biliary strictures
- Eosinophilic gastroenteritis

CLINICAL ISSUES

Presentation

- Eosinophilia
  - Peripheral eosinophilia is frequently but not invariably present
- Presenting signs are similar to other forms of acute and chronic cholecystitis
- Variably present gallstones
  - Although gallbladder calculi are sometimes seen, stones are less commonly seen in EC than in other forms of acute and chronic cholecystitis

Treatment

- Cholecystectomy is standard therapy
  - Diagnosis is invariably made following evaluation of gallbladder specimen
- In rare instances when preoperative diagnosis has been made, steroid therapy is reported to be effective

Prognosis

- Cholecystectomy is curative, and disease does not recur

MACROSCOPIC FEATURES

General Features

- Thickened gallbladder wall
- Gallstones are usually present

MICROSCOPIC PATHOLOGY

Histologic Features

- Thickened and inflamed gallbladder wall
  - Predominantly eosinophilic infiltrate
    - Typically > 50% of inflammatory infiltrate is composed of eosinophils
    - Sheets and clusters of eosinophils infiltrate mucosa, muscularis propria, and subserosa
    - Inflammation at one level, rather than all, may dominate
- Eosinophilic phlebitis may be seen
- Variations
  - In "true" EC, close to 100% of inflammatory component is composed of eosinophils
  - So-called lymphoeosinophilic cholecystitis shows significant component of lymphocytes as well

DIFFERENTIAL DIAGNOSIS

Chronic Cholecystitis

- Subacute phase of acute cholecystitis may show significant tissue eosinophilia

EOSINOPHILIC CHOLECYSTITIS

Key Facts

Terminology

- Inflammatory disease of gallbladder in which inflammatory infiltrate is composed predominantly of eosinophils

Microscopic Pathology

- Dense eosinophilic infiltrate of gallbladder with or without lymphocytic inflammatory component
- Careful evaluation of specimen to exclude parasite
- In "true" EC, close to 100% of inflammatory component is composed of eosinophils
- So-called lymphoeosinophilic cholecystitis shows significant component of lymphocytes as well

Top Differential Diagnoses

- Acute and subacute cholecystitis with cholelithiasis
- Autoimmune pancreatitis-associated cholecystitis

- Dense sheets and significant clustering of eosinophils are not seen in chronic calculous cholecystitis

Acute and Subacute Cholecystitis with Cholelithiasis

- Disease process associated with admixture of neutrophils and eosinophils, particularly in instances of acute cholecystitis in which cholecystectomy is delayed
- Eosinophils do not typically dominate infiltrate

Cholecystitis Associated with Biliary Obstruction

- Diffuse lymphoplasmacytic cholecystitis: Associated with both benign and malignant forms of biliary obstruction, not associated with dominant eosinophil population

Autoimmune Pancreatitis-associated Cholecystitis

- Gallbladder inflammation associated with autoimmune pancreatitis is dominated by lymphocytes and plasma cells
  - Can show significant numbers of eosinophils
- Elevated numbers of IgG4(+) plasma cells help distinguish this entity from EC

DIAGNOSTIC CHECKLIST

Pathologic Interpretation Pearls

- Predominance of eosinophils in inflamed gallbladder
- Variably present gallstones
- May be associated with other eosinophilic diseases or peripheral eosinophilia

SELECTED REFERENCES

1. Wang WL et al: Autoimmune pancreatitis-related cholecystitis: a morphologically and immunologically distinctive form of lymphoplasmacytic sclerosing cholecystitis. Histopathology. 54(7):829-36, 2009
2. Lai CH et al: Clonorchiasis-associated perforated eosinophilic cholecystitis. Am J Trop Med Hyg. 76(2):396-8, 2007
3. Abraham SC et al: Lymphoplasmacytic chronic cholecystitis and biliary tract disease in patients with lymphoplasmacytic sclerosing pancreatitis. Am J Surg Pathol. 27(4):441-51, 2003
4. Vauthey JN et al: Case 57: eosinophilic cholangiopathy. Radiology. 227(1):107-12, 2003
5. Dabbs DJ: Eosinophilic and lymphoeosinophilic cholecystitis. Am J Surg Pathol. 17(5):497-501, 1993
6. Kerstein MD et al: Eosinophilic cholecystitis. Am J Gastroenterol. 66(4):349-52, 1976

IMAGE GALLERY

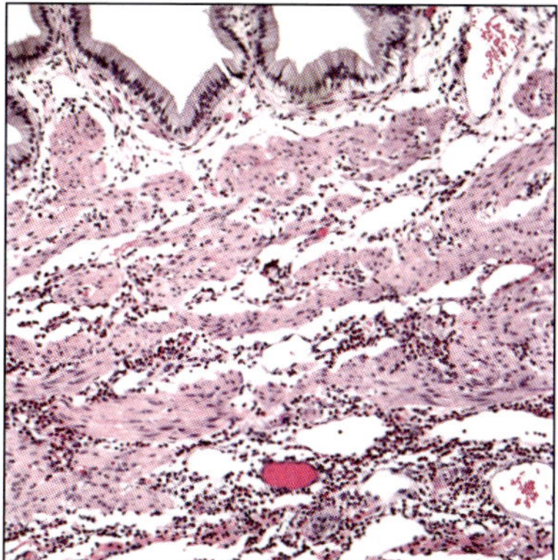

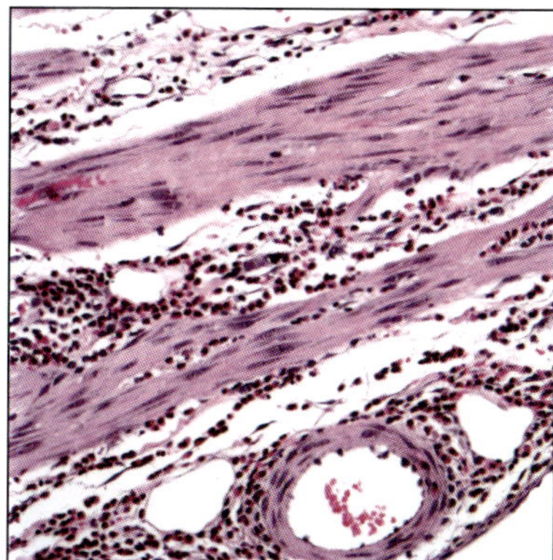

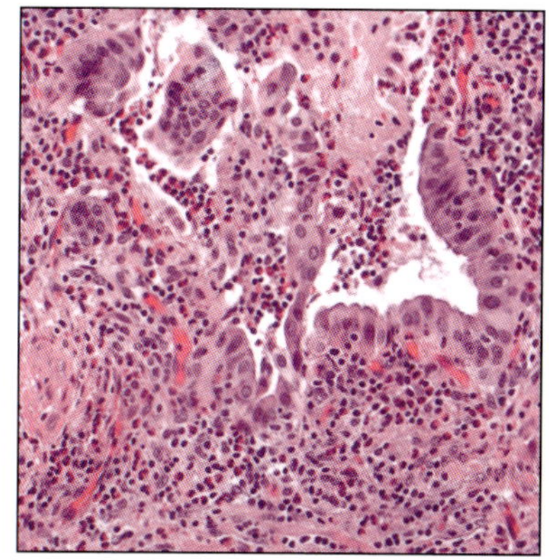

*(**Left**) This case of "pure" eosinophilic cholecystitis shows the exclusively eosinophilic infiltrate extending into the muscular wall of the gallbladder. (**Center**) This high-power view of "pure" eosinophilic cholecystitis shows the eosinophils within the wall of the gallbladder as well as surrounding vessels. (**Right**) Some cases of eosinophilic cholecystitis also have admixed lymphocytes in the inflammatory infiltrate.*

POLYARTERITIS NODOSA AND OTHER VASCULITIDES

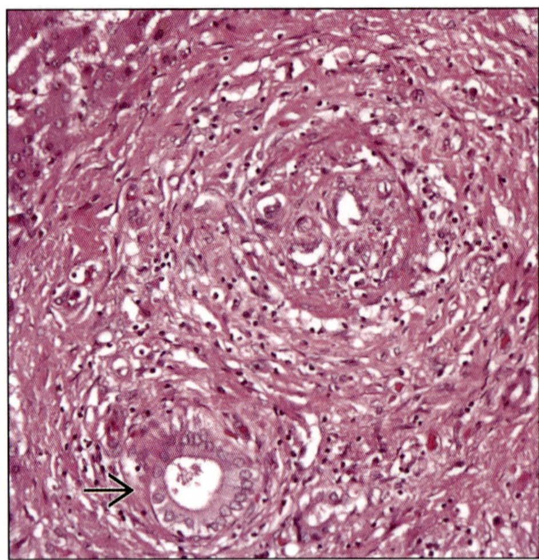

This liver involved by polyarteritis nodosa features a medium-sized artery with fibrinoid necrosis, early fibrosis, and luminal narrowing. Note bile duct ➔.

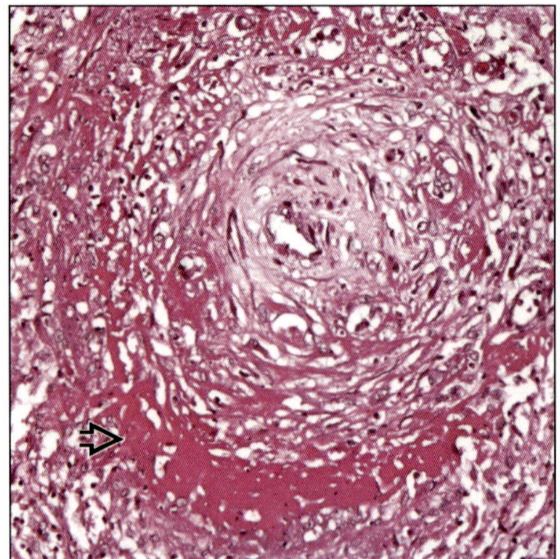

Fibrinoid necrosis ➪ is seen within the wall of a medium-sized artery in the liver. This lesion is the hallmark of polyarteritis nodosa.

TERMINOLOGY

Abbreviations

- Polyarteritis nodosa (PAN)

Definitions

- Involvement of liver &/or gallbladder by vasculitis (inflammation of blood vessels)

ETIOLOGY/PATHOGENESIS

Liver

- Liver involved in > 40% of cases of polyarteritis nodosa (PAN)
  - Associated with hepatitis B (30% of cases)

Gallbladder

- Involved in 2 distinct settings
  - Isolated gallbladder involvement (monoarterial or localized form)
  - Part of systemic disease
    - Most common
    - Gallbladder involved in up to 40% of cases
    - Isolated form rarely progresses to systemic form
    - Systemic form may develop up to 1 year after isolated lesions found in cholecystectomy

CLINICAL ISSUES

Presentation

- Abdominal pain
- Signs and symptoms similar to acute acalculous cholecystitis
- Systemic complaints
  - Malaise/weakness
  - Musculoskeletal pain
  - Fever
  - Renal failure
- Liver/gallbladder involvement may be clinically silent
  - Lesions discovered incidentally in tissue sections
- Sequelae
  - Hepatic infarction
  - Arterial rupture with intraabdominal hemorrhage
  - Nodular regenerative hyperplasia
  - Injury to intrahepatic bile ducts
- Liver and gallbladder rarely involved in vasculitides other than PAN
  - Churg-Strauss syndrome
    - Accompanied by asthma, pulmonary infiltrates, eosinophilia
    - Vasculitis is granulomatous
  - Rheumatoid vasculitis
    - Usually accompanied by severe arthritis, low complement, high levels of circulating antibodies
    - Necrotizing vasculitis resembling PAN
  - Systemic lupus erythematosus
    - Liver and gallbladder affected in persons with severe systemic disease
  - Henoch-Schönlein purpura
    - Accompanied by purpura, arthritis
    - Usually pediatric patients
  - Wegener granulomatosis
  - Temporal arteritis
  - Takayasu arteritis
  - Drug-induced vasculitis

Laboratory Tests

- Laboratory findings usually reflect severe systemic inflammation
  - Elevated ESR
  - Elevated C-reactive protein
  - Elevated white blood cell count
  - Elevated serum immunoglobulins
- Anemia may be present, secondary to blood loss or renal failure

Treatment

- Combination of steroids and immunosuppressive agents

POLYARTERITIS NODOSA AND OTHER VASCULITIDES

Key Facts

Etiology/Pathogenesis

- Liver and gallbladder involved in > 40% of cases of polyarteritis nodosa (PAN)
- Gallbladder involvement occasionally isolated rather than part of systemic process
- Liver and gallbladder rarely involved in vasculitides other than PAN

Clinical Issues

- Common presenting complaints include fever, abdominal pain
- Laboratory findings usually reflect severe systemic inflammation

Microscopic Pathology

- Hallmark lesion of PAN is fibrinoid necrosis involving medium-sized arteries

Prognosis

- Ongoing therapy may be required to maintain remission

IMAGE FINDINGS

Angiography

- May reveal aneurysms, evidence of vasculitis

MACROSCOPIC FEATURES

Liver

- Gross evidence of infarction
- May be normal

Gallbladder

- Thickened, edematous wall

MICROSCOPIC PATHOLOGY

Histologic Features

- Hallmark lesion of PAN is fibrinoid necrosis involving medium-sized arteries
  - Initially involves media, with destruction of elastic laminae and smooth muscle
  - Only segment of wall may be affected
  - In acute phase, endothelial damage may cause thrombosis
  - As healing occurs, bead-like nodular aneurysm (nodose) may form
  - Recanalized thrombi may be seen
  - Usually, temporal mixture of lesions is present, ranging from early to completely scarred
- Often accompanied by mixed inflammatory infiltrate
  - Eosinophils may be prominent
- Infarction, mucosal ulceration (gallbladder) may be present

DIFFERENTIAL DIAGNOSIS

Cholecystitis

- Acute, chronic, and eosinophilic cholecystitis may show perivascular inflammation
  - Lack fibrinoid necrosis

SELECTED REFERENCES

1. Bailey M et al: The effects of vasculitis on the gastrointestinal tract and liver. Gastroenterol Clin North Am. 27(4):747-82, v-vi, 1998
2. Burke AP et al: Localized vasculitis of the gastrointestinal tract. Am J Surg Pathol. 19(3):338-49, 1995
3. Nøhr M et al: Isolated necrotizing panarteritis of the gallbladder. Case report. Acta Chir Scand. 155(9):485-7, 1989

IMAGE GALLERY

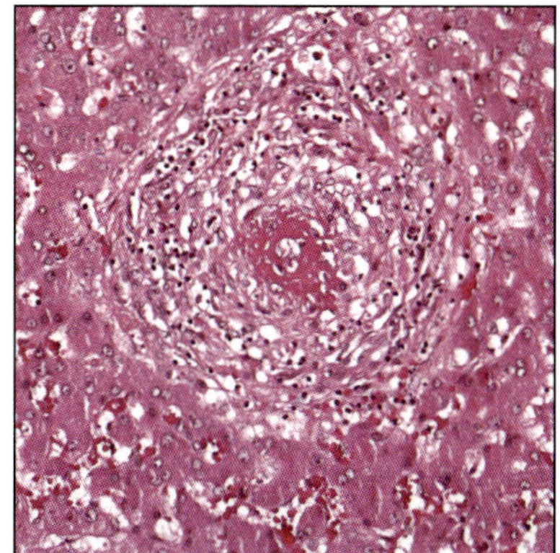

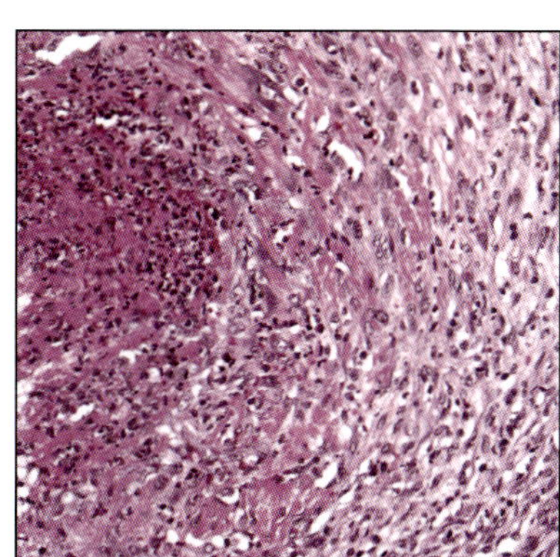

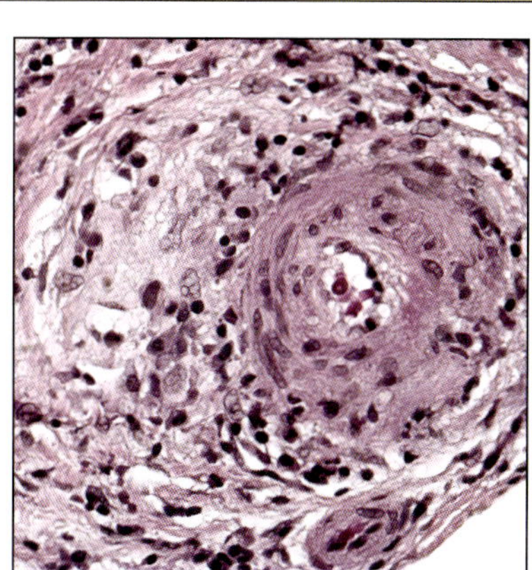

(Left) *A medium-sized artery in the liver shows fibrinoid necrosis and inflammatory destruction of the vessel wall.* ***(Center)*** *This case of polyarteritis nodosa in the gallbladder shows fibrinoid necrosis and destruction of the artery wall with an associated mixed inflammatory infiltrate.* ***(Right)*** *Older lesions in PAN show resolution of the necrosis and scarring of the vessel wall.*

PARASITIC INFECTION

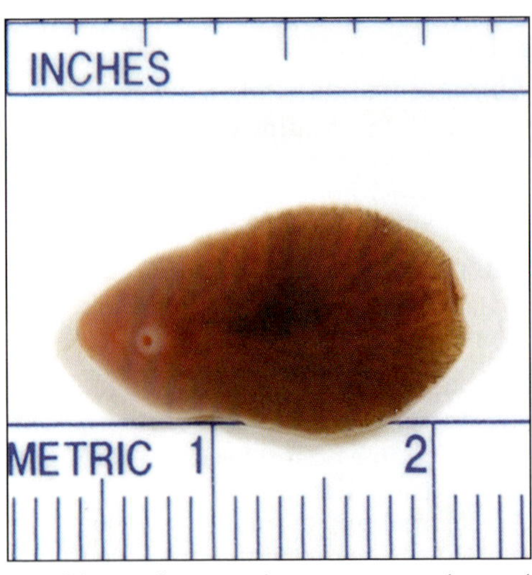

Liver flukes are flat, somewhat transparent, and tapered anteriorly. They have prominent oral and ventral suckers. (Courtesy J. Doss, MD.)

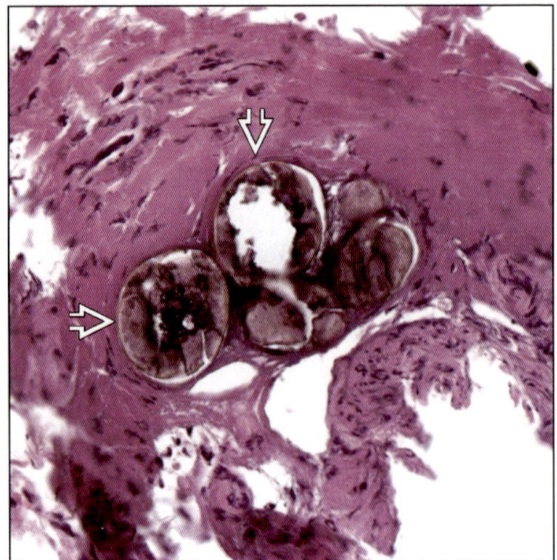

Rarely, calcified schistosomal eggs ⊳ are seen in the periductal connective tissue.

TERMINOLOGY

Definitions

- Infection of bile ducts by a parasite

ETIOLOGY/PATHOGENESIS

Protozoans

- *Cryptosporidium* species
- *Microsporidia* species

Helminths

- Trematodes
  - Liver flukes
    - *Clonorchis sinensis*
    - *Opisthorchis* species
    - *Fasciola* species
  - *Schistosoma* species (blood flukes)
- Nematodes
  - *Ascaris* species

CLINICAL ISSUES

Presentation

- Protozoans
  - Infection is usually seen in context of AIDS (so-called AIDS cholangiopathy)
    - May also be seen in transplant patients
  - Gradual and regular stenosis of common bile duct with dilation of intrahepatic bile ducts
    - Some patients have irregularities of intrahepatic bile ducts that mimic primary sclerosing cholangitis
  - Symptoms
    - Abdominal pain
    - Low-grade fever may be present
    - Jaundice rare
- *Clonorchis* and *Opisthorchis*
  - Endemic in many parts of Asia (*Clonorchis* and *O. viverrini*), Russia and Eastern Europe (*O. felineus*)
  - Infection acquired from eating raw or undercooked fish, crawfish
  - Symptoms
    - Right upper quadrant (RUQ) pain
    - Fatigue
    - Anorexia
    - Diarrhea
    - Growth retardation in children
    - Light infection may be asymptomatic
  - Complications include obstruction, cholangitis
- *Fasciola*
  - Primarily disease of farm animals; human infection acquired from eating contaminated watercress
  - Acute fascioliasis causes
    - Fever
    - Hepatomegaly
    - Blood eosinophilia
  - Chronic infection presents as biliary colic
- *Schistosoma* species (schistosomiasis)
  - May involve both intra- and extrahepatic bile ducts
  - Present with signs and symptoms of portal hypertension
- *Ascaris*
  - Duodenal infection that may involve bile ducts
  - Sudden onset of severe right upper quadrant pain when worm enters duct

Laboratory Tests

- Elevated bilirubin and alkaline phosphatase
- Elevated transaminases

Treatment

- Cholangiopathy due to protozoal infection
  - Sphincterotomy to relieve obstruction and correct stenosis
- Helminths usually treated with medical therapy

Prognosis

- Depends on specific infection and status of host

PARASITIC INFECTION

Key Facts

Terminology
- Infection of bile ducts by parasite
  - Usually protozoan (*Microsporidia*, *Cryptosporidia*) or helminth (liver fluke, schistosomiasis, ascariasis)

Clinical Issues
- Protozoal infection usually seen in context of AIDS (so-called AIDS cholangiopathy)
  - Can mimic PSC radiographically
- Helminths present with fever, RUQ pain, signs of biliary obstruction

Macroscopic Features
- Helminths usually visible to naked eye

Microscopic Pathology
- Protozoa: Epithelial disarray, lymphocytic inflammation, organisms in epithelium
- Flukes: Inflammation of ducts with fibrosis, reactive epithelial changes

- Sequelae of *Clonorchis*, *Opisthorchis* infection include cholangiocarcinoma, Oriental cholangiohepatitis
  - Fasciola not associated with malignancy

MACROSCOPIC FEATURES

General Features
- Protozoans
  - Stenosis of common bile duct
- *Clonorchis*, *Opisthorchis*, *Fasciola*: Variably present dilation of intrahepatic ducts, with mural thickening
  - Worms are visible to naked eye
- *Schistosoma* species: Fibrosis of bile ducts (pipestem fibrosis)
- *Ascaris*: Large worms easily visible to naked eye

MICROSCOPIC PATHOLOGY

Histologic Features
- Protozoans
  - Epithelial disarray, lymphocytic inflammation
  - Organisms present within epithelium
- *Opisthorchis* and *Clonorchis*: Epithelial desquamation followed by hyperplasia of epithelium and periductal mucus glands, periductal fibrosis
- *Fasciola*: Necrosis and hemorrhage of ducts with abscess formation, resulting in fibrosis
- *Schistosoma* species: Vigorous fibroinflammatory response to dead eggs entraps bile ducts
  - Viable and nonviable eggs may rarely be seen in fibrous tissue adjacent to ducts

DIFFERENTIAL DIAGNOSIS

Primary Sclerosing Cholangitis
- Protozoal infection of biliary tree can mimic PSC radiographically

Other Causes of Large Bile Duct Obstruction
- Gallstones
- Tumors

Other Causes of Cholangitis
- Bacterial infection

SELECTED REFERENCES

1. Rana SS et al: Parasitic infestations of the biliary tract. Curr Gastroenterol Rep. 9(2):156-64, 2007
2. Carpenter HA: Bacterial and parasitic cholangitis. Mayo Clin Proc. 73(5):473-8, 1998
3. Pol S et al: Microsporidia infection in patients with the human immunodeficiency virus and unexplained cholangitis. N Engl J Med. 328(2):95-9, 1993
4. Dowsett JF et al: Sclerosing cholangitis in acquired immunodeficiency syndrome. Case reports and review of the literature. Scand J Gastroenterol. 23(10):1267-74, 1988

IMAGE GALLERY

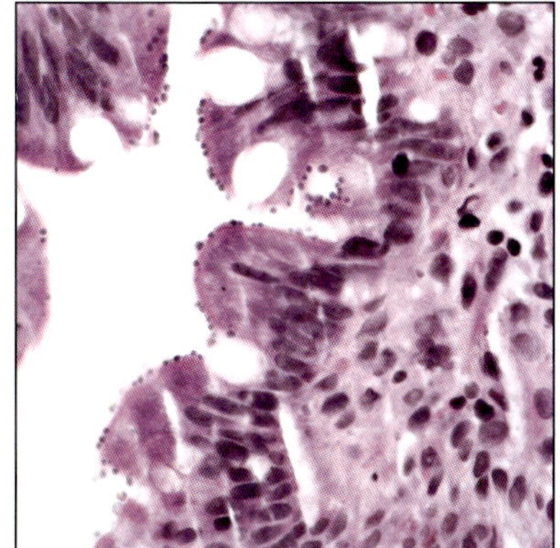

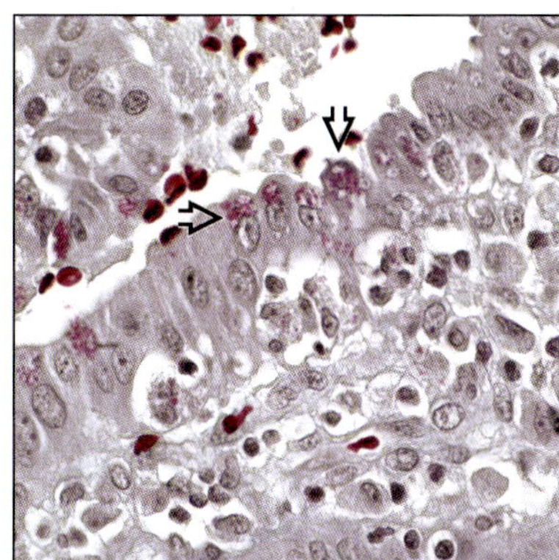

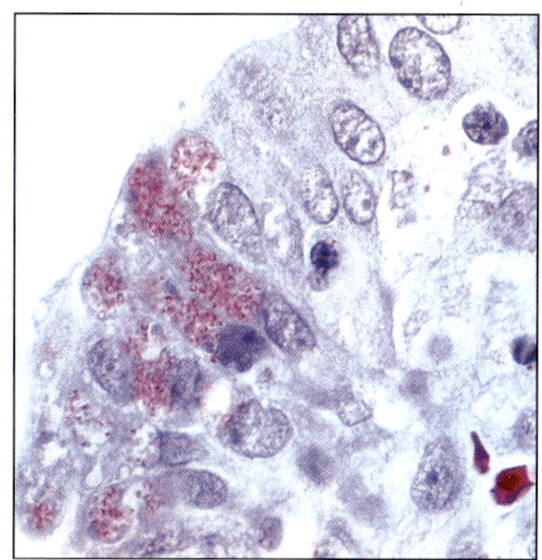

(Left) *Cryptosporidia are round, basophilic protozoa with a unique location within the apical cytoplasm of epithelial cells.* ***(Center)*** *The modified trichrome stain highlights Microsporidia (red) ➡ within the cytoplasm of biliary epithelium.* ***(Right)*** *This high-power view of Microsporidia infection in the biliary tree shows the red spores within the cytoplasm of the epithelial cells.*

Nonneoplastic and Inflammatory Disorders of the Pancreas

ACUTE PANCREATITIS

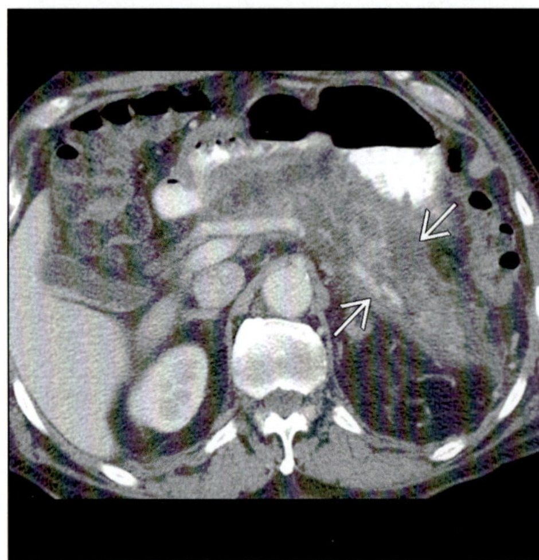

This CT shows severe acute necrotizing pancreatitis with heterogeneous and diminished enhancement of the pancreas ➡.

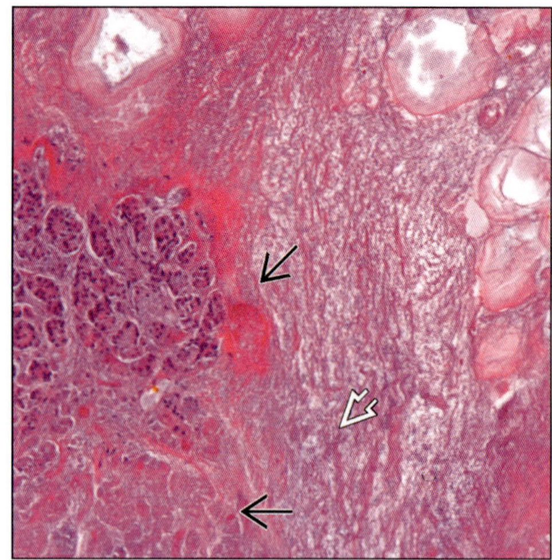

Severe acute necrotizing pancreatitis features necrosis of peripancreatic fat (right) accompanied by basophilic saponification ➡ and patchy hemorrhagic necrosis ➡.

TERMINOLOGY

Definitions

- Acute inflammatory process of pancreas

ETIOLOGY/PATHOGENESIS

Mechanical

- Gallstones, biliary sludge, periampullary diverticulum, neoplasms, duodenal stricture or obstruction
  - Most common cause is gallstones, accounting for 35-60% of cases

Toxic

- Ethanol, methanol, scorpion venom, organophosphate poisoning
  - 2nd most common cause is alcoholism

Trauma

- Blunt or penetrating abdominal injury, iatrogenic injury during procedure

Metabolic

- Hyperlipidemia type V and hypercalcemia

Vascular

- Ischemia, intraoperative hypotension, hemorrhagic shock, atheroembolism, vasculitis

Genetic

- Mutations of serine protease 1 gene (*PRSS1*), serine protease inhibitor Kazal type 1 (*SPINK1*), and cystic fibrosis transmembrane conductance regulator (*CFTR*)

Drug-induced

- Numerous drugs implicated

Infectious Agents

- Virus: Mumps, Coxsackievirus, CMV, varicella-zoster, HSV, HIV
- Bacteria: *Mycoplasma*, *Legionella*, *Leptospira*, *Salmonella*
- Parasites: *Toxoplasma*, *Cryptosporidium*, *Ascaris*

Congenital

- Choledochocele type V

Miscellaneous

- Post ERCP, pregnancy, renal transplant, α-1-antitrypsin deficiency

Idiopathic

- 10-25% of patients have no identifiable cause

CLINICAL ISSUES

Epidemiology

- Age
  - Occurs at any age
    - Most common in adults in 3rd to 6th decade of life
    - 1st decade suggests hereditary cause, infection, or trauma
- Gender
  - Gallstone pancreatitis more common in women between 50-60 years of age
  - Alcoholic pancreatitis more common in men

Presentation

- Acute upper abdominal pain, nausea, vomiting

Laboratory Tests

- Elevated amylase and lipase

Natural History

- Mild cases usually recover within 5-7 days
- Severe necrotizing pancreatitis is associated with high rate of complication and significant mortality
  - Common sequelae are pancreatic abscess and pseudocyst

Treatment

- Supportive care, infection prevention

ACUTE PANCREATITIS

Key Facts

Terminology
- Acute inflammation of pancreas

Etiology/Pathogenesis
- Gallstone and alcoholic pancreatitis account for 70-80% of cases

Clinical Issues
- Abdominal pain
- Elevated serum amylase

Microscopic Pathology
- Severe acute pancreatitis
  - Large areas of fat necrosis along with variable parenchymal necrosis
  - Hemorrhage, vascular thrombosis
- Mild acute pancreatitis is most often a clinical diagnosis

Prognosis
- Mortality in USA ranges from 2-10%
  - Severe disease has higher mortality of 17%

Atlanta Classification
- Clinical classification; utility somewhat controversial
  - Mild (edematous and interstitial)
  - Severe (necrotizing)

MACROSCOPIC FEATURES

Mild Acute Pancreatitis
- Enlarged and swollen
- Foci of fat necrosis (yellow-white, waxy or chalky consistency)
- Hemorrhagic necrosis often absent

Severe Acute Pancreatitis
- Larger confluent areas of fat necrosis and parenchymal necrosis
- Hemorrhage can encase pancreas and simulate hematoma

MICROSCOPIC PATHOLOGY

Histologic Features
- Mild acute pancreatitis
  - Spotty peripancreatic or perilobular fat necrosis
  - Interstitial acute inflammation
  - Usually clinical rather than morphologic diagnosis
- Severe acute pancreatitis
  - Large areas of fat necrosis along with variable pancreatic parenchymal necrosis
    - Necrotic areas may have abundant neutrophils that can involve duct lumens
    - Viable acinar lumens may be widened and contain secretory material
    - Saponification
  - Fat necrosis may extend to omentum, retroperitoneum, bone marrow, subcutaneous tissue
  - Hemorrhage and usually venous thrombosis

DIFFERENTIAL DIAGNOSIS

Chronic Pancreatitis
- Fibrosis, chronic inflammation, lacks inflammatory component

SELECTED REFERENCES

1. Wu BU et al: Update in acute pancreatitis. Curr Gastroenterol Rep. 12(2):83-90, 2010
2. Bradley EL 3rd: A clinically based classification system for acute pancreatitis. Summary of the International Symposium on Acute Pancreatitis, Atlanta, Ga, September 11 through 13, 1992. Arch Surg. 128(5):586-90, 1993

IMAGE GALLERY

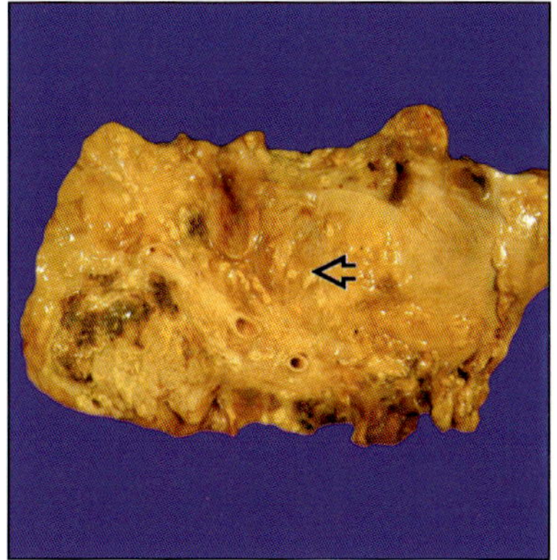

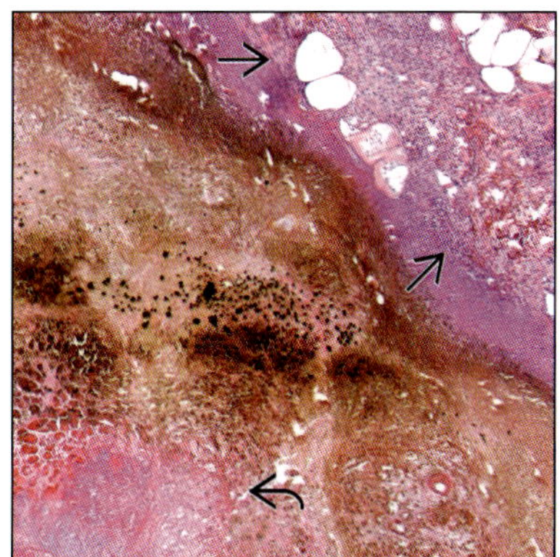

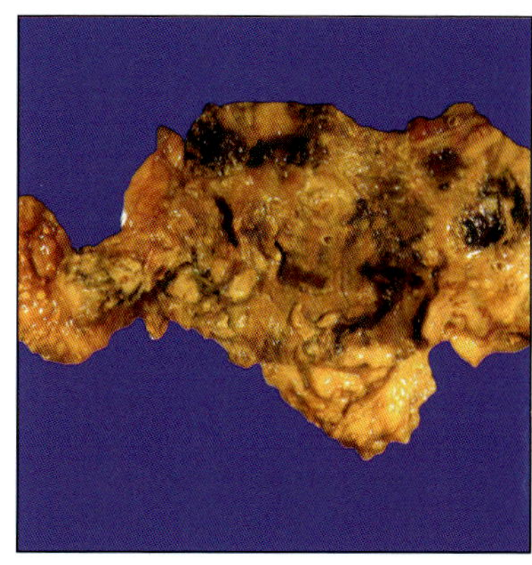

(Left) *This gross specimen shows areas of yellow-white, chalky fat necrosis ⇨.* ***(Center)*** *Trypsinogen activation is a key step in the development of acute pancreatitis. The release of digestive enzymes results in fat necrosis with acute inflammation → and pancreatic parenchymal necrosis ↗.* ***(Right)*** *Severe acute necrotizing pancreatitis shows necrosis and irregular, black foci of hemorrhage.*

CHRONIC PANCREATITIS

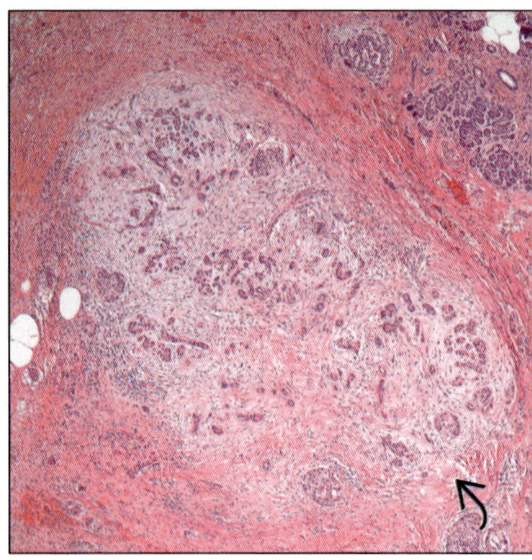

Hematoxylin and eosin demonstrates retention of the normal lobular architecture in chronic pancreatitis. The rounded configuration of the lobule ➚ is apparent at low power.

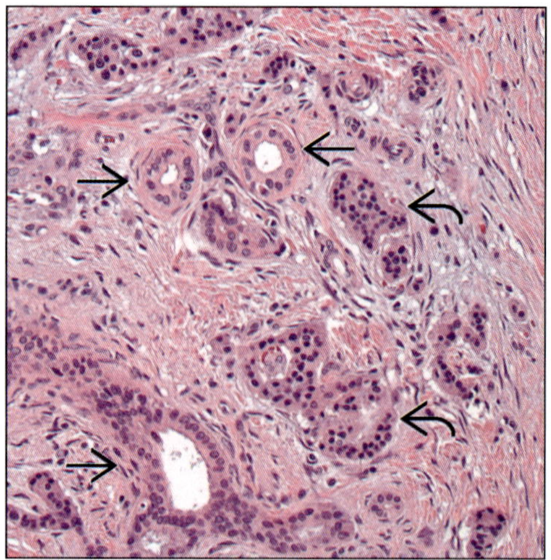

Hematoxylin and eosin demonstrates lobular arrangements of small ducts ➔, fibrous tissue, and residual islet cells ➚ in chronic pancreatitis. No residual acini are seen.

TERMINOLOGY

Abbreviations

- Chronic pancreatitis (CP)

Definitions

- Progressive inflammatory disorder of pancreas resulting in scarring, gland destruction, and functional impairment

ETIOLOGY/PATHOGENESIS

Alcoholic

- By far the most common cause of CP in developed countries

Anatomic

- Obstructive
  - Pancreatic duct obstruction leads to proximal duct dilatation, gland atrophy, and scarring
  - Obstruction may be due to stones or tumors involving head of pancreas
- Paraduodenal or "groove" pancreatitis

Metabolic

- Occurs in patients with hypercalcemia
- Hyperlipidemia is risk factor for CP

Hereditary

- Autosomal dominant form of pancreatitis
- Several associated gene mutations described
  - Trypsinogen gene (*PRSS1*)
  - Cystic fibrosis transmembrane conductance regulator gene (*CFTR*)
  - Serine protease inhibitor Kazal type 1 gene (*SPINK1*)
- Presents during childhood with recurrent attacks of acute pancreatitis
- Affected patients develop complications similar to those seen in alcohol-related CP but at younger age

Eosinophilic

- Rare form of chronic pancreatitis with prominent eosinophilic infiltrate
- May present as mass-forming process or with biliary obstruction
- Patients often have systemic process with blood eosinophilia and eosinophilias in other organs
- May occur as primary disease or with other processes
  - Parasitic infection
  - Allergic process or hypersensitivity reaction
  - Associated with pancreatic carcinoma or inflammatory myofibroblastic tumor
  - Pancreatic allograft rejection

Tropical

- Aggressive form of juvenile pancreatitis occurring in tropical developing countries
- May be related to malnutrition, toxin exposure, &/or genetic predisposition

Idiopathic

- Up to 25% of cases for which no cause can be identified

Other

- Miscellaneous forms related to trauma, radiation injury, or medications

CLINICAL ISSUES

Epidemiology

- Age
  - Alcohol-related CP usually affects adults > 40 years of age
  - Hereditary and tropical forms of CP present during childhood
- Gender
  - Alcohol-related CP is more common in males than in females

CHRONIC PANCREATITIS

Key Facts

Terminology
- Progressive inflammatory disorder of pancreas resulting in scarring, gland destruction, and functional impairment

Etiology/Pathogenesis
- Alcohol is by far the most common cause of CP in developed countries

Clinical Issues
- Chronic progressive disease leading to permanent loss of pancreatic function
- Steatorrhea
- Diabetes mellitus
- Weight loss

Macroscopic Features
- Grossly affected area should be thoroughly sampled to exclude pancreatic adenocarcinoma, which can mimic CP grossly

Microscopic Pathology
- Irregular atrophy and obliteration of pancreatic acini and ducts
- Variable extent and distribution of fibrosis
- Retention of normal lobular pancreatic architecture
- Pancreatic duct alterations related to fibrosis and destruction
- Islets of Langerhans usually preserved

Top Differential Diagnoses
- Pancreatic adenocarcinoma
- Autoimmune pancreatitis

Presentation
- Abdominal pain
  - Most common presenting symptom
- Steatorrhea
  - Associated with malabsorption due to impaired pancreatic enzyme secretion
- Diabetes mellitus
  - Occurs with advanced disease
- Weight loss
- Nausea
- Vomiting
- Often follows recurrent attacks of acute pancreatitis

Laboratory Tests
- May see elevated CA19-9

Natural History
- Chronic, progressive disease leading to permanent loss of pancreatic function
  - Loss of pancreatic enzyme secretions leads to malabsorption and steatorrhea
  - Pancreatic endocrine insufficiency
    - Diabetes more common in late disease
- Symptoms may wax and wane over course of disease
- Complications of advanced disease
  - Portal vein thrombosis
  - Splenic vein thrombosis
  - Jaundice
  - Pancreatic ascites
  - Pancreatic pseudocysts

Treatment
- Surgical approaches
  - Whipple pancreaticoduodenectomy
  - Pancreatic duct drainage procedure
  - Local or duodenum-preserving resection of pancreatic head
- Drugs
  - Pancreatic enzyme replacement aids intestinal absorption
- Pain management
  - Medical therapy
  - Celiac nerve block
- Diabetes treatment as needed with insulin and diet
- Dietary management
  - Low-fat meals
  - Frequent small meals may be better tolerated than less frequent, larger meals
- Stop offending agent (if identifiable)
  - Discontinue alcohol use
  - If obstructive CP, remove source of obstruction
    - Gallstones may be removed by endoscopic retrograde cholangiopancreatography (ERCP)
    - Sphincterotomy or balloon dilatation can relieve duct obstruction
    - Stent may be placed to maintain pancreatic duct opening

Prognosis
- CP is risk factor for pancreatic cancer
  - Lifetime risk varies
  - Patients with hereditary pancreatitis have 40% lifetime risk of pancreatic cancer

IMAGE FINDINGS

Ultrasonographic Findings
- Pancreatic stones evident

CT Findings
- Intrapancreatic calcifications

ERCP Findings
- Irregular, dilated pancreatic duct and branches
- May reveal source of obstructive pancreatitis

MACROSCOPIC FEATURES

General Features
- Findings may be diffuse, focal, or segmental
  - Usually, affected area is enlarged but may be shrunken in advanced CP
- Firm, indurated, and fibrotic pancreas
- Cystically dilated pancreatic ducts

- May contain calcified protein concretions
- Pseudocysts may be evident
  - Variably sized, thick-walled cysts containing blood and necrotic debris

Sections to Be Submitted

- Grossly affected area should be thoroughly sampled to exclude pancreatic adenocarcinoma, which can appear similar grossly

MICROSCOPIC PATHOLOGY

Histologic Features

- Irregular atrophy and obliteration of pancreatic acini and ducts
  - Results in overall loss of acinar tissue
- Retention of normal lobular pancreatic architecture
  - Rounded configuration of lobules is preserved
- Pancreatic duct alterations related to fibrosis and destruction
  - Results in duct ectasia and saccular dilatations
  - Duct epithelium may show atrophy, reactive, or hyperplastic changes
    - Reactive epithelial cells show mild nuclear enlargement
  - Ducts may show spectrum of reactive alterations or metaplasia
    - Squamous metaplasia
    - Mucous cell metaplasia
    - Pyloric gland metaplasia
- Variable extent and distribution of fibrosis
  - Occurs around ducts and within & between lobules
- Chronic inflammation usually mild
- Islets of Langerhans usually relatively well preserved
  - Islets may become lost or atrophic in advanced CP
  - May also show "pseudohyperplasia" as result of parenchymal loss

DIFFERENTIAL DIAGNOSIS

Pancreatic Adenocarcinoma

- Invasive growth pattern indicative of malignancy
  - Malignant glands demonstrate infiltrative growth pattern
    - In adenocarcinoma, glands are more irregularly distributed
  - CP retains lobular pancreatic architecture
  - Perineural invasion is feature of malignancy
  - Angiolymphatic space invasion
- Gland architecture more irregular in adenocarcinoma
  - In CP, glands are rounded or tubular with minimal branching
  - Individual malignant-appearing cells are feature of adenocarcinoma
    - Residual islet cells may appear singly and should not be overinterpreted as evidence of cancer
  - Necrotic debris may be seen in malignant glands but not in ducts in CP
- Cytologic features of malignancy are seen in adenocarcinoma
  - Nuclei are larger, more irregular, and more hyperchromatic in adenocarcinoma than in CP
  - Adenocarcinoma shows greater variation in nuclear size than does CP
  - Mitotic activity and atypical mitotic features are features of adenocarcinoma but not of CP
- Areas of CP are often present in association with pancreatic adenocarcinoma

Autoimmune Pancreatitis

- More densely cellular inflammatory infiltrates than CP
  - Periductal inflammation consisting of large numbers of lymphocytes and plasma cells
    - Inflammatory infiltrates associated with injury and destruction of duct epithelium
    - Plasma cells are IgG4 positive
  - Lymphoid follicles may be seen
  - Obliterative phlebitis of small to medium-sized veins
    - Present in most cases
    - Can be highlighted with elastic stain
- Serum IgG4 level elevated in most patients with autoimmune pancreatitis

DIAGNOSTIC CHECKLIST

Clinically Relevant Pathologic Features

- Most often associated with alcohol consumption
- Abdominal pain is most common presenting symptom

Pathologic Interpretation Pearls

- Dense parenchymal fibrosis may mimic neoplasm
- Lobular architecture aids histologic distinction from pancreatic adenocarcinoma

SELECTED REFERENCES

1. Whitcomb DC: Genetic aspects of pancreatitis. Annu Rev Med. 61:413-24, 2010
2. Gaisano HY et al: New insights into the mechanisms of pancreatitis. Gastroenterology. 136(7):2040-4, 2009
3. Klöppel G et al: Chronic pancreatitis and the differential diagnosis versus pancreatic cancer. Arch Pathol Lab Med. 133(3):382-7, 2009
4. Klöppel G: Chronic pancreatitis, pseudotumors and other tumor-like lesions. Mod Pathol. 20 Suppl 1:S113-31, 2007

CHRONIC PANCREATITIS

Microscopic Features

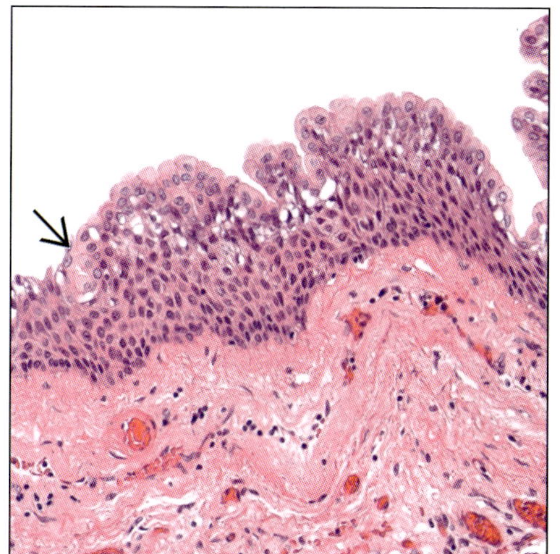
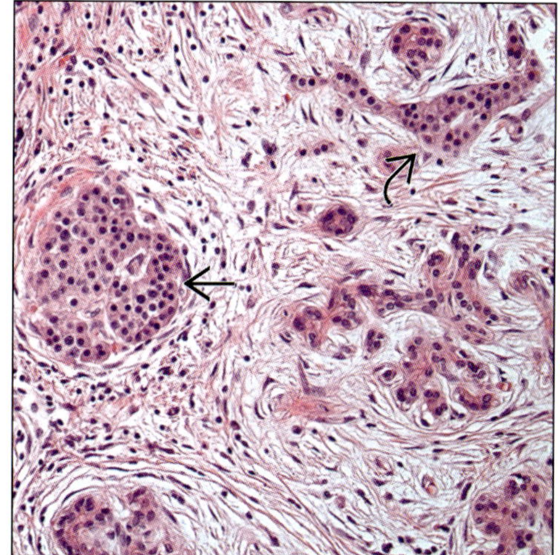

*(**Left**) Hematoxylin and eosin demonstrates a focus of squamous metaplasia → in a pancreatic duct in a patient with chronic pancreatitis. (**Right**) Hematoxylin and eosin demonstrates fibrosis surrounding small pancreatic duct branches ↗ and preserved islets of Langerhans →. No residual acini are seen.*

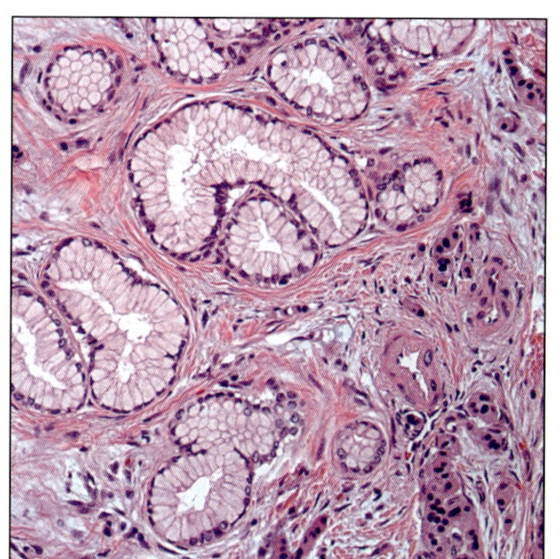
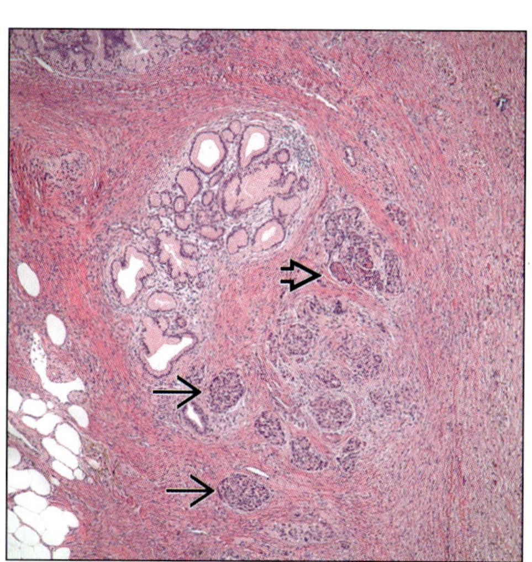

*(**Left**) Hematoxylin and eosin shows mucinous metaplasia in small pancreatic duct branches in a case of chronic pancreatitis. Islet cells are also seen. (**Right**) Hematoxylin and eosin demonstrates retention of the normal lobular architecture in chronic pancreatitis. Residual islets of Langerhans → are present, but there are only focal residual acini ⇨.*

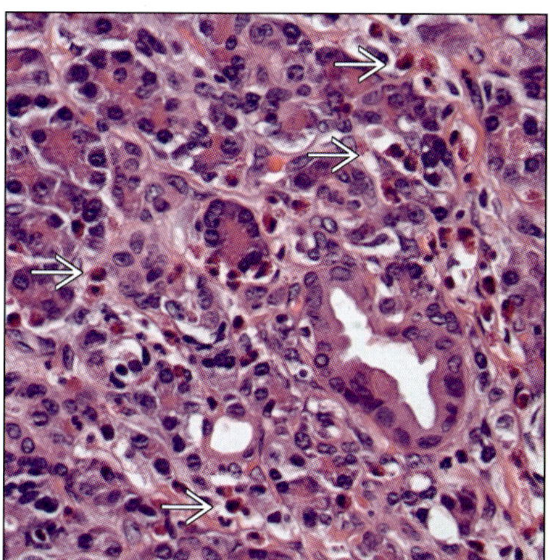
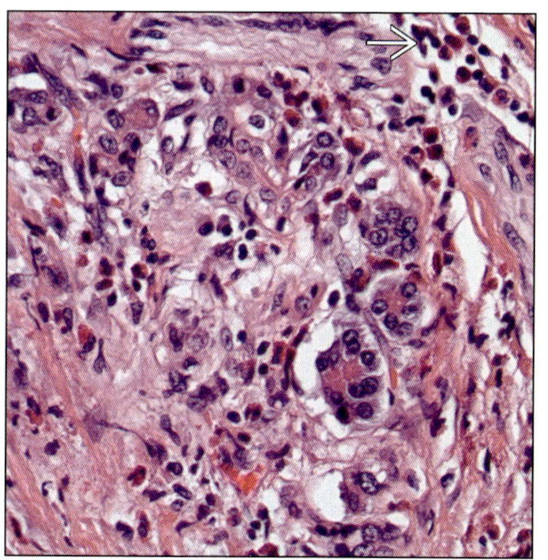

*(**Left**) Hematoxylin and eosin shows eosinophilic infiltrates ➡ and associated acinar injury in eosinophilic pancreatitis. (**Right**) Hematoxylin and eosin demonstrates eosinophilic infiltrates ➡ and acinar injury in eosinophilic pancreatitis.*

AUTOIMMUNE PANCREATITIS

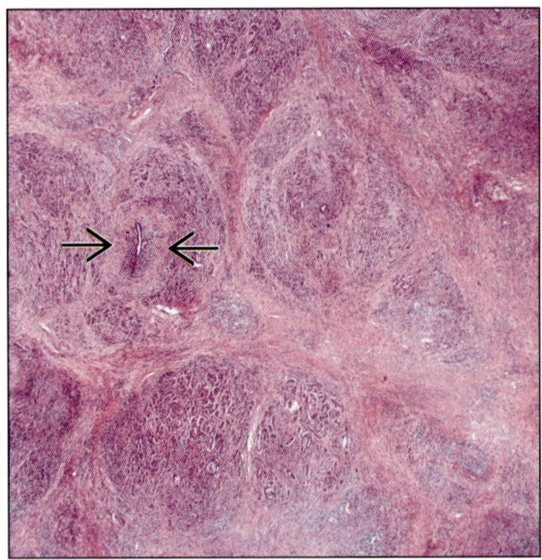

Hematoxylin & eosin section of lymphoplasmacytic sclerosing pancreatitis shows a prominent fibroinflammatory process with a periductal accentuation →.

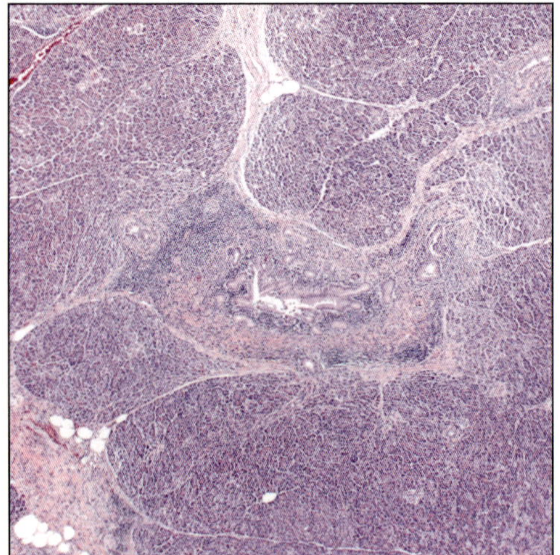

The fibroinflammatory process is limited to the periductal region, without significant lobular destruction or interlobular fibrosis, in idiopathic duct-centric chronic pancreatitis.

TERMINOLOGY

Abbreviations

- Autoimmune pancreatitis (AIP)

Synonyms

- Lymphoplasmacytic sclerosing pancreatitis (LPSP)
- Idiopathic duct-centric chronic pancreatitis (IDCP)
- Primary sclerosing pancreatitis
- Nonalcoholic duct destructive chronic pancreatitis

Definitions

- Fibroinflammatory disease of presumed autoimmune etiology that affects pancreas
  - Similar fibroinflammatory process often affects other organs such as bile ducts, salivary glands, retroperitoneum, and lymph nodes
  - Associated with many other autoimmune diseases
    - Specific antigenic trigger unknown

CLINICAL ISSUES

Presentation

- Jaundice
- Weight loss
- Vague abdominal pain

Laboratory Tests

- Elevated serum IgG4
- Elevated pancreatic enzymes
- ANA often positive

Treatment

- Surgical approaches
  - Surgically resected when differentiation from pancreatic cancer is difficult or impossible
- Drugs
  - Steroids

Prognosis

- Steroid therapy is usually very effective
  - Natural regression seen in some cases
  - Recurrence reported in 6-26%

IMAGE FINDINGS

General Features

- Diffusely or segmentally enlarged gland with delayed enhancement
- Segmental or diffuse, irregular duct with narrowing

MACROSCOPIC FEATURES

General Features

- Markedly firm, enlarged pancreas
  - Usually head is most prominently involved
- Discrete mass lesion variably present
- Stenosis of pancreatic duct and intrapancreatic common bile duct are common

MICROSCOPIC PATHOLOGY

Histologic Features

- Dense lymphoplasmacytic infiltration centered around main and interlobular pancreatic ducts
  - Smaller ducts more involved in advanced disease
- Infiltrate may compress lumen and cause infolding of epithelium
- Ductal epithelium may be detached &/or destroyed
- 2 main histologic types
  - **Lymphoplasmacytic sclerosing pancreatitis (LPSP)**
    - Marked lobular **and** interlobular fibroinflammatory process
    - Infiltrate is composed of plasma cells and eosinophils
    - Venulitis and obliterative phlebitis

AUTOIMMUNE PANCREATITIS

Key Facts

Terminology
- Fibroinflammatory disease of presumed autoimmune etiology that affects pancreas
  - Often elevated serum IgG4
  - Similar fibroinflammatory process often affects other organs such as bile ducts, salivary glands, retroperitoneum, and lymph nodes
  - Associated with many other autoimmune diseases

Image Findings
- Diffusely enlarged gland
- Delayed (rim) enhancement
- Attenuated, irregular main pancreatic duct

Macroscopic Features
- Enlarged, firm pancreas
- Variably present mass lesion
- May mimic adenocarcinoma

Microscopic Pathology
- Dense lymphoplasmacytic infiltration centered around main and interlobular pancreatic ducts
- Periductal, lobular, and perilobular fibrosis
- Obliterative phlebitis and venulitis
- Granulocytic epithelial lesions
- IgG4(+) plasma cells

Top Differential Diagnoses
- Pancreatic cancer
- Other forms of chronic pancreatitis

    - Lymphoid aggregates with variably present germinal centers
    - Process often extends into peripancreatic tissue
    - Numerous IgG4(+) plasma cells (on average > 10/HPF)
  - **Idiopathic duct-centric chronic pancreatitis (IDCP)**
    - Fibroinflammatory process has duct-centric distribution
    - Minimal intralobular fibroblastic proliferation
    - Granulocytic epithelial lesions are frequent, consisting of neutrophilic exocytosis, microabscesses, and ductular destruction with reactive epithelial changes
    - Only rare IgG4 positive plasma cells

Predominant Pattern/Injury Type
- Inflammatory, chronic

Predominant Cell/Compartment Type
- Plasma cell

DIFFERENTIAL DIAGNOSIS

Pancreatic Adenocarcinoma
- Firm, enlarged pancreas with stenotic ducts can mimic adenocarcinoma grossly and radiographically
- Histology usually resolves differential diagnosis

Inflammatory Myofibroblastic Tumor (IMT)
- IMT is ALK1 positive
- Serum IgG4 not elevated

Alcohol-related Chronic Pancreatitis
- Diffuse and intralobular fibrosis, granulocytes rare in alcohol-related chronic pancreatitis
- Serum IgG4 not elevated

Chronic Obstructive Pancreatitis
- Periductal fibrosis rare, no granulocytes
- Serum IgG4 not elevated

DIAGNOSTIC CHECKLIST

Clinically Relevant Pathologic Features
- Often mimics pancreatic adenocarcinoma clinically and radiographically
- Associated with IgG4

Pathologic Interpretation Pearls
- Duct-centric pattern of lymphoplasmacytic inflammation, fibrosis
- Venulitis/phlebitis

SELECTED REFERENCES

1. Sahani DV et al: Autoimmune pancreatitis: disease evolution, staging, response assessment, and CT features that predict response to corticosteroid therapy. Radiology. 250(1):118-29, 2009
2. Sepehr A et al: IgG4+ to IgG+ plasma cells ratio of ampulla can help differentiate autoimmune pancreatitis from other "mass forming" pancreatic lesions. Am J Surg Pathol. 32(12):1770-9, 2008
3. Deshpande V et al: Autoimmune pancreatitis: a systemic immune complex mediated disease. Am J Surg Pathol. 2006 Dec;30(12):1537-45. Erratum in: Am J Surg Pathol. 31(2):328, 2007
4. Chari ST et al: Diagnosis of autoimmune pancreatitis: the Mayo Clinic experience. Clin Gastroenterol Hepatol. 4(8):1010-6; quiz 934, 2006
5. Finkelberg DL et al: Autoimmune pancreatitis. N Engl J Med. 355(25):2670-6, 2006
6. Deshpande V et al: Autoimmune pancreatitis: more than just a pancreatic disease? A contemporary review of its pathology. Arch Pathol Lab Med. 129(9):1148-54, 2005
7. Mino-Kenudson M et al: Histopathology of autoimmune pancreatitis: recognized features and unsolved issues. J Gastrointest Surg. 9(1):6-10, 2005
8. Zamboni G et al: Histopathological features of diagnostic and clinical relevance in autoimmune pancreatitis: a study on 53 resection specimens and 9 biopsy specimens. Virchows Arch. 445(6):552-63, 2004
9. Notohara K et al: Idiopathic chronic pancreatitis with periductal lymphoplasmacytic infiltration: clinicopathologic features of 35 cases. Am J Surg Pathol. 27(8):1119-27, 2003

AUTOIMMUNE PANCREATITIS

Microscopic Features

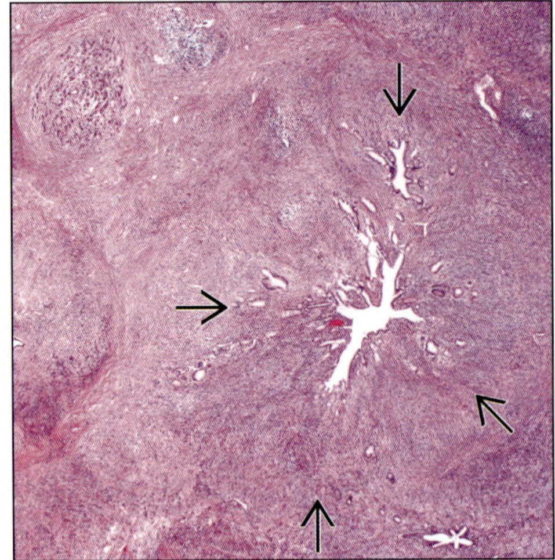

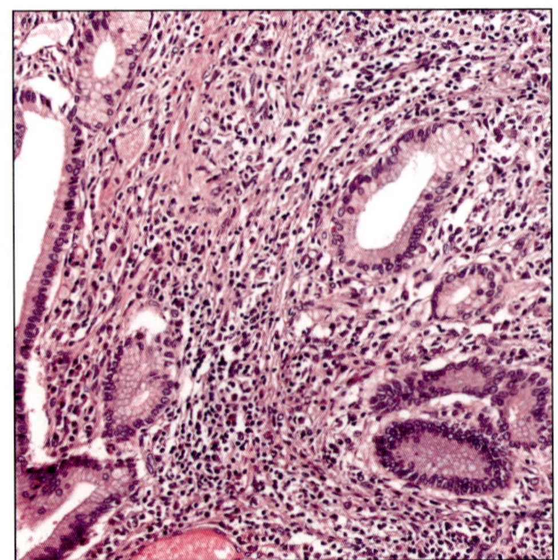

(Left) *Hematoxylin & eosin section of lymphoplasmacytic sclerosing pancreatitis shows marked chronic inflammation involving the periductal stroma* ⇒. ***(Right)*** *Hematoxylin & eosin section of lymphoplasmacytic sclerosing pancreatitis illustrates that the inflammatory component consists of lymphocytes, numerous plasma cells, and eosinophils.*

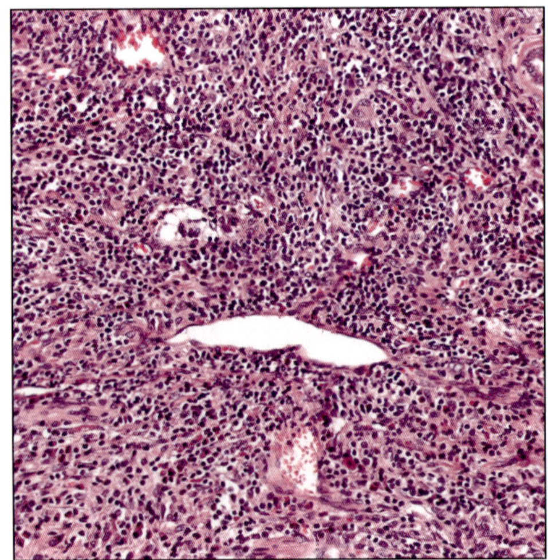

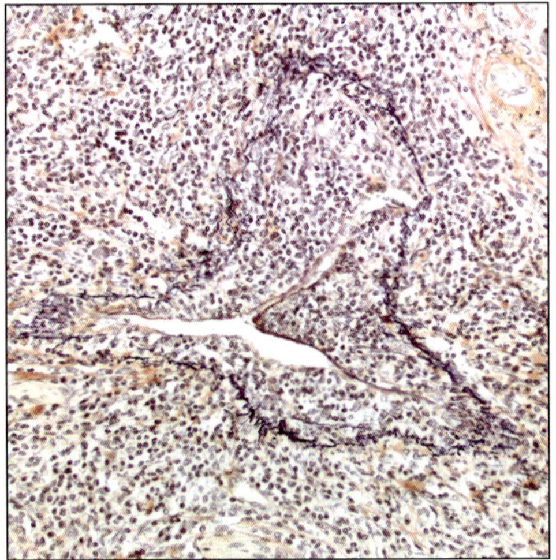

(Left) *Hematoxylin & eosin section of obliterative phlebitis shows marked lymphoplasmacytic infiltration that partially obliterates a vein.* ***(Right)*** *An elastic stain highlights a partially obliterated vein in lymphoplasmacytic sclerosing pancreatitis; obliterative phlebitis.*

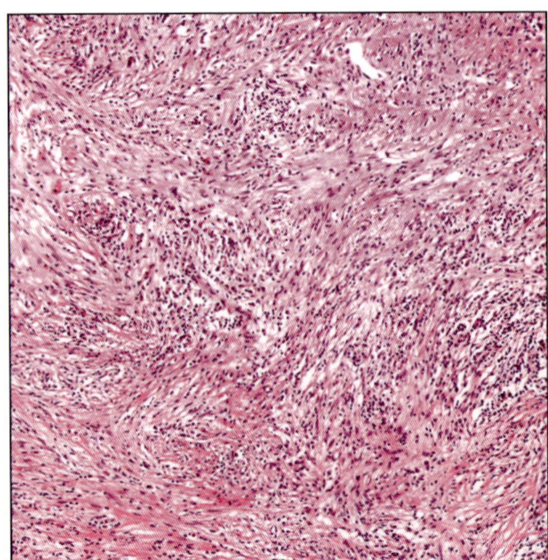

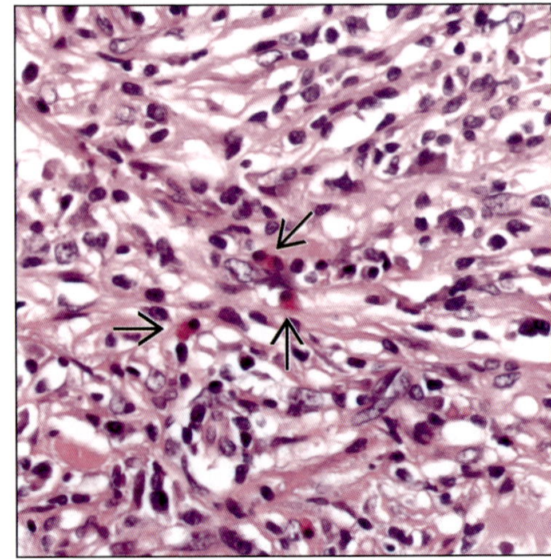

(Left) *Hematoxylin & eosin section of lymphoplasmacytic sclerosing pancreatitis shows that interlobular stroma is replaced by a storiform pattern of fibrosis.* ***(Right)*** *Chronic inflammatory cells, including eosinophils* ⇒*, are seen in the storiform fibrosis.*

Microscopic Features

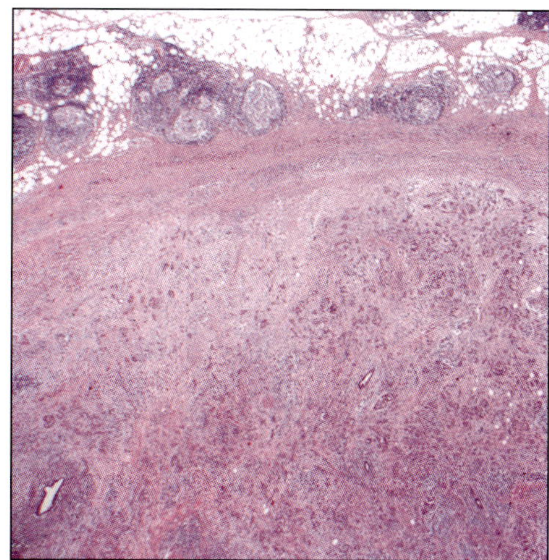

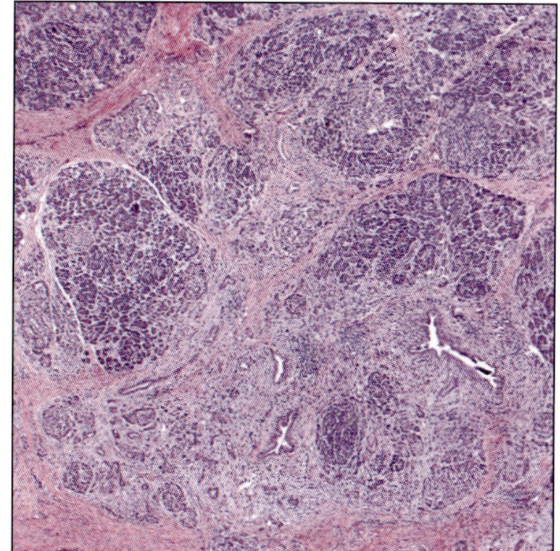

(Left) *The fibroinflammatory process extends into the peripancreatic soft tissue, with lymphoid follicle formation, in lymphoplasmacytic sclerosing pancreatitis.* ***(Right)*** *In comparison with LPSP, destruction of lobules is less prominent in this example of idiopathic duct-centric chronic pancreatitis. Marked edema may be seen within lobules &/or the perilobular interstitium.*

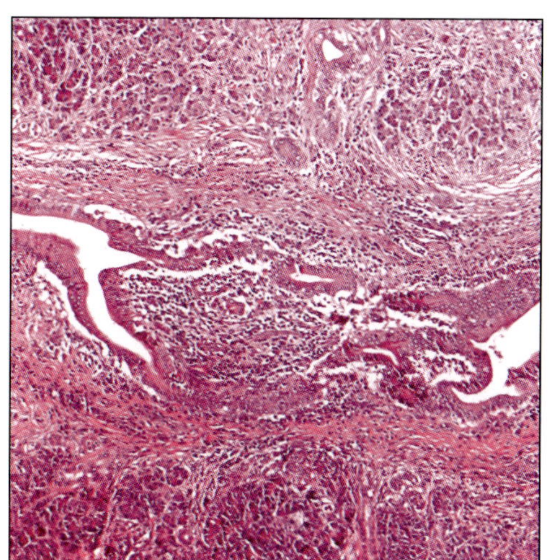

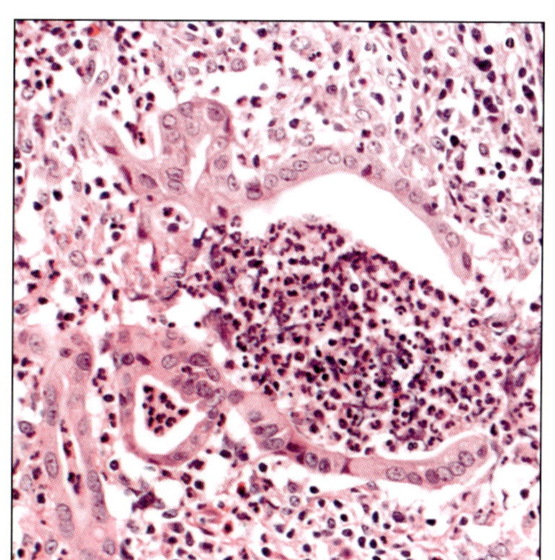

(Left) *An interlobular duct is distorted and stenotic due to marked inflammation and reactive epithelial changes in idiopathic duct-centric chronic pancreatitis.* ***(Right)*** *Numerous neutrophils infiltrate duct epithelium and fill duct lumens, with destruction of epithelium and reactive epithelial atypia, in idiopathic duct-centric chronic pancreatitis. This is known as a granulocytic epithelial lesion (GEL).*

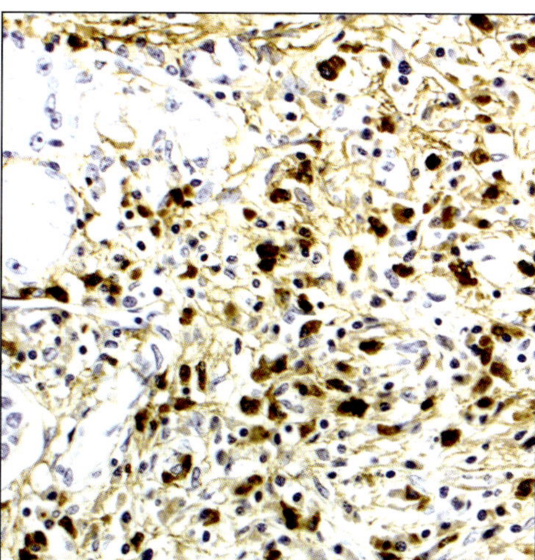

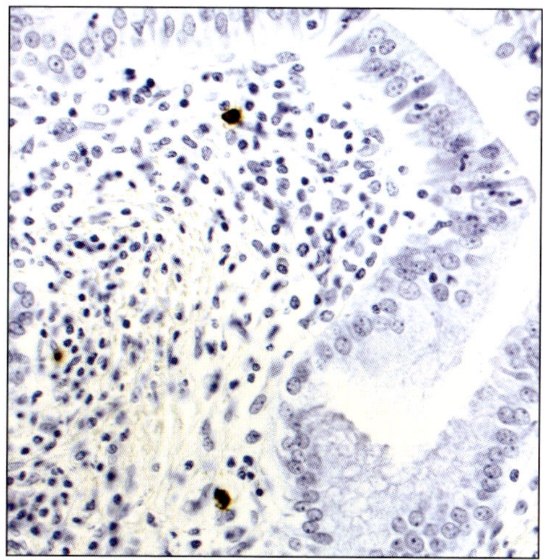

(Left) *IgG4 stain in lymphoplasmacytic sclerosing pancreatitis shows a large number of IgG4(+) plasma cells (> 10/HPF) in the periductal stroma.* ***(Right)*** *IgG4 stain in idiopathic duct-centric sclerosing pancreatitis shows that IgG4(+) cells are scant.*

GROOVE PANCREATITIS

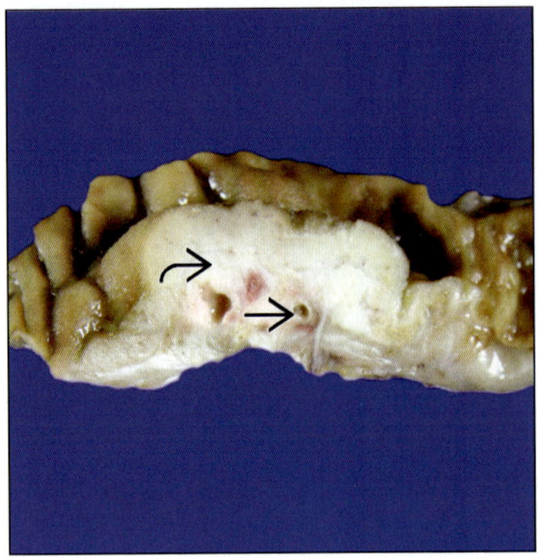

Gross photograph of a pancreaticoduodenectomy specimen shows a mass-like lesion beneath the duodenal mucosa ➚. Note the paraduodenal zone of fibrosis with numerous small cysts ➔.

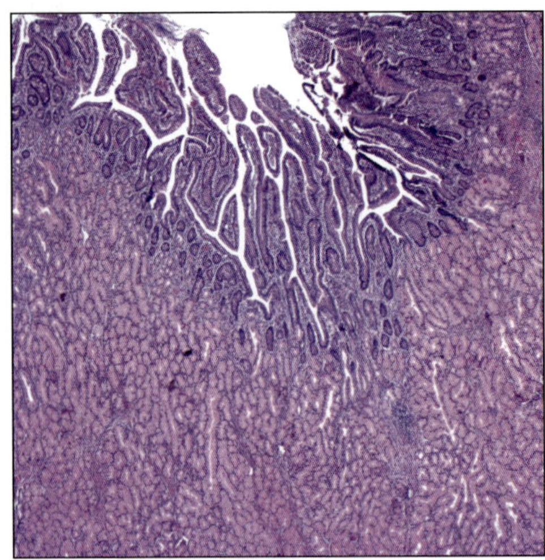

Prominent Brunner gland hyperplasia in the region of the minor ampulla frequently accompanies groove pancreatitis.

TERMINOLOGY

Synonyms

- Paraduodenal pancreatitis
- Cystic dystrophy of heterotopic pancreas
- Paraduodenal wall cyst
- Pancreatic hamartoma of duodenum
- Myoadenomatosis

Definitions

- Distinct form of pancreatitis that results in fibrosis of paraduodenal region in vicinity of minor ampulla

ETIOLOGY/PATHOGENESIS

Combination of Factors

- Developmental anomalies and environmental exposure
  - Anatomical/functional variations in region of minor papilla, such as pancreatic divisum, predispose to development of groove pancreatitis
  - History of alcohol abuse is common
  - Likely that disease develops in individuals with anomalies of minor ampulla, conceivably leading to outflow obstruction, with alcohol as precipitating factor

CLINICAL ISSUES

Epidemiology

- Incidence
  - Uncommon
- Age
  - Middle age
- Gender
  - Predominantly male

Presentation

- Abdominal pain
- Vomiting caused by stenosis of duodenum
- Weight loss
- Jaundice rare

Treatment

- Surgical approaches
  - Whipple resection may be required to exclude malignancy
- Conservative medical treatment in majority of cases

IMAGE FINDINGS

Ultrasonographic Findings

- Hypoechoic area is seen between duodenal wall and pancreatic parenchyma on endoscopic ultrasound
  - Narrowing of duodenal wall &/or common bile duct may be seen

CT Findings

- Hypodense lesion between pancreatic head and duodenum
- Variably present, cyst-like changes in duodenal wall or groove area

MACROSCOPIC FEATURES

General Features

- Changes are centered around minor papilla and involve "groove" between pancreas and duodenum
- Thickening and fibrosis of duodenum and paraduodenal pancreas may be mistaken for pancreatic carcinoma
- Approximately 1/2 of lesions are cystic, and some may mimic pancreatic cystic neoplasm

GROOVE PANCREATITIS

Key Facts

Etiology/Pathogenesis
- Disease develops in individuals with anomalies of minor ampulla
  - Alcohol is a precipitating factor

Clinical Issues
- Whipple resection may be required to exclude malignancy

Macroscopic Features
- Thickening and fibrosis of duodenum wall and paraduodenal pancreas with cyst formation; may mimic pancreatic neoplasm

Microscopic Pathology
- Duodenal wall around minor ampulla is thickened with marked fibrosis involving muscular propria and adjacent head of pancreas
  - Cysts are lined by granulation tissue

MICROSCOPIC PATHOLOGY

Histologic Features
- Duodenal wall around minor ampulla is thickened with marked fibrosis involving muscular propria
- Fibrosis extends into head of pancreas and may involve common bile duct
- Duodenal fibrosis is frequently accompanied by cyst formation
  - Cysts are lined by inflammatory granulation tissue
- Brunner gland hyperplasia is commonly seen
- Nonparaduodenal pancreas frequently shows dilated ducts with inspissated secretions and prominent interlobular fibrosis

DIFFERENTIAL DIAGNOSIS

Chronic Pancreatitis, Alcohol-related
- Alcohol-related pancreatitis diffusely involves pancreas and lacks duodenal wall changes that are characteristic of groove pancreatitis

Autoimmune Pancreatitis
- Lacks paraduodenal accentuation of groove pancreatitis
- Periductal inflammation, obliterative phlebitis, and storiform fibroinflammatory proliferation are characteristic of autoimmune pancreatitis
  - Either entirely absent or only focally seen in groove pancreatitis
- Elevated numbers of IgG4(+) plasma cells (> 10/HPF) are invariably seen in autoimmune pancreatitis

Pancreatic Adenocarcinoma
- Clinically and radiologically, groove pancreatitis may be indistinguishable from pancreatic carcinoma
  - Histologically, lack of malignancy is obvious
  - Although occasional reactive and entrapped ducts may appear worrisome

SELECTED REFERENCES

1. de Tejada AH et al: Endoscopic and EUS features of groove pancreatitis masquerading as a pancreatic neoplasm. Gastrointest Endosc. 68(4):796-8, 2008
2. Klöppel G: Chronic pancreatitis, pseudotumors and other tumor-like lesions. Mod Pathol. 20 Suppl 1:S113-31, 2007
3. Adsay NV et al: Paraduodenal pancreatitis: a clinico-pathologically distinct entity unifying "cystic dystrophy of heterotopic pancreas", "para-duodenal wall cyst", and "groove pancreatitis". Semin Diagn Pathol. 21(4):247-54, 2004

IMAGE GALLERY

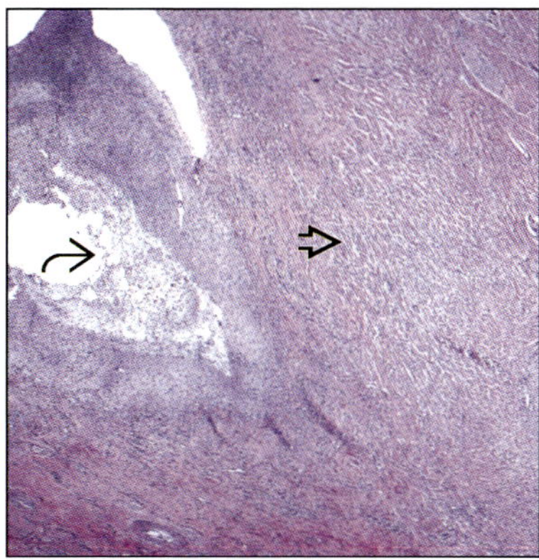

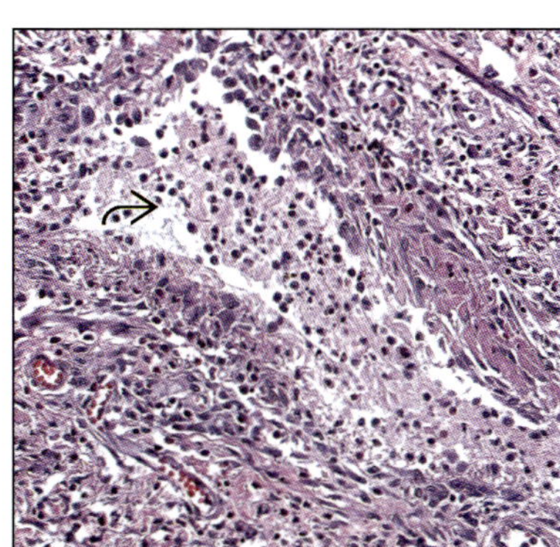

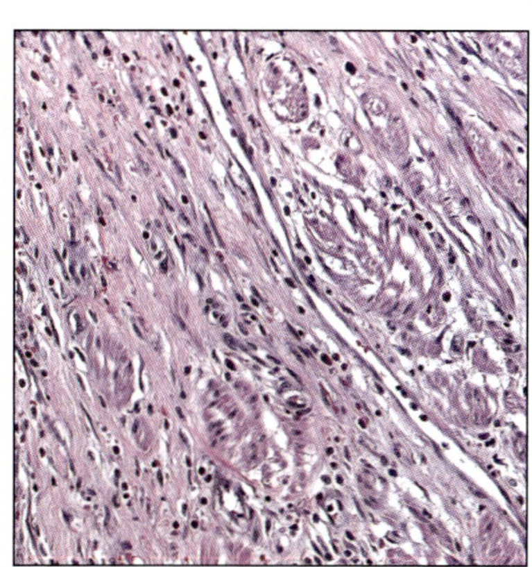

(Left) *Paraduodenal cyst ➔ is seen lined by inflammation and granulation tissue. The paraduodenal "mass" is composed predominantly of a thickened muscularis propria with severe fibrosis ⇨.* ***(Center)*** *Cyst formation ➔ is frequently seen in groove pancreatitis, accounting for one of the plethora of names used for this entity, "paraduodenal wall cyst."* ***(Right)*** *High-power view of groove pancreatitis shows exuberant fibrosis within the muscularis propria.*

INFECTIOUS PANCREATITIS

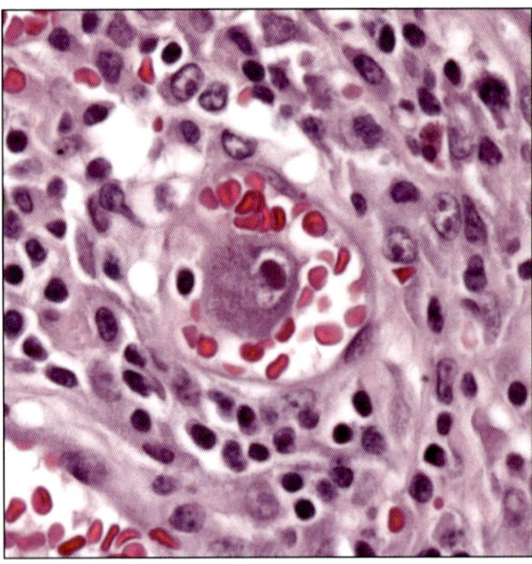

CMV infection of the pancreas is most often seen in immunocompromised patients, especially AIDS patients.

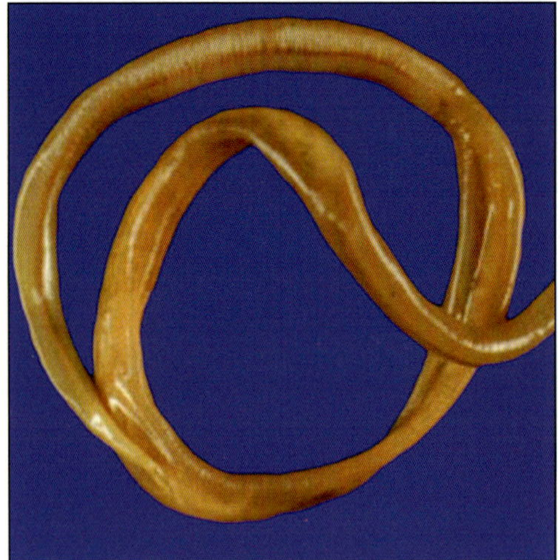

Ascaris lumbricoides can migrate into the pancreatic duct, causing an obstructive pancreatitis.

TERMINOLOGY

Definitions

- Primary infection of pancreas by virus, bacteria, fungus, or parasite
  - Rare
  - Pancreatic involvement is usually not significant in overall context of systemic infection
    - Exception is mumps, which can cause severe pancreatitis
  - Acute bacterial infection of pancreas is usually a secondary event
    - Occurs in 40-70% of patients with necrotizing pancreatitis
    - Usually due to Gram-negative aerobic bacteria

ETIOLOGY/PATHOGENESIS

Infectious Agents

- Viruses
  - Mumps
  - Coxsackievirus B
  - Cytomegalovirus
    - Usually seen in context of immunosuppression (AIDS or other causes) and in neonates
  - EBV
  - Rubella
  - Arbovirus
  - Fulminant hepatitis B
- Parasites
  - *Toxoplasma gondii*
  - *Clonorchis*
    - Migrates to pancreas from liver in about 1/3 of hepatic clonorchiasis cases
  - *Ascaris*
    - Can migrate into pancreatic duct, causing acute obstruction
  - *Echinococcus*
    - Very rare cause of pancreatitis
    - Hydatid cysts rupture in pancreas, leading to inflammation
- Bacteria
  - *Treponema pallidum* (syphilis)
  - *M. tuberculosis*
    - Pancreatic tuberculosis is rare but reported
  - *Leptospira* species (leptospirosis)
- Fungi
  - *Candida*
  - *Aspergillus*

CLINICAL ISSUES

Presentation

- Depends on specific infectious agent
- Patients with viral infections may have prodrome of diarrhea

Laboratory Tests

- Serologies, blood cultures, molecular tests for specific infectious organisms may be useful

Treatment

- Depends on specific infection

Prognosis

- Depends on specific infection
  - Pancreatic involvement is usually mild in cases of systemic infection
    - Mumps can cause severe pancreatitis
    - Abscesses, bacterial superinfection, and parenchymal atrophy are complications of echinococcal infection of pancreas

MACROSCOPIC FEATURES

General Features

- Gross findings are not well described

INFECTIOUS PANCREATITIS

Key Facts

Terminology
- Primary infection of pancreas
- Pancreatic involvement is usually not significant in context of systemic infection

Etiology/Pathogenesis
- May be caused by viruses, parasites, bacteria, and fungi

Microscopic Pathology
- Gross and histologic findings are not well described

Diagnostic Checklist
- Very rare cause of acute pancreatitis, but infection should be considered in immunocompromised patients with pancreatitis

MICROSCOPIC PATHOLOGY

Histologic Features
- Histologic findings are not well described in general
  - Spotty acinar or ductal cell death, without fat necrosis or ductal necrosis, has been described in cases of viral pancreatitis and some bacterial infections
- Viral inclusions, parasites, fungi, or bacteria may be seen in some cases

DIFFERENTIAL DIAGNOSIS

Other Causes of Acute Pancreatitis
- Alcohol
- Gallstones
- Hyperlipidemia
- Drugs
- Anatomic abnormalities
- Neoplasms

DIAGNOSTIC CHECKLIST

Clinically Relevant Pathologic Features
- Clinical signs and symptoms of specific infections may be helpful in making diagnosis of infectious pancreatitis

Pathologic Interpretation Pearls
- Very rare, but infection should be considered in immunocompromised patients with pancreatitis

SELECTED REFERENCES

1. Safioleas MC et al: Clinical considerations of primary hydatid disease of the pancreas. Pancreatology. 5(4-5):457-61, 2005
2. Dalamaga M et al: Leptospirosis presenting as acute pancreatitis and cholecystitis. J Med. 35(1-6):181-5, 2004
3. Dhall JC et al: Tuberculosis of the pancreas: a clinical rarity. Am J Gastroenterol. 92(1):172, 1997
4. Parenti DM et al: Infectious causes of acute pancreatitis. Pancreas. 13(4):356-71, 1996
5. Wilcox CM et al: Cytomegalovirus-associated acute pancreatic disease in patients with acquired immunodeficiency syndrome. Report of two patients. Gastroenterology. 99(1):263-7, 1990
6. Joe L et al: Severe pancreatitis in an AIDS patient in association with cytomegalovirus infection. South Med J. 82(11):1444-5, 1989
7. Renner IG et al: Death due to acute pancreatitis. A retrospective analysis of 405 autopsy cases. Dig Dis Sci. 30(10):1005-18, 1985
8. Imrie CW et al: Coxsackie and mumpsvirus infection in a prospective study of acute pancreatitis. Gut. 18(1):53-6, 1977

IMAGE GALLERY

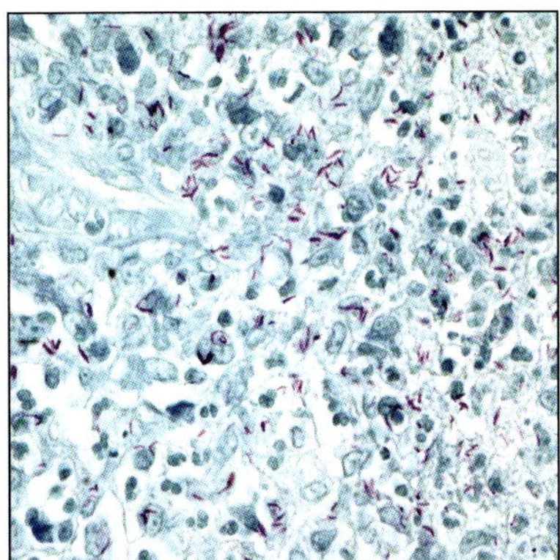
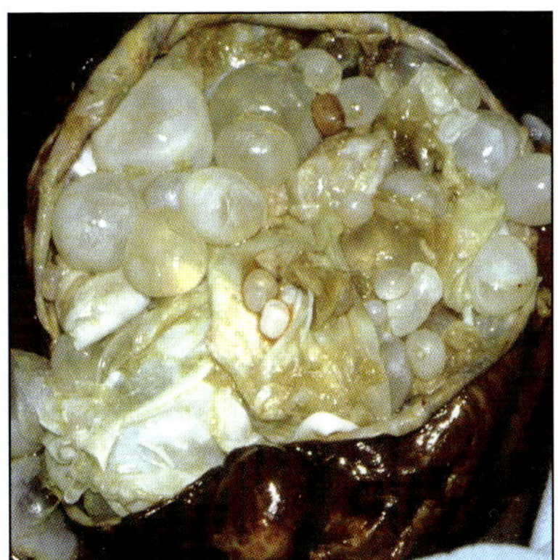
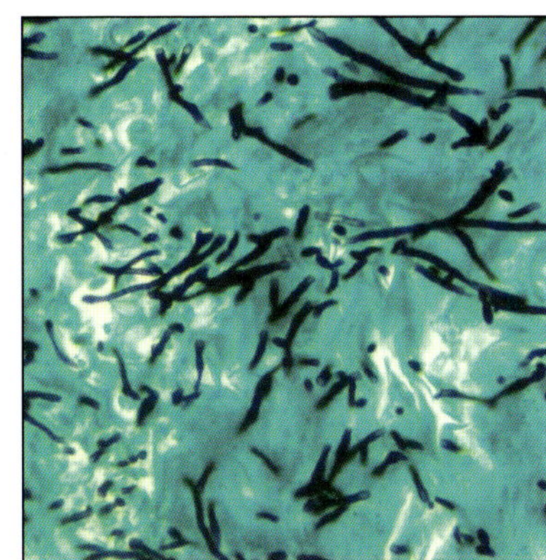

(Left) *M. tuberculosis infection of the pancreas is rare, even in miliary disease.* ***(Center)*** *Acute pancreatitis can follow rupture of a hepatic hydatid cyst into the bile ducts with secondary obstruction of the pancreatic ducts. Rarely, Echinococcus causes primary pancreatic infection.* ***(Right)*** *The pancreas can be involved in systemic candidiasis, or Candida species can superinfect acute necrotizing pancreatitis.*

PSEUDOCYSTS

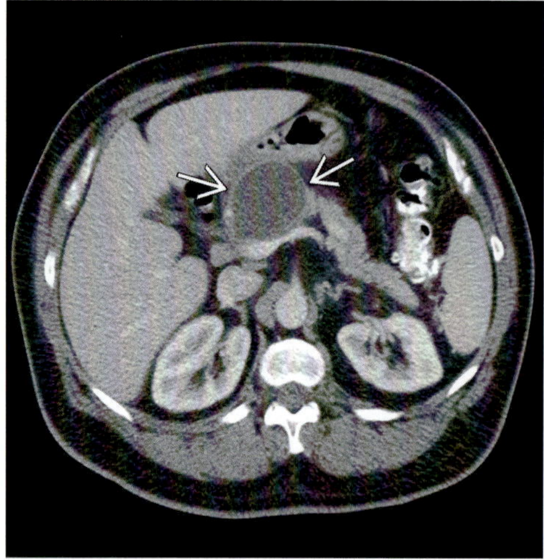

CT image shows a pancreatic pseudocyst ➡. A unilocular cyst is located in the head of the pancreas.

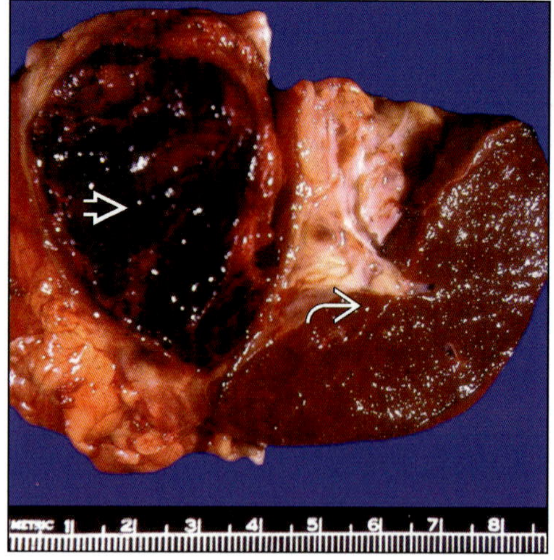

Gross photograph shows a pseudocyst in the tail of the pancreas ➡. The cyst is filled with hemorrhagic fluid. Note the adjacent spleen ➡.

TERMINOLOGY

Definitions

- Pancreatic or peripancreatic collection of fluid rich in pancreatic enzymes

ETIOLOGY/PATHOGENESIS

Risk Factors

- Most common: Acute pancreatitis
- Certain surgical procedures, such as gastrectomy
- Rarely, pseudocyst may develop adjacent to pancreatic mass lesion, including adenocarcinoma

CLINICAL ISSUES

Epidemiology

- Incidence
  - Historically, pseudocysts make up approximately 75% of all pancreatic cysts
  - Increased detection of pancreatic cysts by imaging, often incidentally, has significantly decreased the overall incidence of pseudocysts
- Age
  - Middle age
- Gender
  - Female predominance associated with gallstone-related pancreatitis
  - Male predominance associated with alcohol-related pancreatitis

Presentation

- Abdominal pain
- Established history of acute pancreatitis
  - Clinically, in absence of this history, distinction of pseudocyst from neoplastic cyst is often difficult

Treatment

- Spontaneous resolution is frequent
- Endoscopic, percutaneous drainage or surgical drainage may be necessary

IMAGE FINDINGS

Radiographic Findings

- Unilocular cyst without septations or mural nodule
- Atrophy of background pancreas with calcification is frequently found

MACROSCOPIC FEATURES

General Features

- Unilocular cyst with thick fibrous wall

Sections to Be Submitted

- Histological evaluation of entire cyst wall is required

Size

- Few cm to > 20 cm

MICROSCOPIC PATHOLOGY

Histologic Features

- Wall is composed of granulation tissue and fibrosis
- Lining epithelium is not seen
- Hemosiderin and blood pigments are frequently seen in lumen and wall
- In individuals with alcohol abuse, background pancreas will frequently show acinar atrophy, dense interlobular fibrosis, and dilated pancreatic ducts filled with proteinaceous material

Predominant Pattern/Injury Type

- Cystic

Predominant Cell/Compartment Type

- Inflammatory

PSEUDOCYSTS

Key Facts

Terminology

- Pancreatic or peripancreatic collection of fluid rich in pancreatic enzymes

Etiology/Pathogenesis

- Occurrence parallels that of pancreatitis
- Alcoholic abuse is leading cause

Macroscopic Features

- Histological evaluation of entire cyst wall is required

Microscopic Pathology

- Lining epithelium is not seen

Top Differential Diagnoses

- Intraductal papillary-mucinous neoplasm & mucinous cystic neoplasm
- Unilocular serous cystadenoma

DIFFERENTIAL DIAGNOSIS

Intraductal Papillary-Mucinous Neoplasm & Mucinous Cystic Neoplasm

- Absence of lining epithelium is key to diagnosis of pseudocyst
- Both intraductal papillary-mucinous neoplasm and mucinous cystic neoplasm are lined by mucinous epithelium, at least focally
  - Presence of ovarian-type stroma supports diagnosis of mucinous cystic neoplasm
- On fluid analysis, pseudocysts show elevated levels of amylase (> 250 IU/mL) and low levels of CEA (< 100 ng/mL)
  - Elevated cyst fluid CEA is strongly suggestive of mucinous neoplasm

Other Cystic Tumors

- Serous cystadenoma, solid pseudopapillary tumor, and cystic variant of pancreatic endocrine neoplasm
  - Unilocular serous cystadenomas may be largely denuded of neoplastic cells and mimic pseudocyst
  - Solid pseudopapillary tumors and pancreatic endocrine neoplasms show monotonous round neoplastic cells within cyst

Pseudocyst Adjacent to Pancreatic Neoplasms

- Pancreatic ductal adenocarcinomas can rarely show extensive cystification
- Invasive carcinoma is generally easily recognized within grossly identifiable nodule adjacent to pseudocyst

DIAGNOSTIC CHECKLIST

Clinically Relevant Pathologic Features

- Cystic lesion in background of pancreatitis

Pathologic Interpretation Pearls

- Pseudocysts lack epithelial lining
- Entire cyst wall should be examined histologically before diagnosis of pseudocyst is rendered

SELECTED REFERENCES

1. Basturk O et al: Pancreatic cysts: pathologic classification, differential diagnosis, and clinical implications. Arch Pathol Lab Med. 133(3):423-38, 2009
2. Habashi S et al: Pancreatic pseudocyst. World J Gastroenterol. 15(1):38-47, 2009
3. Kosmahl M et al: Pancreatic ductal adenocarcinomas with cystic features: neither rare nor uniform. Mod Pathol. 18(9):1157-64, 2005
4. Brugge WR et al: Diagnosis of pancreatic cystic neoplasms: a report of the cooperative pancreatic cyst study. Gastroenterology. 126(5):1330-6, 2004
5. Klöppel G: Pseudocysts and other non-neoplastic cysts of the pancreas. Semin Diagn Pathol. 17(1):7-15, 2000
6. Klöppel G et al: Pseudocysts in chronic pancreatitis: a morphological analysis of 57 resection specimens and 9 autopsy pancreata. Pancreas. 6(3):266-74, 1991

IMAGE GALLERY

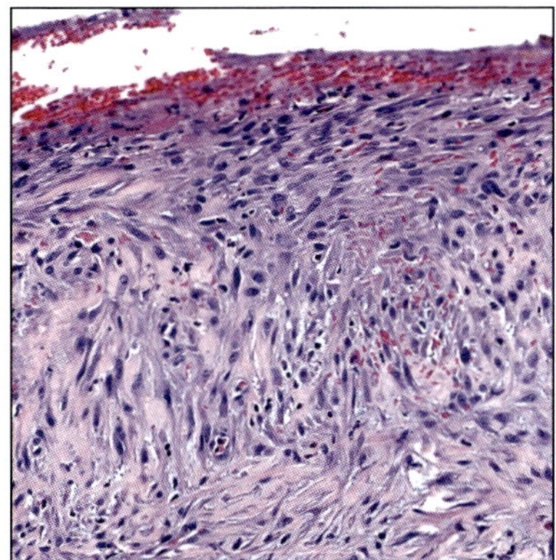

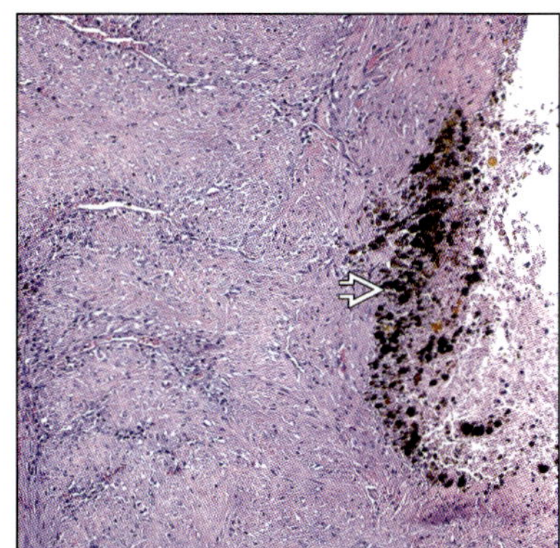

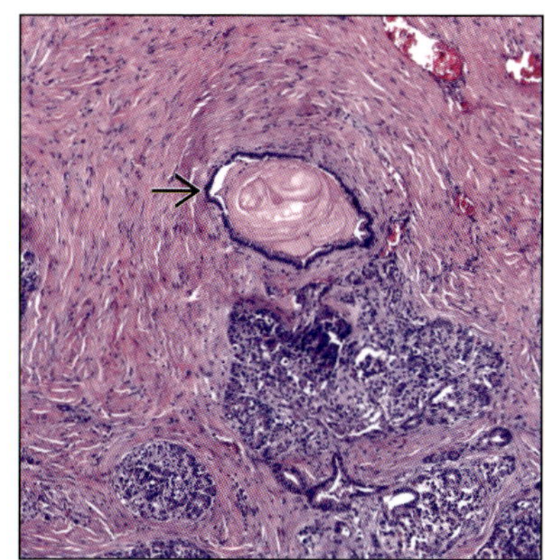

(Left) *Pseudocysts lack a true lining epithelium. The cyst wall shows an exuberant fibroblastic proliferation.* ***(Center)*** *Cyst wall is composed of fibrosis and few scattered inflammatory cells. Note the hemosiderin ⇒ in the lumen of the cyst.* ***(Right)*** *Alcohol-related chronic pancreatitis shows marked interlobular fibrosis, atrophy of the acinar tissue, and a dilated duct → filled with eosinophilic proteinaceous material.*

DIABETES MELLITUS

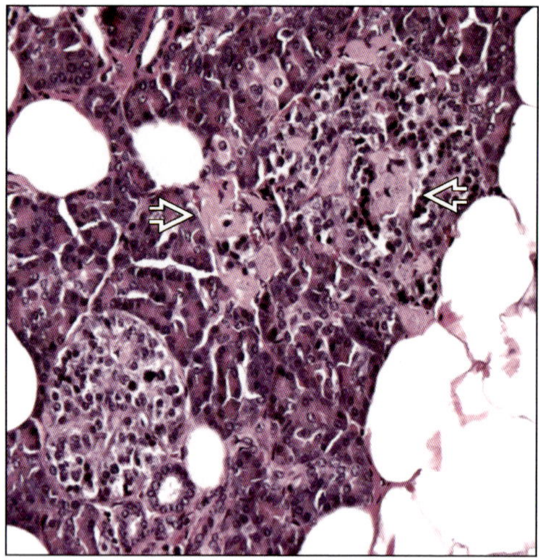

The islet to the left is unremarkable, while the islet to the right shows small nodules of amyloid ➡. There is also fatty infiltration of the pancreas.

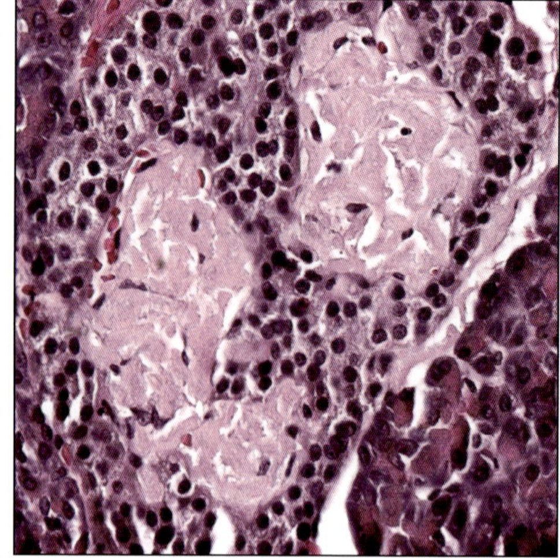

Dense nodules of amyloid are seen within an islet in this case of type 2 diabetes.

TERMINOLOGY

Abbreviations

- Diabetes mellitus (DM)

Definitions

- Heterogeneous group of metabolic diseases characterized by hyperglycemia
  - Result of defects in insulin secretion, insulin activity, or both
- General classification
  - Type 1
    - Absolute insulin deficiency
  - Type 2
    - Insulin resistance and inadequate secretion resulting in relative insulin deficiency

ETIOLOGY/PATHOGENESIS

Unknown and Multifactorial

- Possible autoimmune causes
- Some genetic causes (defects of B-cell function or insulin action)
- Diseases of exocrine pancreas
  - Pancreatitis
  - Trauma/surgery
  - Cystic fibrosis
- Nonpancreatic endocrine diseases
- Drug or chemical-related causes
- Infections
- Gestational diabetes

CLINICAL ISSUES

Presentation

- Polyuria
- Polydipsia
- Unexplained weight loss

Laboratory Tests

- Elevated random plasma glucose (> 200 mg/dL)
- Elevated fasting plasma glucose (> 126 mg/dL)
- Abnormal glucose tolerance test

Treatment

- Drugs
  - Exogenous insulin
  - Oral hypoglycemics
- Other
  - Weight reduction
  - Diet modification

Prognosis

- Chronic, progressive disease with many complications

MACROSCOPIC FEATURES

Type 1 Diabetes

- Early in disease course
  - Normal size, weight, consistency of pancreas
- Later in disease course
  - Decrease in size and weight
    - May decrease by as much as 1/2 of normal
  - Firm consistency due to fibrosis
  - More extreme loss of size than seen in type 2 DM

Type 2 Diabetes

- Reduced size of pancreas
- Reduced weight
  - Sometimes due to fatty infiltration (lipomatosis)

MICROSCOPIC PATHOLOGY

Histologic Features

- Type 1
  - Very variable depending on duration of disease
  - Early in disease course (6 months to 1 year)
    - Variation in islet size and shape

DIABETES MELLITUS

Key Facts

Terminology

- Heterogeneous group of metabolic diseases characterized by hyperglycemia, generally classified as types 1 and 2

Macroscopic Features

- Decreased size and weight (type 1 > type 2)

Microscopic Pathology

- Type 1
  - Variation in islet size and shape
  - Reduced or absent B cells
  - Islet inflammation
- Type 2
  - Islet amyloidosis
  - Reduction in both A and B cells
  - Islets reduced in number but unchanged in size
- Both types
  - Fibrosis, exocrine atrophy

    - Irregularly shaped islets
    - Reduced B cells by immunohistochemistry
    - Lymphocytic inflammation of islets; may be patchy, not always present
  - Later in disease course (1 year and longer)
    - Interlobular and interacinar fibrosis
    - Exocrine atrophy
    - Complete or near absence of B cells
    - Variably present diabetic angiopathy
- Type 2
  - Reduced acinar component
  - Perilobular and intraacinar fibrosis
  - Reduction in number and density of islets
    - Unchanged islet size
  - Reduction in both B and A cells by immunohistochemistry
  - Amyloidosis of islets
    - Increases with length of disease duration, severity of disease, and treatment with insulin
    - Forms cords and nodules in perisinusoidal spaces
    - Represents concentrated form of islet amyloid polypeptide, which appears to be result of, rather than cause of, DM

DIFFERENTIAL DIAGNOSIS

Normal Aging

- Aging also causes decreased size and weight of pancreas
- Islet amyloidosis also present in 4-23% of elderly persons without diabetes
  - These patients may be prediabetic
- Correlates with serum glucose tests, clinical data

DIAGNOSTIC CHECKLIST

Clinically Relevant Pathologic Features

- Aging and type 2 diabetes may have similar pathologic features
- Islet amyloidosis is almost never seen in type 1 diabetes

SELECTED REFERENCES

1. Waguri M et al: Histopathologic study of the pancreas shows a characteristic lymphocytic infiltration in Japanese patients with IDDM. Endocr J. 44(1):23-33, 1997
2. Alzaid A et al: The size of the pancreas in diabetes mellitus. Diabet Med. 10(8):759-63, 1993
3. Pancreatic abnormalities in type 2 diabetes mellitus. Lancet. 2(8574):1497-8, 1987
4. Maloy AL et al: The relation of islet amyloid to the clinical type of diabetes. Hum Pathol. 12(10):917-22, 1981

IMAGE GALLERY

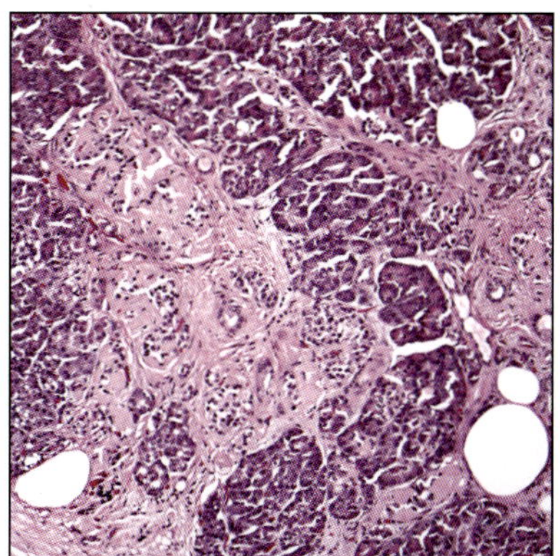

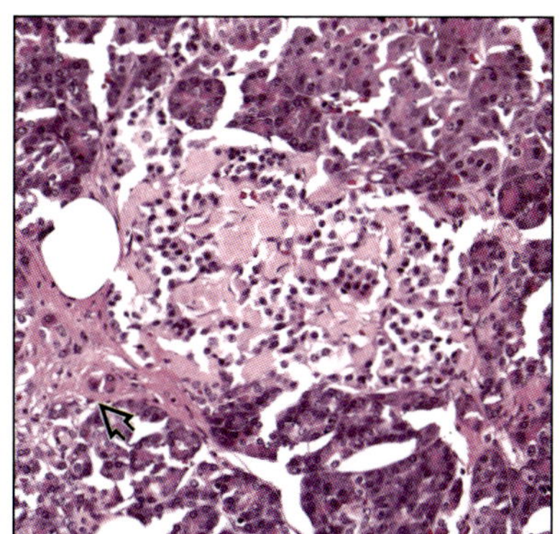

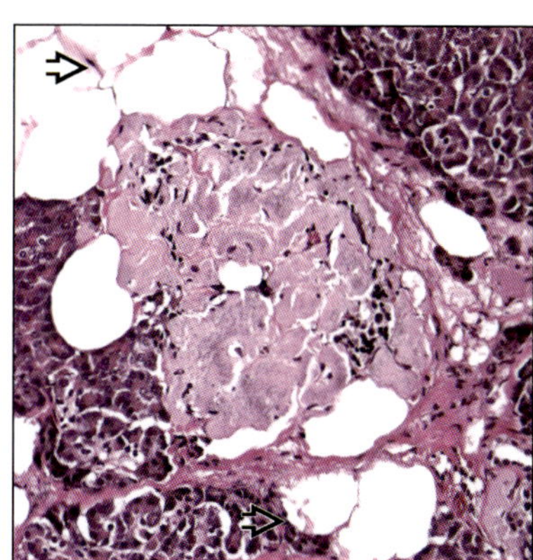

*(**Left**) This case of type 2 diabetes shows intraacinar and perilobular fibrosis. (**Center**) This islet cell contains small ribbons and nodules of amyloid. There is also focal fibrosis at the edge of the islet ⇨. (**Right**) This islet is almost completely replaced by amyloid. There is also fatty infiltration of the pancreas ⇨.*

LYMPHOEPITHELIAL CYSTS

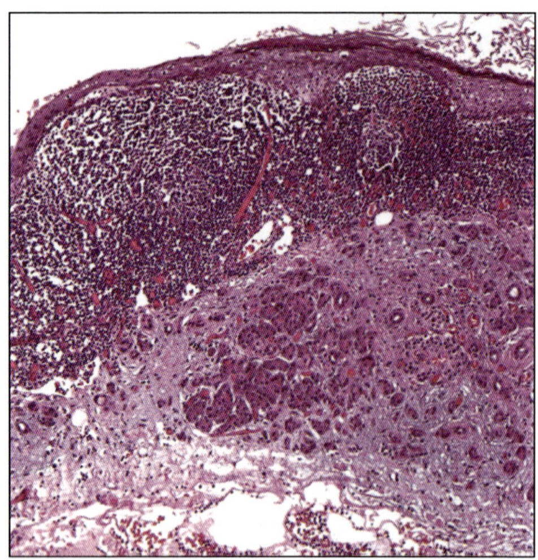

This pancreatic lymphoepithelial cyst shows the prominent lymphoid stroma and overlying keratinizing squamous epithelium. Lymphocytes may extend into the underlying pancreatic parenchyma.

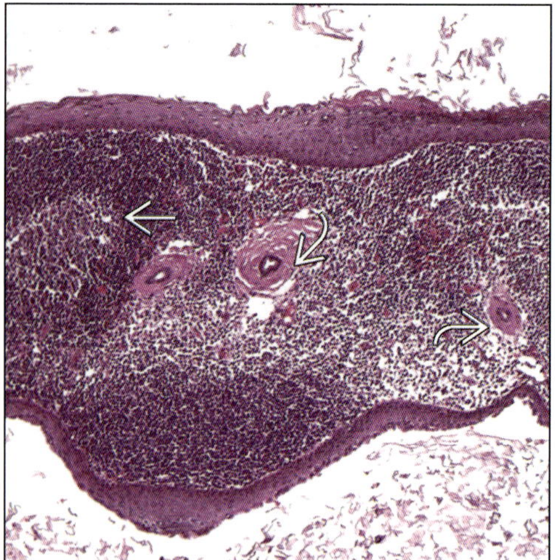

Benign pancreatic ducts ➔ are seen within the lymphoid component in the wall of a lymphoepithelial cyst. Germinal centers may be present ➔.

TERMINOLOGY

Definitions

- Nonneoplastic cyst with lymphoid and squamous epithelial components
  - Somewhat resemble epidermal inclusion cysts

ETIOLOGY/PATHOGENESIS

Uncertain

- Not associated with conditions related to lymphoepithelial cysts of salivary gland

CLINICAL ISSUES

Epidemiology

- Incidence
  - Rare
    - Account for 0.5% of pancreatic cystic lesions
- Age
  - Mean: 56 years
  - Range: 38-82 years
- Gender
  - M:F = 4:1

Presentation

- Vague intermittent abdominal pain
- Nausea/vomiting/diarrhea
- Abdominal mass
- Weight loss
- Often asymptomatic and incidentally discovered

Treatment

- Only symptomatic lymphoepithelial cysts should be resected

Prognosis

- Good
  - Resection is curative
- Malignant transformation has not been described

MACROSCOPIC FEATURES

General Features

- Multilocular (60%) or unilocular (40%) cystic lesion
- Anywhere in pancreas
- Cyst contents
  - Smooth or finely granular lining
  - Serous to cheesy/caseous contents
  - If lymphoid tissue is prominent, may be band of soft tan tissue surrounding cyst wall

Size

- 1.5-17 cm

MICROSCOPIC PATHOLOGY

Histologic Features

- Cyst lining
  - Usually stratified squamous epithelium
    - May show keratinization
  - Cuboidal or transitional-like epithelium may be present
  - Sebaceous and mucinous goblet cells are rarely seen
  - Inflammation, reactive epithelial changes variably present
- Cyst wall &/or trabeculae
  - 1-3 mm in thickness
  - Dense distinct band of lymphoid tissue
    - Composed of mature T cells
    - Intervening germinal center formation by B cells
- Other elements variably present
  - Epithelioid granulomas
  - Foamy histiocytes
  - Fat necrosis
  - Cholesterol clefts
  - Stromal hyalinization
- Adjacent pancreas is often unremarkable

Key Facts

Clinical Issues

- Rare nonneoplastic pancreatic cystic lesions composed of squamous epithelial and lymphoid elements

Macroscopic Features

- Multilocular or unilocular cystic lesions

Microscopic Pathology

- Squamous-lined cysts
- Dense distinct band of lymphoid tissue

Top Differential Diagnoses

- Cystic entities lined by squamous epithelium
  - Epidermoid cyst in intrapancreatic spleen is surrounded by splenic tissue
  - Dermoid cyst has dermal appendages
  - Squamoid cyst is small without associated lymphoid tissue

- Some appear to have arisen in peripancreatic lymph node
  - Presence of thin capsule and subcapsular sinuses

DIFFERENTIAL DIAGNOSIS

Epidermoid Cyst of Intrapancreatic Accessory Spleen or Heterotopic Spleen

- Occurs exclusively in tail of pancreas
- Similarly lined by stratified squamous epithelium, which may be attenuated
- Surrounded by normal-appearing splenic tissue
  - Varying amounts of red and white pulp, latter may be sparse

Dermoid Cyst

- Difficult to distinguish if composed predominately of epidermal elements
  - Presence of dermal appendages or hair shafts
    - Sebaceous glands or hair follicles

Squamoid Cyst of Pancreatic Duct

- Relatively small unilocular cyst
  - Often a cystically dilated duct
- Lined by squamous or transitional epithelium without keratinization
- Surrounded by acinar tissue
- Lumen may contains acidophilic secretions that form concretions

Lymphangioma

- Multilocular cyst with endothelial lining
- Aggregates of lymphoid tissue rather than thick band of lymphoid tissue

Pseudocyst

- No epithelial lining
  - Sample entire cyst wall before rendering this diagnosis

SELECTED REFERENCES

1. Basturk O et al: Pancreatic cysts: pathologic classification, differential diagnosis, and clinical implications. Arch Pathol Lab Med. 133(3):423-38, 2009
2. Adsay NV et al: Lymphoepithelial cysts of the pancreas: a report of 12 cases and a review of the literature. Mod Pathol. 15(5):492-501, 2002
3. Adsay NV et al: Squamous-lined cysts of the pancreas: lymphoepithelial cysts, dermoid cysts (teratomas), and accessory-splenic epidermoid cysts. Semin Diagn Pathol. 17(1):56-65, 2000
4. Truong LD et al: Lymphoepithelial cyst of the pancreas. Am J Surg Pathol. 11(11):899-903, 1987

IMAGE GALLERY

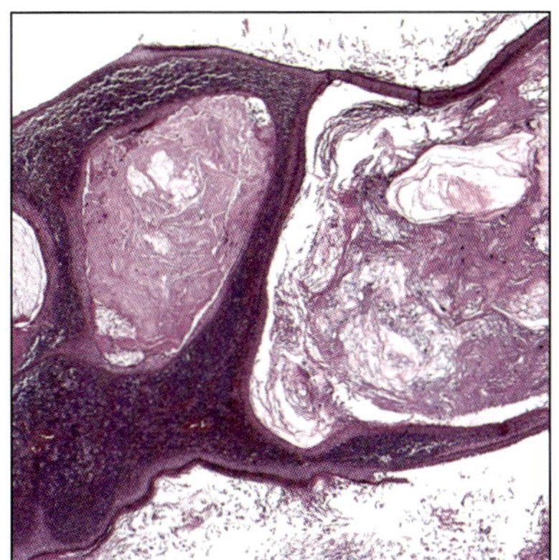
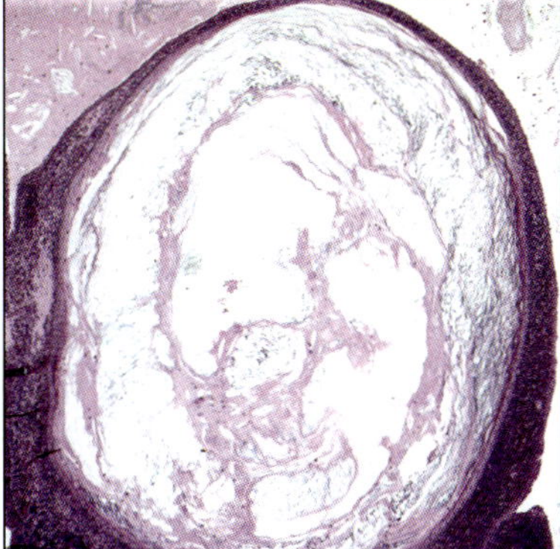
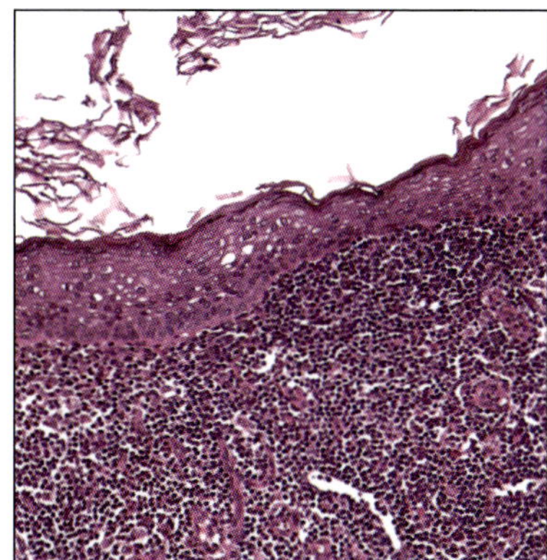

(Left) *60% of lymphoepithelial cysts in the pancreas are multilocular. Note the abundant keratinaceous debris.* ***(Center)*** *Abundant keratinaceous debris is seen within this cyst locule. The cyst wall is composed of lymphoid tissue with a thin squamous epithelial lining.* ***(Right)*** *A high-power view of this lymphoepithelial cyst shows the benign stratified squamous epithelial lining above the prominent lymphoid stroma.*

Tumors of the Gallbladder and Extrahepatic Biliary Tree

PYLORIC GLAND ADENOMA

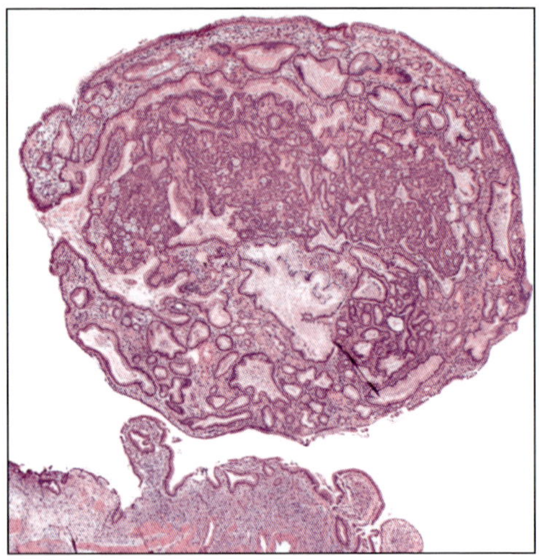

This pyloric gland adenoma forms a polypoid lesion in the lumen of the gallbladder composed of tightly packed pyloric-type glands.

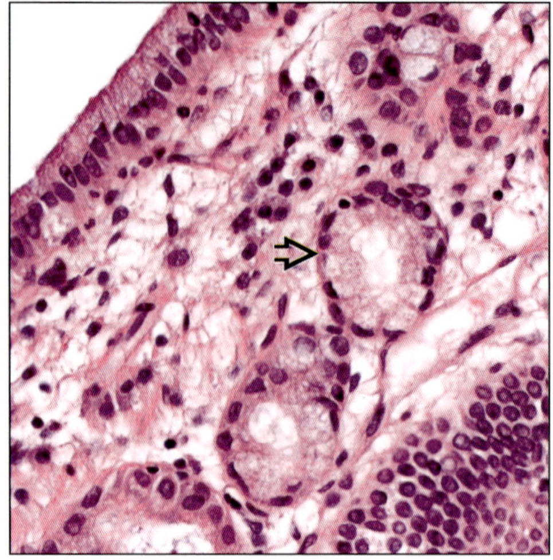

High-power view demonstrates pyloric gland differentiation. Pyloric glands ➡ are lined by cells with basal nuclei and pale cytoplasm.

TERMINOLOGY

Abbreviations

- Pyloric gland adenoma (PGA)

Synonyms

- Tubular adenoma
- Metaplastic adenoma

Definitions

- Benign neoplasm of glandular epithelium showing pyloric gland differentiation

ETIOLOGY/PATHOGENESIS

Etiology Remains Speculative

- Occasional PGAs have been reported in association with Peutz-Jeghers and Gardner syndrome
- Current data suggest that PGAs are not a common pathway for development of gallbladder carcinoma
- Also reported in other sites
  - Stomach
  - Duodenum
  - Pancreas
  - Common bile duct
  - Uterine cervix

CLINICAL ISSUES

Presentation

- Asymptomatic
- Usually discovered incidentally
- When multiple and filling the lumen or at neck of gallbladder, can mimic chronic cholecystitis

Treatment

- Surgical approaches
  - Surgical resection is curative

Prognosis

- Excellent

MACROSCOPIC FEATURES

General Features

- Usually solitary sessile lesions

Size

- Typically measures a few millimeters but can be as large as 2 cm

MICROSCOPIC PATHOLOGY

Histologic Features

- Well-demarcated nodules composed of closely packed pyloric-type glands with little intervening stroma
  - Majority of glands are small and typically round
  - Occasional dilated glands are present
  - Glands composed of epithelial cells with basal nuclei and mucin-containing pale apical cytoplasm
    - Mild nuclear atypia is common
    - Severe cytological atypia or in situ carcinoma are rare in gallbladder
- Squamoid morules composed of spindle-shaped squamous cells are occasionally seen; overt keratinization is infrequent
- Occasional goblet and Paneth cells may be present

ANCILLARY TESTS

Immunohistochemistry

- PGA tumor cells are positive for MUC6 and negative for MUC2
- Intestinal-type adenomas are negative for MUC6 and positive for MUC2

PYLORIC GLAND ADENOMA

Key Facts

Terminology
- Benign neoplasm of glandular epithelium showing pyloric differentiation

Clinical Issues
- Usually discovered incidentally

Macroscopic Features
- Usually solitary sessile lesions

Microscopic Pathology
- Well-demarcated nodules composed of closely packed pyloric-type glands with little intervening stroma
- Lining epithelium shows basal nuclei with mucin-containing pale apical cytoplasm

Top Differential Diagnoses
- Nodular hyperplasia of pseudopyloric glands
- Ectopic gastric mucosa
- Intestinal-type adenoma

Molecular Genetics
- Gallbladder PGAs frequently have β-*catenin* mutations and are negative for *KRAS* mutations
- In contrast, gallbladder carcinomas lack β-*catenin* mutations and frequently show *KRAS* mutations

DIFFERENTIAL DIAGNOSIS

Nodular Hyperplasia of Pseudopyloric Glands
- Pseudopyloric metaplasia is commonly seen in association with chronic cholecystitis
- Pseudopyloric glands may coalesce and produce elevations of gallbladder mucosa, mimicking PGA
- Continuity with adjacent pseudopyloric metaplasia and poor demarcation help distinguish pseudopyloric metaplasia from PGA

Papillary Hyperplasia
- Seen in approximately 5% of gallbladders with chronic cholecystitis
- Well-formed delicate papillary processes lined by epithelium that is similar to that seen in normal gallbladder
  - May be either focal or diffuse

Ectopic Gastric Mucosa
- Parietal and oxyntic cells are invariably present

Intestinal-type Adenoma
- Lining epithelium resembles colonic adenoma and shows numerous goblet cells
- MUC6 staining is negative

Other Gallbladder Polyps
- Cholesterol polyps, lymphoid polyps, and fibrous polyps

DIAGNOSTIC CHECKLIST

Pathologic Interpretation Pearls
- Histologically, cells resemble gastric pyloric gland epithelium and Brunner glands

SELECTED REFERENCES

1. Wani Y et al: Aberrant expression of an "intestinal marker" Cdx2 in pyloric gland adenoma of the gallbladder. Virchows Arch. 453(5):521-7, 2008
2. Vieth M et al: Pyloric gland adenoma: a clinico-pathological analysis of 90 cases. Virchows Arch. 442(4):317-21, 2003
3. Wistuba II et al: Gallbladder adenomas have molecular abnormalities different from those present in gallbladder carcinomas. Hum Pathol. 30(1):21-5, 1999
4. Albores-Saavedra J et al: Non-neoplastic polypoid lesions and adenomas of the gallbladder. Pathol Annu. 28 Pt 1:145-77, 1993

IMAGE GALLERY

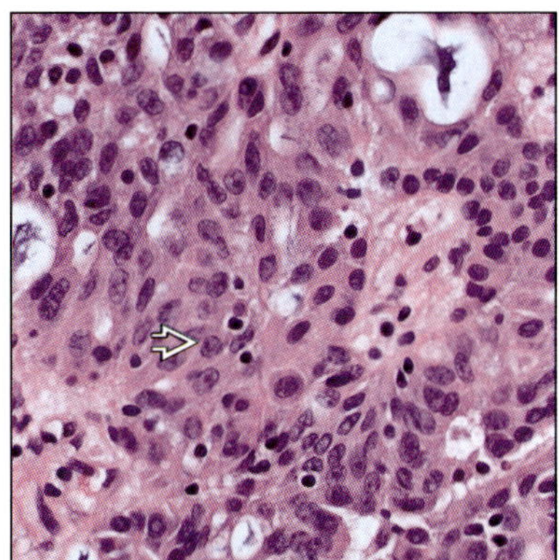

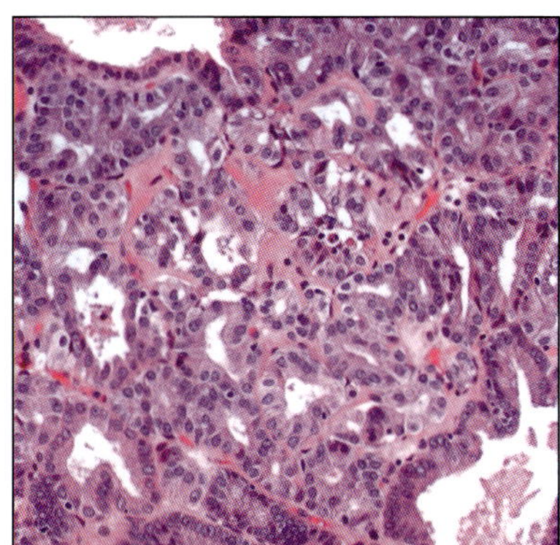

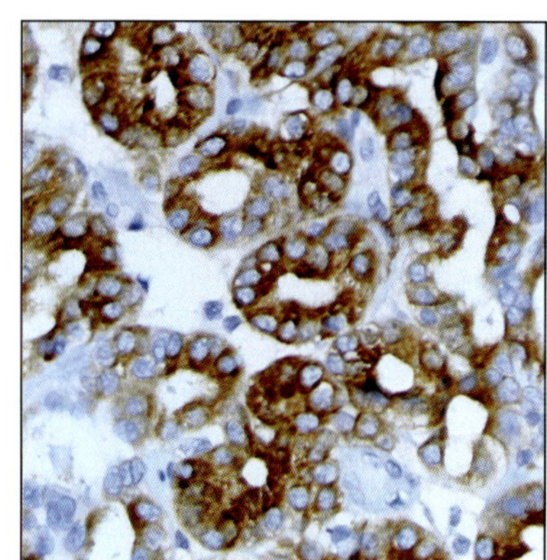

(Left) *Pyloric gland adenomas may show squamous differentiation ⇨.* ***(Center)*** *Pyloric gland adenomas typically feature closely spaced glands with little intervening stroma. The cytoplasm in this example is more deeply eosinophilic. Only mild nuclear atypia is seen.* ***(Right)*** *MUC6 reactivity confirms pyloric gland differentiation.*

INTESTINAL-TYPE ADENOMA

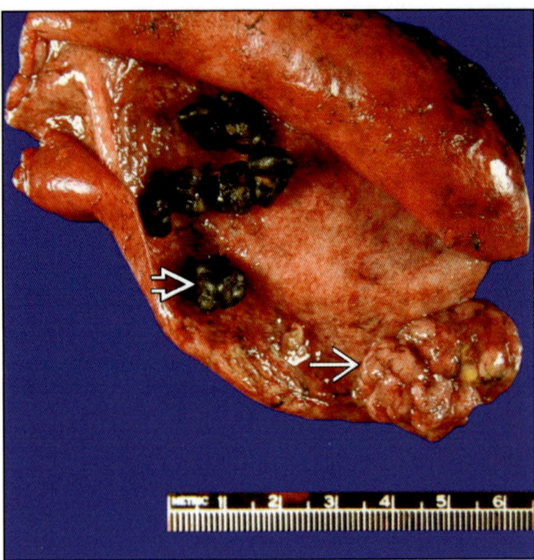

This lobulated intraluminal polypoidal adenoma of the gallbladder ➡ was associated with chronic cholecystitis and gallstones ⇨, as are the majority of intestinal-type adenomas.

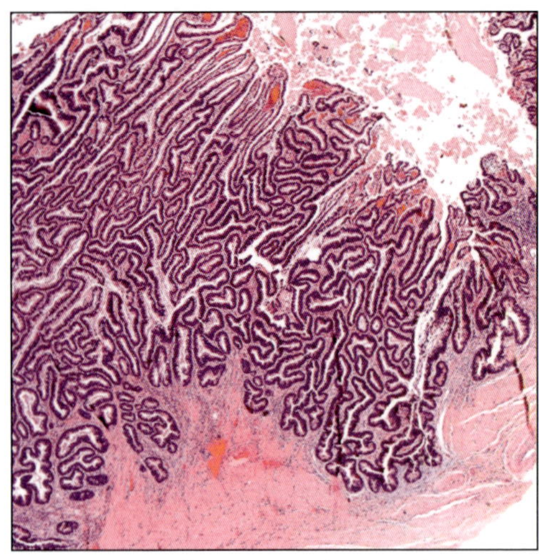

This tubulopapillary intestinal-type adenoma is composed of intestinal-type epithelium that resembles an adenoma of the colon.

TERMINOLOGY

Definitions

- Gallbladder polyp predominantly composed of intestinal-type epithelium

ETIOLOGY/PATHOGENESIS

Unknown

- Associated with chronic cholecystitis and cholelithiasis

CLINICAL ISSUES

Epidemiology

- Incidence
  - Low: 0.3-0.5% of cholecystectomy specimens
- Age
  - Mean age: 58 years
    - Uncommon in children
- Gender
  - Women > men

Presentation

- Asymptomatic and often incidentally detected
- Large lesions may produce symptoms similar to chronic cholecystitis

Treatment

- Surgical approaches
  - Cholecystectomy

Prognosis

- Risk of progression to carcinoma
  - Variable but low
  - Only minority of gallbladder carcinomas arise from preexisting adenomas
  - Risk of invasive carcinoma increases with size and papillary growth pattern

MACROSCOPIC FEATURES

General Features

- Pedunculated or sessile
  - May be papillary or lobulated
  - Red-tan in color
- Most frequently in fundus
- 10% multiple
- Entire adenoma should be submitted to exclude carcinoma

Size

- Usually < 2 cm

MICROSCOPIC PATHOLOGY

Histologic Features

- Resemble colonic adenomas
- Tubular, papillary, or mixed tubulopapillary patterns
  - High-grade dysplasia may be seen
- Predominant cell type is nonmucinous columnar cells with hyperchromatic nuclei
  - Other cell types
    - Goblet cells
    - Neuroendocrine cells
    - Paneth cells

ANCILLARY TESTS

Immunohistochemistry

- MUC2: Diffusely positive
- MUC6: Typically negative
- Neuroendocrine markers reveal scattered neuroendocrine cells

Molecular Genetics

- Mutations in β-*catenin* present
  - Lower frequency than pyloric gland adenoma
- *P53* mutations virtually absent

INTESTINAL-TYPE ADENOMA

Key Facts

Terminology
- Gallbladder polyp composed of intestinal-type epithelium

Clinical Issues
- Progression to carcinoma uncommon

Microscopic Pathology
- Resemble colonic adenomas
- Tubular, papillary to mixed tubulopapillary patterns

Ancillary Tests
- MUC2: Diffusely positive
- Mutations in β-*catenin* present
- *P53* mutations virtually absent

Top Differential Diagnoses
- Pyloric-type adenoma
- Invasive adenocarcinoma

  - *P53* mutations common in flat dysplasia and invasive carcinoma

DIFFERENTIAL DIAGNOSIS

Intestinal Metaplasia
- May form small nodule but not discrete polypoid lesion

Papillary Hyperplasia
- Diffuse mucosal papillary proliferation lined by biliary-type epithelium

Pyloric-type Adenoma
- Small tubules lined by pyloric-type epithelium
- MUC6 positive, MUC2 only focally positive

Biliary-type Adenoma
- Papillary lesion lined by cells resembling gallbladder epithelium

Invasive Carcinoma Arising in Gallbladder Adenoma
- Extension of dysplastic epithelium along Rokitansky-Aschoff sinuses may mimic invasive adenocarcinoma
- Invasive carcinomas show irregularly shaped glands, small infiltrative glands, and high-grade cellular atypia

DIAGNOSTIC CHECKLIST

Clinically Relevant Pathologic Features
- Gallbladder carcinomas often develop from flat dysplasia, and only a minority are associated with adenomas

Pathologic Interpretation Pearls
- Polypoidal adenoma may be detached from lumen and grossly mimic gallstones
- Entire adenoma should be submitted to rule out associated invasive carcinoma

SELECTED REFERENCES

1. Albores-Saavedra J et al: In situ and invasive adenocarcinomas of the gallbladder extending into or arising from Rokitansky-Aschoff sinuses: a clinicopathologic study of 49 cases. Am J Surg Pathol. 28(5):621-8, 2004
2. Wistuba II et al: Gallbladder adenomas have molecular abnormalities different from those present in gallbladder carcinomas. Hum Pathol. 30(1):21-5, 1999
3. Albores-Saavedra J et al: Non-neoplastic polypoid lesions and adenomas of the gallbladder. Pathol Annu. 28 Pt 1:145-77, 1993

IMAGE GALLERY

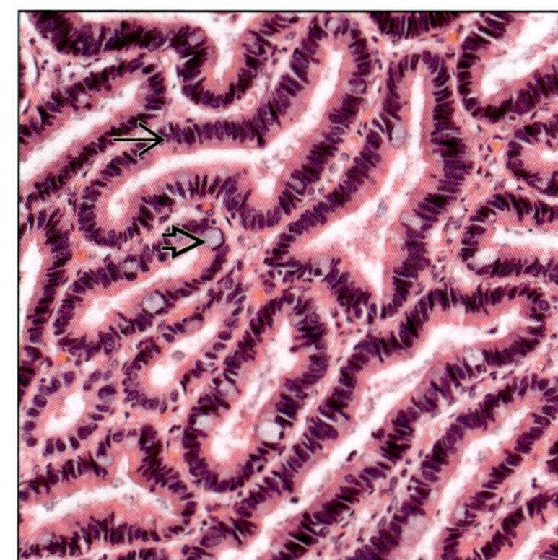

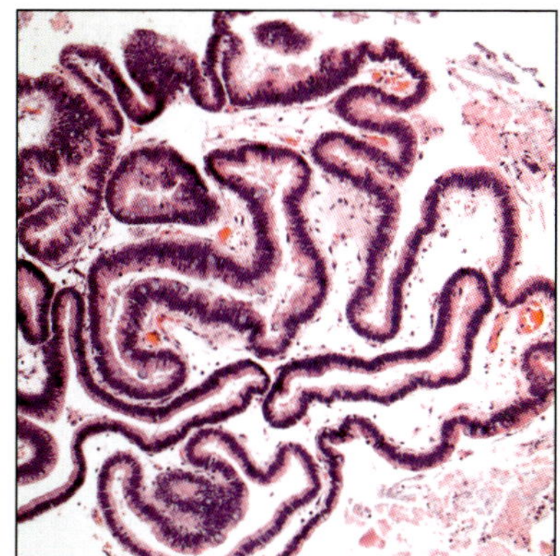

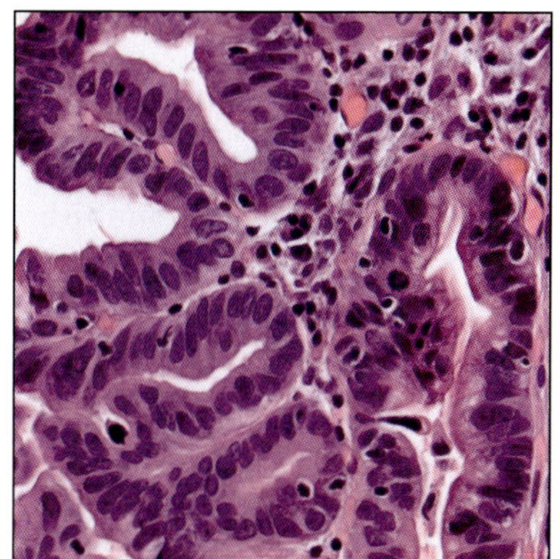

(Left) *This intestinal-type gallbladder adenoma is composed predominantly of mucin-depleted pencil-shaped cells ➙, with scattered goblet cells ➪.* ***(Center)*** *This intestinal-type adenoma of the gallbladder resembles a colorectal adenoma and has only low-grade dysplasia.* ***(Right)*** *This intestinal-type adenoma of the gallbladder has high-grade dysplasia.*

BILIARY PAPILLOMATOSIS

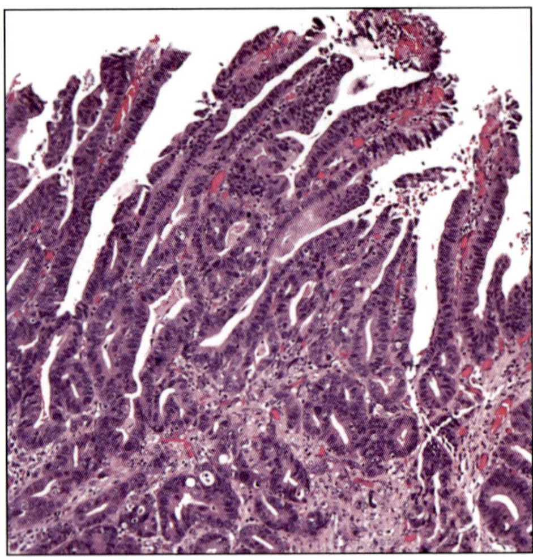

Biliary papillomatosis features numerous polypoid adenomatous lesions of the biliary tract. This one, present in the common bile duct, resembles an intestinal-type tubulovillous adenoma.

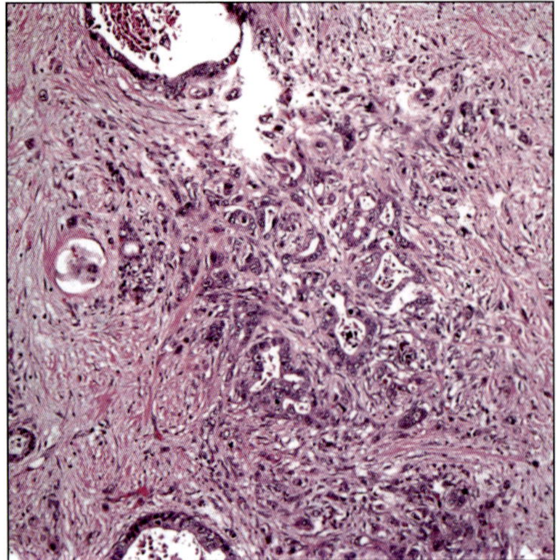

This case of biliary papillomatosis had multiple foci of invasive adenocarcinoma. This poorly differentiated carcinoma arose in the common bile duct.

TERMINOLOGY

Synonyms

- Multiple biliary papillomatosis

Definitions

- Multiple, often numerous adenomas of bile ducts

CLINICAL ISSUES

Epidemiology

- Incidence
  - Extremely rare; minority associated with other diseases, such as
    - Ulcerative colitis
    - Familial adenomatous polyposis
    - Choledochal cyst
- Age
  - Peak incidence in 6th-7th decade of life
- Gender
  - No significant gender predominance
    - Some sources report slight male predominance

Presentation

- Jaundice
- Signs and symptoms of biliary obstruction
- Abdominal pain

Treatment

- Surgical excision if possible
  - Often not possible given multicentricity
- Laser treatment or local excision may be options in some cases
- Even resected lesions are prone to recurrence

Prognosis

- Approximately 50% mortality rate
  - Serious complications
    - Adenocarcinoma
    - Biliary obstruction
    - Cholangitis
  - Very difficult to treat if lesions are multiple and widespread
  - Mean survival after diagnosis is approximately 3 years

IMAGE FINDINGS

General Features

- ERCP may be useful confirmatory test
  - Multiple filling defects within biliary tree
  - Mucosal irregularities within biliary tree

MACROSCOPIC FEATURES

General Features

- Soft, friable, often villiform polypoid masses
  - Red-brown to gray-white in color
  - Pedunculated or sessile
  - May have cauliflower-like appearance
- 0.2-2.0 cm in size
- Often grow circumferentially
- Detached fragments of tumor tissue and associated thrombus may be found in duct lumen

Location

- Most are multicentric throughout biliary tract
- Rarely, lesions are confined to intrahepatic bile ducts
- Occasional involvement of proximal pancreatic duct and gallbladder

MICROSCOPIC PATHOLOGY

Histologic Features

- Multiple complex papillary lesions
  - Architecture may be tubular as well
    - May resemble intestinal-type villous or tubulovillous adenomas

BILIARY PAPILLOMATOSIS

Key Facts

Terminology
- Multiple adenomas of bile ducts

Clinical Issues
- Very rare; some cases associated with familial adenomatous polyposis
- Resection often not possible given multicentricity
- Complications include adenocarcinoma, biliary obstruction

Macroscopic Features
- Soft, friable, often villiform polypoid masses
  - Most are located throughout biliary tract; rarely confined to intrahepatic bile ducts

Microscopic Pathology
- Multiple complex papillary lesions
  - Columnar or cuboidal epithelium
  - Cytoplasmic mucin may be present
  - May resemble intestinal-type adenomas

  - Delicate fibrovascular cores
  - Epithelium can be cuboidal or columnar
  - Cytoplasmic mucin may be present
  - Nuclei are often basally located and uniform
- Associated with noninvasive papillary carcinoma as well as frankly invasive malignancy
  - Malignancy may be multifocal as well
  - Even low-grade, noninvasive lesions have been reported to metastasize

DIFFERENTIAL DIAGNOSIS

Isolated Adenomatous Polyp
- Morphologically may be identical
- Given the difficulty of surveillance and likelihood of recurrence, it is important to note if multiple adenomas are present

Pyloric Adenoma
- Composed of closely packed tubular glands that resemble pyloric epithelium
- Lack papillary architecture
- Lack intestinal-type epithelium

DIAGNOSTIC CHECKLIST

Clinically Relevant Pathologic Features
- Important to recognize this rare entity given serious complications and difficulties with treatment and surveillance
- Minority of cases associated with familial adenomatous polyposis

SELECTED REFERENCES

1. Hubens G et al: Papillomatosis of the intra- and extrahepatic bile ducts with involvement of the pancreatic duct. Hepatogastroenterology. 38(5):413-8, 1991
2. Okulski EG et al: Intrahepatic biliary papillomatosis. Arch Pathol Lab Med. 103(12):647-9, 1979
3. Helpap B: Malignant papillomatosis of the intrahepatic bile ducts. Acta Hepatogastroenterol (Stuttg). 24(6):419-25, 1977
4. Neumann RD et al: Adenocarcinoma in biliary papillomatosis. Gastroenterology. 70(5 PT. 1):779-82, 1976
5. Madden JJ Jr et al: Multiple biliary papillomatosis. Cancer. 34(4):1316-20, 1974
6. Eiss S et al: Multiple papillomas of the entire biliary tract: case report. Ann Surg. 152:320-4, 1960

IMAGE GALLERY

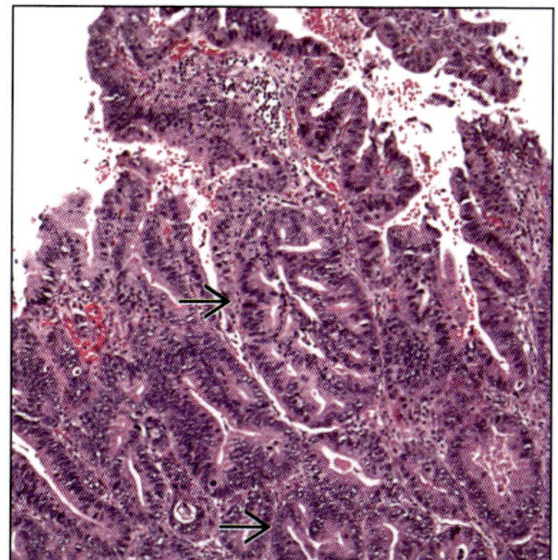
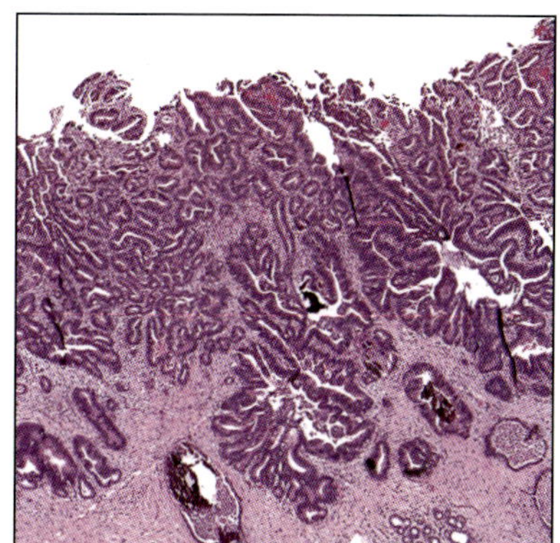
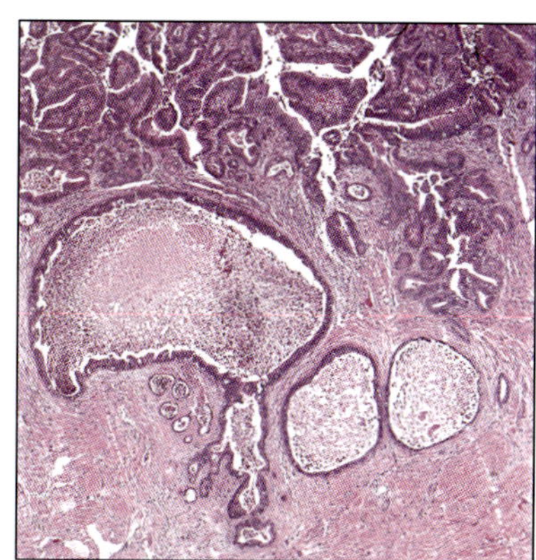

(Left) *This adenoma has papillary fronds lined by dysplastic columnar epithelium. There are cribriformed areas consistent with high-grade dysplasia as well ⇒.* ***(Center)*** *This adenoma in biliary papillomatosis is sessile rather than exophytic. It was present in the distal common bile duct.* ***(Right)*** *A well-differentiated adenocarcinoma arises from the base of this papillary adenoma and infiltrates the wall of the duct.*

ADENOCARCINOMA OF THE GALLBLADDER

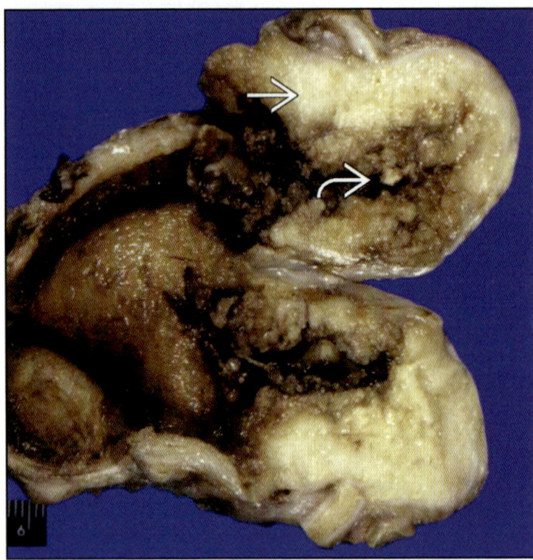

This gross cholecystectomy specimen contains areas of mucosal irregularity associated with thickening of the gallbladder wall in a case of gallbladder adenocarcinoma.

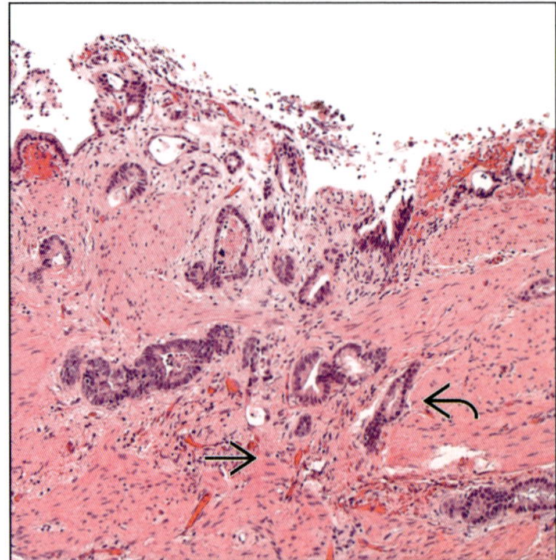

Hematoxylin and eosin stained section demonstrates malignant glands invading the smooth muscle of the gallbladder wall in an irregular and infiltrative pattern.

TERMINOLOGY

Definitions

- Malignant glandular epithelial neoplasm arising in gallbladder

ETIOLOGY/PATHOGENESIS

Developmental Anomaly

- Anomalous junction of pancreatic duct and common bile duct
  - Pancreatic duct and common bile duct meet outside duodenal wall

Chronic Inflammation

- Cholelithiasis
  - > 80% of gallbladder adenocarcinomas are associated with gallstones
- Chronic cholecystitis
- Porcelain gallbladder
  - > 10% of affected patients have or will develop adenocarcinoma
- Primary sclerosing cholangitis
  - Gallbladder adenocarcinoma reported in 14% of patients with primary sclerosing cholangitis undergoing liver transplantation
- Chronic biliary infections
  - *Opisthorchis viverrini*
  - *Salmonella typhi*
- Intestinal and pseudopyloric metaplasia
  - Result from longstanding chronic inflammation

Gastrointestinal Polyposis

- Familial adenomatous polyposis coli (FAP)
- Gardner syndrome
- Peutz-Jeghers syndrome

Molecular Alterations

- Reported *KRAS* mutation rates vary from 0-50%
- *P53* mutations common in late-stage disease

CLINICAL ISSUES

Epidemiology

- Incidence
  - Reported 1.43 cases per 100,000 persons at risk
  - Rates of incidental diagnosis at time of laparoscopic cholecystectomy range from 0.28-2.1%
- Age
  - Predominantly affects elderly patients
  - Mean age: 65 years
- Gender
  - Females more often affected
    - 3:1 female to male ratio
- Ethnicity
  - Most often occurs in India, Chile, Pakistan, and Ecuador
  - In western countries, Latin American and Native American individuals at greatest risk

Presentation

- Symptoms often vague, nonspecific
- Abdominal pain
  - Upper abdomen
- Weight loss
- Fever
- Jaundice, cholestatic
- Asymptomatic
  - May present as incidental finding at examination of cholecystectomy specimen

Laboratory Tests

- Elevated alkaline phosphatase

Treatment

- Options, risks, complications
  - Surgery is most effective and the only potentially curative treatment
    - Not effective for advanced disease
- Surgical approaches
  - Low-stage tumors

ADENOCARCINOMA OF THE GALLBLADDER

Key Facts

Terminology
- Malignant neoplasm of glandular epithelium arising in gallbladder

Etiology/Pathogenesis
- Chronic inflammation of gallbladder
  - Chronic cholecystitis, cholelithiasis, chronic biliary infections

Clinical Issues
- Often incidental finding at cholecystectomy for cholecystitis or cholelithiasis
  - Rates of incidental diagnosis at time of cholecystectomy range from 0.28-2.1%
- Surgery is most effective and the only potentially curative treatment
- Tumor stage is probably most important prognostic factor

Image Findings
- Tumor mass or wall thickening may be seen on imaging

Microscopic Pathology
- Malignant glands, clusters, or individual cells invading gallbladder wall
- Majority of cases associated with epithelial dysplasia &/or carcinoma in situ
- Some extremely well-differentiated tumors are deceptively bland and difficult to recognize

---

      - Often identified incidentally at time of cholecystectomy for cholelithiasis or cholecystitis
      - Simple cholecystectomy may be adequate therapy
  - Advanced tumors
    - Radical cholecystectomy with lymphadenectomy and right hepatic lobectomy
- Drugs
  - Adjuvant chemotherapy
    - Gemcitabine and gemcitabine-based regimens appear to be most effective to date
    - Small molecule growth factor inhibitors are under study and may provide benefit

Prognosis
- Approximately 10% 5-year survival, overall
  - 42% 5-year survival for patients with resectable tumors
- Tumor stage probably most important prognostic factor
- Other prognostic factors
  - Tumor grade
    - Poorly differentiated tumors associated with poor survival
  - Depth of invasion
  - Lymph node metastases
  - Completeness of resection
  - Angiolymphatic space invasion and perineural invasion may represent prognostic factor
    - Variable reports, not predictive of survival in all studies

IMAGE FINDINGS

Radiographic Findings
- Various appearances may be seen on imaging
  - Tumor mass occupying or replacing gallbladder lumen
    - 40-65% of tumors
  - Localized or diffuse wall thickening
  - Polypoid lesion in gallbladder lumen
  - Liver invasion may be seen
- Ultrasound is common first-line test for suspected gallbladder disease
  - High sensitivity for advanced tumors
  - Unreliable for staging and diagnosis or early tumors
- CT and MR provide more detailed information
  - Tumor staging
  - Evaluate for metastases

Ultrasonographic Findings
- Mostly hypoechoic tumor seen in lumen

CT Findings
- Tumor usually hypodense on unenhanced CT

MACROSCOPIC FEATURES

General Features
- Tumors located in fundus (60%), body (30%), or neck (10%) of gallbladder
- Variable gross appearances
  - Area of thickening and induration of gallbladder wall
  - Exophytic or polypoid mucosal mass
- Tumor may not be grossly evident
- Tumors often firm, white, and gritty on cut section

Sections to Be Submitted
- Cystic duct margin
  - Tumors are often incidental and more often located near gallbladder neck
  - Evaluate margin for carcinoma or dysplasia
- Gallbladder dysplasia
  - If identified, extensive sampling warranted to exclude occult carcinoma
  - Dysplasia can cause granular mucosal patches but may not be grossly recognizable

MICROSCOPIC PATHOLOGY

Histologic Features
- Malignant glands, clusters, or individual cells invading gallbladder wall

ADENOCARCINOMA OF THE GALLBLADDER

 - Complex and irregular glands can also be seen
- Wide spectrum of histologic appearances
  - May be extremely well differentiated
    - Some tumors are deceptively bland
    - May exhibit well-formed glands and only minimal cytologic abnormalities
    - Infiltrative growth pattern, nuclear grooves, and mitotic activity are helpful clues
  - Malignant epithelial elements may be rare and widely spaced in abundant desmoplastic stroma
  - Multiple histologic variants of carcinoma recognized by World Health Organization
    - Papillary adenocarcinoma
    - Intestinal-type or gastric foveolar-type adenocarcinoma
    - Mucinous adenocarcinoma
    - Clear cell adenocarcinoma
    - Signet ring cell carcinoma
    - Adenosquamous carcinoma
    - Micropapillary
    - Adenosquamous carcinoma or squamous cell carcinoma
    - Small cell or large cell neuroendocrine carcinoma
    - Undifferentiated carcinoma
    - Biliary cystadenocarcinoma
- Majority of cases associated with epithelial dysplasia &/or carcinoma in situ
  - Dysplasia or carcinoma in situ are usually incidental findings
  - May extend into Rokitansky-Aschoff sinuses
    - Involvement of Rokitansky-Aschoff sinuses does not indicate invasion
  - Lacks perineural invasion

Cytologic Features

- Peritoneal cytology most helpful in patients with advanced tumors

Lymphatic/Vascular Invasion

- Provides evidence of malignancy
- May or may not be independent prognostic factor

Margins

- Evaluation important for prognostication
- Cystic duct margin
- Hepatic resection margin

Lymph Nodes

- Utility of cytokeratin staining is controversial

ANCILLARY TESTS

Immunohistochemistry

- Similar to other adenocarcinomas arising in pancreaticobiliary tree
- Express cytokeratins and CEA
- Most tumors CK7, CK19 positive and may also express CK20

DIFFERENTIAL DIAGNOSIS

Chronic Cholecystitis

- Rokitansky-Aschoff sinuses can mimic invasive adenocarcinoma
  - Usually consist of larger glandular structures that are contiguous with surface epithelium
  - Can extend deeply into and even through gallbladder wall
    - Protrude between smooth muscle bundles but do not invade into smooth muscle
  - May be set in fibrotic stroma that mimics desmoplastic stroma
  - Even more problematic if epithelial dysplasia or carcinoma in situ involves epithelium
    - Adenocarcinoma arising in Rokitansky-Aschoff sinuses reported but extremely rare
- Adenocarcinoma usually comprised of smaller glands with more cytologic atypia
  - Glands usually more crowded than Rokitansky-Aschoff sinuses

Adenomyoma

- Irregular, dilated cystic structures set in hypertrophic smooth muscle
- Bland epithelium and lobular configuration distinguishes adenomyoma from adenocarcinoma

Acute Cholecystitis

- Reactive epithelial alterations may be mistaken for dysplasia or carcinoma
- Use caution when making diagnosis in setting of marked inflammation

Ducts of Luschka

- Groups of small, round, benign ducts often seen at hepatic surface of gallbladder
- Lack invasive growth pattern or cytologic features of malignancy

Metastatic Adenocarcinoma to Gallbladder

- Extremely rare
- Diagnosis based on clinical history or immunohistochemistry

SELECTED REFERENCES

1. Choi SB et al: Incidental gallbladder cancer diagnosed following laparoscopic cholecystectomy. World J Surg. 33(12):2657-63, 2009
2. Goldin RD et al: Gallbladder cancer: a morphological and molecular update. Histopathology. 55(2):218-29, 2009
3. Henson DE et al: Carcinomas of the pancreas, gallbladder, extrahepatic bile ducts, and ampulla of vater share a field for carcinogenesis: a population-based study. Arch Pathol Lab Med. 133(1):67-71, 2009
4. Furlan A et al: Gallbladder carcinoma update: multimodality imaging evaluation, staging, and treatment options. AJR Am J Roentgenol. 191(5):1440-7, 2008
5. Morine Y et al: Surgical strategy for advanced gallbladder carcinoma according to invasive depth of the tumor. Hepatogastroenterology. 55(88):1965-70, 2008

Microscopic Features

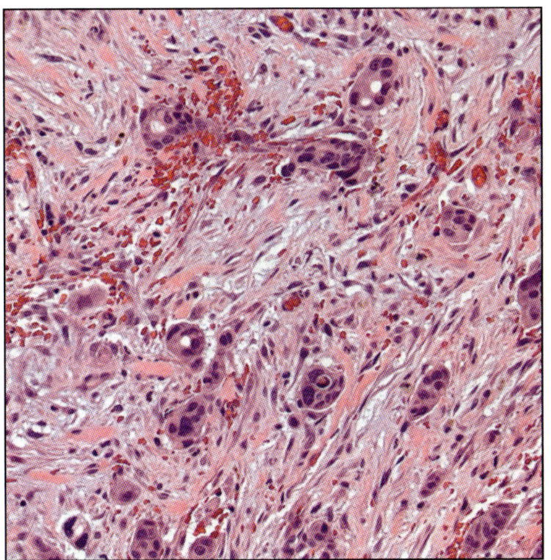

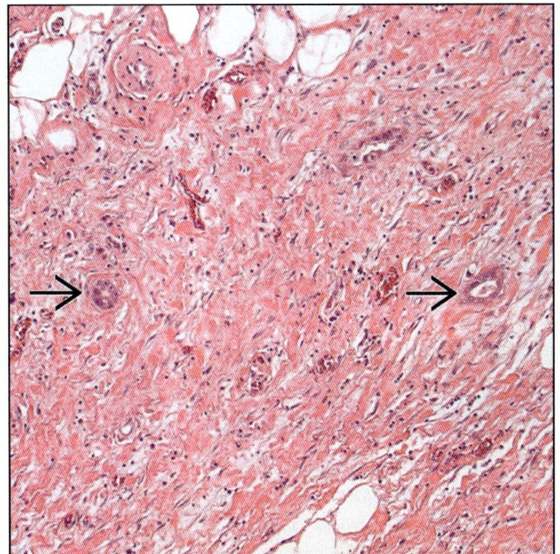

(Left) *Hematoxylin and eosin stained section shows irregular and abortive glands set in prominent desmoplastic stroma in an invasive gallbladder adenocarcinoma.* ***(Right)*** *Hematoxylin and eosin stained slide contains singly dispersed malignant glands penetrating the gallbladder wall ⇒ in an infiltrative pattern in gallbladder adenocarcinoma.*

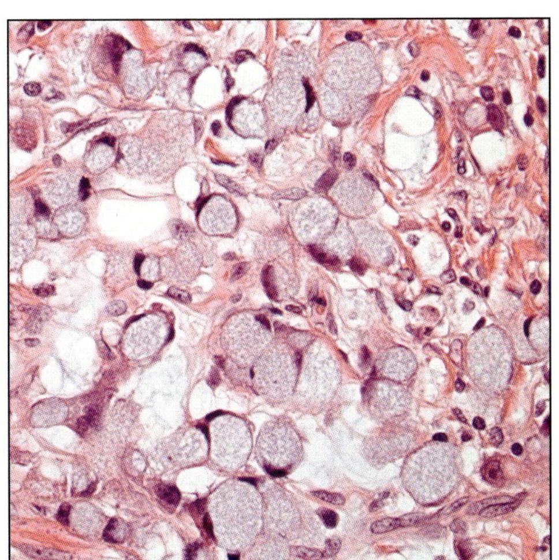

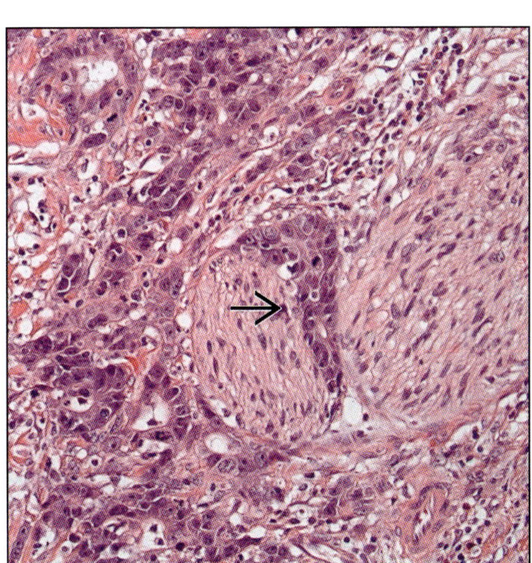

(Left) *This hematoxylin and eosin stained section demonstrates signet ring cell adenocarcinoma of the gallbladder.* ***(Right)*** *Hematoxylin and eosin stained section shows perineural invasion ⇒ in a case of gallbladder carcinoma.*

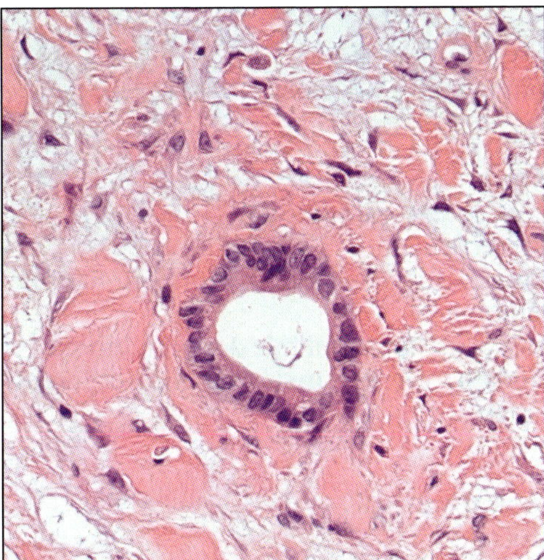

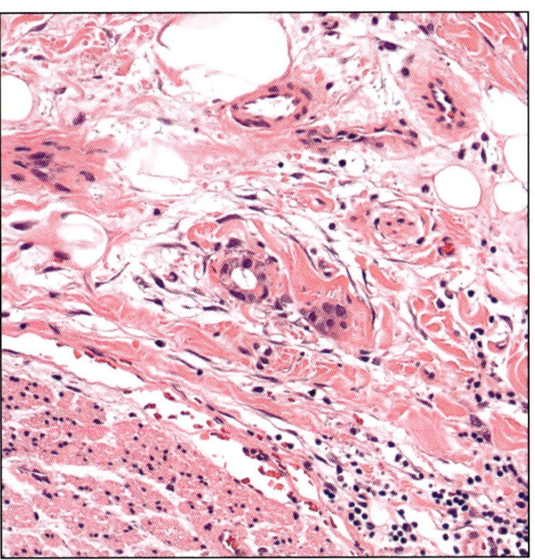

(Left) *Hematoxylin and eosin stained slide demonstrates a relatively well-formed yet malignant gland infiltrating the wall in an example of well-differentiated gallbladder adenocarcinoma.* ***(Right)*** *Hematoxylin and eosin stained section exhibits a few bland-appearing glands in perimuscular connective tissue in a case of well-differentiated gallbladder adenocarcinoma.*

ADENOCARCINOMA OF THE EXTRAHEPATIC BILE DUCTS

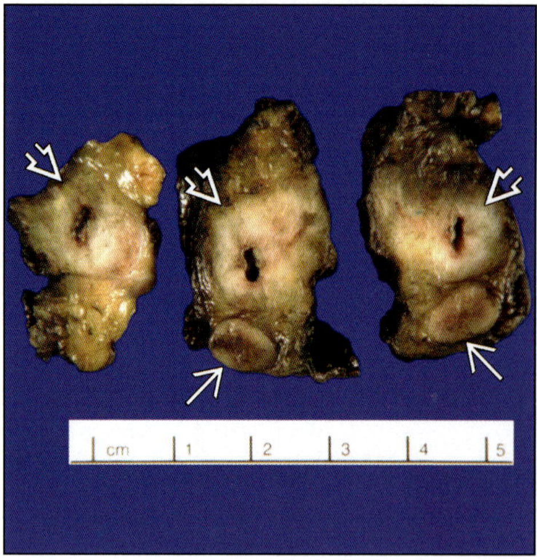

Segmental resection for perihilar bile duct carcinoma shows marked thickening of the common hepatic duct with firm, white cut surfaces ➡. A portion of dilated cystic duct is present ➡.

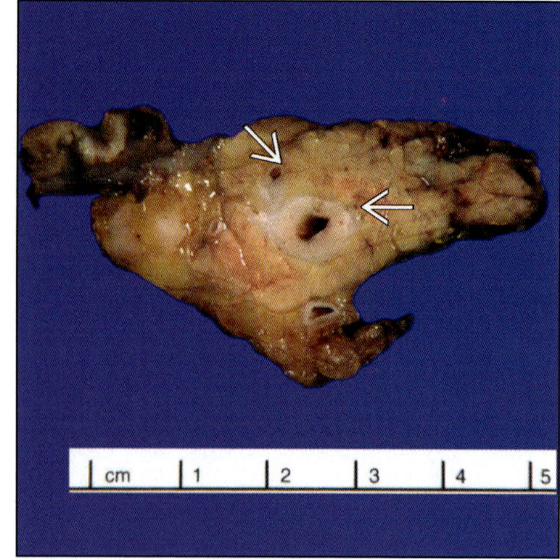

Cross section of a Whipple specimen shows distal bile duct carcinoma involving the intrapancreatic portion of the common bile duct and causing marked thickening of the duct wall ➡.

TERMINOLOGY

Synonyms

- Extrahepatic cholangiocarcinoma

Definitions

- Malignant neoplasm arising from epithelium lining right and left hepatic ducts, common hepatic duct, and common bile duct
- Perihilar bile duct carcinoma
  - Arises in extrahepatic bile ducts upstream to origin of cystic duct
    - Klatskin tumor occurs at confluence of right and left hepatic ducts
  - Comprises 70-80% of extrahepatic cholangiocarcinoma
- Distal bile duct carcinoma
  - Arises in common bile duct (including intrapancreatic portion) above ampulla of Vater
  - Comprises 20-30% of extrahepatic cholangiocarcinoma
- Diffuse involvement of extrahepatic bile ducts is rare, comprising ~ 2% of extrahepatic cholangiocarcinoma

ETIOLOGY/PATHOGENESIS

Developmental Anomaly

- Choledochal cyst
- Abnormal choledochopancreatic junction

Chronic Inflammation

- Primary sclerosing cholangitis
- Cholelithiasis (controversial)

Parasitic Infection (Flukes)

- *Clonorchis sinensis*
- *Opisthorchis viverrini*

Genetic Syndromes

- Familial adenomatous polyposis

Molecular Alterations

- *KRAS* mutations in ~ 30% of cases
- Overexpression of p53 oncoprotein in ~ 50% of cases

CLINICAL ISSUES

Epidemiology

- Incidence
  - 0.53-2 per 100,000 in population
- Age
  - Primarily seen during 6th and 7th decades of life
- Gender
  - Slight male predominance

Presentation

- Nonspecific symptoms and signs
  - Abdominal pain, malaise, anorexia, nausea, vomiting, weight loss
- Symptoms and signs of biliary obstruction
  - Jaundice, pruritus, acholic stools, dark urine

Laboratory Tests

- Elevated serum CA19-9, CEA, and CA125 levels

Treatment

- Surgical resection
  - Only hope for long-term survival
  - Segmental resection
    - May include partial hepatectomy for perihilar bile duct carcinoma
  - Whipple procedure for distal bile duct carcinoma
- Combined modality therapy, including chemotherapy and radiotherapy

Prognosis

- 10% overall 5-year survival
- Prognostic indicators
  - Tumor stage
    - Most important prognostic indicator
  - Tumor location

ADENOCARCINOMA OF THE EXTRAHEPATIC BILE DUCTS

Key Facts

Terminology
- Malignant neoplasm arising from epithelium lining right and left hepatic ducts, common hepatic duct, and common bile duct
  - Perihilar bile duct carcinoma
  - Distal bile duct carcinoma

Etiology/Pathogenesis
- Developmental anomalies
- Primary sclerosing cholangitis

Clinical Issues
- Poor prognosis with 10% overall 5-year survival
- Surgical resection is only hope for long-term survival
- Prognostic indicators include tumor stage, location, histology, and surgical margins

Image Findings
- Biliary stricture, wall thickening, intraluminal mass

Microscopic Pathology
- Wide spectrum of histologic appearance ranging from glandular structures to solid or cord-like clusters to individual tumor cells
- Malignant glands are arranged in haphazard pattern, infiltrating duct wall
- Often associated with desmoplastic stroma
- Nuclear pleomorphism with increased N:C ratio, nuclear grooves, and brisk mitotic activity

Top Differential Diagnoses
- Reactive periductal glands
- Indistinguishable from pancreatic ductal carcinoma histologically and immunophenotypically

    - Better prognosis for distal bile duct carcinoma due to early detection and resectability
  - Histologic grade
    - Poorly differentiated tumors are associated with worse prognosis
  - Histologic variants
    - Poorer prognosis for signet ring cell carcinoma
    - More favorable outcome for papillary adenocarcinoma
  - Surgical resection margins
    - Improved overall survival for those with negative resection margins
  - Lymphovascular invasion
    - Associated with adverse outcome
  - Perineural invasion
    - Associated with adverse outcome

IMAGE FINDINGS

Ultrasonographic Findings
- Duct dilation indicative of downstream obstruction

CT and MR Findings
- Infiltrative pattern
  - Duct wall thickening, obliteration of duct lumen
- Mass-like lesion
  - Distension of duct by intraluminal mass

Cholangiographic (ERCP) Findings
- Bile duct stricture

MACROSCOPIC FEATURES

General Features
- Firm, white, and gritty cut surface
- 4 categories traditionally
  - Polypoid
  - Nodular
  - Scirrhous constricting
  - Diffusely infiltrating

MICROSCOPIC PATHOLOGY

Histologic Features
- Wide variation in histologic appearance overall
- Neoplastic glands with lumina
  - Well-formed, irregular, abortive, cribriforming, or with papilla formation
  - Arranged in random or haphazard pattern, infiltrating duct wall
  - Often widely spaced
  - May form solid or cord-like structures
  - Individual infiltrating cells may be present
- Cytologic features
  - Range from deceptively bland to overtly high-grade nuclei
  - Acidophilic, basophilic, granular, pale, clear, foamy, or microvesicular cytoplasm
- Prominent desmoplastic stroma
- Varying amounts of intraluminal or extracellular mucin
- Frequent lymphovascular &/or perineural invasion
- Varying degree of tumor necrosis
- Frequent association with epithelial dysplasia or carcinoma in situ

Histologic Grade
- Well differentiated: > 95% of tumor volume composed of glands
- Moderately differentiated: 50-95% of tumor volume composed of glands
- Poorly differentiated: < 50% of tumor volume composed of glands

Cytopathology
- Brush cytology
  - Low sensitivity but high specificity
- Fine needle aspiration
  - High sensitivity and high specificity
- Cytologic features
  - Loss of honeycombing pattern
  - Nuclear pleomorphism with increased nuclear to cytoplasmic ratio

- Raisinoid nuclei with nuclear grooves
- Prominent nucleoli
- Frequent mitosis and atypical mitotic figures

Histologic Variants

- Papillary adenocarcinoma, noninvasive or invasive
  - Composed predominantly of papillary structures lined by cuboidal or columnar epithelial cells
- Adenocarcinoma, intestinal type
  - Resembles colonic adenocarcinoma
- Adenocarcinoma, gastric foveolar type
  - Glands lined by layer of tall, columnar, mucin-secreting cells resembling gastric foveolar cells
- Mucinous adenocarcinoma
  - Extracellular mucin is > 50% of tumor volume
    - Neoplastic glands distended with mucin
    - Clusters of tumor cells floating in mucin lakes
- Clear cell adenocarcinoma
  - Composed predominantly of glycogen-rich clear cells with distinct cytoplasmic borders
  - Mimics clear cell carcinoma of kidney
- Signet ring cell carcinoma
  - Signet ring cells constitute > 50% of tumor volume
  - Diffusely infiltrative pattern
- Adenosquamous carcinoma
  - Composed of both glandular and squamous components
    - Squamous component comprises ≥ 25% for a tumor that is predominantly glandular
    - Any degree of glandular differentiation for a tumor that is predominantly squamous
- Biliary cystadenocarcinoma
  - Unilocular or multilocular cystic lesion
  - Likely represents malignant transformation of biliary cystadenoma

Microscopic Tumor Extension (Staging)

- Perihilar bile duct carcinoma
  - pT1: Tumor confined to bile duct, with extension up to muscle layer or fibrous tissue
  - pT2a: Tumor invades beyond wall of bile duct to surrounding adipose tissue
  - pT2b: Tumor invades adjacent hepatic parenchyma
  - pT3: Tumor invades unilateral branches of portal vein or hepatic artery
  - pT4: Tumor invades main portal vein or its branches bilaterally; or common hepatic artery; or 2nd-order biliary radicals bilaterally; or unilateral 2nd-order biliary radicals with contralateral portal vein or hepatic artery involvement
- Distal bile duct carcinoma
  - pT1: Tumor confined to bile duct histologically
  - pT2: Tumor invades beyond wall of bile duct
  - pT3: Tumor invades gallbladder, pancreas, duodenum, or other adjacent organs without involvement of celiac axis or superior mesenteric artery
  - pT4: Tumor involves celiac axis or superior mesenteric artery

Regional Lymph Nodes

- Perihilar bile duct carcinoma
  - pN0: No regional lymph node metastasis
  - pN1: Regional lymph node metastasis (including nodes along cystic duct, common bile duct, hepatic artery, and portal vein)
  - pN2: Metastasis to periaortic, pericaval, superior mesentery artery, &/or celiac artery lymph nodes
- Distal bile duct carcinoma
  - pN0: No regional lymph node metastasis
  - pN1: Regional lymph node metastasis
    - Nodes along common bile duct, hepatic artery, and celiac trunk
    - Posterior and anterior pancreaticoduodenal nodes
    - Nodes along superior mesenteric vein and right lateral wall of superior mesenteric artery

Margins

- Perihilar bile duct carcinoma
  - Bile duct margin(s)
  - Circumferential (radial) soft tissue margin
  - Liver parenchymal margin for cases with partial hepatic resection
- Distal bile duct carcinoma
  - Bile duct margin(s)
  - Gastric &/or duodenal margins
  - Retroperitoneal and distal pancreatic margins

ANCILLARY TESTS

Immunohistochemistry

- Positive for pancytokeratins, CK7, CK19, CEA, CA19-9, MUC1, and MUC5AC
- Positive for CK20 and CDX-2 in < 50% of cases

DIFFERENTIAL DIAGNOSIS

Reactive Periductal Glands

- Preserved lobular architecture with uniform glands
- History of stent
- Immunohistochemical stains can be helpful
  - Negative S100-pla and IMP3, positive pVHL (von Hippel-Lindau protein) in benign duct epithelium
  - Positive S100-pla &/or IMP3, loss of pVHL expression in adenocarcinoma

Secondary Involvement by Pancreatic Ductal Adenocarcinoma

- Indistinguishable histologically and immunophenotypically
- Clinical history, image findings helpful

SELECTED REFERENCES

1. Patel T: Cholangiocarcinoma. Nat Clin Pract Gastroenterol Hepatol. 3(1):33-42, 2006
2. Welzel TM et al: Impact of classification of hilar cholangiocarcinomas (Klatskin tumors) on the incidence of intra- and extrahepatic cholangiocarcinoma in the United States. J Natl Cancer Inst. 98(12):873-5, 2006

ADENOCARCINOMA OF THE EXTRAHEPATIC BILE DUCTS

Imaging and Microscopic Features

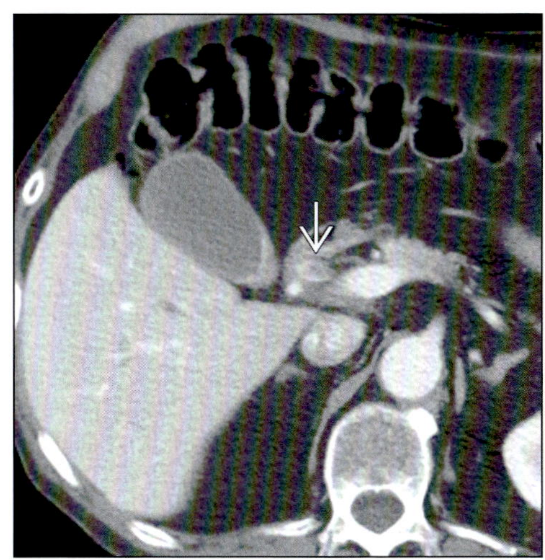

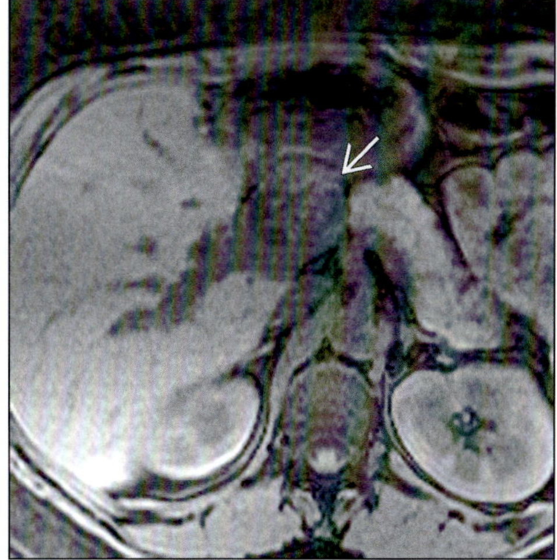

(Left) *Axial contrast-enhanced CT shows thickening and hyperenhancement of the common bile duct ➡. An ill-defined outer duct wall is a concerning feature for invasion beyond duct.* ***(Right)*** *Axial T1WI C+ FS MR image shows an intermediate signal intensity intraluminal solid and polypoid mass in the dilated common bile duct with filling defect ➡. The findings are consistent with distal bile duct carcinoma.*

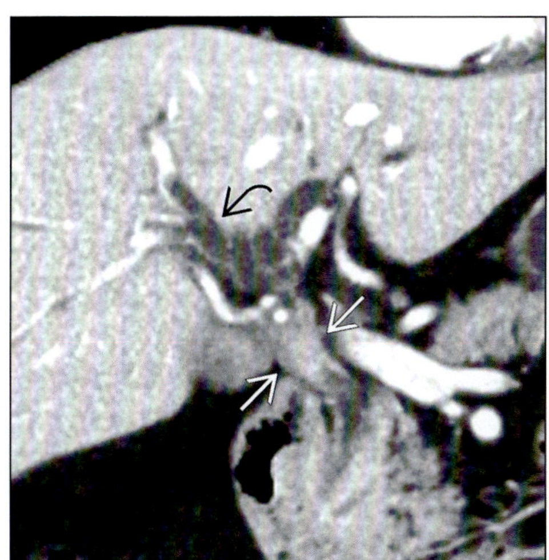

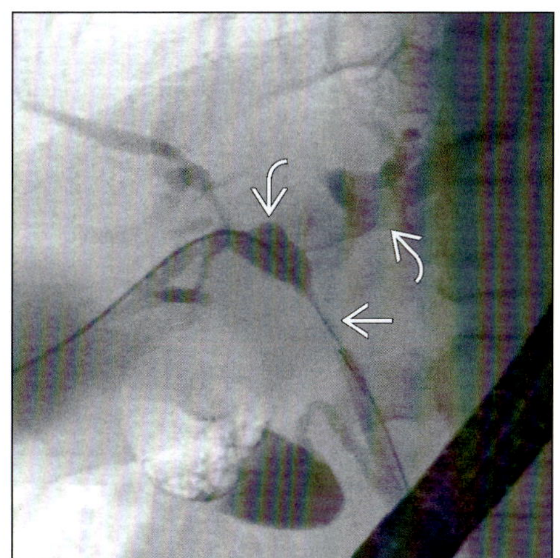

(Left) *A coronal contrast-enhanced CT image shows segmental wall thickening and hyperenhancement of the common bile duct ➡. An ill-defined outer duct wall is suggestive of invasion beyond the duct. Note dilated upstream intrahepatic bile ducts ↗.* ***(Right)*** *Endoscopic retrograde cholangiopancreatography (ERCP) shows obstruction at the confluence ➡ of the right and left hepatic ducts with upstream bile duct dilation ↗, consistent with Klatskin tumor.*

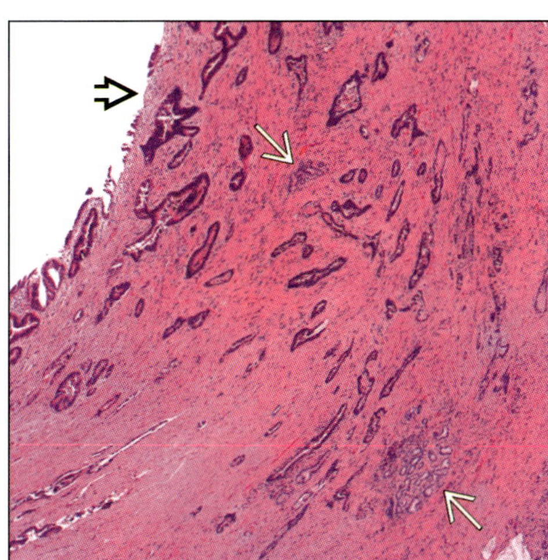

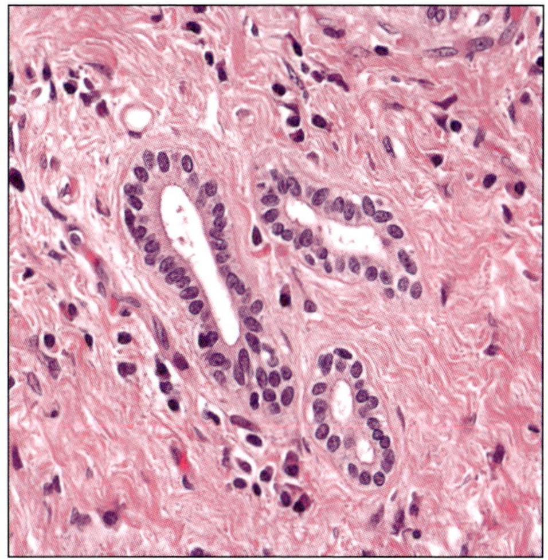

(Left) *Adenocarcinoma of the extrahepatic bile duct shows widely spaced, irregular glands infiltrating the duct wall. Note the presence of residual benign periductal glands arranged in a lobular pattern ➡. The duct lumen is partially denuded ⇨.* ***(Right)*** *A case of well-differentiated adenocarcinoma of the extrahepatic bile duct features well-formed glandular structures lined by a single layer of cuboidal epithelial cells with minimal cytologic atypia.*

ADENOCARCINOMA OF THE EXTRAHEPATIC BILE DUCTS

Microscopic Features

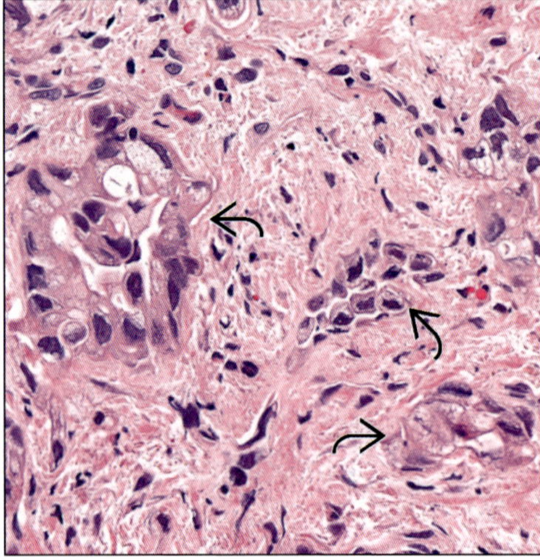

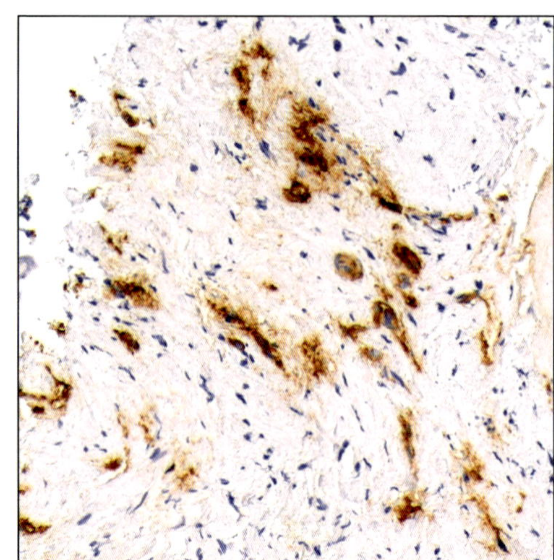

(Left) *A bile duct biopsy shows moderately differentiated adenocarcinoma characterized by scattered glands ➩ infiltrating a fibrotic stroma. The neoplastic glands are lined by pleomorphic tumor cells with foamy cytoplasm.* ***(Right)*** *A bile duct biopsy shows poorly differentiated adenocarcinoma with cord-like clusters and individual cells infiltrating desmoplastic stroma. The tumor cells are highlighted with cytokeratin 7 immunostaining.*

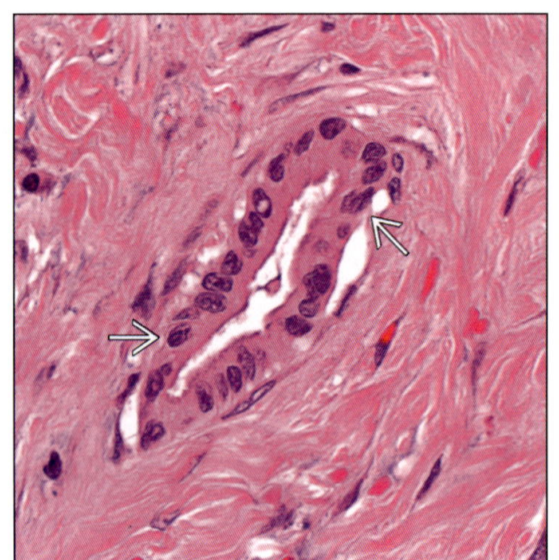

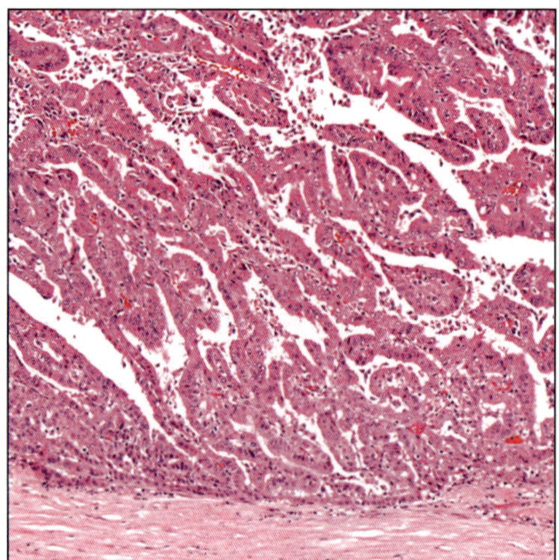

(Left) *A case of well-differentiated adenocarcinoma of the extrahepatic bile duct shows a well-formed gland lined by raisinoid tumor cells with nuclear grooves ➡ and variation in nuclear size and shape.* ***(Right)*** *A case of papillary adenocarcinoma of the common bile duct shows proliferation of complex papillary structures within the lumen of the duct. No invasion is seen in this area.*

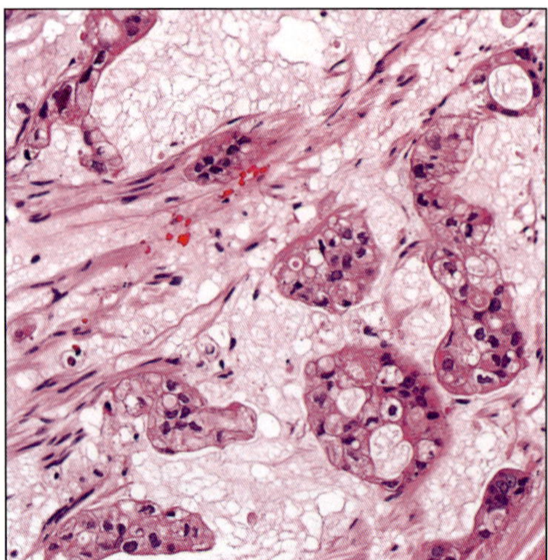

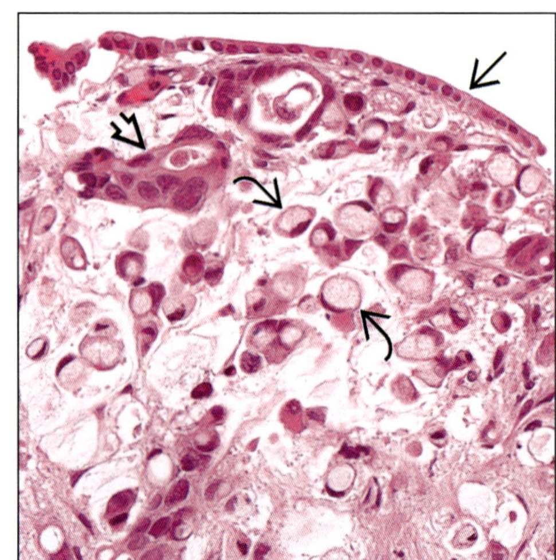

(Left) *A case of mucinous adenocarcinoma of the extrahepatic bile duct shows clusters of tumor cells floating in mucin pools. Tumor cells exhibit raisinoid nuclei and foamy cytoplasm.* ***(Right)*** *A bile duct biopsy shows numerous signet ring cells ➩ infiltrating the duct wall. Poorly formed glandular structures ➩ are only occasionally seen in this case. The overlying biliary epithelium ➡ appears cytologically unremarkable.*

Microscopic and Immunohistochemical Features

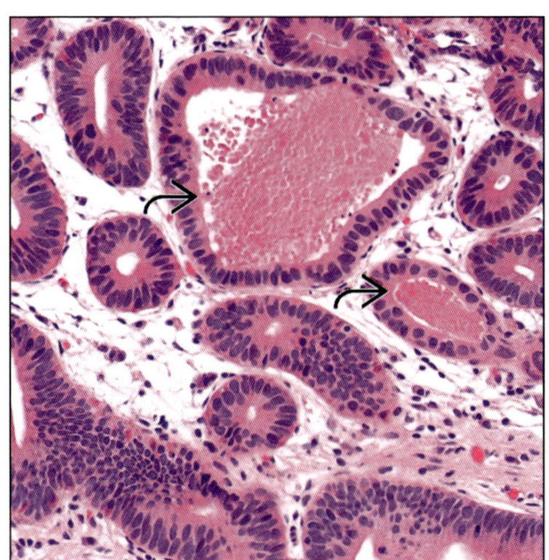

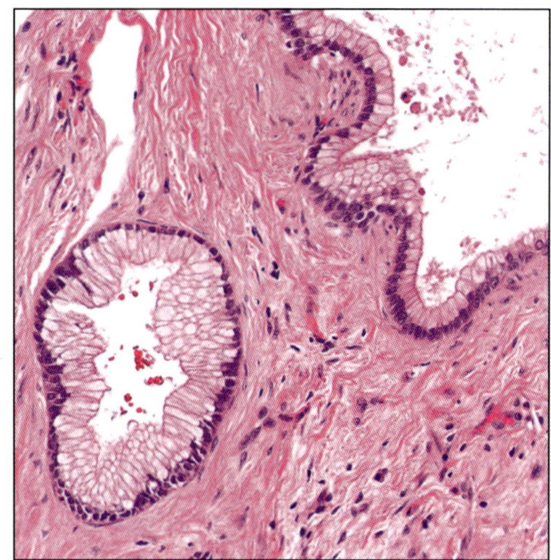

(Left) *A case of intestinal-type adenocarcinoma of the extrahepatic bile duct closely resembles adenocarcinoma of the colon. Note the presence of necrotic debris within the lumens of neoplastic glands ⮫.* ***(Right)*** *A case of adenocarcinoma of the extrahepatic bile duct shows well-formed glands lined by a single layer of tall, columnar, and mucin-secreting epithelial cells with basal nuclei and microvesicular cytoplasm, resembling gastric foveolar epithelium.*

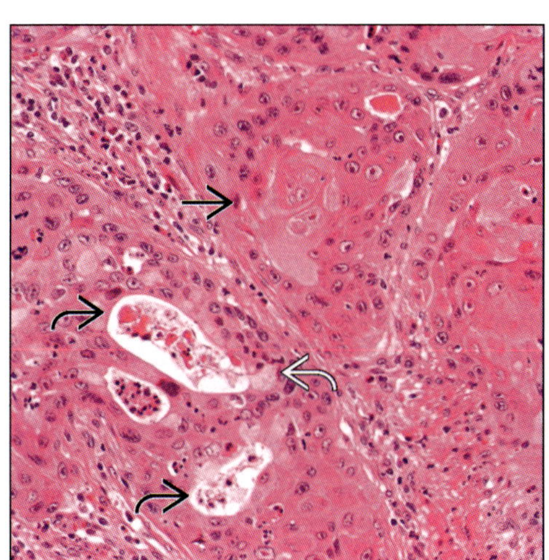

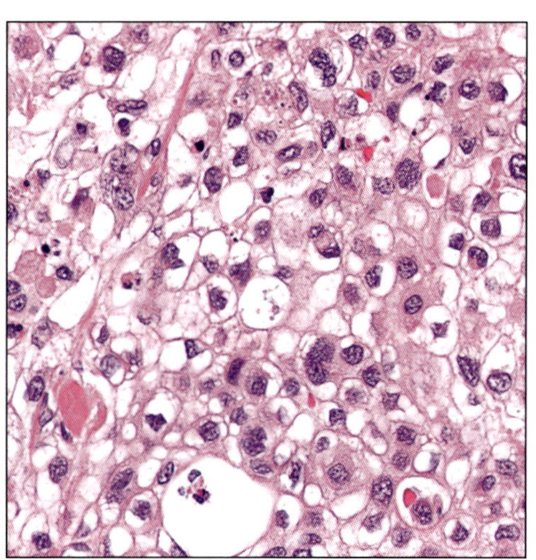

(Left) *A case of adenosquamous carcinoma of the extrahepatic bile duct shows squamous differentiation ➔ and gland formation ⮫ with mucin-producing tumor cells ⮫.* ***(Right)*** *A case of poorly differentiated clear cell adenocarcinoma of the extrahepatic bile duct shows sheets of tumor cells with irregular nuclei, clear cytoplasm, and distinct cell borders, resembling clear cell carcinoma of the kidney.*

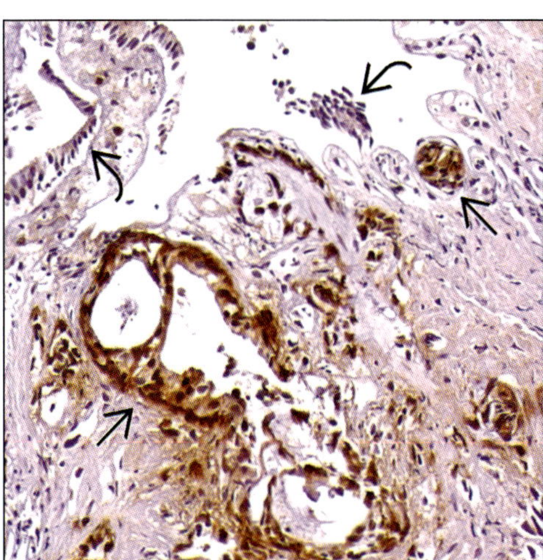

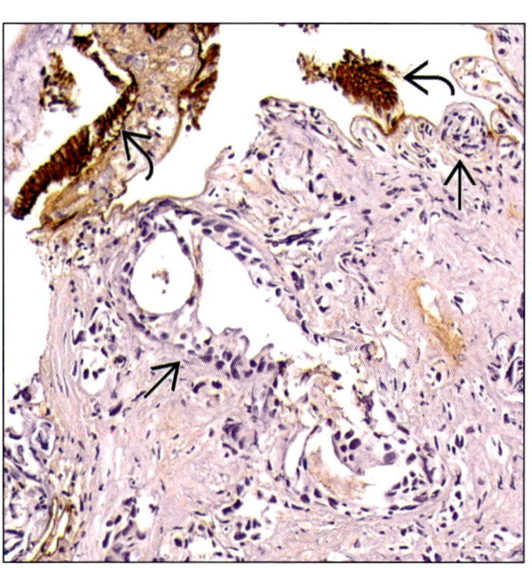

(Left) *Immunohistochemical stain for S100-pla performed on a bile duct biopsy shows nuclear and cytoplasmic positivity in malignant glands ➔. No immunoreactivity is detected in the overlying benign biliary epithelium ⮫.* ***(Right)*** *Immunostaining for von Hippel-Lindau protein (pVHL) performed on the same biopsy shows reciprocal loss of pVHL expression in malignant glands ➔ but membranous immunoreactivity in the overlying benign biliary epithelium ⮫.*

SQUAMOUS/ADENOSQUAMOUS CARCINOMA, GALLBLADDER

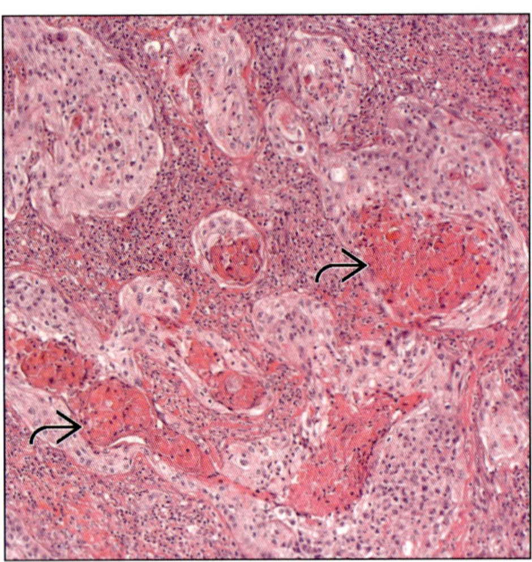

Paraffin section of a primary squamous cell carcinoma of the gallbladder shows islands of malignant squamous cells with keratinization ⮫.

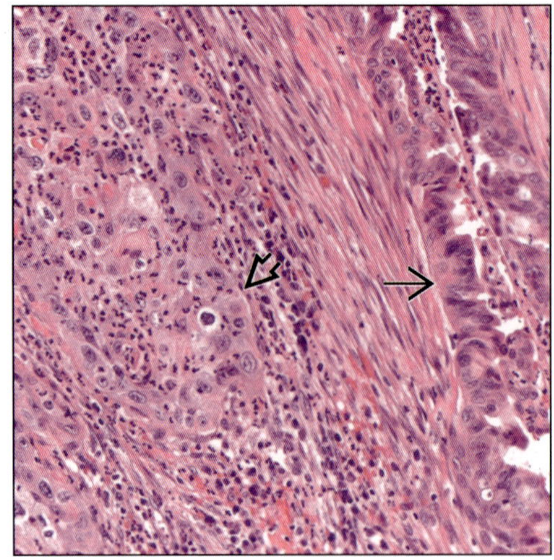

Paraffin section of an adenosquamous carcinoma of the gallbladder shows the squamous cell component ⮚ *adjacent to a malignant gland* →.

TERMINOLOGY

Definitions

- Squamous cell carcinoma of gallbladder is rare variant of gallbladder cancer with only squamous differentiation
- Adenosquamous carcinoma of gallbladder is uncommon variant of gallbladder cancer with both glandular and squamous differentiation

ETIOLOGY/PATHOGENESIS

Neoplastic

- Several theories exist to explain origin of squamous component
  - Squamous metaplasia of gallbladder mucosa
  - Stepwise molecular progression from preexisting adenocarcinoma of gallbladder
    - Mapping of tumors has shown squamous components in deeper portions of tumor
    - Flow cytometric data have demonstrated DNA heterogeneity between glandular and squamous components in over 70% of cases

CLINICAL ISSUES

Epidemiology

- Incidence
  - 1.4-9.6% of gallbladder carcinomas
- Age
  - Range: 5th to 9th decade of life
  - Average: 7th decade of life
- Gender
  - Female predominance

Presentation

- Abdominal pain
- Jaundice, cholestatic
- Weight loss

Treatment

- Surgical approaches
  - Cholecystectomy or cholecystectomy with partial hepatectomy are most common approaches
  - More extensive resections may be necessary depending on size, exact location of tumor, and involvement of adjacent structures

Prognosis

- Generally poor prognosis but depends upon grade, stage, and ability to achieve curative resection
  - Median survival < 1 year
  - Similar to conventional gallbladder adenocarcinoma of same stage

Associations

- Gallstones present in about 40% of cases

MACROSCOPIC FEATURES

General Features

- White-tan, firm tumor
- Nodular configuration or diffusely involving gallbladder wall
- May involve adjacent organs including liver, colon, duodenum, omentum, pancreas, stomach, and extrahepatic bile ducts

Size

- Mean diameter: 5-7 cm

Site

- Most arise in gallbladder fundus but may involve entire gallbladder or arise from gallbladder body
- Less often centered on gallbladder neck

SQUAMOUS/ADENOSQUAMOUS CARCINOMA, GALLBLADDER

Key Facts

Terminology
- Squamous cell carcinoma shows only squamous differentiation whereas adenosquamous carcinoma shows both glandular and squamous differentiation

Clinical Issues
- 1.4-9.6% of gallbladder carcinomas
- Generally poor prognosis but depends upon grade, stage, and ability to achieve curative resection

Macroscopic Features
- Most arise in gallbladder fundus as nodular masses or diffusely involve the gallbladder

Microscopic Pathology
- Glandular component can be intestinal, foveolar, papillary, or other pattern of cholangiocarcinoma
- Squamous component shows whorls, keratin pearls, keratinization, &/or intercellular bridges

MICROSCOPIC PATHOLOGY

Histologic Features
- Adenosquamous carcinoma has malignant glandular and squamous components
  - Glandular component can be intestinal type, foveolar type, papillary type, or other patterns of cholangiocarcinoma
  - Squamous component shows whorls, keratin pearls, individual cell keratinization, &/or intercellular bridges
- Squamous cell carcinoma shows only squamous component

Cytologic Features
- Proportion of cells with glandular or squamous features varies according to amount in tumor and sampling
- Pure squamous cell carcinoma may be undersampling of adenosquamous carcinoma, and metastatic squamous cell carcinoma must be considered

ANCILLARY TESTS

Histochemistry
- Mucicarmine
  - Reactivity: Positive
  - Staining pattern
    - Intracytoplasmic mucin in glandular component

Immunohistochemistry
- p63
  - Positive in squamous component

DIFFERENTIAL DIAGNOSIS

Metastatic Squamous Cell Carcinoma
- History of squamous cell carcinoma, no precursor lesion in gallbladder mucosa, similar morphology to presumptive primary tumor

DIAGNOSTIC CHECKLIST

Clinically Relevant Pathologic Features
- Pure squamous cell carcinoma of gallbladder is rare, and metastasis should be considered

SELECTED REFERENCES

1. Chan KM et al: Adenosquamous/squamous cell carcinoma of the gallbladder. J Surg Oncol. 95(2):129-34, 2007
2. Kondo M et al: Adenosquamous carcinoma of the gallbladder. Hepatogastroenterology. 49(47):1230-4, 2002
3. Oohashi Y et al: Adenosquamous carcinoma of the gallbladder warrants resection only if curative resection is feasible. Cancer. 94(11):3000-5, 2002
4. Nishihara K et al: Adenosquamous carcinoma of the gallbladder: a clinicopathological, immunohistochemical and flow-cytometric study of twenty cases. Jpn J Cancer Res. 85(4):389-99, 1994

IMAGE GALLERY

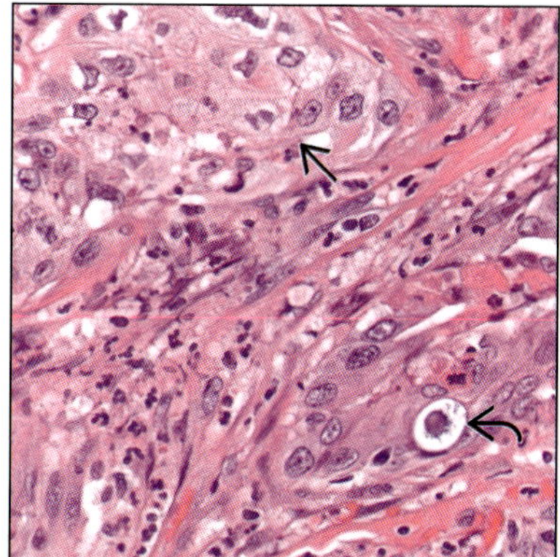

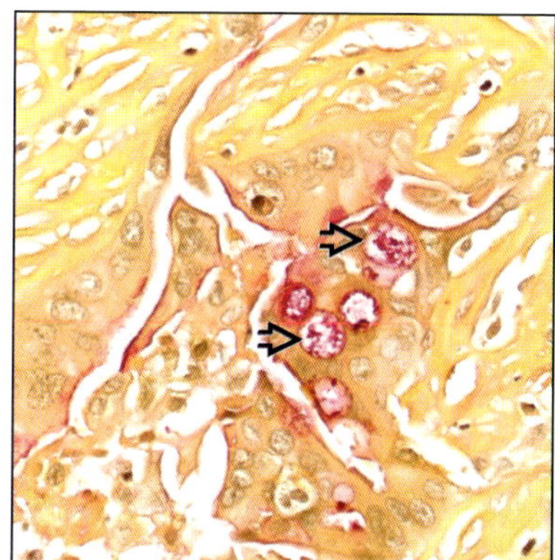

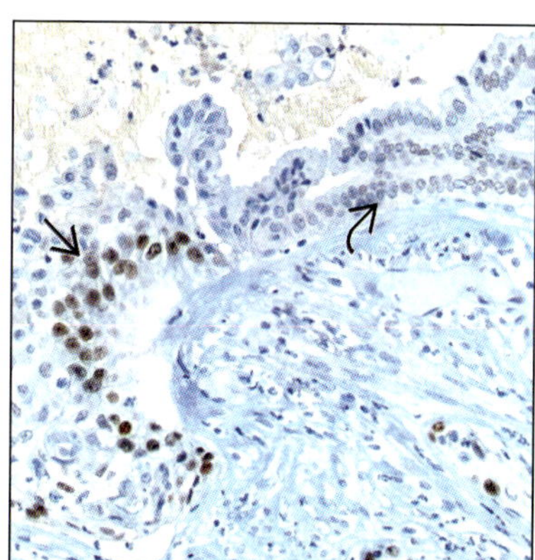

(Left) High-power view shows adenosquamous carcinoma with squamous component ➔ and glandular component with intracytoplasmic mucin ➔. *(Center)* Mucicarmine stain highlights the presence of intracytoplasmic mucin ➔ in the glandular component of an adenosquamous carcinoma. *(Right)* Immunohistochemical stain for p63 shows nuclear staining of the squamous component in adenosquamous carcinoma ➔ and absent staining in the glandular component ➔.

CARCINOID TUMOR

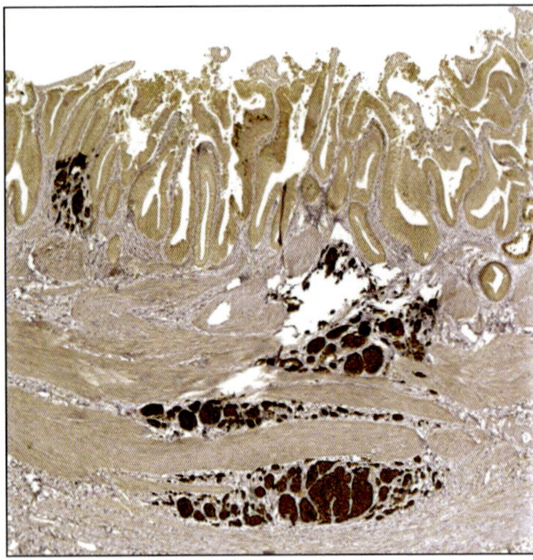

Synaptophysin immunostain highlights a carcinoid tumor of the gallbladder. Note that several foci extend from the mucosa into the wall.

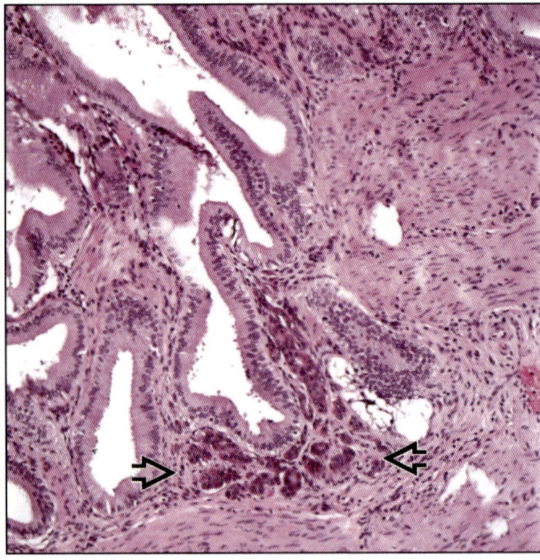

A small focus of carcinoid tumor is present at the base of the gallbladder epithelium ➩.

TERMINOLOGY

Synonyms

- Well-differentiated neuroendocrine tumor

Definitions

- Neoplasm of diffuse endocrine cell system

CLINICAL ISSUES

Epidemiology

- Incidence
  - Rare primary neoplasm of biliary tract
    - Most common location in biliary tract is gallbladder
- Age
  - Mean age at presentation is 60 years
- Gender
  - Slightly more common in females

Presentation

- May have symptoms of biliary obstruction, particularly those arising in extrahepatic bile ducts
- May be discovered incidentally
  - Small tumors may remain undetected for long periods
- Most discovered in patients who present with acute or chronic cholecystitis secondary to cholelithiasis
- Some are associated with von Hippel-Lindau syndrome, multiple endocrine neoplasia syndrome (MEN-1), or Zollinger-Ellison syndrome
- Not typically associated with carcinoid syndrome

Treatment

- Surgical approaches
  - Varied, depending on extent of disease
    - Simple cholecystectomy to extensive surgical resections, including regional lymph node dissections and hepatic lobectomy

Prognosis

- Similar behavior to carcinoid tumors occurring in other parts of GI tract
  - All tumors have metastatic potential
    - Risk is dependent on location in GI tract, size, and depth of invasion
    - Tumors > 2 cm are more likely to metastasize
- Overall 5-year survival rate of patients with biliary carcinoid tumor is around 40%

IMAGE FINDINGS

General Features

- Difficult to detect radiographically, mainly due to small size
- Occasionally discovered by ultrasound or computed tomography (CT) scan
- May be detected by octreotide scan

MACROSCOPIC FEATURES

General Features

- Nodular or polypoid lesions
  - Can arise in any part of gallbladder
- Cut surface usually solid, homogeneous, and white-yellow
- May be infiltrative and extend into adjacent liver

MICROSCOPIC PATHOLOGY

Histologic Features

- Uniform cells in insular, trabecular, and nesting patterns
  - Occasional tubule formation
    - Carcinoid tumors may show pseudogland formation, which should not be interpreted as adenocarcinoma
    - Focal signet ring cell morphology may be seen

CARCINOID TUMOR

Key Facts

Clinical Issues

- Rare primary neoplasm of biliary tract
- All tumors have metastatic potential
- Risk is mostly dependent on location in GI tract, size, and depth of invasion

Microscopic Pathology

- Uniform cells in insular, trabecular, and nesting patterns of growth within fibrous stroma
- Round, uniform nuclei with finely stippled chromatin ("salt and pepper")
- Scant mitoses, ≤ 2 mitotic figures per 10 HPF
- Minimal or no necrosis
- Diffuse reactivity with neuroendocrine markers (chromogranin, synaptophysin, and neuron-specific enolase)

  - Round, uniform nuclei with finely stippled chromatin ("salt and pepper")
    - Inconspicuous nucleoli
    - Small amount of eosinophilic and granular cytoplasm
    - Some may show signet ring cell morphology
    - Minimal nuclear atypia
    - Scant mitoses, ≤ 2 mitotic figures per 10 HPF
    - Minimal or no necrosis
- Prominent fibrous stroma
- Mucosa adjacent to tumor may show hyperplasia
- Variants
  - Tubular variant of carcinoid tumor has been described, similar to that in appendix
  - Clear cell variant, especially those associated with von Hippel-Lindau syndrome
  - Mixed (composite) carcinoid-adenocarcinoma
    - Classic carcinoid tumor mixed with adenocarcinoma

ANCILLARY TESTS

Immunohistochemistry

- Diffuse reactivity with neuroendocrine markers
  - Chromogranin, synaptophysin, and neuron-specific enolase
- Some tumors also express reactivity for serotonin, somatostatin, pancreatic polypeptide, or gastrin
  - Usually, tumors express > 1 substance

DIFFERENTIAL DIAGNOSIS

High-Grade Neuroendocrine Carcinoma

- Increased mitotic activity (> 10 per 10 HPF), necrosis, or both

Well-Differentiated Adenocarcinoma

- Tubular variant of carcinoid tumor should show positive staining with neuroendocrine markers
- Adenocarcinoma strongly keratin positive
  - Some carcinoid tumors show keratin positivity as well

DIAGNOSTIC CHECKLIST

Clinically Relevant Pathologic Features

- Correlation between immunohistochemical expression of peptide hormones and serologic levels has not been determined

SELECTED REFERENCES

1. Anjaneyulu V et al: Carcinoid tumor of the gall bladder. Ann Diagn Pathol. 11(2):113-6, 2007
2. Maitra A et al: Carcinoid tumors of the extrahepatic bile ducts: a study of seven cases. Am J Surg Pathol. 24(11):1501-10, 2000
3. Deehan DJ et al: Carcinoid tumour of the gall bladder: two case reports and a review of published works. Gut. 34(9):1274-6, 1993

IMAGE GALLERY

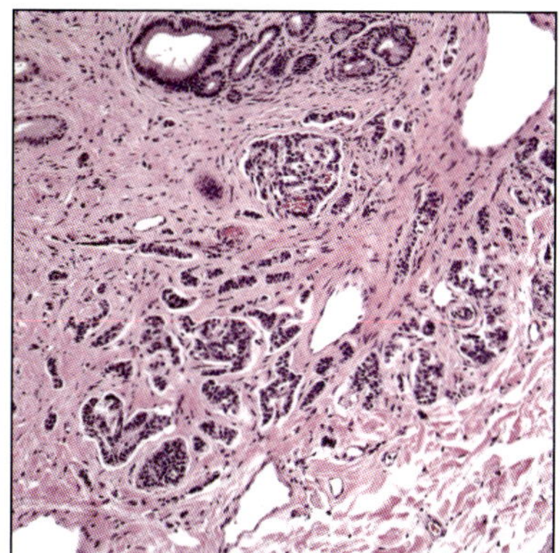

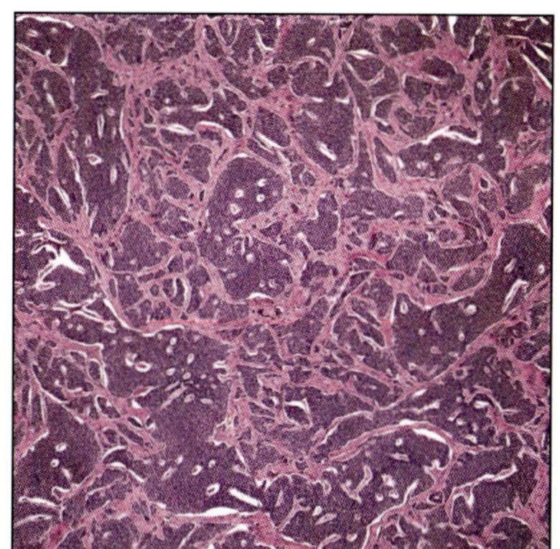

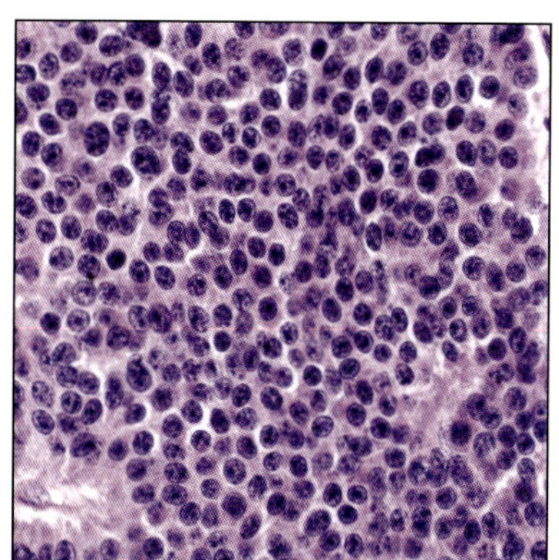

(Left) *This small carcinoid tumor was discovered in the common bile duct after a liver transplant.* ***(Center)*** *Carcinoid tumors typically show nests and trabeculae of uniform cells separated by prominent fibrous stroma.* ***(Right)*** *Carcinoid tumor cells typically have uniform nuclei, eosinophilic cytoplasm, and finely stippled chromatin, sometimes referred to as "salt and pepper" nuclei.*

POORLY DIFFERENTIATED NEUROENDOCRINE CARCINOMA, GALLBLADDER

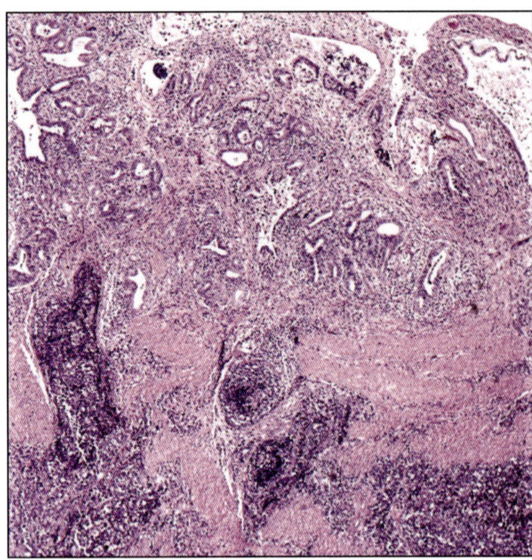

This low-power view of poorly differentiated neuroendocrine carcinoma of the gallbladder shows the characteristic diffuse submucosal growth pattern.

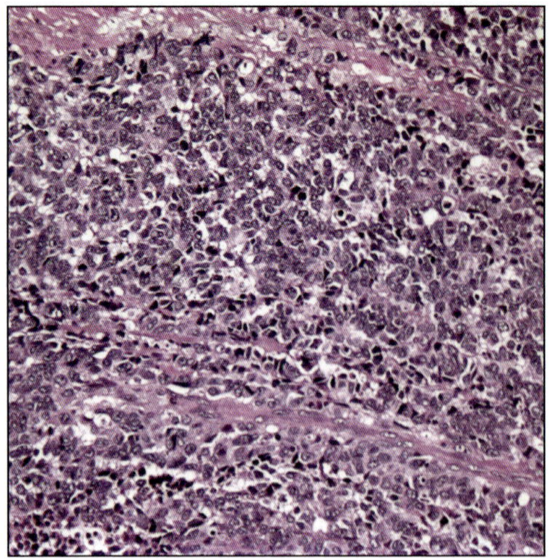

The tumor is composed of sheets of round to spindled small blue cells with finely dispersed chromatin and little cytoplasm.

TERMINOLOGY

Abbreviations

- Poorly differentiated neuroendocrine carcinoma (PDNC)

Synonyms

- Small cell carcinoma
- Small cell undifferentiated carcinoma
- Oat cell carcinoma

Definitions

- Most are similar to small cell counterpart in other organs, but some tumors have a large cell phenotype

ETIOLOGY/PATHOGENESIS

Unknown

- Associated with gallstones

CLINICAL ISSUES

Epidemiology

- Incidence
    - Very rare
        - < 5% of gallbladder carcinomas
        - More common in gallbladder than extrahepatic biliary tree
- Age
    - Older adults (6th to 7th decade of life; mean age at presentation is 67)
- Gender
    - Some sources report female predominance

Presentation

- Similar to other types of gallbladder carcinoma
- Rare syndrome of ectopic hormone production may give rise to Cushing syndrome

Treatment

- Chemotherapy regimen similar to that of PDNC of lung

Prognosis

- Dismal
    - Aggressive neoplasm that behaves similarly to counterparts in other organs
    - Many patients die within 6 months

MACROSCOPIC FEATURES

General Features

- Similar to other invasive carcinomas of gallbladder
    - Range from thickening of wall to bulging nodular mass
- Abundant necrosis is common

MICROSCOPIC PATHOLOGY

Histologic Features

- Similar to PDNC in other organs
    - Small, round to spindled blue cells
        - Hyperchromatic nuclei with finely dispersed chromatin
        - Nuclear moulding
        - Inconspicuous nucleoli
        - Scant eosinophilic cytoplasm
    - Tumor may grow in solid, nested, or trabecular patterns
        - Submucosal rather than mucosal growth is very common
    - Abundant necrosis
        - Viable tumor may be limited to areas around blood vessels
        - Walls of vessels may show deeply basophilic DNA deposition (Azzopardi effect)
    - Numerous mitoses

POORLY DIFFERENTIATED NEUROENDOCRINE CARCINOMA, GALLBLADDER

Key Facts

Terminology

- Similar to small cell carcinomas in other organs

Clinical Issues

- Highly aggressive neoplasm

Microscopic Pathology

- Round to spindled blue cells with hyperchromatic nuclei, finely dispersed chromatin, nuclear moulding
- Abundant necrosis and numerous mitoses
- May have foci of adenocarcinoma, squamous cell carcinoma, &/or mucosal dysplasia/carcinoma in situ
- Cytokeratin positive; many are negative for neuroendocrine markers

Diagnostic Checklist

- Important to make diagnosis so that patients get the correct chemotherapeutic regimen

- May be associated with conventional adenocarcinoma, squamous cell carcinoma, &/or mucosal dysplasia/carcinoma in situ

ANCILLARY TESTS

Immunohistochemistry

- May be positive for synaptophysin, chromogranin, NSE
  - More than half are negative for neuroendocrine markers in some reports; thus morphology is more important than immunophenotype
- Virtually all are cytokeratin positive

DIFFERENTIAL DIAGNOSIS

Metastatic Poorly Differentiated Neuroendocrine Carcinoma

- May require imaging studies to distinguish primary vs. secondary PDNC
- Cannot be distinguished on histologic grounds

Undifferentiated Carcinoma of Gallbladder

- Often consist of poorly differentiated glandular structures combined with spindled cells and giant cells
- Vesicular nuclei and prominent nucleoli

Carcinoid Tumor of Gallbladder

- Lack typical nuclear features of PDNC, necrosis, and mitotic activity
- Usually small submucosal nodules rather than infiltrative, destructive lesions
- Crucial distinction since behavior is very different

Lymphoma

- Marks with B- or T-cell markers; cytokeratin negative
- Lacks characteristic nuclear features, including moulding

DIAGNOSTIC CHECKLIST

Clinically Relevant Pathologic Features

- Important to diagnose this subtype so that patients get correct chemotherapy

SELECTED REFERENCES

1. Albores-Saavedra J et al: Carcinoid tumors and small-cell carcinomas of the gallbladder and extrahepatic bile ducts: a comparative study based on 221 cases from the Surveillance, Epidemiology, and End Results Program. Ann Diagn Pathol. 13(6):378-83, 2009
2. Albores-Saavedra J et al: Unusual malignant epithelial tumors of the gallbladder. Semin Diagn Pathol. 13(4):326-38, 1996
3. Henson DE et al: Carcinoma of the gallbladder. Histologic types, stage of disease, grade, and survival rates. Cancer. 70(6):1493-7, 1992
4. Albores-Saavedra J et al: Unusual types of gallbladder carcinoma. A report of 16 cases. Arch Pathol Lab Med. 105(6):287-93, 1981

IMAGE GALLERY

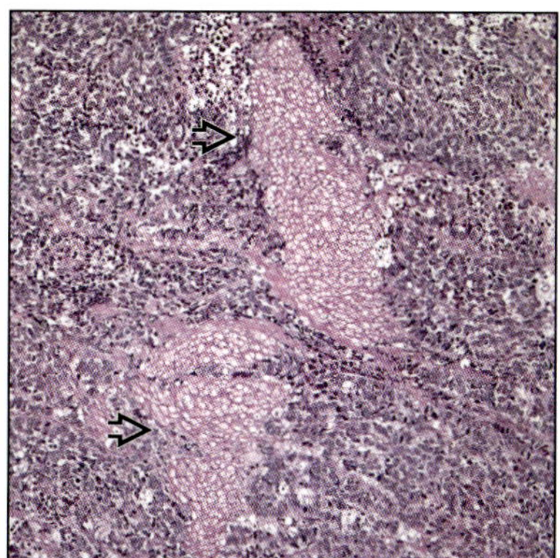

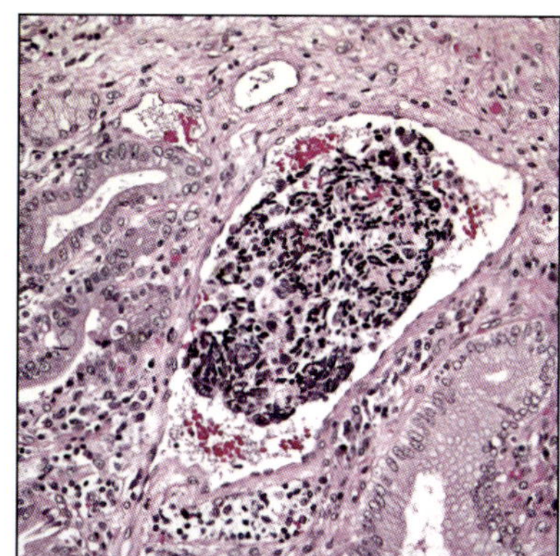

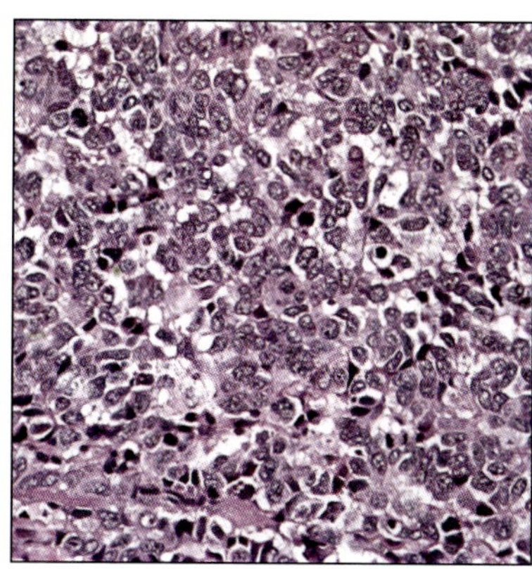

(Left) *Necrosis ➡ is often prominent both grossly and histologically in poorly differentiated neuroendocrine carcinoma of the gallbladder.* ***(Center)*** *Extensive lymphovascular invasion is commonly seen.* ***(Right)*** *The nuclei are typically small and round with finely dispersed chromatin and scant cytoplasm typical of neuroendocrine carcinomas. Nuclear moulding may be seen as well. Nucleoli are indistinct.*

GRANULAR CELL TUMOR

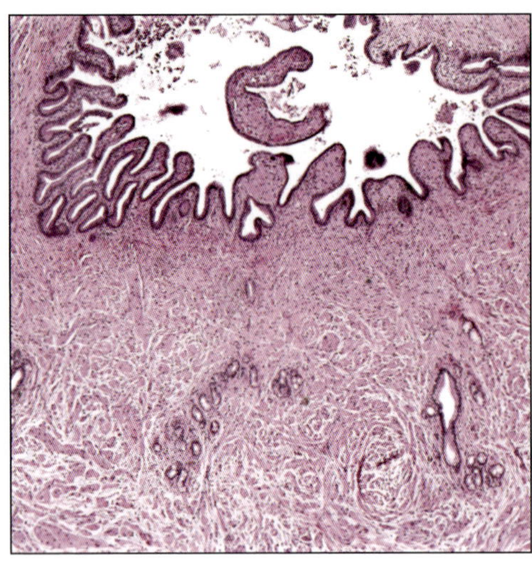

This granular cell tumor is growing concentrically around the common bile duct, compressing the lumen of the duct.

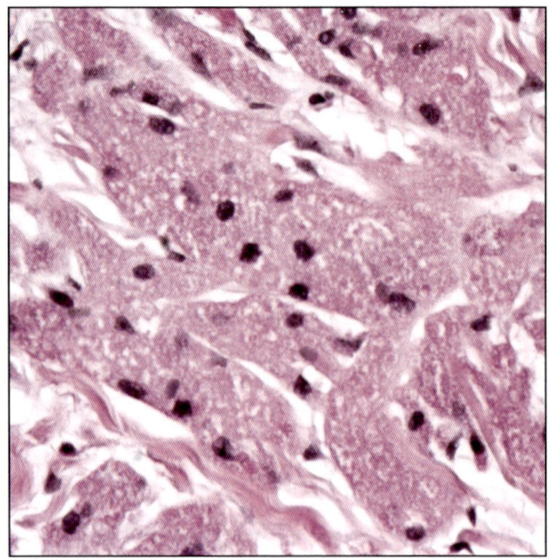

The tumor cells have abundant pink granular cytoplasm and small hyperchromatic nuclei.

TERMINOLOGY

Abbreviations

- Granular cell tumor (GCT)

Synonyms

- Granular cell myoblastoma

Definitions

- Benign neural tumor composed of large, granular, eosinophilic cells
  - Immunohistochemistry and electron microscopy have shown schwannian differentiation

CLINICAL ISSUES

Epidemiology

- Age
  - Young patients
    - Mean age: 34.7 years
    - Range: 11-61 years
- Gender
  - More common in women
- Ethnicity
  - More common in African-American population

Site

- Occurs most frequently in common bile duct
  - Majority of tumors at or near confluence of cystic (37%), hepatic (15%), and common bile ducts (50%)
  - Rarely (4%) involves gallbladder
- Most common nonepithelial tumor of extrahepatic bile ducts
- May be multicentric in the biliary tract or at other sites in body

Presentation

- Common bile duct or hepatic duct tumors
  - Obstructive symptoms such as
    - Jaundice
    - Hepatomegaly
    - Right upper quadrant pain
- Cystic duct tumors
  - Recurrent biliary colic and occasionally cholecystitis
- Often discovered incidentally

Treatment

- Surgical approaches
  - Cured by adequate excision
    - Location usually makes them amenable to simple excision
    - Recurrence is rare

Prognosis

- Benign
  - Malignant granular cell tumors have not been documented in the biliary tract

IMAGE FINDINGS

General Features

- Ultrasound, percutaneous transhepatic cholangiography, or endoscopic retrograde cholangiopancreatography
  - Obstruction or area of stricture
  - May mimic cholangiocarcinoma or sclerosing cholangitis radiographically

MACROSCOPIC FEATURES

General Features

- Firm, yellow-tan to yellow-white, ill-defined mass
  - Often grows concentrically around bile duct, compressing lumen
- Usually < 3 cm in greatest dimension

GRANULAR CELL TUMOR

Key Facts

Terminology
- Benign neural tumor with schwannian differentiation

Clinical Issues
- Occur most often in young African-American women
- Most common site is common bile duct

Macroscopic Features
- Often grows concentrically around bile duct

Microscopic Pathology
- Nests or sheets of infiltrating cells
  - Cells may be separated by collagenous bands
  - Abundant pink granular cytoplasm with small hyperchromatic nuclei
- Can be associated with marked atypia of overlying biliary surface epithelium

MICROSCOPIC PATHOLOGY

Histologic Features
- Nests or sheets of cells infiltrating soft tissue
  - Cells may be separated by collagenous bands
    - Older lesions may contain more connective tissue than tumor cells
  - May cluster around or infiltrate peripheral nerves
- Large oval to polygonal cells
  - Abundant acidophilic (pink) granular cytoplasm with occasional globules
  - Small hyperchromatic nuclei
  - Occasionally, spindled granular cells may be seen
- May be associated with marked proliferation and atypia of overlying biliary surface epithelium
  - Epithelial reaction can mimic dysplasia or carcinoma

ANCILLARY TESTS

Immunohistochemistry
- Shows immunoreactivity to S100, CD68, myelin proteins, and inhibin

DIFFERENTIAL DIAGNOSIS

Cholangiocarcinoma
- GCT may have a striking associated overlying epithelial cell proliferation with atypia
- Important to recognize underlying associated granular cell tumor and lack of invasive glandular component

Rhabdomyoma
- Pediatric patients
- Cells have cross striations
- Lacks granular cytoplasm

Sclerosing Cholangitis
- GCT can mimic sclerosing cholangitis radiographically
- Histologic appearance of sclerosing cholangitis very different from granular cell tumor

Leiomyoma
- Spindled cells with fascicular growth pattern
- Positive smooth muscle immunohistochemical markers

SELECTED REFERENCES

1. Patel AJ et al: Granular cell tumor of the biliary tract. Gastroenterol Hepatol (N Y). 6(5):331-6, 2010
2. Karakozis S et al: Granular cell tumors of the biliary tree. Surgery. 128(1):113-5, 2000
3. te Boekhorst DS et al: Granular cell tumor at the hepatic duct confluence mimicking Klatskin tumor. A report of two cases and a review of the literature. Dig Surg. 17(3):299-303, 2000
4. Butler JD Jr et al: Granular cell tumor of the extrahepatic biliary tract. Am Surg. 64(11):1033-6, 1998
5. Eisen RN et al: Granular cell tumor of the biliary tree. A report of two cases and a review of the literature. Am J Surg Pathol. 15(5):460-5, 1991

IMAGE GALLERY

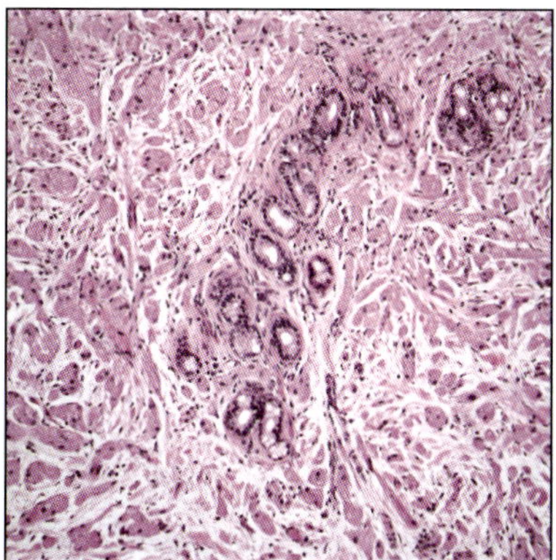

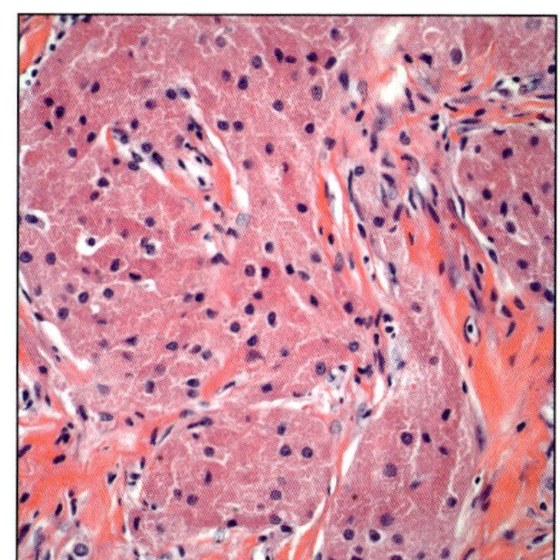

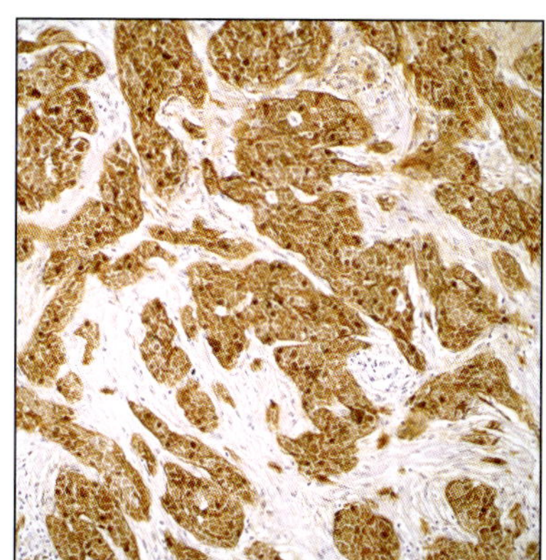

(Left) *The tumor cells can have a very infiltrative growth pattern. Here they surround and infiltrate small peribiliary radicals.* ***(Center)*** *The granular, pink, polygonal tumor cells are often interspersed with bands of collagen.* ***(Right)*** *S100 immunohistochemical stain is strongly positive within the tumor cells. (Courtesy J. McKenney, MD.)*

EMBRYONAL RHABDOMYOSARCOMA

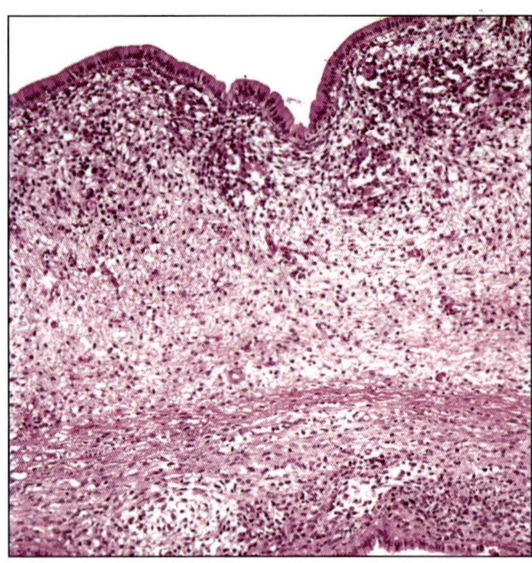

Closely packed neoplastic cells of rhabdomyosarcoma (RMS) form a dense "cambium layer" beneath a single layer of intact biliary epithelium. Deep to this are spindled tumor cells within a myxoid stroma.

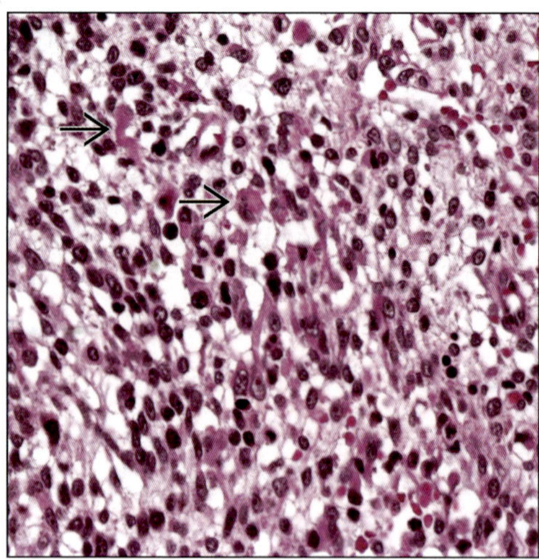

The tumor cells are typically small and hyperchromatic. Some cells have abundant eosinophilic cytoplasm →.

TERMINOLOGY

Abbreviations

- Rhabdomyosarcoma (RMS)

Definitions

- Primary rhabdomyosarcoma, embryonal type, arising in biliary tree or gallbladder
  - Botryoid rhabdomyosarcoma is most common neoplasm of extrahepatic biliary tree in childhood

CLINICAL ISSUES

Epidemiology

- Age
  - Most frequently described in children, in extrahepatic biliary tree
    - Range: 16 months to 11 years; mean age: 4.5 years
  - Occasionally seen in adults
    - Usually in gallbladder (rather than biliary tree) of elderly patients
- Gender
  - No gender predilection

Presentation

- Signs of progressive biliary obstruction
  - Jaundice
  - Acholic stools
- Hepatomegaly
- Abdominal pain
- Fever

Treatment

- Surgery, often followed by chemotherapy and radiation

Prognosis

- Generally poor
  - Tumor has propensity for both local invasion and widespread metastasis
  - Better survival data with use of combined modality therapy including surgery, chemotherapy, radiation

MACROSCOPIC FEATURES

General Features

- More common in biliary tree than gallbladder
  - Common bile duct most frequent location
    - Also reported in hepatic ducts, cystic duct, ampulla of Vater
- Grape-like (botryoid) gelatinous masses in lumen of bile duct
  - May be only loosely attached to wall
    - Wall may be thickened
  - Duct often dilated
- Gallbladder may be distended
  - Biliary RMS may extend to involve gallbladder as well

MICROSCOPIC PATHOLOGY

Histologic Features

- Resembles botryoid-type embryonal RMS elsewhere in the body
  - Single layer of biliary epithelium covering tumor
    - Epithelium may be intact, ulcerated, or inflamed
  - Tumor cells are small and hyperchromatic with variable amounts of eosinophilic cytoplasm
    - Tumor cells densely packed beneath epithelium to form characteristic "cambium layer"
    - Tumor cells within loose myxoid stroma deeper in lesion
  - Spindled cells, strap cells may be seen
  - Cross striations can be seen in approximately 1/2 of cases
- Mitotic count may be very high

EMBRYONAL RHABDOMYOSARCOMA

Key Facts

Terminology

- Botryoid rhabdomyosarcoma is most common pediatric neoplasm of extrahepatic biliary tree

Macroscopic Features

- More common in biliary tree than gallbladder
- Grape-like gelatinous masses in lumen of bile duct

Microscopic Pathology

- Resembles botryoid-type embryonal RMS elsewhere in the body
- Tumor cells densely packed beneath single layer of biliary epithelium to form characteristic "cambium layer"
- Newer myogenic markers such as myogenin, MYOD1 very helpful

ANCILLARY TESTS

Immunohistochemistry

- Positive for desmin, muscle specific actin, myoglobin
- Newer myogenic markers, such as myogenin, MYOD1 very helpful

DIFFERENTIAL DIAGNOSIS

Sarcomatoid Carcinoma

- Cytokeratin positive
- Lacks immunohistochemical demonstration of myogenic marking
- Lacks cambium layer
- Rare in children

Inflammatory Pseudotumor

- More inflammation than RMS
- Lacks desmin, myogenin, MYOD1 positivity

Other Sarcomas

- Leiomyosarcoma
  - Does not mark with myogenin, MYOD1
  - Lacks cambium layer
  - Exceedingly rare in biliary tree of children
- Angiosarcoma
  - Marks with vascular markers
- Kaposi sarcoma
  - Marks with vascular markers, HHV8
  - Present in immunocompromised persons

Primitive Neurectodermal Tumors

- CD99 positive (RMS usually negative)
- Has *EWSR-1* translocation
- Often has pseudorosette formation
- Lacks cambium layer, cross striations
- Very rare in biliary tree/gallbladder

DIAGNOSTIC CHECKLIST

Pathologic Interpretation Pearls

- Small hyperchromatic cells forming "cambium" layer beneath biliary epithelium

SELECTED REFERENCES

1. al-Jaberi TM et al: Adult rhabdomyosarcoma of the gall bladder: case report and review of published works. Gut. 35(6):854-6, 1994
2. Aldabagh SM et al: Rhabdomyosarcoma of the common bile duct in an adult. Arch Pathol Lab Med. 110(6):547-50, 1986
3. Mihara S et al: Botryoid rhabdomyosarcoma of the gallbladder in a child. Cancer. 49(4):812-8, 1982
4. Lack EE et al: Botryoid rhabdomyosarcoma of the biliary tract. Am J Surg Pathol. 5(7):643-52, 1981
5. Davis GL et al: Embryonal rhabdomyosarcoma (sarcoma botryoides) of the biliary tree. Report of five cases and a review of the literature. Cancer. 24(2):333-42, 1969

IMAGE GALLERY

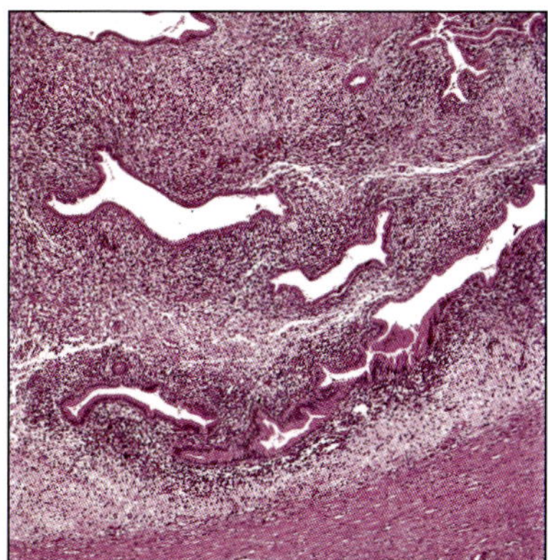

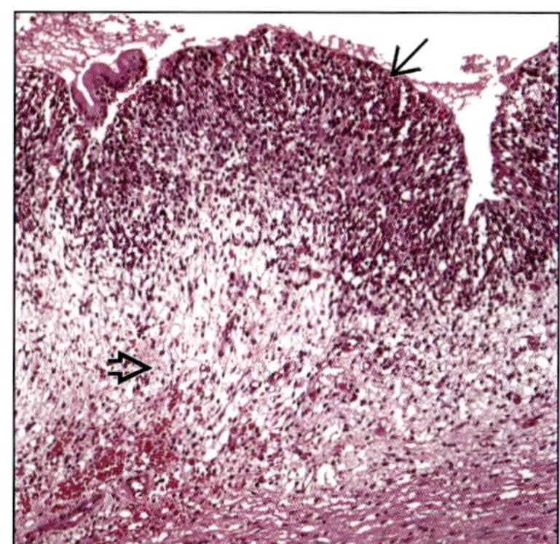

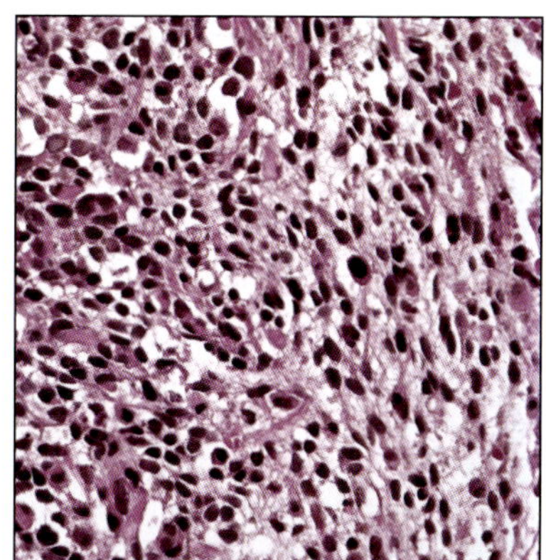

(Left) *This embryonal RMS of the bile duct in a child forms a polypoid mass beneath the biliary epithelium.* ***(Center)*** *The characteristic "cambium layer" consists of densely packed tumor cells beneath the epithelium ⇒, which is disrupted in this case. The deeper tumor cells are spindled and present within a myxoid stroma ⇨.* ***(Right)*** *The tumor cells in embryonal RMS are typically small and hyperchromatic with a variable amount of eosinophilic cytoplasm.*

ADENOMYOMA

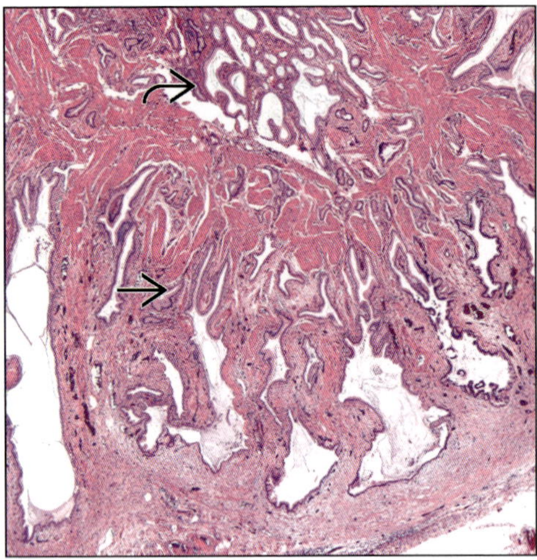

A section of adenomyoma shows irregular invaginations of biliary epithelium extending down from the surface ⇗ and through the smooth muscle ⇒ of the gallbladder wall.

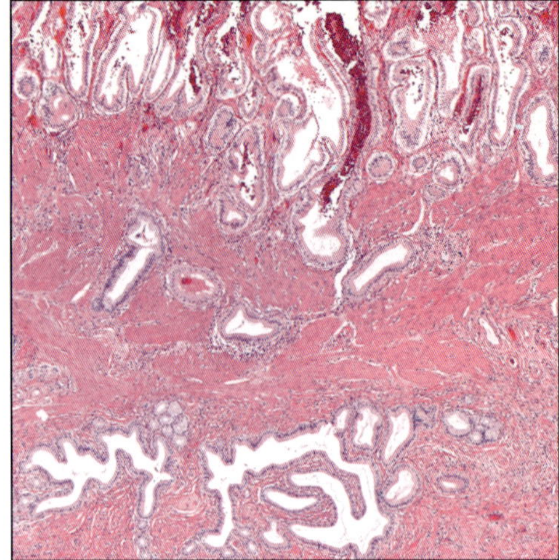

H&E section of adenomyomatous hyperplasia demonstrates Rokitansky-Aschoff sinuses extending downward from the overlying mucosa into the smooth muscle of the gallbladder wall.

TERMINOLOGY

Synonyms

- Adenomyomatous polyp
- Localized adenomyomatous hyperplasia
- Adenomyosis
- Adenomyomatous hyperplasia
- Adenomyomatosis
- Diverticular disease of the gallbladder
- Intramural diverticulosis
- Cholecystitis cystica
- Cholecystitis glandularis proliferans

Definitions

- Acquired lesion of gallbladder with invaginations of surface epithelium into thickened muscular wall

ETIOLOGY/PATHOGENESIS

Acquired Lesion

- Most cases are associated with chronic cholecystitis
- 90% of affected individuals also have cholelithiasis

CLINICAL ISSUES

Epidemiology

- Incidence
  - Present in approximately 10% of cholecystectomy specimens
  - Represents 15-25% of benign gallbladder polyps
  - Approximately 4,500 cases diagnosed in USA each year
- Age
  - Predominantly affects adults although also reported in children
- Gender
  - More common in women than in men

Site

- Most often occurs in fundus of gallbladder
- Present within muscular wall of gallbladder

Presentation

- Usually asymptomatic
  - Often incidental finding at cholecystectomy
- Associated with cholecystitis, so patients may present with symptoms of cholecystitis
  - Persistent right upper quadrant pain

Natural History

- Benign

Treatment

- Cholecystectomy

Prognosis

- Cholecystectomy is curative

IMAGE FINDINGS

Radiographic Findings

- Diffuse or focal gallbladder wall thickening seen on ultrasound, abdominal CT, or MRCP
- Accurate diagnosis relies on identification of diverticula or cystic spaces within lesion

MACROSCOPIC FEATURES

General Features

- Firm area of thickening of gallbladder wall
  - May be diffuse, segmental, or localized lesion
- Gray or gray-white, trabecular appearance
- May form polyp or pseudotumor
- May be mistaken for malignant neoplasm
- Cut surface reveals multiple cysts representing dilated biliary glands

ADENOMYOMA

Key Facts

Terminology
- Acquired lesion of gallbladder with invaginations of surface epithelium into thickened muscular wall

Etiology/Pathogenesis
- Most cases are associated with chronic cholecystitis
- 90% of affected individuals also have cholelithiasis

Microscopic Pathology
- Hypertrophic or cystically dilated glands set in hyperplastic smooth muscle

Top Differential Diagnoses
- Adenocarcinoma
- Chronic cholecystitis

  - Cysts often contain inspissated bile and bile concretions

Size
- 0.5-2.5 cm

MICROSCOPIC PATHOLOGY

Histologic Features
- Hypertrophic or cystically dilated glands set in hyperplastic smooth muscle
  - Glands represent extensions of Rokitansky-Aschoff sinuses, which are invaginations or diverticula of biliary epithelium
- Epithelium usually identical to that seen in normal biliary mucosa but may show metaplasia, dysplasia, or carcinoma
  - May show reactive changes
- Rarely, glands are seen in close proximity to nerves and should not be interpreted as feature of malignancy in adenomyoma

Cytologic Features
- No cytologic atypia or features of malignancy

DIFFERENTIAL DIAGNOSIS

Adenocarcinoma
- Epithelial elements penetrating smooth muscle may be confused with adenocarcinoma
- Cytologic features of malignancy are lacking in adenomyoma

Chronic Cholecystitis
- Mild chronic inflammation with Rokitansky-Aschoff sinuses and smooth muscle hypertrophy
- Chronic cholecystitis shows less prominent wall thickening than adenomyoma
- Most patients with adenomyoma also have chronic cholecystitis

DIAGNOSTIC CHECKLIST

Pathologic Interpretation Pearls
- Bland-appearing epithelium and cystically dilated glands set in thickened smooth muscle
- Associated with chronic cholecystitis and cholelithiasis

SELECTED REFERENCES

1. Albores-Saavedra J et al: Adenomyomatous hyperplasia of the gallbladder with perineural invasion: revisited. Am J Surg Pathol. 31(10):1598-604, 2007
2. Ching BH et al: CT differentiation of adenomyomatosis and gallbladder cancer. AJR Am J Roentgenol. 189(1):62-6, 2007
3. Owen CC et al: Gallbladder polyps, cholesterolosis, adenomyomatosis, and acute acalculous cholecystitis. Semin Gastrointest Dis. 14(4):178-88, 2003

IMAGE GALLERY

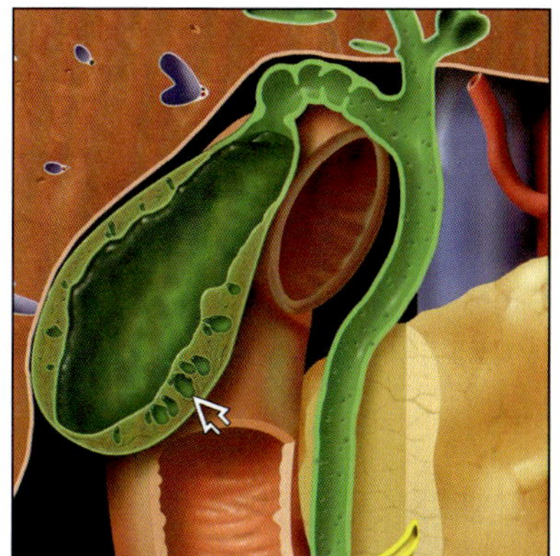

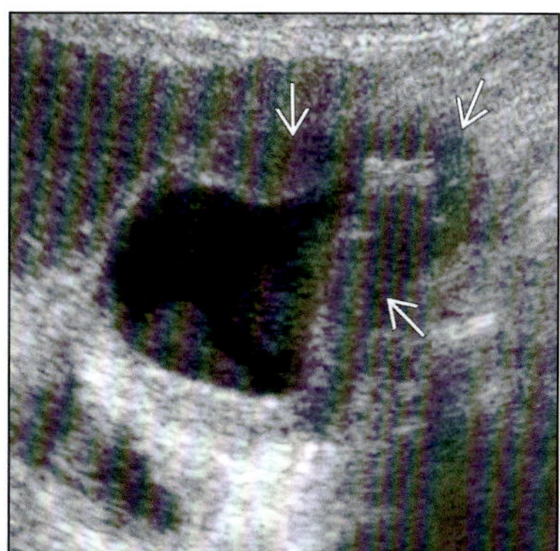

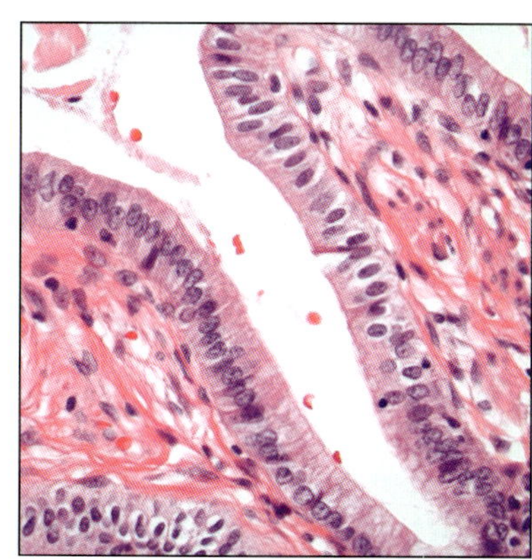

(Left) *Graphic shows characteristic features of adenomyomatosis. Note the thickened gallbladder wall with multiple intramural cystic spaces ➡.* ***(Center)*** *Ultrasound of the gallbladder shows focal mural thickening in the fundus ➡ with no invasion of adjacent structures. This is the typical appearance of adenomyomatosis.* ***(Right)*** *H&E section shows benign biliary epithelium in an adenomyoma. The epithelium lacks nuclear enlargement, hyperchromasia, or pleomorphism.*

INFLAMMATORY POLYPS

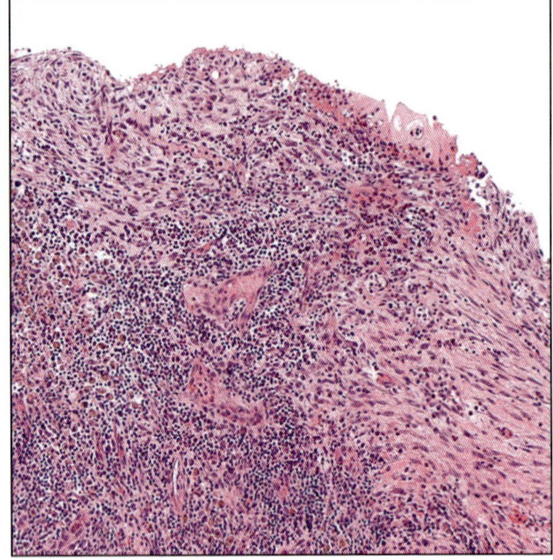

Inflammatory polyps of the gallbladder are composed of inflammation and a proliferation of organizing granulation tissue.

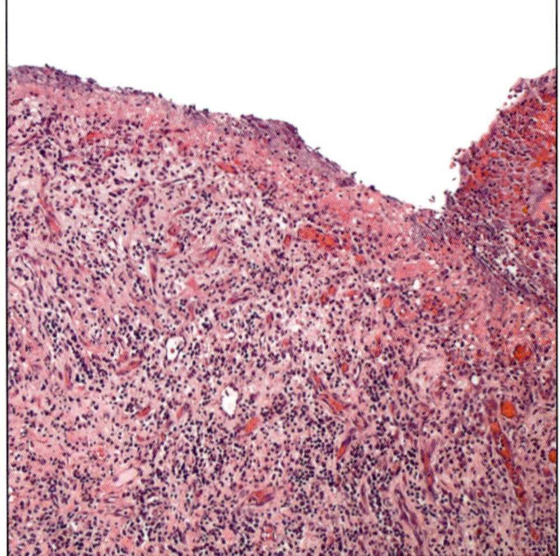

Granulation tissue and overlying fibrinoinflammatory exudate are present at the surface of an inflammatory polyp of the gallbladder.

TERMINOLOGY

Synonyms

- Fibroinflammatory polyp
- Fibroepithelial polyp
- Granulation tissue polyp

Definitions

- Nonneoplastic gallbladder mucosal projections characterized by
  - Granulation tissue
  - Chronic inflammation
  - Edema

ETIOLOGY/PATHOGENESIS

Mucosal Inflammation

- Associated with chronic cholecystitis
- Likely develop as result of mucosal injury

CLINICAL ISSUES

Epidemiology

- Incidence
  - Represent 15% of all benign gallbladder polyps
- Gender
  - Affect females and males

Presentation

- Usually asymptomatic
- Abnormal imaging finding
  - Often incidental
- Often incidental finding seen at gross examination at time of cholecystectomy

Treatment

- Surgical approaches
  - Cholecystectomy recommended for symptomatic or large (> 10 millimeters) lesions identified on imaging
    - For larger polyps, surgery performed to exclude possibility of malignancy
  - Cholecystectomy is curative

Prognosis

- Benign lesions with no malignant potential
- Prognosis is excellent

IMAGE FINDINGS

General Features

- Polypoid lesion may be seen on ultrasound or computed-tomography (CT) scan
- May be difficult to distinguish from gallstones

MACROSCOPIC FEATURES

General Features

- Red-gray or brown mucosal projections
- Usually sessile
- Often solitary

Size

- Typically range from 3-15 mm

MICROSCOPIC PATHOLOGY

Histologic Features

- Composed of inflamed, edematous, granulation tissue-type stroma and benign epithelium
  - Contains chronic inflammatory cells
- Single layer of epithelial cells may cover &/or form invaginations set within fibrous stroma
  - Typical columnar gallbladder-type epithelium
  - Epithelium may show reactive changes
- Clusters of pyloric-type glands may be present

INFLAMMATORY POLYPS

Key Facts

Terminology
- Nonneoplastic gallbladder mucosal projections characterized by granulation tissue, chronic inflammation, and edema

Etiology/Pathogenesis
- Associated with chronic cholecystitis

Clinical Issues
- Usually asymptomatic

Macroscopic Features
- Usually solitary, sessile, red-gray or brown mucosal projections

Microscopic Pathology
- Composed of inflamed, edematous, granulation tissue-type stroma and benign epithelium
- Single layer of epithelial cells may cover or comprise elements set within fibrous stroma

DIFFERENTIAL DIAGNOSIS

Pyloric Gland Adenoma
- Lesion composed of pyloric-type glands

Cholesterol Polyp
- Localized form of cholesterolosis
- Collection of lipid-laden macrophages form polypoid mucosal lesion
- Appears yellow at gross examination
- Stroma filled with lipid-laden macrophages
- Lacks chronic inflammation and granulation tissue-type stroma of inflammatory polyp

Villous Papilloma
- Papillary epithelial hyperplasia
- Can occur in association with metachromatic leukodystrophy
  - Lamina propria expansion by macrophages containing abnormal metachromatic material

Intestinal-type Adenoma
- Exhibits at least low-grade epithelial dysplasia
- Epithelium resembles that of typical colonic adenomas with enlarged, hyperchromatic nuclei showing pseudostratification

Adenomyoma
- Characterized by gallbladder wall thickening and irregular, ectatic invagination of mucosal lining into smooth muscle of gallbladder wall

Hyperplastic Polyp
- Thickened gallbladder mucosa lined by normal-appearing epithelial cells

Biliary-type Adenoma
- Also lined by biliary-type epithelium
  - Lacks inflamed, edematous, granulation-type stroma

SELECTED REFERENCES

1. Sun XJ et al: Diagnosis and treatment of polypoid lesions of the gallbladder: report of 194 cases. Hepatobiliary Pancreat Dis Int. 3(4):591-4, 2004
2. Owen CC et al: Gallbladder polyps, cholesterolosis, adenomyomatosis, and acute acalculous cholecystitis. Semin Gastrointest Dis. 14(4):178-88, 2003
3. Levy AD et al: From the archives of the AFIP. Benign tumors and tumorlike lesions of the gallbladder and extrahepatic bile ducts: radiologic-pathologic correlation. Armed Forces Institute of Pathology. Radiographics. 22(2):387-413, 2002
4. Terzi C et al: Polypoid lesions of the gallbladder: report of 100 cases with special reference to operative indications. Surgery. 127(6):622-7, 2000

IMAGE GALLERY

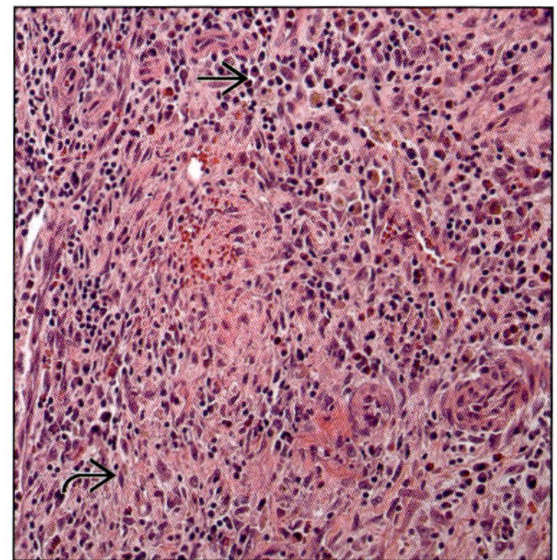

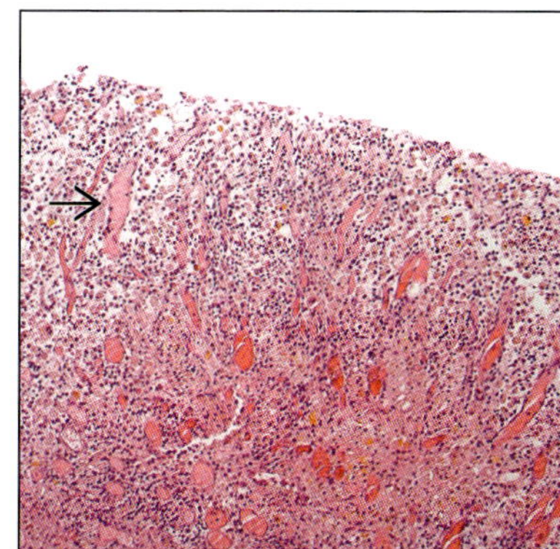

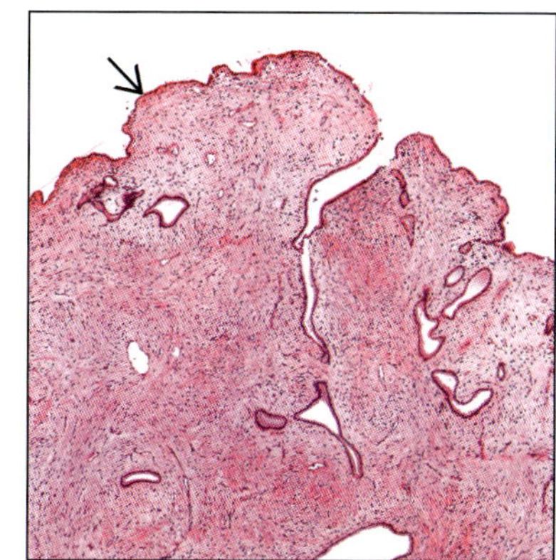

(Left) *This hematoxylin and eosin stained slide of an inflammatory polyp shows organizing granulation tissue ⇨ and inflammation ⇨.* ***(Center)*** *Proliferating capillaries ⇨ and acute and chronic inflammatory cells are present near the surface of an inflammatory polyp.* ***(Right)*** *Hematoxylin and eosin stained slide shows stromal edema in an inflammatory polyp of the gallbladder. The polyp is covered by benign gallbladder epithelium ⇨.*

HYPERPLASTIC POLYPS

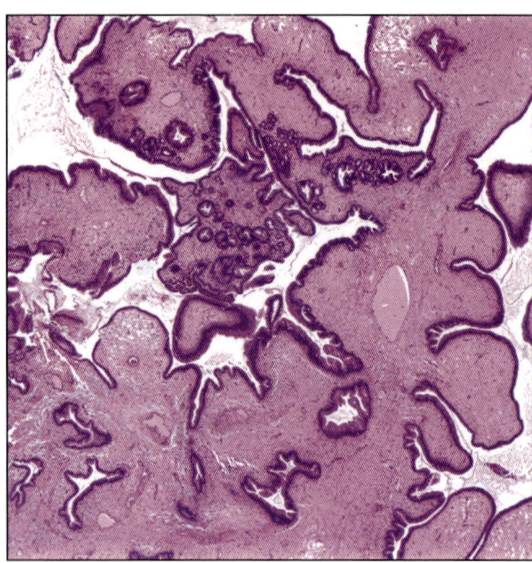

This low-power view of a hyperplastic polyp of the gallbladder illustrates the prominent mucosal folds and papillae with abundant intervening stroma.

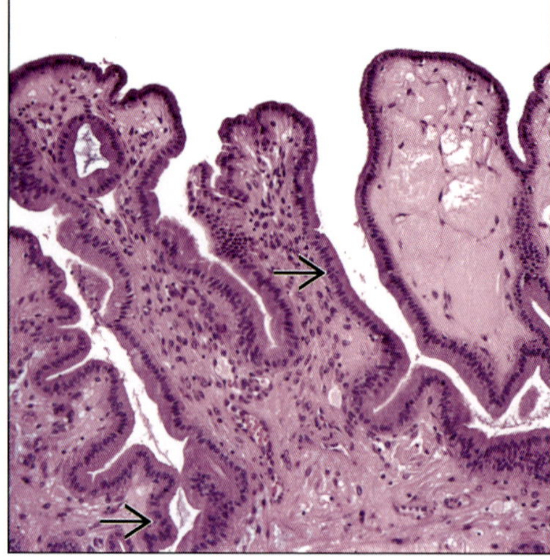

Hematoxylin & eosin section of a hyperplastic polyp at high power shows that the polyp surface is lined by normal-appearing gallbladder mucosa ⇒.

TERMINOLOGY

Abbreviations

- Hyperplastic polyp (HP)

Synonyms

- Metaplastic polyp
- Localized papillary hyperplasia

Definitions

- Polypoid growth of hyperplastic gallbladder mucosa

ETIOLOGY/PATHOGENESIS

Reactive/Inflammatory

- Most occur in setting of cholecystitis or cholelithiasis
- Rarely occur in association with chronic ulcerative colitis or metachromatic leukodystrophy

CLINICAL ISSUES

Epidemiology

- Incidence
  - 2nd most common type of gallbladder polyp
  - Accounts for approximately 20% of cases
- Age
  - No age predilection
    - Documented in both children and adults

Presentation

- Usually incidental finding at time of cholecystectomy
  - May present with symptoms secondary to background cholecystitis &/or cholelithiasis

Treatment

- Surgical approaches
  - Cholecystectomy recommended if patient is symptomatic or if polyp is ≥ 1 cm in diameter on imaging

Prognosis

- Currently regarded as benign lesion with no risk of progression to dysplasia or malignancy
- Cholecystectomy is curative

IMAGE FINDINGS

Radiographic Findings

- Larger lesions may be detected radiographically with ultrasound or computed-tomography (CT) scan

MACROSCOPIC FEATURES

General Features

- Small polypoid mucosal lesions
  - Usually < 0.5 cm in diameter
- May be multiple
- May be either sessile or pedunculated

MICROSCOPIC PATHOLOGY

Histologic Features

- Prominent hyperplastic mucosal folds and papillae
- Mucosa consists of typical columnar-type gallbladder epithelium
- Metaplastic changes are common
  - Gastric-type foveolar mucosa
  - Gastric pyloric-type mucus-secreting glands
  - Intestinal-type mucosa with goblet cells, possible Paneth cells, and endocrine cells
- May show focal inflammation, especially at surface
  - Usually nonspecific chronic inflammation
    - Consists predominantly of lymphocytes with smaller numbers of plasma cells, histiocytes, eosinophils, and neutrophils
  - May be associated with reactive epithelial changes
    - May be confused with dysplasia

HYPERPLASTIC POLYPS

Key Facts

Terminology
- 2nd most common type of gallbladder polyp

Etiology/Pathogenesis
- Most occur secondary to cholecystitis or cholelithiasis

Clinical Issues
- Usually incidental finding

Macroscopic Features
- Small polyps, usually < 5 mm in diameter

Microscopic Pathology
- Prominent hyperplastic mucosal folds and papillae
- Mucosa on surface resembles normal gallbladder epithelium
- Metaplastic changes are common
- May show focal inflammation, especially at surface
- May be associated with reactive epithelial changes that may be confused with dysplasia

    - Reactive changes should be focal and accompanied by inflammation
    - Nuclei are enlarged and vesicular
    - Occasionally, nuclei may be focally pseudostratified or crowded

DIFFERENTIAL DIAGNOSIS

Adenoma, Intestinal Type
- Entire polyp composed of dysplastic intestinal-type epithelium
    - Similar to colonic adenomas
- Absent or minimal inflammation
- Nuclei are hyperchromatic, cigar-shaped, pseudostratified, and show loss of polarity

Adenoma, Pyloric Gland Type
- Discrete lesion
- > 0.5 cm
- Composed of tightly packed, pyloric-type glands
- Minimal cytologic atypia

Cholesterol Polyp
- Formed by multiple lipid-laden foamy macrophages within stroma

Mucus Gland Polyp
- Predominantly in neck region
- Usually < 0.5 cm
- Consists of hyperplastic mucinous glands, not hyperplastic surface epithelium

Diffuse Mucosal Hyperplasia
- Widespread nonpolypoid hyperplasia; not a discrete lesion

Adenomyoma
- Irregular invaginations of mucosa into smooth muscle of gallbladder wall

Gastric Heterotopia
- Composed of pyloric-type glands with parietal and chief cells

SELECTED REFERENCES

1. Mainprize KS et al: Surgical management of polypoid lesions of the gallbladder. Br J Surg. 87(4):414-7, 2000
2. Kubota K et al: Giant hyperplastic polyp of the gallbladder: a case report. J Clin Ultrasound. 24(4):203-6, 1996
3. Albores-Saavedra J et al: Non-neoplastic polypoid lesions and adenomas of the gallbladder. Pathol Annu. 28 Pt 1:145-77, 1993
4. Warfel KA et al: Villous papilloma of the gallbladder in association with leukodystrophy. Hum Pathol. 15(12):1192-4, 1984
5. Christensen AH et al: Benign tumors and pseudotumors of the gallbladder. Report of 180 cases. Arch Pathol. 90(5):423-32, 1970

IMAGE GALLERY

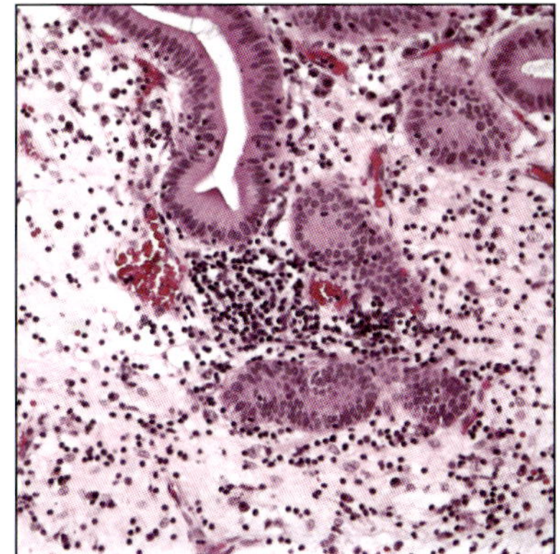

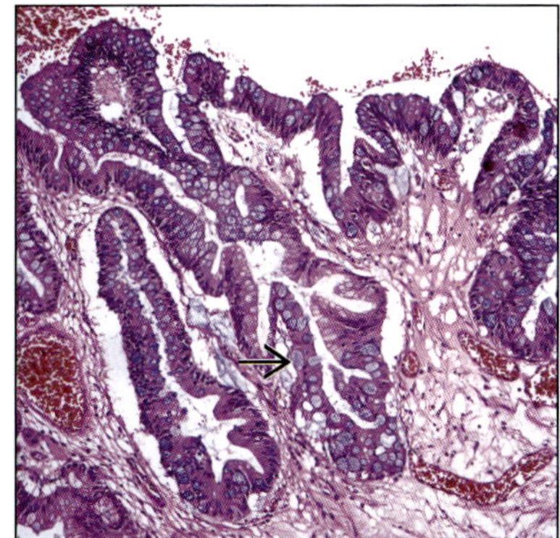

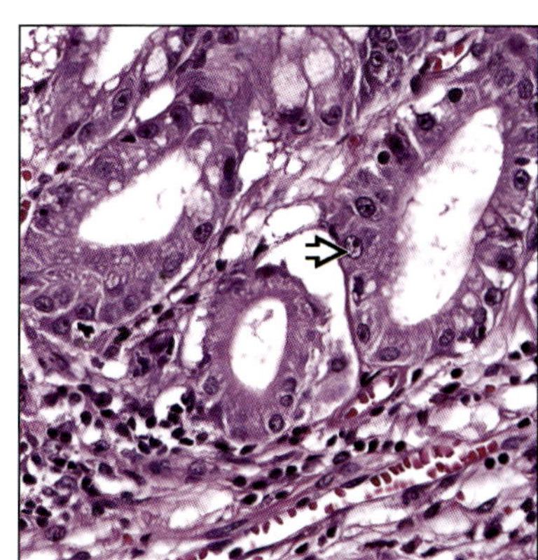

(Left) *Hyperplastic polyps often have focal inflammation consisting predominantly of lymphocytes and plasma cells. Inflammation is most commonly found at the polyp surface.* ***(Center)*** *Metaplastic changes are very common in hyperplastic polyps. This section shows intestinal-type metaplasia with many goblet cells ⇒.* ***(Right)*** *Reactive epithelial changes in a hyperplastic polyp include vesicular nuclei and prominent nucleoli ⇨ associated with inflammation.*

CHOLESTEROL POLYPS AND CHOLESTEROLOSIS

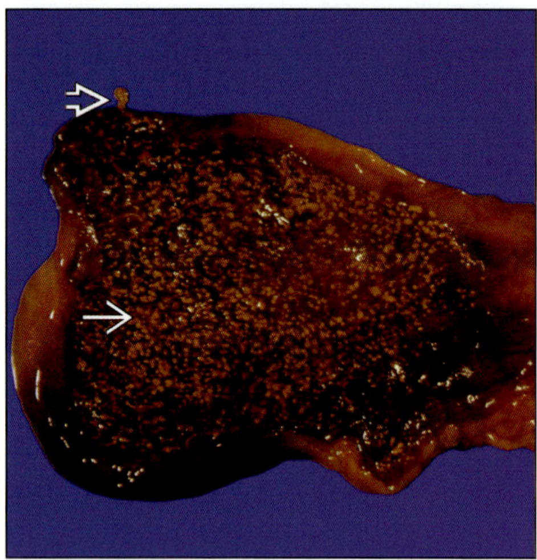

Gross photograph of a gallbladder with cholesterolosis shows numerous yellow dots with a red-brown background ➡, somewhat resembling a strawberry. In addition, there is a cholesterol polyp ➡.

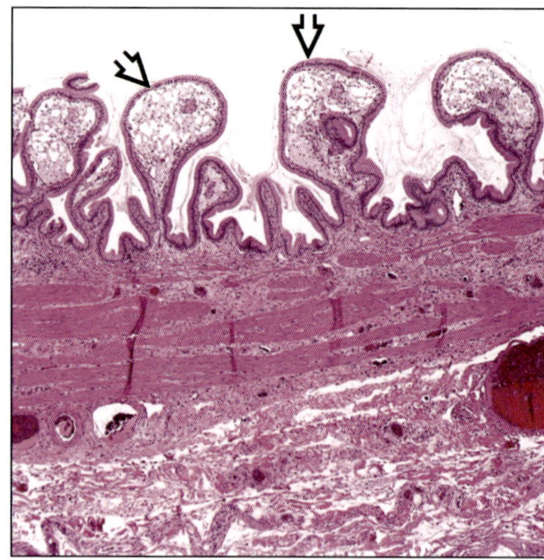

Hematoxylin and eosin section shows multiple villi with expansion of the lamina propria by numerous foamy macrophages, characteristic of cholesterolosis ➡.

TERMINOLOGY

Definitions

- Accumulation of neutral lipid within macrophages of lamina propria of gallbladder

ETIOLOGY/PATHOGENESIS

Pathogenesis

- Poorly understood
- May reflect increased hepatic synthesis of lipids or increased absorption and esterification by gallbladder
- Frequently occurs with cholesterol gallstones in setting of supersaturated bile

CLINICAL ISSUES

Epidemiology

- Incidence
  - Cholesterol polyps account for 50-60% of all gallbladder polyps
  - Prevalence rate of 12% in autopsy studies and from 9-26% in surgical studies
    - More prevalent in patients with morbid obesity
  - Reports of possible association with acute pancreatitis
- Age
  - Usually patients between ages of 20 and 70
  - Peak in 5th and 6th decades of life

Presentation

- May be asymptomatic and discovered incidentally
- Also associated with abdominal pain and postprandial symptoms
- Occasional reports of cholesterol polyps becoming detached and impacted in distal bile duct, resulting in jaundice

Treatment

- Surgical approaches
  - Cholecystectomy

Prognosis

- Cholecystectomy is curative

IMAGE FINDINGS

Radiographic Findings

- Cholesterol polyps may be diagnosed, but diffuse form of cholesterolosis is infrequently recognized

MACROSCOPIC FEATURES

General Features

- Cholesterolosis: Yellow flecks or streaks against green or red background
  - Flecks composed of lipid droplets, usually < 1 mm in diameter
  - Appearance has been compared with that of a strawberry
- Cholesterol polyps: Polypoid excrescences composed of lipid droplets that project into lumen
  - Small pedunculated lesions measuring 0.4-1.0 cm
  - Connected to mucosa by a fine stalk, which can be easily disrupted
- 4 different patterns may be seen
  - Diffuse type (majority of cases, up to 80%)
  - Polypoid pattern with 1 or more small mucosal polyps
    - Polyps in absence of diffuse pattern in approximately 10% of cases
  - Mixed pattern with cholesterol polyps present within background of diffuse cholesterolosis (about 10% of cases)
  - Focal type: Cholesterolosis is limited to small area of gallbladder mucosa only

CHOLESTEROL POLYPS AND CHOLESTEROLOSIS

Key Facts

Terminology
- Accumulation of neutral lipid within macrophages of lamina propria of gallbladder

Macroscopic Features
- Lipid droplets appear as yellow flecks or streaks against green or red background ("strawberry" gallbladder)
- Lipid droplets may form polypoid excrescences, called cholesterol polyps, that project into lumen
- May contain cholesterol gallstones

Microscopic Pathology
- Foamy macrophages with small dark nuclei within lamina propria of gallbladder mucosa
- Cholesterol polyps have vascular stalk and villous projections
  - Lamina propria of polyp is filled with foamy lipid containing macrophages

- Associated with cholesterol gallstones
- Cholesterolosis usually ends at start of cystic duct, but involvement of cystic or common ducts has been reported
- Bile may be thick and tarry with detached yellow flecks consisting of masses of foam cells (lipoidic corpuscles)

MICROSCOPIC PATHOLOGY

Histologic Features
- Foamy macrophages with small dark nuclei within lamina propria
  - May result in thickened folds &/or polyps
  - Adjacent mucosa may be normal or inflamed
    - Inflammation almost exclusively occurs in patients with gallstones
  - Extracellular deposits of lipid are rare
  - Clear spaces in histiocytes are PAS(-), consistent with absence of mucus
- Cholesterol polyps
  - Vascular connective tissue stalk
  - Variable number of branching villous projections
  - Packed with numerous foamy macrophages of type seen in diffuse form of cholesterolosis
  - Covered by histologically unremarkable biliary epithelium
- Lipofuscin pigment may be present in small number of patients
  - Can be within histiocytes as well as adjacent gallbladder epithelium
  - Brownish, granular pigment that is weakly PAS(+)
  - Most likely related to leakage of bile into mucosa

DIFFERENTIAL DIAGNOSIS

Metachromic Leukodystrophy
- Macrophages contain brown-tan material, not cholesterol

Hyperplastic or Inflammatory Polyp
- Do not contain lipid-filled macrophages

SELECTED REFERENCES

1. Sandri L et al: Gallbladder cholesterol polyps and cholesterolosis. Minerva Gastroenterol Dietol. 49(3):217-24, 2003
2. Jacyna MR et al: Cholesterolosis: a physical cause of "functional" disorder. Br Med J (Clin Res Ed). 295(6599):619-20, 1987
3. Salmenkivi K: Cholesterosis of the gallbladder. Surgical considerations. Int Surg. 45(3):304-9, 1966
4. Salmenkivi K: Cholersterosis of the gall-bladder. A clinical study based on 269 cholecystectomies. Acta Chir Scand Suppl. 105: suppl 324: 1-93, 1964
5. Feldman M et al: Cholesterosis of the gallbladder; an autopsy study of 165 cases. Gastroenterology. 27(5):641-8, 1954

IMAGE GALLERY

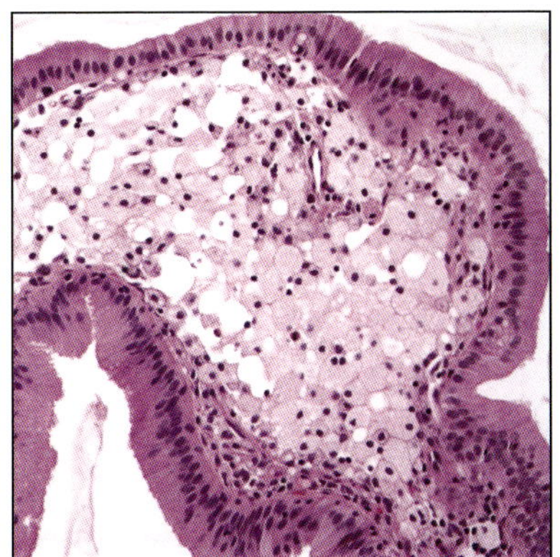

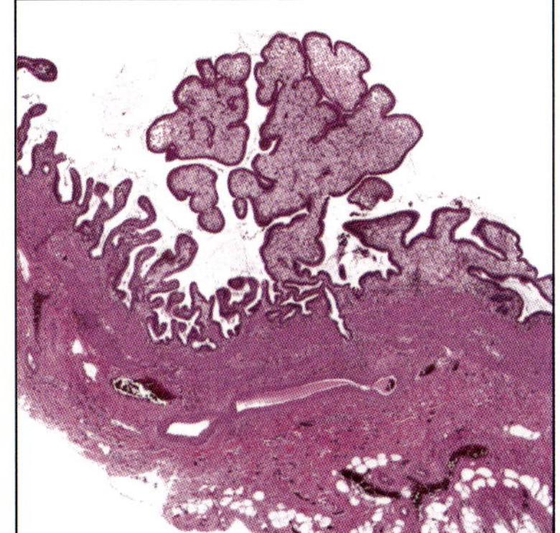

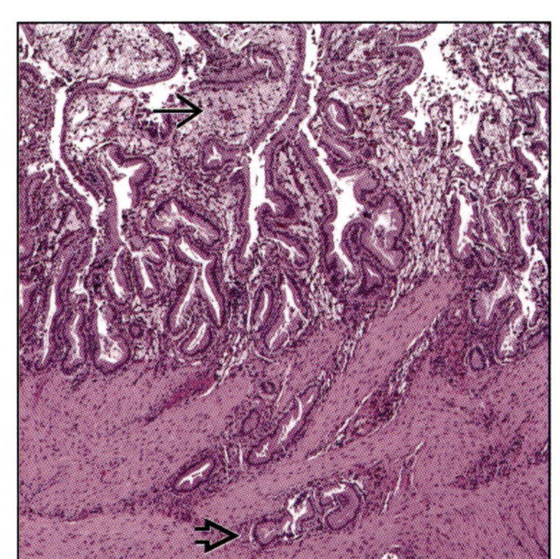

*(**Left**) Hematoxylin and eosin section at high power shows expansion of a villous tip by numerous macrophages with expanded foamy clear cytoplasm. (**Center**) Low-power hematoxylin and eosin section shows a lobulated cholesterol polyp. (**Right**) Hematoxylin and eosin section shows cholesterosis and chronic cholecystitis. There is thickening of the wall, Rokitansky-Aschoff sinuses ⇒, mild chronic inflammation, and villi expanded by foamy macrophages →.*

GALLBLADDER CARCINOMA CANCER PROTOCOL

Gallbladder: Resection/Cholecystectomy

Surgical Pathology Cancer Case Summary (Checklist)

Specimen (select all that apply)

___ Gallbladder
___ Liver
___ Extrahepatic bile duct
___ Other (specify): ___________________________
___ Not specified

Procedure

___ Simple cholecystectomy (laparoscopic or open)
___ Radical cholecystectomy (with liver resection and lymphadenectomy)
___ Other (specify): ___________________________
___ Not specified

Tumor Site (select all that apply)

___ Fundus
___ Body
___ Neck
___ Cystic duct
___ Free peritoneal side of gallbladder
___ Hepatic side of gallbladder
___ Cannot be determined
___ Other (specify): ___________________________
___ Not specified

Tumor Size

Greatest dimension: _________ cm
*Additional dimensions: _________ x _________ cm
___ Cannot be determined

Histologic Type

___ Adenocarcinoma, not otherwise specified
___ Papillary adenocarcinoma
___ Adenocarcinoma, intestinal type
___ Mucinous carcinoma
___ Signet ring cell carcinoma
___ Clear cell carcinoma
___ Squamous cell carcinoma
___ Adenosquamous carcinoma
___ Small cell carcinoma
___ Undifferentiated carcinoma
___ Carcinoma, not otherwise specified
___ Carcinosarcoma
___ Other (specify): ___________________________

Microscopic Tumor Extension

___ Tumor invades lamina propria
___ Tumor invades muscle layer
___ Tumor invades perimuscular connective tissue; no extension beyond serosa or into liver
___ Tumor perforates serosa (visceral peritoneum)
___ Tumor directly invades liver
___ Tumor directly invades extrahepatic bile ducts
___ Tumor directly invades other adjacent organ or structure, such as stomach, duodenum, colon, pancreas, or omentum (specify): ___________________________

GALLBLADDER CARCINOMA CANCER PROTOCOL

Margins (select all that apply)

___ Cannot be assessed

___ Margins uninvolved by invasive carcinoma

Distance of invasive carcinoma from closest margin: ________ mm

Specify margin: ____________________________

___ Margins involved by invasive carcinoma

Specify margin(s): ____________________________

___ Cystic duct margin uninvolved by intramucosal carcinoma

___ Cystic duct margin involved by intramucosal carcinoma

***Lymph-Vascular Invasion**

*___ Not identified

*___ Present

***Perineural Invasion**

*___ Not identified

*___ Present

Pathologic Staging (pTNM)

TNM descriptors (required only if applicable) (select all that apply)

___ m (multiple primary tumors)

___ r (recurrent)

___ y (post-treatment)

Primary tumor (pT)

___ pTX: Cannot be assessed

___ pT0: No evidence of primary tumor

___ pTis: Carcinoma in situ

pT1: Tumor invades lamina propria or muscular layer

___ pT1a: Tumor invades lamina propria

___ pT1b: Tumor invades muscle layer

___ pT2: Tumor invades perimuscular connective tissue; no extension beyond serosa or into liver

___ pT3: Tumor perforates serosa (visceral peritoneum) &/or directly invades liver &/or 1 other adjacent organ or structure, such as the stomach, duodenum, colon, pancreas, omentum, or extrahepatic bile ducts

___ PT4: Tumor invades main portal vein or hepatic artery or invades 2 or more extrahepatic organs or structures

Regional lymph nodes (pN)

___ pNX: Cannot be assessed

___ pN0: No regional lymph node metastasis

___ pN1: Metastases to nodes along cystic duct, common bile duct, hepatic artery, &/or portal vein

Specify: Number examined: ________

Number involved: ________

___ pN2: Metastases to periaortic, cervical, superior mesentery artery, &/or celiac artery lymph nodes

Specify: Number examined: ________

Number involved: ________

Distant metastasis (pM)

___ Not applicable

___ pM1: Distant metastasis

*Specify site(s), if known: ____________________________

**Data elements with asterisks are not required. However, these elements may be clinically important but are not yet validated or regularly used in patient management. Adapted with permission from College of American Pathologists, "Protocol for the Examination of Specimens from Patients with Carcinoma of the Gallbladder." Web posting date October 2009, www.cap.org. Protocol applies to all invasive carcinomas of the gallbladder and cystic duct, including those showing focal endocrine differentiation. Well-differentiated neuroendocrine neoplasms (carcinoid tumors) are not included.*

GALLBLADDER CARCINOMA CANCER PROTOCOL

Stage Groupings

Stage	Tumor	Node	Metastasis
0	Tis	N0	M0
I	T1	N0	M0
II	T2	N0	M0
IIIA	T3	N0	M0
IIIB	T1, T2, or T3	N1	M0
IVA	T4	Any N	M0
IVB	Any T	N2	Any M
	Any T	Any N	M1

Adapted from 7th edition AJCC Staging Forms.

GALLBLADDER CARCINOMA CANCER PROTOCOL

KEY STAGING PARAMETERS

Primary Tumor

- Depth of invasion
- Extent of spread to other structures
  - Liver is common site of involvement
    - Not considered distant metastasis
  - Invasion of hilar structures (common bile duct, hepatic artery, portal vein) renders tumors locally unresectable
  - Duodenum, transverse colon also at risk for direct invasion
  - Direct invasion of adjacent organs (colon, duodenum, stomach, common bile duct, abdominal wall, diaphragm) not considered distant metastasis but rather T3 or T4 stage depending on number of organs/structures involved
    - T3: 1 organ/structure involved
    - T4: ≥ 2 organs/structures involved

Lymph Node Status

- Regional nodes
  - Hepatic hilum
    - Including those along common bile duct, hepatic artery, portal vein, cystic duct
- Distant nodes
  - Celiac
  - Periduodenal
  - Peripancreatic
  - Superior mesenteric artery

IMPORTANT PROGNOSTIC FACTORS

T1 Tumors

- 50% 5-year survival

T2 Tumors

- 29% 5-year survival
  - T2 and T3 tumors usually offered 2nd operation to resect involved liver and achieve negative cystic duct margin status

Lymph Node Metastases or Locally Advanced Tumors

- Very low long-term survival
  - Site-specific prognostic features
    - Histologic type
    - Grade
    - Vascular invasion

Histologic Tumor Types

- Papillary carcinoma: Best prognosis
- Small cell carcinoma, undifferentiated carcinoma: Worst prognosis

SELECTED REFERENCES

1. American Joint Committee on Cancer: AJCC Cancer Staging Manual. 7th ed. New York: Springer. 219-25, 2010
2. Kohya N et al: Rational therapeutic strategy for T2 gallbladder carcinoma based on tumor spread. World J Gastroenterol. 16(28):3567-72, 2010
3. Jensen EH et al: Lymph node evaluation is associated with improved survival after surgery for early stage gallbladder cancer. Surgery. 146(4):706-11; discussion 711-3, 2009
4. Gourgiotis S et al: Gallbladder cancer. Am J Surg. 196(2):252-64, 2008
5. Balachandran P et al: Predictors of long-term survival in patients with gallbladder cancer. J Gastrointest Surg. 10(6):848-54, 2006
6. Fong Y et al: Evidence-based gallbladder cancer staging: changing cancer staging by analysis of data from the National Cancer Database. Ann Surg. 243(6):767-71; discussion 771-4, 2006
7. Yagi H et al: Retrospective analysis of outcome in 63 gallbladder carcinoma patients after radical resection. J Hepatobiliary Pancreat Surg. 13(6):530-6, 2006
8. Wakabayashi H et al: Analysis of prognostic factors after surgery for stage III and IV gallbladder cancer. Eur J Surg Oncol. 30(8):842-6, 2004

GALLBLADDER CARCINOMA CANCER PROTOCOL

Staging Parameters

(Left) *In T1a gallbladder carcinoma, the tumor is limited to the lamina propria* ➩. ***(Right)*** *T1a disease is defined as invasion of the lamina propria of the gallbladder. Note the overlying adenocarcinoma in situ.*

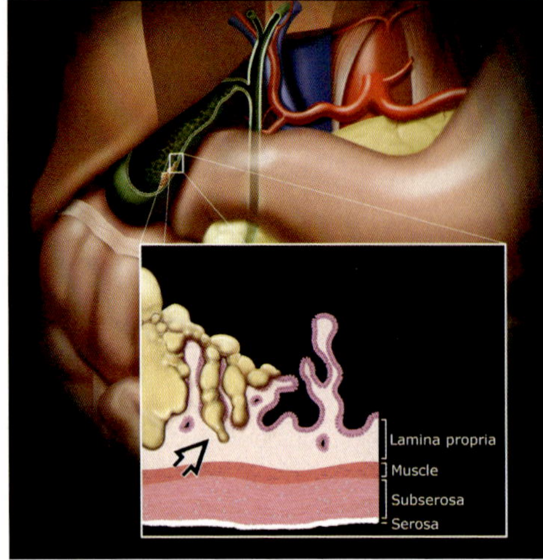

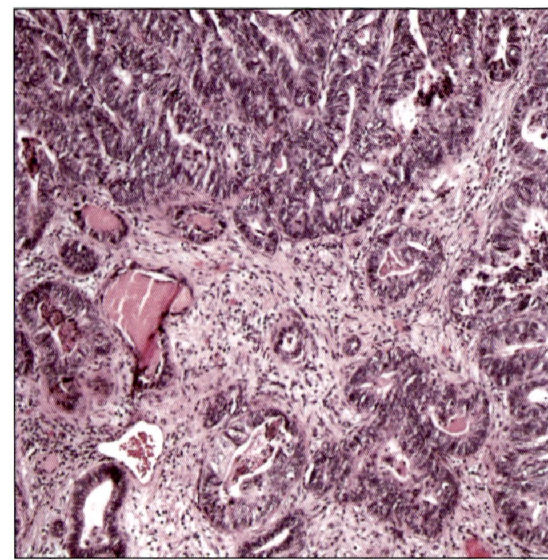

(Left) *In T1b gallbladder carcinoma, the tumor invades the muscular wall of the gallbladder* ↩. ***(Right)*** *This gallbladder adenocarcinoma invades the muscular wall of the gallbladder, consistent with T1b disease. Note the malignant glands infiltrating the muscle bundles.*

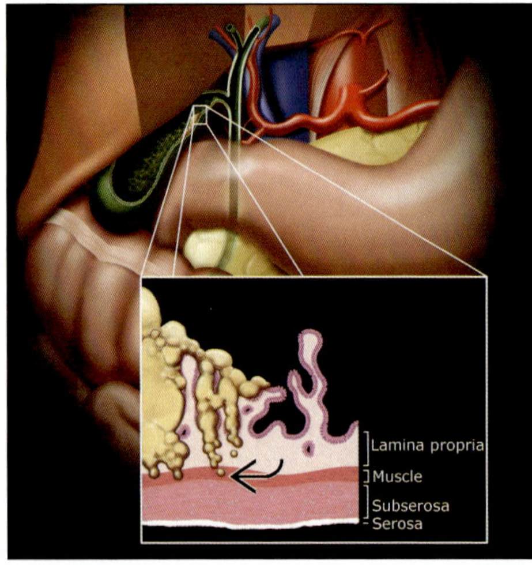

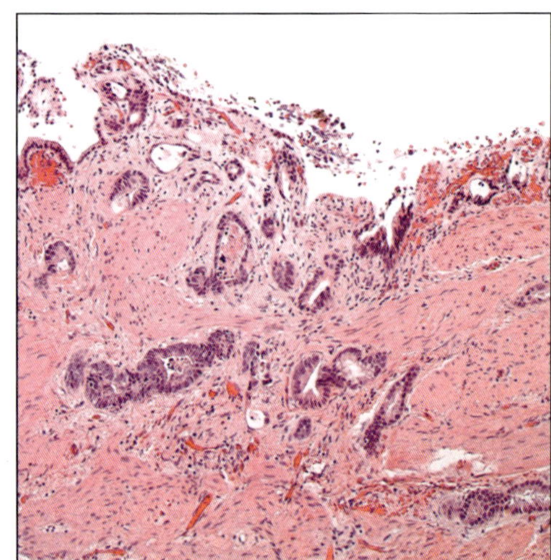

(Left) *In T2 gallbladder carcinoma, the tumor invades the perimuscular connective tissue but does not extend beyond the serosa or into the liver.* ***(Right)*** *This well-differentiated gallbladder adenocarcinoma infiltrates through the muscular layer* → *and into the perimuscular connective tissue* ➩.

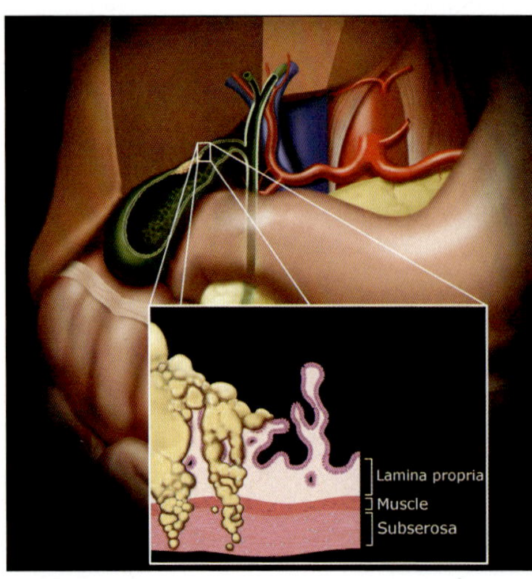

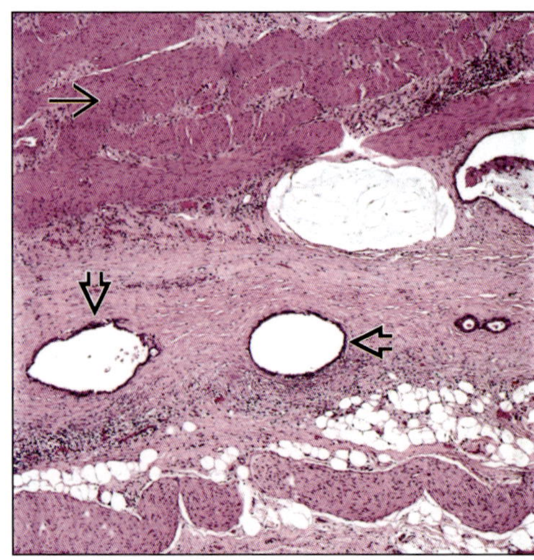

Staging Parameters

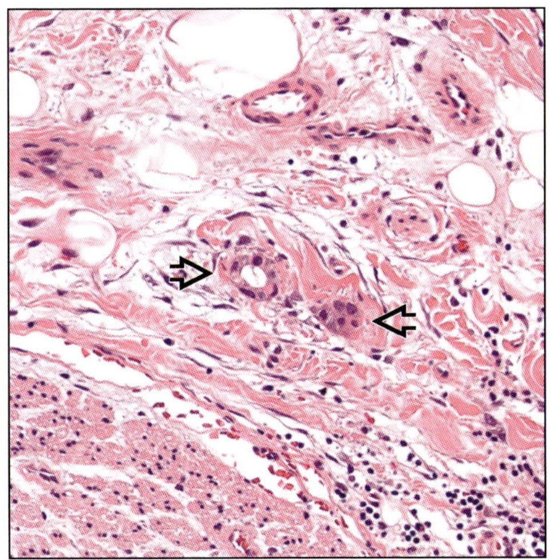

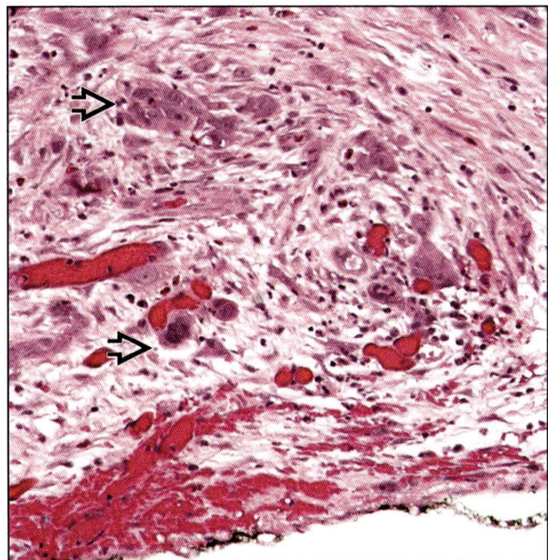

(Left) *This high-power photomicrograph illustrates a gallbladder adenocarcinoma that focally extends into perimuscular connective tissue ➩, consistent with T2 disease.* ***(Right)*** *This poorly differentiated tumor ➩ is within less than a millimeter of the visceral peritoneum but does not invade it; therefore, it is still regarded as T2 disease.*

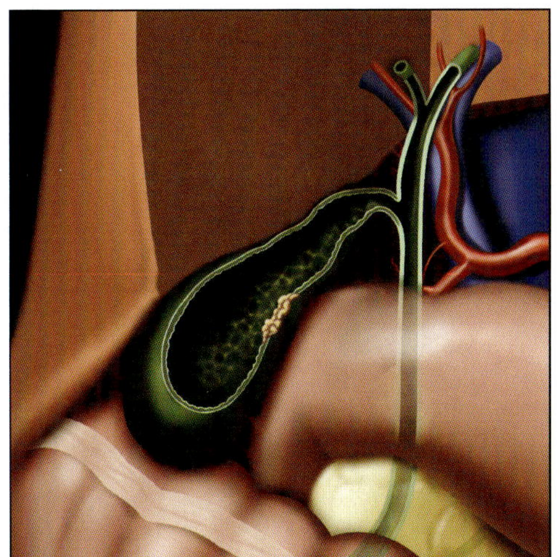

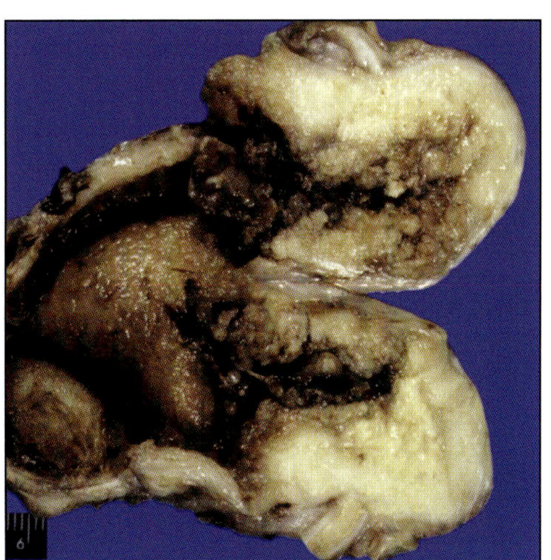

(Left) *This gallbladder carcinoma is arising from the part of the gallbladder with a serosal covering (away from the liver bed). It perforates the serosa (visceral peritoneum), consistent with T3 disease.* ***(Right)*** *This adenocarcinoma extensively involves the wall of the gallbladder as well as the serosa, consistent with T3 disease.*

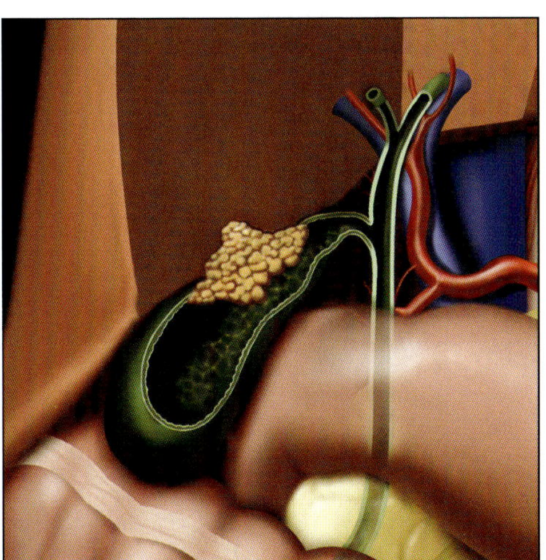

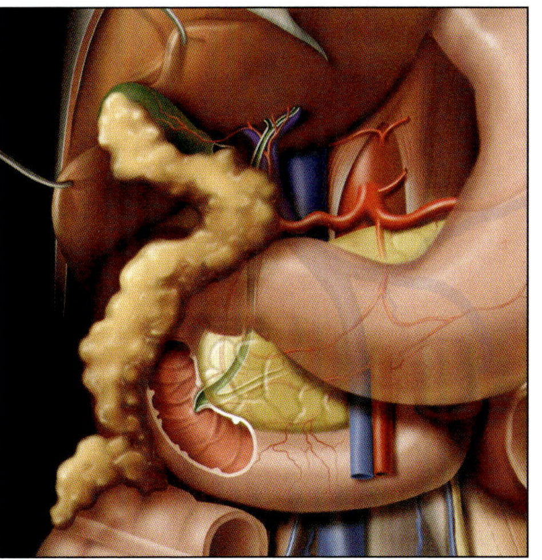

(Left) *Tumors that directly invade the liver &/or 1 other adjacent organ or structure, such as the stomach, duodenum, colon, pancreas, omentum, or extrahepatic bile ducts, are also classified as T3 disease.* ***(Right)*** *This graphic illustrates gallbladder carcinoma infiltrating the duodenum and the colon, consistent with T4 disease. Tumors that invade 2 or more extrahepatic organs or structures, or that invade the main portal vein or main hepatic artery, are all considered T4 disease.*

PERIHILAR BILE DUCT CANCER PROTOCOL

Perihilar Bile Ducts: Local or Segmental Resection, Hilar Resection With or Without Hepatic Resection

Surgical Pathology Cancer Case Summary (Checklist)

Specimen (select all that apply)

___ Common bile duct
___ Right hepatic duct
___ Left hepatic duct
___ Junction of right and left hepatic ducts
___ Common hepatic duct
___ Cystic duct

Other organs received

___ Liver
___ Gallbladder
___ Other (specify): ____________________________

Procedure

___ Hilar and hepatic resection
___ Segmental resection of bile ducts(s)
___ Choledochal cyst resection
___ Total hepatectomy
___ Other (specify): ____________________________
___ Not specified

Tumor Site

___ Right hepatic duct
___ Left hepatic duct
___ Junction of right and left hepatic ducts
___ Cystic duct
___ Common hepatic duct
___ Common bile duct
___ Not specified

Tumor Size

Greatest dimension: _________ cm
*Additional dimensions: _________ x _________ cm
___ Cannot be determined

Histologic Type

___ Adenocarcinoma (not otherwise characterized)
___ Papillary adenocarcinoma
___ Mucinous adenocarcinoma
___ Clear cell adenocarcinoma
___ Signet ring cell carcinoma
___ Adenosquamous carcinoma
___ Squamous cell carcinoma
___ Small cell carcinoma
___ Biliary cystadenocarcinoma
___ Other (specify): ____________________________
___ Carcinoma, not otherwise specified

Histologic Grade

___ Not applicable
___ GX: Cannot be assessed
___ G1: Well differentiated
___ G2: Moderately differentiated
___ G3: Poorly differentiated

___ G4: Undifferentiated

Microscopic Tumor Extension (select all that apply)

___ Carcinoma in situ
___ Tumor confined to bile duct histologically
___ Tumor invades beyond wall of bile duct into surrounding connective tissue
___ Tumor invades adjacent liver parenchyma
___ Tumor invades gallbladder
___ Tumor invades unilateral branches of portal vein (right or left)
___ Tumor invades unilateral branches of hepatic artery (right or left)
___ Tumor invades main portal vein or its branches bilaterally
___ Tumor invades common hepatic artery
___ Tumor invades second-order biliary radicals
  ___ Unilateral
  ___ Bilateral

Margins (select all that apply)

Segmental resection specimen

___ Cannot be assessed
___ Margins uninvolved by invasive carcinoma
  Distance of invasive carcinoma from closest margin: ________ mm or ________ cm
  Specify margin: ____________________________
___ Margins involved by invasive carcinoma
  ___ Proximal bile duct margin
  ___ Distal bile duct margin
  ___ Hepatic parenchymal margin
  ___ Other (specify): ____________________________
___ Dysplasia/carcinoma in situ not identified at bile duct margin
___ Dysplasia/carcinoma in situ present at bile duct margin

Lymph-Vascular Invasion

___ Not identified
___ Present
___ Indeterminate

Perineural Invasion

___ Not identified
___ Present
___ Indeterminate

Pathologic Staging (pTNM)

TNM descriptors (required only if applicable) (select all that apply)

___ m (multiple primary tumors)
___ r (recurrent)
___ y (post-treatment)

Primary tumor (pT)

___ pTX: Cannot be assessed
___ pT0: No evidence of primary tumor
___ pTis: Carcinoma in situ
___ pT1: Tumor confined to bile duct, with extension up to muscle layer or fibrous tissue
___ pT2a: Tumor invades beyond wall of bile duct to surrounding adipose tissue
___ pT2b: Tumor invades adjacent hepatic parenchyma
___ pT3: Tumor invades unilateral branches of portal vein or hepatic artery
___ PT4: Tumor invades main portal vein or its branches bilaterally; or common hepatic artery; or second-order biliary radicals bilaterally; or unilateral second-order biliary radicals with contralateral portal vein or hepatic artery involvement

Regional lymph nodes (pN)

___ pNX: Cannot be assessed
___ pN0: No regional lymph node metastasis

PERIHILAR BILE DUCT CANCER PROTOCOL

___ pN1: Regional lymph node metastasis (including nodes along cystic duct, common bile duct, hepatic artery, and portal vein)

___ pN2: Metastasis to periaortic, pericaval, superior mesentery artery, &/or celiac artery lymph nodes

Specify: Number examined: ________

Number involved: ________

Distant metastasis (pM)

___ Cannot be assessed

*Specify site(s), if known: ________________

*Additional Pathologic Findings (select all that apply)

*___ None identified

*___ Choledochal cyst

*___ Dysplasia

*___ Primary sclerosing cholangitis (PSC)

*___ Biliary stones

*___ Other (specify): ____________________

*Ancillary Studies

*Specify: ____________________

*Clinical History (select all that apply)

*___ PSC

*___ Inflammatory bowel disease

*___ Biliary stones

*___ Other (specify): ____________________

*___ Not known

**Data elements with asterisks are not required. However, these elements may be clinically important but are not yet validated or regularly used in patient management. Adapted with permission from College of American Pathologists, "Protocol for the Examination of Specimens from Patients with Carcinoma of the Perihilar Bile Ducts." Web posting date October 2009, www.cap.org. Protocol applies to all invasive carcinomas of the perihilar bile ducts. Carcinomas of the distal extrahepatic bile ducts, intrahepatic bile ducts, and well-differentiated neuroendocrine neoplasms (carcinoid tumors) are not included.*

Stage Groupings

Stage	Tumor	Node	Metastasis
0	Tis	N0	M0
I	T1	N0	M0
II	T2a or T2b	N0	M0
IIIA	T3	N0	M0
IIIB	T1, T2, or T3	N1	M0
IVA	T4	N0 or N1	M0
IVB	Any T	N2	M0 or M1
	Any T	Any N	M1

Adapted from 7th edition AJCC Staging Forms.

PERIHILAR BILE DUCT CANCER PROTOCOL

DEFINITIONS

Proximal or Perihilar Carcinomas (Klatskin Tumor)

- Involve confluence of right &/or left hepatic ducts at hilum of liver
- Perihilar is defined as proximal to origin of cystic duct
  - May extend to involve right or left hepatic duct or both
  - 50-70% of biliary carcinomas
- In most patients, tumor is unresectable at diagnosis and thus is not pathologically staged
  - TNM classification therefore applies to clinical, radiographic, and pathologic variables

PROGNOSTIC INDICATORS

Adverse Indicators

- High histologic tumor grade
- Vascular invasion
- Lymph node metastasis
- Elevated CA19-9
- Elevated bilirubin
- Lobar atrophy

Positive Indicators

- Complete resection with negative margins is best predictor of long-term survival
  - Often difficult given proximity to hepatic artery, portal vein, and liver parenchyma at hilum
- Papillary tumors have better prognosis than nodular or sclerosing carcinomas
- Patients with liver parenchymal involvement (T2) now believed to have better survival than those with unilateral vascular invasion (T3)

LYMPH NODES

General

- Frequency of lymph node metastases increases with T classification
  - Occur in approximately 30-50% of patients overall
  - Hilar, pericholedochal nodes in hepatoduodenal ligament most often involved

Regional Nodes (N1)

- Cystic duct
- Common bile duct
- Hepatic artery
- Portal vein nodes

Distant Nodes (N2)

- Periaortic, pericaval, superior mesenteric, celiac artery nodes

METASTASES

Liver Most Common Site

- Tumor spreads through
  - Bile duct radicals
  - Lymphatics
  - Nerves
- Spread to other organs rare, especially outside abdomen

SELECTED REFERENCES

1. American Joint Committee on Cancer: AJCC Cancer Staging Manual. 7th ed. New York: Springer. 219-25, 2010
2. Gatto M et al: Cholangiocarcinoma: update and future perspectives. Dig Liver Dis. 42(4):253-60, 2010
3. Giuliante F et al: Liver resections for hilar cholangiocarcinoma. Eur Rev Med Pharmacol Sci. 14(4):368-70, 2010
4. Singal AG et al: The clinical presentation and prognostic factors for intrahepatic and extrahepatic cholangiocarcinoma in a tertiary care centre. Aliment Pharmacol Ther. 31(6):625-33, 2010
5. Blechacz B et al: Cholangiocarcinoma: advances in pathogenesis, diagnosis, and treatment. Hepatology. 48(1):308-21, 2008
6. Baton O et al: Major hepatectomy for hilar cholangiocarcinoma type 3 and 4: prognostic factors and longterm outcomes. J Am Coll Surg. 2007 Feb;204(2):250-60. Epub 2006 Dec 27. Erratum in: J Am Coll Surg. 204(6):1304, 2007
7. Cheng Q et al: Predictive factors for prognosis of hilar cholangiocarcinoma: postresection radiotherapy improves survival. Eur J Surg Oncol. 33(2):202-7, 2007
8. Hemming AW et al: Surgical management of hilar cholangiocarcinoma. Ann Surg. 241(5):693-9; discussion 699-702, 2005
9. Hong SM et al: Analysis of extrahepatic bile duct carcinomas according to the New American Joint Committee on Cancer staging system focused on tumor classification problems in 222 patients. Cancer. 104(4):802-10, 2005
10. Jarnagin WR et al: Staging, resectability, and outcome in 225 patients with hilar cholangiocarcinoma. Ann Surg. 234(4):507-17; discussion 517-9, 2001
11. Kitagawa Y et al: Lymph node metastasis from hilar cholangiocarcinoma: audit of 110 patients who underwent regional and paraaortic node dissection. Ann Surg. 233(3):385-92, 2001
12. Nakeeb A et al: Cholangiocarcinoma. A spectrum of intrahepatic, perihilar, and distal tumors. Ann Surg. 224(4):463-73; discussion 473-5, 1996
13. Su CH et al: Factors influencing postoperative morbidity, mortality, and survival after resection for hilar cholangiocarcinoma. Ann Surg. 223(4):384-94, 1996

PERIHILAR BILE DUCT CANCER PROTOCOL

Staging Parameters

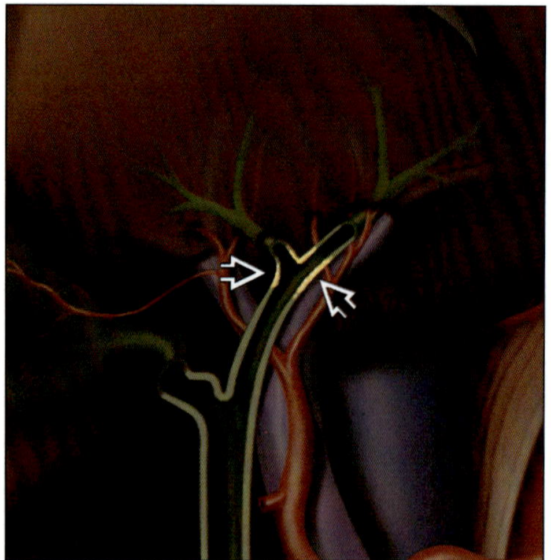

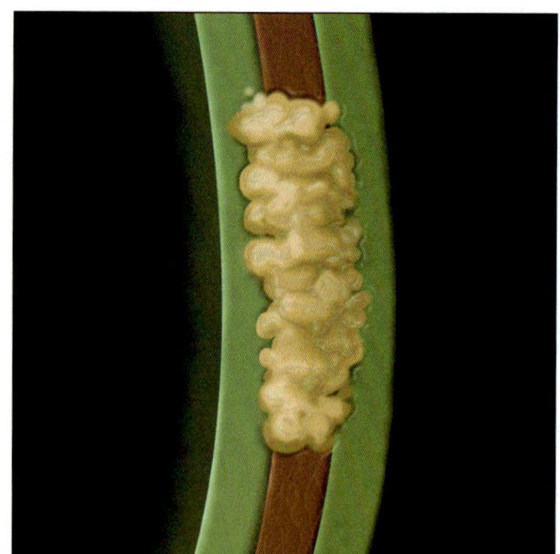

(Left) *This graphic depicts an infiltrative tumor* ➡ *at the confluence of the right and left hepatic ducts at the hepatic hilum. Tumor confined to the bile duct wall is classified as T1 disease.* ***(Right)*** *The wall of the bile duct is composed of the lamina propria, the fibromuscular wall, and the connective tissue that surrounds the fibromuscular wall. T1 tumors are defined as confined to the bile duct, with extension up to the muscle layer or the fibrous tissue.*

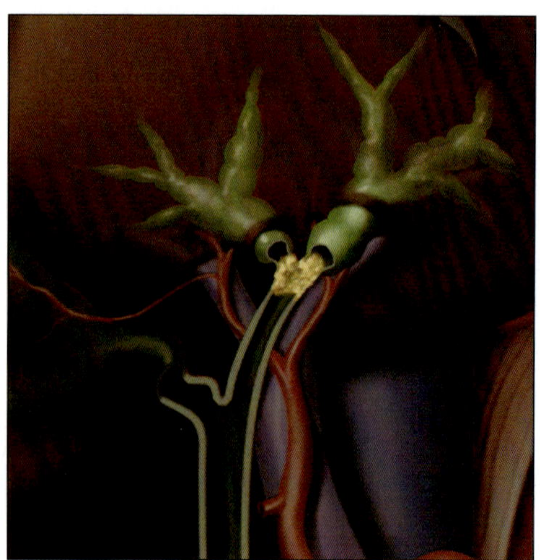

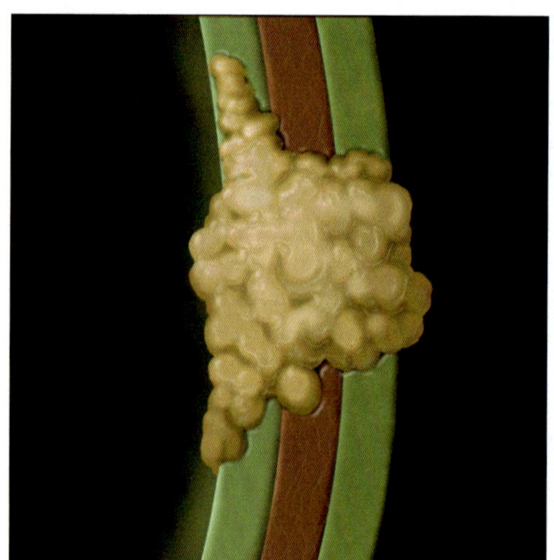

(Left) *This graphic illustrates a tumor at the hepatic hilum at the confluence of the right and left hepatic ducts. The tumor extends beyond the bile duct into the surrounding adipose tissue, consistent with T2a disease.* ***(Right)*** *This graphic illustrates a high-power view of a T2a tumor extending out of the bile duct into the surrounding adipose tissue.*

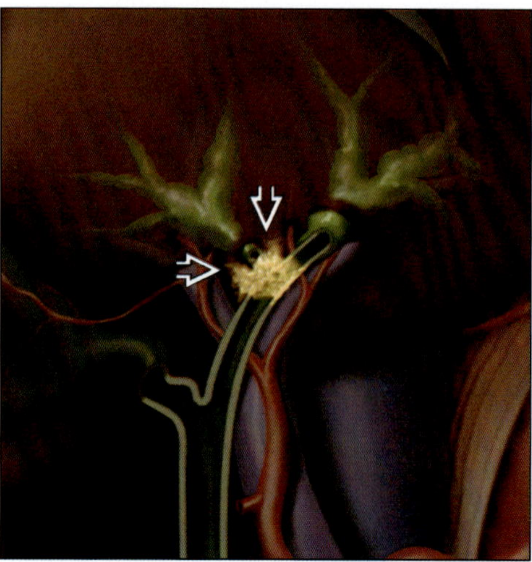

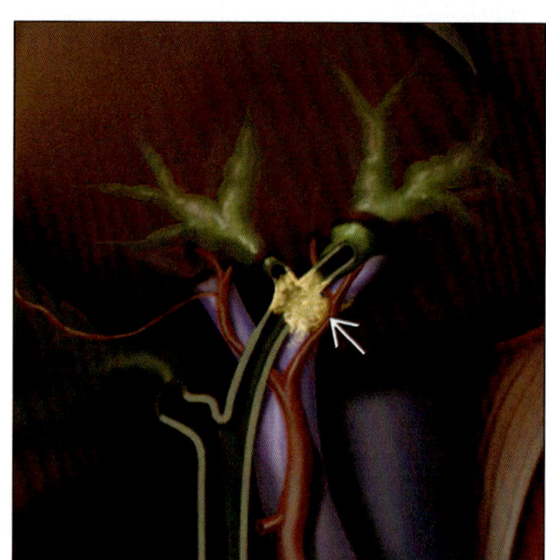

(Left) *T2b disease is defined as invading the adjacent hepatic parenchyma. This graphic illustrates a tumor at the confluence of the right and left hepatic ducts that extends into the adjacent hepatic tissue* ➡. ***(Right)*** *This graphic illustrates T3 disease, defined as invading unilateral branches of the portal vein or hepatic artery. This tumor at the confluence of the right and left hepatic ducts invades the left portal vein* ➡.

Staging Parameters

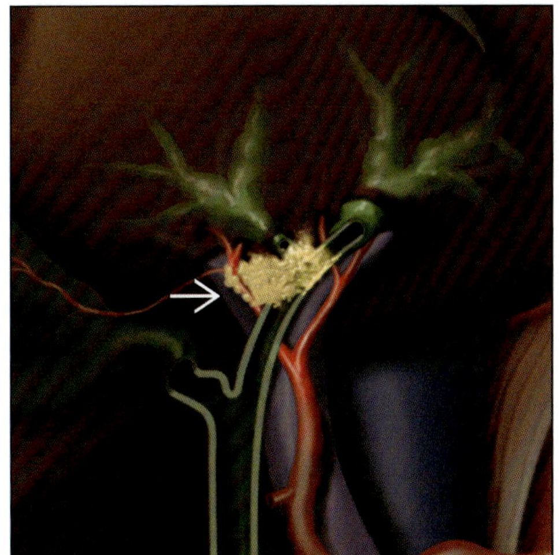

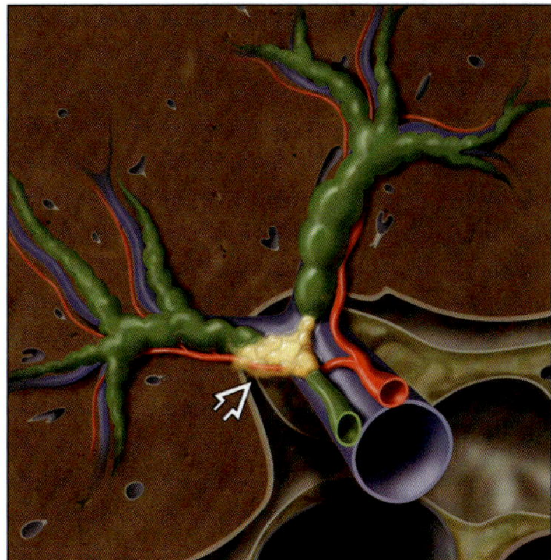

(Left) *This tumor is also classified as T3 disease because it invades the right hepatic artery ➔. T3 tumors can unilaterally invade the portal vein, hepatic artery, or both.* ***(Right)*** *This axial graphic depicts a biliary carcinoma at the hilum with tumor encasing the right hepatic artery ➔ (T3 disease).*

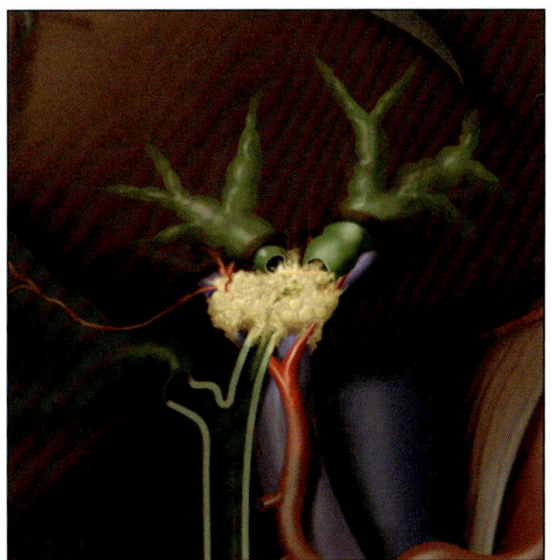

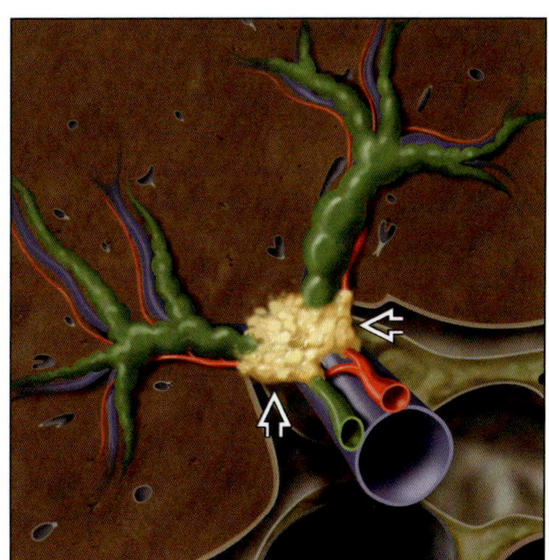

(Left) *Invasion of the common hepatic artery, main portal vein, or bilateral branches is classified as a T4 tumor. This tumor at the confluence of the right and left hepatic ducts forms a mass that invades the bilateral portal veins and hepatic arteries.* ***(Right)*** *This axial graphic illustrates a tumor at the hilum that encases the right and left hepatic arteries ➔.*

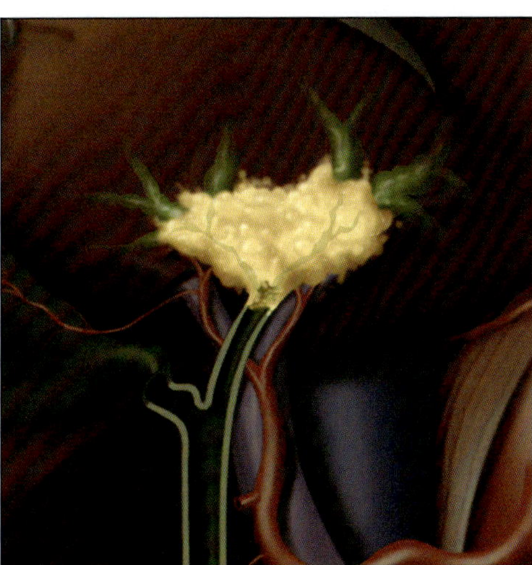

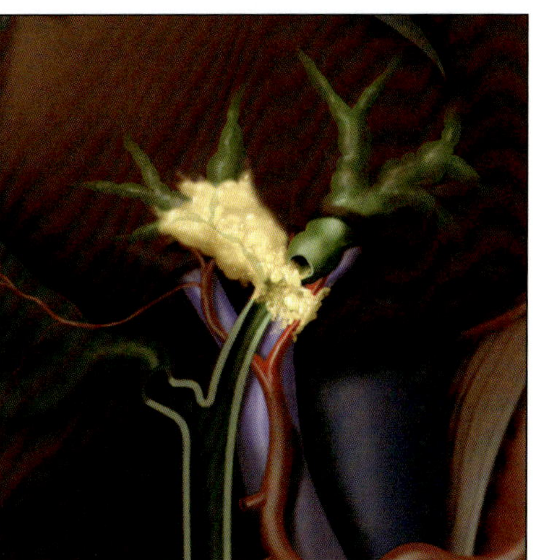

(Left) *Bilateral tumor involvement of the secondary biliary radicals is classified as T4 regardless of vascular involvement. This tumor at the confluence of the right and left hepatic ducts forms a mass that extends to involve the secondary biliary branches bilaterally.* ***(Right)*** *Unilateral secondary biliary radical involvement (shown on the right) with contralateral portal vein or hepatic artery involvement (shown on the left) is also classified as T4 disease.*

DISTAL EXTRAHEPATIC BILE DUCT CANCER PROTOCOL

Distal Extrahepatic Bile Ducts: Local or Segmental Resection, Pancreaticoduodenectomy

Surgical Pathology Cancer Case Summary (Checklist)

Specimen (select all that apply)

___ Common bile duct
___ Right hepatic duct
___ Left hepatic duct
___ Junction of right and left hepatic ducts
___ Common hepatic duct
___ Cystic duct
___ Not specified

Other organs received

___ Stomach
___ Duodenum
___ Pancreas
___ Ampulla
___ Gallbladder
___ Other (specify): ___________________________

Procedure

___ Pancreaticoduodenectomy
___ Segmental resection of bile duct(s)
___ Choledochal cyst resection
___ Other (specify): ___________________________
___ Not specified

Tumor Site (select all that apply)

___ Common bile duct
  ___ Extrapancreatic
  ___ Intrapancreatic
___ Other (specify): ___________________________
___ Not specified

Tumor Size

Greatest dimension: _________ cm
*Additional dimensions: _________ x _________ cm
___ Cannot be determined

Histologic Type

___ Adenocarcinoma (not otherwise characterized)
___ Papillary adenocarcinoma
___ Mucinous adenocarcinoma
___ Clear cell adenocarcinoma
___ Signet ring cell carcinoma
___ Adenosquamous carcinoma
___ Squamous cell carcinoma
___ Small cell carcinoma
___ Large cell neuroendocrine carcinoma
___ Biliary cystadenocarcinoma
___ Other (specify): ___________________________
___ Carcinoma, type cannot be determined

Histologic Grade

___ Not applicable
___ GX: Cannot be assessed
___ G1: Well differentiated

___ G2: Moderately differentiated
___ G3: Poorly differentiated
___ G4: Undifferentiated

Microscopic Tumor Extension (select all that apply)

___ Carcinoma in situ
___ Tumor confined to bile duct histologically
___ Tumor invades beyond wall of bile duct
___ Tumor invades duodenum
___ Tumor invades pancreas
___ Tumor invades gallbladder
___ Tumor invades other adjacent structures (specify): ____________________

Margins (select all that apply)

Segmental resection specimen

___ Cannot be assessed
___ Margins uninvolved by invasive carcinoma
Distance of invasive carcinoma from closest margin: _______ mm
Specify margin: ____________________
___ Margins involved by invasive carcinoma
___ Proximal bile duct margin
___ Distal bile duct margin
___ Other (specify): ____________________
___ Dysplasia/carcinoma in situ not identified at bile duct margin
___ Dysplasia/carcinoma in situ present at bile duct margin

Pancreaticoduodenal resection specimen

Proximal margin (gastric or duodenal)
___ Cannot be assessed
___ Uninvolved by invasive carcinoma
___ Involved by invasive carcinoma

Distal margin (distal duodenal)
___ Cannot be assessed
___ Uninvolved by invasive carcinoma
___ Involved by invasive carcinoma

Pancreatic retroperitoneal margin
___ Not applicable
___ Cannot be assessed
___ Uninvolved by invasive carcinoma
___ Involved by invasive carcinoma (tumor present 0-1 mm from margin)

Bile duct margin
___ Not applicable
___ Cannot be assessed
___ Margin uninvolved by invasive carcinoma
___ Margin involved by invasive carcinoma

Distal pancreatic margin
___ Not applicable
___ Cannot be assessed
___ Margin uninvolved by invasive carcinoma
___ Margin involved by invasive carcinoma

If all margins uninvolved by invasive carcinoma
distance of invasive carcinoma from closest margin: _______ mm OR _______ cm
Specify margin: ____________________

Lymph-Vascular Invasion

___ Not identified
___ Present

DISTAL EXTRAHEPATIC BILE DUCT CANCER PROTOCOL

___ Indeterminate

Perineural Invasion

___ Not identified

___ Present

___ Indeterminate

Pathologic Staging (pTNM)

TNM descriptors (required only if applicable (select all that apply)

___ m (multiple primary tumors)

___ r (recurrent)

___ y (post-treatment)

Primary tumor (pT)

___ pTX: Cannot be assessed

___ pT0: No evidence of primary tumor

___ pTis: Carcinoma in situ

___ pT1: Tumor confined to bile duct histologically

___ pT2: Tumor invades beyond wall of bile duct

___ pT3: Tumor invades gallbladder, pancreas, duodenum, or other adjacent organs without involvement of celiac axis or superior mesenteric artery

___ Tumor involves celiac axis or superior mesenteric artery

Regional lymph nodes (pN)

___ pNX: Cannot be assessed

___ pN0: No regional lymph node metastasis

___ pN1: Regional lymph node metastasis

Specify: Number examined: ________

Number involved: ________

Distant metastasis (pM)

___ Not applicable

___ pM1: Distant metastasis

*Specify site(s), if known: ________________________

**Additional Pathologic Findings (select all that apply)*

*___ None identified

*___ Choledochal cyst

*___ Dysplasia

*___ Primary sclerosing cholangitis (PSC)

*___ Stones

*___ Other (specify): ________________________

**Ancillary Studies*

*Specify: ________________________

**Clinical History (select all that apply)*

*___ Primary sclerosing cholangitis

*___ Inflammatory bowel disease

*___ Biliary stones

*___ Other (specify): ________________________

**Data elements with asterisks are not required. However, these elements may be clinically important but are not yet validated or regularly used in patient management. Adapted with permission from College of American Pathologists, "Protocol for the Examination of Specimens from Patients with Carcinoma of the Distal Extrahepatic Bile Ducts." Web posting date October 2009, www.cap.org. Protocol applies to all invasive carcinomas of the distal extrahepatic bile ducts. Well-differentiated neuroendocrine neoplasms (carcinoid tumors) are not included. Carcinomas of the perihilar bile ducts are not included.*

DISTAL EXTRAHEPATIC BILE DUCT CANCER PROTOCOL

Stage Groupings

Stage	Tumor	Node	Metastasis
0	Tis	N0	M0
IA	T1	N0	M0
IB	T2	N0	M0
IIA	T3	N0	M0
IIB	T1	N1	M0
	T2	N1	M0
	T3	N1	M0
III	T4	Any N	M0
IV	Any T	Any N	M1

Adapted from 7th edition AJCC Staging Forms.

DISTAL EXTRAHEPATIC BILE DUCT CANCER PROTOCOL

GENERAL COMMENTS

Anatomic Considerations

- 20-30% of extrahepatic bile duct malignancies are distal
  - Staged separately from perihilar and intrahepatic malignancies
  - Distal tumors defined as those arising between junction of cystic duct/common bile duct (CBD) and ampulla of Vater
  - Includes tumors arising in choledochal cysts and the intrapancreatic portion of common bile duct
    - May be grossly difficult to determine if tumors arise from the intrapancreatic CBD, pancreas, or ampulla; distinction important for staging
- Distal bile duct anatomy
  - Wall composed of submucosal connective tissue and muscle
  - Muscle fibers most prominent in distal bile duct
  - Extrahepatic ducts lack serosa but are surrounded by variable amounts of periductal adipose tissue
    - Invasion of this adipose tissue is considered T2 disease

Staging

- Usually occurs following surgery and pathologic examination
  - Minority of patients deemed unresectable due to local extension
  - Treated without pathologic staging

Prognostic Factors

- Extent of resection and margin status is most important stage-independent prognostic factor
  - Should be carefully documented in report
- Adverse prognostic factors
  - Histologic type
    - Papillary carcinomas have more favorable outcome
  - Tumor grade
  - Vascular invasion
  - Lymphatic invasion
  - Perineural invasion
  - Lymph node metastases
  - Elevated CEA and CA19-9

Lymph Nodes

- Need minimum of 12 lymph nodes
- Regional nodes
  - Common bile duct
  - Hepatic artery
  - Celiac trunk
  - Posterior pancreaticoduodenal
  - Anterior pancreaticoduodenal
  - Superior mesenteric vein
  - Right lateral wall of superior mesenteric artery

Metastases

- Regional spread
  - Pancreas
  - Duodenum
  - Stomach
  - Colon
  - Omentum
- Distant metastases
  - Liver, lungs, peritoneum
  - Usually late in course of disease

SELECTED REFERENCES

1. American Joint Committee on Cancer: AJCC Cancer Staging Manual. 7th ed. New York: Springer. 227-33, 2010
2. DeOliveira ML et al: Cholangiocarcinoma: thirty-one-year experience with 564 patients at a single institution. Ann Surg. 245(5):755-62, 2007
3. Murakami Y et al: Prognostic significance of lymph node metastasis and surgical margin status for distal cholangiocarcinoma. J Surg Oncol. 95(3):207-12, 2007
4. Hong SM et al: Analysis of extrahepatic bile duct carcinomas according to the New American Joint Committee on Cancer staging system focused on tumor classification problems in 222 patients. Cancer. 104(4):802-10, 2005
5. He P et al: Multivariate statistical analysis of clinicopathologic factors influencing survival of patients with bile duct carcinoma. World J Gastroenterol. 8(5):943-6, 2002

Tumors of the Pancreas

PANCREATIC INTRAEPITHELIAL NEOPLASIA

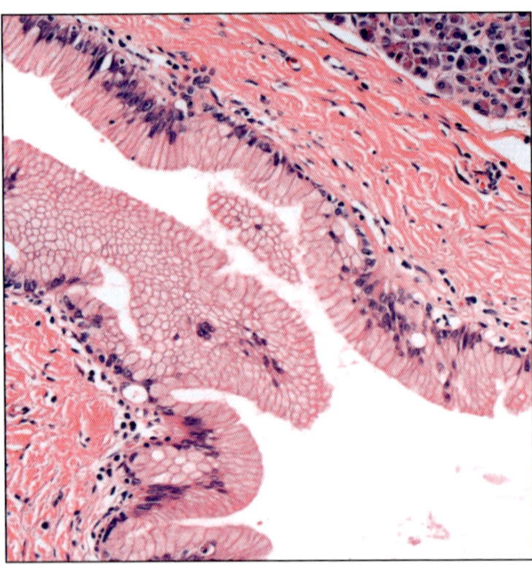

This example of PanIN-1 shows a pancreatic duct lined by a single layer of epithelium with abundant apical mucinous cytoplasm and basal nuclei that lack atypia.

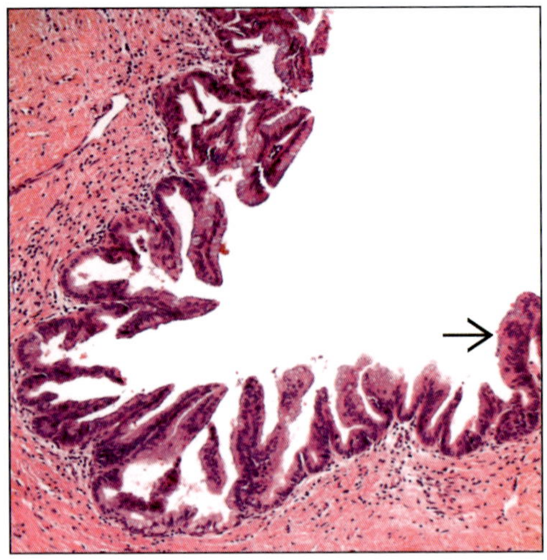

This example of PanIN-2 shows a pancreatic duct lined by a micropapillary proliferation of mucinous epithelial cells. Focally, a loss of nuclear polarity is present →.

TERMINOLOGY

Abbreviations

- Pancreatic intraepithelial neoplasia (PanIN)

Synonyms

- Metaplasia, dysplasia, carcinoma in situ

Definitions

- Noninvasive pancreatic ductal epithelial proliferations that are associated with pancreatic ductal adenocarcinoma

CLINICAL ISSUES

Natural History

- PanIN-1: Commonly found in resected pancreata; significance unclear
- PanIN-3: Associated with significant risk of progression to pancreatic ductal adenocarcinoma

Treatment

- High-grade PanIN, particularly PanIN-3, indicates elevated risk for pancreatic adenocarcinoma
  - Surveillance of these patients is warranted
  - Appropriate management of isolated presence of PanIN-3 has not been established
  - High-grade PanIN at a surgical margin may warrant the resection of more tissue

Incidence

- Frequency of low-grade PanIN correlates with age; sharply increases after age 40
- PanIN-3 is most often found in pancreata with concurrent pancreatic ductal adenocarcinoma and only rarely (< 5%) in association with chronic pancreatitis and benign cysts

IMAGE FINDINGS

General Features

- PanIN lesions are typically very small and thus radiologically undetectable

MACROSCOPIC FEATURES

General Features

- Not visible grossly

MICROSCOPIC PATHOLOGY

Histologic Features

- PanIN typically involves the epithelium of ducts < 5 mm in diameter
  - Both the main pancreatic duct and peripheral pancreatic lobules may be involved
  - Invariably multifocal with varying grades found within a single pancreas
- Lining epithelium can be either flat or papillary and occasionally shows complex architectural patterns
- Often abundant supranuclear mucin without intraluminal mucin

Grading PanIN

- PanIN-1
  - Flat (PanIN-1A) or papillary/micropapillary (PanIN-1B)
  - Tall columnar epithelium with basal nuclei and abundant supranuclear mucin
  - Nuclei are small, lack nuclear atypia
- PanIN-2
  - Generally papillary, occasionally flat
  - Nuclear atypia is always present
    - Loss of nuclear polarity, nuclear crowding, enlarged nuclei, pseudostratification, and hyperchromasia are seen in varying combinations

PANCREATIC INTRAEPITHELIAL NEOPLASIA

Key Facts

Terminology

- Noninvasive ductal epithelial proliferations associated with pancreatic ductal adenocarcinoma

Clinical Issues

- High-grade PanIN, particularly PanIN-3, indicates elevated risk for pancreatic adenocarcinoma

Microscopic Pathology

- Ducts are lined by mucinous epithelium, either flat or papillary
  - PanIN-1: Lacks cytologic atypia
  - PanIN-2: Nuclear atypia is always present
  - PanIN-3: Atypia parallels that seen in pancreatic ductal adenocarcinoma

    - Mitoses are rare; when present, they are not atypical
- PanIN-3
  - Usually papillary and micropapillary
  - Architectural abnormalities including cribriforming, budding, and luminal necrosis
  - Cytologic abnormalities including irregular nuclear contours, macronucleoli, and frequent (often abnormal) mitoses

DIFFERENTIAL DIAGNOSIS

Intraductal Papillary Mucinous Neoplasm

- Usually > 0.5 cm
- Papillae taller and more complex than PanIN
- Abundant luminal mucin
- MUC2 positive

Reactive Ductal Epithelial Changes

- Associated with inflammation
- Usually lack significant architectural atypia

Cancerization of Ducts

- Spread of invasive carcinoma along preexisting ducts may be difficult to distinguish from PanIN-3
- Abrupt transition from normal to markedly atypical epithelium, and continuity of carcinoma with involved duct, favor cancerization

DIAGNOSTIC CHECKLIST

Pathologic Interpretation Pearls

- Many experts do not report PanIN-1 in their surgical pathology reports
- At frozen section, it is not essential to report PanIN-1 lesions, whereas communicating the presence of PanIN-2 and PanIN-3 lesions is essential
  - Presence of low-grade PanIN will not change surgical management

SELECTED REFERENCES

1. Sipos B et al: Pancreatic intraepithelial neoplasia revisited and updated. Pancreatology. 9(1-2):45-54, 2009
2. Brune K et al: Multifocal neoplastic precursor lesions associated with lobular atrophy of the pancreas in patients having a strong family history of pancreatic cancer. Am J Surg Pathol. 30(9):1067-76, 2006
3. Hruban RH et al: An illustrated consensus on the classification of pancreatic intraepithelial neoplasia and intraductal papillary mucinous neoplasms. Am J Surg Pathol. 28(8):977-87, 2004
4. Andea A et al: Clinicopathological correlates of pancreatic intraepithelial neoplasia: a comparative analysis of 82 cases with and 152 cases without pancreatic ductal adenocarcinoma. Mod Pathol. 16(10):996-1006, 2003
5. Hruban RH et al: Pancreatic intraepithelial neoplasia: a new nomenclature and classification system for pancreatic duct lesions. Am J Surg Pathol. 25(5):579-86, 2001

IMAGE GALLERY

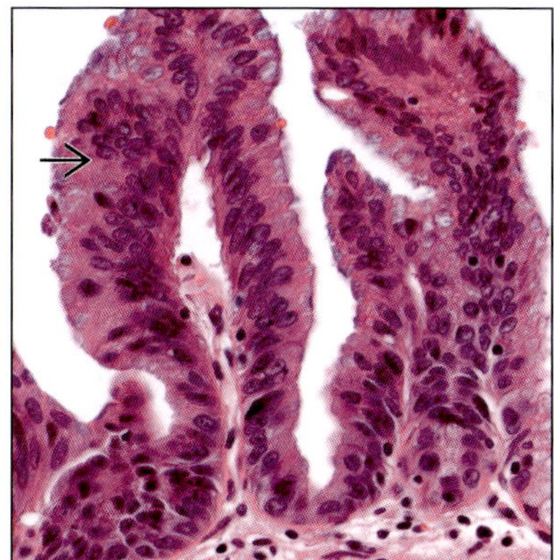

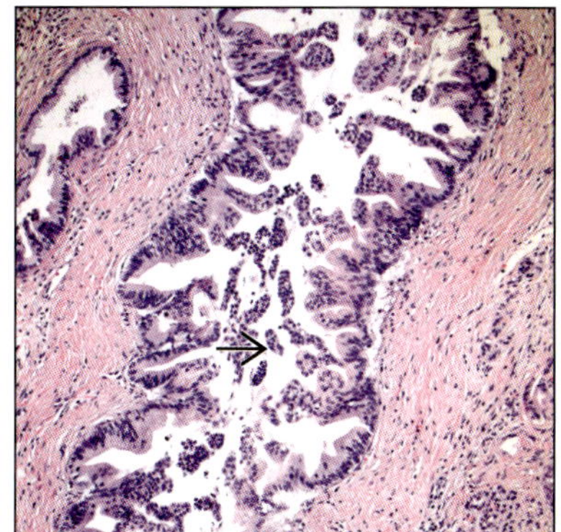

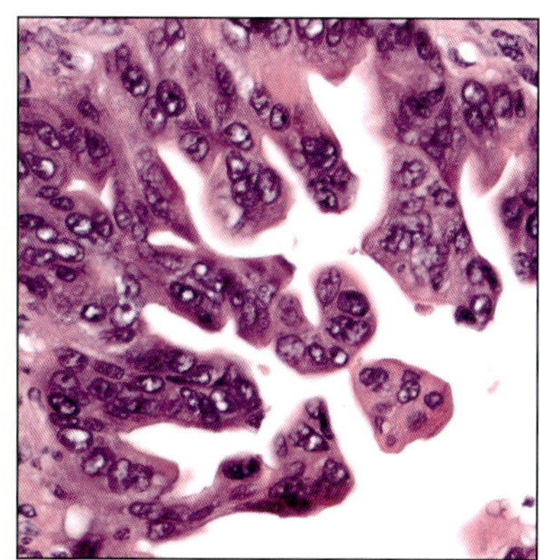

(Left) *The presence of cytologic atypia in PanIN-2, as demonstrated here, distinguishes it from PanIN-1. Note the enlarged hyperchromatic nuclei and the slight loss of nuclear polarity* ⇒. ***(Center)*** *This example of PanIN-3 shows a duct with micropapillary architecture and epithelial budding* ⇒. ***(Right)*** *In PanIN-3, ducts are lined by epithelial cells with cytologic atypia that is severe enough to warrant classification as noninvasive carcinoma.*

DUCTAL ADENOCARCINOMA, INCLUDING VARIANTS

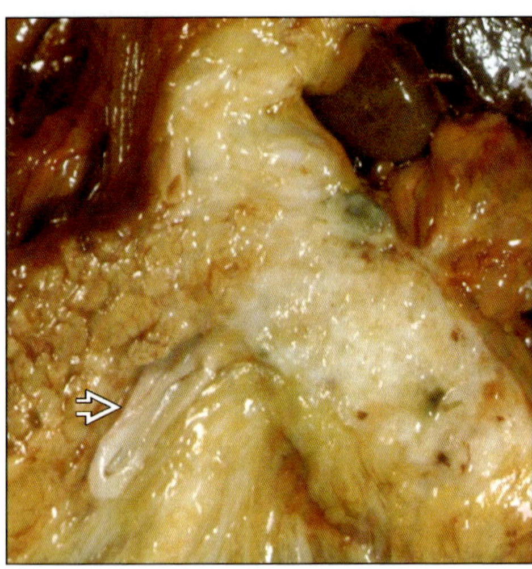

This gross photograph shows the cut surface of a large pancreatic adenocarcinoma. The surface is firm, white, and gritty. Note the dilated pancreatic duct ➔.

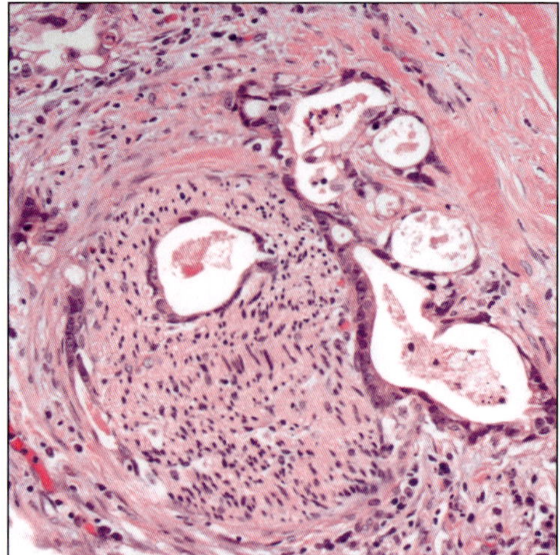

Perineural invasion is a common feature of pancreatic ductal adenocarcinoma.

TERMINOLOGY

Abbreviations

- Pancreatic ductal adenocarcinoma (PDAC)

Synonyms

- Pancreatic adenocarcinoma
- Duct cell adenocarcinoma

Definitions

- Malignant epithelial neoplasm arising in pancreatic ductal system
  - 85-90% of all pancreatic neoplasms
- Predominantly glandular differentiation

ETIOLOGY/PATHOGENESIS

Hereditary Risk Factors

- Family history of pancreatic cancer
- Hereditary pancreatitis
- Peutz-Jeghers syndrome
- Familial atypical multiple mole melanoma syndrome
- *BRCA2* and *BRCA1* mutations

Medical Risk Factors

- Chronic pancreatitis
- Diabetes mellitus
- Previous cholecystectomy or partial gastrectomy

Environmental and Occupational Risk Factors

- Cigarette smoking approximately doubles risk
- Diet high in meat, fat, nitrates, and pork products increases risk
- Obesity
- Chemicals (solvents, DDT, gasoline)
- Occupational (coal gas workers, metal working, hide tanning, dry cleaning)

Precursor Lesions

- Pancreatic intraepithelial neoplasia

CLINICAL ISSUES

Epidemiology

- Age
  - Peak incidence in 7th and 8th decades of life
    - Rare before age 40
    - Majority of cases occur between age 60-80
- Gender
  - More common in men than in women (1.3:1)
- Ethnicity
  - More common in Maoris, native Hawaiians, and African-Americans in USA

Presentation

- Very nonspecific symptoms may result in delay in diagnosis
  - Epigastric pain radiating to the back
  - Weight loss
  - Painless jaundice
  - Signs of biliary obstruction
- Disease associations
  - Trousseau syndrome (migratory thrombophlebitis)
  - Diabetes mellitus
  - Sister Mary Joseph sign (palpable periumbilical nodules)
  - Courvoisier sign (distended, palpable gallbladder)

Treatment

- Resection
  - Only 10-20% of cases resectable at diagnosis
- Chemotherapy before resection, after resection, or both
  - Gemcitabine seems most promising

Prognosis

- Dismal
  - Overall 5-year survival less than 5%

DUCTAL ADENOCARCINOMA, INCLUDING VARIANTS

Key Facts

Terminology
- Adenocarcinoma arising in pancreatic ductal system
  - Comprises 85-90% of all pancreatic neoplasms

Clinical Issues
- Most cases unresectable at presentation
- Nonspecific symptoms often mean delay in diagnosis

Macroscopic Features
- Majority in head of pancreas
- Poorly defined, firm mass with intense fibrotic reaction
  - Carcinoma may be difficult to distinguish from background pancreatitis

Microscopic Pathology
- Small, haphazardly infiltrating glands embedded in dense desmoplastic stroma
- Perineural and angiolymphatic invasion and associated chronic pancreatitis are very common
- Many histologic patterns and variants
  - Foamy gland pattern
  - Clear cell pattern
  - Colloid carcinoma
  - Adenosquamous
- Immunopositive for many antigens
  - Cytokeratins 7, 8, 18, 19
  - CEA, CA19-9, CA125, B72.3
  - MUC1, MUC4, MUC5AC, and MUC6 (25%)

IMAGE FINDINGS

General Features
- CT scan is most commonly used radiological method for diagnosis and staging
- Magnetic resonance angiography can be used to examine vascular anatomy and determine resectability
- Endoscopic ultrasound also very reliable for diagnosis and staging
- ERCP/MRCP help visualize ductal system

MACROSCOPIC FEATURES

General Features
- Majority in head of pancreas
  - Minority in body or tail
  - Minority diffusely involves whole gland
- Solitary (majority) or multifocal
- Firm, solid, poorly defined, white-yellow mass
  - May have cystic degeneration
- Usually intense fibrotic reaction
  - May make carcinoma difficult to distinguish from background pancreatitis
- Pancreatic duct may be dilated
- May cause stenosis of common bile duct
- Tumors often grossly extend beyond pancreas

MICROSCOPIC PATHOLOGY

Histologic Features
- Invasive malignant glands
  - Range from very well-differentiated to very poorly differentiated
  - Glands grow in haphazard fashion and are very infiltrative
- Nuclear features
  - Nuclear crowding and overlapping
  - Nuclei vary in size, shape, and intracellular location from cell to cell within a given neoplastic gland
  - Loss of polarity
  - Irregular chromatin distribution
  - Irregular nuclear contour
- Dense desmoplastic stroma
  - Fibroblasts and other inflammatory cells
  - Neoplastic tumor cells may represent only small component of tumor mass with the rest made up of desmoplastic reaction
- Mucin production
- Perineural invasion is very common
  - Present in > 75% of cases
- Angiolymphatic invasion is common
- Tumor may infiltrate larger blood vessels and cause thrombi
- Tumor cells may grow along basement membrane of adjacent intact epithelium such as in pancreatic ducts (cancerization), bile duct, and duodenum
- Associated pancreatitis is common
  - Parenchymal atrophy
  - Fibrosis
  - Islet cell clustering ("pseudohyperplasia")

ANCILLARY TESTS

Immunohistochemistry
- Positive for cytokeratins 7, 8, 18, 19
- Positive for CEA, CA19-9, CA125, B72.3
- Positive for MUC1, MUC4, MUC5AC, and MUC6 (25%)
- Positive for claudin-4, fascin, mesothelin, PSCA (60%), S100 proteins
- Loss of nuclear expression of p16 (> 90%) and SMAD4 (55%)
- Overexpression of p53 (50-75%)

Histologic Patterns and Variants
- Foamy gland pattern
  - Deceptively bland, benign-appearing cells with microvesicular cytoplasm
  - Mimics PanIN, benign glands, or histiocytes
- Clear cell pattern
  - Clear cytoplasm resembles renal cell carcinoma

  - Common focal finding in conventional ductal adenocarcinoma
- Colloid carcinoma
  - Neoplastic epithelial cells suspended in large pools of extracellular mucin
  - Colloid component must comprise at least 80% of tumor
  - Almost always arises in association with intraductal papillary mucinous neoplasm (IPMN)
- Signet ring cell carcinoma
  - At least 50% of tumor composed of infiltrating, noncohesive cells with intracytoplasmic mucin
- Adenosquamous carcinoma
  - Squamous differentiation in at least 30% of entire lesion
- Large duct adenocarcinoma
  - Composed of large, dilated, invasive glands, often with simple architecture
  - May simulate (dilated) PanIN
- Microadenocarcinoma pattern
  - Small uniform cells arranged in microglandular structures
  - Represents a mix of ductal adenocarcinoma, endocrine neoplasm, and acinar cell carcinoma
- Medullary carcinoma
  - Poorly differentiated carcinoma with pushing rather than infiltrating borders
  - Associated with microsatellite instability, hereditary nonpolyposis colorectal cancer (HNPCC)
- Undifferentiated carcinoma with or without osteoclastic-like giant cells
  - May have giant cell, spindle cell, or glandular component
- Hepatoid carcinoma
  - Significant component demonstrates hepatocellular differentiation
  - Mark with Hep-Par1, CD10, polyclonal CEA, AFP

DIFFERENTIAL DIAGNOSIS

Chronic Pancreatitis

- Often involves younger patients (< 40 years)
- Diffuse scarring of gland without a discrete mass
- Relatively preserved lobular architecture

Normal/Reactive Duct Changes

- Very well-differentiated tumors may mimic normal or reactive pancreatic ducts but can be distinguished from the latter by the following features
  - Small glands immediately adjacent to muscular arteries without intervening stroma or acini
  - Incomplete gland formation
  - Disorganized, haphazard growth of neoplastic glands
  - 4x variation in nuclear size within single gland

Ampullary/Periampullary Carcinomas

- Differentiation from PDAC is based on epicenter of mass grossly and presence of precursor lesions

Acinic Cell Carcinoma

- Highly cellular carcinoma with acinar, trabecular, &/or solid patterns
- Eosinophilic granular cytoplasm
- Basally located nuclei with single prominent nucleolus
- Positive for trypsin and chymotrypsin
- Negative for CK7

Neuroendocrine Neoplasms

- Nesting &/or trabecular patterns
- Often have hyalinized stroma
- Uniform nuclei with "salt and pepper" chromatin
- Positive for chromogranin, synaptophysin

DIAGNOSTIC CHECKLIST

Clinically Relevant Pathologic Features

- Perineural or angiolymphatic invasion in retroperitoneal soft tissue margin is underrecognized basis for surgical failure
  - More than half of patients have extrapancreatic nerve involvement in this area
- Lymph node metastases present at time of surgery in 70-80% of patients

SELECTED REFERENCES

1. Shi C et al: Familial pancreatic cancer. Arch Pathol Lab Med. 133(3):365-74, 2009
2. Hruban RH et al: Pancreatic adenocarcinoma: update on the surgical pathology of carcinomas of ductal origin and PanINs. Mod Pathol. 20 Suppl 1:S61-70, 2007
3. Adsay NV et al: Ductal neoplasia of the pancreas: nosologic, clinicopathologic, and biologic aspects. Semin Radiat Oncol. 15(4):254-64, 2005
4. Forrester DW et al: Carcinoma of the pancreas: a review of 342 cases. J R Coll Surg Edinb. 25(6):436-43, 1980
5. Cubilla AL et al: Classification of pancreatic cancer (nonendocrine). Mayo Clin Proc. 54(7):449-58, 1979
6. Cubilla A et al: Pancreas cancer. I. Duct adenocarcinoma. A clinical-pathologic study of 380 patients. Pathol Annu. 13 Pt 1:241-89, 1978
7. Kissane JM: Carcinoma of the exocrine pancreas: pathologic aspects. J Surg Oncol. 7(2):167-74, 1975

Microscopic Features

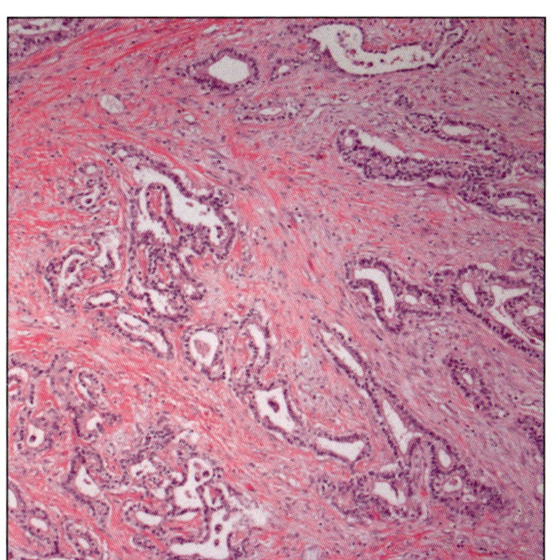

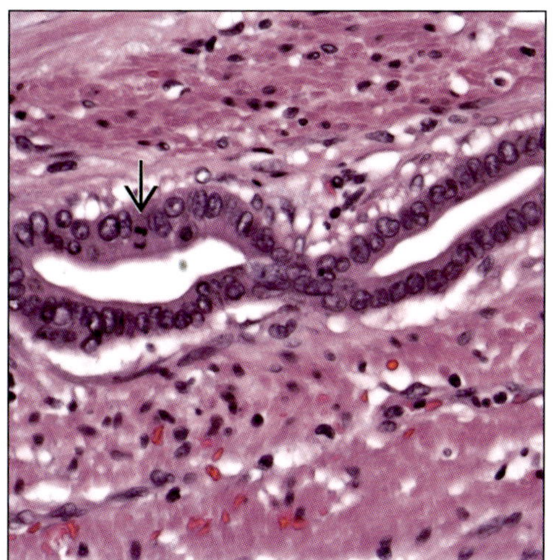

(Left) *Ductal adenocarcinoma typically features small to medium-sized glands with haphazard growth embedded in dense desmoplastic stroma.* ***(Right)*** *Cytologic clues to the diagnosis of well-differentiated pancreatic adenocarcinoma include variation in nuclear size, haphazard arrangement of nuclei, irregular nuclear membranes, and mitoses* ➔.

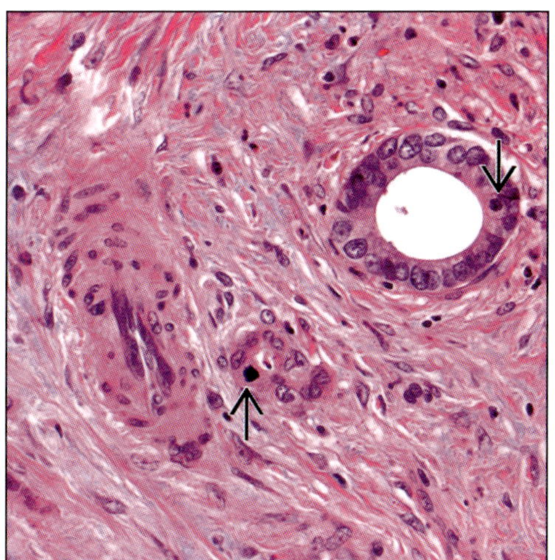

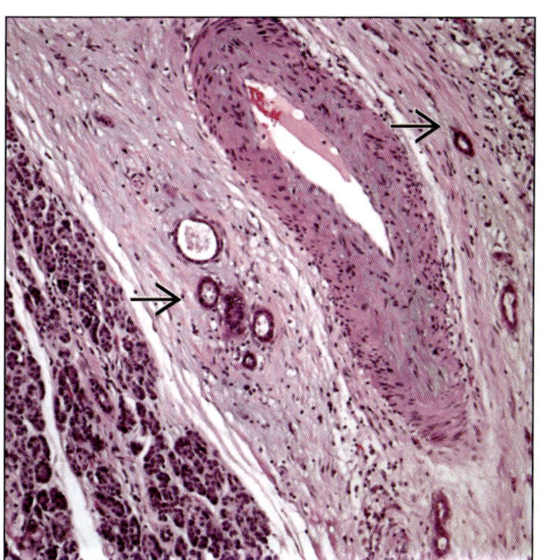

(Left) *Glands directly adjacent to a muscular artery are a clue to malignancy. Note the prominent mitoses* ➔ *and irregular nuclear membranes in these neoplastic glands as well.* ***(Right)*** *This photograph shows small infiltrating malignant glands* ➔ *directly adjacent to a muscular artery without intervening acinar parenchyma. This abnormal growth pattern is a sign of malignancy.*

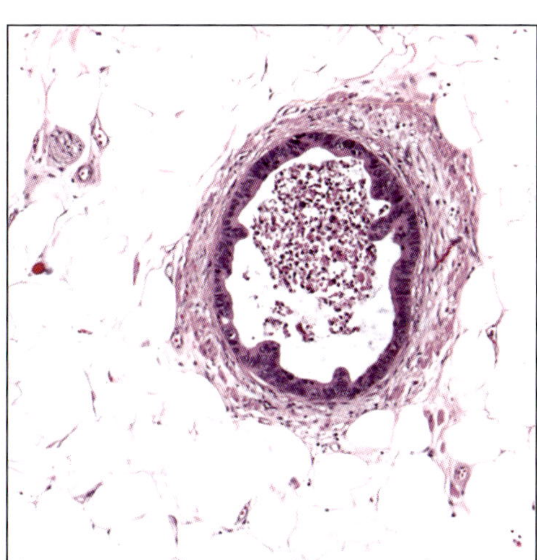

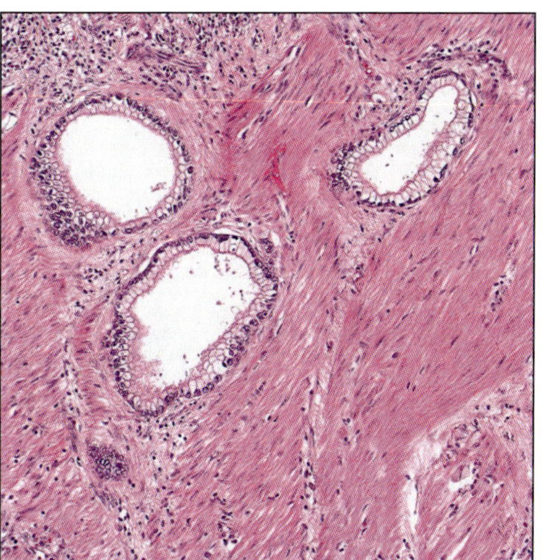

(Left) *This well-differentiated malignant gland is present within the peripancreatic fat.* ***(Right)*** *The foamy gland pattern features well-formed glands with clear foamy cytoplasm. In this case, the tumor infiltrates the muscularis propria of the duodenum.*

DUCTAL ADENOCARCINOMA, INCLUDING VARIANTS

Microscopic Features

(Left) **The foamy gland pattern features basally located round nuclei, microvesicular cytoplasm, and distinctive cytoplasmic condensation ("brush border-like zone") ➡. The cytology is deceptively bland and mimics pancreatic intraepithelial neoplasm (PanIN) 1A.** *(Right)* **This high-power photograph of the foamy gland pattern shows a group of cells with microvesicular cytoplasm, raisinoid nuclei, and a low nuclear to cytoplasmic ratio. This pattern may mimic a collection of foamy histiocytes.**

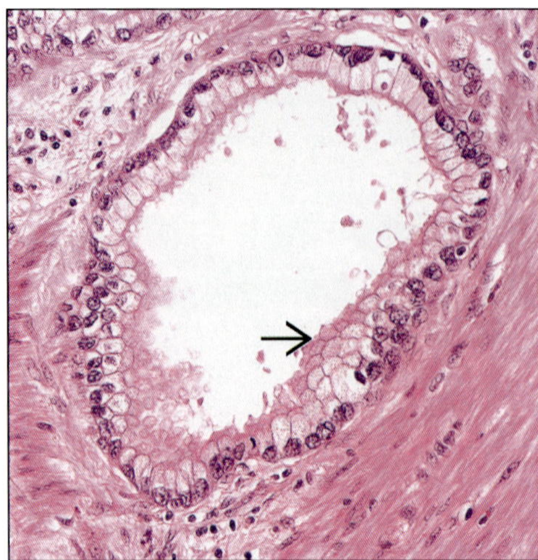

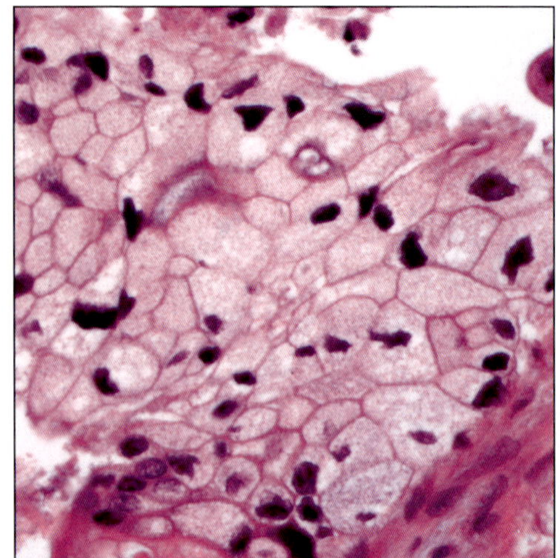

(Left) The mucinous or colloid pattern of pancreatic adenocarcinoma features neoplastic epithelium that is suspended in, or partially lines, large pools of extracellular mucin. *(Right)* A high-power view of the mucinous (colloid) pattern shows detached clusters of malignant cells floating in pools of mucin. Colloid carcinomas are almost always associated with intraductal papillary mucinous neoplasm, especially of the intestinal type.

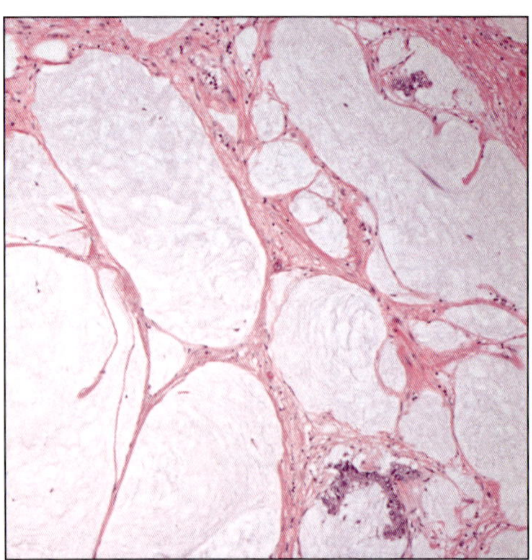

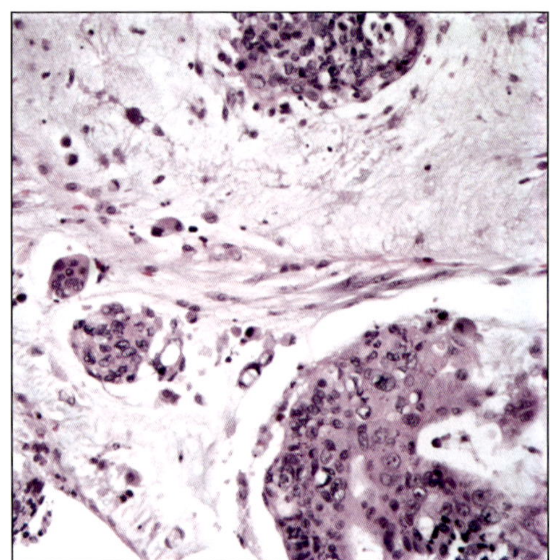

(Left) A large component of the tumor cells have signet ring cell morphology in this signet ring cell variant of pancreatic ductal adenocarcinoma. *(Right)* This example of poorly differentiated adenocarcinoma lacks well-formed glands. The tumor is composed of sheets of poorly differentiated tumor cells as well as single malignant cells. Heterogeneous morphology, encompassing well, moderate, and poor differentiations, is often seen in pancreatic ductal adenocarcinoma.

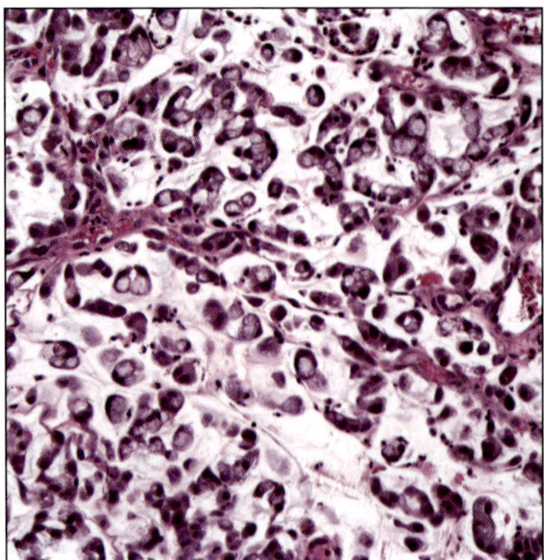

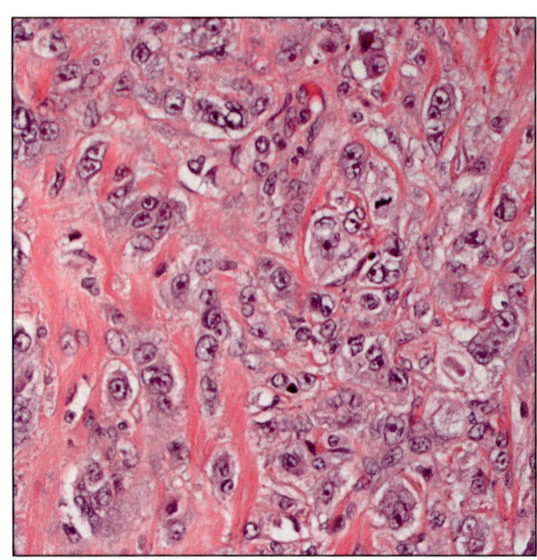

Microscopic Features

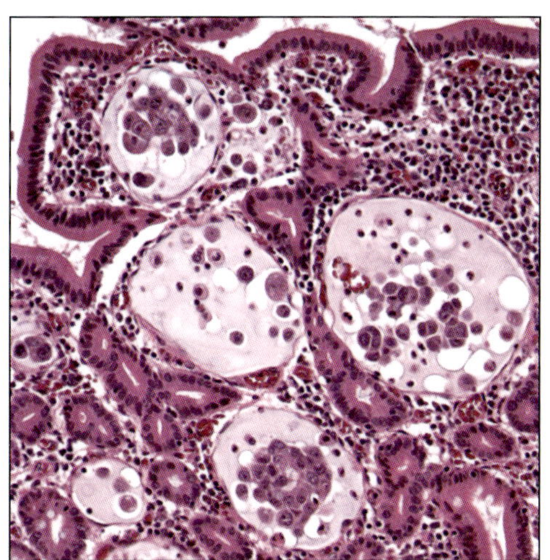

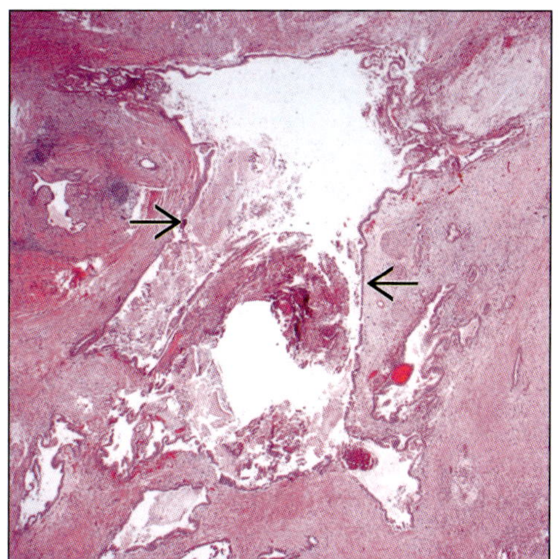

(Left) *This photograph shows extensive involvement of the duodenal lymphovascular spaces by pancreatic ductal adenocarcinoma.* ***(Right)*** *Ductal adenocarcinoma, large duct type, is characterized by cystically dilated neoplastic ducts ⇒ that can mimic PanIN or branch-duct IPMN. It can be differentiated from the latter based on the absence of low-grade epithelium in the duct lining.*

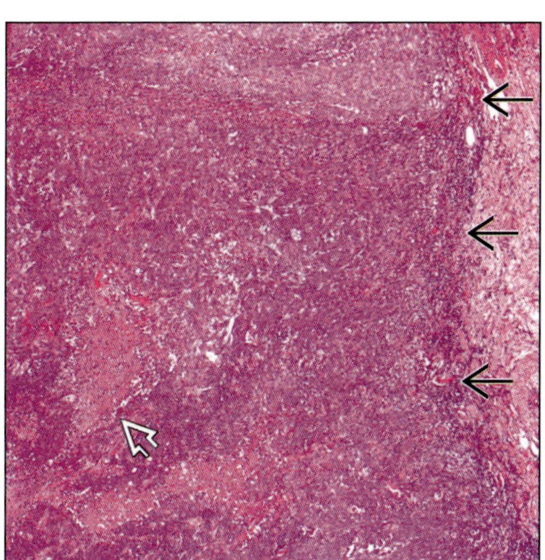

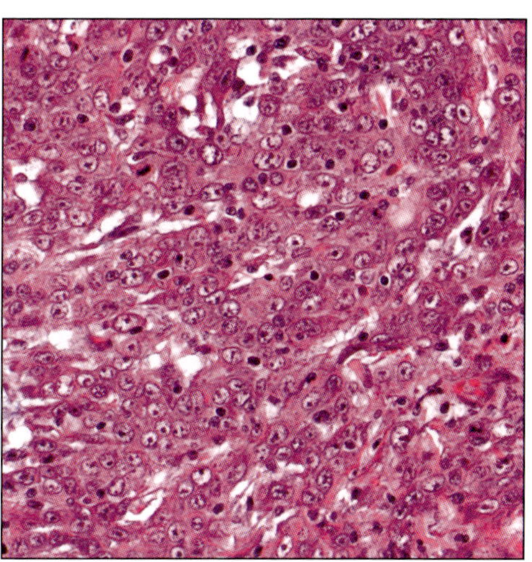

(Left) *This example of the medullary variant of pancreatic ductal carcinoma has well-defined borders ⇒ and foci of necrosis ➢.* ***(Right)*** *Medullary pancreatic carcinoma features a syncytial growth pattern containing poorly differentiated cells with scattered tumor-infiltrating lymphocytes.*

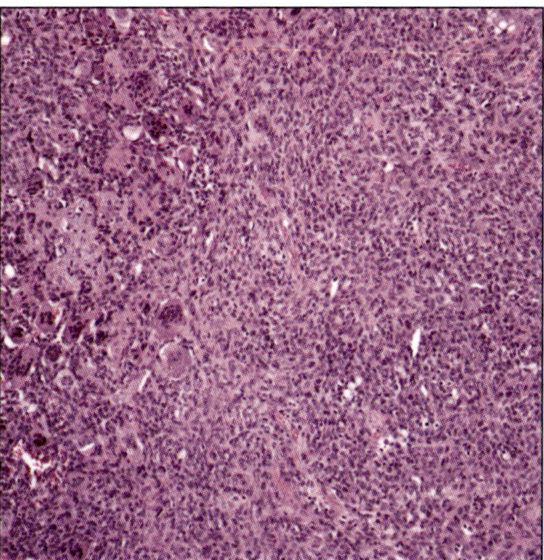

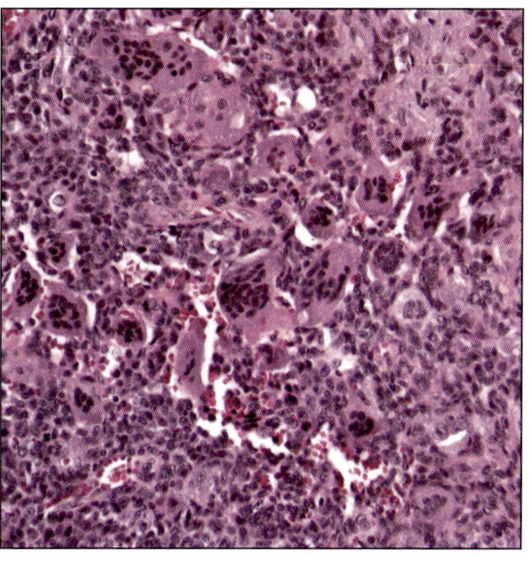

(Left) *This case of undifferentiated pancreatic ductal adenocarcinoma shows clusters of giant cells on the left and a poorly differentiated, spindled pattern on the right. The undifferentiated variant may or may not have giant cells.* ***(Right)*** *This high-power photomicrograph highlights the numerous giant cells in this case of undifferentiated pancreatic ductal adenocarcinoma.*

UNDIFFERENTIATED CARCINOMA

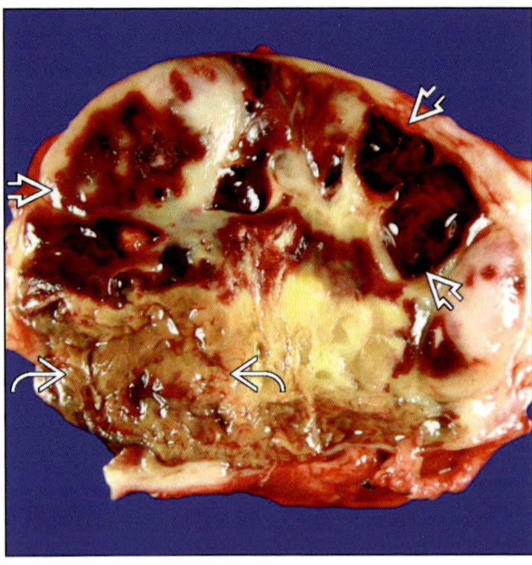

This gross photograph of an undifferentiated carcinoma with osteoclast-like giant cells has a soft, fleshy cut surface with prominent hemorrhage ➡ and necrosis ➡.

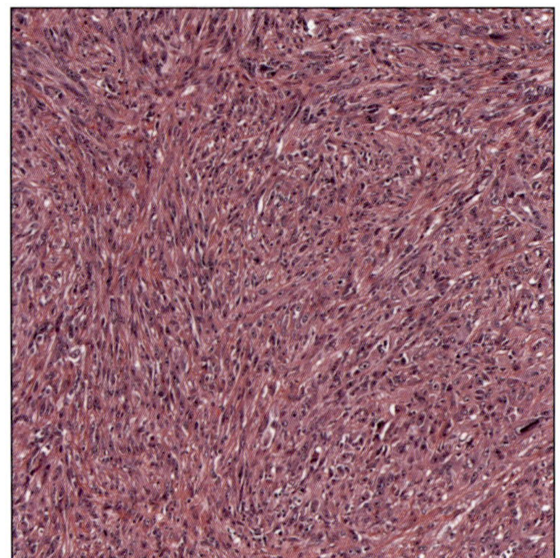

This undifferentiated carcinoma has a prominent sarcomatoid component featuring plump spindle cells in a fascicular pattern.

TERMINOLOGY

Synonyms

- Pleomorphic carcinoma, pleomorphic large cell carcinoma, pleomorphic giant cell carcinoma
- Undifferentiated carcinoma with osteoclast-like giant cells
  - Giant cell tumor of pancreas
  - Osteoclast-like giant cell tumor of pancreas

Definitions

- Malignant epithelial neoplasm with significant component showing no definite differentiation
  - Wide range of morphologic findings ranging from pleomorphic epithelioid cells to multinucleated giant cells to spindle cells
  - Multiple patterns often present within same tumor

CLINICAL ISSUES

Epidemiology

- Incidence
  - Rare, < 1% of pancreatic neoplasms
- Age
  - Range: 25-96 years; average: 60s
- Gender
  - Undifferentiated carcinoma: 3:1 male predominance
  - Undifferentiated carcinoma with osteoclast-like giant cells: Slight female predominance

Presentation

- Abdominal pain
- Weight loss, fatigue, nausea, vomiting
- Palpable mass
- Jaundice is infrequent

Treatment

- Surgical resection with curative intent is treatment of choice
  - Vast majority present at inoperative stage

Prognosis

- Dismal, often < 1 year

MACROSCOPIC FEATURES

General Features

- Very large, fleshy mass with hemorrhage and necrosis
  - Average: 9-10 cm; anywhere in pancreas
- Often infiltrates adjacent organs

MICROSCOPIC PATHOLOGY

Histologic Features

- Heterogeneous features including anaplastic giant cell and spindle cell (sarcomatoid) components in varying proportions
  - Anaplastic component
    - Relatively monotonous, pleomorphic mononuclear cells admixed with multinucleated giant cells exhibiting bizarre nuclei and abundant eosinophilic cytoplasm
    - Numerous mitoses
    - May be associated with dense neutrophilic infiltrate, cannibalism/emperipolesis of tumor cells
    - Scant desmoplastic stroma, extensive necrosis and hemorrhage
  - Sarcomatoid component
    - Proliferation of plump spindle cells in fascicular or herringbone pattern with relatively minimal stroma
    - Significant atypia, mitoses, and extensive necrosis
    - Heterologous elements such as bone, cartilage, and striated muscle may be seen in some cases
  - More than 1/2 of undifferentiated carcinomas contain a glandular component, and 1/4 to 1/3 have focal squamous differentiation

UNDIFFERENTIATED CARCINOMA

Key Facts

Terminology

- Malignant epithelial neoplasm with significant component showing no definite differentiation
  - Wide range of morphologic findings ranging from pleomorphic epithelioid cells to multinucleated giant cells to spindle cells

Clinical Issues

- Rare
- Prognosis is dismal

Macroscopic Features

- Large, fleshy mass, often with hemorrhage and necrosis, that invades adjacent organs

Microscopic Pathology

- Heterogeneous features consisting of anaplastic giant cell and spindle cell components in varying proportions
- Variably present large, benign-appearing, multinucleated osteoclast-like giant cells

---

- Undifferentiated carcinoma with osteoclast-like giant cells
  - Mixture of osteoclast-like giant cells composed of benign-appearing multinucleated giant cells admixed with highly atypical neoplastic cells
    - Benign-appearing multinucleated osteoclast-like giant cells may have phagocytotic activity
    - Undifferentiated round to spindled atypical mononuclear cells have mitotic activity
  - May contain osteoid or focal chondroid differentiation
  - Often associated with mucinous cystic neoplasm or conventional adenocarcinoma

ANCILLARY TESTS

Immunohistochemistry

- Often mark with cytokeratins, including CK7, CK8, CK18, and CK19, although staining may be very focal
- Majority also express CEA, CA19-9, MUC1
- Neoplastic spindle cells may express smooth muscle actin but not desmin
- CD68, KP1, CD45, and α-1-antitrypsin expression are seen in osteoclast-like giant cells

DIFFERENTIAL DIAGNOSIS

Melanoma

- When anaplastic large cell component is prominent
- S100, HMB-45, Melan-A positive

Choriocarcinoma

- When anaplastic large cell component is prominent
- β-HCG positive
- Affects younger patients

Metastatic Undifferentiated Carcinoma

- Less often associated with other pancreatic tumors, such as mucinous cystic neoplasm
- Imaging may be required to resolve differential dx

Other Causes of Multinucleated Giant Cells

- Pseudocysts
- Infection
- Reaction to tumor
- Other malignant neoplasms (i.e., lymphoma, sarcoma)
- Above conditions are composed of only 1 population (benign or malignant) of giant cells, rather than a mix

DIAGNOSTIC CHECKLIST

Clinically Relevant Pathologic Features

- Helpful to include pertinent descriptors (i.e., pleomorphic or giant cell) when making this diagnosis

SELECTED REFERENCES

1. Yonemasu H et al: Phenotypical characteristics of undifferentiated carcinoma of the pancreas: a comparison with pancreatic ductal adenocarcinoma and relevance of E-cadherin, alpha catenin and beta catenin expression. Oncol Rep. 8(4):745-52, 2001

IMAGE GALLERY

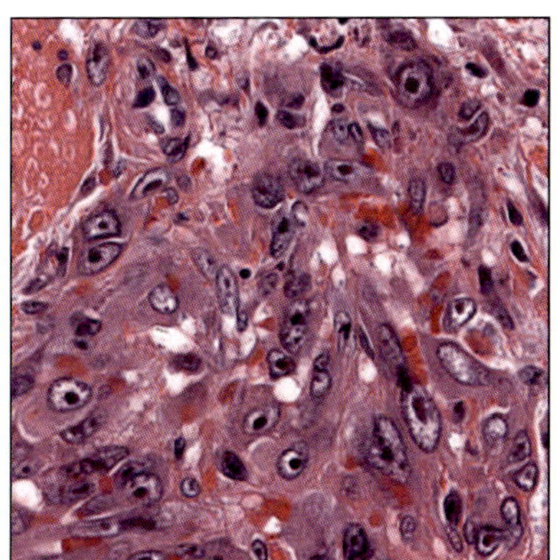

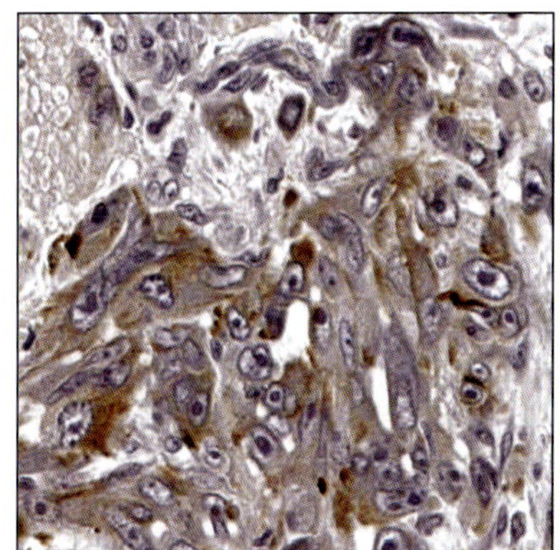

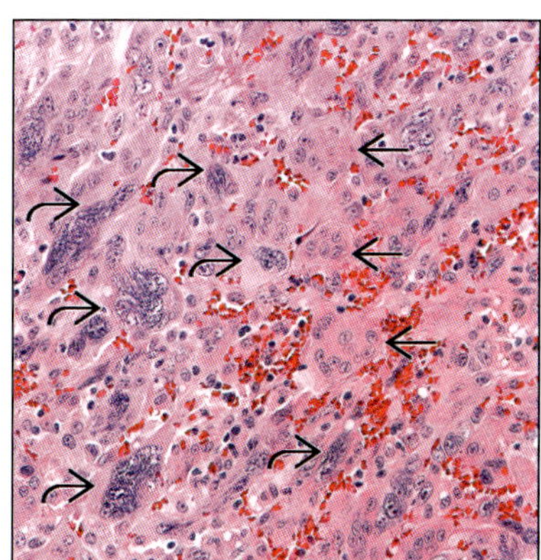

(Left) *This undifferentiated carcinoma contains large, atypical mononuclear cells without glandular differentiation.* ***(Center)*** *Undifferentiated carcinoma frequently demonstrates pankeratin expression in the large, atypical mononuclear cells.* ***(Right)*** *Undifferentiated carcinoma with osteoclast-like giant cells contains 2 cell populations: Large atypical multinucleated or mononuclear malignant cells ↪ and benign osteoclast-like giant cells →.*

SQUAMOUS/ADENOSQUAMOUS CARCINOMA, PANCREAS

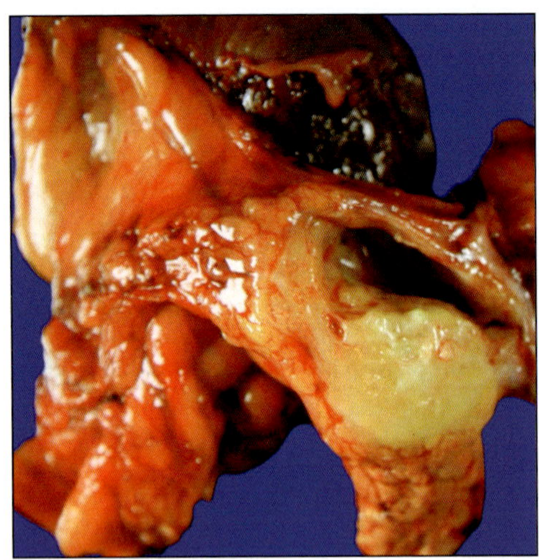

A primary adenosquamous cell carcinoma in the tail of the pancreas shows a relatively well-demarcated tan-white to yellow solid mass with a cystic component.

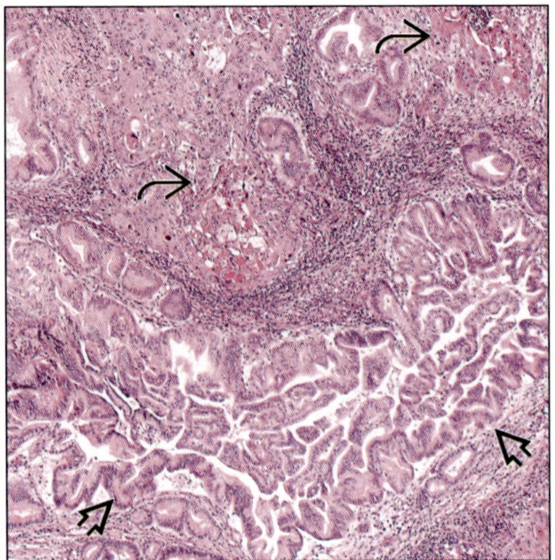

Adenosquamous cell carcinoma of the pancreas demonstrates islands of malignant squamous cells with keratinization ➩ adjacent to PanIN-3 involving an interlobular duct ➪.

TERMINOLOGY

Definitions

- Uncommon variant of pancreatic cancer with both glandular and squamous differentiation
  - Pure squamous cell carcinoma of pancreas is vanishingly rare

ETIOLOGY/PATHOGENESIS

Neoplastic

- A few hypotheses attempt to explain origin of squamous component
  - Squamous metaplasia of pancreatic duct epithelium
  - Both components derive from common progenitor

CLINICAL ISSUES

Epidemiology

- Incidence
  - Adenosquamous carcinoma accounts for 3-4% of malignancies of exocrine pancreas
  - Pure squamous cell carcinoma reportedly accounts for up to 0.7% of pancreatic carcinoma
- Age
  - Mean: 63 years
  - Range: 28-86 years
- Gender
  - Male to female ratio is 1.5 to 1.0

Presentation

- Similar to conventional ductal adenocarcinoma of pancreas
  - Weight loss
  - Painless jaundice
  - Other abdominal symptoms

Treatment

- Surgical resection

Prognosis

- Extremely poor with median survival period of 6 months
- Mean survival of 11 months even in patients with surgically resectable tumors

IMAGE FINDINGS

General Features

- Similar to conventional pancreatic ductal adenocarcinoma

MACROSCOPIC FEATURES

General Features

- Firm, ill-defined, tan to white mass with or without cystic component
- Most arise in head of pancreas but can also arise in body or tail or even diffusely involve entire gland

Size

- Large
- Mean size: ~ 6 cm

MICROSCOPIC PATHOLOGY

Histologic Features

- Squamous cell carcinoma exhibits only squamous component
- Adenosquamous carcinoma has malignant glandular and squamous components
  - Glandular component usually consists of conventional adenocarcinoma
    - But may have clear cell or signet ring cell components
  - Squamous cell carcinoma shows nests or sheets of neoplastic cells with whorls, keratin pearls,

SQUAMOUS/ADENOSQUAMOUS CARCINOMA, PANCREAS

Key Facts

Terminology
- Pure squamous or mixed glandular and squamous carcinoma of pancreas

Clinical Issues
- Adenosquamous carcinoma accounts for 3-4% of exocrine pancreas malignancies
- Pure squamous cell carcinoma is vanishingly rare
- Extremely poor survival

Microscopic Pathology
- Squamous cell carcinoma exhibits only squamous component
- Adenosquamous carcinoma has malignant glandular and squamous components
  - Glandular component may contain conventional ductal-type, clear cell, or signet ring cell components

individual cell keratinization, &/or intercellular bridges
  - 2 components can be intimately admixed or topographically separate within tumor

Cytologic Features
- Various proportions of cells with glandular or squamous features on smear
- Pure squamous cell carcinoma may be undersampling of adenosquamous cell carcinoma or metastatic squamous cell carcinoma from another organ

ANCILLARY TESTS

Histochemistry
- Mucicarmine
  - Reactivity: Positive in glandular component
  - Staining pattern
    - Intracytoplasmic mucin

Immunohistochemistry
- p63
  - Positive in squamous component
- CK7, CK20, CEA, and CA19-9
  - Often restricted to glandular component

DIFFERENTIAL DIAGNOSIS

Metastatic Squamous Cell Carcinoma
- Clinical history of extrapancreatic squamous cell carcinoma
- Absence of glandular differentiation

Pancreatoblastoma
- Predominant acinar component in addition to squamoid nests with or without glandular elements

DIAGNOSTIC CHECKLIST

Clinically Relevant Pathologic Features
- Pure squamous cell carcinomas of pancreas are extremely rare
- Adequate sectioning may reveal glandular component in tumors with dominant squamous morphology

SELECTED REFERENCES

1. Voong KR et al: Resected pancreatic adenosquamous carcinoma: clinicopathologic review and evaluation of adjuvant chemotherapy and radiation in 38 patients. Hum Pathol. 41(1):113-22, 2010
2. Brody JR et al: Adenosquamous carcinoma of the pancreas harbors KRAS2, DPC4 and TP53 molecular alterations similar to pancreatic ductal adenocarcinoma. Mod Pathol. 22(5):651-9, 2009

IMAGE GALLERY

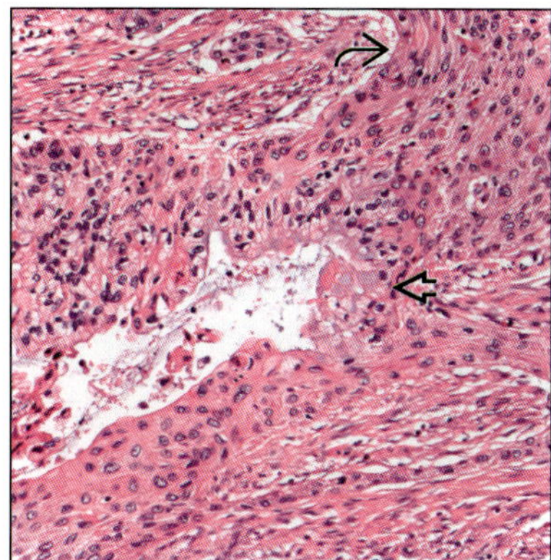

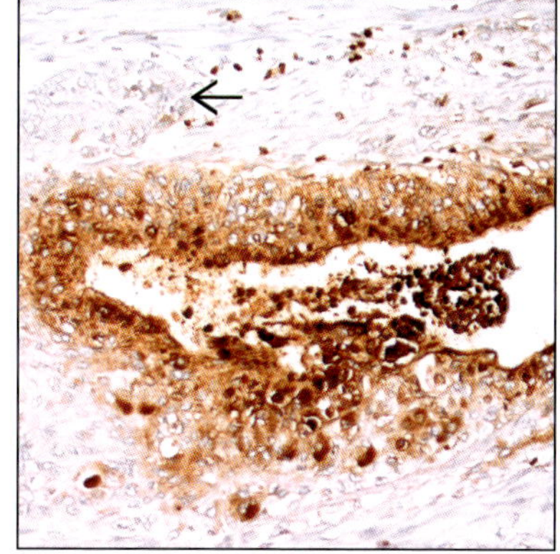

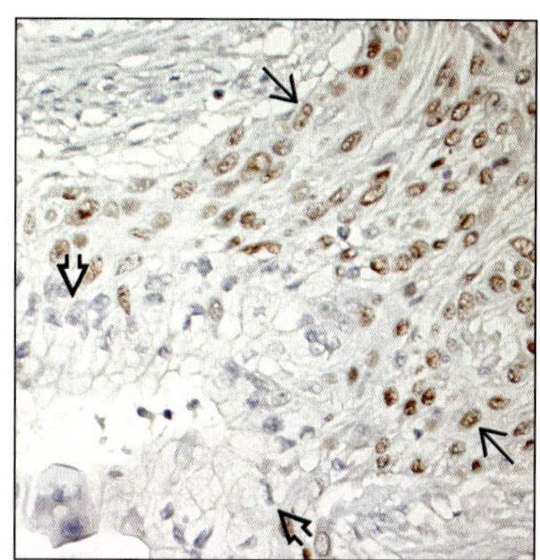

(Left) *High-power view of pancreatic adenosquamous cell carcinoma shows both a squamous component ⇨ and a glandular component with intracytoplasmic mucin ⇨.* ***(Center)*** *Immunohistochemical stain for CEA highlights the glandular component but not the squamous component →.* ***(Right)*** *Immunohistochemical stain for p63 shows nuclear staining in the squamous component → of adenosquamous cell carcinoma and absent staining in the glandular component ⇨.*

SEROUS CYSTADENOMA

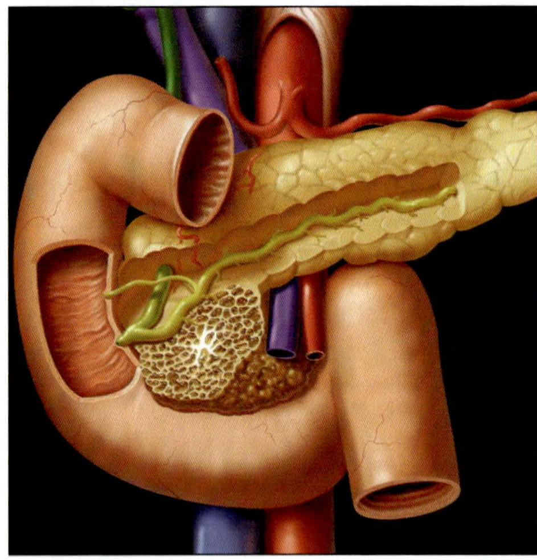

Graphic shows a sponge-like or "honeycomb" mass in the pancreatic head. Note the presence of innumerable small cysts and central scar. The pancreatic duct is not obstructed.

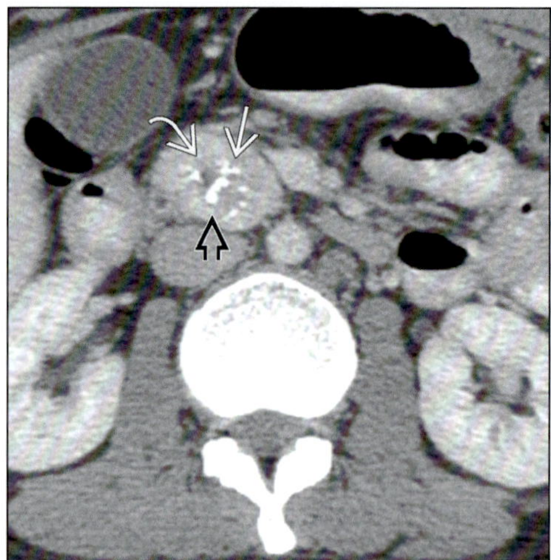

Transverse CECT shows a well-defined enhancing mass ➔ in the pancreatic head. Foci of calcification ⇒ and a hypodense center (scar/cystic component) ↷ are noted within the lesion.

TERMINOLOGY

Abbreviations

- Serous cystadenoma (SCA)

Synonyms

- Serous microcystic adenoma
- Clear cell or glycogen-rich adenoma

Definitions

- Benign cystic epithelial neoplasm
  - Presumably originates from centroacinar cell/ intercalated duct system

ETIOLOGY/PATHOGENESIS

No Uniform Consensus on Cellular Origin

- Acinar, centroacinar, and ductal have all been considered
  - Some immunohistochemical and ultrastructural features suggest centroacinar cell origin

CLINICAL ISSUES

Epidemiology

- Incidence
  - Accounts for 10% of surgically resected cystic pancreatic lesions
- Age
  - Mean age: 66 years
    - Range: 18-91 years
    - Rarely reported in infants (oligocystic variant)
- Gender
  - Female predominance
    - F:M ratio ranges from 3:1 to 7:3

Site

- Anywhere in pancreas

Presentation

- Abdominal mass &/or pain
  - 2/3 of patients
  - Larger SCA (> 4 cm) more likely to give rise to symptoms
- Asymptomatic, incidentally discovered
  - 1/3 of patients

Treatment

- Surgically resect if symptomatic
  - Complete resection usually curative
  - Recurs in < 2% of cases

Prognosis

- Excellent

IMAGE FINDINGS

Radiographic Findings

- Grayscale ultrasound and contrast-enhanced computed tomography (CECT) are best imaging modalities
  - Well-defined mass
  - Microlacunae separated by delicate septa
    - Enhancement of septa on computed tomography
  - Central stellate scar
    - Echogenic area that may be calcified resulting in "sunburst" appearance on ultrasound

MACROSCOPIC FEATURES

General Features

- Discrete, well-demarcated, slightly bosselated tumor
  - Variably sized, thin-walled cysts
    - Filled with clear, watery, or straw-colored fluid
  - No communication of cyst to pancreatic ductal system
- Microcystic (most common growth pattern)
  - Sponge-like or "honeycomb" appearance

SEROUS CYSTADENOMA

Key Facts

Terminology
- Benign cystic epithelial neoplasm

Clinical Issues
- Discovered because of abdominal mass &/or pain or incidentally
- Most likely in female in 6th decade of life

Macroscopic Features
- Discrete, well-demarcated cystic tumor
  - Numerous thin-walled cysts filled with serous fluid

Microscopic Pathology
- Cysts typically lined by single layer of cuboidal to flat epithelial cells
  - Clear to pale cytoplasm with sharp cell border
  - Small, round to oval, uniform nuclei
  - Periodic acid-Schiff without diastase has granular cytoplasmic staining
- Exuberant rich capillary network immediately adjacent to epithelium
- May have stellate scar that can be calcified

Ancillary Tests
- Immunohistochemical reactivity
  - Positive for cytokeratin, α-inhibin, calponin, GLUT1, MUC6
- von Hippel-Lindau (*VHL*) gene alteration detected even in sporadic cases

Top Differential Diagnoses
- von Hippel-Lindau-associated pancreatic cysts
- Serous cystadenocarcinoma

    - Numerous tightly packed cysts
    - Diameter of most cysts 0.1 to < 1 cm
  - Often has central stellate fibrous scar
    - May become calcified

Size
- Usually < 5 cm but can be up to 25 cm

Variants
- Solid variant
  - Well-demarcated, solid mass with thick fibrous bands
- Oligocystic (macrocystic, megacystic) variant (20% of cases)
  - Locules are larger with fewer septations
    - Larger cysts (peripheral) admixed with smaller cysts (central)
  - No central scar
  - Often in pancreatic head

MICROSCOPIC PATHOLOGY

Histologic Features
- Variably sized cysts lined by single layer of cuboidal to flat epithelial cells
  - Rarely, microscopic papillary tufts without fibrovascular cores or true papillae with fibrovascular cores
  - Solid variant can have solid nests of cells and small acini
- Cells are uniform and lack atypia and mitotic activity
  - Clear to pale cytoplasm
  - Well-defined cytoplasmic borders
  - Abundant intracytoplasmic glycogen
  - Rarely have eosinophilic (oncocyte-like) cytoplasm
  - Small, round to oval, uniform nuclei
    - Dense homogeneous chromatin
    - Can have nuclear enlargement
    - Inconspicuous nucleoli
- Rich capillary network intimately admixed with epithelium
  - Red blood cells seem to be interspersed between epithelial cells
- Can have stellate scar composed of collagen, which may become calcified
- No necrosis

Cytologic Features
- Microcystic, oligocystic, and solid variants are cytologically similar
  - No atypia, necrosis, or mitotic activity

Predominant Pattern/Injury Type
- Cystic

Predominant Cell/Compartment Type
- Epithelial
  - Serous cells

ANCILLARY TESTS

Cytology
- Clear, thin fluid; may be bloody
- Generally paucicellular or acellular
- Epithelial cells form small sheets and flat sheets
  - Important to distinguish from gastrointestinal epithelium

Histochemistry
- Granular cytoplasmic positivity for periodic acid-Schiff without diastase (PAS) stain
- Negative for periodic acid-Schiff with diastase (PASD) stain

Immunohistochemistry
- Uniformly negative for vimentin, CEA, HMB-45, Melan-A, MUC5, chromogranin, and trypsin
  - Generally negative for MUC2 and synaptophysin, but report of positive staining in < 5% of SCA cases
  - Cytokeratin positive

Molecular Genetics
- von Hippel-Lindau (*VHL*) gene alteration detected in 40-70% of sporadic cases

SEROUS CYSTADENOMA

Immunohistochemistry

Antibody	Reactivity	Staining Pattern	Comment
AE1/AE3	Positive	Cytoplasmic	
CK7	Positive	Cytoplasmic	
CK8/18/CAM5.2	Positive	Cytoplasmic	
CK19	Positive	Cytoplasmic	
Inhibin-α	Positive	Cytoplasmic	76-92%
Calponin	Positive	Cytoplasmic	85%
MUC6	Positive	Cytoplasmic	60-85%
GLUT1	Positive	Cell membrane & cytoplasm	94%, but may not have diffuse staining
EMA	Positive	Cytoplasmic	33%
MUC1	Positive	Cytoplasmic	24-38%

  - Loss of heterozygosity at chromosome 3p25
  - *VHL* gene germline mutation

DIFFERENTIAL DIAGNOSIS

von Hippel-Lindau-associated Pancreatic Cysts

- Autosomal dominant disorder characterized by clear cell neoplasms
- Histologically identical to SCA, but distribution differs
  - Does not form distinct lesion
    - Irregularly scattered cysts in pancreas, multifocal or diffuse
- Some authorities classify these together with nonsyndromic SCA; others designate them separately

Serous Cystadenocarcinoma

- Extremely rare and morphologically indistinguishable from SCA
- Serous cystic neoplasm with extrapancreatic involvement
  - Spleen, stomach, duodenum, liver, lymph node, and peritoneum

Pseudocyst

- Unilocular cyst with thick fibrous wall
- If epithelial lining is not identified, sample entire cyst before rendering this diagnosis
- Epithelial denudation of oligocystic variant can occur if previously biopsied

Mucinous Cystic Neoplasm

- Often in females in pancreatic tail
- Multilocular thick-walled cyst with mucoid material
- Ovarian-type stroma with overlying mucinous epithelium with variable degree of cytologic atypia
- Serous macrocystic adenoma can radiographically resemble mucinous cystic neoplasm

Lymphangioma

- Multilocular cyst lined by endothelial cells and lymphoid aggregates
  - If SCA has attenuated epithelial lining, it may mimic this entity
- Immunoreactive for CD34, CD31, and D2-40

Metastatic Renal Cell Carcinoma

- Has glycogen-rich clear cells but is cytologically atypical
- Positive immunohistochemical staining for clear cell type of renal cell carcinoma
  - RCC, pax-2, and pax-8

Combined Well-Differentiated Endocrine Neoplasm/Serous Cystadenoma

- Occurs in patients with von Hippel-Lindau syndrome
- Neoplasm with well-differentiated pancreatic endocrine neoplasm and serous cystadenoma
  - 2 entities can be adjacent to one another or intermixed

SELECTED REFERENCES

1. Marsh WL et al: Calponin is expressed in serous cystadenomas of the pancreas but not in adenocarcinomas or endocrine tumors. Appl Immunohistochem Mol Morphol. 17(3):216-9, 2009
2. Thirabanjasak D et al: Is serous cystadenoma of the pancreas a model of clear-cell-associated angiogenesis and tumorigenesis? Pancreatology. 9(1-2):182-8, 2009
3. Wargo JA et al: Management of pancreatic serous cystadenomas. Adv Surg. 43:23-34, 2009
4. Reese SA et al: Solid serous adenoma of the pancreas: a rare variant within the family of pancreatic serous cystic neoplasms. Pancreas. 33(1):96-9, 2006
5. Matsumoto T et al: Malignant serous cystic neoplasm of the pancreas: report of a case and review of the literature. J Clin Gastroenterol. 39(3):253-6, 2005
6. Kosmahl M et al: Serous cystic neoplasms of the pancreas: an immunohistochemical analysis revealing alpha-inhibin, neuron-specific enolase, and MUC6 as new markers. Am J Surg Pathol. 28(3):339-46, 2004
7. Perez-Ordonez B et al: Solid serous adenoma of the pancreas. The solid variant of serous cystadenoma? Am J Surg Pathol. 20(11):1401-5, 1996
8. George DH et al: Serous cystadenocarcinoma of the pancreas: a new entity? Am J Surg Pathol. 13(1):61-6, 1989
9. Alpert LC et al: Microcystic adenoma (serous cystadenoma) of the pancreas. A study of 14 cases with immunohistochemical and electron-microscopic correlation. Am J Surg Pathol. 12(4):251-63, 1988
10. Compagno J et al: Microcystic adenomas of the pancreas (glycogen-rich cystadenomas): a clinicopathologic study of 34 cases. Am J Clin Pathol. 69(3):289-98, 1978

Gross and Microscopic Features

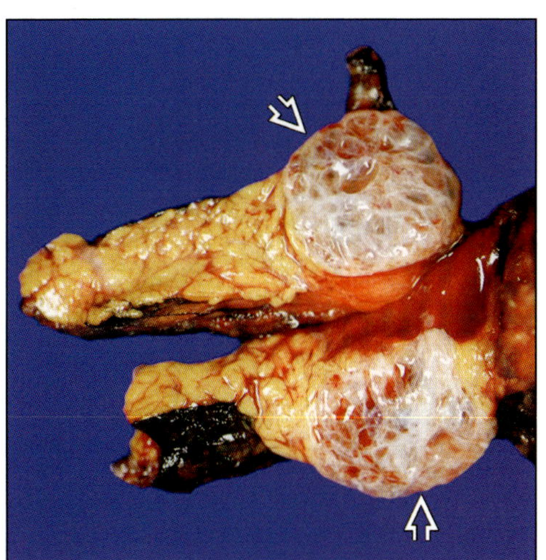

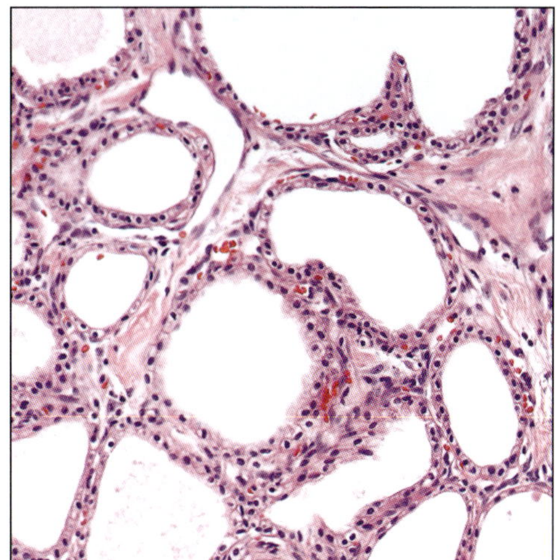

(Left) *This round, well-circumscribed mass ➡ in the tail of the pancreas has been bivalved to reveal compact, small, thin, smooth-walled cysts containing clear serous fluid. This mass lacked a stellate central scar, and the cyst did not communicate with the pancreatic duct.* ***(Right)*** *These microcysts are lined by bland cuboidal epithelium with pale cytoplasm and have congested capillaries immediately adjacent to the epithelial cells.*

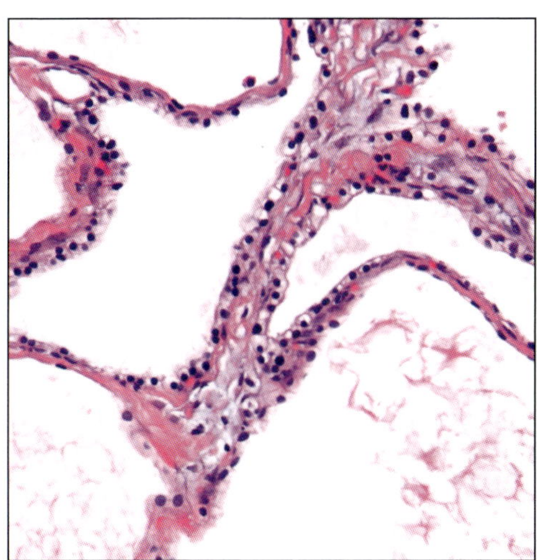

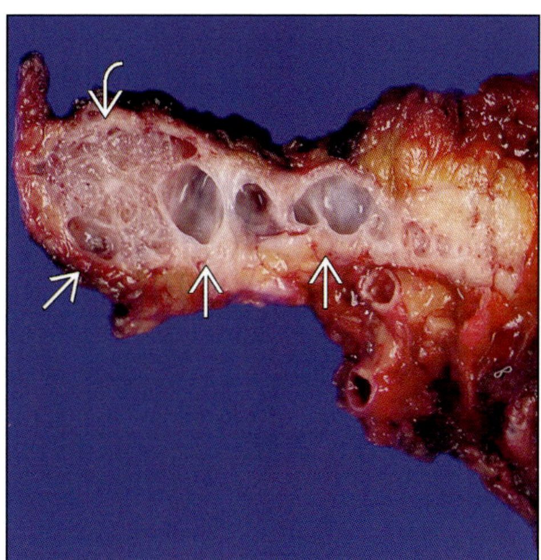

(Left) *These small cysts containing proteinaceous fluid are lined by cuboidal cells that typically have clear cytoplasm. The subjacent rich capillary network can be better appreciated at higher magnification.* ***(Right)*** *This distal (body and tail) pancreatic resection specimen contains a cystic mass containing smaller cysts around a central scar ➡ and larger peripheral cysts ➡.*

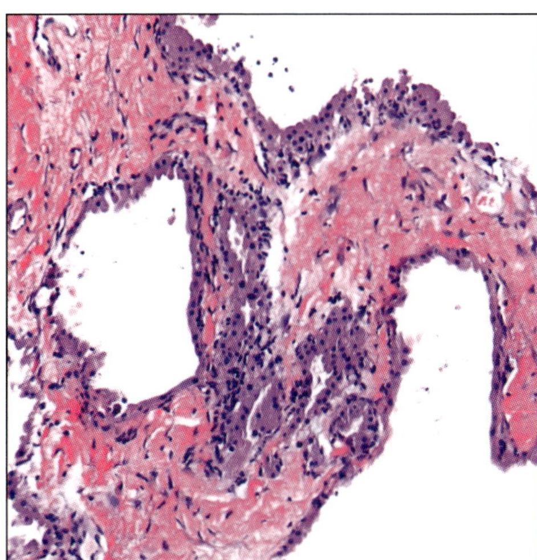

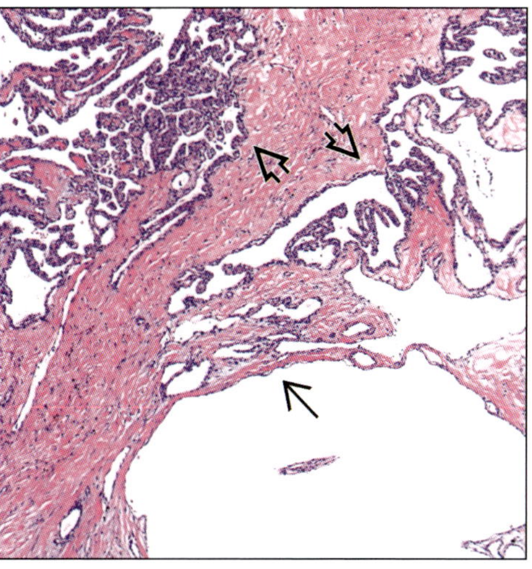

(Left) *In addition to the typically cuboidal cells with clear or pale cytoplasm, serous cystadenomas can have abundant granular eosinophilic (oncocyte-like) cytoplasm, but the nuclei maintain their small bland appearance.* ***(Right)*** *In most serous cystadenomas, the bland epithelial lining is composed of a single layer of cuboidal cells ➡. Rarely, microscopic papillary tufts without fibrovascular cores ➡ can occur that project into the cyst lumens.*

ACINAR CELL CYSTADENOMA

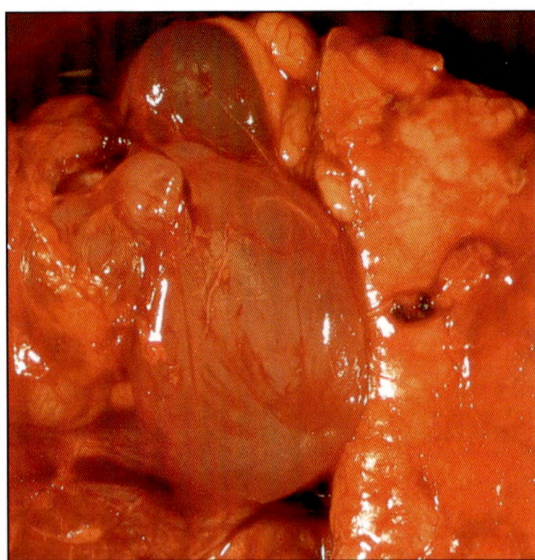

This acinar cell cystadenoma shows multiple unilocular thin-walled cysts. The cysts are filled with clear fluid and lack a mural nodule.

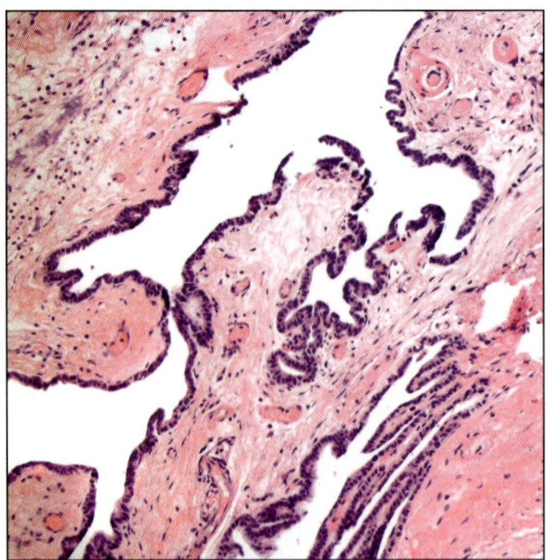

Acinar cell cystadenomas are lined by a single layer of cuboidal epithelium and could easily be mistaken for a serous cystadenomas.

TERMINOLOGY

Definitions

- Benign pancreatic cyst lined by cells with acinar cell differentiation

CLINICAL ISSUES

Epidemiology

- Age
  - Young to middle-aged
  - Reported range: 16-66 years
- Gender
  - More common in women

Presentation

- Abdominal pain
- Incidentally detected by imaging

Natural History

- Benign cyst without risk of malignant transformation

Treatment

- Surgical resection is curative

Prognosis

- Benign tumor with excellent prognosis

IMAGE FINDINGS

General Features

- Unilocular to multilocular cyst without solid areas or papillary projections
- Occasionally multiple cysts could involve entire pancreas

MACROSCOPIC FEATURES

General Features

- Unilocular to multilocular thin-walled cyst(s) filled with serous fluid
- No dilatation of main pancreatic duct
- Both pancreatic head and body/tail are involved

Sections to Be Submitted

- Entire cyst should be submitted for histological evaluation

Size

- Range from 1.5-10 cm
- Incidentally detected cysts identified during pathologic examination may measure < 1 cm

MICROSCOPIC PATHOLOGY

Histologic Features

- Cyst lined by single layer of cuboidal epithelium without multilayering or pseudostratification
  - In areas, lining epithelium may be flattened and resemble ductal epithelium
- Budding/incipient acinar structures frequently seen, providing evidence of acinar differentiation
  - Smaller acinar structures may surround dominant cyst
  - Apical cytoplasmic compartment shows deeply eosinophilic granules
- Eosinophilic intraluminal concretions are frequently seen
- Bland, basally placed nuclei with small nucleoli
- Mitoses are absent

ANCILLARY TESTS

Histochemistry

- PAS-diastase

ACINAR CELL CYSTADENOMA

Key Facts

Terminology
- Benign pancreatic cyst lined by acinar cells

Clinical Issues
- Young to middle-aged
- Benign cyst without risk of malignant transformation

Macroscopic Features
- Unilocular to multilocular thin-walled cyst(s) filled with serous fluid

Microscopic Pathology
- Cysts lined by single layer of cuboidal epithelium without multilayering
- Budding/incipient acinar structures frequently seen, providing evidence of acinar differentiation

Ancillary Tests
- Lining cells are positive for trypsin &/or lipase

 - Reactivity: Positive
 - Staining pattern
   - Apical cytoplasmic compartment

Immunohistochemistry
- Lining cells are focally positive for trypsin &/or lipase
- Cells are positive for CAM5.2 and negative for chromogranin and synaptophysin

Electron Microscopy
- Transmission
  - Cyst lining cells show apical, round, electron-dense granules measuring 200-800 nm that resemble normal pancreatic zymogen granules

DIFFERENTIAL DIAGNOSIS

Serous Cystadenoma
- Also lined by single layer of cuboidal epithelium
  - Cytoplasm of lining cells is clear and filled with glycogen
- On PAS-D stain, cells of serous cystadenoma lack intracellular granules, and apical PAS-D granules are seen in acinar cell cystadenomas
- Lacks incipient acinar structures, and on immunohistochemistry, cells are negative for trypsin

Retention Cyst
- Lacks morphological or immunohistochemical evidence of acinar cell differentiation

Intraductal Papillary-Mucinous Neoplasm & Mucinous Cystic Neoplasm
- Neoplastic cysts lined by mucinous epithelium
  - Mucinous lining epithelium excludes diagnosis of acinar cell cystadenoma

Acinar Cell Cystadenocarcinoma & Acinar Cell Carcinoma
- Both lesions show sheets of neoplastic cells with nuclear atypia and many mitoses

SELECTED REFERENCES

1. Albores-Saavedra J: Acinar cystadenoma of the pancreas: a previously undescribed tumor. Ann Diagn Pathol. 6(2):113-5, 2002
2. Chatelain D et al: Unilocular acinar cell cystadenoma of the pancreas an unusual acinar cell tumor. Am J Clin Pathol. 118(2):211-4, 2002
3. Couvelard A et al: [Acinar cystic transformation of the pancreas (or acinar cell cystadenoma), a rare and recently described entity.] Ann Pathol. 22(5):397-400, 2002
4. Zamboni G et al: Acinar cell cystadenoma of the pancreas: a new entity?. Am J Surg Pathol. 26(6):698-704, 2002

IMAGE GALLERY

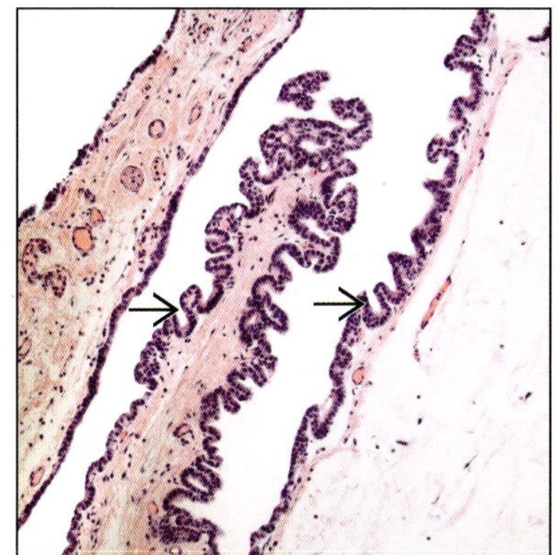

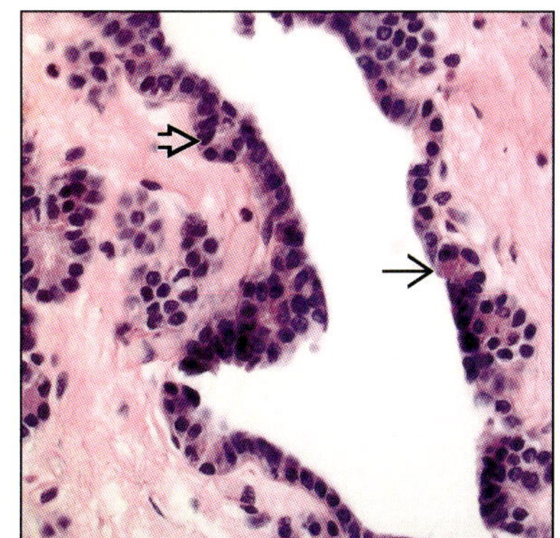

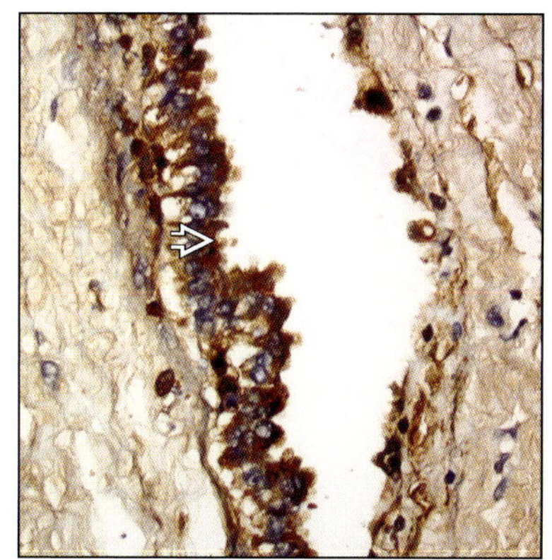

(Left) *Papillary structures are occasionally seen. The formation of buds or incipient acinar structures ⇒ is strong evidence of acinar cell differentiation.* ***(Center)*** *Incipient acinar structures ⇨ are seen on this H&E section. Some of the cells lining these structures show apical eosinophilic granules ⇒. These granules are PAS positive and diastase resistant and represent zymogen granules.* ***(Right)*** *The apical cytoplasmic compartment of the cyst lining cells is positive for trypsin ⇨.*

MUCINOUS CYSTIC NEOPLASM

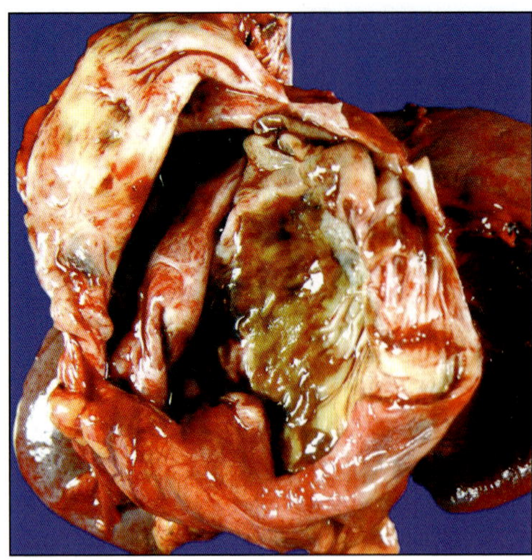

Gross photograph of a mucinous cystic neoplasm features a unilocular cyst with a smooth, partially discolored lining located in the tail of the pancreas.

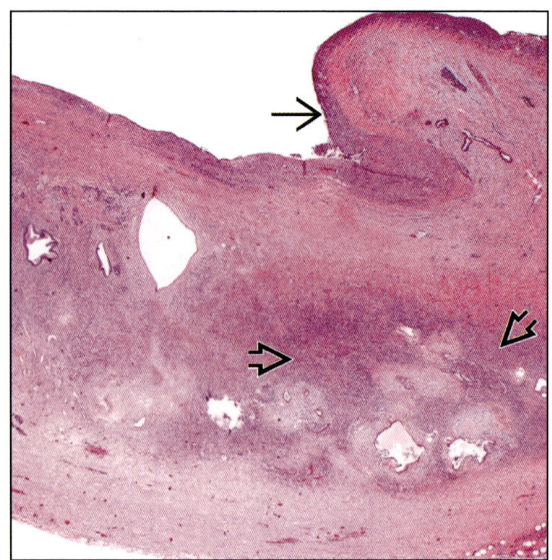

This mucinous cystic neoplasm contains a thick fibrous wall with ovarian-type stroma located underneath the epithelial lining ➔ and extending into the periductal regions ➲.

TERMINOLOGY

Abbreviations

- Mucinous cystic neoplasm (MCN)

Definitions

- Neoplasm composed of mucin-producing epithelial cells associated with ovarian-type stroma

ETIOLOGY/PATHOGENESIS

Developmental Anomaly

- May develop from endodermal immature stroma (periductal stroma) stimulated by female hormones
- May develop from primary yolk cells implanted in pancreas during embryogenesis

CLINICAL ISSUES

Epidemiology

- Incidence
  - 10% of cystic lesions in pancreas
- Age
  - Average age at diagnosis: 40-50 years
  - Range: 14-95 years
- Gender
  - Predominantly female (female to male ratio is 20:1)

Presentation

- Vague abdominal symptoms associated with compression of adjacent organs and tissues; may include epigastric pain and abdominal fullness

Prognosis

- Excellent prognosis for patients with benign MCN and MCN with noninvasive carcinoma
- 5-year survival rate of 50% for invasive MCN
  - Extent of invasion (confined to pancreas vs. beyond tumor capsule) and age of patient (lower survival rate > 50 years) correlates with survival

IMAGE FINDINGS

CT Findings

- Usually large, well-demarcated, thick-walled multilocular cystic mass with peripheral calcification (present in 20% of cases)
- Mural nodules and papillary excrescences are more common in mucinous cystic neoplasms with invasive component

ERCP Findings

- Main pancreatic duct and large interlobular ducts do not communicate with cysts in majority of cases

MACROSCOPIC FEATURES

General Features

- 90% in body or tail of pancreas
- Usually solitary and quite large
  - Mean: 7-10 cm
- Usually multiloculated with thick walls; filled with thick, tenacious mucoid material
- Intracystic papillary excrescences &/or mural nodules suggestive of high-grade dysplasia or invasive carcinoma

MICROSCOPIC PATHOLOGY

Histologic Features

- Usually surrounded by thick band of heavily collagenized tissue that separates cysts from adjacent nonneoplastic pancreatic parenchyma
- Ovarian-type stroma is required for diagnosis of mucinous cystic neoplasm

MUCINOUS CYSTIC NEOPLASM

Key Facts

Terminology
- Neoplasm composed of mucin-producing epithelial cells associated with ovarian-type stroma

Clinical Issues
- Comprises 10% of cystic lesions of pancreas
- Average age at diagnosis: 40-50 years
  - Range: 14-95 years
- Predominantly female
  - Female to male ratio is 20:1

Macroscopic Features
- 90% of mucinous cystic neoplasms arise in body or tail of pancreas
- Usually solitary and large
  - Mean: 7-10 cm
- Usually multiloculated with thick walls; filled with thick, tenacious mucoid material

Microscopic Pathology
- Tall, columnar, mucin-producing epithelium with varying degrees of cellular atypia
  - Invasive components can be very focal
  - Recommended to submit entire lesion for microscopic evaluation
- Ovarian-type stroma is required for diagnosis
  - Broad areas of stroma may be hyalinized

  - Ovarian-type stroma may be replaced by broad zones of hyalinization; multiple sections may be required to demonstrate cellular stroma
  - Stroma often expresses estrogen &/or progesterone receptors, supporting role of female hormones in its pathogenesis
  - Calretinin and inhibin expression seen in leutenized cells in ovarian stroma
  - CD10 immunostain may highlight hyalinized ovarian-type stroma
- Lined, at least focally, by tall, columnar, mucin-producing epithelium
  - Epithelium is often focally denuded; several histologic sections may be needed to demonstrate epithelial lining
  - May be focally lined by flat &/or cuboidal cells of pancreatobiliary type
  - Varying degrees of cellular atypia
    - Low-grade dysplasia
    - Moderate dysplasia
    - High-grade dysplasia

DIFFERENTIAL DIAGNOSIS

Pseudocyst
- More common in men than women; typically associated with history of pancreatitis and elevated serum amylase levels

Intraductal Papillary Mucinous Neoplasms (Branch Duct Type)
- More common in men than women; present in head of gland more frequently than body/tail
- Often demonstrate communication with pancreatic duct system and lack ovarian-type stroma

Serous Cystic Neoplasm
- Smaller cysts, central stellate scar, and glycogen-rich cuboidal lining cells

Solid-Pseudopapillary Neoplasm
- Areas of necrosis and hemorrhage associated with dropout of dyshesive tumor cells

DIAGNOSTIC CHECKLIST

Clinically Relevant Pathologic Features
- Presence or absence of associated invasive carcinoma is best predictor of survival following surgical resection
- Invasive components can be very focal, thus submission of entire neoplasm is recommended
- Staging of mucinous cystic neoplasms with associated invasive carcinoma follows the same staging system applied to carcinomas of exocrine pancreas

Pathologic Interpretation Pearls
- Ovarian-type stroma required for diagnosis of MCN

SELECTED REFERENCES

1. Nishigami T et al: Comparison between mucinous cystic neoplasm and intraductal papillary mucinous neoplasm of the branch duct type of the pancreas with respect to expression of CD10 and cytokeratin 20. Pancreas. 38(5):558-64, 2009
2. Crippa S et al: Mucinous cystic neoplasm of the pancreas is not an aggressive entity: lessons from 163 resected patients. Ann Surg. 247(4):571-9, 2008
3. Wilentz RE et al: Mucinous cystic neoplasms of the pancreas. Semin Diagn Pathol. 17(1):31-42, 2000
4. Thompson LD et al: Mucinous cystic neoplasm (mucinous cystadenocarcinoma of low-grade malignant potential) of the pancreas: a clinicopathologic study of 130 cases. Am J Surg Pathol. 23(1):1-16, 1999
5. Wilentz RE et al: Pathologic examination accurately predicts prognosis in mucinous cystic neoplasms of the pancreas. Am J Surg Pathol. 23(11):1320-7, 1999
6. Shyr YM et al: Mucin-producing neoplasms of the pancreas. Intraductal papillary and mucinous cystic neoplasms. Ann Surg. 223(2):141-6, 1996

MUCINOUS CYSTIC NEOPLASM

Microscopic Features

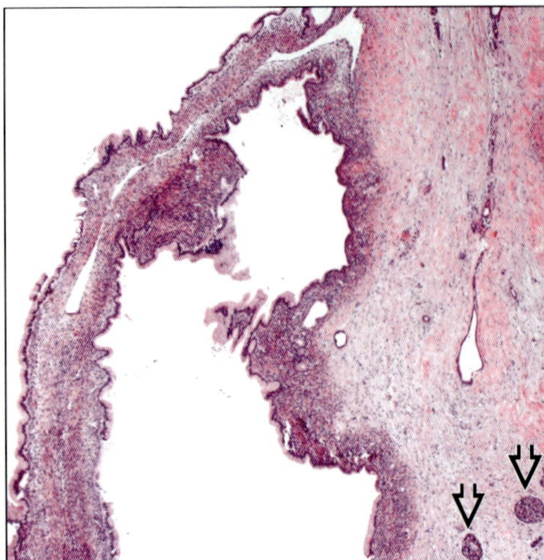

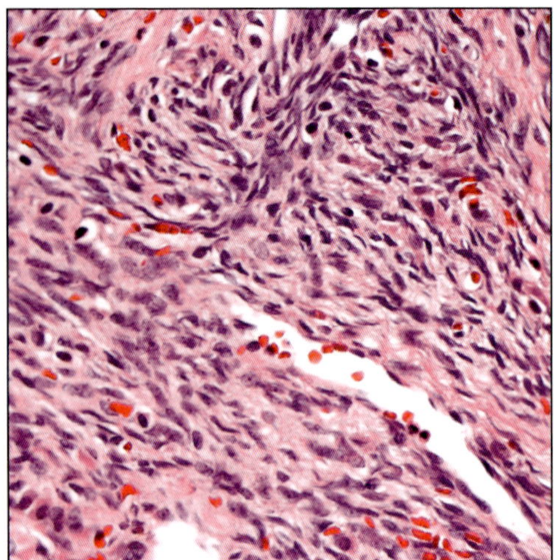

(Left) *A mucinous cystic neoplasm with low-grade dysplasia features a cyst lined by tall, columnar mucinous cells with underlying ovarian-type stroma. The adjacent pancreatic parenchyma is fibrotic with a few residual islets ⮚.* ***(Right)*** *Ovarian-type stroma consists of densely packed spindle cells with scant cytoplasm and uniform, elongated wavy nuclei. Mitoses are rare to absent.*

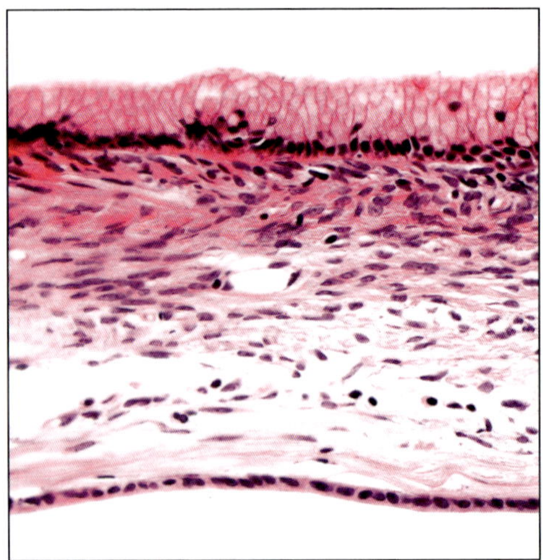

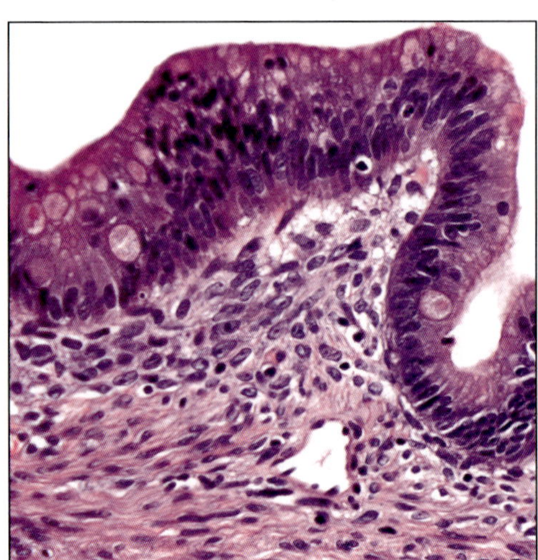

(Left) *Epithelium with low-grade dysplasia can consist of flat, cuboidal, or mucinous columnar epithelial cells without significant atypia.* ***(Right)*** *This mucinous cystic neoplasm with moderate dysplasia contains epithelium with more hyperchromatic, stratified nuclei.*

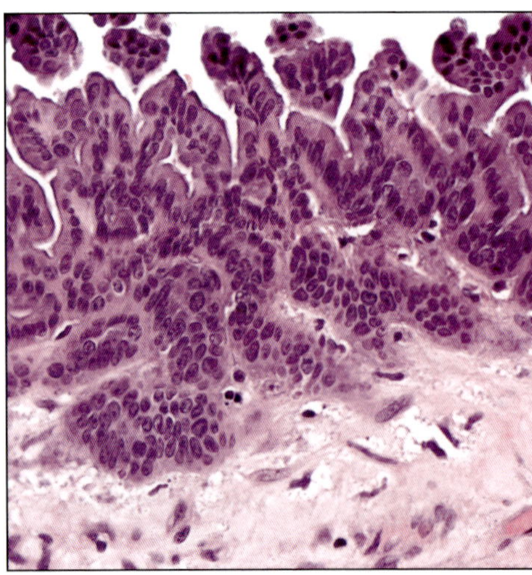

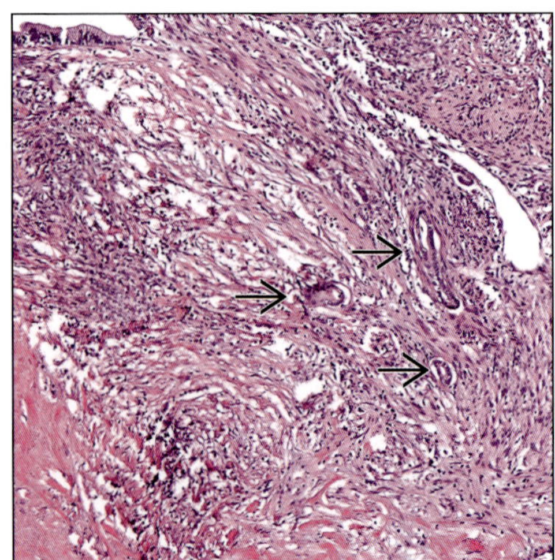

(Left) *A mucinous cystic neoplasm with high-grade dysplasia contains epithelium with papillary to micropapillary architecture and significant cytologic atypia.* ***(Right)*** *Minimally invasive adenocarcinoma arising in a mucinous cystic neoplasm features a few infiltrating malignant glands → within the ovarian-type stroma. This is the only focus of invasive carcinoma in this particular case.*

Microscopic and Immunohistochemical Features

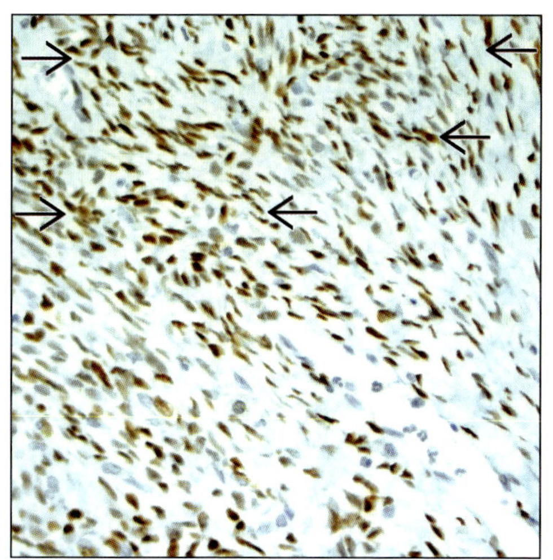

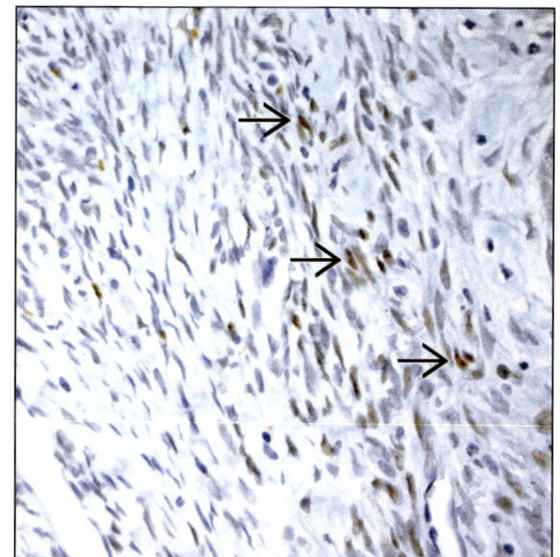

(Left) *Some subepithelial spindle cells are reactive to an antibody against progesterone receptor ➙ in 50-75% of mucinous cystic neoplasms.* ***(Right)*** *Estrogen receptors are expressed in subepithelial spindle cells ➙ in 25% of MCNs, less extensively than progesterone receptor. These spindle cells also label with antibodies to vimentin, smooth muscle actin, desmin, CD99, and Bcl-2; this immunophenotype is strikingly similar to that of normal ovarian stroma.*

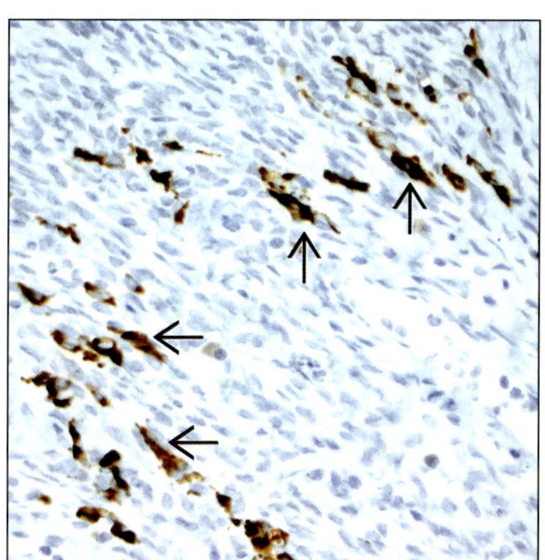

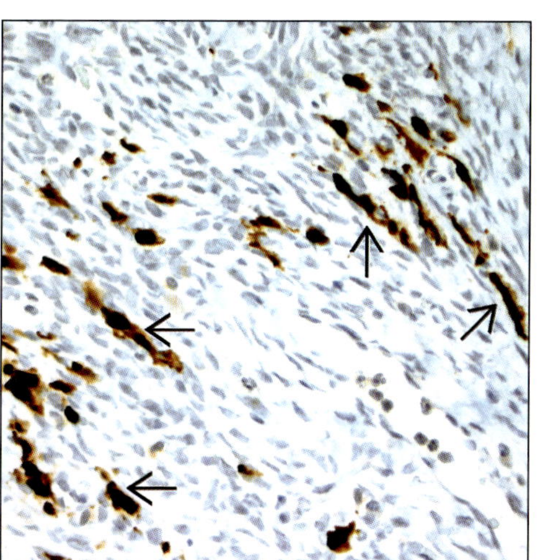

(Left) *The luteinized cells of the ovarian-type stromal cells label with an antibody to α-inhibin ➙.* ***(Right)*** *The luteinized cells also label with an antibody to calretinin ➙ along with tyrosine hydroxylase and Melan-A, markers that are reactive to normal hilar cells of the ovary. Labeling for S100 and CD34 is usually negative.*

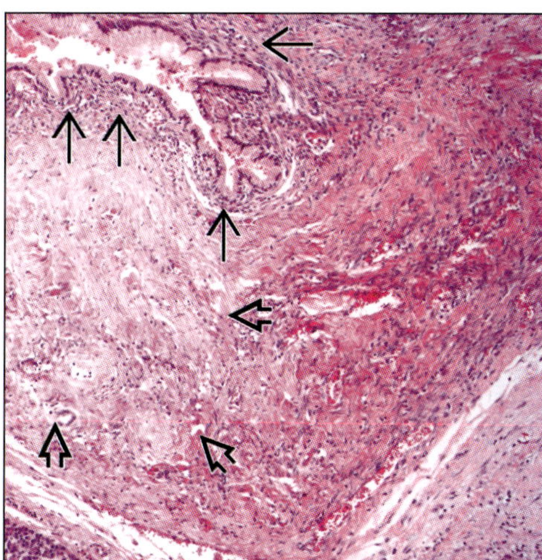

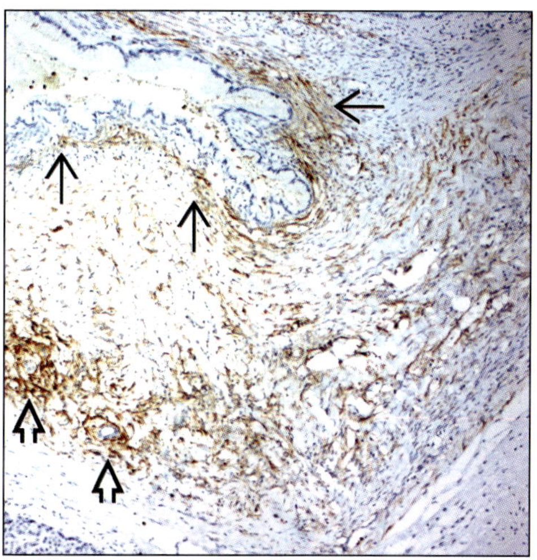

(Left) *Some mucinous cystic neoplasms have markedly hyalinized stroma ⇨ and scant ovarian-type stroma ➙. Multiple sections may be required to demonstrate the ovarian-type stroma required for diagnosis.* ***(Right)*** *The hyalinized stroma is reactive to an antibody against CD10 ⇨ with some accentuation in the subepithelial region ➙. When the ovarian-type stroma is indiscernible, CD10 expression may suggest the possibility of its hyalinization.*

INTRADUCTAL PAPILLARY MUCINOUS NEOPLASM

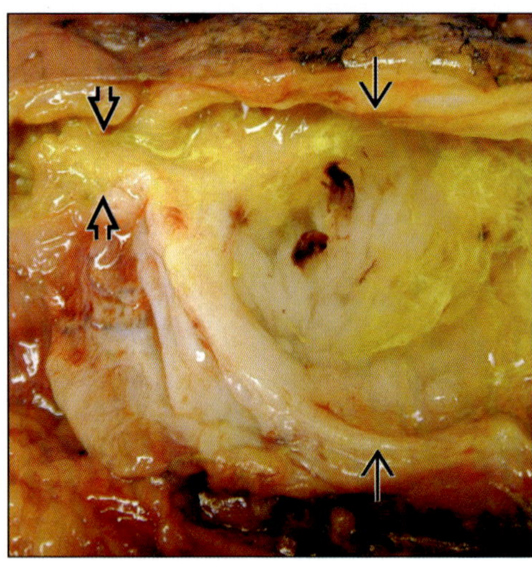

In IPMN, main-duct type, the markedly dilated main duct ➔ shows nodular mucosa with abundant mucin (stained with yellow dye). The ampullary orifice is indicated ➲.

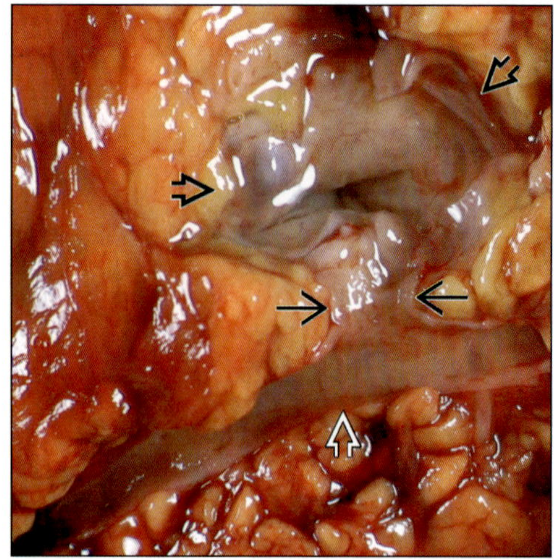

IPMN, branch-duct type, features a small cyst with a smooth lining ➲ connected to the main pancreatic duct ➲ through a dilated branch duct ➔.

TERMINOLOGY

Abbreviations

- Intraductal papillary mucinous neoplasm (IPMN)

Definitions

- Grossly visible, mucin-producing epithelial neoplasm that primarily grows within main duct &/or its branches
- Subclassification based on type of duct involvement
  - Main-duct type
    - Mucinous epithelium confined to main pancreatic duct
  - Combined type
    - Mucinous epithelium involving both main duct and branch ducts
  - Branch-duct type
    - Mucinous epithelium confined to branch ducts

CLINICAL ISSUES

Epidemiology

- Incidence
  - Most common cystic tumor of pancreas
    - Approximately 8-20% of all resected pancreatectomy specimens
- Age
  - Range: 25-94 years
    - Average: 63 years
- Gender
  - Slightly more common in men

Presentation

- Symptoms associated with intermittent pancreatic ductal obstruction
  - Abdominal pain
  - Back pain
  - Anorexia
  - Weight loss
  - Recurrent episodes of pancreatitis
- Symptoms often present for months to years before diagnosis is established
- Growing number of cases discovered incidentally during imaging for another indication

Endoscopic Findings

- Mucin extravasation from patulous ampulla of Vater

Treatment

- Surgical resection is treatment of choice
  - 80-98% of IPMNs are surgically resectable

Prognosis

- Noninvasive tumors: 5-year survival rate > 75%
- Invasive tumors: 5-year survival rate is significantly lower (34-62%) than for noninvasive tumors
  - Still significantly better than that of conventional pancreatic ductal adenocarcinoma

IMAGE FINDINGS

CT Findings

- Main-duct or combined type
  - Markedly dilated main duct often associated with dilated large branch ducts
- Branch-duct type
  - Single or numerous cysts that represent dilated branch ducts

ERCP Findings

- Dilated main pancreatic duct &/or branch ducts in absence of stricture
- Filling defects due to papillary projections of neoplasm &/or mucous plugs

MRCP Findings

- In addition to dilated ducts, mural nodules are better visualized
  - Indicative of higher grade lesion

INTRADUCTAL PAPILLARY MUCINOUS NEOPLASM

Key Facts

Terminology

- Grossly visible, mucin-producing epithelial neoplasm
- Predominantly grows within main duct &/or its branches
  - Classified into main duct, combined, or branch duct type

Clinical Issues

- Most frequent cystic tumor of pancreas
- Symptoms associated with intermittent pancreatic ductal obstruction by tenacious mucin
- Classic endoscopic finding: Mucin extravasation from patulous ampulla of Vater
- Prognosis better than conventional ductal adenocarcinoma
  - Noninvasive tumors: 5-year survival rate > 75%
  - Invasive tumors: 5-year survival rate is 34-62%
  - Invasive components may be very focal, requiring submission of the entire lesion

Microscopic Pathology

- Composed of mucin-secreting columnar epithelial cells with varying degrees of atypia
- Classified as having low-grade dysplasia, moderate dysplasia, high-grade dysplasia, or invasive carcinoma arising in IPMN
- 4 epithelial subtypes
  - Gastric
  - Intestinal
  - Pancreatobiliary
  - Oncocytic

MACROSCOPIC FEATURES

General Features

- Most common in pancreatic head
  - Often involve only a portion of pancreatic duct
  - Some are multifocal
  - Entire gland may be involved
- Main-duct and combined types
  - Florid papillary projections, often in background of dilated ducts
- Branch-duct type
  - Single or multiple peripheral cysts that connect to main duct, often with smooth lining
- Mural nodules &/or solid components may be seen in IPMNs with invasion

MICROSCOPIC PATHOLOGY

Histologic Features

- Usually have papillary architecture
- Do not have ovarian-type stroma
- 4 epithelial subtypes of mucin-secreting columnar epithelium
  - **Gastric (null) type**
    - Histologically low grade
    - Basally located nuclei
    - Slightly eosinophilic cytoplasm
    - Abundant apical cytoplasmic mucin
    - Usually sole epithelial type in branch duct IPMNs, mixed with other epithelial types in main/combined types
  - **Intestinal type**
    - Villous papillae with basophilic cytoplasm
    - Enlarged, oval, hyperchromatic nuclei with pseudostratification
  - **Pancreatobiliary type**
    - Thin, branching papillae
    - Amphophilic cytoplasm
    - Enlarged, hyperchromatic nuclei
  - **Oncocytic type**
    - Thick branching papillae with intracellular and intraepithelial lumina
    - Abundant eosinophilic cytoplasm
    - Large round nuclei with prominent nucleoli
    - Some consider these to be separate type of neoplasm (intraductal oncocytic papillary neoplasm)
  - Some authorities classify intraductal tubular adenoma as pyloric-gland-type IPMN
    - Closely packed glands with minimal cytologic atypia
    - Reminiscent of pyloric gland adenoma of gallbladder
- Varying degrees of atypia; grading based on highest degree of epithelial atypia
  - Low-grade dysplasia
    - Uniform cells
    - Only mild atypia
    - No architectural complexity
  - Moderate dysplasia
    - Nuclear stratification
    - High nuclear to cytoplasmic ratio
    - Nuclear pleomorphism
  - High-grade dysplasia/carcinoma in situ
    - Marked architectural complexity
    - Marked nuclear atypia
    - Loss of nuclear polarity
    - Increased mitoses
  - Different grades of dysplasia are often mixed in single IPMN
- 35% of IPMN have associated invasive component
  - Invasive carcinomas arising in IPMN often have tubular features, reminiscent of pancreatic ductal adenocarcinoma, or colloid features
    - Intestinal-type IPMNs associated with colloid carcinoma
    - Pancreatobiliary-type IPMNs associated with tubular adenocarcinoma
    - Invasive carcinoma arising in association with gastric-type IPMN is rare; if present, has tubular features

INTRADUCTAL PAPILLARY MUCINOUS NEOPLASM

Epithelial Subtypes of Intraductal Papillary Neoplasms

Subtype	MUC1 Expression	MUC2 Expression	MUC5AC Expression	MUC6 Expression	CDX2 Expression	Associated Invasive Carcinoma
Gastric	-	-	+	+	-	Rare (ductal)
Intestinal	-	+	+	-	+	Colloid
Pancreatobiliary	+	-	-	+ (weak)	-	Ductal
Oncocytic (IOPN)	- (variable)	+ (variable)	+	+	+ (variable)	Oncocytic

IOPN = intraductal oncocytic papillary neoplasm.

Cytologic Features

- Small clusters and flat sheets of glandular epithelial cells
  - ± intracytoplasmic mucin

DIFFERENTIAL DIAGNOSIS

Mucinous Cystic Neoplasm (MCN)

- Usually involves body/tail of pancreas
- Does not communicate with pancreatic ducts
- Younger women
- Presence of ovarian-like stroma is required for diagnosis of MCN

Pancreatic Intraepithelial Neoplasm (PanIN)

- Does not produce grossly visible lesion
- Smaller than IPMN (usually < 5 mm in diameter)

Serous Cystic Neoplasm

- Often seen in women
- Microcysts lined by bland cuboidal epithelial cells with cytoplasmic glycogen
- Central scar seen in majority
- Does not communicate with pancreatic ducts

Retention Cyst

- Usually unilocular and lined by nonmucinous, pancreatic duct epithelium

Solid-Pseudopapillary Neoplasm

- Usually in younger women
- Contains areas of necrosis and hemorrhage
- Composed of poorly cohesive, uniform neoplastic cells that form pseudopapillae
- Does not communicate with pancreatic ducts

DIAGNOSTIC CHECKLIST

Clinically Relevant Pathologic Features

- Invasive components may be very focal
  - Thus submission of entire lesion is necessary
- Careful gross examination to document communication between tumor and pancreatic ductal system is essential
- Predictors of recurrence
  - Main duct resection margin involved by any grade of IPMN
  - Branch duct involvement by moderate or high-grade dysplasia at resection margin
    - Presence of either of these requires excision of additional tissue if present on frozen section

Pathologic Interpretation Pearls

- Mucinous intraductal neoplasm that may contain several types of epithelium
- Must communicate with main &/or branch ducts
- Invasive component may be very focal
- Does not have ovarian-like stroma

SELECTED REFERENCES

1. Basturk O et al: Preferential expression of MUC6 in oncocytic and pancreatobiliary types of intraductal papillary neoplasms highlights a pyloropancreatic pathway, distinct from the intestinal pathway, in pancreatic carcinogenesis. Am J Surg Pathol. 34(3):364-70, 2010
2. Sahani DV et al: Multidisciplinary approach to diagnosis and management of intraductal papillary mucinous neoplasms of the pancreas. Clin Gastroenterol Hepatol. 7(3):259-69, 2009
3. Ishida M et al: Characteristic clinicopathological features of the types of intraductal papillary-mucinous neoplasms of the pancreas. Pancreas. 35(4):348-52, 2007
4. Tanaka M et al: International consensus guidelines for management of intraductal papillary mucinous neoplasms and mucinous cystic neoplasms of the pancreas. Pancreatology. 6(1-2):17-32, 2006
5. Furukawa T et al: Classification of types of intraductal papillary-mucinous neoplasm of the pancreas: a consensus study. Virchows Arch. 447(5):794-9, 2005
6. Adsay NV et al: Pathologically and biologically distinct types of epithelium in intraductal papillary mucinous neoplasms: delineation of an "intestinal" pathway of carcinogenesis in the pancreas. Am J Surg Pathol. 28(7):839-48, 2004
7. Hruban RH et al: An illustrated consensus on the classification of pancreatic intraepithelial neoplasia and intraductal papillary mucinous neoplasms. Am J Surg Pathol. 28(8):977-87, 2004

Microscopic Features

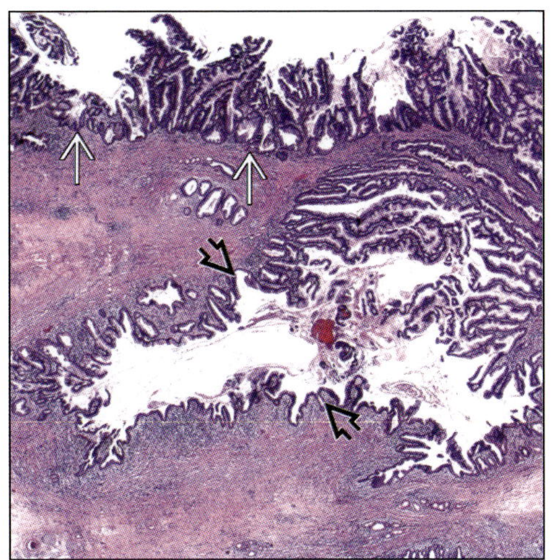

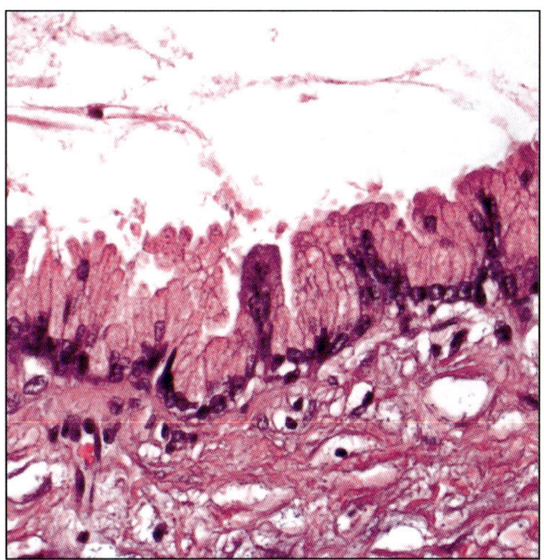

*(**Left**) IPMN combined type features an intraductal papillary proliferation in both the main duct ➔ and a large branch duct ⇨. (**Right**) IPMN with low-grade dysplasia shows columnar cells with intracytoplasmic mucin and basally located small nuclei.*

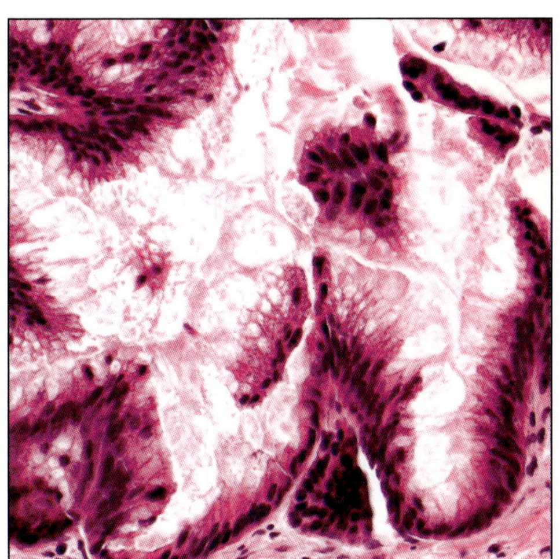

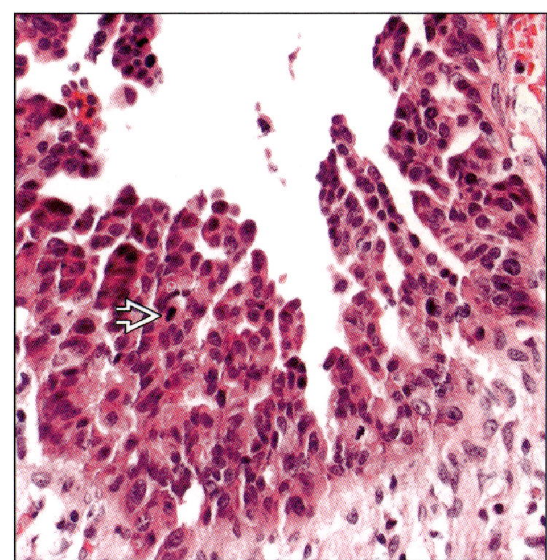

*(**Left**) IPMN with moderate dysplasia is characterized by mucinous columnar cells with elongated, hyperchromatic nuclei with stratification. (**Right**) IPMN with high-grade dysplasia demonstrates a micropapillary proliferation of tumor cells with a high nuclear to cytoplasmic ratio. Scattered mitoses ➔ are present.*

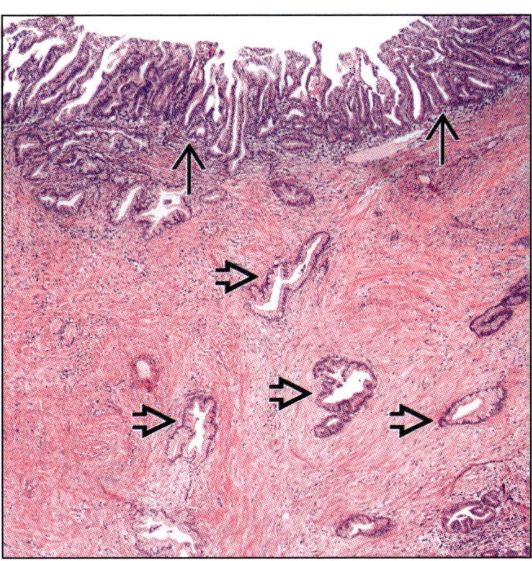

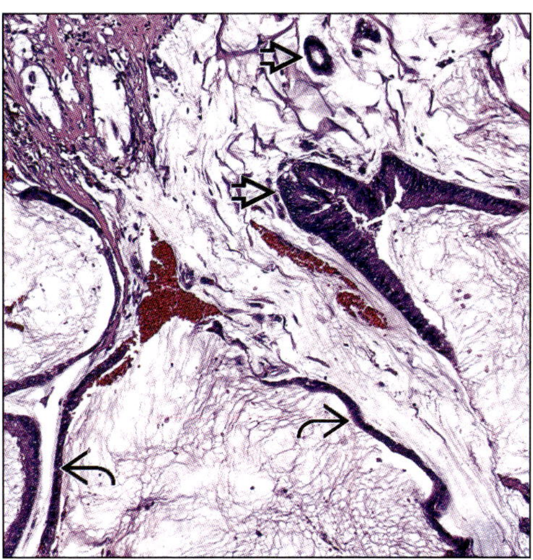

*(**Left**) Invasive tubular adenocarcinoma arising in association with IPMN combined type is shown. The main duct is replaced by moderate- to high-grade dysplastic epithelium →. The infiltrating ducts ⇨ resemble pancreatic ductal adenocarcinoma. (**Right**) Colloid carcinoma arising in association with intestinal-type IPMN features strips ↗ or nests ⇨ of neoplastic cells present within mucin pools.*

INTRADUCTAL PAPILLARY MUCINOUS NEOPLASM

Microscopic and Immunohistochemical Features

*(**Left**) IPMN, gastric (null) type is characterized by low-grade mucinous epithelium with abundant apical cytoplasmic mucin and small, basally located nuclei, reminiscent of gastric epithelium. (**Right**) IPMN gastric type demonstrates negative immunoreactivity to MUC2. CDX2 and MUC1 core are also negative in gastric-type IPMN.*

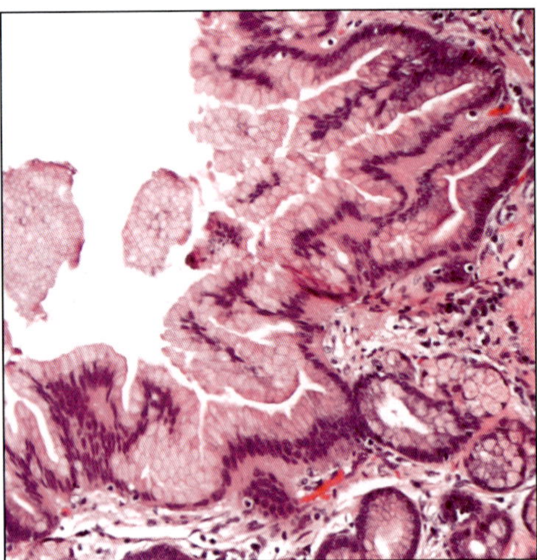

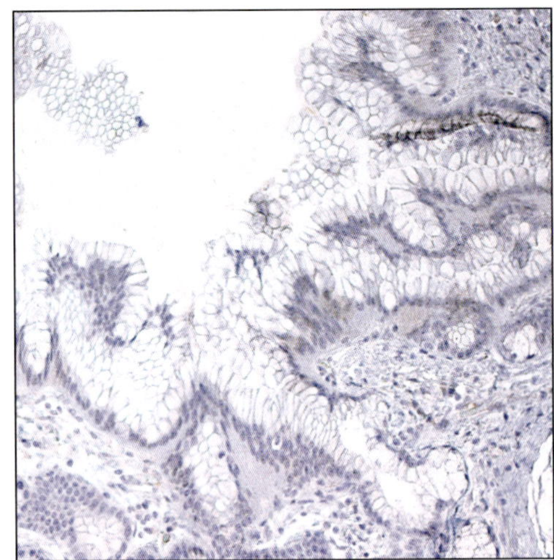

*(**Left**) IPMN gastric type demonstrates diffuse MUC5AC expression. (**Right**) IPMN gastric type demonstrates MUC6 expression in basal glands ➔ that resemble gastric pyloric glands. The combination of foveolar epithelium (MUC5AC) and pyloric gland (MUC6) type morphology and mucin phenotypes is reminiscent of gastric antrum.*

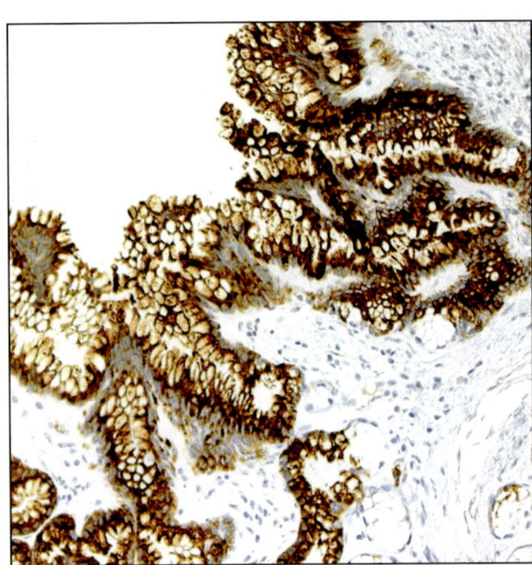

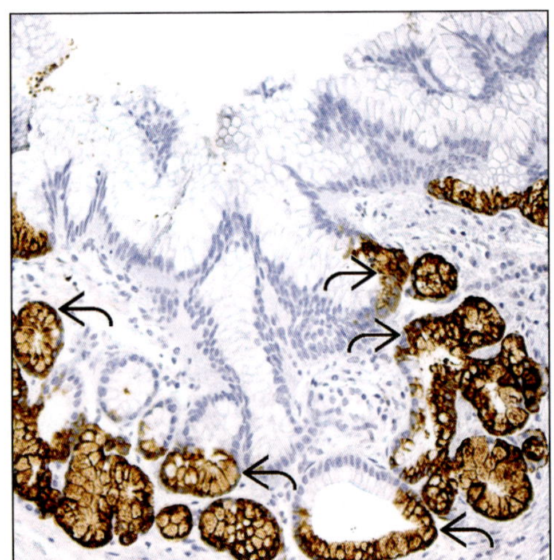

*(**Left**) IPMN intestinal type is characterized by villous papillae with basophilic cytoplasm and elongated nuclei with pseudostratification. Slightly amphophilic, apical mucin ➩ is characteristic of the intestinal type. (**Right**) IPMN intestinal type demonstrates diffuse MUC2 expression. This type is also characterized by nuclear expression of CDX2.*

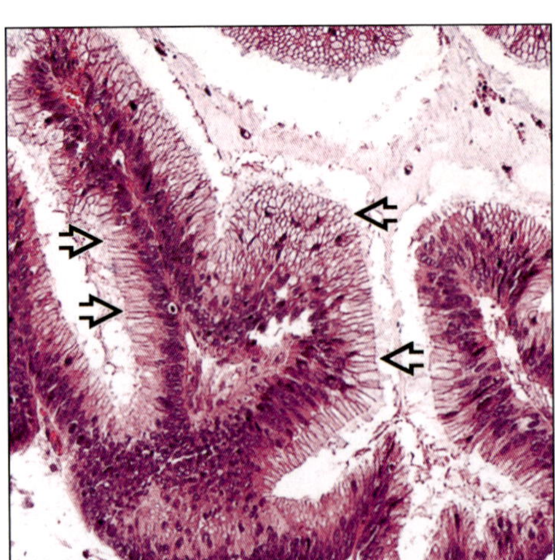

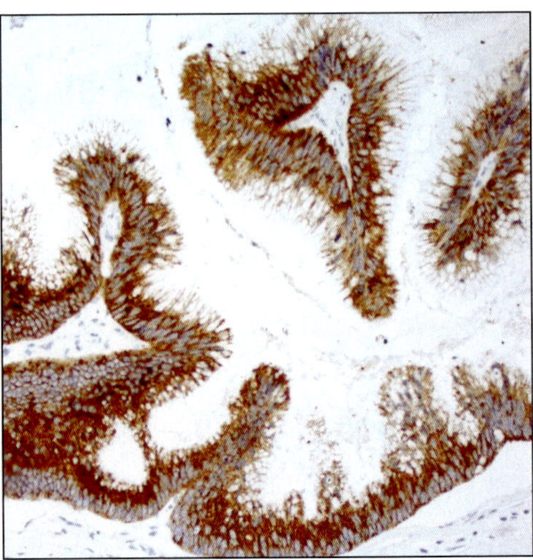

Microscopic and Immunohistochemical Features

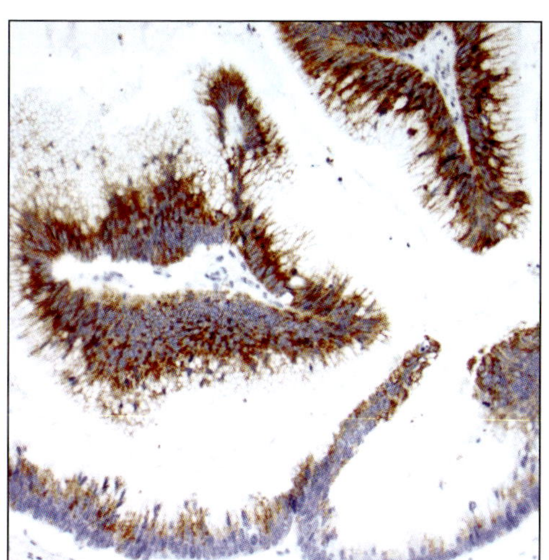
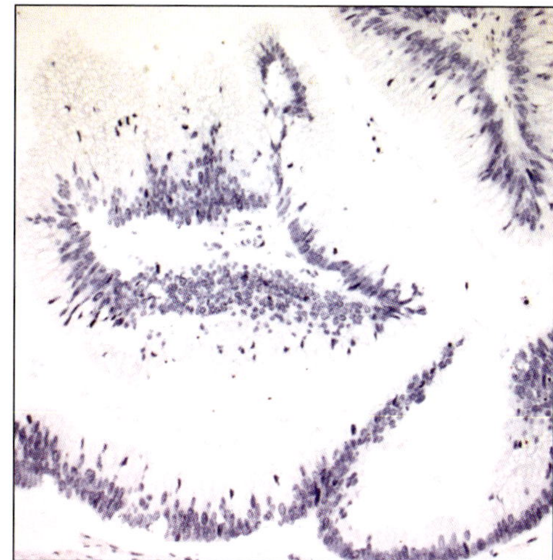

(Left) *IPMN intestinal type demonstrates MUC5AC expression in the majority of neoplastic cells.* ***(Right)*** *IPMN intestinal type shows negative MUC6 expression. MUC1 core expression (in an apical membranous pattern) may be seen in high-grade lesions but is usually negative in intestinal-type IPMN.*

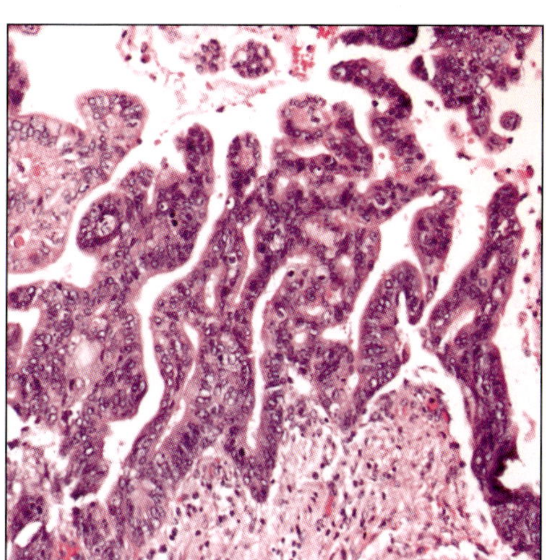
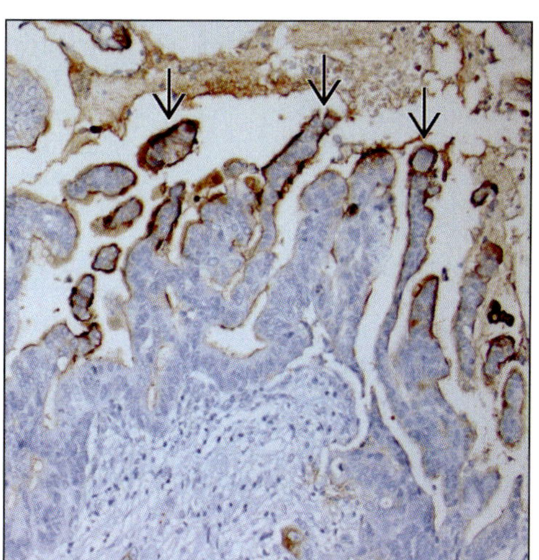

(Left) *IPMN pancreatobiliary type is characterized by thin branching complex papillae with moderate amphophilic cytoplasm and round, vesicular nuclei.* ***(Right)*** *IPMN pancreatobiliary type demonstrates MUC1 core expression in an apical cytoplasmic membranous pattern ➔.*

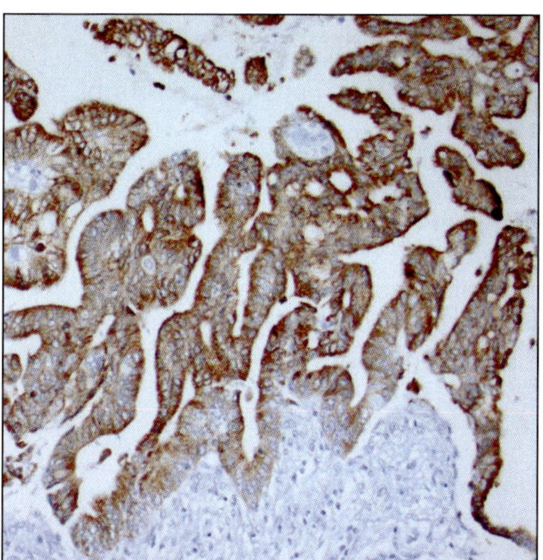
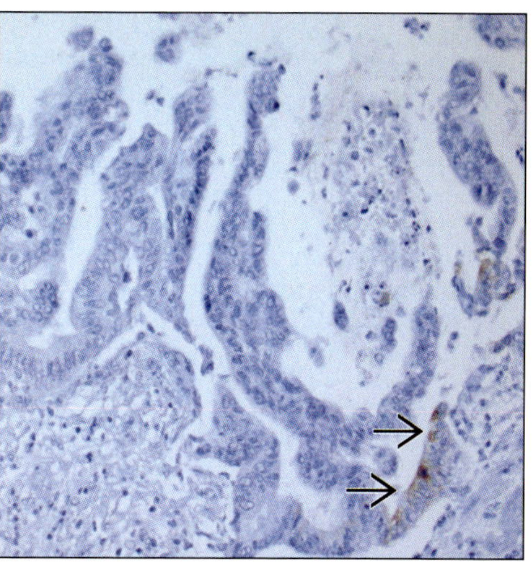

(Left) *IPMN pancreatobiliary type shows diffuse MUC5AC expression.* ***(Right)*** *IPMN pancreatobiliary type exhibits focal MUC6 expression ➔. MUC2 and CDX2 are usually negative in pancreatobiliary-type IPMN.*

INTRADUCTAL ONCOCYTIC PAPILLARY NEOPLASM

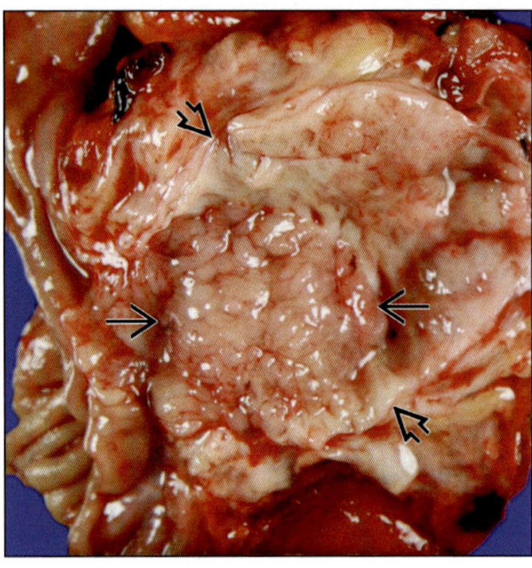

A tan-red luminal papillary mass ➔ partially involves the dilated main pancreatic duct ⊳.

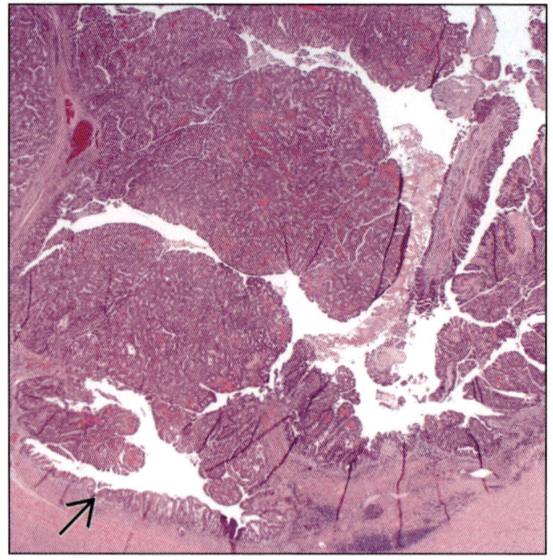

IOPNs consist of architecturally complex, thick papillae, seen here growing in a dilated branch duct that is, in part, lined by relatively flat epithelium ➔.

TERMINOLOGY

Abbreviations

- Intraductal oncocytic papillary neoplasm (IOPN)
- Intraductal papillary mucinous neoplasm (IPMN)

Definitions

- Grossly cystic neoplasm consisting of architecturally complex papillary **intraductal** growth of oncocytic (oxyntic) epithelium
- Grouped with IPMN in most recent WHO classification but considered a distinct entity by other groups

CLINICAL ISSUES

Epidemiology

- Incidence
  - Rare entity with approximately 40 cases reported in literature
- Age
  - Ranging from 20-80 years; average 60s
- Gender
  - Affects men and women equally

Presentation

- Similar to IPMNs
- Majority present with nonspecific symptoms or are discovered incidentally during imaging study for another indication

Treatment

- Surgical resection is treatment of choice

Prognosis

- 5-year survival rate of noninvasive IOPN: Approaches 100%
- 5-year survival rate of invasive IOPN: > 70%

IMAGE FINDINGS

General Features

- Large masses within cystic lesion connected to dilated main pancreatic duct
  - Similar to combined-type IPMN

MACROSCOPIC FEATURES

General Features

- Usually unilocular or multilocular and cystic, with soft red-brown or tan-red papillary masses

Size

- Range: 1.6-15 cm
- Average: 4-6 cm

MICROSCOPIC PATHOLOGY

Histologic Features

- Architecturally complex intraductal epithelial proliferation with arborizing papillae, cribriforming, and solid nests
  - Often classified as having high-grade dysplasia given architectural complexity
- Neoplastic epithelial cells exhibit abundant granular eosinophilic cytoplasm with large nuclei and prominent nucleoli
- Both intracytoplasmic and intercellular lumens are found, many containing mucin, with scattered goblet cells
- Stroma can be edematous or myxoid at tip &/or base of papillae
- Invasive carcinomas, often minimally invasive, are found in 25-50% of reported cases, and some retain oncocytic features

Immunohistochemistry

- Stain strongly with MUC6

INTRADUCTAL ONCOCYTIC PAPILLARY NEOPLASM

Key Facts

Terminology
- Grossly cystic neoplasm with intraductal growth pattern and oncocytic epithelium

Clinical Issues
- Rare entity with ~ 40 cases reported in literature
- Majority present with nonspecific symptoms or are discovered incidentally
- 5-year survival rate of noninvasive IOPN approaches 100%; invasive IOPN > 70%

Microscopic Pathology
- Oncocytic epithelium that forms architecturally complex papillary growth pattern as well as areas of cribriforming and solid growth
- Neoplastic cells have abundant granular eosinophilic cytoplasm with large nuclei, prominent nucleoli
- Invasive carcinoma, often minimally invasive, present in 25-50%

- Variable staining with MUC1, MUC2, MUC5AC, CEA, CA19-9
- May have focal chromogranin, chymotrypsin positivity
- Hepatocyte antigen positive

DIFFERENTIAL DIAGNOSIS

Other Types of IPMN
- Complex architecture and eosinophilic cytoplasm are distinct from gastric- or intestinal-type epithelium
- Overlap with pancreatobiliary-type IPMN, but abundant granular eosinophilic cytoplasm should be prominent feature in cases designated IOPN

Other Solid Pancreatic Neoplasms
- If solid growth pattern predominates
  - Pancreatic endocrine neoplasm
    - Diffusely positive for chromogranin, synaptophysin
  - Acinar cell carcinoma
    - Immunoreactivity to trypsin and chymotrypsin
    - Periodic acid-Schiff with diastase (dPAS) positive granules may be seen in apical aspect of gland-forming cells
  - Solid-pseudopapillary neoplasm
    - Typically in young females
    - Mark with CD10, vimentin, and nuclear expression of β-catenin

DIAGNOSTIC CHECKLIST

Pathologic Interpretation Pearls
- Similar to IPMN in many aspects but with prominent oncocytic features

SELECTED REFERENCES

1. Basturk O et al: Preferential expression of MUC6 in oncocytic and pancreatobiliary types of intraductal papillary neoplasms highlights a pyloropancreatic pathway, distinct from the intestinal pathway, in pancreatic carcinogenesis. Am J Surg Pathol. 34(3):364-70, 2010
2. Patel SA et al: Genetic analysis of invasive carcinoma arising in intraductal oncocytic papillary neoplasm of the pancreas. Am J Surg Pathol. 26(8):1071-7, 2002
3. Nobukawa B et al: Intraductal oncocytic papillary carcinoma with invasion arising from the accessory pancreatic duct. Gastrointest Endosc. 50(6):864-6, 1999
4. Jyotheeswaran S et al: A newly recognized entity: intraductal "oncocytic" papillary neoplasm of the pancreas. Am J Gastroenterol. 93(12):2539-43, 1998
5. Adsay NV et al: Intraductal oncocytic papillary neoplasms of the pancreas. Am J Surg Pathol. 20(8):980-94, 1996

IMAGE GALLERY

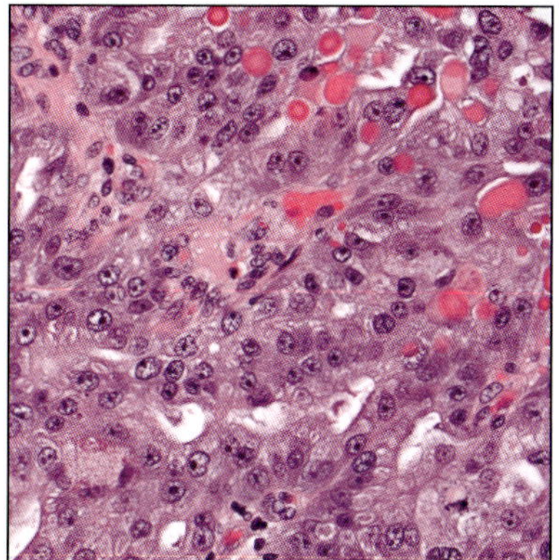
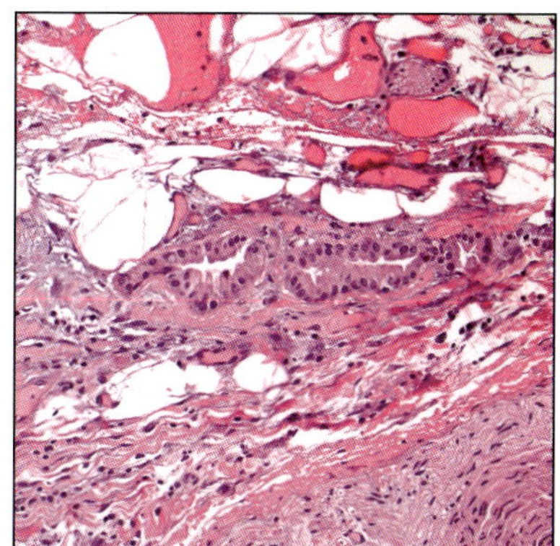
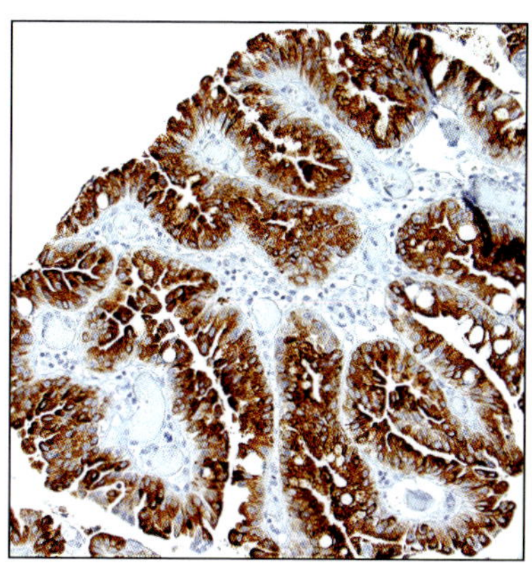

(Left) *IOPN typically exhibits architecturally complex growth with cribriforming &/or solid nests. The neoplastic epithelial cells have abundant granular eosinophilic cytoplasm and large nuclei with prominent nucleoli.* ***(Center)*** *An invasive carcinoma arising in IOPN has glands with similar oncocytic features infiltrating the peripancreatic soft tissue.* ***(Right)*** *IOPNs demonstrate strong MUC6 expression.*

INTRADUCTAL TUBULOPAPILLARY NEOPLASM

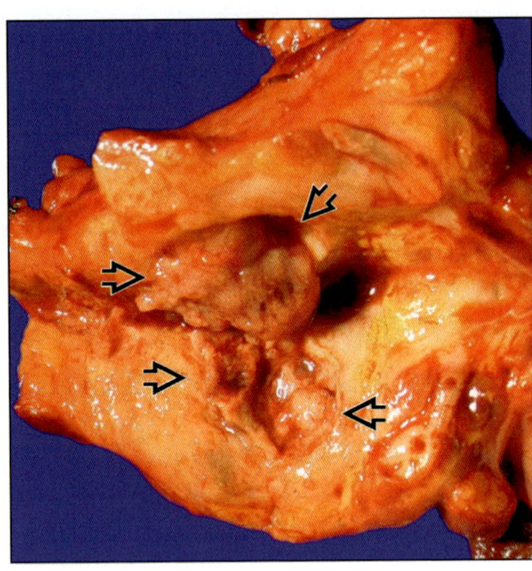

This ITPN is forming solid nodules ➾ that obstruct the dilated pancreatic duct. There is no grossly visible mucin.

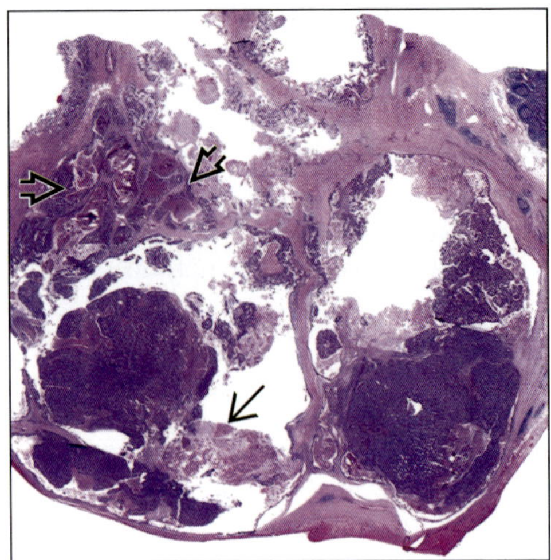

This low-power view shows an ITPN with stromal invasion. Note the solid masses with focal necrosis → within a dilated duct. A focus of invasion is also seen ➾.

TERMINOLOGY

Abbreviations

- Intraductal tubulopapillary neoplasm (ITPN)
- Intraductal tubular carcinoma (ITC)
- Intraductal tubular adenoma (ITA)
- Intraductal papillary mucinous neoplasm (IPMN)

Definitions

- ITPN: Solid epithelial neoplasm composed of back-to-back tubular glands and papillae that grows within and obstructs pancreatic ducts
  - No visible mucin
- Some authorities group ITC and ITA together as a separate diagnostic classification known as intraductal tubular neoplasms
- Others group ITC and ITPN together but classify ITA as pyloric-type IPMN

CLINICAL ISSUES

Epidemiology

- Incidence
  - Rare entity (< 20 cases reported in literature)
- Age
  - Range: 36-79 years
  - Average: 59 years
- Gender
  - Equal gender distribution

Presentation

- Similar to IPMNs
  - Symptomatic cases present with abdominal pain
  - Majority are discovered incidentally

Treatment

- Surgical approaches
  - Pancreatectomy with curative intent is treatment of choice

Prognosis

- Limited follow-up data suggest relatively indolent course, especially if there is no invasive component

MACROSCOPIC FEATURES

General Features

- Solid nodules obstructing dilated pancreatic ducts
  - Sessile or pedunculated
  - No visible mucin

Size

- Range: 1-15 cm
- Average: 4.2 cm

MICROSCOPIC PATHOLOGY

Histologic Features

- Tubulopapillary (ITPN) or tubular (ITC, ITA) growth patterns
  - Closely packed glands may resemble pyloric gland adenomas
    - Cuboidal to columnar cells with enlarged nuclei and eosinophilic to amphophilic cytoplasm
  - Solid &/or cribriform areas may be seen in some cases
  - Scarce or absent cytoplasmic mucin
- May have low- or high-grade dysplasia
  - Cases with high-grade dysplasia have unequivocal architectural and cytologic evidence of malignancy, abundant mitoses, and necrosis
- Invasive component, if present, may resemble intraductal components (tubulopapillary pattern) or may be composed of infiltrating ducts

INTRADUCTAL TUBULOPAPILLARY NEOPLASM

Key Facts

Terminology

- Solid epithelial neoplasm composed of back-to-back tubular glands and papillae that grows within and obstructs pancreatic ducts
  - No grossly visible mucin

Clinical Issues

- Very rare entity
- Majority are discovered incidentally

Microscopic Pathology

- Tubulopapillary or tubular growth
  - Some may resemble pyloric gland adenomas
  - Scant or absent mucin
- Cases with high-grade dysplasia have marked architectural and cytologic atypia, mitoses, necrosis
- Invasive component may be similar to intraductal component or highly infiltrative

ANCILLARY TESTS

Immunohistochemistry

- CK7 and CK19 positive; CK20 negative
- Focal MUC1 positivity
- Variable marking with MUC6
- ITA (a.k.a. pyloric gland-type IPMN) is MUC5AC positive; ITPN and ITC are MUC5AC negative
- Markers for pancreatic acinar differentiation, such as trypsin and chymotrypsin, are negative

DIFFERENTIAL DIAGNOSIS

Intraductal Papillary Mucinous Neoplasm

- Dilated pancreatic ducts filled with mucin grossly
- Tall columnar epithelium with obvious cytoplasmic mucin
- Well-developed papillae with no necrosis
- Consistent marking with MUC5AC

Acinar Cell Carcinoma, Intraductal Variant

- Usually positive for exocrine markers, including trypsin
- Solid nesting pattern with granular cytoplasm

Pancreatic Ductal Adenocarcinoma

- Does not have prominent intraductal growth pattern
- Is very infiltrative and destructive
- Has marked desmoplastic stroma
- Transition to normal ductal epithelium may help confirm intraductal location of ITC

DIAGNOSTIC CHECKLIST

Pathologic Interpretation Pearls

- Intraductal growth is similar to IPMNs, but lack of mucin and presence of tubulopapillary patterns is distinct from IPMN
- Important to note intraductal growth pattern grossly

SELECTED REFERENCES

1. Chetty R et al: Intraductal tubular adenoma (pyloric gland-type) of the pancreas: a reappraisal and possible relationship with gastric-type intraductal papillary mucinous neoplasm. Histopathology. 55(3):270-6, 2009
2. Yamaguchi H et al: Intraductal tubulopapillary neoplasms of the pancreas distinct from pancreatic intraepithelial neoplasia and intraductal papillary mucinous neoplasms. Am J Surg Pathol. 33(8):1164-72, 2009
3. Königsrainer I et al: Intraductal and cystic tubulopapillary adenocarcinoma of the pancreas--a possible variant of intraductal tubular carcinoma. Pancreas. 36(1):92-5, 2008
4. Tajiri T et al: Intraductal tubular neoplasms of the pancreas: histogenesis and differentiation. Pancreas. 30(2):115-21, 2005
5. Albores-Saavedra J et al: Intraductal tubular adenoma, pyloric type, of the pancreas: additional observations on a new type of pancreatic neoplasm. Am J Surg Pathol. 28(2):233-8, 2004

IMAGE GALLERY

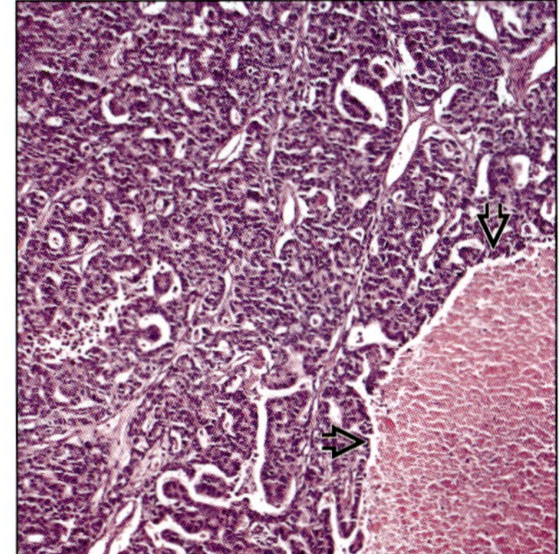

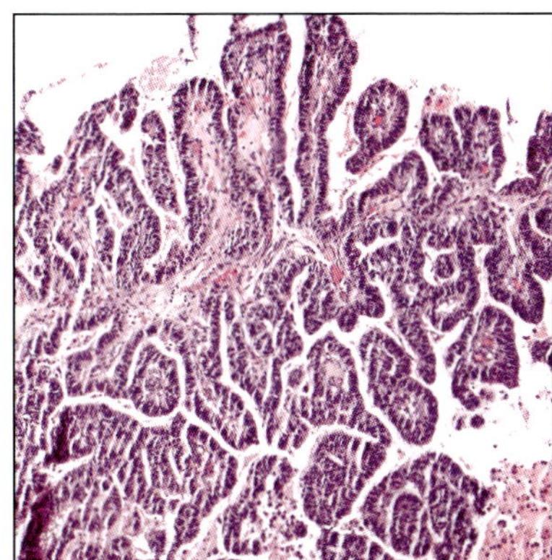

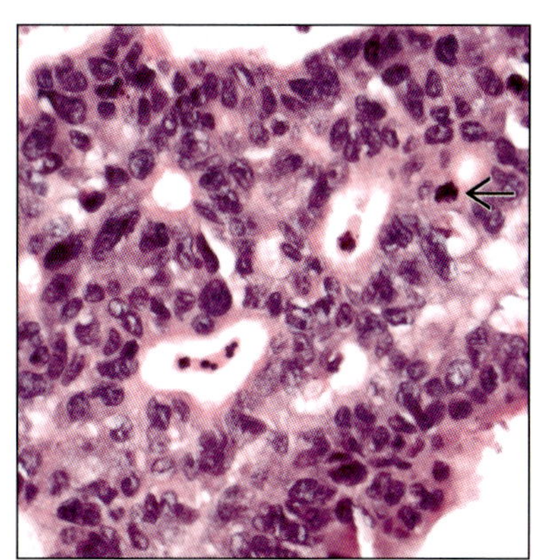

(Left) *ITPN typically exhibits a cellular, tubulopapillary growth pattern with high-grade cytologic atypia and easily identifiable necrosis ⇨.* ***(Center)*** *This area of an ITPN has a well-developed papillary architectural pattern.* ***(Right)*** *ITPNs may contain back to back tubules. The neoplastic cells have eosinophilic cytoplasm and enlarged, irregular nuclei with scattered mitoses →. There is no mucinous epithelium.*

ACINAR CELL CARCINOMA

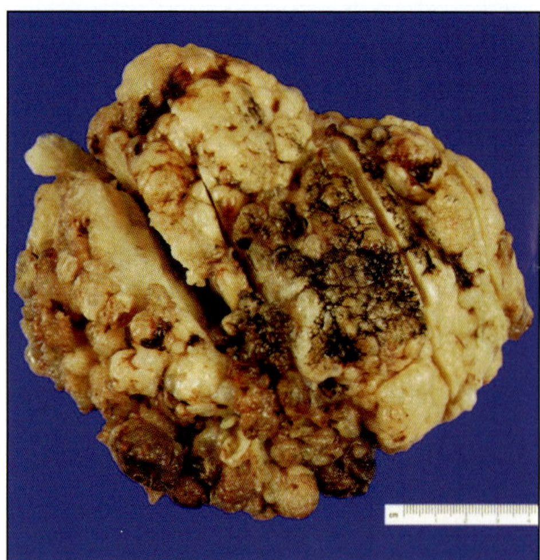

This relatively well-circumscribed acinar cell carcinoma is large, fleshy, and white-tan with a lobular configuration and easily identifiable necrosis.

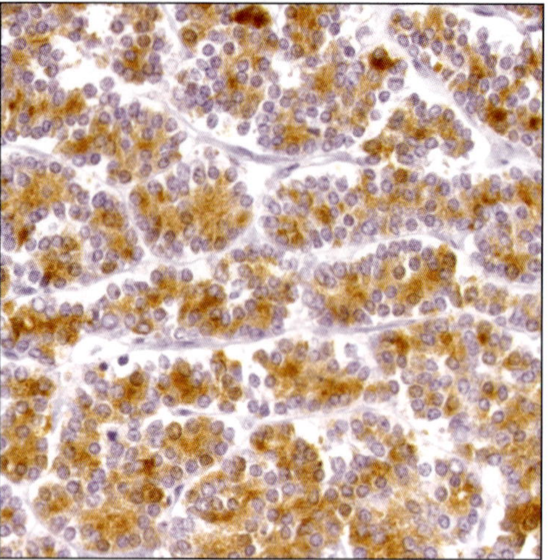

Antibodies against pancreatic exocrine enzymes are most sensitive. Note the cytoplasmic staining for trypsin. Chymotrypsin can be equally beneficial, and lipase is detected slightly less often.

TERMINOLOGY

Abbreviations

- Acinar cell carcinoma (ACC)

Definitions

- Malignant exocrine carcinoma with acinar differentiation
  - Production of pancreatic exocrine enzymes in zymogen granules

CLINICAL ISSUES

Epidemiology

- Incidence
  - 1-2% of primary pancreatic neoplasms
- Age
  - Between 5th and 7th decade of life
  - Rarely documented in children
    - Youngest reported patient was 3 years old
- Gender
  - Male predominance

Presentation

- Nonspecific symptoms
  - Abdominal pain and weight loss
- Lipase hypersecretion paraneoplastic syndrome (10-15%)
  - Subcutaneous fat necrosis and polyarthralgia

Laboratory Tests

- ↑ serum lipase in lipase hypersecretion syndrome
- Elevated α-fetoprotein in younger patients

Natural History

- Most patients have metastatic disease at presentation, usually to lymph nodes and liver

Prognosis

- 5-year survival of 6%

MACROSCOPIC FEATURES

General Features

- Solid, circumscribed mass
  - Capsular invasion common
- Solid, soft-fleshy, lobulated, tan to red cut surface
  - Rare cystic variant with innumerable variably sized cysts is known as acinar cell cystadenocarcinoma

Size

- Large, average of 10 cm in diameter (range: 2-30 cm)

MICROSCOPIC PATHOLOGY

Histologic Features

- Densely cellular
- Several architectural patterns
  - Acinar: Minute lumens with basally located nuclei and apical cytoplasm
  - Solid
    - Sheets and nests of cells without lumen formation
    - Basal nuclear palisading along the stromal interface
  - Glandular: Dilated acinar lumens
  - Trabecular: Interlacing ribbons of cells with nuclei oriented toward the periphery
- Typically, a paucity of stroma
  - Desmoplastic stromal response is absent
- Uniform nuclei with vesicular chromatin
  - Often single prominent central nucleoli
- Minimal to moderate amounts of finely granular, eosinophilic to amphophilic cytoplasm
- Mitotic rate variable, but most have easily identifiable mitoses
- Vascular invasion common
- Variants
  - Cystic growth pattern (acinar cell cystadenocarcinoma)
  - Intraductal or papillocystic growth

ACINAR CELL CARCINOMA

Key Facts

Terminology

- Rare, highly aggressive malignant epithelial neoplasm
  - Acinar differentiation with zymogen granules

Clinical Issues

- Minority of patients have lipase hypersecretion paraneoplastic syndrome

Macroscopic Features

- Solid, well circumscribed, and fleshy

Microscopic Pathology

- Multiple architectural patterns, most commonly acinar or solid
- Uniform nuclei with central prominent nucleoli
  - Eosinophilic, finely granular cytoplasm
- Typically, a paucity of stroma
- Immunoreactive for trypsin or chymotrypsin
- PASD stain may be negative

    - Can mimic intraductal neoplasm
  - Oncocytic ACC
    - Have abundant eosinophilic cytoplasm, may not mark with trypsin
  - Signet ring or clear cell features

ANCILLARY TESTS

Histochemistry

- Positive for periodic acid-Schiff and resistant to diastase digestion
  - Many ACC have insufficient quantities of zymogen granules, resulting in negative stain

Immunohistochemistry

- Pancreatic exocrine enzymes: Trypsin (97%), chymotrypsin (66-95%), and lipase (70-84%)
- Positive for cytokeratin 8 and 18
- Focal staining for synaptophysin or chromogranin (35-54%)
- Amylase, CK7, CK20, and α-fetoprotein are less commonly positive

Molecular Genetics

- Allelic loss of chromosome arm 11p (50% of ACC)
- Alterations in *APC/β-catenin* pathway (24% of ACC)

Electron Microscopy

- 2 forms of zymogen granules

DIFFERENTIAL DIAGNOSIS

Pancreatic Endocrine Neoplasm

- "Salt and pepper" chromatin
- Diffusely positive for synaptophysin and chromogranin

Mixed Endocrine/Acinar Neoplasm

- > 25% endocrine differentiation as well as acinar cell differentiation
  - Extent of differentiation is determined by immunohistochemical reactivity

Pancreatoblastoma

- Bimodal age distribution
  - 2/3 occurs in early childhood
  - 1/3 occurs in adults
- Predominantly acinar but also has distinctive squamoid nests

Solid-Pseudopapillary Neoplasm

- Solid areas with uniform cells but has characteristic degenerative pseudopapillary formation
- Immunoreactive for β-catenin, not trypsin or chymotrypsin

SELECTED REFERENCES

1. Stelow EB et al: Pancreatic acinar cell carcinomas with prominent ductal differentiation: Mixed acinar ductal carcinoma and mixed acinar endocrine ductal carcinoma. Am J Surg Pathol. 34(4):510-8, 2010

IMAGE GALLERY

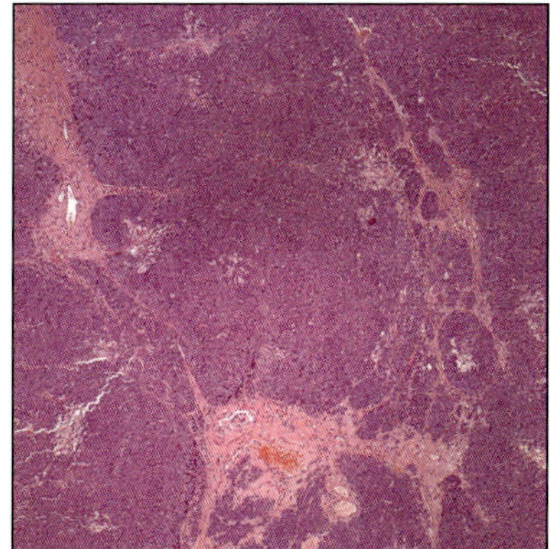

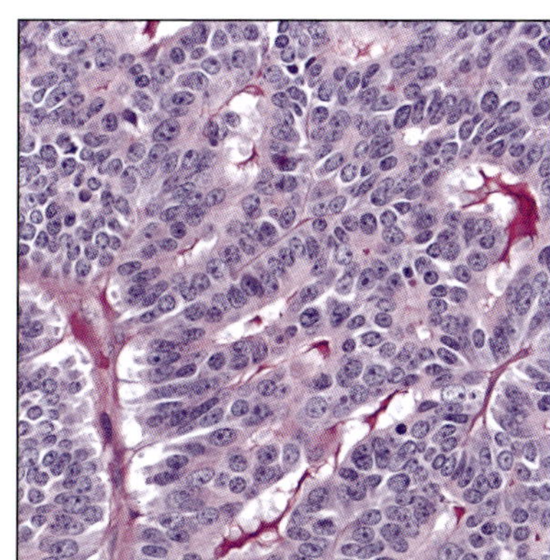

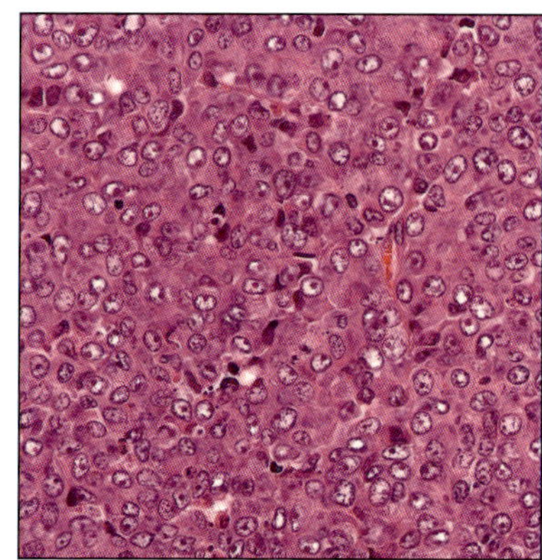

(Left) *At low power, acinar cell carcinomas are densely cellular with a relatively minimal stromal component.* ***(Center)*** *The lack of sufficient cytoplasmic zymogen granules in these neoplastic ACC cells results in a negative PASD stain. Note the acinar growth pattern with small lumens and nuclei that are polarized in the acini.* ***(Right)*** *This ACC with the solid growth pattern shows solid sheets of neoplastic cells with characteristic prominent nucleoli.*

PANCREATOBLASTOMA

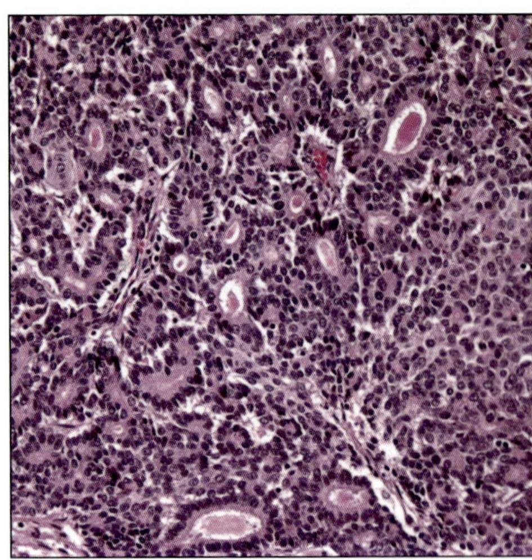

The acinar pattern is one of the most common patterns of differentiation in pancreatoblastoma.

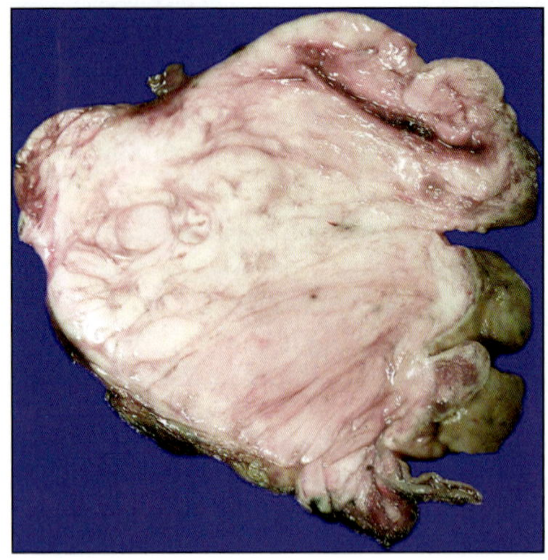

This gross photograph of a pancreatoblastoma shows a lobulated, well-circumscribed mass with a fleshy, white-tan cut surface.

TERMINOLOGY

Abbreviations

- Pancreatoblastoma (PB)

Definitions

- Malignant epithelial neoplasm with multiple lines of differentiation
  - Acinar, squamous, endocrine, ductal, or mesenchymal components may be seen
- Many are associated with mutations in β-*catenin/APC* pathway
- Minority associated with *SMAD4/DPC4* alterations

CLINICAL ISSUES

Epidemiology

- Incidence
  - Rare overall but is most common malignant pancreatic neoplasm of childhood
    - 25% of pancreatic tumors in pediatric population
- Age
  - 2/3 of PB occur in children, 1/3 in adults
    - Bimodal distribution; mean age at diagnosis is 2.4 years in children and 40 years in adults
- Gender
  - No gender predominance
- Ethnicity
  - More common in Asians

Presentation

- Upper abdominal mass
  - Large and often palpable in children
- Abdominal pain
- Weight loss
- Jaundice is rare
- May be associated with Beckwith-Wiedemann syndrome
  - Often cystic in this context

Laboratory Tests

- 25-30% have elevated α-fetoprotein

Treatment

- Surgery is treatment of choice
- Chemotherapy and radiation have been used for unresectable disease or recurrence

Prognosis

- Aggressive neoplasm
  - 1/3 have metastases at time of diagnosis
    - Liver
    - Lymph nodes
    - Lungs
    - Peritoneum
  - Prognosis worse for adults than children

MACROSCOPIC FEATURES

General Features

- Usually solitary
- Equally distributed between head and tail
- Well circumscribed and at least partially encapsulated
- Lobulated
- Gray, tan, or yellow cut surface with variably present necrosis

Size

- Large; mean: 10-11 cm

MICROSCOPIC PATHOLOGY

Histologic Features

- Lobular growth pattern with distinct fibrous bands
- Multiple histologic patterns
  - Acinar pattern
    - Usually predominant
    - Cells polarized around small lumens
    - Basal nuclei with single nucleolus

PANCREATOBLASTOMA

Key Facts

Clinical Issues

- Rare overall but most common malignant pancreatic neoplasm of childhood
- 2/3 of PB occur in children, 1/3 in adults
  - Mean age at diagnosis is 2.4 years in children and 40 years in adults
- 25-30% have elevated α-fetoprotein

Macroscopic Features

- Usually solitary, well-circumscribed, lobulated neoplasm

Microscopic Pathology

- Lobular growth pattern with distinct fibrous bands
- Multiple histologic patterns including acinar, squamoid nests, endocrine, ductal, primitive

---

- Squamoid nests
  - Virtually always present, usually in center of tumor lobules
  - Whorled, plump, sometimes spindled cells with eosinophilic cytoplasm
  - Variably present keratinization
- Endocrine component
  - Present in 1/2-2/3 of tumors
  - Endocrine cells either scattered within acini or form trabeculae or nests
- Stromal component
  - Ranges from paucicellular to highly cellular
  - May contain foci of cartilage or osseous differentiation
- Primitive component: Variably present, composed of monotonous immature small blue cells
- Ductal component: Rare and usually focal

ANCILLARY TESTS

Immunohistochemistry

- Acinar component stains with keratins (7, 8, 18, 19, CAM5.2, AE1/AE3), pancreatic enzymes
  - May stain with AFP
- Endocrine component stains with synaptophysin, chromogranin, NSE; does not stain with insulin, glucagon, or somatostatin
- Squamoid nests are often not immunoreactive

DIFFERENTIAL DIAGNOSIS

Acinar Cell Carcinoma

- Lacks squamoid nests and prominent stromal component
- Usually in older patients

Well-Differentiated Pancreatic Endocrine Tumor

- Uniform endocrine differentiation, negative for acinar markers
- Lacks squamoid nests

Solid-Pseudopapillary Neoplasm

- Pseudopapillary pattern, foamy macrophages, cholesterol clefts
- Usually in young adult females
- Stains with CD10; negative for pancreatic enzyme stains

SELECTED REFERENCES

1. Hua C et al: Pancreatoblastoma: a histochemical and immunohistochemical analysis. J Clin Pathol. 49(11):952-4, 1996
2. Levey JM et al: Adult pancreatoblastoma: a case report and review of the literature. Am J Gastroenterol. 91(9):1841-4, 1996
3. Klimstra DS et al: Pancreatoblastoma. A clinicopathologic study and review of the literature. Am J Surg Pathol. 19(12):1371-89, 1995

IMAGE GALLERY

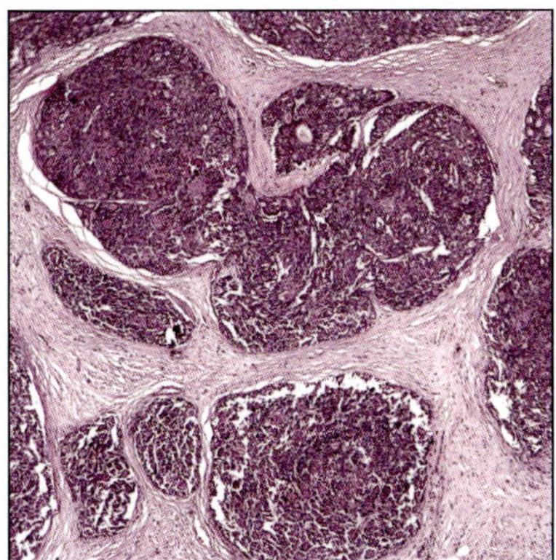

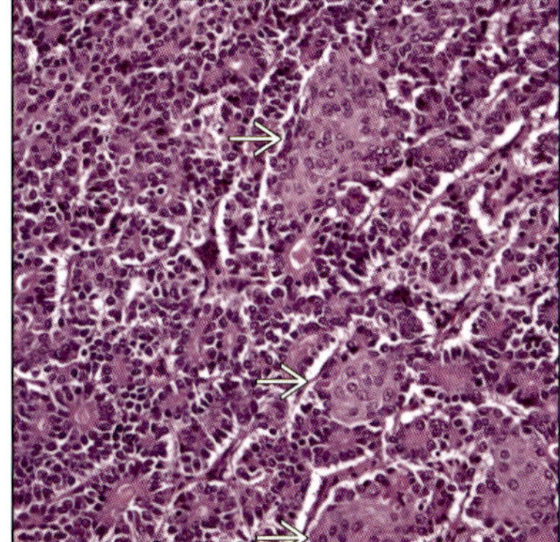

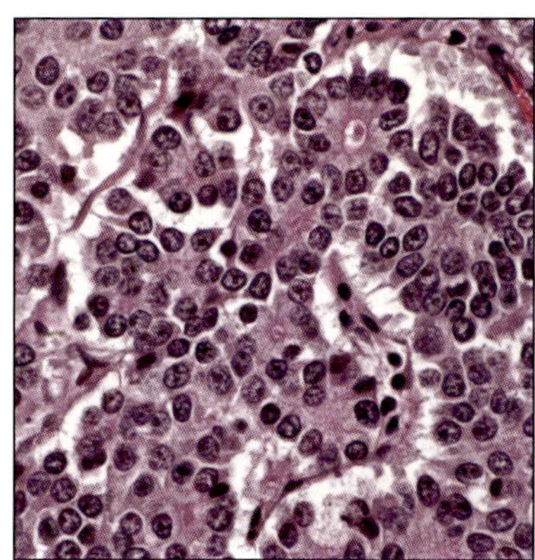

(Left) *This low-power photomicrograph illustrates the lobular growth pattern of pancreatoblastoma as well as the prominent fibrous stroma.* ***(Center)*** *Squamoid nests ➡ are invariably present in pancreatoblastoma, seen here admixed with areas of acinar differentiation.* ***(Right)*** *The acinar pattern is characterized by acinar structures with small lumens and basally located nuclei.*

DERMOID CYST

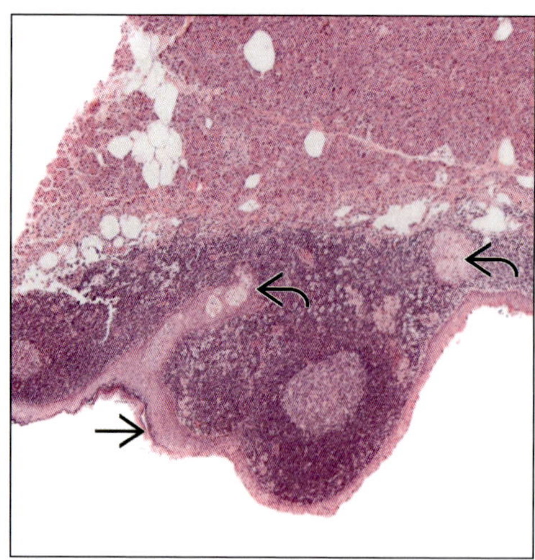

This pancreatic dermoid cyst is lined by squamous epithelium ➡ and a rind of lymphoid tissue. There is extensive sebaceous differentiation ↪.

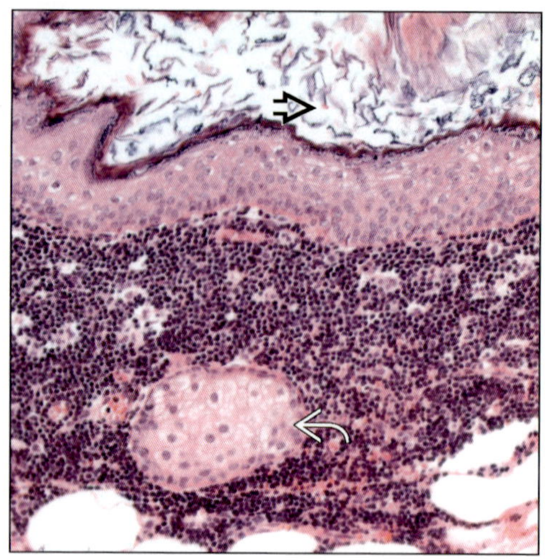

The squamous lining epithelium is mature and shows surface keratinization ⇨. Sebaceous differentiation is evident ↪.

TERMINOLOGY

Synonyms

- Mature cystic teratoma

Definitions

- Squamous-lined cyst with differentiation along 1 or more germ cell layers

CLINICAL ISSUES

Epidemiology

- Incidence
  - Extremely rare
    - Only a handful of cases reported
- Age
  - Range: 2-53 years
    - Mean: 29 years

Presentation

- Nonspecific gastrointestinal symptoms
  - Nausea and vomiting
  - Malaise
  - Epigastric pain
  - Weight loss
  - Dyspepsia
- Palpable mass

Treatment

- Surgical approaches
  - May include pancreaticoduodenectomy, distal pancreatectomy, or enucleation
  - Nonoperative management is feasible in cases with firm preoperative diagnosis

Prognosis

- Benign tumor

MACROSCOPIC FEATURES

General Features

- Unilocular tumor
  - Often variegated solid and cystic
  - Contents appear pasty or "cheesy"
  - Involves head, body, or tail of pancreas
  - Main pancreatic duct typically uninvolved with no communication with cystic tumor

MICROSCOPIC PATHOLOGY

Histologic Features

- Similar to dermoid cysts of other organs
  - Multilayered mature squamous epithelium without atypia
  - Adnexal structures present such as sebaceous glands and hair follicles
  - Mucinous metaplasia has been reported
- Pancreatic dermoid cysts are predominantly monodermal
  - Mesodermal tissue, such as cartilage, is only rarely present

Cytologic Features

- Anucleated squamous cells
- Necrotic debris
- May have prominent lymphoid component

DIFFERENTIAL DIAGNOSIS

Lymphoepithelial Cyst

- Lined by squamous epithelium with prominent layer of lymphoid tissue
- Occasionally, sebaceous glands may be found, but other adnexal structures are absent
- Nonetheless, there exists an overlap between lymphoepithelial cysts and dermoid cysts

DERMOID CYST

Key Facts

Terminology
- Squamous-lined cyst with differentiation along 1 or more germ cell layers

Clinical Issues
- Extremely rare

Macroscopic Features
- Unilocular tumor, often variegated solid and cystic

Microscopic Pathology
- Similar to dermoid cysts of other organs
  - Multilayered mature squamous epithelium without atypia
  - Adnexal structures present such as sebaceous glands and hair follicles
  - Mesodermal tissue, such as cartilage, is only rarely present in pancreas

  - Extensive sebaceous differentiation may indicate dermoid cyst

Epidermoid Cyst in Intrapancreatic Splenic Tissue
- Splenic pulp is present

Pancreatic Squamous Cyst
- Lined by squamous epithelium but lacks adnexal structures

Serous Cystadenoma
- Lined by single, occasionally multilayered, epithelium with clear cytoplasm
- Lacks adnexal structures, lymphoid tissue, and mesodermal elements

Mucinous Cystadenoma and Intraductal Papillary Mucinous Neoplasm
- Mucin-producing cells dominate epithelium lining
- Lacks squamous, adnexal, and lymphoid components
- Intraductal papillary mucinous neoplasm communicates with pancreatic duct

Retention Cyst
- Lined by simple cuboidal epithelium
- When present, squamous differentiation is focal
- Lacks lymphoid stroma, adnexal structures

DIAGNOSTIC CHECKLIST

Clinically Relevant Pathologic Features
- Solid, fleshy, or necrotic areas should be carefully sampled for the possibility of carcinoma arising within dermoid cyst

SELECTED REFERENCES

1. Othman M et al: Squamoid cyst of pancreatic ducts: A distinct type of cystic lesion in the pancreas. Am J Surg Pathol. 31(2):291-7, 2007
2. Tucci G et al: Dermoid cyst of the pancreas: presentation and management. World J Surg Oncol. 5:85, 2007
3. Adsay NV et al: Lymphoepithelial cysts of the pancreas: a report of 12 cases and a review of the literature. Mod Pathol. 15(5):492-501, 2002
4. Adsay NV et al: Squamous-lined cysts of the pancreas: lymphoepithelial cysts, dermoid cysts (teratomas), and accessory-splenic epidermoid cysts. Semin Diagn Pathol. 17(1):56-65, 2000
5. Mandavilli SR et al: Lymphoepithelial cyst (LEC) of the pancreas: cytomorphology and differential diagnosis on fine-needle aspiration (FNA). Diagn Cytopathol. 20(6):371-4, 1999

IMAGE GALLERY

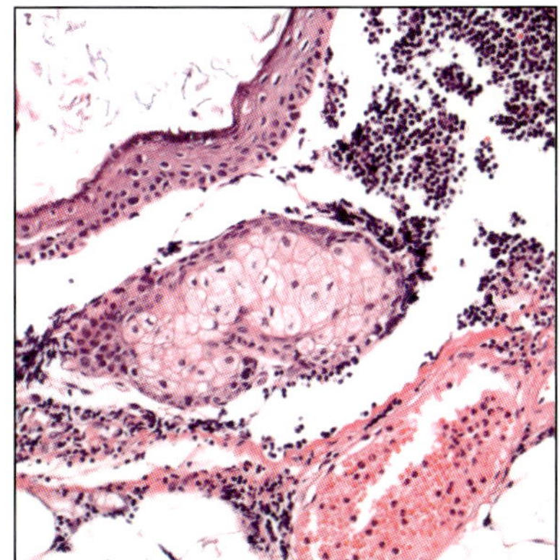
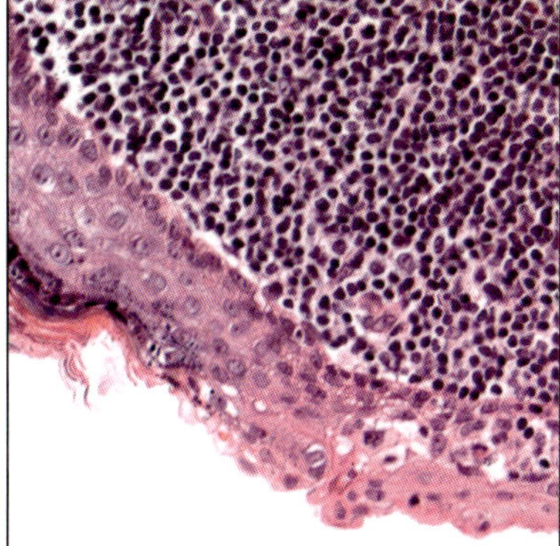
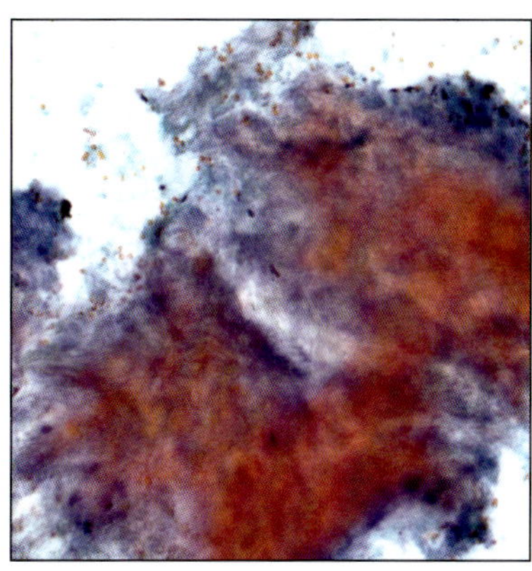

(Left) *This dermoid cyst contains mature squamous epithelium with underlying sebaceous differentiation and lymphoid tissue. Mesodermal differentiation is only rarely present in dermoid cysts of the pancreas.* ***(Center)*** *This high-power view shows mature keratinizing squamous epithelium with underlying lymphoid stroma in a dermoid cyst.* ***(Right)*** *This aspirate from a lymphoepithelial cyst shows anucleate squamous cells. A dermoid cyst would have a similar appearance.*

WELL-DIFFERENTIATED NEUROENDOCRINE NEOPLASM, PANCREAS

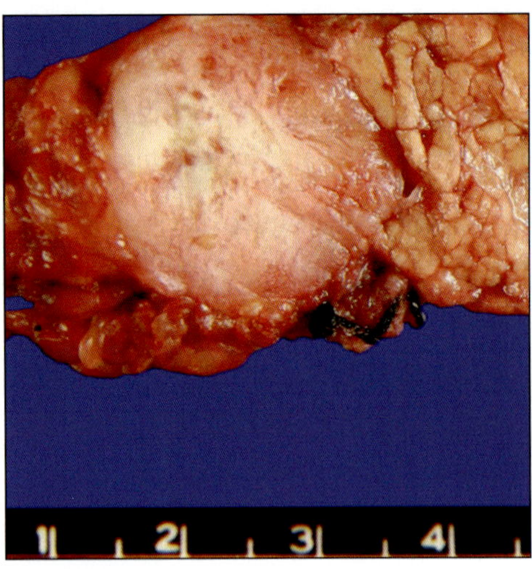

This well-circumscribed solid mass in the pancreas is typical of a well-differentiated neuroendocrine tumor.

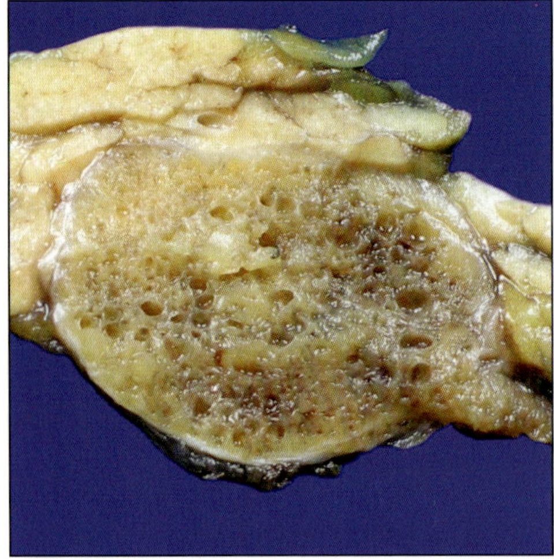

This pancreatic endocrine neoplasm has a microcystic appearance that mimics a serous cystadenoma.

TERMINOLOGY

Abbreviations

- Pancreatic endocrine neoplasm (PEN)

Synonyms

- Pancreatic endocrine tumor
- Islet cell tumor
- Pancreatic neuroendocrine tumor

Definitions

- Low- to intermediate-grade neuroendocrine neoplasm of pancreas

ETIOLOGY/PATHOGENESIS

Syndromic

- Multiple endocrine neoplasia syndrome (MEN1)
- von Hippel-Lindau syndrome
- Tuberous sclerosis

Sporadic

- Majority of cases are nonsyndromic and sporadic

CLINICAL ISSUES

Presentation

- Epidemiology
  - Peak incidence between 30-60 years
  - No significant gender predilection
- Presenting symptoms
  - Abdominal pain
  - Jaundice
  - Asymptomatic, detected by imaging
    - Such incidentally detected pancreatic endocrine neoplasms are increasingly common
- Endocrine function
  - Functioning tumors
    - Insulinoma
    - Glucagonoma
    - Somatostatinoma
    - Gastrinoma
    - Vipomas
  - Nonfunctional tumors
    - More common than functional tumors

Treatment

- Surgical approaches
  - Surgical resection remains mainstay of therapy for tumors confined to pancreas
    - Enucleation is restricted to small tumors (typically < 2 cm)
  - Options for tumors metastatic to liver
    - Resection of primary and surgical debulking of metastatic tumor
    - Long-acting somatostatin analogs (octreotide and lanreotide)
    - Liver-directed therapy including embolization, chemoembolization, radiofrequency ablation
    - Novel agents such as inhibitor of VEGF, inhibitor of tyrosine kinase, and mTOR pathway

Prognosis

- Outcome is variable
  - Histological and immunohistochemical features help estimate risk of aggressive behavior
- Features associated with adverse outcome include
  - Mitosis > 2/10 HPF
  - Tumor necrosis
  - Vascular invasion
  - Perineural invasion
  - High Ki-67 labeling index
  - Cytokeratin 19 positive tumor
  - Size > 2 cm

WELL-DIFFERENTIATED NEUROENDOCRINE NEOPLASM, PANCREAS

Key Facts

Etiology/Pathogenesis
- MEN1
- von Hippel-Lindau syndrome
- Tuberous sclerosis
- Sporadic

Clinical Issues
- Surgical resection remains mainstay of therapy for tumors confined to pancreas
- Features associated with adverse outcome include
  - Mitosis > 2/10 HPF
  - Tumor necrosis
  - Vascular invasion
  - High Ki-67 labeling index

Microscopic Pathology
- Monotonous population of round cells arranged in wide range of patterns including nested, trabecular, glandular, and solid

Ancillary Tests
- Chromogranin and synaptophysin
  - Diffusely and strongly positive
- Ki-67

Top Differential Diagnoses
- Acinar cell carcinoma
- Solid pseudopapillary neoplasm
- Poorly differentiated endocrine carcinoma

IMAGE FINDINGS

CT Findings
- Solid, or less commonly, solid and cystic, well-circumscribed, enhancing lesion

MACROSCOPIC FEATURES

General Features
- Solid, round to oval, well-circumscribed mass
- Approximately 5% of tumors are cystic
  - Either multilocular or unicystic

Size
- Tumors < 0.5 cm are termed microadenomas

MICROSCOPIC PATHOLOGY

Histologic Features
- Monotonous population of round cells
  - Wide range of patterns including nested, trabecular, glandular, and solid
- Nuclear chromatin is typically coarse with "salt and pepper" appearance
- Less common cytoplasmic variations include oncocytic, vacuolated lipid-rich variant, and rhabdoid
- Morphological appearance generally does not predict functional status
  - Exceptions to this rule
    - Amyloid deposits are indicative of insulinoma
- Large nucleoli may be present

ANCILLARY TESTS

Immunohistochemistry
- Chromogranin and synaptophysin
  - Diffusely and strongly positive
  - Recommended for confirmation of diagnosis
- Other neuroendocrine markers, such as CD56, CD57, and NCAM are not specific for neuroendocrine differentiation
- Cytokeratins
  - Positive for keratin 8 and 18
- Ki-67
  - Along with mitotic counts, it is the only widely accepted predictive marker
- Immunohistochemistry for peptide hormones
  - Rarely required for diagnosis
  - Nonfunctional tumors may stain for multiple peptides
- Marker for PENs in metastatic setting
  - ISL1 positivity would support primary endocrine tumor in pancreas

DIFFERENTIAL DIAGNOSIS

Acinar Cell Carcinoma
- Acinar pattern suggests acinar cell carcinoma
- Intracytoplasmic PAS-positive diastase-resistant granules are present
- Immunohistochemistry: Tumor cells are positive for trypsin

Solid-Pseudopapillary Neoplasm
- Pseudopapillary pattern is only rarely observed in PENs
- Nuclear features are distinctive
  - Oval nuclei with fine, evenly distributed chromatin and longitudinal nuclear grooves
- Immunohistochemistry
  - β-catenin: Intranuclear reactivity
  - E-cadherin: Total loss of membrane staining

Poorly Differentiated Endocrine Carcinoma
- Show > 10 mitoses per HPF

WELL-DIFFERENTIATED NEUROENDOCRINE NEOPLASM, PANCREAS

Immunohistochemistry

Antibody	Reactivity	Staining Pattern	Comment
Chromogranin-A	Positive	Cytoplasmic	SPT negative; ACC may be focally positive
Synaptophysin	Positive	Cytoplasmic	Both SPT (weak) and ACC may be positive
E-cadherin	Positive	Cell membrane	SPT negative; ACC positive
Trypsin	Negative	Cytoplasmic	ACC positive; SPT negative
β-catenin-nuclear	Negative	Nuclear	SPT positive; ACC negative

WHO Criteria for Clinicopathological Classification of Pancreatic Endocrine Tumors

WHO Tumor Type	Criteria
Well-differentiated endocrine tumor: Benign	Confined to pancreas, no angioinvasive, no perineural invasion, < 2 cm in diameter, < 2 mitoses/10 HPF, and < 2% Ki-67 positive cells
Well-differentiated endocrine tumor: Uncertain behavior	Confined to pancreas and 1 or more of the following features: Angioinvasive, perineural invasion, ≥ 2 cm in diameter, 2-10 mitoses/10 HPF, and > 2% Ki-67 positive cells
Well-differentiated endocrine carcinoma	Gross local invasion &/or metastasis
Poorly differentiated endocrine carcinoma	> 10 mitoses/10 HPF

Minimal Data Set

Required Data - 1	Required Data - 2
Size	*Neuroendocrine markers: Chromogranin, synaptophysin
Presence of unusual histologic features (oncocytic, clear cell, gland forming, etc.)	*Ki-67 labeling index (count multiple regions with highest labeling density, report average percentage; "eyeballed" estimate is adequate)
Grade (specify grading system used)	Mitotic rate
Extent of invasion (use anatomic landmarks for the AJCC T-staging of analogous carcinomas of the same anatomic sites)	Presence of vascular and perineural invasion
	Resection margins, lymph node metastasis

Optional data. However, these are encouraged on biopsy material.

DIAGNOSTIC CHECKLIST

Clinically Relevant Pathologic Features

- Functional tumors are defined on basis of clinical symptoms and not immunohistochemical findings

Pathologic Interpretation Pearls

- Multiple endocrine tumors suggest syndrome, such as MEN1 and VHL syndrome
- Rarely, tumors < 2 cm and without aggressive features may metastasize
- Morphologically PENs and SPNs may be indistinguishable
  - Tumors negative for chromogranin may represent solid-pseudopapillary tumors
  - β-catenin and E-cadherin should be performed on such cases

GRADING

Grade 1

- Mitosis < 2 per 10 HPF, Ki-67 ≤ 2

Grade 2

- Mitosis 2-20 per 10 HPF, Ki-67 > 2-20

Grade 3

- Mitosis > 20 per 10 HPF, Ki-67 > 20
  - Mitotic count should be based upon counting 50 high-power (40x objective) fields in area of highest mitotic activity and reported as number of mitoses per 10 HPF
  - Ki-67 index reported as percentage of positive tumor cells in area of highest nuclear labeling; recommendation is to count 2,000 tumor cells to determine Ki-67 index, but this may not be practical for routine clinical purposes

STAGING

AJCC Cancer Staging Manual 7th Edition

- Use AJCC staging for pancreatic ductal adenocarcinomas

SELECTED REFERENCES

1. Klimstra DS et al: Pathology reporting of neuroendocrine tumors: application of the Delphic consensus process to the development of a minimum pathology data set. Am J Surg Pathol. 34(3):300-13, 2010

Microscopic Features

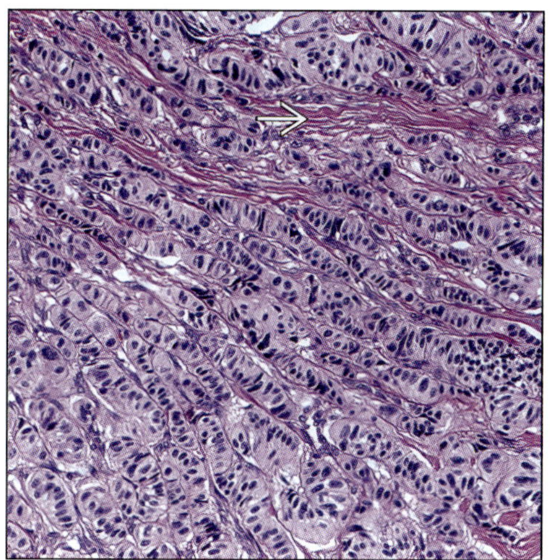

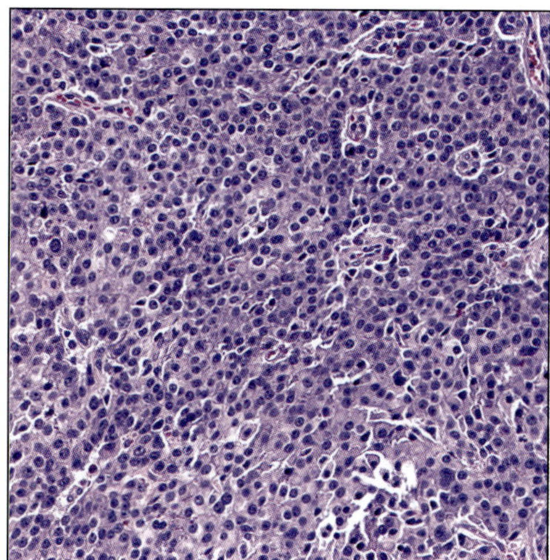

(Left) *This pancreatic endocrine tumor shows prominent trabecular architecture. The monotony of the cells suggest neuroendocrine cell differentiation. Scant collagenous stroma is present ➡. Some pancreatic endocrine neoplasms may show abundant stroma.* ***(Right)*** *This pancreatic endocrine neoplasm has a solid pattern of growth.*

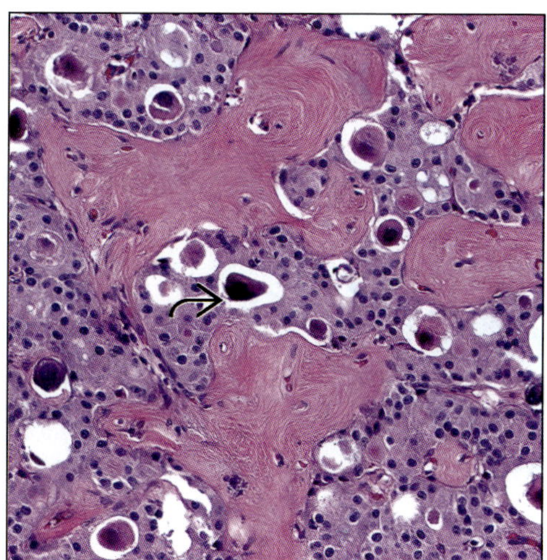

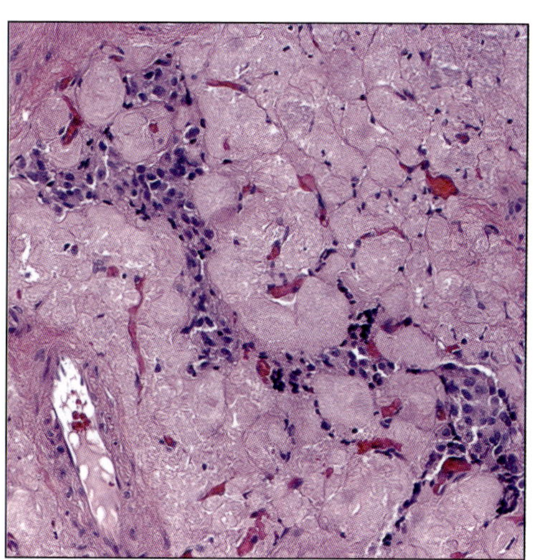

(Left) *This pancreatic endocrine tumor shows a prominent acinar pattern and intraluminal calcifications ➡. On immunohistochemistry, the tumor was positive for insulin.* ***(Right)*** *This well-differentiated endocrine tumor contains abundant amyloid. The amyloid is composed of islet amyloid polypeptide.*

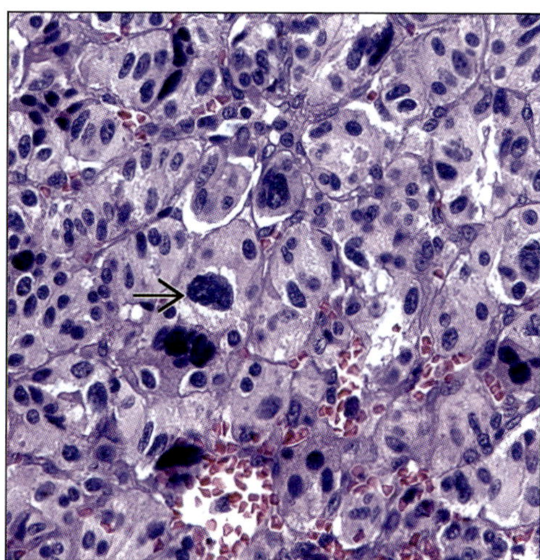

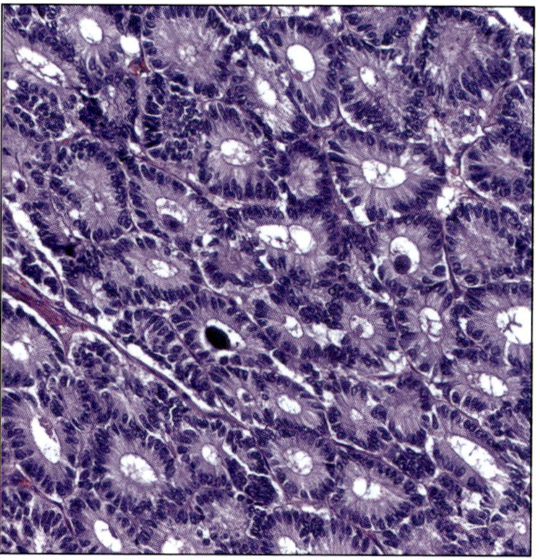

(Left) *Marked pleomorphism ➡ is occasionally seen in pancreatic endocrine tumors. This finding does not affect patient survival.* ***(Right)*** *This pancreatic endocrine tumor has a predominantly glandular/acinar pattern of growth. This appearance may mimic an acinar cell carcinoma.*

Microscopic Features

*(**Left**) Punctate foci of necrosis ⇨ are seen in a well-differentiated endocrine tumor. (**Right**) Perineural invasion ↷, like tumor necrosis, is predictive of aggressive behavior.*

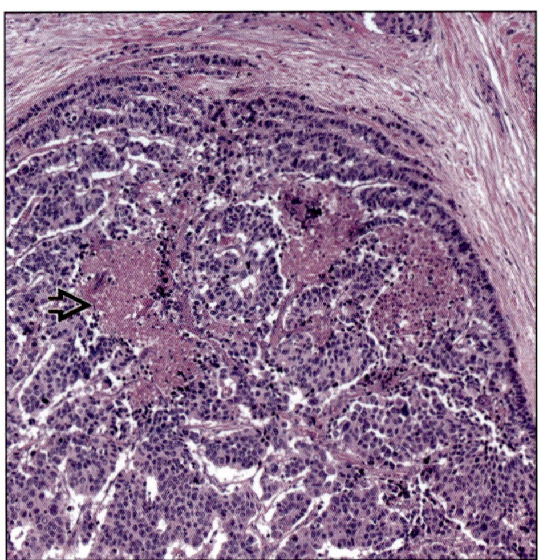

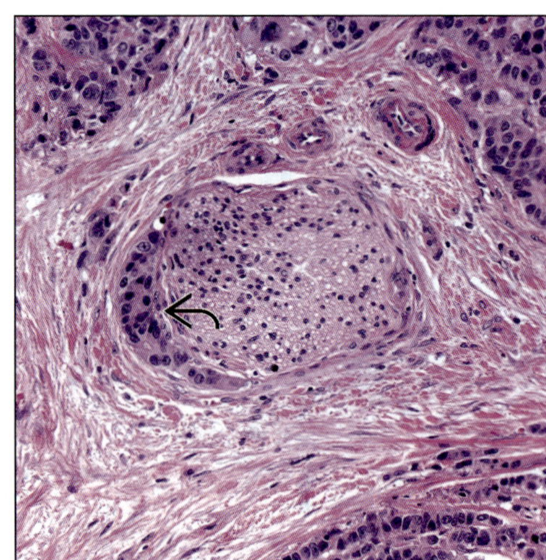

*(**Left**) This pancreatic endocrine tumor presented as a unilocular cyst without a mural nodule. A thin layer of tumor ⇨ is compressed along the fibrous cyst wall. (**Right**) This pancreatic endocrine tumor contains entrapped ductules →. This does not indicate a mixed ductal-endocrine tumor.*

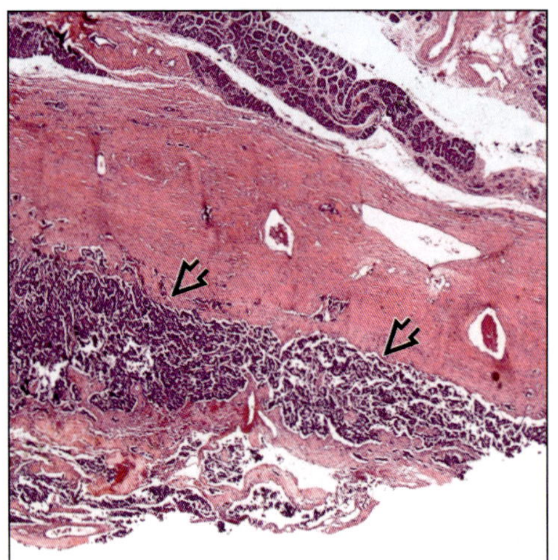

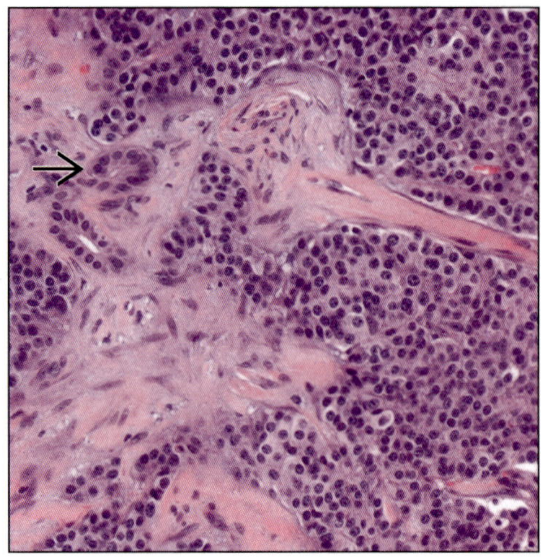

*(**Left**) Pancreatic endocrine tumors are diffusely positive for chromogranin. Absence of reactivity for chromogranin should prompt reevaluation of the diagnosis (**Right**) This is a pancreatic microadenoma ↷ from an individual with MEN1 syndrome. In contrast to normal islets →, microadenomas either show absence of insulin staining or only focal insulin reactivity. Pancreata resected from individuals with MEN1 show large numbers of microadenomas.*

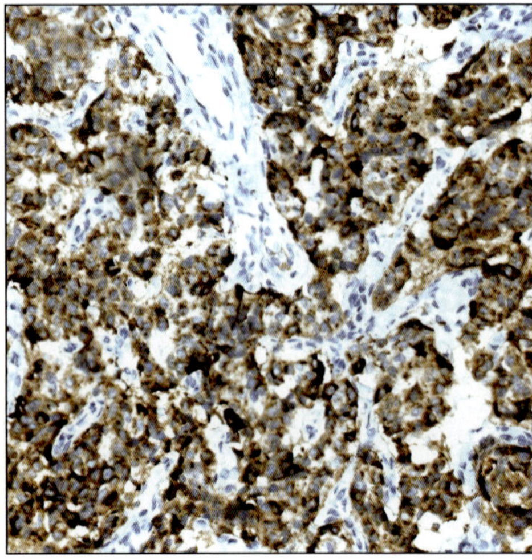

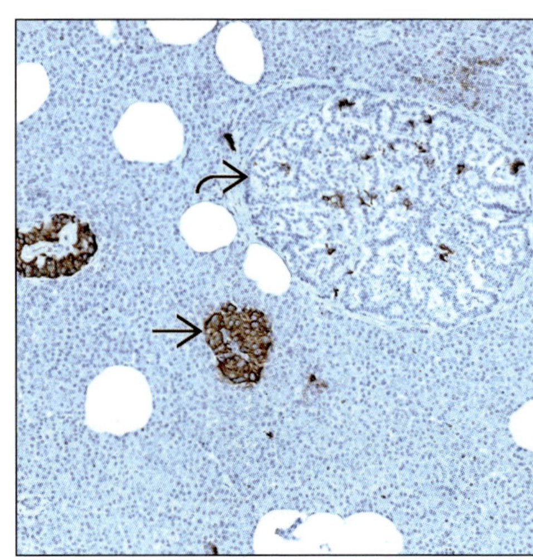

Microscopic Features

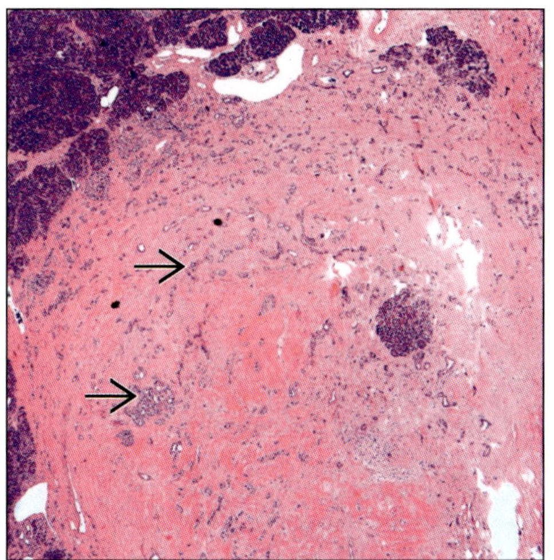

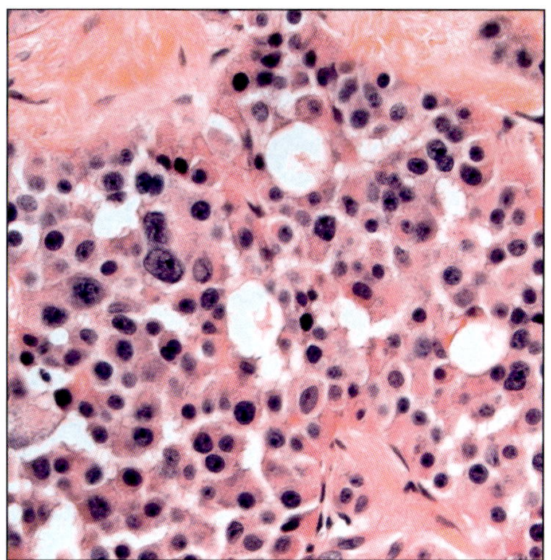

*(**Left**) In this pancreatic endocrine neoplasm with abundant hyalinized stroma, a small percentage of endocrine tumors show extensive hyalinization. Note the entrapped nests of tumor cells ⇒. (**Right**) In this pancreatic endocrine tumor with abundant eosinophilic cytoplasm, these tumors may be referred to as endocrine tumors with oncocytic change.*

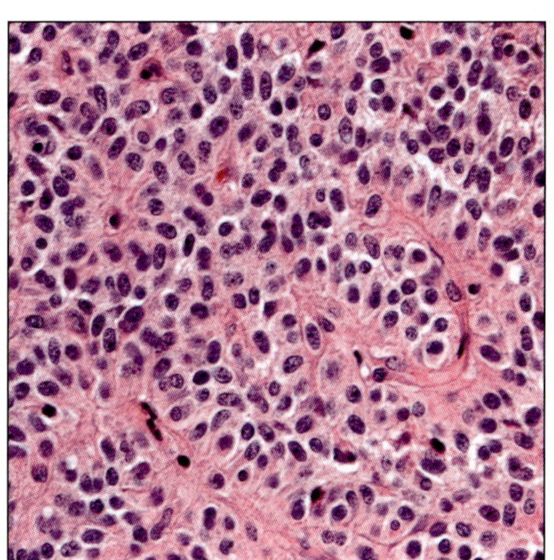

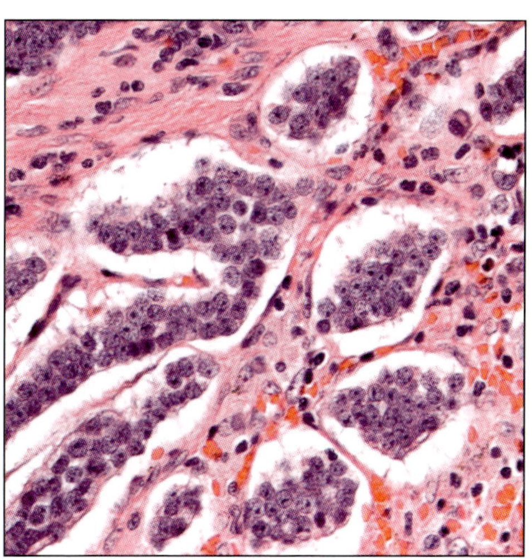

*(**Left**) This solid-pseudopapillary tumor of the pancreas closely mimics a endocrine tumor. However, oval nuclei are seldom seen in pancreatic endocrine tumors. (**Right**) In this pancreatic endocrine tumor with a nested pattern of growth, the nuclei are essentially all round.*

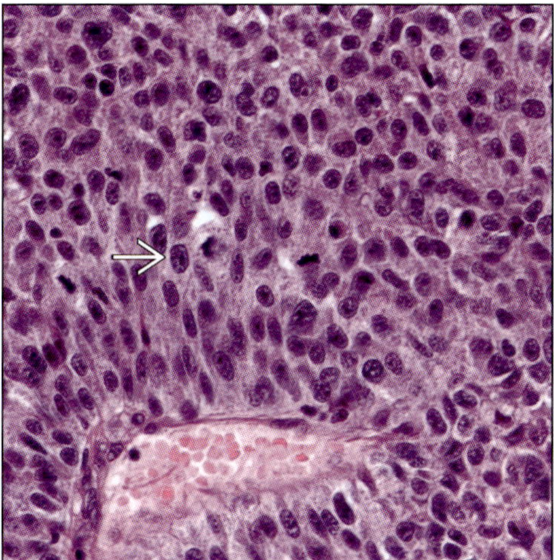

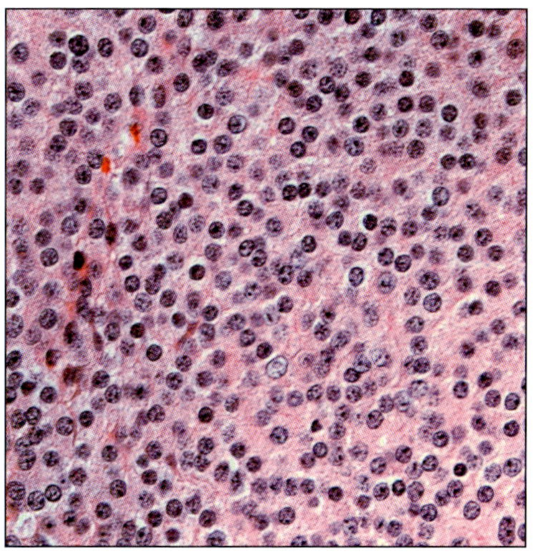

*(**Left**) Acinar cell carcinoma with a solid growth pattern may mimic a pancreatic endocrine tumor. The large and prominent nucleoli ➡ would favor acinar cell carcinoma. However, immunohistochemical analysis is required to make this distinction. (**Right**) The round monotonous nuclei support a diagnosis of PEN, seen here with a solid growth pattern. However, immunohistochemical analysis to exclude solid-pseudopapillary tumor and acinar cell carcinoma may be required.*

POORLY DIFFERENTIATED NEUROENDOCRINE CARCINOMA, PANCREAS

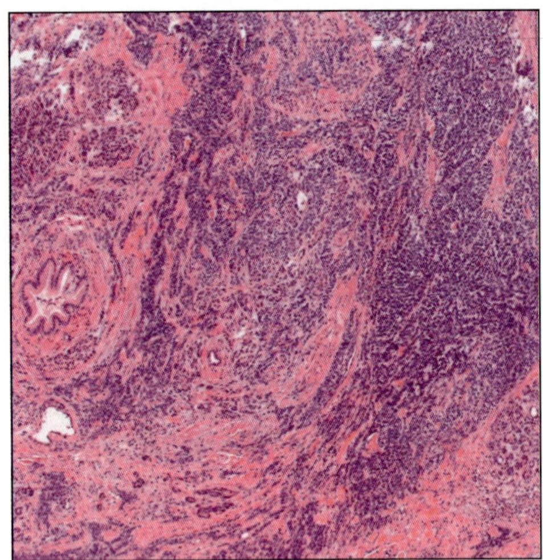

The pancreatic parenchyma is replaced by a poorly differentiated neuroendocrine carcinoma, featuring small round blue tumor cells organized in sheets and trabeculae.

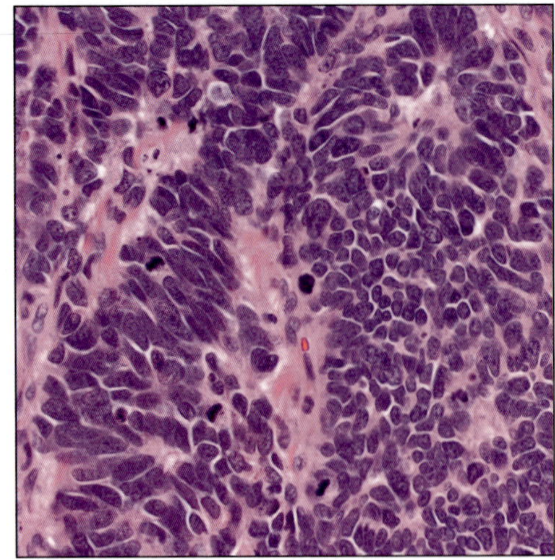

Most poorly differentiated neuroendocrine carcinomas of the pancreas are virtually identical to small cell carcinoma of the lung. Note the hyperchromatic nuclei with moulding and prominent apoptosis.

TERMINOLOGY

Synonyms

- Small cell carcinoma
- High-grade neuroendocrine carcinoma
- Poorly differentiated endocrine carcinoma

Definitions

- Clinically aggressive carcinoma of pancreas with morphological features suggestive of neuroendocrine differentiation and high proliferation (> 10 mitotic figures/10 HPF)

ETIOLOGY/PATHOGENESIS

Unknown

- No unequivocal evidence that well-differentiated endocrine neoplasms progress to poorly differentiated carcinomas

CLINICAL ISSUES

Epidemiology

- Incidence
  - Rare, constituting 2-3% of all pancreatic endocrine neoplasms

Presentation

- Jaundice
- Back pain
- Some patients present with hormonal symptoms including Cushing syndrome and hypercalcemia

Treatment

- Surgical approaches
  - Radical pancreatic surgery
    - Many patients unresectable at diagnosis
  - Platinum-based chemotherapy similar to that used with small cell carcinoma of lung

Prognosis

- Aggressive neoplasms
  - Survival typically a few months, less than ductal adenocarcinoma of pancreas
- Occasional cases have responded to cisplatin-based chemotherapy

MACROSCOPIC FEATURES

Size

- Typically large tumors
  - Solid white to tan

MICROSCOPIC PATHOLOGY

Histologic Features

- Small cell variant
  - Resembles small cell carcinoma of lung
  - Diffuse sheet-like arrangement of cells
    - Small to medium-sized cells with scant cytoplasm, hyperchromatic nuclei, gritty chromatin, and prominent nuclear moulding
  - Necrosis invariably seen; varies from punctate foci to geographic necrosis
  - Extensive vascular and perineural invasion is common
  - Mitotic figures typically > 50/HPF
    - By definition, at least 10 mitotic figures/HPF are required
- Large cell neuroendocrine variant
  - Resembles large cell neuroendocrine carcinoma of lung
  - Pronounced neuroendocrine architecture seen, most commonly tumor nests and trabeculae
    - Abundant eosinophilic cytoplasm, vesicular nuclei, and prominent nucleoli
    - Gland formation is not a feature

Key Facts

Clinical Issues

- Very aggressive neoplasms
- Patients may benefit from platinum-based chemotherapy

Microscopic Pathology

- Small cell variant
  - Resembles small cell carcinomas of lung
  - Scant cytoplasm, hyperchromatic nuclei, prominent nuclear moulding
  - At least 10 mitotic figures/HPF are required
- Large cell variant
  - Resembles large cell neuroendocrine carcinoma of lung
  - Frequent mitoses (> 10/10 HPF), vascular invasion, necrosis

Ancillary Tests

- Positive for neuroendocrine markers, keratin

- Aggressive cytologic features, including frequent mitoses (> 10/10 HPF), vascular invasion, and necrosis, invariably seen

ANCILLARY TESTS

Immunohistochemistry

- Chromogranin and synaptophysin
  - Positive but reactivity may be focal &/or weak
  - Documenting immunohistochemical evidence of neuroendocrine differentiation not required with small cell carcinoma variant
  - Positive reactivity with synaptophysin or chromogranin is required for diagnosis of large cell carcinoma variant
- Cytokeratin positive

DIFFERENTIAL DIAGNOSIS

Well-Differentiated Neuroendocrine Neoplasm

- Lack brisk mitotic activity and typically show < 10 mitoses/10HPF
- Lack nuclear features of small cell carcinoma

Poorly Differentiated Adenocarcinoma

- Lacks histologic and immunohistochemical evidence of neuroendocrine differentiation
- Gland formation invariably noted

Metastatic Small Cell Carcinomas from Lung

- TTF-1 positive
  - Rare extrapulmonary small cell carcinomas: TTF-1(+)

Other Malignant Round Cell Tumors

- Rhabdomyosarcoma, desmoplastic round cell tumor, and primitive neuroectodermal tumor (PNET)
- Desmin, WT1, and CD99 positive

DIAGNOSTIC CHECKLIST

Clinically Relevant Pathologic Features

- Important to make diagnosis as patients may benefit from platinum-based chemotherapy

Pathologic Interpretation Pearls

- Tumors resemble their pulmonary counterparts

SELECTED REFERENCES

1. Sakamoto H et al: Small cell carcinoma of the pancreas: role of EUS-FNA and subsequent effective chemotherapy using carboplatin and etoposide. J Gastroenterol. 44(5):432-8, 2009
2. Bismar TA et al: Desmoplastic small cell tumor in the pancreas. Am J Surg Pathol. 28(6):808-12, 2004
3. Movahedi-Lankarani S et al: Primitive neuroectodermal tumors of the pancreas: a report of seven cases of a rare neoplasm. Am J Surg Pathol. 26(8):1040-7, 2002
4. Reyes CV et al: Undifferentiated small cell carcinoma of the pancreas: a report of five cases. Cancer. 47(10):2500-2, 1981

IMAGE GALLERY

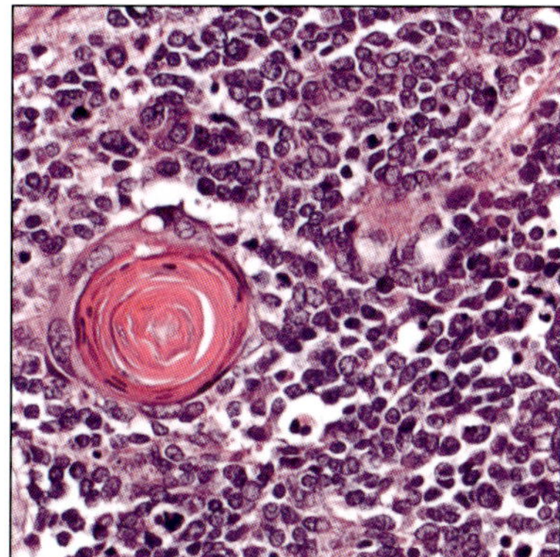

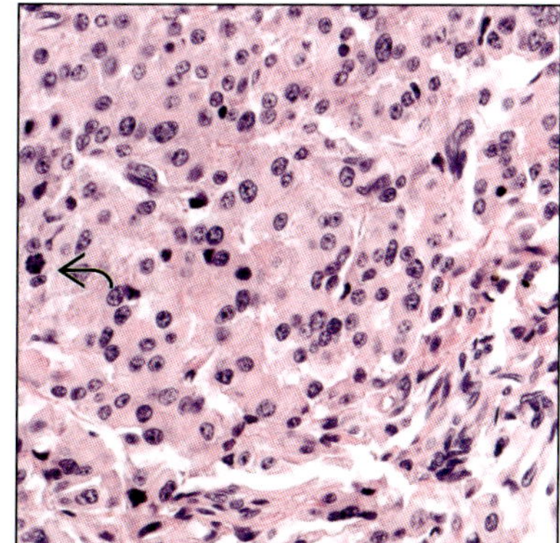

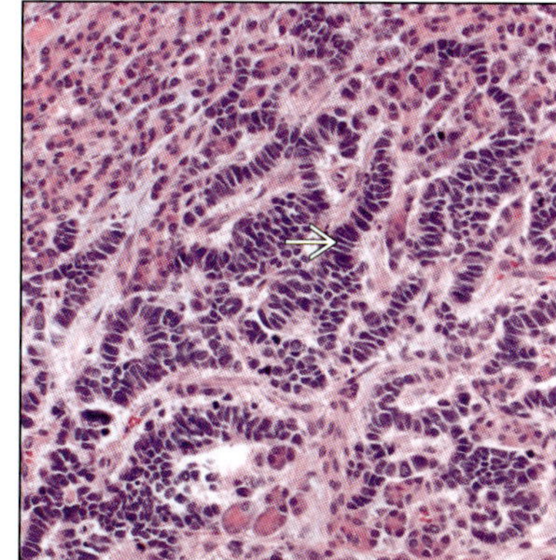

(Left) *Focal squamous differentiation is present in an otherwise typical poorly differentiated neuroendocrine carcinoma.* ***(Center)*** *This poorly differentiated neuroendocrine carcinoma, large cell variant, showed 30 mitoses/10 HPF ➔ and large areas of necrosis.* ***(Right)*** *This poorly differentiated neuroendocrine carcinoma of the pancreas was metastatic to the liver. The tumor shows prominent nuclear moulding ➔.*

SOLID-PSEUDOPAPILLARY TUMORS

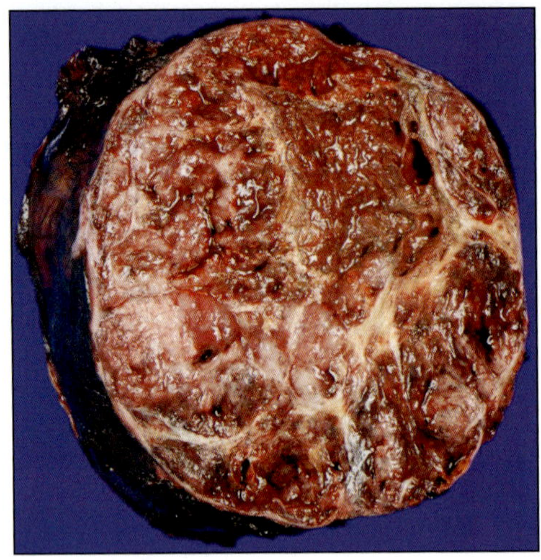

This well-demarcated tumor has a soft and friable solid surface with hemorrhagic areas. Grossly, this could mimic a pancreatic endocrine tumor.

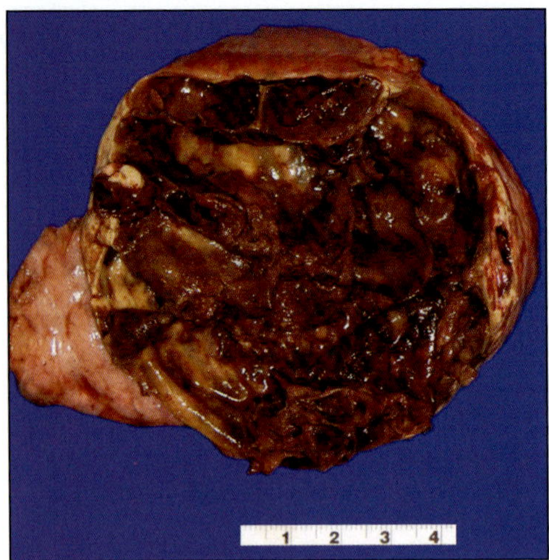

An SPT can also present as a well-demarcated hemorrhagic cystic mass that could, on imaging or gross examination, mimic a pseudocyst.

TERMINOLOGY

Abbreviations

- Solid-pseudopapillary tumor (SPT)
- Solid-pseudopapillary neoplasm (SPN)

Synonyms

- Plethora of descriptive names
  - Solid and papillary epithelial neoplasm
  - Solid cystic tumor
  - Papillary and cystic neoplasm
  - Frantz tumor

Definitions

- Low-grade malignant neoplasm of uncertain cellular differentiation
- Originally described in 1959

ETIOLOGY/PATHOGENESIS

Cellular Lineage

- Uncertain
  - Electron microscopy shows evidence of epithelial differentiation

Molecular

- 90-100% harbor mutations in β-catenin gene

CLINICAL ISSUES

Epidemiology

- Incidence
  - Uncommon
  - 1-2% of all exocrine pancreatic tumors
- Age
  - Most patients in 20s and 30s
    - Mean: 25-35 years
    - Overall age range: 7-79 years
- Gender
  - Female predominance
    - Male to female ratio 1:9-20

Site

- Evenly distributed throughout pancreas

Presentation

- Nonspecific symptoms related to intraabdominal mass
  - Vague abdominal pain
  - Weight loss
  - Anorexia
- May have palpable abdominal mass
- Up to 1/3 of cases discovered incidentally
- Complications
  - Rupture
  - Hemoperitoneum

Laboratory Tests

- Serum oncomarkers, laboratory tests usually normal

Natural History

- Most are indolent, slow-growing, and nonaggressive
- May directly invade stomach, duodenum, spleen
- Metastasis
  - 10-15% of cases
  - Liver, peritoneum, lymph nodes
    - Peritoneal metastases more common in patients with trauma, rupture, or drainage of neoplasm
- Rare, clinically aggressive variant

Treatment

- Surgical resection is treatment of choice
- Can recur if incompletely resected

Prognosis

- Excellent
  - > 80% cured with surgical resection
  - 10-15% of cases have metastases or recurrence
  - Even patients with metastases have favorable long-term survival
- No proven morphologic predictors of outcome

SOLID-PSEUDOPAPILLARY TUMORS

Key Facts

Terminology
- Solid-pseudopapillary tumor (SPT)
- Low-grade malignant neoplasm of uncertain cellular differentiation

Etiology/Pathogenesis
- 90-100% harbor mutations in β-*catenin* gene

Clinical Issues
- Occurs predominately in young females
- Presents with nonspecific symptoms related to intraabdominal mass
- Can be located in head, body, or tail of pancreas
- Indolent and nonaggressive behavior
- Metastasis in 10-15% of cases to liver, peritoneum, and lymph node
- > 80% are cured with surgical resection

Microscopic Pathology
- Well-demarcated large mass
- Solid monomorphic sheets of polygonal cells
- Delicate vessels surrounded by hyalinized or myxoid stroma
- Characteristic degenerative change
  - Pseudopapillae formation
- Intracytoplasmic eosinophilic hyaline globules (PASD positive)
- Uniform round to oval nuclei with finely dispersed chromatin
- Neoplastic cells often have nuclear grooves
- Immunoreactivity for β-catenin (nuclear staining)

Top Differential Diagnoses
- Pancreatic endocrine tumor

IMAGE FINDINGS

General Features
- Radiographic features reflect variable gross findings
  - Well-circumscribed neoplasm with solid and cystic components
  - Calcifications in approximately 30%

Ultrasonographic Findings
- Well-demarcated heterogeneous mass
- Variable echo texture

CT Findings
- Heterogeneous, well-circumscribed mass
- Areas with differing attenuation
- Variably present fluid/debris levels
- Pancreatic and bile ducts not dilated

MACROSCOPIC FEATURES

General Features
- Large solitary mass
  - Rarely multiple
  - Well circumscribed, can be encapsulated
  - Solid to cystic, usually mixed
    - Cystic areas often contain friable, necrotic material
    - Minority of tumors are almost completely solid or completely cystic
  - White-gray to yellow cut surface
- Evenly distributed throughout pancreas

Size
- Range: 1.5-25 cm
- Mean diameter: 9-10 cm

MICROSCOPIC PATHOLOGY

Histologic Features
- Solid monomorphic sheets of polygonal cells
  - Admixed delicate vessels surrounded by hyalinized or myxoid stroma
  - True glandular lumina not present
- Infrequent mitotic figures
- Perineural and true vascular invasion are quite rare
- Marked degenerative changes
  - Pseudopapillae formation
  - Foamy macrophages
  - Cholesterol clefts
  - Hemorrhage
  - Lipofuscin or melanin pigment
  - Calcification/ossification
  - Areas of infarction
    - Although true tumor necrosis is rare
- Interface with normal pancreas
  - Infiltration of adjacent parenchyma is common
  - "Blood lakes" common at periphery of neoplasm
  - May have fibrous capsule

Cytologic Features
- Nuclei can be oriented away from vessels, with zone of cytoplasm separating nuclei from capillaries
  - Uniform and round to oval with finely dispersed nuclear chromatin
  - Often with longitudinal nuclear grooves
- Moderate amount of eosinophilic cytoplasm but can be clear with vacuoles
- Intracytoplasmic eosinophilic hyaline globules

ANCILLARY TESTS

Histochemistry
- PASD positive intracytoplasmic eosinophilic hyaline globules

Molecular Genetics
- β-*catenin* mutational analysis
  - Missense mutations in > 83% of cases
  - Mutation inactives glycogen synthase kinase-3 β
    - Results in cytoplasmic accumulation of β-catenin protein that translocates into the nucleus

SOLID-PSEUDOPAPILLARY TUMORS

Immunohistochemistry

Antibody	Reactivity	Staining Pattern	Comment
β-catenin	Positive	Nuclear & cytoplasmic	> 90% of tumors
Vimentin	Positive	Cytoplasmic	Diffuse and strong
α-1-antitrypsin	Positive	Cytoplasmic	In tumor cells and hyaline globules
CD10	Positive	Cytoplasmic	
PR	Positive	Nuclear	
NSE	Positive	Cytoplasmic	Diffuse
CD56	Positive	Cytoplasmic	Variable intensity
Cyclin-D1	Positive	Nuclear	> 70% of tumors
FLI-1	Positive	Nuclear	38-63%
CD117	Positive	Cytoplasmic	50% of tumors
Synaptophysin	Positive	Cytoplasmic	Diffuse to focal and weak
ERP-β	Positive	Nuclear	
Chromogranin-A	Negative		
E-cadherin	Negative		Loss of membranous staining with antibody to extracellular domain
CD34	Negative		
CK7	Negative		
CK19	Negative		
EMA	Negative		
CK8/18/CAM5.2	Equivocal	Cytoplasmic	Mostly negative, focal weak in < 20% of tumors
AE13	Equivocal	Cytoplasmic	Focal weak, 50% of tumors

DIFFERENTIAL DIAGNOSIS

Pseudocyst

- No epithelial lining
  - Submit entire cyst before rendering this diagnosis
- More common in men
- History of pancreatitis, elevated amylase
- High levels of amylase in cyst fluid

Pancreatic Endocrine Tumor

- Well-differentiated endocrine tumors classically have nuclei with "salt and pepper" chromatin pattern
- Synaptophysin and chromogranin positive
- β-catenin and CD10 negative

Acinar Cell Carcinoma

- Typically, a solid neoplasm
- Cytologically different
  - Cohesive cells
    - Granular cytoplasm
    - More nuclear pleomorphism and mitoses
    - Prominent nucleoli
  - Lumen formation is present
- Trypsin &/or chymotrypsin positive; negative for β-catenin
- However, both neoplasms can be positive for α-1-antitrypsin

DIAGNOSTIC CHECKLIST

Clinically Relevant Pathologic Features

- Typically in young women
- Solid and cystic gross appearance

Pathologic Interpretation Pearls

- Nuclear staining for β-catenin
- Nuclear grooves, pseudopapillae are characteristic

SELECTED REFERENCES

1. Basturk O et al: Pancreatic cysts: pathologic classification, differential diagnosis, and clinical implications. Arch Pathol Lab Med. 133(3):423-38, 2009
2. Comper F et al: Expression pattern of claudins 5 and 7 distinguishes solid-pseudopapillary from pancreatoblastoma, acinar cell and endocrine tumors of the pancreas. Am J Surg Pathol. 33(5):768-74, 2009
3. Adsay NV: Cystic neoplasia of the pancreas: pathology and biology. J Gastrointest Surg. 12(3):401-4, 2008
4. Klimstra DS: Nonductal neoplasms of the pancreas. Mod Pathol. 20 Suppl 1:S94-112, 2007
5. Tang LH et al: Clinically aggressive solid pseudopapillary tumors of the pancreas: a report of two cases with components of undifferentiated carcinoma and a comparative clinicopathologic analysis of 34 conventional cases. Am J Surg Pathol. 29(4):512-9, 2005
6. Kosmahl M et al: Cystic neoplasms of the pancreas and tumor-like lesions with cystic features: a review of 418 cases and a classification proposal. Virchows Arch. 445(2):168-78, 2004
7. Abraham SC et al: Solid-pseudopapillary tumors of the pancreas are genetically distinct from pancreatic ductal adenocarcinomas and almost always harbor beta-catenin mutations. Am J Pathol. 160(4):1361-9, 2002

Microscopic and Immunohistochemical Features

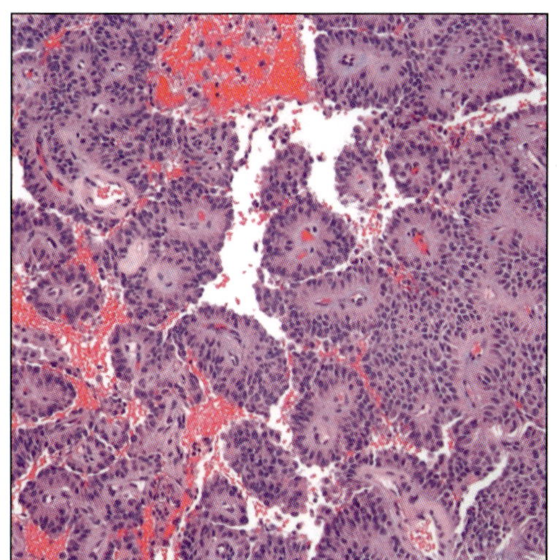

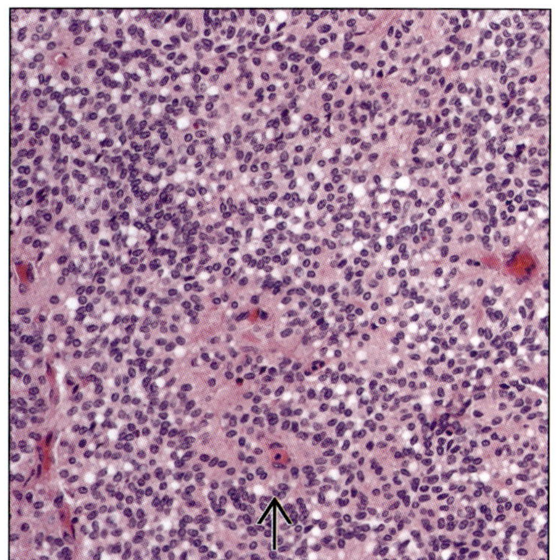

(Left) *Solid sheets of tumor cells become discohesive and result in a characteristic feature of SPT, pseudopapillary formation with a central fibrovascular-like core surrounded by neoplastic cells.* ***(Right)*** *The sheets of tumor cells have overlapping, round to oval nuclei that are oriented away from the vessels ➔ with a rim of cytoplasm toward the capillary. There is lumen formation.*

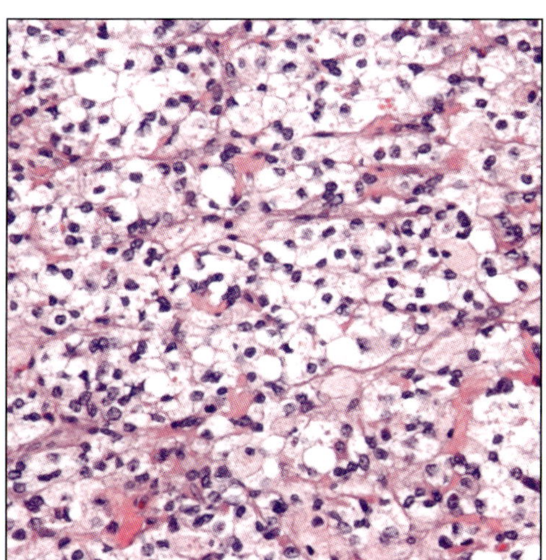

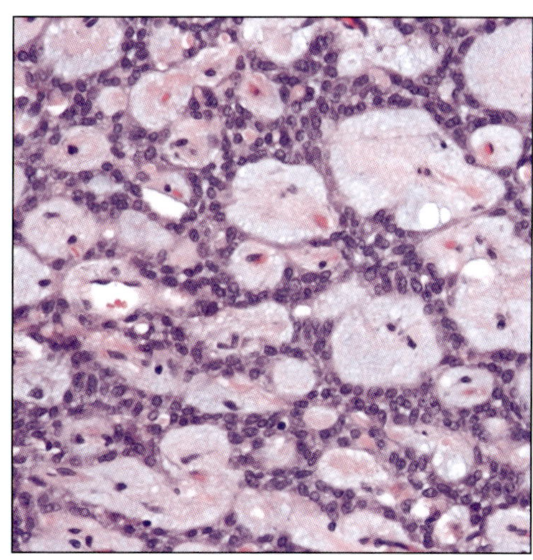

(Left) *Typically the neoplastic cells are polygonal with eosinophilic cytoplasm, but these tumors can also have clear cytoplasm or, rarely, be composed of monomorphic spindle cells. The cytological features can overlap those of a pancreatic endocrine tumor; thus, immunohistochemical stains are useful in distinguishing these entities.* ***(Right)*** *The delicate vessels within an SPT can have myxoid stroma, as displayed in this case, or may be hyalinized.*

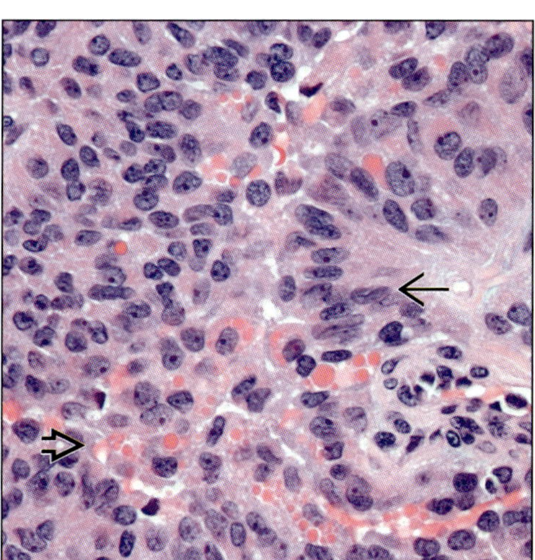

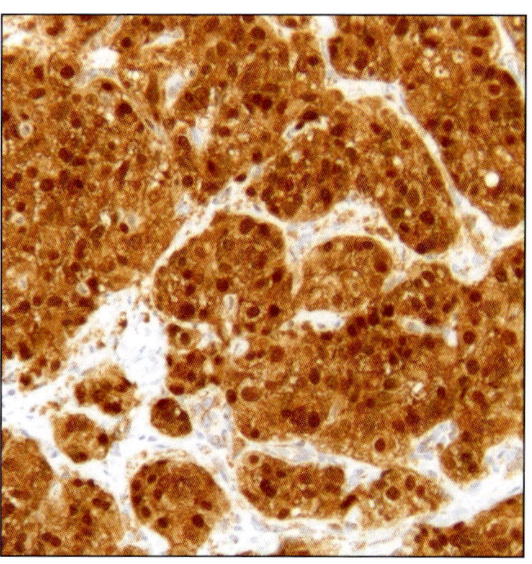

(Left) *Tumor cells have round to oval nuclei and sometimes exhibit longitudinal nuclear grooves ➔. These intra- and extracytoplasmic eosinophilic hyaline globules ⇨ stain positive for PASD and α-1-antitrypsin.* ***(Right)*** *A valuable immunohistochemical stain for the diagnosis is β-catenin since > 90% of SPTs display an abnormal nuclear and cytoplasmic staining pattern rather than cell membrane reactivity.*

ENDOCRINE PANCREAS CANCER PROTOCOL

Pancreas (Endocrine): Resection

Surgical Pathology Cancer Case Summary (Checklist)

Specimen

___ Head of pancreas
___ Body of pancreas
___ Tail of pancreas
___ Stomach
___ Common bile duct
___ Gallbladder
___ Spleen
___ Adjacent large vessels
 ___ Portal vein
 ___ Superior mesenteric vein
___ Other larger vessel (specify): ___________________________
___ Other (specify): ___________________________
___ Not specified
___ Cannot be determined

Procedure

___ Excisional biopsy (enucleation)
___ Pancreaticoduodenectomy (Whipple resection), partial pancreatectomy
___ Pancreaticoduodenectomy (Whipple resection), total pancreatectomy
___ Partial pancreatectomy, pancreatic tail
___ Other (specify): ___________________________
___ Not specified

Tumor Site (select all that apply)

___ Pancreatic head
___ Uncinate process
___ Pancreatic tail
___ Other (specify): ___________________________
___ Cannot be determined
___ Not specified

Tumor Size

Greatest dimension: _________ cm (specify size of largest tumor if multiple tumors are present)
*Additional dimensions: _________ x _________ cm
___ Cannot be determined

Tumor Focality

___ Unifocal
___ Multifocal (specify number of tumors): ___________________________
___ Cannot be determined
___ Not specified

Histologic Type

___ Well-differentiated endocrine neoplasm
___ Poorly differentiated endocrine carcinoma
 *___ Small cell carcinoma
 *___ Large cell endocrine carcinoma
___ Other (specify): ___________________________
___ Carcinoma, type cannot be determined

**World Health Organization Classification*

*___ Well-differentiated endocrine tumor, benign behavior
*___ Well-differentiated endocrine tumor, uncertain behavior
*___ Poorly differentiated endocrine carcinoma

ENDOCRINE PANCREAS CANCER PROTOCOL

*Functional Type (select all that apply)

*___ Cannot be assessed
*___ Pancreatic endocrine tumor, functional
(Correlation with clinical syndrome and elevated serum levels of hormone product)
*___ Insulin-producing (insulinoma)
*___ Glucagon-producing (glucagonoma)
*___ Somatostatin-producing (somatostatinoma)
*___ Gastrin-producing (gastrinoma)
*___ Vasoactive intestinal polypeptide (VIP)-producing (VIP-oma)
*___ Other (specify): ___________________________
*___ Pancreatic endocrine tumor, nonfunctional
*___ Pancreatic endocrine tumor, functional status unknown

Mitotic Activity (select all that apply)

___ Not applicable
___ < 2 mitoses/10 high-power fields (HPF)
Specify mitoses per 10 HPF: _________
___ 2-10 mitoses/10 HPF
Specify mitoses per 10 HPF: _________
___ > 10 mitoses per 10 HPF
___ Cannot be determined
*Ki-67 labeling index
*___ ≤ 2% Ki-67-positive cells
*___ 3-20% Ki-67-positive cells
*___ > 20% Ki-67-positive cells

*Tumor Necrosis

*___ Not identified
*___ Present
*___ Not applicable
*___ Cannot be determined

Microscopic Tumor Extension (select all that apply)

___ Cannot be determined
___ No evidence of primary tumor
___ Tumor is confined to pancreas
___ Tumor invades ampulla of Vater
___ Tumor invades common bile duct
___ Tumor invades duodenal wall
___ Tumor invades peripancreatic soft tissues
___ Tumor invades other adjacent organs or structures (specify): ___________________________

Margins (select all that apply)

___ Cannot be assessed
___ Margins uninvolved by tumor
Distance of tumor from closest margin: _________ mm
*Specify margin (if possible): ___________________________
___ Margin(s) involved by tumor
___ Uncinate process (retroperitoneal) margin (nonperitonealized surface of the uncinate process)
___ Distal pancreatic margin
___ Common bile duct margin
___ Proximal pancreatic margin
___ Other (specify): ___________________________
*___ Tumor involves posterior retroperitoneal surface of pancreas

Lymph-Vascular Invasion

___ Not identified

ENDOCRINE PANCREAS CANCER PROTOCOL

___ Present

___ Indeterminate

Pathologic Staging (pTNM)

TNM descriptors (required only if applicable) (Select all that apply)

___ m (multiple descriptors)

___ r (recurrent)

___ y (post-treatment)

Primary tumor (pT)

___ pTX: Cannot be assessed

___ pT0: No evidence of primary tumor

___ pT1: Tumor limited to pancreas, ≤ 2 cm in greatest dimension

___ pT2: Tumor limited to pancreas, > 2 cm in greatest dimension

___ pT3: Tumor extends beyond pancreas but without involvement of celiac axis or superior mesenteric artery

___ pT4: Tumor involves celiac axis or superior mesenteric artery

Regional lymph nodes (pN)

___ pNX: Cannot be assessed

___ pN0: No regional lymph node metastasis

___ pN1: Regional lymph node metastasis

Specify: Number examined: ________

Number involved: ________

Distant metastasis (pM)

___ Not applicable

___ pM1: Distant metastasis

*Specify site(s), if known: ____________________

*Additional Pathologic Findings (select all that apply)

*___ None identified

*___ Chronic pancreatitis

*___ Acute pancreatitis

*___ Adenomatosis (multiple endocrine tumors, each < 5 mm in greatest dimension)

*___ Other (specify): ____________________

*Clinical History (select all that apply)

*___ von Hippel-Lindau disease

*___ Multiple endocrine neoplasia type 1

*___ Familial pancreatic cancer syndrome

*___ Hypoglycemic syndrome

*___ Necrolytic migratory erythema

*___ Watery diarrhea

*___ Hypergastrinemia

*___ Zollinger-Ellison syndrome

*___ Other (specify): ____________________

*___ Not specified

**Data elements with asterisks are not required. However, these elements may be clinically important but are not yet validated or regularly used in patient management. Adapted with permission from College of American Pathologists, "Protocol for the Examination of Specimens from Patients with Carcinoma of the Endocrine Pancreas." Web posting date October 2009, www.cap.org.*

ENDOCRINE PANCREAS CANCER PROTOCOL

Anatomic Stage/Prognostic Groupings

Stage	Tumor	Node	Metastasis
IA	T1	N0	M0
IB	T2	N0	M0
IIA	T3	N0	M0
IIB	T1	N1	M0
	T2	N1	M0
	T3	N1	M0
III	T4	Any N	M0
IV	Any T	Any N	M1

Adapted from 7th edition AJCC Staging Forms.

ENDOCRINE PANCREAS CANCER PROTOCOL

PANCREATIC NEUROENDOCRINE TUMORS

Staging

- Same staging protocol as pancreatic exocrine tumors
  - Prognostic significance of tumor size, presence of lymph node metastases remains unclear
  - Use of this staging system will allow standardization of reporting and collection of survival data for these tumors
- Histologic prognostic factors
  - Tumor differentiation
  - Mitotic count
- Clinical prognostic factors
  - Distant metastases
  - Tumor functional status
  - Patient age

SELECTED REFERENCES

1. American Joint Committee on Cancer: AJCC Cancer Staging Manual. 7th ed. New York: Springer. 241-49, 2010
2. Ito H et al: Surgery and staging of pancreatic neuroendocrine tumors: a 14-year experience. J Gastrointest Surg. 14(5):891-8, 2010
3. Klimstra DS et al: The pathologic classification of neuroendocrine tumors: a review of nomenclature, grading, and staging systems. Pancreas. 39(6):707-12, 2010
4. Scarpa A et al: Pancreatic endocrine tumors: improved TNM staging and histopathological grading permit a clinically efficient prognostic stratification of patients. Mod Pathol. 23(6):824-33, 2010
5. Bilimoria KY et al: Application of the pancreatic adenocarcinoma staging system to pancreatic neuroendocrine tumors. J Am Coll Surg. 205(4):558-63, 2007

Staging Parameters

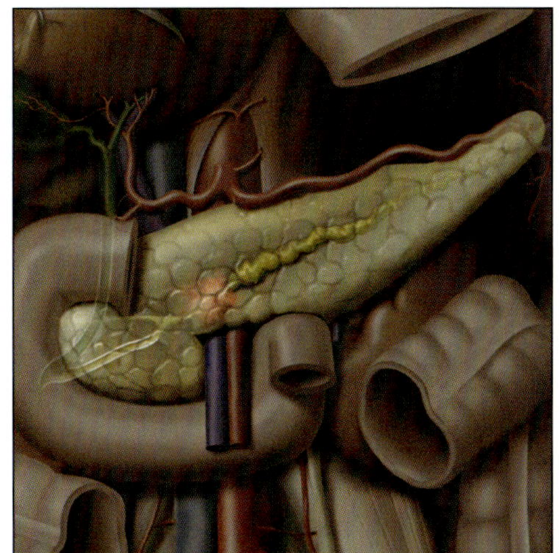

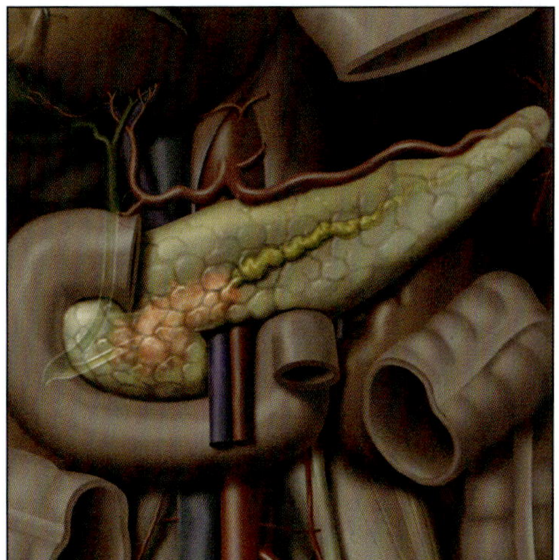

(Left) *Similar to exocrine pancreatic carcinoma, T1 disease is defined as tumor confined to the pancreas and measuring 2.0 cm or less in greatest dimension.* ***(Right)*** *T2 disease is defined as tumor confined to the pancreas but larger than 2.0 cm in greatest dimension.*

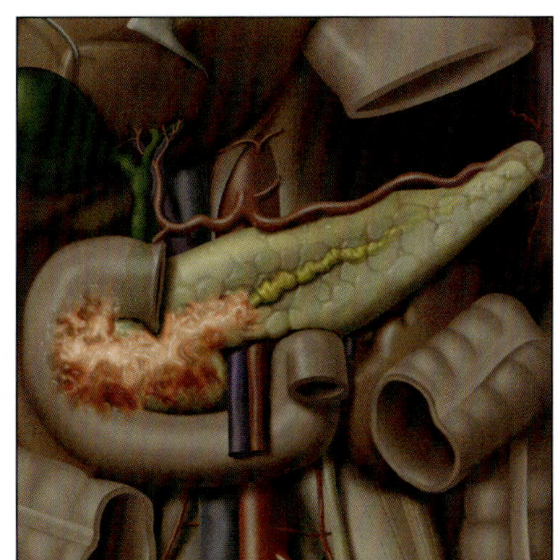

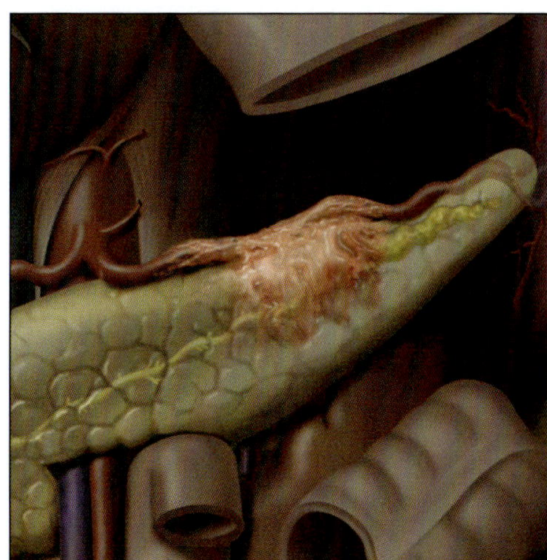

(Left) *In T3 disease, tumor extends beyond the pancreas but does not involve the celiac axis or superior mesenteric artery. This graphic illustrates tumor involving the duodenum but without involvement of the celiac axis or superior mesenteric artery.* ***(Right)*** *Involvement of the splenic artery is also classified as T3 disease.*

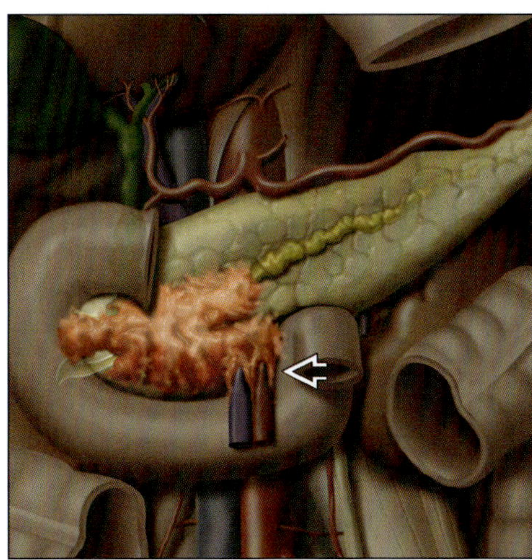

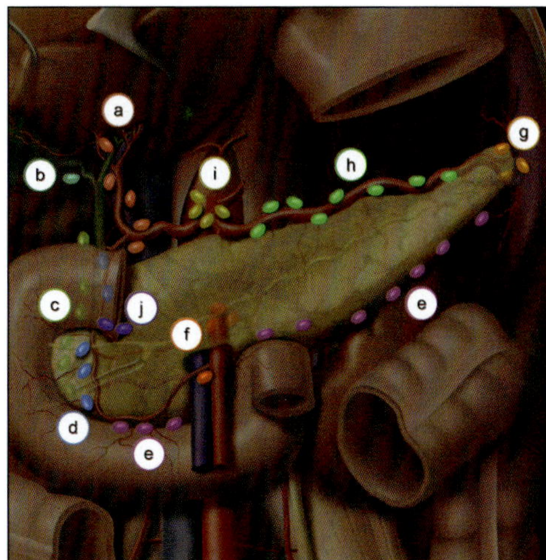

(Left) *This tumor involves the superior mesenteric artery ➔. Tumors that involve the celiac axis or superior mesenteric artery are classified as T4.* ***(Right)*** *Important regional peripancreatic lymph node groups include: a) hepatic, b) cystic duct, c) posterior pancreaticoduodenal, d) anterior pancreaticoduodenal, e) inferior, f) superior mesenteric, g) splenic hilar, h) superior, i) celiac, and j) pyloric. A minimum of 12 nodes are needed for adequate staging.*

EXOCRINE PANCREAS CANCER PROTOCOL

Pancreas (Exocrine): Resection

Surgical Pathology Cancer Case Summary (Checklist)

Specimen (select all that apply)

___ Head of pancreas
___ Body of pancreas
___ Tail of pancreas
___ Duodenum
___ Stomach
___ Common bile duct
___ Gallbladder
___ Spleen
___ Adjacent large vessels
  ___ Portal vein
  ___ Superior mesenteric vein
  ___ Other large vessel (specify): ____________________
___ Other (specify): ____________________
___ Not specified
___ Cannot be determined

Procedure

___ Pancreaticoduodenectomy (Whipple resection), partial pancreatectomy
___ Pancreatoduodenectomy (Whipple resection), total pancreatectomy
___ Partial pancreatectomy, pancreatic body
___ Partial pancreatectomy, pancreatic tail
___ Other (specify): ____________________
___ Not specified

Tumor Site (select all that apply)

___ Pancreatic head
___ Uncinate process
___ Pancreatic body
___ Other (specify): ____________________
___ Not specified

Tumor Size

Greatest dimension: ________ cm
*Additional dimensions: ________ x ________ cm
___ Cannot be determined

Histologic Type (select all that apply)

___ Ductal adenocarcinoma
___ Mucinous noncystic carcinoma
___ Signet ring cell carcinoma
___ Adenosquamous carcinoma
___ Undifferentiated (anaplastic) carcinoma
___ Undifferentiated carcinoma with osteoclast-like giant cells
___ Mixed ductal-endocrine carcinoma
___ Serous cystadenocarcinoma
  ___ Noninvasive
  ___ Invasive
___ Intraductal papillary-mucinous carcinoma
  ___ Noninvasive
  ___ Invasive
___ Acinar cell carcinoma
___ Acinar cell cystadenocarcinoma
___ Mixed acinar-endocrine carcinoma

EXOCRINE PANCREAS CANCER PROTOCOL

___ Other (specify): ___

Histologic Grade (ductal carcinoma only)

___ Not applicable
___ GX: Cannot be assessed
___ G1: Well differentiated
___ G2: Moderately differentiated
___ G3: Poorly differentiated
___ G4: Undifferentiated
___ Other (specify): ___

Microscopic Tumor Extension (select all that apply)

___ Cannot be assessed
___ No evidence of primary tumor
___ Carcinoma in situ
___ Tumor is confined to pancreas
___ Tumor invades ampulla of Vater or sphincter of Oddi
___ Tumor invades duodenal wall
___ Tumor invades peripancreatic soft tissues
  *___ Tumor invades retroperitoneal soft tissue
  *___ Tumor invades mesenteric adipose tissue
  *___ Tumor invades mesocolon
  *___ Tumor invades other peripancreatic soft tissue (specify): ___
  ___ Tumor invades extrapancreatic common bile duct
___ Tumor invades other adjacent organs or structures (specify): ___

Margins (select all that apply)

___ Cannot be assessed
___ Margins uninvolved by invasive carcinoma
  Distance of invasive carcinoma from closest margin: ___ mm
  *Specify margin (if possible): ___
___ Margins uninvolved by carcinoma in situ
___ Margin(s) involved by carcinoma in situ
  ___ Carcinoma in situ present at common bile duct margin
  ___ Carcinoma in situ present at pancreatic parenchymal margin
___ Margin(s) involved by invasive carcinoma
  ___ Uncinate process (retroperitoneal) margin (nonperitonealized surface of uncinate process)
  ___ Distal pancreatic margin
  ___ Common bile duct margin
  ___ Proximal pancreatic margin
  ___ Other (specify): ___
*___ Invasive carcinoma involves posterior retroperitoneal surface of pancreas

Treatment Effect (applicable to carcinomas treated with neoadjuvant therapy) (select all that apply)

___ No prior treatment
___ Present
  *___ No residual tumor (complete response, grade 0)
  *___ Marked response (grade 1, minimal residual cancer)
  *___ Moderate response (grade 2)
___ No definite response identified (grade 3, poor or no response)
___ Not known

Lymph-Vascular Invasion

___ Not identified
___ Present
___ Indeterminate

EXOCRINE PANCREAS CANCER PROTOCOL

Pathologic Staging (pTNM)

TNM descriptors (required only if applicable) (select all that apply)

___ m (multiple primary tumors)

___ r (recurrent)

___ y (post-treatment)

Primary tumor (pT)

___ pTX: Cannot be assessed

___ pT0: No evidence of primary tumor

___ pTis: Carcinoma in situ

___ pT1: Tumor limited to pancreas, ≤ 2 cm in greatest dimension

___ pT2: Tumor limited to pancreas, > 2 cm in greatest dimension

___ pT3: Tumor extends beyond pancreas but without involvement of celiac axis or superior mesenteric artery

___ pT3: Tumor involves celiac axis or superior mesenteric artery

Regional lymph nodes (pN)

___ pNX: Cannot be assessed

___ pN0: No regional lymph node metastasis

___ pN1: Regional lymph node metastasis

Specify: Number examined: _________

Number involved: _________

Distant metastasis (pM)

___ Not applicable

___ pM1: Distant metastasis

*Specify site(s), if known: ___________________________

**Additional Pathologic Findings (select all that apply)*

*___ None identified

*___ Pancreatic intraepithelial neoplasia (highest grade: PanIN _________)

*___ Chronic pancreatitis

*___ Acute pancreatitis

*___ Other (specify): ___________________________

**Ancillary Studies*

*Specify: ___________________________

**Clinical History (select all that apply)*

*___ Neoadjuvant therapy

*___ Familial pancreatitis

*___ Familial pancreatic cancer syndrome

*___ Other (specify): ___________________________

*___ Not specified

**Data elements with asterisks are not required. However, these elements may be clinically important but are not yet validated or regularly used in patient management. Adapted with permission from College of American Pathologists, "Protocol for the Examination of Specimens from Patients with Carcinoma of the Exocrine Pancreas." Web posting date October 2009, www.cap.org. Protocol applies to all epithelial tumors of the exocrine pancreas. Endocrine tumors and tumors of the ampulla of Vater are not included.*

EXOCRINE PANCREAS CANCER PROTOCOL

Stage Groupings

Stage	Tumor	Node	Metastasis
0	Tis	N0	M0
IA	T1	N0	M0
IB	T2	N0	M0
IIA	T3	N0	M0
IIB	T1	N1	M0
	T2	N1	M0
	T3	N1	M0
III	T4	Any N	M0
IV	Any T	Any N	M1

Adapted from 7th edition AJCC Staging Forms.

EXOCRINE PANCREAS CANCER PROTOCOL

ANATOMIC SITE OF TUMOR

Head of Pancreas

- Tumors arise to right of confluence of superior mesenteric vein and portal vein
- Includes tumors of uncinate process
- Most pancreatic carcinomas arise in this location
- Tumors often present with obstructive jaundice

Body of Pancreas

- Tumors located between left edge of superior mesenteric vein/portal vein confluence and left edge of aorta
- Often present late in course of disease

Tail of Pancreas

- Those tumors arising to left of left edge of aorta
- Often present late in course of disease

STAGING

Clinical

- Usually based on CT or MR findings
- Endoscopic ultrasound may also be helpful

Pathologic

- Depending on surgical procedure performed, evaluation of margins (bile duct, pancreatic duct, and superior mesenteric artery [retroperitoneal or uncinate]) is critical
- Most local recurrences are in soft tissue of pancreatic bed along retroperitoneal margin

Lymph Nodes

- Tumors of pancreatic head and neck
  - Regional nodes include those along common bile duct, hepatic artery, portal vein, superior mesenteric vein, right lateral wall of superior mesenteric artery, and posterior and anterior pancreaticoduodenal arcades
- Tumors of pancreatic body and tail
  - Regional nodes include those along hepatic artery, celiac axis, splenic artery, and splenic hilum
- Minimum of 12 lymph nodes required for staging

Vascular Involvement

- Superior mesenteric vein or portal vein
  - Usually T3
    - Resectable at some centers
    - Prognostic significance unknown
- Celiac axis or superior mesenteric artery
  - Classified as T4
  - Unresectable

Metastases

- Distant spread
  - Common at presentation
    - Liver, peritoneal cavity, lungs are common sites
    - Positive peritoneal cytology also considered M1 disease

SELECTED REFERENCES

1. American Joint Committee on Cancer: AJCC Cancer Staging Manual. 7th ed. New York: Springer. 29-40, 2010
2. Adsay NV et al: The number of lymph nodes identified in a simple pancreatoduodenectomy specimen: comparison of conventional vs orange-peeling approach in pathologic assessment. Mod Pathol. 22(1):107-12, 2009
3. Sohn TA et al: Resected adenocarcinoma of the pancreas-616 patients: results, outcomes, and prognostic indicators. J Gastrointest Surg. 4(6):567-79, 2000
4. Millikan KW et al: Prognostic factors associated with resectable adenocarcinoma of the head of the pancreas. Am Surg. 65(7):618-23; discussion 623-4, 1999
5. Conlon KC et al: Long-term survival after curative resection for pancreatic ductal adenocarcinoma. Clinicopathologic analysis of 5-year survivors. Ann Surg. 223(3):273-9, 1996
6. Staley CA et al: The need for standardized pathologic staging of pancreaticoduodenectomy specimens. Pancreas. 12(4):373-80, 1996
7. Hermreck AS et al: Importance of pathologic staging in the surgical management of adenocarcinoma of the exocrine pancreas. Am J Surg. 127(6):653-7, 1974

Staging Parameters

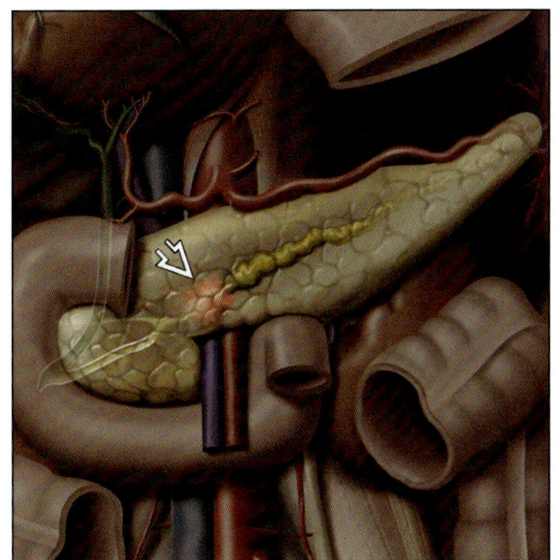

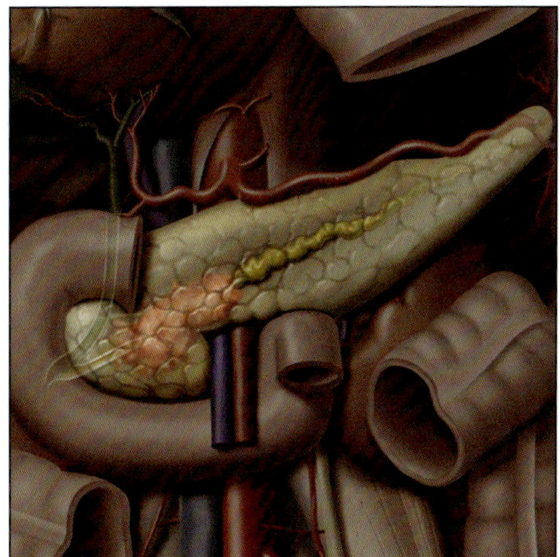

(Left) *This graphic illustrates T1 disease, defined as tumor* ➡ *limited to the pancreas and ≤ 2.0 cm in greatest dimension. There is upstream pancreatic ductal dilation. This is a resectable tumor.* ***(Right)*** *Tumors limited to the pancreas but > 2.0 cm in greatest dimension are defined as T2 disease, as seen in this graphic. Note the upstream pancreatic ductal dilation. This is a resectable tumor.*

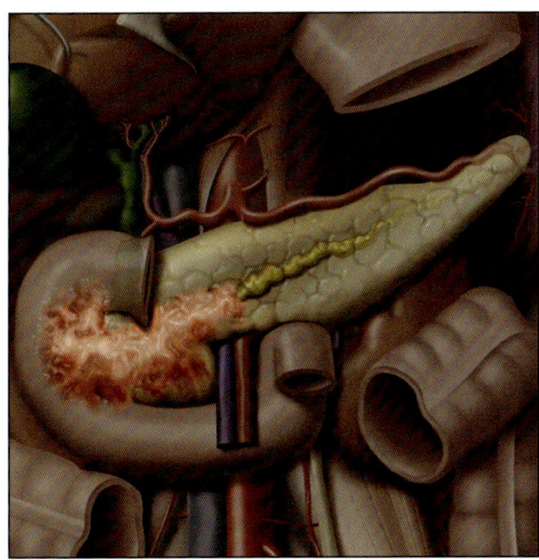

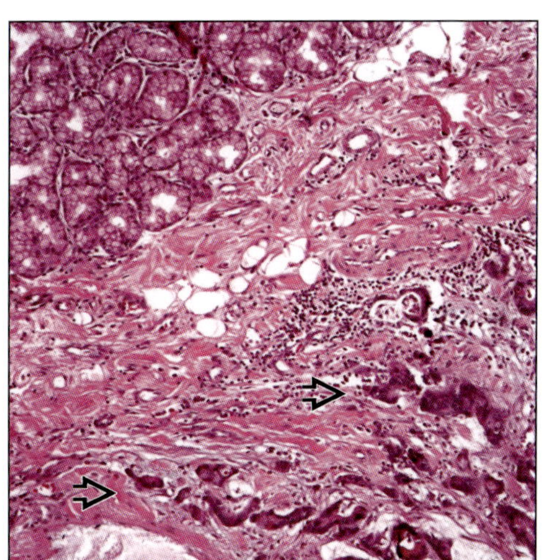

(Left) *T3 disease is defined as tumor extending beyond the pancreas but without involving the celiac axis or superior mesenteric artery. This graphic depicts involvement of the duodenum with obstruction of the pancreatic and common bile ducts. This would be a resectable tumor.* ***(Right)*** *This poorly differentiated pancreatic adenocarcinoma extends into the submucosa of the duodenum* ➡*. Note the Brunner glands in the upper left-hand corner.*

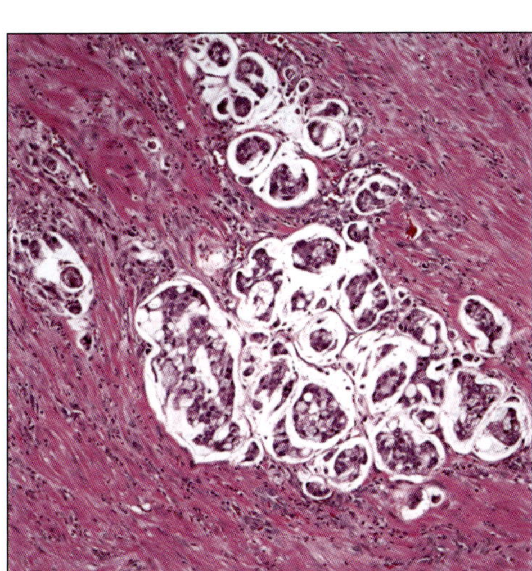

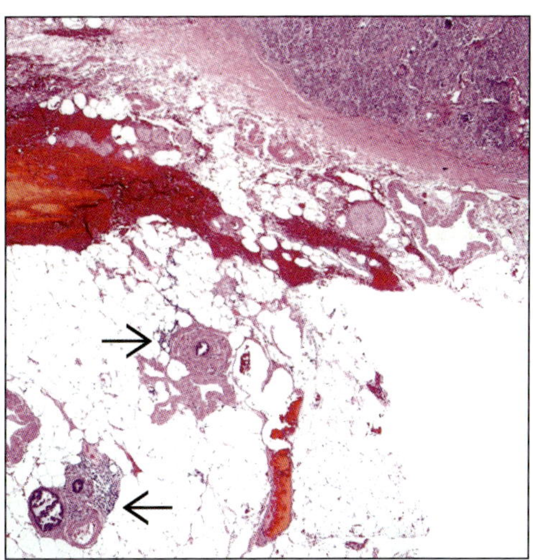

(Left) *This mucinous (colloid) carcinoma of the pancreas invades the muscular wall of the duodenum. Involvement of the duodenum is classified as T3 disease.* ***(Right)*** *This low-power photomicrograph shows tumor extending into the peripancreatic soft tissue* →*. This is classified as T3 disease, since the celiac axis and superior mesenteric artery were not involved.*

Staging Parameters

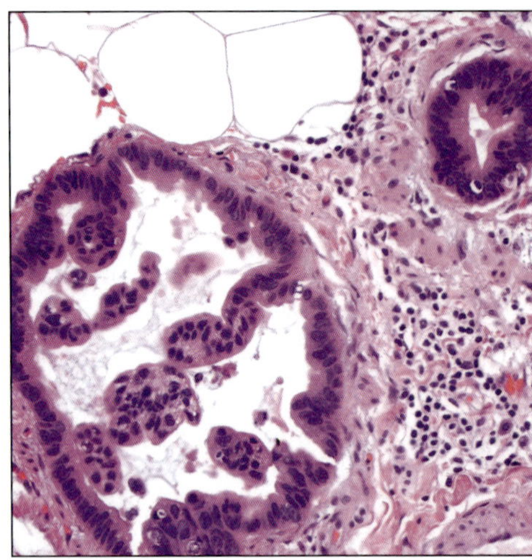

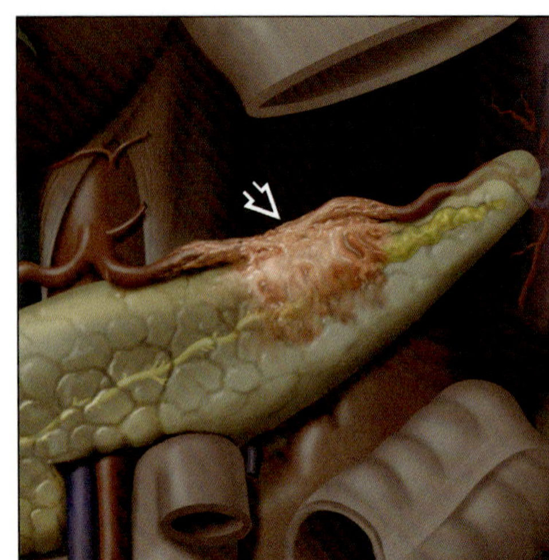

(Left) *This high-power photomicrograph shows pancreatic adenocarcinoma in the peripancreatic adipose tissue in a case of T3 disease.* ***(Right)*** *This T3 pancreatic tail tumor extends beyond the pancreas and invades the splenic artery ⇨. There is upstream pancreatic ductal dilation.*

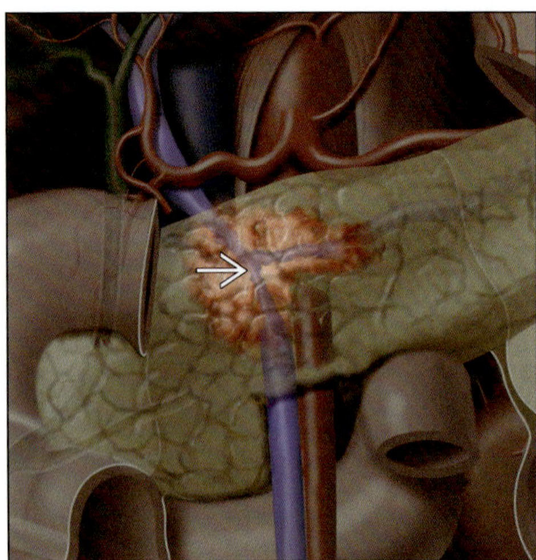

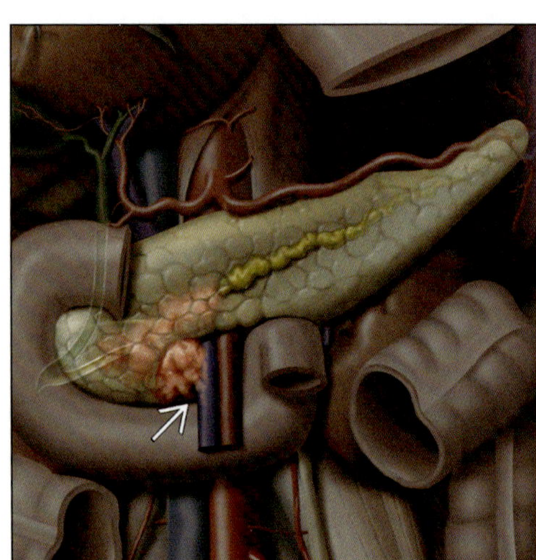

(Left) *This tumor extends beyond the pancreas posteriorly to invade the confluence of the superior mesenteric, splenic, and main portal veins ➔. Since it does not involve the superior mesenteric artery or celiac axis, it is still designated T3.* ***(Right)*** *This pancreatic head tumor invades the upper superior mesenteric vein ➔. However, because the superior mesenteric and celiac arteries are spared, this borderline resectable tumor is classified as T3.*

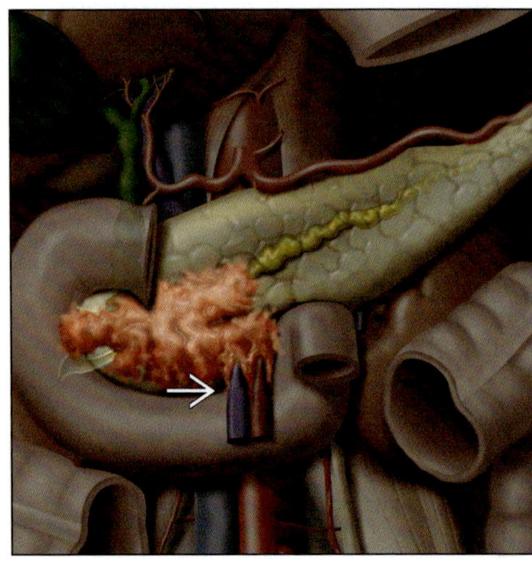

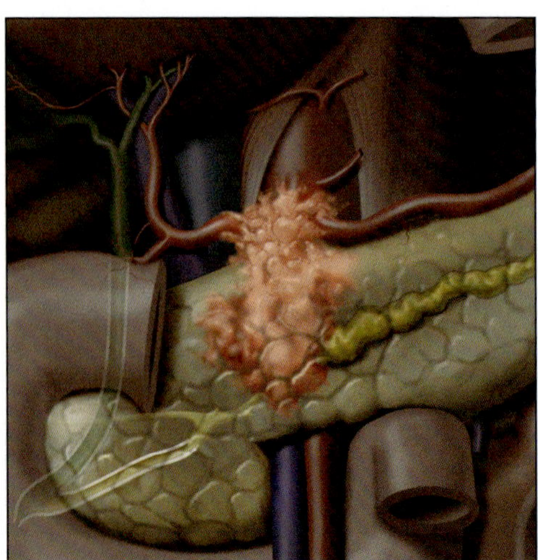

(Left) *This graphic depicts tumor invading the superior mesenteric artery and vein ➔, thus it is classified as T4. In addition, there is invasion of the duodenum. Any tumors that invade the superior mesenteric artery or celiac axis are designated T4.* ***(Right)*** *This tumor extends beyond the pancreas and invades the celiac axis as well as the proximal common hepatic and splenic arteries. Involvement of the celiac axis results in a T4 classification. This is an unresectable tumor.*

Tumors of the Ampulla

AMPULLARY ADENOMA

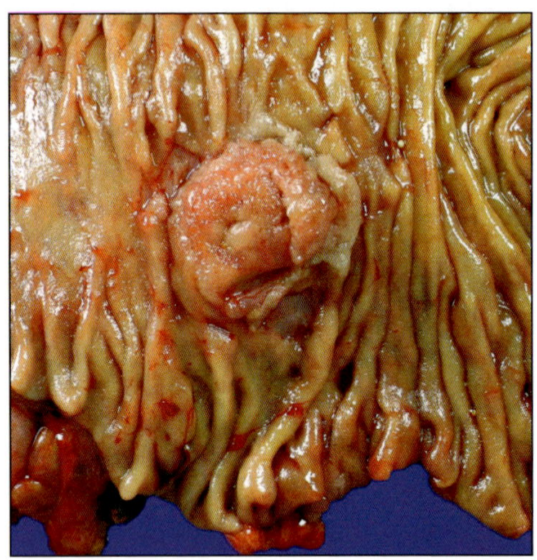

A single circumscribed mass with a nodular surface occupies the ampulla. The histology of this lesion showed a tubulopapillary adenoma with invasive adenocarcinoma.

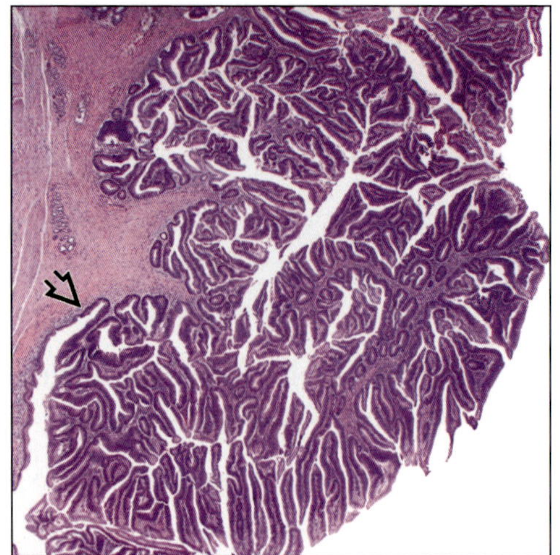

This ampullary papillary adenoma focally extends into the distal common bile duct epithelium ⇨.

TERMINOLOGY

Definitions

- Intestinal-type adenoma of ampullary or periampullary region
  - Resembles adenomas of small and large bowel

CLINICAL ISSUES

Epidemiology

- Incidence
  - 55% of small intestinal adenomas
    - Most are sporadic
  - Seen in 50-95% of patients with familial adenomatous polyposis (FAP) and Gardner syndrome
    - Most common site of extracolonic polyps in FAP patients
- Age
  - Range: 30-80 years
    - Average: 60s
  - Polyposis syndrome patients develop them at younger age
- Gender
  - M:F ratio = 1:2.6 in sporadic setting
  - No gender predominance in polyposis syndromes

Presentation

- Symptoms associated with biliary obstruction
  - Jaundice variably present
- Usually detected during screening endoscopy in polyposis patients

Treatment

- Complete endoscopic excision including ampullectomy
- Pancreatoduodenectomy for large lesions

Prognosis

- Cured by complete excision
- May recur after local excision
- Precursor lesion of ampullary adenocarcinoma

MACROSCOPIC FEATURES

General Features

- Polypoid or papillary growths
- Subtle prominence/thickening of ampulla
- Velvety, flat, sessile lesions
- Often involves one or more parts of periampullary region
  - Intraduodenal ampulla
  - Ampullary or periampullary duodenal mucosa
  - Extension into distal bile duct &/or pancreatic duct

Size

- Usually 1-3 cm in symptomatic cases

MICROSCOPIC PATHOLOGY

Histologic Features

- 3 histologic categories
  - Tubular adenoma
    - Least common
    - Often exophytic
    - Has some villous configurations due to normal villous architecture of ampulla
  - Tubulopapillary (tubulovillous) adenoma
    - > 25 % of both tubular and papillary elements
    - Feathery, frond-like, or papillary appearance
  - Papillary (villous) adenoma
    - Usually sessile
    - Simple &/or branching papillae
    - Often contains foci of high-grade dysplasia &/or intramucosal carcinoma
    - Majority (if not virtually all) are associated with invasive carcinoma
- Adenomatous epithelium

AMPULLARY ADENOMA

Key Facts

Clinical Issues

- Most are sporadic
- Seen in 50-95% of patients with (FAP) and Gardner syndrome

Macroscopic Features

- May involve one or more parts of ampullary/ periampullary region
- Polypoid, sessile, or subtle mucosal thickening

Microscopic Pathology

- 3 histologic categories: Tubular, tubulopapillary (tubulovillous), and papillary (villous)
  - Papillary almost always associated with invasive adenocarcinoma
- Extension of adenomatous epithelium into periductal glands of bile &/or pancreatic ducts or into submucosal glands may mimic invasion

---

  - Elongated columnar cells with basally located, pseudostratified, elongated, hyperchromatic nuclei
  - Paneth cells, goblet cells, neuroendocrine cells are common
- Dysplasia
  - By definition, all are dysplastic
  - Similar to colon, dysplasia is classified as low or high grade
    - Depends on degree of cytologic atypia and architectural complexity
- Pseudoinvasion with acellular mucin extravasation may be present

DIFFERENTIAL DIAGNOSIS

Reactive Epithelial Atypia

- Large nuclei with open chromatin pattern and visible nucleoli
  - No nuclear pseudostratification
- Presence of inflammation
  - Differential may be especially problematic if biliary stent has been present

Invasive Ampullary Carcinoma

- Extension of adenomatous epithelium into periductal glands of bile &/or pancreatic ducts or submucosal glands can mimic invasion

Invasive Pancreaticobiliary Carcinoma

- Colonization of mucosal basement membrane by underlying carcinoma can mimic adenoma

Ampullary Adenomyoma

- Glands are intermingled with smooth muscle fascicles

DIAGNOSTIC CHECKLIST

Pathologic Interpretation Pearls

- Degree of dysplasia may vary in different areas within 1 tumor, and invasive carcinoma, if present, may be focal
  - Extensive sampling of the lesion is warranted to exclude carcinoma

SELECTED REFERENCES

1. Noda Y et al: Histologic follow-up of ampullary adenomas in patients with familial adenomatosis coli. Cancer. 70(7):1847-56, 1992
2. Alexander JR et al: High prevalence of adenomatous polyps of the duodenal papilla in familial adenomatous polyposis. Dig Dis Sci. 34(2):167-70, 1989
3. Rosenberg J et al: Benign villous adenomas of the ampulla of Vater. Cancer. 58(7):1563-8, 1986
4. Oh C et al: Benign adenomatous polyps of the papilla of Vater. Surgery. 57:495-503, 1965

IMAGE GALLERY

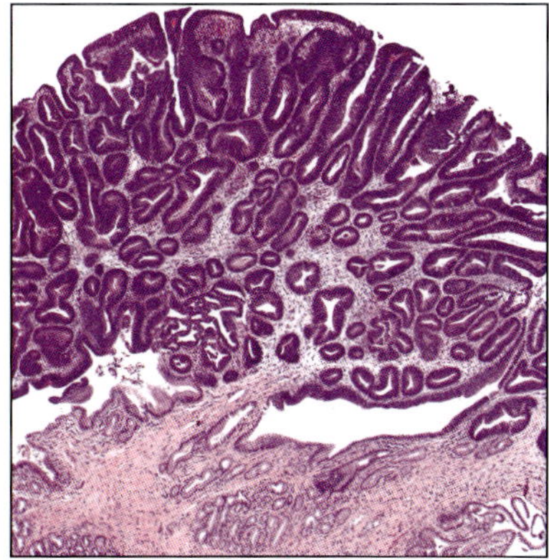

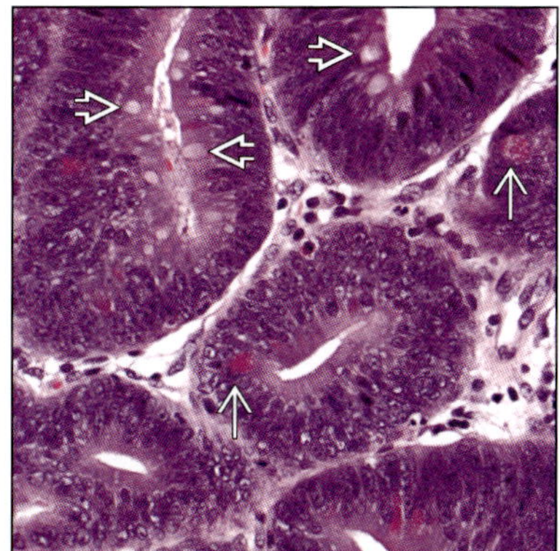

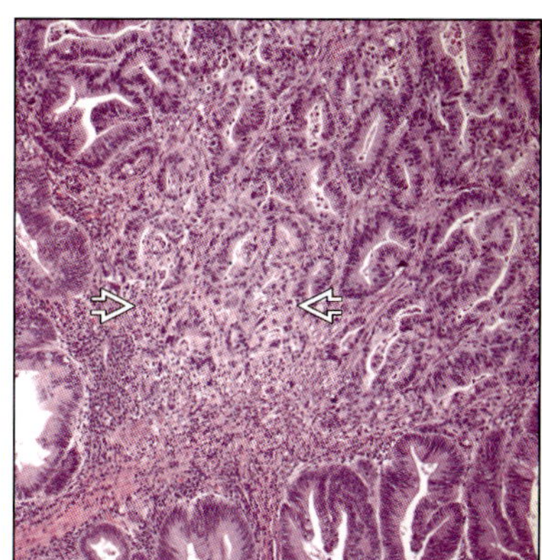

*(**Left**) This polypoid ampullary tubular adenoma is attached to the ampullary channel by a short stalk. (**Center**) Goblet cells ➡ and Paneth cells ➡ are quite common in ampullary adenomas. They are usually present in areas with low-grade dysplasia. (**Right**) This ampullary papillary adenoma contains a focus of intramucosal adenocarcinoma ➡ at the base.*

AMPULLARY ADENOCARCINOMA AND VARIANTS

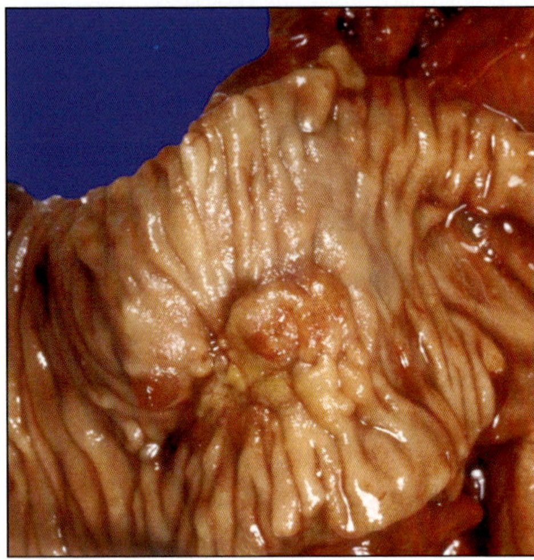

From the luminal aspect of this resection specimen, the ampulla is replaced by a protruding tumor grossly involving the duodenal mucosa of the papilla and periampullary duodenum.

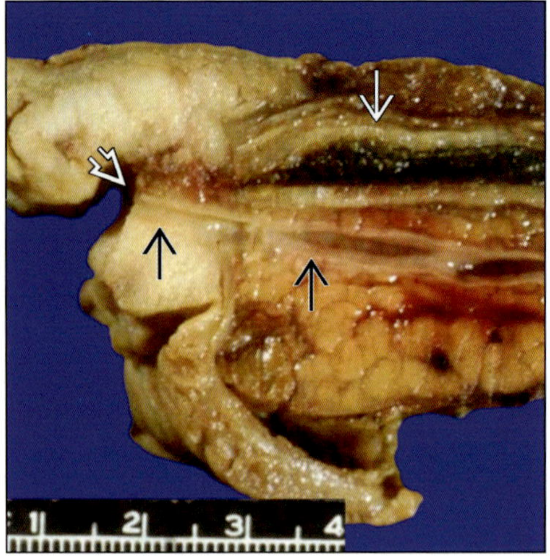

This ampullary adenocarcinoma consists of an exophytic white tumor involving the orifice ➡ of the common bile duct ➡, but not invading the pancreatic duct ➡.

TERMINOLOGY

Synonyms

- Periampullary adenocarcinoma

Definitions

- Adenocarcinoma arising in ampullary region and periampullary duodenal adenocarcinoma are collectively termed "ampullary adenocarcinoma"
  - Approximately 90% of all carcinomas of region

CLINICAL ISSUES

Epidemiology

- Incidence
  - Relatively uncommon
    - Approximately 0.2% of GI tract malignancies
    - Ampulla is most common site of small bowel adenocarcinoma
- Age
  - Most common in 7th-8th decade of life
  - Patients with familial adenomatous polyposis develop ampullary carcinoma at younger age than patients with sporadic cases
- Gender
  - Slightly more common in men (M:F = 1.48:1)

Presentation

- Jaundice
- Weight loss
- Abdominal pain
- Distended, palpable gallbladder (Courvoisier sign)

Treatment

- Resection (Whipple procedure)
  - Resectability is approximately 60%
- Role of adjuvant chemoradiation therapy (5-FU based) is controversial

Prognosis

- 5-year survival rate after surgical resection is approximately 50%
  - Significantly better than that of pancreatic adenocarcinoma
  - Comparable to that of duodenal adenocarcinoma

IMAGE FINDINGS

Endoscopic Findings

- Exophytic or ulcerated mass
- Tumors contained within ampulla appear as prominent submucosal bulge

MACROSCOPIC FEATURES

General Features

- Variable gross appearance
  - Intraampullary: Arise within ampulla itself
  - Periampullary duodenal: Arise from duodenal mucosa surrounding ampulla
  - Mixed ampullary/duodenal
- Majority arise from preexisting adenomas
- May be exophytic, ulcerated, or mixture of both

Size

- Often small
  - Approximately 20% are < 1 cm in diameter, and 75% are < 4 cm

MICROSCOPIC PATHOLOGY

Histologic Features

- Intestinal-type adenocarcinoma
  - Most common type (> 50%)
  - Histologically indistinguishable from tumors of colorectum
- Pancreatobiliary-type adenocarcinoma

AMPULLARY ADENOCARCINOMA AND VARIANTS

Key Facts

Terminology
- Ampullary adenocarcinoma comprises both adenocarcinomas arising in ampullary region and periampullary duodenal adenocarcinomas

Clinical Issues
- 5-year survival rate after surgical resection is approximately 50%
  - Significantly better than that of pancreatic adenocarcinoma

Macroscopic Features
- Tumors may be intraampullary, periampullary duodenal, mixed exophytic, or mixed ulcerated

Microscopic Pathology
- Intestinal type
- Pancreatobiliary type
- Papillary carcinoma (noninvasive)
- Invasive papillary carcinoma
- Mucinous (colloid) carcinoma
- Adenosquamous carcinoma

Ancillary Tests
- Intestinal type usually positive for CK20 and CDX2; often negative for CK7
- Pancreatobiliary type usually positive for CK7; often negative for CK20 and CDX2

Diagnostic Checklist
- Intestinal type of histologic differentiation is associated with favorable outcome in comparison to pancreatobiliary type

  - 2nd most common type
  - Closely resembles primary tumors of pancreas or extrahepatic bile ducts
  - High-grade nuclear pleomorphism in presence of architecturally well-formed glands
  - Desmoplastic stroma
  - Perineural invasion is common
- Papillary carcinoma (noninvasive)
  - Exophytic tumor arising in intraampullary mucosa
  - Resembles similar papillary neoplasms of pancreas or bile ducts
  - Does not invade stroma
- Invasive papillary carcinoma
  - < 10% of ampullary adenocarcinomas
  - Complex, branching papillary structures with fibrovascular cores or micropapillae
    - Diagnosis is based on papillary architecture rather than cytologic appearance
- Mucinous (colloid) carcinoma
  - < 10% of ampullary adenocarcinomas
  - Consists predominantly (> 50%) of extracellular mucin pools with floating carcinoma cells
  - Often associated with adenomatous component
- Adenosquamous carcinoma
  - < 3% of ampullary carcinomas
  - Exhibits both glandular and squamous differentiation
  - Squamous component should be significant (> 25%), but focal glandular differentiation is sufficient for diagnosis
- Other rare histologic types
  - Signet ring cell carcinoma
  - Clear cell carcinoma
  - Adenocarcinoma with hepatoid differentiation

ANCILLARY TESTS

Immunohistochemistry
- CEA and CA19-9 positive
- Intestinal type
  - Positive for CK20 and CDX2; often negative for CK7
- Pancreatobiliary type
  - Positive for CK7; often negative for CK20, CDX2

DIFFERENTIAL DIAGNOSIS

Distal Bile Duct Carcinoma
- Majority exhibit pancreatobiliary-type histology
- Fusiform growth pattern along bile duct

Pancreatic Adenocarcinoma
- Vast majority exhibit pancreatobiliary-type histology
- Pancreatic adenocarcinoma usually arises from main pancreatic duct; ampullary involvement represents peripheral extension
- No associated ampullary adenoma

DIAGNOSTIC CHECKLIST

Clinically Relevant Pathologic Features
- Important to distinguish ampullary from pancreatic or biliary adenocarcinoma because ampullary adenocarcinomas have better prognosis

Pathologic Interpretation Pearls
- Thorough sampling to rule out invasion is warranted in noninvasive papillary carcinomas

SELECTED REFERENCES

1. Sommerville CA et al: Survival analysis after pancreatic resection for ampullary and pancreatic head carcinoma: an analysis of clinicopathological factors. J Surg Oncol. 100(8):651-6, 2009
2. Schirmacher P et al: Ampullary adenocarcinoma - differentiation matters. BMC Cancer. 8:251, 2008
3. Westgaard A et al: Pancreatobiliary versus intestinal histologic type of differentiation is an independent prognostic factor in resected periampullary adenocarcinoma. BMC Cancer. 8:170, 2008
4. Fischer HP et al: Pathogenesis of carcinoma of the papilla of Vater. J Hepatobiliary Pancreat Surg. 11(5):301-9, 2004

Microscopic and Immunohistochemical Features

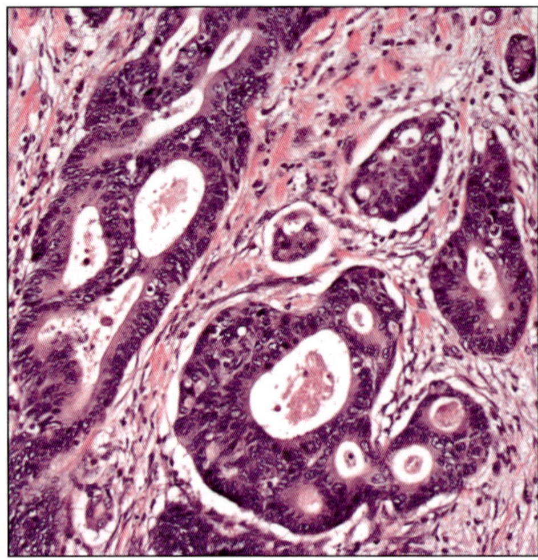

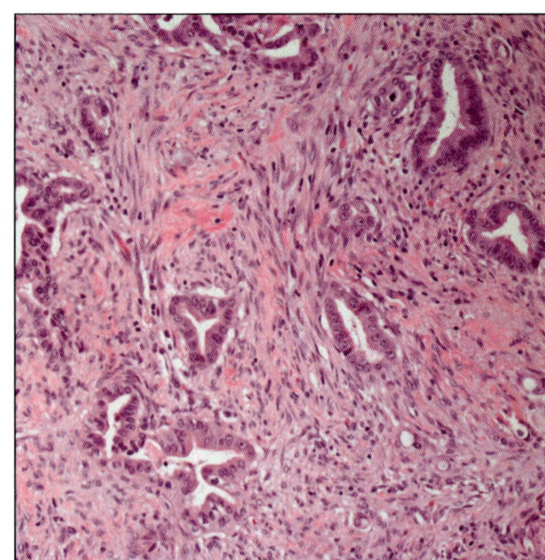

(Left) *In the intestinal type, the tumor consists of columnar cells with stratified, elongated nuclei and a cribriform pattern with luminal necrosis. This type resembles colonic adenocarcinoma.* ***(Right)*** *Pancreatobiliary-type adenocarcinomas consist of well-formed tubules with a single layer of cuboidal to low-columnar cells in a background of prominent desmoplastic stroma.*

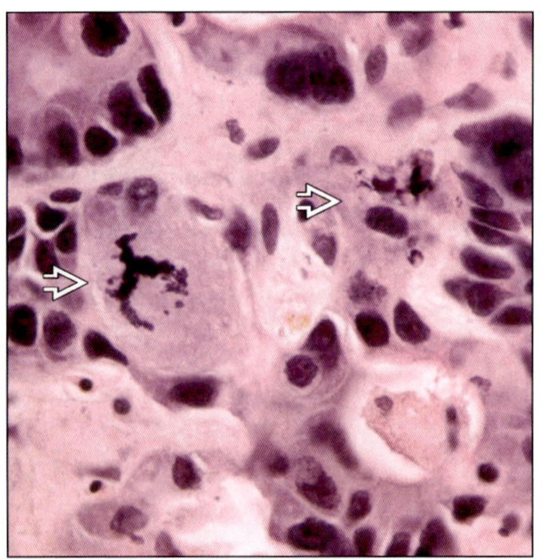

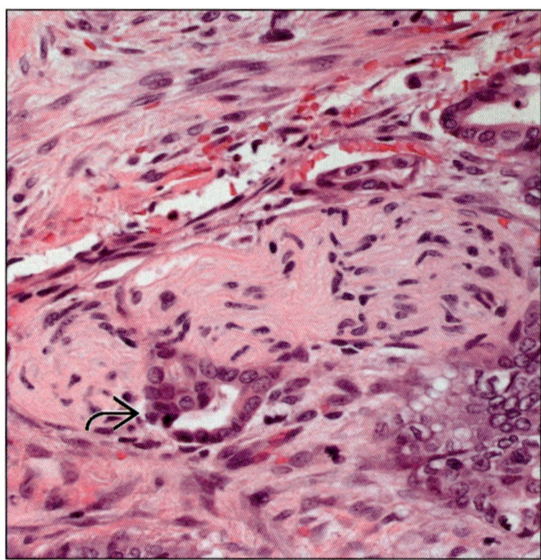

(Left) *Pancreatobiliary-type adenocarcinoma often features nuclear pleomorphism and atypical mitoses ➔ within architecturally well-formed glands.* ***(Right)*** *This nerve is partially wrapped by malignant glands ➔. Prominent perineural invasion is a characteristic feature of pancreatobiliary-type ampullary adenocarcinomas.*

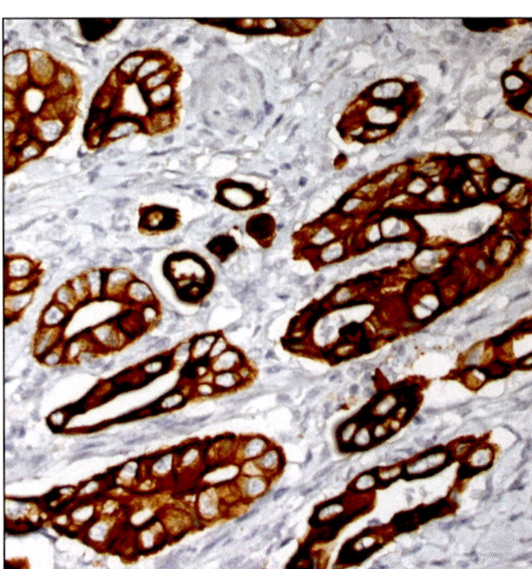

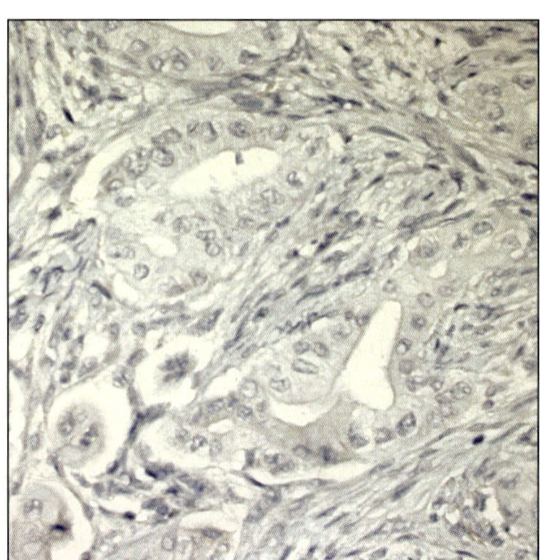

(Left) *This pancreatobiliary-type adenocarcinoma shows infiltrating well-formed glands that strongly express CK7. These tumors also express moderate to intense marking with CEA and CA19-9.* ***(Right)*** *Pancreatobiliary-type ampullary adenocarcinoma demonstrates negative expression of CK20. This type is often negative for CK20 and CDX2. Conversely, the intestinal-type adenocarcinoma usually stains positively with CK20 and CDX2 and is negative for CK7.*

Variant Microscopic Features

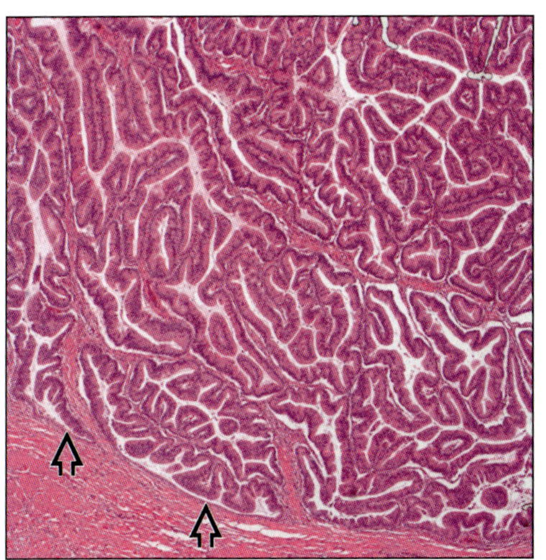

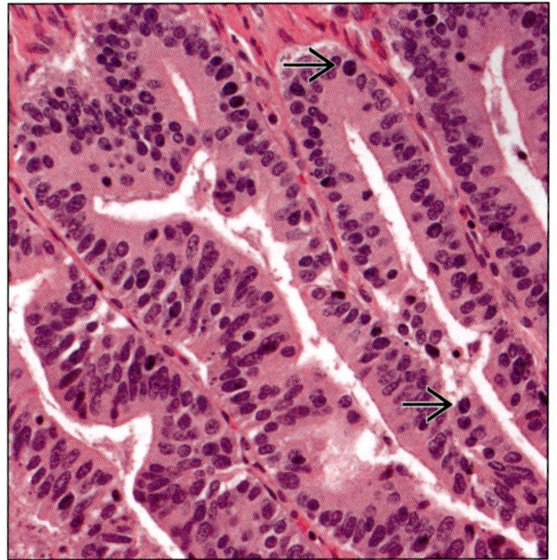

(Left) *Noninvasive papillary carcinomas of the ampulla are exophytic tumors resembling similar papillary neoplasms of the pancreas or bile ducts. They have a pushing border ⇨ and no submucosal invasion.* ***(Right)*** *In some areas, this noninvasive papillary tumor exhibits enlarged nuclei with nuclear stratification, scattered mitoses →, and micropapillary architecture.*

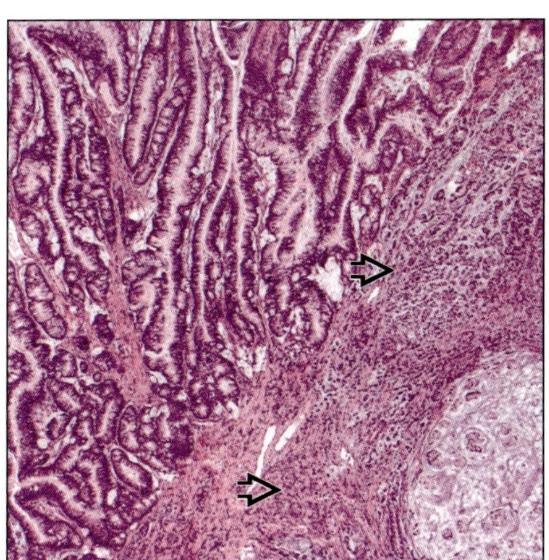

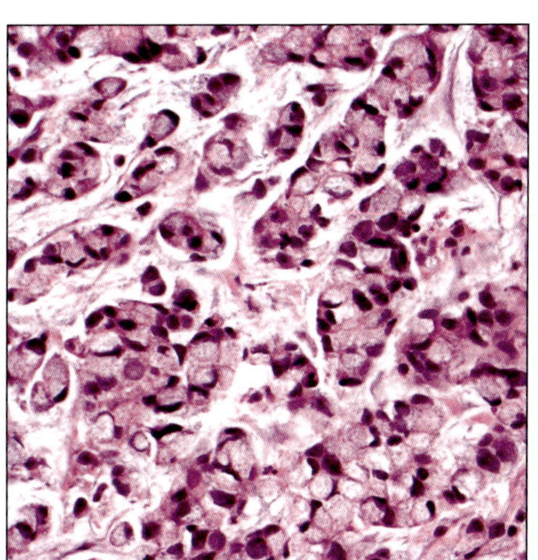

(Left) *This signet ring cell adenocarcinoma ⇨ is associated with a large tubulovillous adenoma with high-grade dysplasia.* ***(Right)*** *The infiltrating component consists of clusters of single signet ring cells in a background of mucinous or desmoplastic stroma. Although pure signet ring cell carcinoma is rare in the ampulla, the presence of signet ring cells as a minor component is not uncommon.*

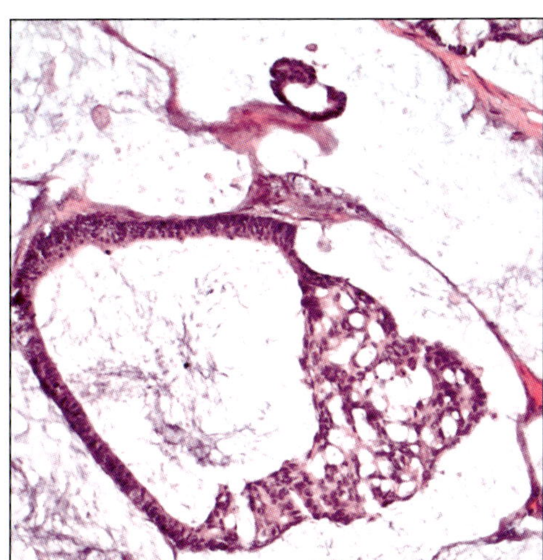

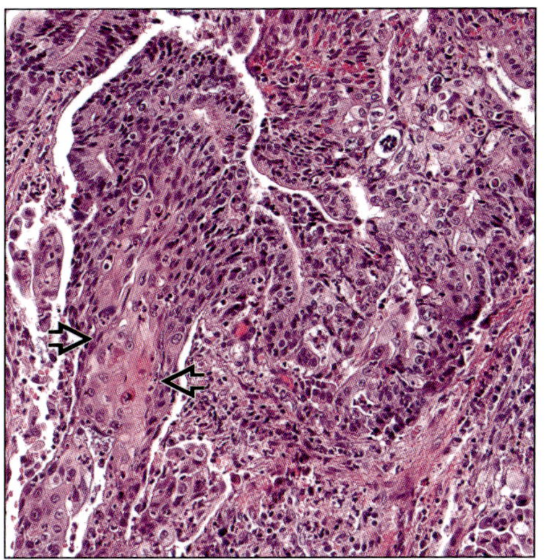

(Left) *This mucinous carcinoma shows a strip of malignant cells and a cluster of malignant cells with a cribriform pattern suspended in extracellular mucin pools.* ***(Right)*** *This adenosquamous carcinoma contains a component of keratinizing squamous cell carcinoma ⇨ as well as a glandular component. The squamous component should be significant (> 25%) to support the diagnosis of adenosquamous cell carcinoma.*

WELL-DIFFERENTIATED NEUROENDOCRINE NEOPLASM, AMPULLA

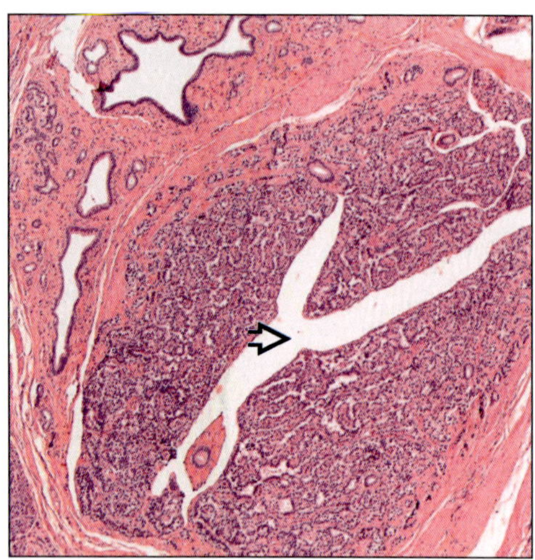

A well-circumscribed, well-differentiated neuroendocrine tumor is seen involving the distal portion of the bile duct. The lumen of the bile duct ⇨ is narrowed.

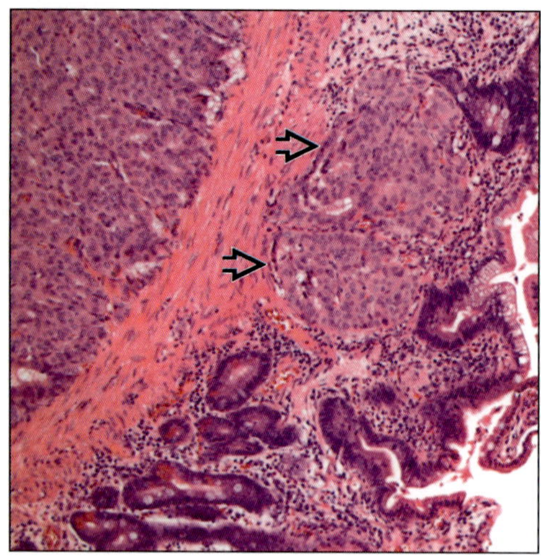

A gastrinoma of the periampullary region infiltrates the overlying duodenal mucosa ⇨. The neoplastic cells in this neuroendocrine tumor are monotonous.

TERMINOLOGY

Abbreviations

- Well-differentiated neuroendocrine neoplasm (WDNEN)

Synonyms

- Carcinoid tumor

ETIOLOGY/PATHOGENESIS

Syndromic Cases

- Neurofibromatosis
  - Majority are somatostatinomas
- MEN1 and Zollinger-Ellison syndrome
  - Gastrinoma or nonfunctional tumor

Nonsyndromic Cases

- Unknown

CLINICAL ISSUES

Epidemiology

- Gender
  - Male predominance

Presentation

- Somatostatinoma syndrome
  - Diabetes mellitus
  - Diarrhea
  - Cholecystitis
  - Extremely rare; somatostatinomas almost always nonfunctional
- Jaundice

Treatment

- Surgical approaches
  - Pancreaticoduodenectomy
  - Local excision in selected cases

Prognosis

- Difficult to predict
  - Size, mitotic rate are poor predictors of prognosis
- 20% of patients with somatostatinomas die of disease

MACROSCOPIC FEATURES

General Features

- Ampullary submucosal nodules, typically < 2 cm

MICROSCOPIC PATHOLOGY

Histologic Features

- Somatostatinoma
  - Gland formation common, some with psammoma bodies in lumen
  - Shares common cytologic features with other neuroendocrine neoplasms
    - Monotonous cells, round nuclei with "salt and pepper" chromatin
  - Widely infiltrative into duodenal wall and pancreas
  - Lymph node metastasis in 50% of cases
- Gastrinoma
  - Insular and trabecular growth patterns
  - Share common cytologic features with other neuroendocrine neoplasms

ANCILLARY TESTS

Immunohistochemistry

- Neuroendocrine stains
  - Chromogranin: Somatostatinomas are variably positive
  - Synaptophysin: Diffusely positive
- Peptide hormones
  - Majority stain for 1 or more of peptides
    - Somatostatin
    - Gastrin

WELL-DIFFERENTIATED NEUROENDOCRINE NEOPLASM, AMPULLA

Key Facts

Etiology/Pathogenesis

- Syndromic cases associated with neurofibromatosis, MEN1, Zollinger-Ellison syndrome

Clinical Issues

- Behavior/prognosis difficult to predict
  - Size, mitotic rate are poor predictors of prognosis

Microscopic Pathology

- Similar to well-differentiated neuroendocrine neoplasms of other sites
- Somatostatinoma
  - Gland formation common, some with psammoma bodies in lumen

Ancillary Tests

- Majority stain for one or more peptides

- Serotonin: Occasional tumor cells only

DIFFERENTIAL DIAGNOSIS

Adenocarcinoma

- Morphologic overlap caused by high proportion of gland-forming neuroendocrine tumors
- Presence of nuclear atypia, mitotic activity suggest adenocarcinoma
- Negative neuroendocrine markers
  - Somatostatinoma may stain weakly for chromogranin
  - Synaptophysin uniformly positive in WDNEN
- Desmoplastic stroma is invariably seen
  - Such stroma is typically absent in WDNEN

Gangliocytic Paraganglioma

- Ganglion-like elements and Schwann cells admixed with neuroendocrine cells

Adenocarcinoid

- Mixed adenocarcinoma/WDNEN tumor
- Entrapped ductules in WDNEN may mimic adenocarcinoid

DIAGNOSTIC CHECKLIST

Pathologic Interpretation Pearls

- Somatostatin-producing endocrine cells are normally present in ampullary region

GRADING

Low Grade

- Grade 1
  - Mitosis < 2/10 per HPF, Ki-67 ≤ 2

Intermediate Grade

- Grade 2
  - Mitosis 2-20 per HPF, Ki-67 = 2-20

High Grade

- Grade 3
  - Mitosis > 20 per HPF, Ki-67 > 20

SELECTED REFERENCES

1. Washington MK et al: Protocol for the examination of specimens from patients with neuroendocrine tumors (carcinoid tumors) of the small intestine and ampulla. Arch Pathol Lab Med. 134(2):181-6, 2010
2. Makhlouf HR et al: Carcinoid tumors of the ampulla of Vater: a comparison with duodenal carcinoid tumors. Cancer. 85(6):1241-9, 1999
3. Burke AP et al: Carcinoids of the duodenum. A histologic and immunohistochemical study of 65 tumors. Am J Surg Pathol. 13(10):828-37, 1989
4. Dayal Y et al: Psammomatous somatostatinomas of the duodenum. Am J Surg Pathol. 7(7):653-65, 1983

IMAGE GALLERY

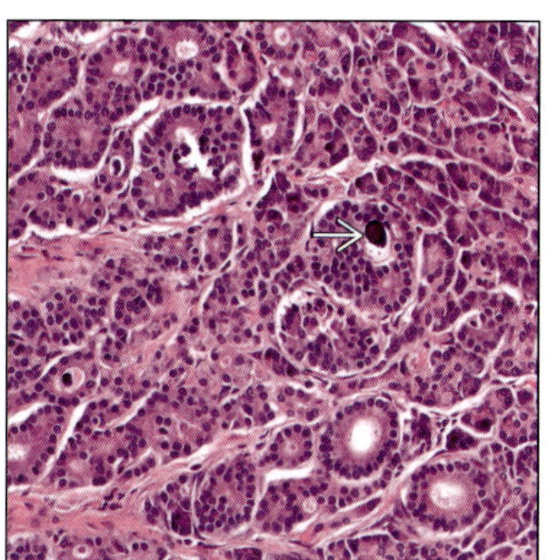

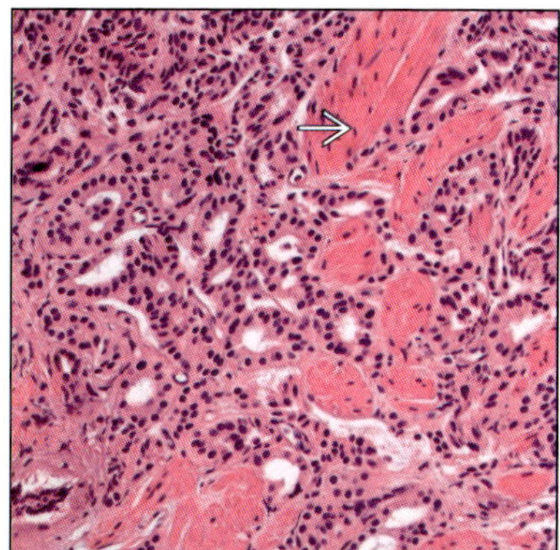

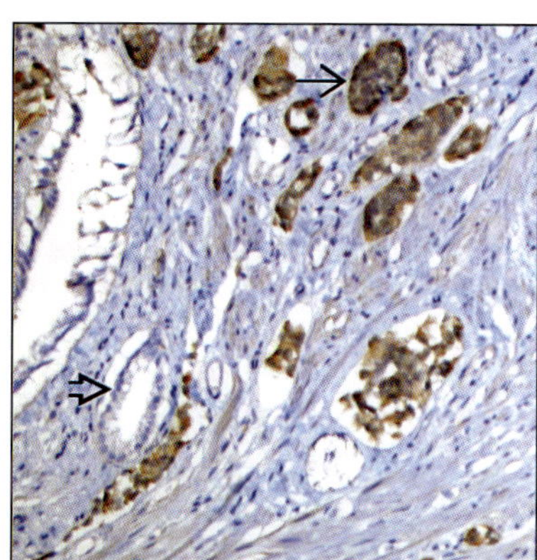

(Left) *This ampullary somatostatinoma has extensive gland formation and psammomatous calcification within some of the lumens ➡.* ***(Center)*** *This somatostatinoma infiltrates the muscularis propria of the duodenum ➡. Extensive gland formation may mimic invasive adenocarcinoma. Note the lack of a desmoplastic stromal reaction.* ***(Right)*** *This WDNEN of the ampulla is positive for somatostatin ➡. Note that the entrapped ducts are negative for this peptide ➡.*

POORLY DIFFERENTIATED NEUROENDOCRINE CARCINOMA, AMPULLA

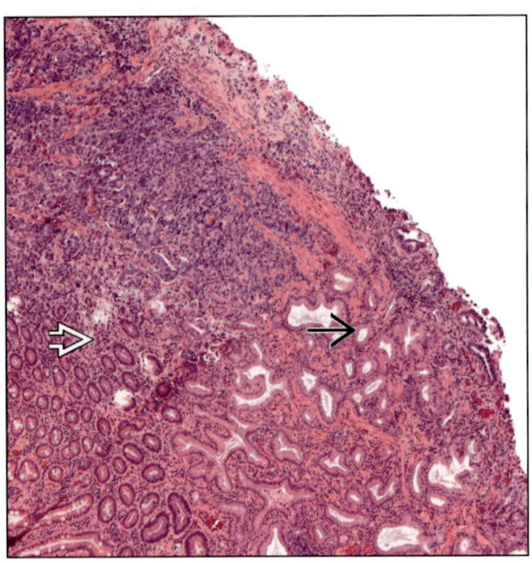

This poorly differentiated neuroendocrine carcinoma involves the ampulla ➔ and the duodenum ➔.

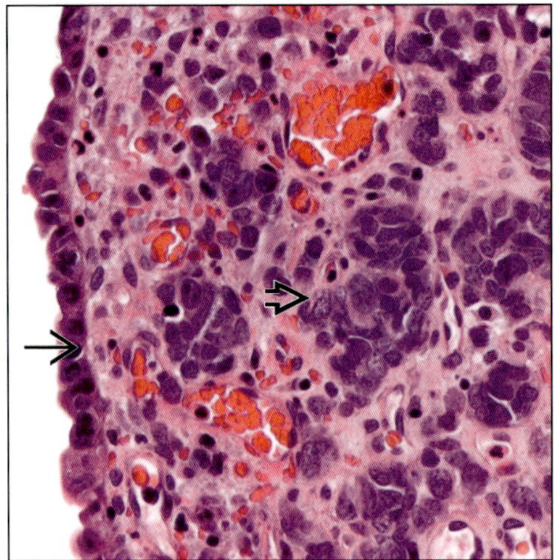

The neoplastic cells ➔ of this poorly differentiated neuroendocrine carcinoma show scant cytoplasm, hyperchromatic nuclei, and nuclear moulding. Note the overlying reactive biliary-type epithelium ➔.

TERMINOLOGY

Synonyms

- High-grade neuroendocrine carcinoma
- Small cell carcinoma
- Poorly differentiated endocrine carcinoma

Definitions

- Clinically aggressive carcinoma of ampulla with neuroendocrine features and high proliferation rate

ETIOLOGY/PATHOGENESIS

Unknown

- Association with conventional adenocarcinomas of ampulla suggests that at least initial pathogenetic mechanisms are similar

CLINICAL ISSUES

Presentation

- Jaundice

Treatment

- Surgical approaches
  - Pancreaticoduodenectomy for resectable tumors
- Adjuvant therapy
  - Platinum-based chemotherapy
    - Favorable but short-lived response

Prognosis

- Aggressive tumors with mean survival of 14.5 months
- Lymph node metastasis is invariably seen, and distant metastasis is frequent

MACROSCOPIC FEATURES

General Features

- Tumor is centered on major papilla
  - With large tumors, it may be difficult to assign site of origin

Size

- 0.8-2.5 cm

MICROSCOPIC PATHOLOGY

Histologic Features

- Tumors resemble either
  - Small cell carcinoma
  - Large cell neuroendocrine carcinoma of lung
- Associated adenoma or conventional adenocarcinoma seen in 1/2 of cases
  - Small cell carcinoma
    - Diffuse sheet-like growth with high mitotic activity (> 10/10 HPF) and abundant apoptosis
    - Cells with high nuclear to cytoplasmic ratios and nuclear moulding
    - Finely granular chromatin, inconspicuous nucleoli
  - Large cell neuroendocrine carcinoma
    - Presence of neuroendocrine architecture essential for diagnosis; organoid, palisading, rosettes, or trabecular pattern
    - Monotonous cells with moderate to abundant cytoplasm
    - Vesicular nuclei and prominent nucleoli
    - Brisk mitotic activity (> 10/10 HPF)
  - Occasional tumors show features intermediate between small cell and large cell neuroendocrine carcinoma

Lymphatic/Vascular Invasion

- Widespread lymphatic invasion is invariably present

POORLY DIFFERENTIATED NEUROENDOCRINE CARCINOMA, AMPULLA

Key Facts

Clinical Issues

- Aggressive tumors with mean survival of 14.5 months

Microscopic Pathology

- Tumors resemble either small cell carcinoma or large cell neuroendocrine carcinoma of lung

Ancillary Tests

- Positive for chromogranin and synaptophysin
  - Reactivity may be focal
- For large cell neuroendocrine pattern, immunohistochemical proof of neuroendocrine differentiation is essential

Top Differential Diagnoses

- Well-differentiated neuroendocrine carcinoma
- High-grade lymphoma
- Metastatic pulmonary small cell carcinoma

ANCILLARY TESTS

Immunohistochemistry

- Positive for chromogranin and synaptophysin
  - Small cell carcinoma pattern invariably positive for these markers
    - Although such reactivity is not an absolute requirement
  - In large cell neuroendocrine pattern, immunohistochemical proof of neuroendocrine differentiation is required
    - In addition to the appropriate histologic features
- Keratin
  - Tumors consistently positive for AE1/AE3
    - Cytokeratin 7-87% positive
    - Cytokeratin 20-38% positive
- Ki-67
  - Labeling index is high
    - Typically > 50%

DIFFERENTIAL DIAGNOSIS

Well-Differentiated Neuroendocrine Carcinoma

- Lack high-grade cellular atypia
- Mitotic count < 10/10 HPF

High-Grade Lymphoma

- Consistently negative for cytokeratin and positive for lymphoid markers

Metastatic Pulmonary Small Cell Carcinoma

- Presence of adenoma or conventional adenocarcinoma would support ampullary primary
- TTF-1 reactivity supports metastasis from lung
  - Rarely, primary gastrointestinal high-grade neuroendocrine carcinomas may be TTF-1 positive
- Presence of lung mass helpful

SELECTED REFERENCES

1. Shia J et al: Is nonsmall cell type high-grade neuroendocrine carcinoma of the tubular gastrointestinal tract a distinct disease entity? Am J Surg Pathol. 32(5):719-31, 2008
2. Nassar H et al: High-grade neuroendocrine carcinoma of the ampulla of vater: a clinicopathologic and immunohistochemical analysis of 14 cases. Am J Surg Pathol. 29(5):588-94, 2005
3. Zamboni G et al: Small-cell neuroendocrine carcinoma of the ampullary region. A clinicopathologic, immunohistochemical, and ultrastructural study of three cases. Am J Surg Pathol. 14(8):703-13, 1990

IMAGE GALLERY

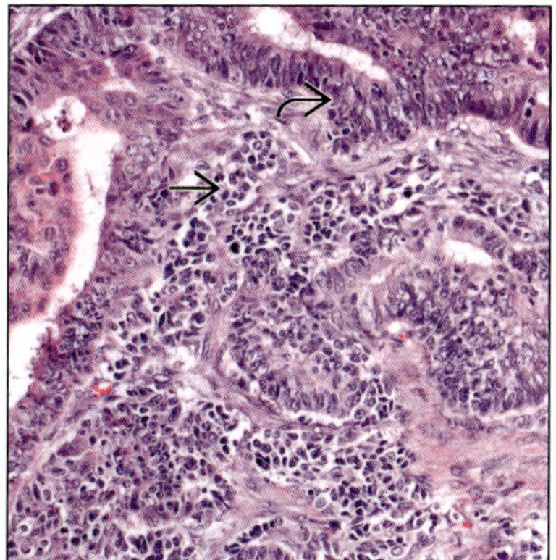

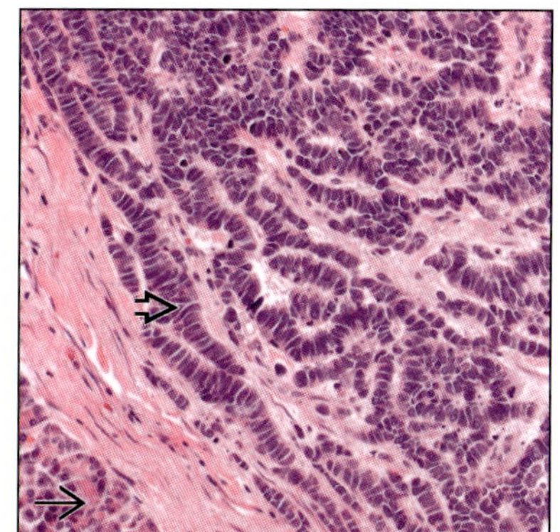

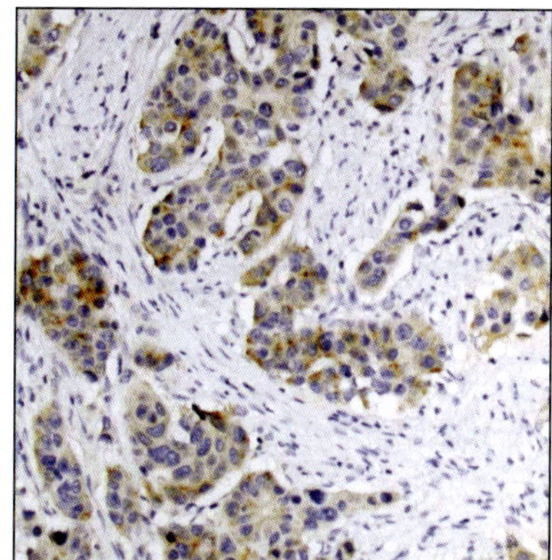

*(**Left**) The neuroendocrine component resembles a small cell carcinoma ➔. Foci of a conventional adenocarcinoma were also noted in this tumor ➔. (**Center**) High-grade neuroendocrine carcinoma shows ribbons of neoplastic cells ➔ focally infiltrating the pancreas ➔. (**Right**) This poorly differentiated endocrine carcinoma is focally positive for chromogranin.*

PARAGANGLIOMA

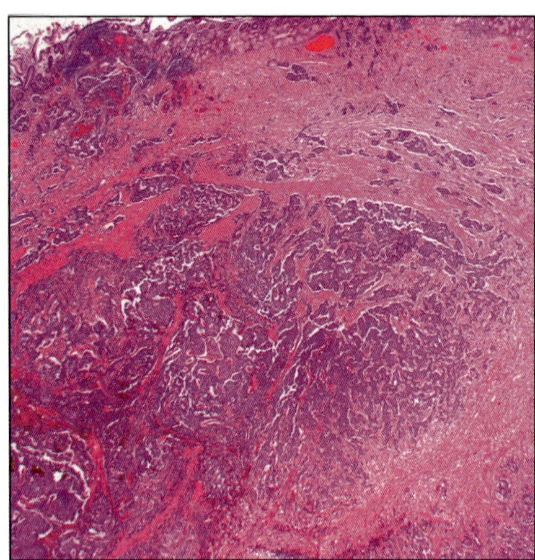

Periampullary gangliocytic paragangliomas often have an infiltrating pattern at the periphery. The lesion is centered in the submucosa with extension into the overlying mucosa.

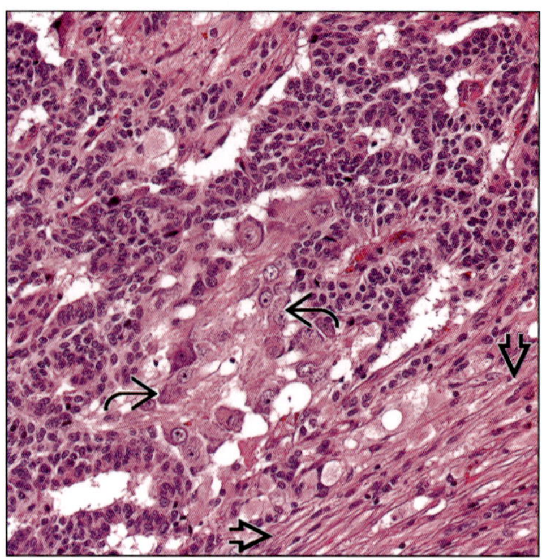

Gangliocytic paragangliomas consisting of a mixture of epithelioid cells, ganglion-like cells ⮫, and nerve sheath elements ⮚.

TERMINOLOGY

Synonyms

- Gangliocytic paraganglioma
- Nonchromaffin paraganglioma

Definitions

- Neoplasm consisting of epithelioid, ganglion-like cells, and nerve sheath elements
  - Associated with neurofibromatosis type 1 (NF1) in some cases

ETIOLOGY/PATHOGENESIS

Origin

- Several theories
  - Progenitor neural crest cells
  - Embryonic celiac ganglion
  - Endodermally derived epithelial cells originating from the ventral primordium of pancreas (hamartomatous proliferation)
  - Pancreatic tumor composed of ganglion-islet cell complexes

CLINICAL ISSUES

Epidemiology

- Incidence
  - Uncommon (1.2 % of ampullary neoplasms in 1 series)
    - Associated with neurofibromatosis 1
- Age
  - 3rd to 9th decades with mean age in 50s
- Gender
  - Males slightly outnumber females (1.7 to 1)

Site

- Vast majority involve 2nd portion of duodenum (periampullary duodenum)
  - Extraduodenal sites include jejunum, pylorus, and lung

Presentation

- GI bleeding
- Abdominal pain
- Obstructive jaundice (less frequent)

Treatment

- Snare polypectomy or ampullectomy for smaller lesions
- Surgical resection (Whipple procedure) for larger lesions

Prognosis

- Vast majority benign
  - Few reports of regional lymph node metastases &/or recurrence
- No distant metastases or death associated with disease has been reported

MACROSCOPIC FEATURES

General Features

- Sessile or pedunculated, centered in submucosa
- Ulceration of overlying mucosa is common
- Tan to white and moderately firm

Size

- 1-4 cm, although larger tumors are occasionally seen

MICROSCOPIC PATHOLOGY

Histologic Features

- 3 elements in varying proportions
  - **Epithelioid cells**
    - Anastomosing cords and trabeculae
    - Small, monotonous cells with round nuclei, stippled chromatin, eosinophilic cytoplasm, small nucleoli

PARAGANGLIOMA

Key Facts

Terminology

- Gangliocytic paraganglioma
- Uncommon (approximately 1% of ampullary neoplasms)
- Some cases associated with NF-1

Clinical Issues

- Most commonly involve periampullary duodenum
- Clinically benign

Microscopic Pathology

- Epithelioid, spindled, and ganglion-like cells present in varying proportions
- Endocrine cells may also be present
- S100 may reveal sustentacular-like cells surrounding nests of epithelioid cells
- No mitoses or necrosis

    - Positive for NSE, chromogranin, synaptophysin, somatostatin; variable marking with keratin, pancreatic polypeptide, somatostatin
  - **Ganglion-like cells**
    - Abundant eosinophilic cytoplasm with large eccentric nuclei and prominent nucleoli
    - Can look like normal ganglion cells or transitional epithelioid cells with less cytoplasm and inconspicuous nucleoli
    - Positive for neurofilament markers, NSE; variably present endocrine-associated hormones
  - **Spindled cells**
    - Indistinguishable from Schwann cells
    - Elongated cells with tapered ends, faintly eosinophilic cytoplasm, elongated nuclei
    - Positive for neurofilament markers, S100, NSE
  - Endocrine cells may also be present
  - S100 may reveal sustentacular-like cells surrounding nests of epithelioid cells
- Growth pattern is infiltrative with entrapment of smooth muscle or ductular structures
- No mitoses or necrosis

DIFFERENTIAL DIAGNOSIS

Low-Grade Neuroendocrine Tumor

- Positive for pancreatic polypeptide, keratins
- Lacks ganglion-like and spindled cells

Ampullary Carcinoma

- Strongly positive for keratins
- Nuclear atypia, mitoses, necrosis, and architectural complexity
- Lacks ganglion-like and spindled cells

Ganglioneuroma

- Lacks epithelioid component

Neurofibroma

- Lacks epithelioid and ganglion-like cells

Gastrointestinal Stromal Tumor

- C-Kit or DOG-1 positive

DIAGNOSTIC CHECKLIST

Pathologic Interpretation Pearls

- Periampullary tumors with any of 3 elements should be carefully examined for others

SELECTED REFERENCES

1. Sundararajan V et al: Duodenal gangliocytic paraganglioma with lymph node metastasis: a case report and review of the literature. Arch Pathol Lab Med. 127(3):e139-41, 2003
2. Sakhuja P et al: Periampullary gangliocytic paraganglioma. J Clin Gastroenterol. 33(2):154-6, 2001

IMAGE GALLERY

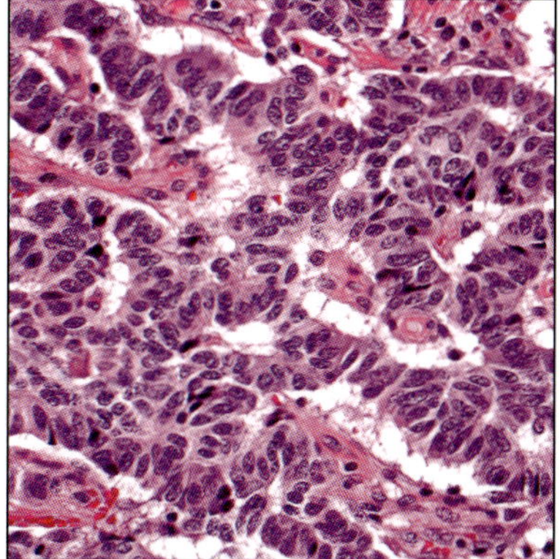

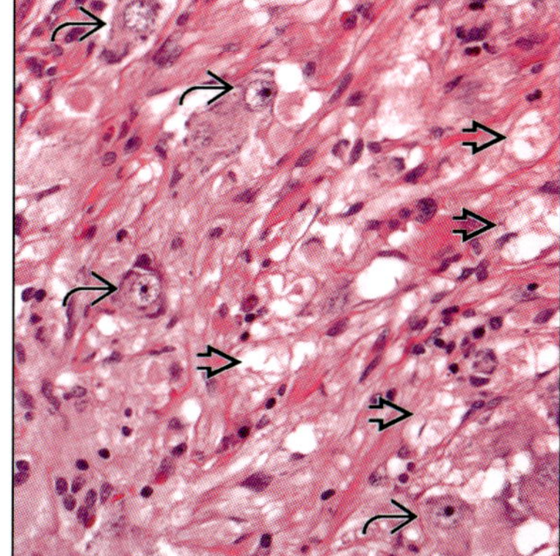

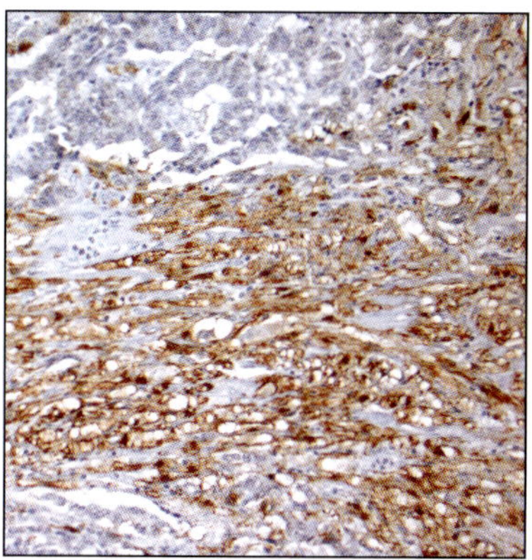

(Left) *The epithelioid cells with amphophilic cytoplasm and fine chromatin are arranged in trabeculae, resembling a carcinoid tumor.* ***(Center)*** *Ganglion-like cells ⮫ with dense cytoplasm, open chromatin, and prominent nucleoli are indistinguishable from normal ganglion cells. Nerve sheath elements ⮚ contain Schwann cells with elongated nuclei and vacuolated cytoplasm. Neural filaments are not well visualized.* ***(Right)*** *The Schwann cell component is positive for S100.*

AMPULLA OF VATER CANCER PROTOCOL

Ampulla of Vater: Ampullectomy, Pancreaticoduodenectomy (Whipple Resection)

Surgical Pathology Cancer Case Summary (Checklist)

Specimen (select all that apply)

___ Ampulla of Vater
___ Stomach
___ Head of pancreas
___ Duodenum
___ Common bile duct
___ Gallbladder
___ Other (specify): ____________________
___ Not specified

Procedure

___ Ampullectomy
___ Pancreaticoduodenectomy (Whipple resection)
___ Other (specify): ____________________
___ Not specified

Tumor Site

___ Intraampullary
___ Periampullary
___ Papilla of Vater (junction of ampullary and duodenal mucosa)
___ Other (specify): ____________________
___ Cannot be determined
___ Not specified

****Tumor Size***

Greatest dimension: _______ x _______ cm
*Additional dimensions: ___ x ___ cm
___ Cannot be determined

Histologic Type

___ Adenocarcinoma (not otherwise characterized)
___ Papillary adenocarcinoma
___ Adenocarcinoma, intestinal type
___ Mucinous adenocarcinoma
___ Clear cell adenocarcinoma
___ Signet ring cell carcinoma
___ Adenosquamous carcinoma
___ Squamous cell carcinoma
___ Small cell carcinoma
___ Other (specify): ____________________
___ Carcinoma, not otherwise specified

Histologic Grade

___ Not applicable (histologic type not usually graded)
___ GX: Cannot be assessed
___ G1: Well differentiated
___ G2: Moderately differentiated
___ G3: Poorly differentiated
___ G4: Undifferentiated
___ Other (specify): ____________________

Microscopic Tumor Extension (select all that apply)

___ Cannot be assessed
___ No evidence of primary tumor

AMPULLA OF VATER CANCER PROTOCOL

____ Carcinoma in situ
____ Tumor limited to ampulla of Vater or sphincter of Oddi
____ Tumor invades duodenal wall
____ Tumor invades pancreas
____ Tumor invades peripancreatic soft tissues
____ Tumor invades extrapancreatic common bile duct
____ Tumor invades other adjacent organs or structures other than pancreas
(specify): ____________________________

Margins (select all that apply)

Ampullectomy specimen

____ Cannot be assessed
____ Margins uninvolved by invasive carcinoma
Distance of invasive carcinoma from closest margin: _________ mm
Specify margin (if possible): ____________________________
____ Margins involved by invasive carcinoma
Specify margin (if possible): ____________________________
____ Not applicable

Pancreaticoduodenal resection specimen

Proximal mucosal margin (gastric or duodenal)
____ Cannot be assessed
____ Uninvolved by invasive carcinoma
____ Involved by invasive carcinoma
____ Intramucosal carcinoma/adenoma not identified at proximal margin
____ Intramucosal carcinoma/adenoma present at proximal margin

Distal margin (distal duodenal or jejunal)
____ Cannot be assessed
____ Uninvolved by invasive carcinoma
____ Involved by invasive carcinoma
____ Intramucosal carcinoma/adenoma not identified at distal margin
____ Intramucosal carcinoma/adenoma present at distal margin

Pancreatic retroperitoneal (uncinate) margin
____ Not applicable
____ Cannot be assessed
____ Uninvolved by invasive carcinoma
____ Involved by invasive carcinoma (tumor present 0-1 mm from margin)

Bile duct margin
____ Not applicable
____ Cannot be assessed
____ Margin uninvolved by invasive carcinoma
____ Margin involved by invasive carcinoma

Distal pancreatic resection margin
____ Not applicable
____ Cannot be assessed
____ Margin uninvolved by invasive carcinoma
____ Margin involved by invasive carcinoma

If all margins uninvolved by invasive carcinoma
Distance of invasive carcinoma from closest margin: ____ mm OR ____ cm
Specify margin: ____________________________

Lymph-Vascular Invasion

____ Not identified
____ Present
____ Indeterminate

AMPULLA OF VATER CANCER PROTOCOL

*Perineural Invasion

*____ Not identified

*____ Present

*____ Indeterminate

Pathologic Staging (pTNM)

TNM descriptors (required only if applicable) (select all that apply)

____ m (multiple primary tumors)

____ r (recurrent)

____ y (post-treatment)

Primary tumor (pT)

____ pTX: Cannot be assessed

____ pT0: No evidence of primary tumor

____ pTis: Carcinoma in situ

____ pT1: Tumor limited to ampulla of Vater or sphincter of Oddi

____ pT2: Tumor invades duodenal wall

____ pT3: Tumor invades pancreas

____ pT4: Tumor invades peripancreatic soft tissues or other adjacent organs or structures

Regional lymph nodes (pN)

____ pNX: Cannot be assessed

____ pN0: No regional lymph node metastasis

____ Regional lymph node metastasis

Specify: Number examined: ________

Number involved: ________

Distant metastasis (pM)

____ Not applicable

____ pM1: Distant metastasis

*Specify sites (if known): ________________________

*Additional Pathologic Findings (select all that apply)

*____ None identified

*____ Dysplasia/adenoma

*____ Other (specify): ________________________

*Ancillary Studies

*Specify: ________________________

*____ Not performed

*Clinical History (select all that apply)

*____ Familial adenomatous polyposis coli

*____ Other (specify): ________________________

*____ Not known

**Data elements with asterisks are not required. However, these elements may be clinically important but are not yet validated or regularly used in patient management. Adapted with permission from College of American Pathologists, "Protocol for the Examination of Specimens from Patients with Carcinoma of the Ampulla of Vater." Web posting date October 2009, www.cap.org. Protocol applies to all intra-ampullary, periampullary, and mixed intra- and periampullary carcinomas. Well-differentiated neuroendocrine neoplasms (carcinoid tumors) are not included.*

PROGNOSTIC FEATURES

Survival

- Ampullary/periampullary adenocarcinoma has superior survival when compared to pancreatic or common bile duct adenocarcinoma
  - Obstruction of bile duct and jaundice tend to occur early due to strategic location of ampulla
- Because of superior prognosis, ampullary adenocarcinoma must be distinguished from pancreatic ductal, common bile duct, and duodenal adenocarcinomas
  - May be very difficult to determine exact primary site in large tumors

Primary Tumor

- Assessment based on surgical resection
  - Completeness of resection has significant prognostic implications
  - Positive resection margin(s) associated with less favorable outcome
- Local extension
  - Main staging parameters depend on extension into the duodenal wall, pancreas, or peripancreatic soft tissue and other organs
    - Even T4 tumors are usually resectable
- Other adverse prognostic factors
  - Poorly differentiated histology
    - Papillary tumors associated with better prognosis, conversely
  - Perineural invasion
  - Prognostic significance of CEA and CA19-9 unclear, but can be used to monitor treatment

Lymph Nodes

- Regional lymph nodes
  - Peripancreatic
    - Include nodes along hepatic artery, portal vein
  - Positive regional nodes have significant negative affect on survival
  - Minimum of 12 nodes should be examined

Distant Metastases

- Most common sites are liver, peritoneum
- Less common sites include lung, pleura

SELECTED REFERENCES

1. American Joint Committee on Cancer: AJCC Cancer Staging Manual. 7th ed. New York: Springer. 219-25, 2010
2. Heinrich S et al: Ampullary cancer. Curr Opin Gastroenterol. 26(3):280-5, 2010
3. Hurtuk MG et al: Does lymph node ratio impact survival in resected periampullary malignancies? Am J Surg. 197(3):348-52, 2009
4. Lowe MC et al: Important prognostic factors in adenocarcinoma of the ampulla of Vater. Am Surg. 75(9):754-60; discussion 761, 2009
5. Carter JT et al: Tumors of the ampulla of vater: histopathologic classification and predictors of survival. J Am Coll Surg. 207(2):210-8, 2008
6. Sudo T et al: Prognostic impact of perineural invasion following pancreatoduodenectomy with lymphadenectomy for ampullary carcinoma. Dig Dis Sci. 53(8):2281-6, 2008
7. Sakata J et al: Number of positive lymph nodes independently affects long-term survival after resection in patients with ampullary carcinoma. Eur J Surg Oncol. 33(3):346-51, 2007
8. Bettschart V et al: Presentation, treatment and outcome in patients with ampullary tumours. Br J Surg. 91(12):1600-7, 2004
9. Bakkevold KE et al: Staging of carcinoma of the pancreas and ampulla of Vater. Tumor (T), lymph node (N), and distant metastasis (M) as prognostic factors. Int J Pancreatol. 17(3):249-59, 1995

AMPULLA OF VATER CANCER PROTOCOL

Staging Parameters

*(**Left**) This graphic illustrates a tumor confined to the ampulla (T1 disease) ➡. T1 disease is defined as tumor limited to the ampulla of Vater or the sphincter of Oddi. (**Right**) This nodular tumor was limited to the ampulla of Vater.*

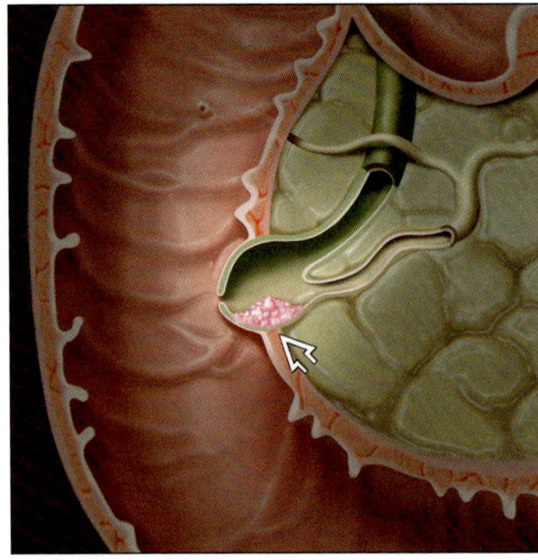

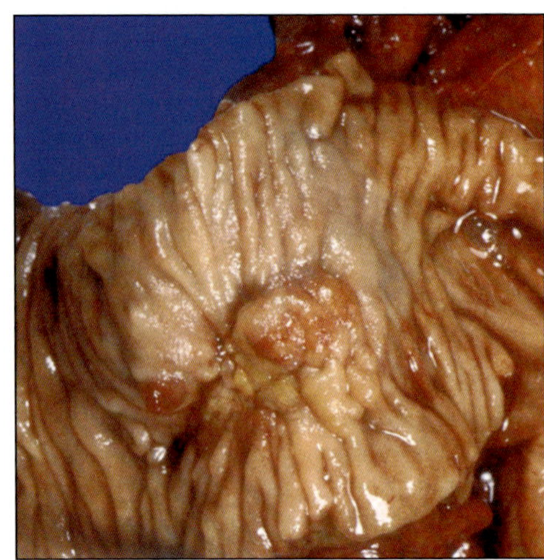

*(**Left**) This ampullary adenocarcinoma consists of an exophytic white tumor involving the orifice ➡ of the common bile duct but not invading the pancreas. (**Right**) T2 disease is defined as tumor that invades the duodenal wall, as illustrated in this graphic.*

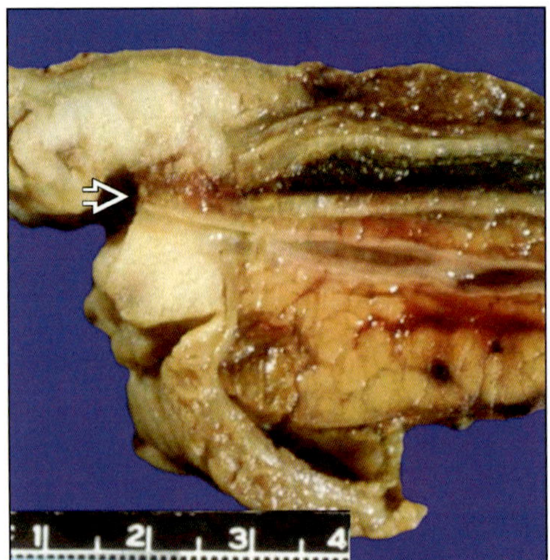

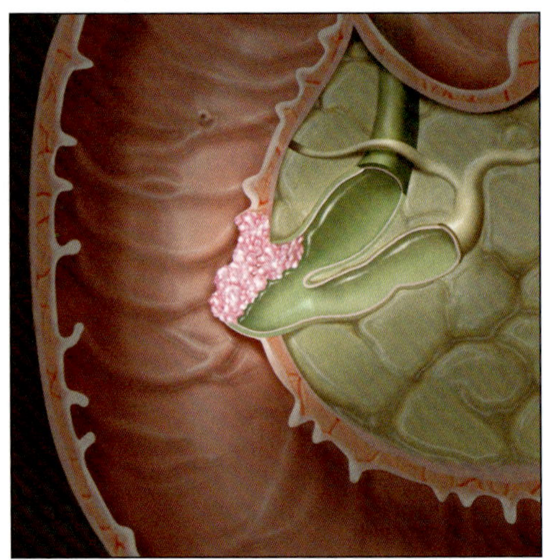

*(**Left**) This axial graphic shows an ampullary tumor involving the duodenal wall ➡, consistent with T2 disease. (**Right**) This tumor arises from the ampulla and invades the muscular wall → of the duodenum (T2 disease).*

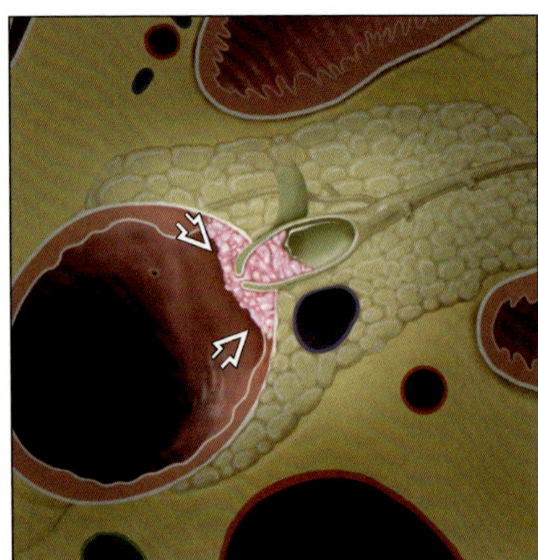

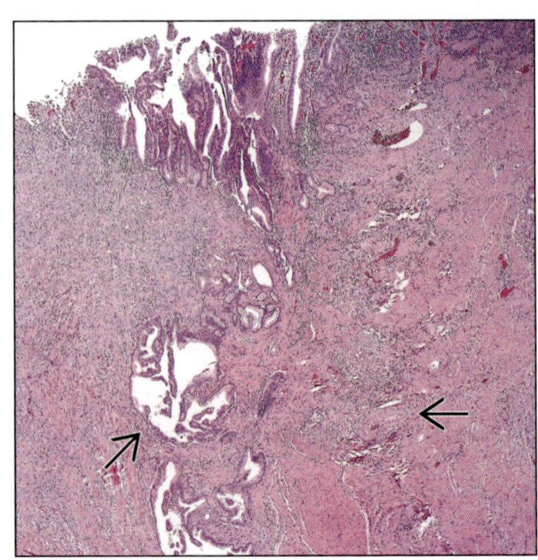

Staging Parameters

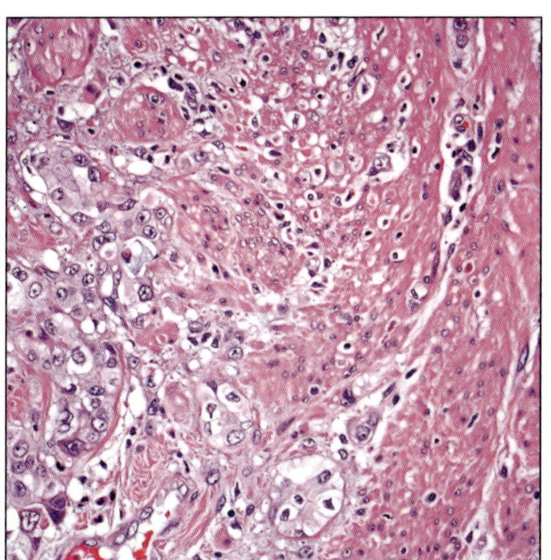

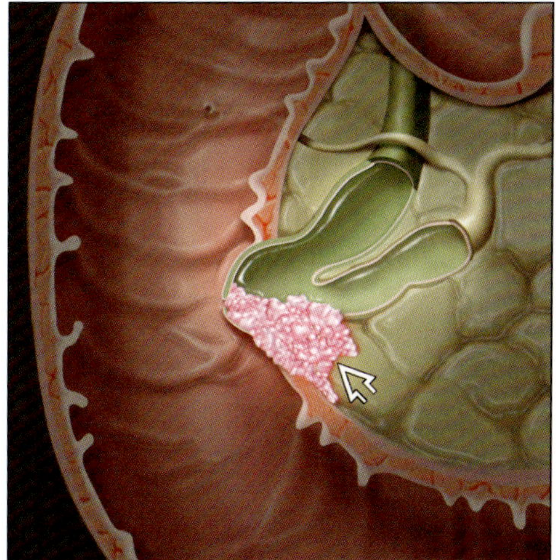

(Left) *This high-power photomicrograph shows adenocarcinoma of the ampulla invading the muscular wall of the duodenum.* ***(Right)*** *This graphic illustrates an ampullary tumor invading the pancreas ➲, consistent with T3 disease.*

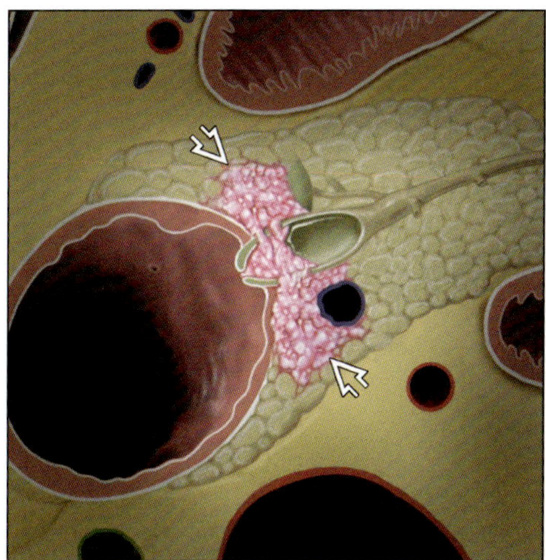

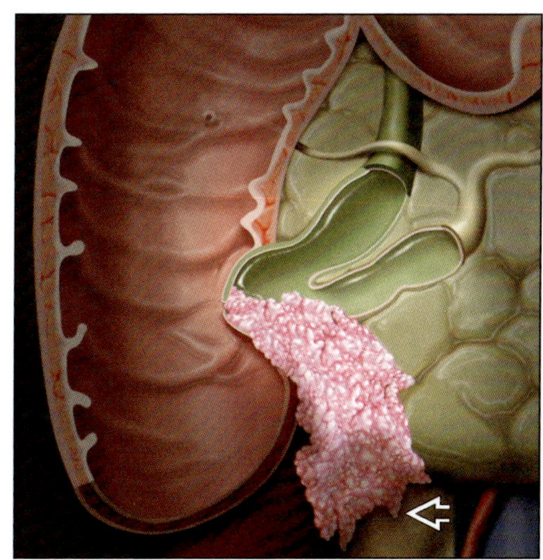

(Left) *This axial graphic shows an ampullary tumor invading the pancreas ➲, consistent with T3 disease.* ***(Right)*** *This graphic illustrates T4 disease, defined as ampullary tumor that invades through the pancreas into the peripancreatic soft tissues ➲.*

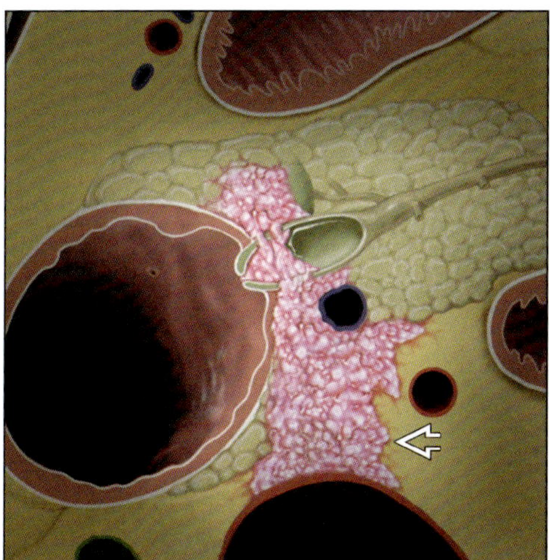

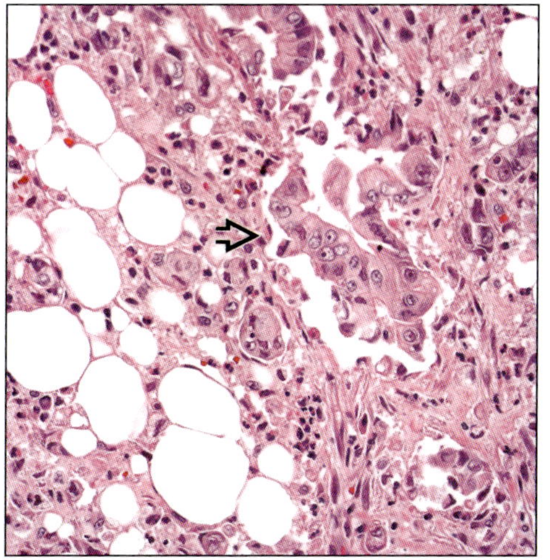

(Left) *This axial graphic also illustrates an ampullary tumor invading through the pancreas into the peripancreatic tissues ➲, consistent with T4 disease. T4 disease also includes tumors that invade adjacent organs or structures other than the pancreas.* ***(Right)*** *This photomicrograph shows ampullary adenocarcinoma within the peripancreatic adipose tissue, consistent with T4 disease ➲.*

Specimen Handling, Whipple II-7-2

SPECIMEN HANDLING, WHIPPLE

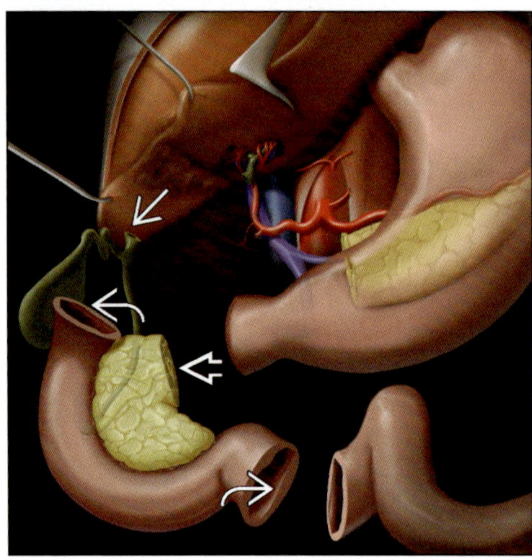

This illustration shows the Whipple (pancreaticoduodenectomy) procedure. Note the common bile duct margin ➡, the pancreatic margin ⇨, and the intestinal margins ↪.

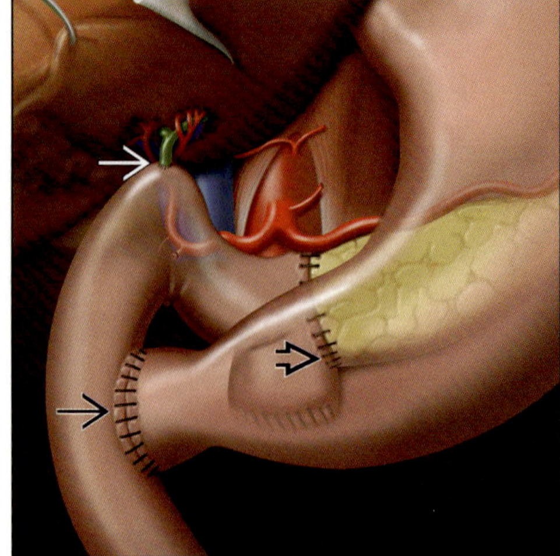

This graphic depicts the reanastomoses after a Whipple procedure, including the anastomoses between the small bowel and the stomach →, the pancreas ⇨, and the bile duct ➡.

WHIPPLE (PANCREATICODUODENECTOMY)

Major Components

- Duodenum
  - May or may not include pylorus depending on whether it was a pylorus-sparing procedure
- Ampulla of Vater
- Common bile duct
- Pancreas

Anatomic Orientation

- Duodenum
  - Free proximal end usually shorter than free distal segment
  - Small portion of stomach usually attached to proximal end
  - Distal end may be either duodenum or jejunum
- Common bile duct
  - Sometimes greenish in color
  - Posterior and superior to pancreas
  - May be easier to identify from ampulla than from transected end
  - If gallbladder is present, can identify insertion of cystic duct and follow to common bile duct
- Ampulla of Vater
  - Usually obvious within duodenum if not obscured by tumor
  - Some patients have an accessory ampulla that drains accessory duct of Santorini
- Pancreas
  - General anatomic features
    - Retroperitoneal organ located in C-groove of 2nd part of duodenum
    - Anterior to pancreas is free space (omental bursa/ lesser sac) and then posterior aspect of stomach
  - Anatomic divisions of pancreas
    - Head: To right of superior mesenteric vein/portal vein confluence; includes uncinate process
    - Neck: Constricted region to left of head
    - Body: Between superior mesenteric vein/portal vein confluence and aorta
    - Tail: Between aorta and splenic hilum
  - Pancreatic duct
    - Usually main pancreatic duct drains bulk of gland into duodenum at major duodenal papilla (ampulla) along with common bile duct
    - Normal diameter is < 1 cm

Specimen Handing

- Identify proximal end of intestines
  - Usually shorter than distal end
- Head of pancreas sits in duodenal C-loop
  - Neck margin can be identified as oval-cut pancreatic surface with central duct
- Determine anterior vs. posterior pancreatic surface
  - Anterior pancreatic surface bulges
  - Posterior pancreatic surface is flat
    - Common bile duct is superior to pancreas near 1st part of duodenum
- Adsay trapezoid method of orientation
  - Useful method to identify essential margins/surfaces
  - Place proximal intestinal margin to left, distal intestinal margin to right, and medial aspect of pancreas facing toward you
  - Visualize a trapezoid
    - Left nonparallel side represents pancreatic neck margin
    - Right nonparallel side is uncinate margin
    - Space between sides is vascular groove
    - Anterior surface is base, and posterior surface is parallel opposite side
- Hand method of orientation
  - Curled left hand resembles pancreas enveloping superior mesenteric artery and portal vein
  - Thumb is uncinate process; flat fingers are neck, body, tail

SPECIMEN HANDLING, WHIPPLE

Surgical Margins

- Common bile duct (shave margin)
- Pancreatic resection (shave margin to include duct)
  - CAP calls this the distal margin
  - AJCC calls this the pancreatic neck
- Uncinate/retroperitoneal (perpendicular margin)
  - CAP: Uncinate
  - AJCC: Retroperitoneal
  - Should be inked, sectioned perpendicularly, and entire area submitted
  - Additional lymph nodes often found if this method is used
- Proximal and distal intestinal (or gastric)
  - Can be shave or perpendicular depending on distance from lesion
- Anterior surface is **not** a surgical margin (because it is covered by smooth layer of peritoneum)
- Posterior surface: Controversial as to whether it is a surgical margin
  - Consists of soft tissue between anterior surface of inferior vena cava and posterior aspect of pancreatic head and duodenum
  - During surgery, this is peeled off the anterior surface of inferior vena cava
- Vascular groove or bed: Controversial as to whether it is a surgical margin
  - Defined as indentation of superior mesenteric vein to portal vein confluence
  - Concave and smooth and glistening aspect of specimen between pancreatic neck and uncinate margins
- Note if tumor involves any margins grossly

Dissection

- Measure dimensions of important structures
- Ink surface of pancreas and uncinate/retroperitoneal margin area
- Take margins, as above
- Open duodenum along side opposite pancreas
  - Document any lesions
  - If tumor involves ampulla, determine epicenter of tumor
    - Is papilla or adjacent duodenal mucosa involved by tumor?
    - Does tumor expand ampulla or form thick rind-like mass along duct?
  - Note presence of tenacious mucin extruding through papilla (diagnostic of intraductal papillary mucinous tumor)
- Open common bile duct with small scissors
  - May be easier to start at proximal end since duct is often dilated
  - Extend incision down through ampulla of Vater
  - Note any strictures or masses in bile duct or ampulla
  - Ink common bile duct with colored ink to distinguish it from pancreatic duct on microscopic sections
  - Alternative method: Cannulate common bile duct and pancreatic duct with probes, then make single cut that bivalves pancreas and ducts
- Examine pancreas
  - "Bread-loaf" pancreas into thin slides perpendicular to long axis of duodenum
    - Leave each slide thinly attached to duodenum for orientation
  - Ascertain if ducts are dilated, stenotic, or thickened
  - Note if there is a cystic tumor communicating with pancreatic duct (main or branch ducts)
  - Note luminal contents of ducts
  - Note if tumor extends into peripancreatic soft tissue grossly
- Find lymph nodes
- Main questions to answer during dissection
  - Is there a tumor?
  - Where is tumor?
    - What is site of origin, and what structures are involved?
  - How big is tumor?
  - What is appearance of tumor (solid, cystic, etc.)?
    - If tumor is cystic, document cyst contents: If multi- or unilocular, size of cysts, and presence of mural nodules
    - If cystic tumor is mucinous, entire tumor should be submitted
  - How many lymph nodes are there, and what is their gross appearance?

Histologic Sections

- Margins, as detailed above
- Tumor
  - Demonstrate relationship to ampulla, pancreas, pancreatic duct, common bile duct, duodenum
    - Sections parallel to long axis of bile duct including duodenum, ampulla, bile duct, and pancreas all in 1 section can be very helpful
  - Posterior surface of pancreas
    - Palpate, if tumor appears close, ink, and take perpendicular sections
  - Anterior surface of pancreas
  - Sections of interface between tumor and normal
  - Sections of normal uninvolved parenchyma
    - At least 1 section from anterior and posterior halves
  - Sections of ampulla and accessory ampulla if present

SELECTED REFERENCES

1. Adsay NV et al: The number of lymph nodes identified in a simple pancreatoduodenectomy specimen: comparison of conventional vs orange-peeling approach in pathologic assessment. Mod Pathol. 22(1):107-12, 2009
2. Riediger H et al: The lymph node ratio is the strongest prognostic factor after resection of pancreatic cancer. J Gastrointest Surg. 13(7):1337-44, 2009
3. Freelove R et al: Pancreatic cancer: diagnosis and management. Am Fam Physician. 73(3):485-92, 2006
4. Westra WH et al: Surgical Pathology Dissection: An Illustrated Guide. 2nd ed. New York: Springer, 2002
5. Strasberg SM et al: Evolution and current status of the Whipple procedure: an update for gastroenterologists. Gastroenterology. 113(3):983-94, 1997

SPECIMEN HANDLING, WHIPPLE

Specimen Orientation

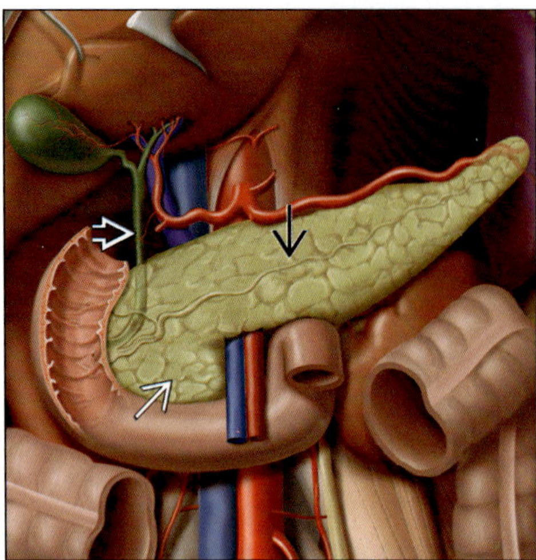

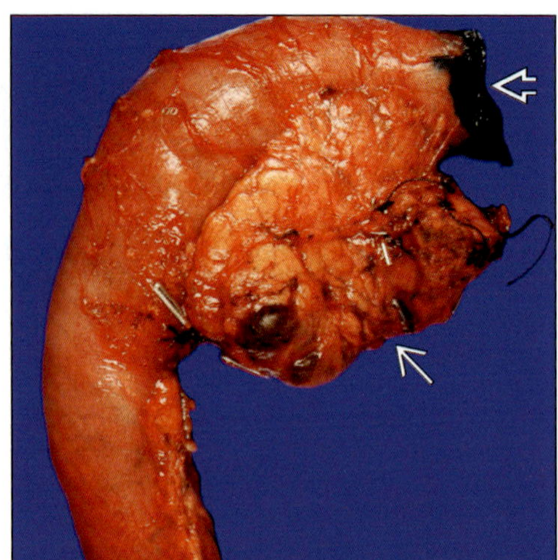

(Left) *The pancreas lies within the C-loop of the duodenum. The head of the pancreas is nearest to the duodenum ➡. The main pancreatic duct ➡ and the common bile duct ➡ converge at the ampulla.* ***(Right)*** *The pancreas ➡ lies within the C-loop of the duodenum. The shorter segment of bowel is the proximal end ➡, and the longer segment of bowel is the distal end.*

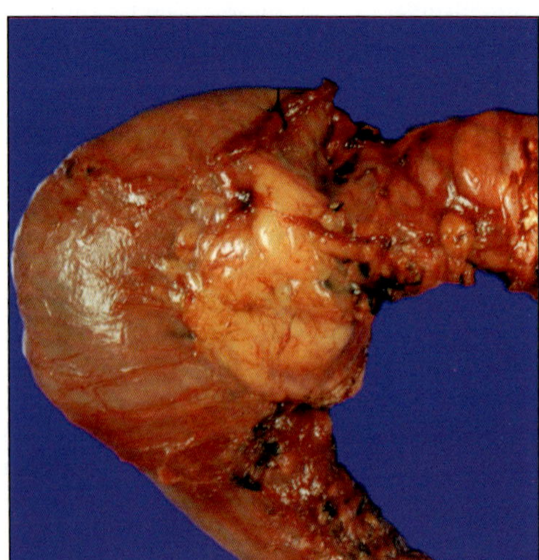

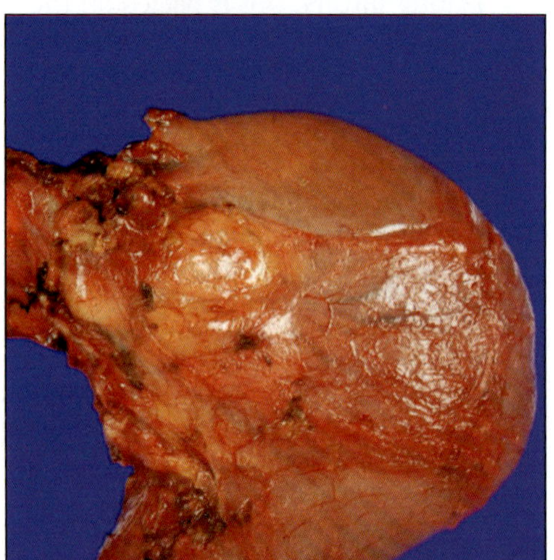

(Left) *The anteromedial surface of the pancreas bulges and is fatty.* ***(Right)*** *The posterior surface of the pancreas is flat.*

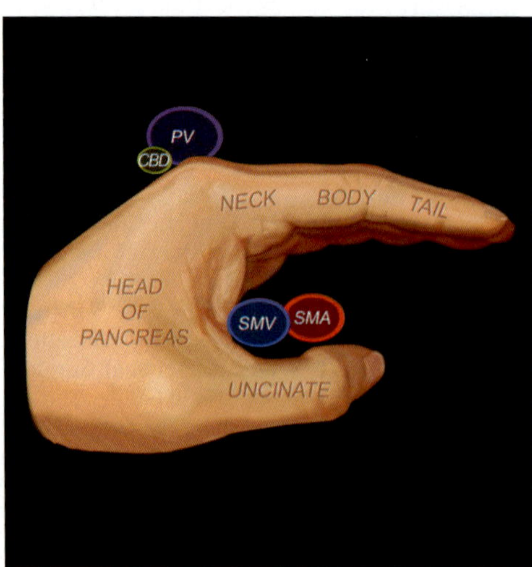

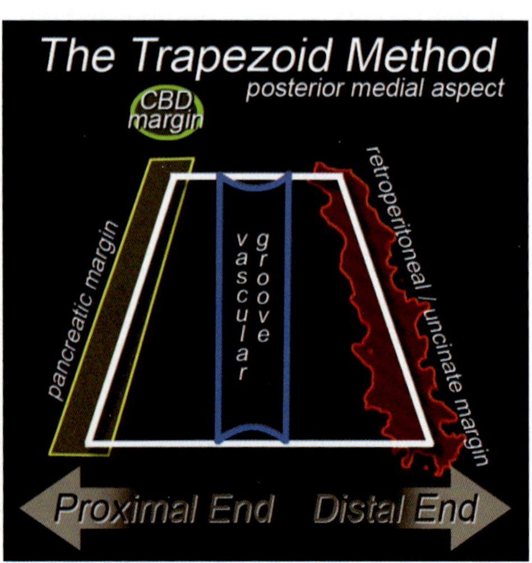

(Left) *You can use your left hand to help orient the anterior view of the pancreas. The hooked thumb is the uncinate process, and the superior mesenteric vein and superior mesenteric artery rest in the vascular groove. The flattened fingers represent the neck, body, and tail of the pancreas.* ***(Right)*** *This graphic illustrates the Adsay "trapezoid" method of orienting a Whipple specimen.*

Specimen Orientation

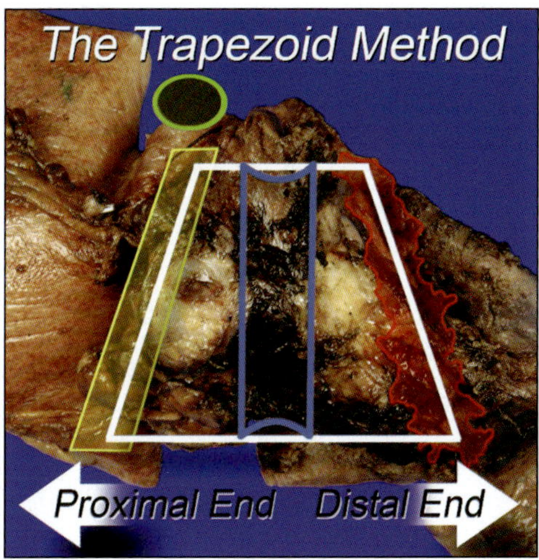

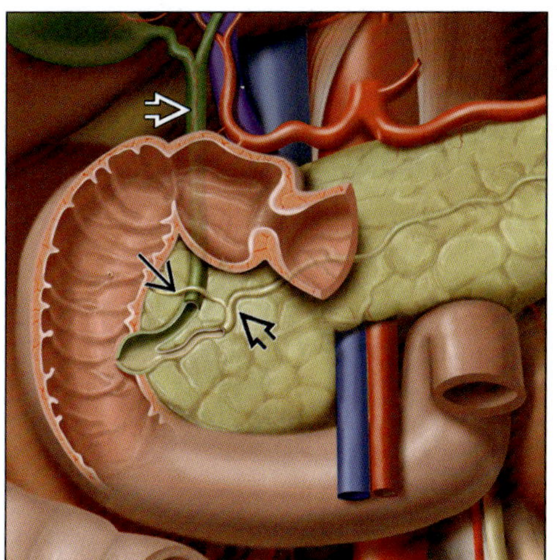

(Left) *Superimposing the trapezoid graphic on a gross specimen, the vascular groove is within the blue lines, the retroperitoneal margin within the red lines, and the pancreatic margin within the yellow lines.* ***(Right)*** *This graphic illustrates the anatomy of the common bile duct ➡ and the pancreatic duct. The pancreatic duct makes a right-angle turn ➡ with the head of the pancreas. Note the accessory pancreatic duct ➡ that enters the duodenum at the minor papilla.*

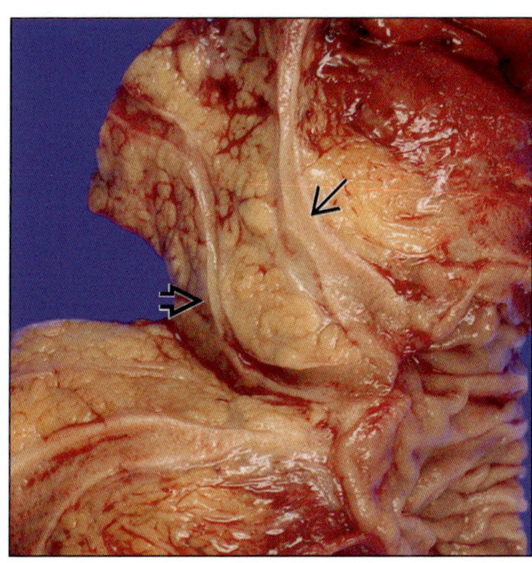

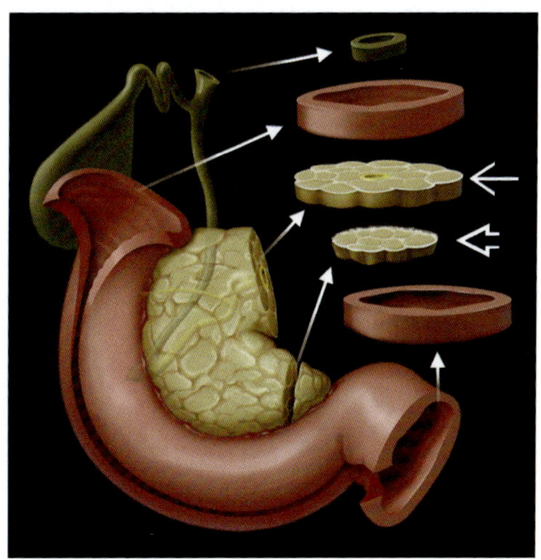

(Left) *This photo of a bivalved pancreas illustrates the pancreatic duct ➡ and the common bile duct ➡ entering the duodenum together at the ampulla. The pancreatic duct makes a right-angle turn with the head of the pancreas.* ***(Right)*** *The important margins include the common bile duct, proximal and distal intestinal, pancreatic neck ➡, and uncinate ➡. The uncinate (retroperitoneal) margin should be inked, sectioned perpendicularly, and entirely submitted.*

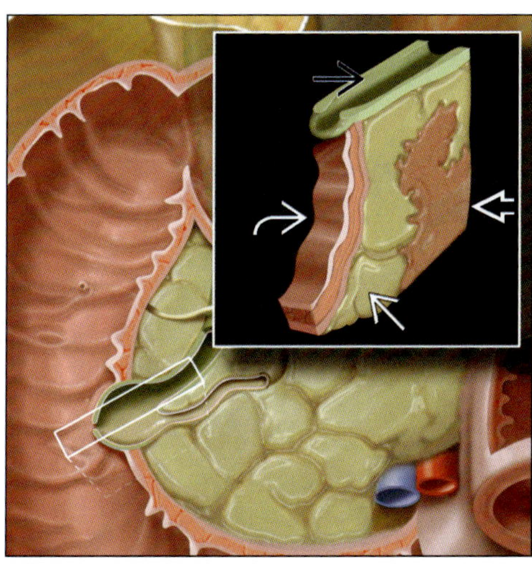

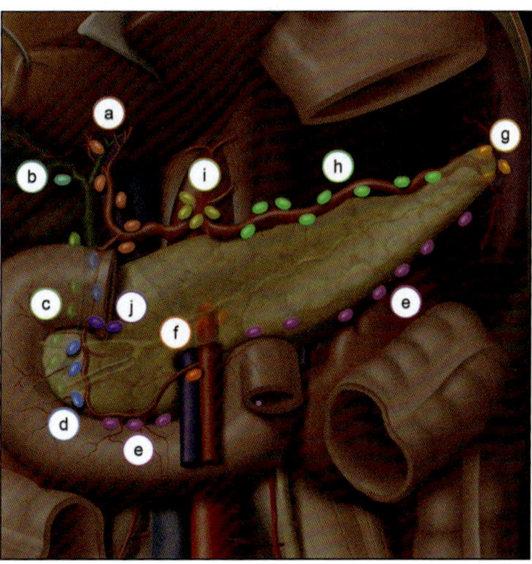

(Left) *A single section demonstrating the tumor ➡ in relationship to pancreas ➡, common bile duct ➡, and duodenum ➡ is often helpful.* ***(Right)*** *This graphic depicts the important peripancreatic lymph node groups: a) hepatic, b) cystic duct, c) posterior pancreaticoduodenal, d) anterior pancreaticoduodenal, e) inferior, f) superior mesenteric, g) splenic hilar, h) superior, i) celiac, and j) pyloric. A minimum of 12 nodes is required for adequate staging.*

Antibody Index

ANTIBODY INDEX

Antibodies Discussed

Antibody Name/Symbol	Antibody Description	Clones/Alternative Names
α-1-antitrypsin	alpha-1-antitrypsin	A1AT
α-fetoprotein	alpha 1 fetoprotein	AFP, Z5A06, clone C3
β-catenin	beta catenin; involved in regulation of cell adhesion and in signal transduction through Wnt pathway	B-catenin, clone 14, e-5, RB-9035Po, 17C2, 5H10
β-catenin-nuclear	beta catenin, nuclear	B-CATEN-NUC
λ light chain	lambda light chain	lambda
12C3	early malignant change in ovary-non-commercial	
1F6	CD 4 (T-cell surface glycoprotein, L3T4, T helper cells)	1290, 4B12, CD4, CD04
AE1/AE3	AE1/AE3; mixuture of 2 anticytokeratin clones that detect a variety of both high-and low-molecular weight cytokeratins	
AE13	AE13 (pilar-type keratin)	
ALK1	anaplastic lymphoma kinase-1	5A4, ALK, ALKC
Amylase	enzyme present in saliva and pancreas, involved in digestion of carbohydrates	
B72.3	tumor-associated glycoprotein-72	TAG72, CC49,TAG-72, BRST-3
Bartonella henselae	*B. henselae*	B-henselae, cat scratch fever agent
BSEP (N16)	bile salt exporter pump	
C4d	clinically useful marker for humoral rejection. A degradation product of activated complement factor C4b	
CA19-9	carbohydrate antigen 19-9; prognostic tumor marker that may be elevated in certain cancers and noncancerous conditions	1116NS19-9, sialylated Lewis (a) antigen
CA125	mucin 16	OV185:1, OC125, MUC16
Calponin	thin filament-associated protein that is implicated in regulation and modulation of smooth muscle contraction	N3, 26A11, CALP, CNN1, SMCC, SmCalp
Calretinin	29 kDa calcium binding protein that is expressed in central and peripheral nervous system and in many normal and pathological tissues	DAK-CALRET, 5A5, CAL 3F5, DC8, AB149
CD1a	T-cell surface glycoprotein	JPM30, CD1A, O10, NA1/34
CD4	T-cell surface glycoprotein L3T4	IF6, 1290, 4B12
CD10	neutral endopeptidase	CALLA, neprilysin, NEP
CD31	platelet endothelial cell adhesion molecule	JC/70, JC/70A, PECAM-1
CD34	hematopoieteic progenitor cell antigen	MY10, IOM34, QBEND10, 8G12, 1309, HPCA-1, NU-4A1, TUK4, clone 581, BI-3c5
CD56	NCAM (neutral cellular adhesion molecule)	MAB735, ERIC-1, 25-KD11, 123C3, 24-MB2, BC56C04, 1B6, 14-MAB735, NCC-LU-243, MOC-1, NCAM
CD63	tetraspan intracellular granule protein	NKI/C3, basophil activation test in allergy
CD68	cytoplasmic granule protein of monocytes, macrophages	PG-M1, KP-1, LN5
CD99	cell surface glycoprotein for migration, T cell adhesion, MIC2	CD99-MEMB, MIC2, 12E7, HBA71, O13, P30/32MIC2, M3601
CD117	C-kit, tyrosine-protein kinase activity	C-19 (C-KIT), 104D2, 2E4, C-KIT, A4502, H300, CMA-767
CD163	macrophage hemoglobin scavenging system	10D6
CDX-2	caudal-type homeobox transcription factor 2	AMT28, 7C7/D4, CDX-2-88
CEA-P	carcinoembryonic antigen, polyclonal	
Chromogranin-A	pituitary secretory protein 1	PHE-5, PHE5, E001, DAK-A3
Chymotrypsin	digestive enzyme synthesized in pancreas, involved in proteolysis	
CK1	cytokeratin 1	CK 01, 34BB4
CK7	cytokerating 7, low molecular weight cytokeratin	K72.7, KS7.18, OVTL 12/30, LDS-68, CK 07
CK8	cytokeratin 8	K8.8, 4.1.18, TS1, C-51, M20
CK19	cytokeratin 19, low molecular weight cytokeratin	BA17, RCK108, LP2K, B170, A53-BA2, KS19.1, 170.2.14
CK20	cytokeratin 20, low molecular weight cytokeratin	KS20.8
CK8/18/CAM5.2	cytokeratin 8/18; simple epithelial-type cytokeratins	5D3, Zym5.2, CAM 5.2, KER 10.11, NCL-5D3, cytokeratin LMW

ANTIBODY INDEX

CK-PAN	cytokeratin-pan (AE1/AE3/LP34); cocktail of high and low molecular weight cytokeratins	keratin pan, MAK-6, K576, LU-5, KL-1, KC-8, MNF 116, pankeratin, pancytokeratin
CMV	cytomegalovirus	
Cyclin-D1	protein with important cell cycle regulatory functions	bcl-1 (cyclin D1) A-12, PRAD1, AM29, DCS-6, SP4, D1GM, P2D11F11, CCND1cyl-1
D2-40	lymphatic epithelial marker	podoplanin, D2-40 clone, M2A
Desmin	class III intermediate filaments found in muscle cells	M760, DE-R-11, D33, DE5, DE-U-10, ZC18
DPC4	mothers against DPP homolog 4	MADR1 JV4-1, DPC4_SMAD4, SMAD4, B-8
EBER	Epstein-Barr virus encoded RNA	
EBV-LMP	Epstein-Barr virus latent membrane protein	LMP1, CS 1-4
E-cadherin	epithelial calcium dependent adhesion molecule	36B5, ECH-6, ECCD-2, CDH1, 5H9, NCH 38, Clone 36, 4A2 C7, E9, 67A4, HECD-1, SC-8426
EMA	epithelial membrane agent	GP1.4, 214D4, MC5, E29
ER	estrogen receptor protein	1D5, 6F11, SP1, 15D, H222, TE111, ERP, ER1D5, NCLER611, NCL-ER-LH2, PGP-1A6
ERP-β	estrogen receptor protein beta	ER-BETA, 14C8, 57/3, PPG5/10
FLI-1	Friend leukemia virus integration 1	G1146-222, SC356
FVIIIRAg	factor VIII-related antigen	F8/86, von Willebrand factor
Gastrin	hormone released by G cells in stomach, duodenum, and pancreas that stimulates secretion of gastric acid (HCl) by parietal cells of stomach	
GFAP	glial fibrillary acidic protein	6F2, M761, GA-51, GFP-8A
GGT	gamma glutamyltransferase	Gamma-glutamyl transpeptidase, GGT 129
GLUT1	glucose transporter 1	
Glutamine synthetase	polyclonal antibody that highlights glutamine synthetasin in liver and brain	
Glypican 3	heparan sulfate proteoglycan with elevated expression in hepatocellular carcinoma	1G12, GPC3
HBcAg	hepatitis B core antigen	HBCAG
HBsAg	hepatitis B surface antigen	HBSAG, 3E7
Hep-Par1	hepatocyte paraffin 1	OCH1E5.2.10, HEPPAR1
HHV8	human herpes virus 8	13B10, LNA-1
HMB-45	monoclonal antibody that reacts against an antigen present in melanocytic tumors	
HSP70	heat shock protein 70	C92F3A-5
HSV1/2	herpes simplex virus 1/2	HSV1&2, HSV1/HSV2
IgG	immunoglobulin G	IGG
IgM	immunoglobulin M	IGM
inhibin	hormone released from testes or ovaries that down-regulates FSH synthesis and secretion	R1, beta A subunit, alpha subunit, INHIBIN
Inhibin-α	produced by ovarina granulosa cells; inhibits production or secretion of pituitary gonadotropins, a sensitive marker for majority of sex cord-stromal tumors	
insulin	peptide hormone produced in islets of Langerhans in pancreas	HB125
ISL1	insulin-related protein	Islet 1, 30.3A4
Ki-67	marker of cell proliferation	MM1, KI88, IVAK-2, MIB1
LF	lactoferrin	
LH	lutenizing hormone	beta-LH
Lipase	pancreatic lipase	
Melan-A	melanoma antigen recognized by T cells 1 (MART-1); protein found on melanocytes; melanocyte differentiation antigen	M2-7C10, CK-MM
Metallothionein	cysteine-rich, low molecular weight protein	Clone E9, MT
MK	neurite growth promoting factor 2	Midkine, G2a
MUC1	epithelial membrane antigen	LICR-LON-M8, BC3, DF3, VU3D1, MUSEII, RD-1, MA695, MA552, PS2P446, 115D8

ANTIBODY INDEX

MUC2	mucin 1, intestinal	CCP58, MUC2-P, M53, MRP, LUM2-3, LDQ10
MUC5AC	mucin 5AC, tracheobronchial, gastric	MUC5, CLH2 2, 45M1, CLH2
MUC6	mucin 6, gastric	CLH5
MYOD1	myogenic differentiation 1	5.8A, 5.2F
Myoglobin	iron- and oxygen-binding protein found in myocytes	MG-1
NCAM	neural cellular adhesion molecule	CD56, MAB735, ERIC-1, 25-KD11, 123C3, 24-MB2, BC56C04, 1B6, 14-MAB735, NCC-LU-243, MOC-1
NSE	neuron specific enolase	BSS/H14
p16	cyclin dependent kinase 4 inhibitor 2A	P16_INK4A, E6H4, sc1661, JC8, Zj11, G175-405, F-12, DCS-50, 6H12, 16P07, 16P04
p53	p53 tumor supressor gene protein	D07, 21N, BP53-12-1, AB6, CM1, PAB1801, DO1, BP53-11, PAP240, RSP53, MU195, P53
p63	tumor protein p63	H137, 7JUL, 4A4
pax-8	paired box gene 8	PAX-8
Podoplanin	lymphatic epithelial marker	D2-40 clone, M2A, D2-40
PR	progesterone receptor protein	10A9, PGR-1A6, KD68, PGR-ICA, PRP-P, PRP, PRI, 1A6, 1AR, HPRA3, PGR-636, 636, PR88, NCL-PGR
PSCA	prostate stem cell antigen	1G8, pro 232
pVHL	von Hippel-Lindau tumor suppressor protein	Ig33
S100	Low molecular weight protein normally present in cells derived from neural crest (Schwwann cells, meloanocytes, and glial cells), chondrocytes, adipocytes, myoepithelial cells, macrophages, Langerhans cells, dendritic cells, and keratinocytes	S-100, A6, 15E2E2, Z311, 4C4.9
S100-pla	S100 placental	S100P, S100PL, placental S100, S0084, 16
SMAD4	Similar to Mothers Against Decapentaplegic (MAD); mothers against DPP homolog 4	MADR1 JV4-1, DPC4_SMAD4, B-8
Somatostatin	somatotropin release-inhibiting factor	
Synaptophysin	major synaptic vesicle protein p38 antibody	SVP38, SY38, SNP-88, SYP, SYPH, Sypl, Syn p38
TPA	tissue plasminogen activator	tPA
Trypsin	digestive serine protease produced in pancreas in the inactive proenzyme form trypsinogen	
Trypsinogen	digestive serine protease produced in pancreas and activated by enteropeptidase in small intestine	
TTF-1	transcripton termination factor	8G7G3/1, SPT-24, SC-13040
TYH	tyrosine hydroxylase	TYR HYDROXY
VCA	Epstein-Barr virus: Viral capsid antigen	EBV-VCA
Vimentin	major subunit protein of indeterminate filaments of mesenchymal cells	43BE8, 3B4, V10, V9, VIM-B34, VIM

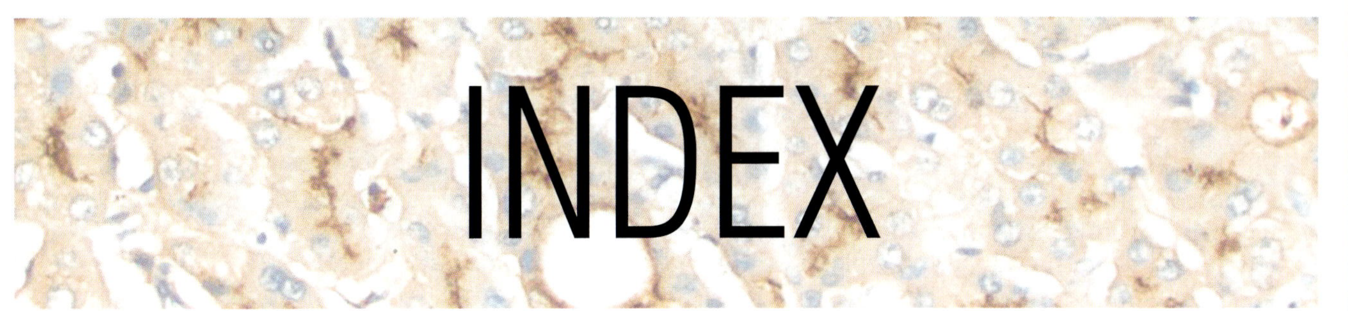

INDEX

A

INDEX

INDEX

B

INDEX

C

INDEX

INDEX

INDEX

D

INDEX

INDEX

INDEX

INDEX

INDEX

INDEX

INDEX

INDEX

M

INDEX

N

INDEX

O

P

INDEX

INDEX

INDEX

Q

R

INDEX

S

T

INDEX

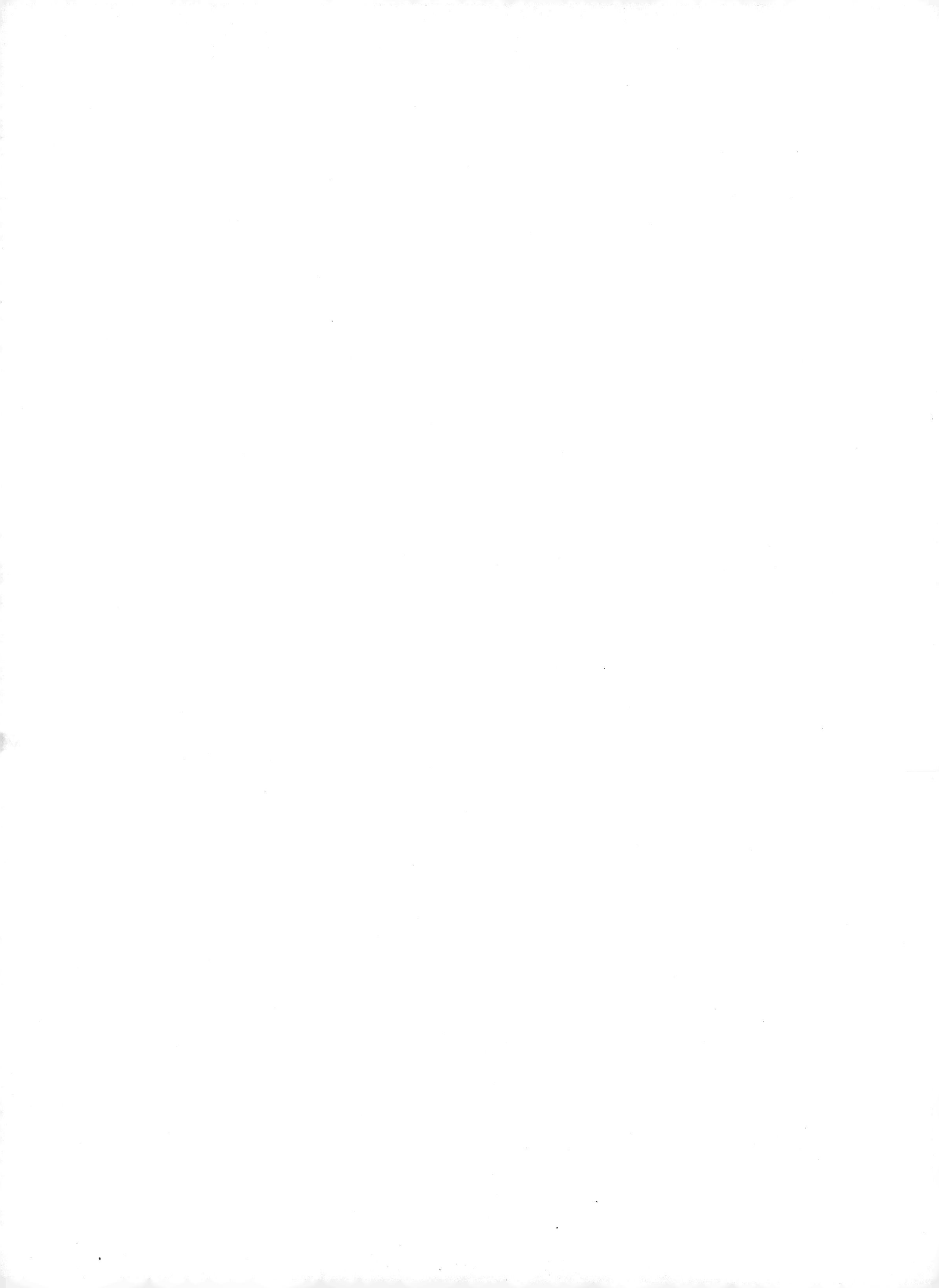